Encyclopedia of Clinical Neuropsychology

Jeffrey S. Kreutzer • John DeLuca
Bruce Caplan

Editors

Encyclopedia of Clinical Neuropsychology

Second Edition

Volume 1

A–B

With 230 Figures and 197 Tables

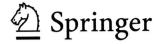 Springer

Editors
Jeffrey S. Kreutzer
Department of Physical
Medicine and Rehabilitation
Virginia Commonwealth University
Richmond, VA, USA

John DeLuca
Kessler Foundation
Pleasant Valley Way
West Orange, NJ, USA

Bruce Caplan
Independent Practice
Wynnewood, PA, USA

ISBN 978-3-319-57110-2 ISBN 978-3-319-57111-9 (eBook)
ISBN 978-3-319-57112-6 (print and electronic bundle)
https://doi.org/10.1007/978-3-319-57111-9

Library of Congress Control Number: 2018945469

This Springer imprint is published by Springer Nature, under the registered company Springer International Publishing AG
The registered company address is: Gewerbestrasse 11, 6330 Cham, Switzerland

Preface

Neuropsychology is a rapidly evolving field with inspiring advances in neurotechnology, assessment, and intervention occurring regularly. An act of labor and love, the conceptualization, compilation, and production of the *Encyclopedia of Clinical Neuropsychology* (2nd ed.) spanned more than 4 years. Building on the foundation of the first edition, the editors-in-chief sought to provide a current corpus of content of empirically based, relevant, and practical information. To this end, we added three new topical sections: neuroimaging, military neuropsychology, and DSM-5 and enlisted the help of three superb new section editors: Erin Bigler, Ph.D., Risa Nakase-Richardson, Ph.D., and Ana Mills, Psy.D, respectively, to orchestrate the new sections. An immense project, the encyclopedia now contains more than 2,200 entries. More than 1,600 first edition entries were updated and 230 new entries were added. The newest edition of the encyclopedia now reflects the work of nearly 900 authors.

As with the first edition, we have aimed to create a comprehensive reference for professionals involved in the evaluation, diagnosis, and rehabilitation of children and adults with neurological disorders. We have also provided students and researchers with the breadth of knowledge to facilitate success in evaluating and treating these patients. Suggested readings and cross references direct readers to additional information on the various topics. We anticipate that the *Encyclopedia of Clinical Neuropsychology* will be the first place readers turn for factual, relevant, and comprehensive information.

August 2018

Jeffrey S. Kreutzer
John DeLuca
Bruce Caplan

Acknowledgment

We are indebted to our cadre of esteemed Associate Editors for helping to develop their sections, recruit contributors, and ensure the presence of consistently high quality entries. We express our utmost appreciation to the brilliant group of authors whose efforts form the core of our project. We are immensely indebted to the superb Springer Major reference works team including Janice Stern, Michael Hermann, and Sonja Peterson. They taught us, encouraged us, kept us organized and on track, and helped us in every step of the way. We are also grateful to our students, patients and their families from whom we learned much about facing challenges and the value of being practical.

List of Topics

Forensics–Jeff Kreutzer

Section Editor: *Julie K. Lynch*

Movement–Jeff Kreutzer

Section Editor: *Douglas I. Katz*

CNS–John Deluca

Section Editor: *Randall E. Merchant* and *John DeLuca*

Cognitive Rehabilitation–John Deluca

Section Editor: *Sarah A. Raskin*

General/Historical–Bruce Caplan

Section Editor: *Anthony Y. Stringer*

Genetics

Section Editor: *John DeLuca*

Illness or Disease–John Deluca

Section Editor: *Susan K. Johnson*

Presenile Dementia
Primacy Effect
Proactive Interference
Procedural Memory
Prospective Memory
Pseudodementia
Recency Effect
Recent Memory
Recognition Memory Test
Remote Memory
Retrieval Techniques
Retroactive Interference
Retrograde Amnesia
Rey Auditory Verbal Learning Test,
    Rey AVLT
Rivermead Behavioral Memory Test
Selective Reminding Test
Semantic Memory
Serial Recall
Short-Term Memory
Source Memory
Subcortical Dementia
Transient Global Amnesia
Warrington Recognition Memory Test
Wechsler Memory Scale All Versions
Wernicke-Korsakoff Syndrome
Wide Range Assessment of Memory and
    Learning
Serial Position Effect
Memory for Intentions Screening Test

Miscellaneous–Jeff Kreutzer

Section Editor: *Stephanie A. Kolakowsky-Hayner*

Anticholinergic
Anticonvulsants
Antihistamines
Antihypertensives
Antipsychotics
Anxiolytics
Autoreceptor
Behavior Modification
Compensation Neurosis
Corticotropin-Releasing Hormone
Dysexecutive Index (DEX)
Dysexecutive Syndrome

Dysphoria
Frontal Behavioral Inventory
Frontal Eye Fields
Glucocorticoids
Hormones
Hyperbaric Therapy
Impersistence
Impulsivity
Inhibition
Irritability
Job Restructuring
Neuroleptic Malignant Syndrome
Neuroleptics
Pharmacodynamics
Pharmacokinetics
Phenobarbital
Projective Technique
Psychopharmacology
Psychotropic
Qualitative Data
Qualitative Neuropsychological Assessment
Reuptake
Reuptake Inhibition
Route Finding
Sedative Hypnotic Drugs
Social Skills Training
Steroids
Stimulants
Stimulus-Bound Behavior
Substance Abuse
Supplementary Motor Area (SMA)
Symmetril (Amantadine)
Tinkertoy Test
Tolerance
Vocational Counseling
Wisconsin Card Sorting Test

Neuropsychological Evaluation–Jeff Kreutzer

Section Editor: *Yana Suchy*

Agitated Behavior Scale
Behavioral Assessment of the Dysexecutive
    Syndrome
Boston Process Approach
Brief Cognitive Rating Scale
Cambridge Neuropsychological Testing
    Automated Battery

Psychological Conditions–Bruce Caplan

Section Editor: *Robert G. Frank*

Seizure–John Deluca

Section Editor: *Nancy D. Chiaravalloti*

Sensory–Bruce Caplan

Section Editor: *John E. Mendoza* and *Bruce Caplan*

Military Neuropsychology–Jeff Kreutzer

Section Editor: *Risa Nakase-Richardson*

About the Editors

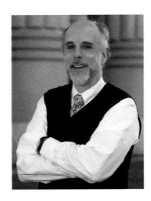

Jeffrey S. Kreutzer Department of Physical Medicine and Rehabilitation, Virginia Commonwealth University, Richmond, VA, USA

Dr. Jeffrey S. Kreutzer is the Rosa Schwarz Cifu Professor in the Department of Physical Medicine and Rehabilitation (PM&R) at Virginia Commonwealth University's Medical College of Virginia Campus in Richmond. He first came to VCU as a postdoctoral fellow in 1982 after completing an internship in Neuropsychology and Family Therapy with Muriel Lezak at the Portland, Oregon VA Medical Center. He joined Virginia Commonwealth University's medical school faculty in the Fall of 1983.

Board certified in rehabilitation psychology (ABPP), Dr. Kreutzer has more than three decades of experience as a brain injury rehabilitation specialist. He was a founding member of the Virginia Head Injury Foundation, now known as BIAV. Since 1987, he has served as the Director of VCU's federally designated Traumatic Brain Injury Model System (TBIMS). As a clinician, Dr. Kreutzer provides neuropsychological and family support services to persons with a wide variety of neurological disabilities. His practice is holistic, emphasizing skills training, psychological support, and patient education.

Throughout his career, Dr. Kreutzer has been involved in developing empirically based intervention programs for persons with brain injury. For example, in 1986 he and Dr. Paul Wehman received a federal grant to adapt supported employment methods for persons with brain injury. Their successful program development along with very positive outcome data has helped make supported employment the current "standard of care" for TBI employment services. More recently, Dr. Kreutzer is developing empirically based programs to enhance resilience, couples' relationships, and family functioning.

Dr. Kreutzer has received numerous awards. In 1994, he received the *Sheldon Berrol Clinical Service Award* from The National Head Injury Foundation. In 2002, he received the *Robert L. Moody Prize for Distinguished Initiatives in Brain Injury Research and Rehabilitation* from the University of Texas. He has received two awards from the American Psychological Association, the *Roger Barker Distinguished Research Contribution Award* (2003) and the *Diller Award for Demonstrated Excellence in the Field of Neurorehabilitation* (2005). In 2010, he received the *Distinguished Lifetime Contribution to Neuropsychology Award* from the National Academy of Neuropsychology. In 2012, he received the McCollom Research Award from the Foundation for Life Care Planning Research, and in 2013 he received the *Innovations in Treatment Award* from the North American Brain Injury Society. In 2017, he was presented with the *Jennett Plum Award for Clinical Achievement in the Field of Brain Injury Medicine* by the International Brain Injury Association.

A frequent speaker at national and international meetings, he has given more than 500 invited presentations. A Fellow in the American Congress of Rehabilitation Medicine (FACRM), National Academy of Neuropsychology, and the American Psychological Association, Dr. Kreutzer has co-authored more than 170 publications, mostly in the area of traumatic brain injury and rehabilitation. Editor-in-Chief of two international journals, *Brain Injury* and *NeuroRehabilitation*, he has also published more than 15 books covering topics such as family intervention, vocational rehabilitation, community reintegration, behavior management, and cognitive rehabilitation.

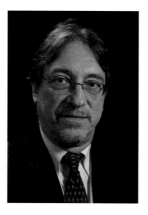

John DeLuca is the Senior Vice President for Research and Training at Kessler Foundation, a Professor in the Department of Physical Medicine and Rehabilitation, and the Department of Neurology at Rutgers, New Jersey

Medical School. He is a licensed Psychologist in New Jersey and New York and is board certified in Rehabilitation Psychology by the American Board of Professional Psychology. Dr. DeLuca has been involved in neuropsychology and rehabilitation research for over 25 years. He is internationally known for his research on disorders of memory and information processing in a variety of clinical populations, including multiple sclerosis, traumatic brain injury, aneurysmal subarachnoid hemorrhage, and chronic fatigue syndrome. Dr. DeLuca has published over 300 articles and chapters in these areas; has edited 5 books in neuropsychology, neuroimaging, and rehabilitation; and is a co-editor for the *Encyclopedia of Clinical Neuropsychology*. He has received over 32 million dollars in grant support for his research. Dr. DeLuca's most recent research ventures include the cerebral mapping of human cognitive processes using functional neuroimaging, as well as the development of research-based techniques to improve cognitive impairment. He serves as an Associate Editor of several journals and is on the editorial boards of many other journals. He is the recipient of several awards in recognition of his work including the 2015 Arthur Benton Award from the International Neuropsychological Society and 2012 Rodger G. Barker Distinguished Research Contribution Award from Division 22 (Rehabilitation Psychology) of the American Psychological Association. Dr. DeLuca has been very involved for many years in the training of postdoctoral fellows in neuropsychology and rehabilitation and has directed several advanced research and training programs sponsored by NIDRR, the National MS Society, and NIH since 1990.

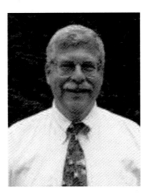

Bruce Caplan is board certified in clinical neuropsychology and rehabilitation psychology by the American Board of Professional Psychology and is a Fellow of the American Psychological Association (APA), National Academy of Neuropsychology, and American Congress of Rehabilitation Medicine. Dr. Caplan serves as Senior Editor of *Journal of Head Trauma Rehabilitation*, is a member of the Editorial Board of *Topics in Stroke Rehabilitation*, and previously served as Editor of *Rehabilitation Psychology*. In 1987, Dr. Caplan published *Rehabilitation Psychology Desk Reference*, the first edited textbook in the specialty. He is past President of the Philadelphia Neuropsychology Society and of Division 22 (Rehabilitation Psychology) of the APA. He is the recipient of two Distinguished Service Awards and the Lifetime Achievement

Award from Division 22. Dr. Caplan was a founding member of the American Board of Rehabilitation Psychology. Currently in independent practice, he was formerly Professor and Chief Psychologist in the Department of Rehabilitation Medicine at Jefferson Medical College in Philadelphia.

Contributors

Galya Abdrakhmanova University of Richmond, Richmond, VA, USA

Thomas M. Achenbach Department of Psychiatry, University of Vermont, Burlington, VT, USA

Russell Adams Department of Psychiatry and Behavioral Science, University of Oklahoma Health Sciences Center, Oklahoma City, OK, USA

Adrienne Adler Department of Neurobiology and Anatomy, Wake Forest School of Medicine, Winston-Salem, NC, USA

Adrienne Adler-Neal Department of Neurobiology and Anatomy, Wake Forest School of Medicine, Winston-Salem, NC, USA

Amma A. Agyemang Department of Physical Medicine and Rehabilitation, Virginia Commonwealth University Medical Center, Richmond, VA, USA

Cristy Akins Mercy Family Center, Metarie, LA, USA

Amy Alderson Department of Rehabilitation Medicine, Emory University, Atlanta, GA, USA

Brittany J. Allen Cox Health System, Springfield, MO, USA

Daniel N. Allen Department of Psychology, University of Nevada, Las Vegas, NV, USA

H. Allison Bender Department of Neurology, Icahn School of Medicine at Mount Sinai, New York, NY, USA

Ahmad Alsemari Psychology, Edgewood College, Madison, WI, USA

Karin Alterescu Department of Psychology, Queens College of the City University of New York (CUNY), Flushing, NY, USA

Robert A. Altmann A-PsychEd Publication Services, Minneapolis, MN, USA

Akshay Amaraneni Department of Pharmacology, Virginia Commonwealth University, Richmond, VA, USA

Melissa Amick Department of Psychiatry and Human Behavior, Brown University, Providence, RI, USA

Aaron Andersen Utah State University, Logan, UT, USA

Heather Anderson Department of Neurology, University of Kansas School of Medicine, Kansas City, KS, USA

Steven W. Anderson University of Iowa Hospitals and Clinics, Iowa City, Iowa, USA

Kevin M. Antshel Department of Psychology, Syracuse University, Syracuse, NY, USA

Jennifer Ann Niskala Apps Department of Psychiatry and Behavioral Medicine, Children's Hospital of Wisconsin/Medical College of Wisconsin, Milwaukee, WI, USA

Juan Carlos Arango-Lasprilla IKERBASQUE, Basque Foundation for Science, Biocruces Research Institute, Bilbao, Spain

Amy J. Armstrong Department of Rehabilitation Counseling, Virginia Commonwealth University, Richmond, VA, USA

Carol L. Armstrong Child and Adolescent Psychiatry and Behavioral Sciences, The Children's Hospital of Philadelphia, Philadelphia, PA, USA

Glenn S. Ashkanazi Department of Clinical and Health Psychology, Clinical and Health Psychology Clinic, College of Public Health and Health Professions, University of Florida, Gainesville, FL, USA

Jane Austin Department of Psychology, William Paterson University, Wayne, NJ, USA

Bradley N. Axelrod John D. Dingell VA Medical Center, Psychology Section (11MHPS), Detroit, MI, USA

Lindsay E. Ayearst Multi-Health Systems Inc., Toronto, ON, Canada

Glen P. Aylward SIU School of Medicine- Developmental-Behavioral Pediatrics, Springfield, IL, USA

Samantha Backhaus Department of Neuropsychology, Rehabilitation Hospital of Indiana, Indianapolis, IN, USA

Erin Bailey Department of Psychology, Miami VA Healthcare System, Miami, FL, USA

Maya Balamane Mount Sinai Brain Injury Research Center, San Francisco, CA, USA

Angel Ball Department of Clinical Health Sciences, Texas A&M University – Kingsville, Kingsville, TX, USA

Sandra Banks Department of Psychiatry, Allegheny General Hospital, Pittsburgh, PA, USA

James H. Baños Department of Medical Education, University of Alabama School of Medicine, Birmingham, AL, USA

Russell A. Barkley Virginia Treatment Center for Children and Virginia Commonwealth University Medical Center, Richmond, VA, USA

Ida Sue Baron Potomac, MD, USA

Erika M. Baron Pace University, New York, NY, USA

Mark S. Baron Department of Neurology, Virginia Commonwealth University Parkinson's and Movement Disorders Center, Richmond, Virginia, USA

Walter Barr Department of Psychology, William Paterson University, Wayne, NJ, USA

William B. Barr NYU Langone Medical Center, Comprehensive Epilepsy Center, New York, NY, USA

Joseph Barrash Department of Neurology, University of Iowa, Iowa City, IA, USA

Russell M. Bauer Department of Clinical and Health Psychology, University of Florida, Gainesville, FL, USA

Allison Baylor Virginia Commonwealth University, Richmond, VA, USA

Jessica Bean Department of Psychology, University of Connecticut, Storrs, CT, USA

Megan Becker Department of Psychology, University of Nevada, Las Vegas, NV, USA

James T. Becker Department of Psychiatry, University of Pittsburgh School of Medicine, WPIC, Pittsburgh, PA, USA

Pélagie M. Beeson Department of Speech, Language, and Hearing Sciences, The University of Arizona, Tucson, AZ, USA

Jay Behel Department of Behavioral Sciences, Rush University Medical Center, Chicago, IL, USA

Stephanie Behrens Department of Psychology, Utah State University, Logan, UT, USA

Stacy Belkonen Salem VA Medical Center, Salem, VA, USA

Department of Psychiatry and Behavioral Medicine, Virginia Tech Carilion School of Medicine, Roanoke, VA, USA

Andrew Bell Department of Anatomy and Neurobiology, Virginia Commonwealth University, Richmond, VA, USA

Brian D. Bell Department of Neurology, University of Wisconsin, Madison, WI, USA

Heidi A. Bender Department of Neurology, Icahn School of Medicine at Mount Sinai, New York, NY, USA

Daniel B. Berch Curry School of Education, University of Virginia, Charlottesville, VA, USA

Brianne Magouirk Bettcher Department of Neurosurgery and Neurology, University of Colorado School of Medicine, Denver, CO, USA
Rocky Mountain Alzheimer's Disease Center, Aurora, CO, USA

Alyssa Beukema School Psychology, The Chicago School of Professional Psychology, Chicago, IL, USA

John Bigbee Anatomy and Neurobiology, Virginia Commonwealth University, Richmond, VA, USA

Erin D. Bigler Department of Psychology and the Neuroscience Center, Brigham Young University, Provo, UT, USA

Rebecca Bind Department of Neurology, Mount Sinai Medical Center, New York, NY, USA

J. Audie Black Allegheny General Hospital, Pittsburgh, PA, USA
Department of Psychiatry; Neuropsychology Section, Allegheny Health Network, Pittsburgh, PA, USA

Margaret Lehman Blake Communication Sciences and Disorders, University of Houston, Houston, TX, USA

Michelle L. Block Stark Neuroscience Research Institute, Indiana University, Indianapolis, IN, USA

Henrike K. Blumenfeld School of Speech, Language and Hearing Sciences, San Diego State University, San Diego, CA, USA

Ty Bodily Psychology Department and the Neuroscience Center, Brigham Young University, Provo, UT, USA

Doug Bodin Department of Pediatrics, Nationwide Children's Hospital and The Ohio State University, Columbus, OH, USA

Angela M. Bodling Center for Health Care Quality, University of Missouri—Columbia, Columbia, MO, USA

Jennifer Bogner Department of Physical Medicine and Rehabilitation, Ohio State University, Columbus, OH, USA

Robert J. Boland Department of Psychiatry, Brigham and Women's Hospital/Harvard Medical School, Boston, MA, USA

Mark W. Bondi University of California San Diego School of Medicine, La Jolla, CA, USA
Neuropsychological Assessment Unit, VA San Diego Healthcare System, San Diego, CA, USA

Amanda D. Bono Department of Psychology, Queens College and The Graduate Center of the City University of New York, Flushing, NY, USA

John G. Borkowski Department of Psychology, University of Notre Dame, Notre Dame, IN, USA

Joan C. Borod Department of Psychology, Queens College and The Graduate Center of the City University of New York (CUNY), New York, NY, USA

Department of Neurology, Icahn School of Medicine at Mount Sinai, New York, NY, USA

Beth Borosh Cognitive/Behavioral Neurology Center Northwestern Feinburg School of Medicine, Chicago, IL, USA

Carley Borza University of Alberta, Edmonton, AB, Canada

Dawn E. Bouman Neuropsychology and Medical Psychology, University of Cincinnati, Department of Neurology and Rehabilitation Medicine, Cincinnati, OH, USA

Isabelle Bourdeau Division of Endocrinology, Department of Medicine, Research Centre, Centre hospitalier de l'université de Montréal (CHUM), Montreal, QC, Canada

Jessica Bove Emory University, Atlanta, GA, USA

Dawn Bowers Department of Clinical and Health Psychology, University of Florida, Gainesville, FL, USA

Mary Boyle The College of Humanities and Social Sciences, Montclair State University, Montclair, NJ, USA

Lauren E. Bradley Department of Behavioral Sciences, Rush University Medical Center, Chicago, IL, USA

Natalie Brei Department of Psychology, University of Wisconsin-Milwaukee, Milwaukee, WI, USA

Lisa A. Brenner Rocky Mountain Mental Illness Research Education and Clinical Center, Denver, CO, USA

University of Colorado, Anschutz Medical Campus, Aurora, CO, USA

Rachel M. Bridges Department of Psychology, University of South Carolina, Columbia, SC, USA

Andrew Brodbelt The Walton Centre NHS Foundation Trust, Liverpool, UK

Justine S. Broecker The Westminster Schools, Atlanta, GA, USA

Alyssa M. Broomfield School of Psychology, The Chicago School of Professional Psychology, Chicago, IL, USA

John Brown Medical College of Georgia, Augusta, GA, USA

Margaret Brown Mount Sinai School of Medicine, New York, NY, USA

Racine Brown Center of Innovation on Disability and Rehabilitation Research, James A. Haley Veterans' Hospital, Tampa, FL, USA

Martha Brownlee-Duffeck Harry S. Truman Memorial, Columbia, MO, USA

Kelly Broxterman School Psychology, The Chicago School of Professional Psychology, Chicago, IL, USA

Hugh W. Buckingham Department of Communication Sciences and Disorders, College of Allied Health Sciences, University of Oklahoma Health Sciences Center, Oklahoma City, OK, USA

Ashley Bujalski Department of Psychology, William Paterson University, Wayne, NJ, USA

Rebecca Burger-Caplan Yale Child Study Center, Yale University School of Medicine, New Haven, CT, USA

Department of Pediatrics, Emory University School of Medicine, Atlanta, GA, USA

Jeffrey M. Burns Department of Neurology, University of Kansas School of Medicine, Kansas City, KS, USA

Thomas G. Burns Department of Neuropsychology, Children's Healthcare of Atlanta, Atlanta, GA, USA

Shane S. Bush Long Island Neuropsychology, P.C., Lake Ronkonkoma, NY, USA

Tamara Bushnik Inter-Hospital Research and Knowledge Translation, Rusk Rehabilitation, New York, NY, USA

Melissa Buttaro Department of Psychiatry, The Miriam Hospital, Providence, RI, USA

Meryl A. Butters Department of Psychiatry, University of Pittsburgh School of Medicine, WPIC, Pittsburgh, PA, USA

Xavier E. Cagigas UCLA Semel Institute for Neuroscience and Human Behavior, Los Angeles, CA, USA

Medical Psychology Assessment Center, Resnick Neuropsychiatric Hospital at UCLA, Los Angeles, CA, USA

Department of Psychiatry and Biobehavioral Sciences, David Geffen School of Medicine at UCLA, Los Angeles, CA, USA

Deborah A. Cahn-Weiner Department of Neurology, University of California, Davis, Davis, CA, USA

Rebecca M. Cain Fairfax Neonatal Associates, Fredericksburg, VA, USA

Charles D. Callahan Memorial Health System, Springfield, IL, USA

Jonathan Campbell Neurology, Virginia Commonwealth University, Richmond, VA, USA

Bruce Caplan Independent Practice, Wynnewood, PA, USA

Jessica A. Carboni Counseling and Psychological Services, Georgia State University, Atlanta, GA, USA

Noelle E. Carlozzi Physical Medicine and Rehabilitation, University of Michigan, Ann Arbor, MI, USA

Helen M. Carmine ReMed, Paoli, PA, USA

Dominic A. Carone University Hospital – Neuropsychology Assessment Program, SUNY Upstate Medical University, Syracuse, NY, USA

Janessa O. Carvalho Department of Psychology, Bridgewater State University, Bridgewater, MA, USA

Jennifer Cass Department of Pediatrics, Nationwide Children's Hospital and The Ohio State University, Columbus, OH, USA

Adam Cassidy Harvard University, Cambridge, MA, USA

Eric Catlin Physical Medicine and Rehabilitation, University of South Florida, Tampa, FL, USA

Amiram Catz Department of Spinal Rehabilitation, Loewenstein Rehabilitation Hospital, Raanana, Israel

Tel-Aviv University, Tel-Aviv, Israel

Jessica Chaiken HeiTech Services, Inc., National Rehabilitation Information Center, Landover, MD, USA

Grace-Anna Chaney Department of Psychology, Towson University, Towson, MD, USA

Lanshin Chang University of Macau, Taipa, Macau SAR, China

Sandra Bond Chapman Center for BrainHealth, The University of Texas at Dallas' school of Behavioral and Brain Sciences, Dallas, TX, USA

Jesse Chasman Department of Psychology, University of Connecticut, Storrs, CT, USA

Sandy Sut Ieng Cheang Department of Psychology, University of Macau, Taipa, Macau, SAR, China

Colby Chlebowski Department of Psychiatry, University of California, San Diego, USA

Woon N. Chow Department of Pathology, Microbiology, and Immunology, Vanderbilt University Medical Center, Nashville, TN, USA

Shawn E. Christ University of Missouri, Columbia, MO, USA

Sarah S. Christman Buckingham Department of Communication Sciences and Disorders, The University of Oklahoma Health Sciences Center, Oklahoma City, OK, USA

Severn B. Churn Neurology, Virginia Commonwealth University, Richmond, VA, USA

Angela Hein Ciccia Department of Psychological Sciences, Program in Communication Sciences, Case Western Reserve University, Cleveland, OH, USA

Elaine Clark Department of Educational Psychology, The University of Utah, Salt Lake City, UT, USA

Lee Anna Clark Department of Psychology, University of Notre Dame, Notre Dame, IN, USA

Robert Clark School Psychology, The Chicago School of Professional Psychology, Chicago, IL, USA

Uraina S. Clark Department of Neurology, Icahn School of Medicine at Mount Sinai, New York, NY, USA

Dave Clarke Comprehensive Epilepsy Program, Dell Children's Medical Center of Central Texas, Austin, TX, USA

Department of Pediatrics, Dell Medical School, The University of Texas at Austin, Austin, TX, USA

Lauren Clevenger University of Iowa, Iowa City, IA, USA

Derin Cobia Department of Psychology and Neuroscience Center, Brigham Young University, Provo, UT, USA

Melanie M. Cochrane Department of Psychology, University of Victoria, Victoria, BC, Canada

Ronald A. Cohen Department of Clinical and Health Psychology, College of Public Health and Health Professions, University of Florida, Gainesville, FL, USA

Center for Cognitive Aging and Memory, McKnight Brain Institute, University of Florida, Gainesville, FL, USA

Morris J. Cohen Neurology, Pediatrics and Psychiatry, Pediatric Neuropsychology, Medical College of Georgia and BT-2601 Children's Medical Center, Augusta, GA, USA

Raymond J. Colello Anatomy and Neurobiology, Virginia Commonwealth University, Richmond, VA, USA

G. Combs Legal Psychology (Psychology and Law), Neuropsychology, Clinical Psychology, Chicago School of Professional Psychology, Chicago, IL, USA

Brian Comly Magee Rehabilitation Hospital, Philadelphia, PA, USA

Adam Conley Virginia Commonwealth University Medical Center, Richmond, VA, USA

Lori G. Cook Center for BrainHealth, The University of Texas at Dallas, Dallas, TX, USA

Andrea Coppens Division of Neurology and Department of Psychology, Sick Kids-Centre for Brain and Mental Health, Toronto, ON, Canada

Patrick Coppens Communication Sciences and Disorders, SUNY Plattsburgh, Plattsburgh, NY, USA

Melinda A. Cornwell Department of Psychology, Queens College and The Graduate Center of the City University of New York, Flushing, NY, USA

Stephen Correia Department of Psychiatry and Human Behavior, Alpert Medical School, Brown University, Providence, USA

John D. Corrigan Department of Physical Medicine and Rehabilitation, Ohio State University, Columbus, OH, USA

Joyce A. Corsica Department of Behavioral Sciences, Rush University Medical Center, Chicago, IL, USA

H. Branch Coslett Department of Neurology, University of Pennsylvania, HUP, Philadelphia, PA, USA

Kelly Coulehan Health Psychology, Neuropsychology, Clinical Psychology, Fordham University, New York, NY, USA

John C. Courtney Socorro Mental Health, Presbyterian Medical Services, Socorro, NM, USA

David R. Cox Neuropsychology and Rehabilitation Consultants, P.C., Chapel Hill, NC, USA

Laura Cramer-Berness Department of Psychology, William Paterson University, Wayne, NJ, USA

Chava Creque Department of Psychology and Neuroscience, University of Colorado Boulder, Boulder, CO, USA

Savannah Crippen Department of Psychology, William Paterson University, Wayne, NJ, USA

Jessica Cruz School Psychology, The Chicago School of Professional Psychology, Chicago, IL, USA

Yenisel Cruz-Almeida Pain Research and Intervention Center of Excellence Clinical and Translational Science Institute, University of Florida, Gainesville, FL, USA

Carter M. Cunningham Fairfax Neonatal Associates, Falls Church, VA, USA

Jacqueline L. Cunningham Department of Psychology, Children's Hospital of Philadelphia, Philadelphia, PA, USA

Sean Cunningham Department of Educational Psychology, University of Utah, Salt Lake City, UT, USA

Cody Curatolo Department of Psychology, William Paterson University, Wayne, NJ, USA

Cherina Cyborski National Intrepid Center of Excellence, Walter Reed National Military Medical Center, Bethesda, MD, USA

Rik Carl D'Amato School Psychology, Clinical Neuropsychology, Clinical Psychology, The Chicago School of Professional Psychology, Chicago, IL, USA

Kristen Dams-O'Connor Department of Rehabilitation Medicine, Mount Sinai School of Medicine, New York, NY, USA

Natalie Dattilo Department of Psychiatry, Indiana University School of Medicine, Indianapolis, IN, USA

Andrew S. Davis Department of Educational Psychology, Ball State University, Muncie, IN, USA

Marcus Ponce de Leon Madigan Army Medical Center, Tacoma, WA, USA

Ashley de Marchena Department of Psychology, University of Connecticut, Storrs, CT, USA

Scott L. Decker Department of Psychology, University of South Carolina, Columbia, SC, USA

Nathalie DeFabrique Cook County Department of Corrections, Chicago, IL, USA

Nick A. DeFilippis Georgia School of Professional Psychology, Atlanta Psychological Associates, Atlanta, GA, USA

Kathleen K. M. Deidrick Neuro- and Behavioral Psychology, St. Luke's Children's Hospital, Boise, ID, USA

Lisa Delano-Wood Memory, Aging and Resilience Clinic (MARC), Department of Psychiatry, University of California, San Diego, La Jolla, CA, USA
VA San Diego Healthcare System, San Diego, CA, USA

Dean C. Delis School of Medicine, University of California-San Diego, La Jolla, CA, USA

John DeLuca Research Department, Kessler Foundation, West Orange, NJ, USA

George J. Demakis Department of Psychology, University of North Carolina at Charlotte, Charlotte, NC, USA

Theslee Joy DePiero Braintree Rehabilitation Hospital, Boston University School of Medicine, Boston, MA, USA

Roberta DePompei School of Speech-Language Pathology and Audiology, University of Akron, Akron, OH, USA

Emily Desbiens Department of Psychology, William Paterson University, Wayne, NJ, USA

Krista Dettle Department of Psychology, William Paterson University, Wayne, NJ, USA

Bruce J. Diamond Department of Psychology, William Paterson University, Wayne, NJ, USA

Aimee Dietz Communication Sciences and Disorders, University of Cincinnati, Cincinnati, OH, USA

María Díez-Cirarda Department of Methods and Experimental Psychology, Faculty of Psychology and Education, University of Deusto, Bilbao, Spain

Marcel P. J. M. Dijkers American Congress of Rehabilitation Medicine, Reston, VA, USA

Department of Rehabilitation Medicine, Icahn School of Medicine at Mount Sinai, New York, NY, USA

Ekaterina Dobryakova Traumatic Brain Injury Research, Kessler Foundation, West Orange, NJ, USA

Carl B. Dodrill Department of Neurology, University of Washington School of Medicine, Seattle, WA, USA

Ben Dodsworth PM&R, University of South Florida, Tampa, FL, USA

Peter Dodzik Fort Wayne Neurological Center, Fort Wayne, IN, USA

Christopher H. Domen School of Medicine, Department of Neurosurgery, University of Colorado, Aurora, CO, USA

Jacobus Donders Mary Free Bed Rehabilitation Hospital, Grand Rapids, MI, USA

Kerry Donnelly VA WNY Healthcare System, University of Buffalo (SUNY) Behavioral Health Careline (116B), Buffalo, NY, USA

Jennifer M. Doran VA Connecticut Healthcare System, Yale School of Medicine, Newington, CT, USA

Vonetta Dotson Department of Psychology, Georgia State University, Atlanta, GA, USA

Department of Clinical and Health Psychology College of Public Health and Health Professions, University of Florida, Gainesville, FL, USA

Lauren R. Dowell Laboratory for Neurocognitive and Imaging Research, Kennedy Krieger Institute, Baltimore, MD, USA

Leah Drasher-Phillips Center of Innovation on Disability and Rehabilitation Research, James A. Haley Veterans' Hospital, Tampa, FL, USA

Elena Harlan Drewel Neuro- and Behavioral Psychology, St. Luke's Children's Hospital, Boise, ID, USA

Tina Drossos Departments of Psychiatry and Behavioral Neuroscience, and Pediatrics, Section of Child and Adolescent Psychiatry, The University of Chicago, Chicago, IL, USA

Lindsey Duca Department of Orthopedics and Rehabilitation, University of Wisconsin School of Medicine and Public Health, Madison, WI, USA

Nicole M. Dudukovic Department of Psychology, University of Oregon, Eugene, OR, USA

Mary Dunkle National Organization for Rare Disorders (NORD), Danbury, CT, USA

Kari Dunning Department of Rehabilitation Sciences, University of Cincinnati, Cincinnati, OH, USA

Jeff Dupree Anatomy and Neurobiology, Virginia Commonwealth University, Richmond, VA, USA

Ana Durand Sanchez Physical Medicine and Rehabilitation, Baylor College of Medicine, Houston, TX, USA

Moira C. Dux US Department of Veteran Affairs, Baltimore, MD, USA

Blessen C. Eapen Polytrauma Rehabilitation Center, South Texas Veterans Health Care System, San Antonio, TX, USA

Department of Rehabilitation Medicine, UT Health San Antonio, San Antonio, TX, USA

Angela Eastvold Department of Neurology, The University of Utah, Salt Lake City, UT, USA

Natalie C. Ebner Department of Psychology, University of Florida, Gainesville, FL, USA

Department of Aging and Geriatric Research, Institute on Aging, University of Florida, Gainesville, FL, USA

Lisa Edmonds Communication Sciences and Disorders, Teachers College Columbia University, New York, NY, USA

Dawn M. Ehde Department of Rehabilitation Medicine, University of Washington, Seattle, WA, USA

Alyssa Eidson Emory University/Rehabilitation Medicine, Atlanta, GA, USA

Donovan Ellis Department of Psychology, University of Florida, Gainesville, FL, USA

Erin E. Emery-Tiburcio Department of Behavioral Sciences, Rush University Medical Center, Chicago, IL, USA

Joel Eppig Joint Doctoral Program in Clinical Psychology, University of California, San Diego State University, San Diego, CA, USA

Jacqueline Estrada School of Psychology, The Chicago School of Professional Psychology, Chicago, IL, USA

Eleazar Eusebio School Psychology, The Chicago School of Professional Psychology, Chicago, IL, USA

Allison S. Evans Concord Comprehensive Neuropsychological Services, Concord, MA, USA

Daniel Erik Everhart Department of Psychology, Eastern Carolina University, Greenville, NC, USA

Nathan Ewigman Mental Health Service Line, San Francisco VA Health Care System, San Francisco, CA, USA

Joseph E. Fair Brigham Young University, Provo, UT, USA

Jacob Faltin School Psychology, The Chicago School of Professional Psychology, Chicago, IL, USA

Jaelyn R. Farris Department of Psychology, Youngstown State University, Youngstown, OH, USA

Khan Fary Department of Medicine, University of Melbourne and the Royal Melbourne Hospital, Parkville, VA, Australia

Deborah Fein Department of Psychological Sciences, University of Connecticut, Storrs, CT, USA

Leilani Feliciano Department of Psychology, University of Colorado at Colorado Springs, Colorado Springs, CO, USA

Aaron Feliu James A Haley Veterans Hospital, Tampa, FL, USA

Warren L. Felton Department of Neurology, Virginia Commonwealth University Medical Center, Richmond, VA, USA

Kyle E. Ferguson University of British Columbia, Vancouver, BC, Canada

Robert Fieo Department of Aging and Geriatric Research, College of Medicine, Institute on Aging, University of Florida, Gainesville, FL, USA

Christina Figueroa Memory and Aging Program, Butler Hospital, Providence, RI, USA

Carole M. Filangieri Department of Behavioral Health, NYU Winthrop Hospital, Mineola, NY, USA

Eric M. Fine Department of Neurology, University of California, San Francisco, CA, USA

Jessica Fish Medical Research Council Cognition and Brain Sciences Unit, Cambridge, UK

Julie Testa Flaada Rochester, MN, USA

Jennifer Fleming School of Health and Rehabilitation Sciences, The University of Queensland, Brisbane, QLD, Australia

Kimberly Fleming Department of Psychiatry and Behavioral Sciences, The University of Kansas KU Medical Center, Kansas City, KS, USA

James R. Flynn Department of Politics, The University of Otago, Dunedin, New Zealand

Kristin Joan Flynn Peters Department of Health Sciences, University of Missouri, Columbia, MO, USA

Nancy S. Foldi Department of Psychology, Queens College and The Graduate Center, The City University of New York, New York, NY, USA

Department of Medicine, Winthrop University Hospital, Stony Brook School of Medicine, Mineola, NY, USA

Samantha Foreman Immaculata University, Immaculata, PA, USA

Hélène Forget Département de psychoéducation et de psychologie, Université du Québec en Outaouais, Gatineau, QC, Canada

Bonny J. Forrest Independent Practice, San Diego, CA, USA

Lisa M. Fox NYU Langone Medical Center, Department of Psychology, Rusk Institute of Rehabilitation Medicine, New York, NY, USA

Michael A. Fox Anatomy and Neurobiology, Virginia Commonwealth University Medical Center, Richmond, VA, USA

Laura L. Frakey Memorial Hospital of Rhode Island and Alpert Medical School of Brown University, Pawtucket, RI, USA

Robert G. Frank University of New Mexico, Albuquerque, NM, USA

Michael Franzen Allegheny General Hospital, Pittsburgh, PA, USA

Stacy Frauwirth Academic Therapy Publications, Novato, CA, USA

Ian Frazier Department of Psychology, University of Florida, Gainesville, FL, USA

Kathleen L. Fuchs Department of Neurology, University of Virginia Health System, Charlottesville, VA, USA

Shawn Gale Department of Psychology and Neuroscience Center, Brigham Young University, Provo, UT, USA

Kristin Galetta Department of Neurology, Brigham and Women's Hospital, Boston, MA, USA

Steven Galetta Department of Neurology, New York University of Medicine, New York, NY, USA

Sherri Gallagher Wellness PSI, LLC Private Practice, Flagstaff, AZ, USA

Frank J. Gallo Department of Psychology, University of Wisconsin-Milwaukee, Milwaukee, WI, USA

Emnet Gammada Department of Psychology, Queens College and The Graduate Center, The City University of New York, New York, NY, USA

Sarah Garcia Department of Psychiatry- Neuropsychology, University of Michigan Health System, Ann Arbor, MI, USA

Pamela Garn-Nunn Department of Pharmacology, Virginia Commonwealth University, Richmond, VA, USA

Kelly Davis Garrett Intermountain Healthcare and University of Utah Center on Aging, Salt Lake City, UT, USA

Kelli Williams Gary Department of Occupational Therapy, Virginia Commonwealth University, Richmond, VA, USA

Brandon E. Gavett Department of Psychology, University of Colorado Colorado Springs, Colorado Springs, CO, USA

Helen M. Genova Neuropsychology and Neuroscience Laboratory, Kessler Foundation Research Center, West Orange, NJ, USA

Savannah J. Geske Department of Psychiatry and Behavioral Sciences, University of Kansas Medical Center, Kansas City, KS, USA

Glen E. Getz Department of Psychiatry, Allegheny General Hospital, Pittsburgh, PA, USA

Neuropsychology Specialty Care, LLC, Pittsburgh, PA, USA

Christine Ghilain Department of Neuropsychology, Children's Healthcare of Atlanta, Atlanta, Georgia, USA

Gerard A. Gioia Children's National Medical Center, Rockville, MD, USA

Elizabeth Louise Glisky Department of Psychology, University of Arizona, Tucson, AZ, USA

Emilie Godwin Virginia Commonwealth University, Richmond, VA, USA

Gary Goldberg Hunter Holmes McGuire Veterans Administration Medical Center, Department of Physical Medicine and Rehabilitation, Virginia Commonwealth University School of Medicine/Medical College of Virginia, Richmond, VA, USA

Myron Goldberg Department of Rehabilitation Medicine, University of Washington Medical Center, Seattle, WA, USA

Diane Cordry Golden Association of Assistive Technology Act Programs, Delmar, NY, USA

Charles J. Golden Center for Psychological Studies, Nova Southeastern University, Fort Lauderdale, FL, USA

Amy S. Goldman Association of Assistive Technology Act Programs (ATAP), Springfield, IL, USA

Bram Goldstein Department of Gynecologic Oncology, Hoag Hospital Cancer Center, Newport Beach, CA, USA

Assawin Gongvatana Department of Psychiatry, University of California, San Diego, San Diego, CA, USA

Efrain Antonio Gonzalez College of Psychology, Nova Southeastern University, Fort Lauderdale, FL, USA

Utah State University, Logan, UT, USA

Matthew E. Goodwin Central Arkansas Veterans Healthcare System, Little Rock, AR, USA

Robert M. Gordon Rusk Rehabilitation, New York University Langone Medical Center, New York, NY, USA

Kimberly A. Gorgens Graduate School of Professional Psychology, University of Denver, Denver, CO, USA

Janet Grace Psychiatry and Human Behavior, Alpert Medical School of Brown University, Providence, RI, USA

Martin R. Graf Department of Neurosurgery, Virginia Commonwealth University Medical Center, Richmond, VA, USA

Lori Grafton Carolinas Rehabilitation Carolinas HealthCare System, Charlotte, NC, USA

Kristin M. Graham Department of Physical Medicine and Rehabilitation, Virginia Commonwealth University, Richmond, VA, USA

Michael R. Greher School of Medicine, Department of Neurosurgery, University of Colorado, Aurora, CO, USA

Sarah Griffin Virginia Commonwealth University, Richmond, VA, USA

Julie Griffith Department of Speech Pathology and Audiology, Ball State University, Muncie, IN, USA

Stephanie Griffiths Simon Fraser University, Burnaby, BC, Canada

Elizabeth S. Gromisch Psychology Service, VA Connecticut, West Haven, CT, USA

Benjamin Grover-Manthey Department of Physical Medicine and Rehabilitation, Indiana University, Indianapolis, IN, USA

William Guido Anatomy and Neurobiology, Virginia Commonwealth University Medical Center, Richmond, VA, USA

Desiree Gulliford Department of Psychology, University of Florida, Gainesville, FL, USA

Carly Gundrum Legal Psychology (Psychology and Law), Neuropsychology, Clinical Psychology, The Chicago School of Professional Psychology, Chicago, IL, USA

Audrey H. Gutherie Rehabilitation Research and Development Center of Excellence Atlanta Veterans Administration Medical Center, Decatur, GA, USA

Karl Haberlandt Department of Psychology, Trinity College, Hartford, CT, USA

Martin Hahn Department of Biology, William Paterson University, Wayne, NJ, USA

Kathrine Hak Applied Psychology and Counselor Education, University of Northern Colorado, Greeley, CO, USA

Katherine Hallahan University of Cincinnati, Cincinnati, OH, USA

John Halperin Overlook Medical Center, Atlantic Health System, Summit, NJ, USA

Marla J. Hamberger Department of Neurology, Columbia University Medical Center, New York, NY, USA

Flora M. Hammond Department of Physical Medicine and Rehabilitation, Indiana University School of Medicine, Indianapolis, IN, USA

Benjamin Hampstead Department of Pharmacology, Virginia Commonwealth University, Richmond, VA, USA

Department of Psychiatry, University of Michigan, Michigan Alzheimer's Disease Center, Ann Arbor, MI, USA

Sarah Hannigen Department of Psychology, Allegheny Health Network, Pittsburgh, PA, USA

Stephanie L. Hanson College of Public Health and Health Professions, University of Florida, Gainesville, FL, USA

Keith Happawana Department of Psychology, William Paterson University, Wayne, NJ, USA

Janna L. Harris Department of Anatomy and Cell Biology, University of Kansas Medical Center, Kansas City, KS, USA

Hoglund Brain Imaging Center, University of Kansas Medical Center, Kansas City, KS, USA

Patti L. Harrison School Psychology, The University of Alabama, Tuscaloosa, AL, USA

Eric S. Hart University of Missouri Center for Health Care Quality, Columbia, MO, USA

Michael J. Hartman Department of Psychology, University of Wisconsin-Milwaukee, Milwaukee, WI, USA

Kari Hawkins Neuropsychology Department, Addenbrooke's Hospital, Cambridge, UK

Amy Heffelfinger Medical College of Wisconsin, Milwaukee, WI, USA

Robert L. Heilbronner Chicago Neuropsychology Group, Chicago, IL, USA

Kenneth M. Heilman Department of Neurology, University of Florida College of Medicine, Center for Neurological Studies and the Research Service of the Malcom Randall Veterans Affairs Medical Center, Gainesville, FL, USA

Nancy Helm-Estabrooks Department of Communication Disorders and Sciences, College of Health and Human Sciences, Western Carolina University, Cullowhee, NC, USA

Nathan Henninger Department of Pediatrics, Nationwide Children's Hospital College of Medicine, Ohio State University, Columbus, OH, USA

Mary Hibbard Department of Rehabilitation Medicine, New York School of Medicine, New York, NY, USA

Ashley K. Hill Nationally Certified School Psychologist, Chicago, IL, USA

Tanisha G. Hill-Jarrett Division of Rehabilitation Neuropsychology, Department of Rehabilitation Medicine, Emory University, Atlanta, GA, USA

Yvonne Hindes Division of Applied Psychology, Faculty of Education, University of Calgary, Calgary, AB, Canada

Merrill Hiscock Department of Psychology, University of Houston, Houston, TX, USA

G. Alex Hishaw Neurology Section, Southern Arizona VA Healthcare System, Tucson, AZ, USA

Department of Neurology, University of Arizona, Tucson, AZ, USA

Elise K. Hodges Department of Psychiatry, Neuropsychology Division, University of Michigan Health System, Ann Arbor, MI, USA

Anna DePold Hohler Boston University Medical Center, Boston, MA, USA

Matthew H. Holcomb Department of Pharmacology, Virginia Commonwealth University, Richmond, VA, USA

Tracey Hollingsworth Developmental Assessment Program, Nationwide Children's Hospital, Columbus, OH, USA

Stephanie Hooker Department of Behavioral Sciences, Rush University Medical Center, Chicago, IL, USA

Kelly L. Hoover Department of Educational Psychology, Ball State University, Muncie, IN, USA

Crista A. Hopp Connected Pathways Coaching, Herndon, VA, USA

Karin F. Hoth Department of Medicine, University of Iowa, Iowa City, IA, USA

Gillian Hotz Department of Neurosurgery/The Miami Project to Cure Paralysis, University of Miami Miller School of Medicine, Miami, FL, USA

Marianne Hrabok Department of Psychology, Addiction and Mental Health, Alberta Health Services, Edmonton, AB, Canada

Gabrielle Hromas Department of Clinical and Health Psychology, University of Florida, Gainesville, FL, USA

Leesa V. Huang Department of Psychology, California State University, Chico, CA, USA

Dawn H. Huber Department of Health Psychology, University of Missouri, Columbia, MO, USA

Adam Hudepohl Georgia State University, Atlanta, GA, USA

Trevor Huff Department of Psychology and Neuroscience Center, Brigham Young University, Provo, UT, USA

Bradley J. Hufford Neuropsychology, Rehabilitation Hospital of Indiana, Indianapolis, IN, USA

Candace Hughes School of Psychology, The Chicago School of Professional Psychology, Chicago, IL, USA

Joel W. Hughes Department of Psychology, Kent State University, Kent, OH, USA

David Hulac Department of School Psychology, College of Education and Behavioral Sciences, University of Northern Colorado, Greeley, CO, USA

Faiza Humayun Inpatient Traumatic Brain Injury Unit, James Haley VA Hospital, Tampa, FL, USA

Edward E. Hunter Department of Psychiatry and Behavioral Sciences, University of Kansas Medical Center, Kansas City, KS, USA

Scott J. Hunter Departments of Psychiatry and Behavioral Neuroscience, and Pediatrics, Pediatric Neuropsychology, Section of Child and Adolescent Psychiatry, The University of Chicago, Chicago, IL, USA

Julia Hussey Department of Psychology, University of Nevada, Las Vegas, Las Vegas, NV, USA

R. Matthew Hutchison Biogen Inc., Cambridge, MA, USA

Karen Hux Quality Living, Omaha, NE, USA

Summer Ibarra Rehabilitation Hospital of Indiana, Indianapolis, IN, USA

Naroa Ibarretxe-Bilbao Department of Methods and Experimental Psychology, Faculty of Psychology and Education, University of Deusto, Bilbao, Spain

Jean Ikanga Division of Rehabilitation Neuropsychology, Department of Rehabilitation Medicine, Emory University, Atlanta, GA, USA

Matilde Inglese Department of Neurology, Radiology and Neuroscience, Icahn School of Medicine at Mount Sinai, New York, NY, USA

Farzin Irani Psychology Department, West Chester University of Pennsylvania, West Chester, PA, USA

Rubyat Islam Department of Psychology, Queens College of the City University of New York, Flushing, NY, USA

Peter K. Isquith Dartmouth Medical School, Lebanon, NH, USA

Cindy B. Ivanhoe Neurorehabilitation Specialists Baylor College of Medicine, The Institute for Rehabilitation and Research, Houston, TX, USA

Grant L. Iverson Department of Psychiatry, British Columbia Mental Health and Addictions, University of British Columbia, Vancouver, BC, Canada

Colleen E. Jackson VA Boston Healthcare System, Boston, MA, USA

Kimberle M. Jacobs Department of Anatomy and Neurobiology, Virginia Commonwealth University, Richmond, VA, USA

Mathew Jacobs Pennsylvania State University, University Park, PA, USA

Lisa A. Jacobson Department of Neuropsychology, Kennedy Krieger Institute, Baltimore, MD, USA

Department of Psychiatry and Behavioral Sciences, Johns Hopkins University School of Medicine, Baltimore, MD, USA

Kelly M. Janke Columbia University Medical Center, New York, NY, USA

Nicholas Jasinski Division of Neuropsychology, Henry Ford Health System, Detroit, MI, USA

Beth A. Jerskey Department of Psychiatry and Human Behavior, Alpert Medical School of Brown University, Providence, RI, USA

Amitabh Jha TBIMS National Data and Statistical Center, Craig Hospital, Englewood, CO, USA

Mi-Yeoung Jo Sherman Oaks, CA, USA

Joshua Johnson Department of Psychiatry (MC-2103), UConn Health Center, Farmington, CT, USA

Judy A. Johnson Special Education Department, Aldine Independent School District, Houston, TX, USA

Julene K. Johnson Center for Aging in Diverse Communities, University of California, San Francisco, San Francisco, CA, USA

Kristin L. Johnson Applied Psychology and Counselor Education, University of Northern Colorado, Greeley, CO, USA

Nancy Johnson Cognitive/Behavioral Neurology Center Northwestern Feinburg School of Medicine, Chicago, IL, USA

Susan K. Johnson Department of Psychology, University of North Carolina at Charlotte, Charlotte, NC, USA

Taylor Johnson School of Psychology, The Chicago School of Professional Psychology, Chicago, IL, USA

Brick Johnstone Intrepid Spirit Center, Fort Belvoir, VA, USA

Robert D. Jones Department of Neurology, The University of Iowa, Iowa City, USA

Aaron N. Juni Neuropsychology Center of Maryland, LLC, Owings Mills, MD, USA

Solomon Kalkstein Psychiatry, University of Pennsylvania, Philadelphia, PA, USA

Randy W. Kamphaus College of Education, The University of Oregon, Eugene, OR, USA

Stephen M. Kanne Thompson Center for Autism and Neurodevelopmental Disorders, University of Missouri, Columbia, MO, USA

Edith Kaplan Department of Psychology, Suffolk University, Boston, MA, USA

Erica Kaplan Rehabilitation Medicine, Brain Injury Research Center, Icahn School of Medicine at Mount Sinai, New York, NY, USA

Paul E. Kaplan Capitol Clinical Neuroscience, Folsom, CA, USA

Richard F. Kaplan Department of Psychiatry (MC-2103), UConn Health Center, Farmington, CT, USA

Narinder Kapur Research Department of Clinical, Educational and Health Psychology, University College London, London, UK

Ninad Karandikar RAC, Department of PM&R AND Physiatrist, Polytrauma Transitional Rehabilitation Program, VA Palo Alto, Palo Alto, California, USA
Department of Orthoedics, Stanford University, Palo Alto, California, USA

Stella Karantzoulis Modern Brain Center, New York, NY, USA

Nadine J. Kaslow Department of Psychiatry and Behavioral Sciences, Emory University School of Medicine, APA, Atlanta, GA, USA

Sheryl Katta-Charles Department of Physical Medicine and Rehabilitation, Indiana University School of Medicine, Indianapolis, IN, USA

Douglas I. Katz Department of Neurology, Boston University School of Medicine, Braintree, MA, USA

Michael Kaufman Department of Neurology, Carolinas Medical Center, Charlotte, NC, USA

Edith Kaplan: deceased.

Margarita Kaushanskaya University of Wisconsin-Madison, Madison, WI, USA

Jacqueline M. Kawa Psychiatry and Behavioral Medicine, Children's Hospital of Wisconsin, Milwaukee, WI, USA

Jaeson Kaylegian Departments of Psychiatry and Behavioral Neuroscience, and Pediatrics, Pediatric Neuropsychology, Section of Child and Adolescent Psychiatry, The University of Chicago, Chicago, IL, USA
Neuropsychology Technician III, University of Chicago Medicine, Chicago, IL, USA

Jacob Kean Department of Physical Medicine and Rehabilitation, Indiana University School of Medicine, Indianapolis, IN, USA

C. Keith Conners Duke University Medical School, Durham, NC, USA

Avril J. Keller Alberta Children's Hospital, University of Calgary, Calgary, AB, Canada

Kristy K. Kelly Educational Psychology, University of Wisconsin-Madison, Madison, WI, USA

Sally L. Kemp University of Missouri, Columbia, MO, USA

Thomas R. Kerkhoff College of Public Health and Health Professions, University of Florida, Gainesville, FL, USA

Kimberly A. Kerns Department of Psychology, University of Victoria, Victoria, BC, Canada

So Hyun Kim Yale Child Study Center, Yale School of Medicine, New Haven, CT, USA

Sangsun Kim Psychological Sciences, University of Missouri, Columbia, MO, USA

Sun Mi Kim Department of Psychology, Queens College of the City University of New York, Flushing, NY, USA

Tricia Z. King Department of Psychology and the Neuroscience Institute, Georgia State University, Atlanta, GA, USA

Brock Kirwan Psychology Department and the Neuroscience Center, Brigham Young University, Provo, UT, USA

Bonita P. "Bonnie" Klein-Tasman Department of Psychology, University of Wisconsin-Milwaukee, Milwaukee, WI, USA

Jennifer Sue Kleiner Department of Psychology, University of Arkansas for Medical Sciences Blandford Physician Center, Little Rock, AR, USA

Daniel W. Klyce Virginia Commonwealth University – School of Medicine, Richmond, VA, USA

C. Keith Conners: deceased.

Samantha Knight Medicine, Royal College of Surgeons in Ireland, Dublin, Ireland

Kelly Knollman-Porter Department of Speech Pathology and Audiology, Miami University, Oxford, OH, USA

Tiffany Kodak Department of Psychology, University of Wisconsin-Milwaukee, Milwaukee, WI, USA

Julia Kolak Department of Psychology, William Paterson University, Wayne, NJ, USA

Stephanie A. Kolakowsky-Hayner Department of Rehabilitation Medicine, Icahn School of Medicine at Mount Sinai, New York, NY, USA

Dan Koonce The Chicago School of Psychology, Chicago, IL, USA

Paul T. Korte Harry S. Truman Memorial Veterans' Hospital, Columbia, MO, USA

Kathleen A. Koth Department of Psychiatry and Behavioral Medicine, Medical College of Wisconsin, Milwaukee, WI, USA

Zhifeng Kou Biomedical Engineering and Radiology, Wayne State University, Detroit, MI, USA

Rothem Kovner Department of Psychiatry, University of Wisconsin-Madison, Madison, WI, USA

Elizabeth Kozora Department of Medicine, National Jewish Medical and Research Center, National Jewish Health, Denver, CO, USA

Joel H. Kramer UCSF Memory and Aging Center UCSF Med Ctr, 0984-8AC, San Francisco, CA, USA

Matthew Kraybill Neuropsychology, Cottage Rehabilitation Hospital, Santa Barbara, CA, USA

Denise Krch Kessler Foundation, East Hanover, NJ, USA

Kate Krival Speech Pathology, School of Health Sciences, Edinboro University of Pennsylvania, Edinboro, PA, USA

Lauren B. Krupp Department of Neuropsychology Research, Stony Brook University SUNY Stony Brook, Stony Brook, NY, USA

Nuri Erkut Kucukboyaci Clinical Psychology, Rusk Institute – NYU Langone Health, New York, NY, USA

Beth Kuczynski Imaging of Dementia and Aging (IDeA) Laboratory, Department of Neurology and Center for Neuroscience, University of California, Davis, CA, USA

Jeffrey G. Kuentzel Wayne State University, Detroit, MI, USA

Richard Kunz Department of Physical Medicine and Rehabilitation, Virginia Commonwealth University, Richmond, VA, USA

Brad Kurowski Department of Physical Medicine and Rehabilitation, Spaulding Rehabilitation Hospital, Massachusetts General Hospital, Brigham and Women's Hospital, Harvard Medical School, Cincinnati, OH, USA

Matthew M. Kurtz Department of Psychology, Wesleyan University, Middletown, CT, USA

Monica Kurylo Departments of Psychiatry and Rehabilitation Medicine, University of Kansas Medical Center, Kansas City, KS, USA

Christina Kwasnica Barrow Neurological Institute, Phoenix, AZ, USA

David Lachar University of Texas Houston Health Science Center, Houston, TX, USA

Susan Ladley Department of Physical Medicine and Rehabilitation, University of Colorado, Denver Health Medical Center, Denver, CO, USA

Ginette Lafleche Memory Disorders Research Center, VA Boston Healthcare System and Boston University School of Medicine, Boston, MA, USA

Audrey Lafrenaye Department of Anatomy and Neurobiology, Virginia Commonwealth University, Richmond, VA, USA

Sarah K. Lageman Parkinson's and Movement Disorders Center, Department of Neurology, School Of Medicine, Virginia Commonwealth University, Richmond, VA, USA

Melissa Lamar Rush Alzheimer's Disease Center, Chicago, IL, USA

Damon G. Lamb Department of Clinical and Health Psychology, University of Florida, Gainesville, FL, USA

Center for Cognitive Aging and Memory, McKnight Brain Institute, University of Florida, Gainesville, FL, USA

Department of Neurology, University of Florida, Gainesville, FL, USA

Brain Rehabilitation Research Center, Malcom Randall VAMC, Gainesville, FL, USA

Gudrun Lange Pain and Fatigue Study Center, New York, NY, USA

Mount Sinai Beth Israel Medical Center, New York, NY, USA

Rael T. Lange Defense and Veterans Brain Injury Center, Walter Reed National Military Medical Center, Bethesda, MD, USA

Karen G. Langer Department of Rehabilitation Medicine, Rusk Rehabilitation, NYU Langone Medical Center, New York, NY, USA

Kayla LaRosa Educational and Psychological Studies/TBI Model Systems, University of South Florida/J.A. Haley VA, Tampa, FL, USA

Michael J. Larson Brigham Young University, Provo, UT, USA

Jennifer C. G. Larson Department of Physical Medicine and Rehabilitation, University of Michigan, Ann Arbor, MI, USA

Adele A. Larsson Department of Educational Psychology, Ball State University, Muncie, IN, USA

Javier Peña Lasa Department of Psychology, Deusto University, Bilbao, Spain

Thomas M. Laudate Department of Adult Neurology, Tufts Medical Center, Boston, MA, USA

Ronald M. Lazar Department of Neurology, University of Alabama at Birmingham, Birmingham, AL, USA

Victoria M. Leavitt Cognitive Neuroscience Division, Columbia University Medical School, New York, NY, USA

Sophie Lebrecht Visual Neuroscience Laboratory, Brown University, Providence, RI, USA

Kangmin D. Lee Department of Neurosurgery, Virginia Commonwealth University, Richmond, VA, USA

Sing Lee Department of Psychiatry, The Chinese University of Hong Kong, Shatin, Hong Kong SAR, China

Stacie A. Leffard Behavioral Medicine and Psychiatry, West Virginia University, Morgantown, WV, USA

George Leichnetz Virginia Commonwealth University, Richmond, VA, USA

Hoyle Leigh Department of Psychiatry, University of California, San Francisco, CA, USA

Sarah J. Leinen Institute for Graduate Clinical Psychology, Widener University, Chester, PA, USA

Jeannie Lengenfelder Kessler Foundation Research Center, West Orange, NJ, USA

José León-Carrión Human Neuropsychology Laboratory, School of Psychology, Department of Experimental Psychology, University of Seville, Seville, Spain

Center for Brain Injury Rehabilitation (CRECER), Seville, Spain

Umberto León-Domínguez Health Sciences Vice-Chancellor, Department of Psychology, University of Monterrey, Monterrey, Mexico

Human Neuropsychology Laboratory, School of Psychology, Department of Experimental Psychology, University of Seville, Seville, Spain

Pierre A. Leon Department of Psychology, William Paterson University, Wayne, NJ, USA

Vanesa C. Lerma Department of Neurological Surgery, Weill Cornell Medicine, New York, NY, USA

Holly Levin-Aspenson Department of Psychology, University of Notre Dame, Notre Dame, IN, USA

Brian Levine Rotman Research Institute at Baycrest, Toronto, ON, Canada

Allen N. Lewis Jr. School of Health and Rehabilitation Science, University of Pittsburgh, Pittsburgh, PA, USA

Pamela H. Lewis Department of Rehabilitation Counseling, School of Allied Health Professions, Virginia Commonwealth University, Richmond, VA, USA

David J. Libon Departments of Geriatrics, Gerontology, and Psychology, Rowan University, New Jersey Institute for Successful Aging, School of Osteopathic Medicine, Stratford, NJ, USA

Edward Liebmann Department of Psychology, The University of Kansas, Lawrence, KS, USA

Tanya P. Lin Neurology Section, Southern Arizona VA Healthcare System, Tucson, AZ, USA

Department of Neurology, University of Arizona, Tucson, AZ, USA

Sara M. Lippa Defense and Veterans Brain Injury Center, Walter Reed National Military Medical Center, Bethesda, MD, USA

Hayley Loblein Department of Educational Psychology, The University of Texas at Austin, Austin, TX, USA

Dona Locke Psychiatry and Psychology, Mayo Clinic, Scottsdale, AZ, USA

Chris Loftis National Council for Community Behavioral Healthcare, Alexandria, VA, USA

Kenneth J. Logan Department of Speech, Language, and Hearing Sciences, University of Florida, Gainesville, FL, USA

Michelle Loman Department of Neurology, Medical College of Wisconsin, Milwaukee, WI, USA

Eduardo Lopez Rehabilitation Medicine, New York Medical College, Metropolitan Hospital, New York, NY, USA

Catherine Lord Center for Autism and the Developing Brain, New York-Presbyterian Hospital/Westchester Division, White Plains, NY, USA

Janis Lorman School of Speech–Language Pathology and Audiology, The University of Akron, Akron, OH, USA

Rachel Losoff School Psychology, The Chicago School of Professional Psychology, Chicago, IL, USA

John A. Lucas Department of Psychiatry and Psychology, Mayo Clinic, Jacksonville, FL, USA

Stephen D. Luke National Dissemination Center for Children with Disabilities (NICHCY), Washington, DC, USA

Jacob T. Lutz Department of Special Education, Ball State University, Muncie, IN, USA

Jon G. Lyon Mazomanie, WI, USA

Paige Lysne Department of Aging and Geriatric Research, Institute of Aging, University of Florida – College of Medicine, Gainesville, FL, USA

Kelly Teresa Macdonald Department of Psychology, University of Houston, Houston, TX, USA

Anna MacKay-Brandt Nathan S. Kline Institute for Psychiatric Research, Orangeburg, NY, USA

Taub Institute for Research on Alzheimer's Disease and the Aging Brain, Columbia University, New York, NY, USA

Stephanie Magou Department of Psychology, William Paterson University, Wayne, NJ, USA

E. Mark Mahone Department of Neuropsychology, Kennedy Krieger Institute, Baltimore, MD, USA

Department of Psychiatry and Behavioral Sciences, Johns Hopkins University School of Medicine, Baltimore, MD, USA

B. Makofske Legal Psychology (Psychology and Law), Neuropsychology, Clinical Psychology, Chicago School of Professional Psychology, Chicago, IL, USA

James F. Malec Department of Physical Medicine and Rehabilitation, Indiana University School of Medicine and the Rehabilitation Hospital of Indiana, Indianapolis, IN, USA

Amit X. Malhotra Department of Pediatric Specialty, Division of Neurology, TPMG, Kaiser Permanente East Bay Medical Center, Oakland, CA, USA

Paul Malloy Department of Psychiatry and Human Behavior, Brown University, Providence, RI, USA

William Victor Maloy The Virginia Institute of Pastoral Care, Richmond, VA, USA

Gail Malvestuto School of Psychology, The Chicago School of Professional Psychology, Chicago, IL, USA

Carlye B. G. Manna Department of Psychology, Queens College of the City University of New York (CUNY), Flushing, NY, USA

Bernice A. Marcopulos Department of Graduate Psychology, James Madison University, Harrisonburg, VA, USA

Christina R. Marmarou Neurosurgery, Virginia Commonwealth University, Richmond, VA, USA

Patrick Marsh Department of Psychiatry and Behavioral Sciences, University of South Florida College of Medicine, Tampa, FL, USA

Matthew P. Martens University of Missouri, Columbia, MO, USA

Thomas Martin Center for Health Care Quality, University of Missouri—Columbia, Columbia, MO, USA

Jairo Enrique Martinez Columbia University, New York, NY, USA

Guido Mascialino Department of Rehab Medicine Brain Injury Research, Mount Sinai School of Medicine, New York, NY, USA

Joshua M. Matyi Department of Psychology, Utah State University, Logan, UT, USA

Micah O. Mazurek Curry School of Education, University of Virginia, Charlottesville, VA, USA

Michèle M. M. Mazzocco Institute of Child Development, University of Minnesota, Minneapolis, MN, USA

David L. McCabe Department of Psychology, Rusk Rehabilitation, NYU Langone Medical Center, New York, NY, USA

Marissa McCarthy Department of Neurology, James A Haley Veterans Hospital, University of South Florida, Tampa, FL, USA

Rebecca McCartney Department of Behavioral Health, Kaiser Permenante, Atlanta, GA, USA

Rehabilitation Medicine, Emory University, Atlanta, GA, USA

Katherine S. McClellan Rehabilitation Research and Development Center, Atlanta Veterans Affairs Medical Center, Decatur, GA, USA

Dalene McCloskey Centennial Board of Cooperative Educational Services, Greeley, CO, USA

Erica McConnell Jefferson County Public Schools, School Psychologist, Golden, CO, USA

Michael McCrea Departments of Neurosurgery and Neurology, Medical College of Wisconsin, Milwaukee, WI, USA

Jacinta McElligott Rehabilitation Medicine, National Rehabilitation Hospital, Dun Laoghaire Co Dublin, Ireland

Melissa J. McGinn Anatomy and Neurobiology, Virginia Commonwealth University School of Medicine, Richmond, VA, USA

Pip McGirl The Chicago School of Professional Psychology, School Psychology Department, Chicago, IL, USA

Amanda McGovern Psychiatry, Columbia University Medical Center, New York, NY, USA

David E. McIntosh Department of Special Education, Teachers College, Bell State University, Muncie, IN, USA

Thomas Martin: deceased.

Micchelle McKelvey Department of Communication Disorders, COE B141, University of Nebraska Kearney, Kearney, NE, USA

Tamara McKenzie-Hartman Defense and Veterans Brain Injury Center, James A. Haley, VA Hospital, Tampa, FL, USA

Molly E. McLaren Center for Cognitive Aging and Memory, Department of Clinical and Health Psychology, University of Florida, Gainesville, FL, USA

Nicole C. R. McLaughlin Butler Hospital Alpert Medical School of Brown University, Providence, RI, USA

Brian T. McMahon Department of Rehabilitation Counseling, Virginia Commonwealth University, Richmond, VA, USA

Lemmietta McNeilly Speech-Language Pathology, American Speech-Language-Hearing Association, Rockville, MD, USA

Rory McQuiston Anatomy and Neurobiology, Virginia Commonwealth University, Richmond, VA, USA

Linda McWhorter Department of Psychology, University of North Carolina at Charlotte, Charlotte, NC, USA

Mary-Ellen Meadows Division of Cognitive and Behavioral Neurology, Brigham and Women's Hospital, Boston, MA, USA

Stephanie Mears MHS Inc, Toronto, ON, Canada

Michael S. Mega Center for Cognitive Health, Portland, OR, USA

Stephen S. Meharg Center for Memory and Learning, Longview, WA, USA

Erica P. Meltzer Department of Psychology, Queens College and The Graduate Center of the City University of New York, Flushing, NY, USA

Patricia Melville Department of Neuropsychology Research, Stony Brook University SUNY Stony Brook, Stony Brook, NY, USA

Andrew Menatti Neuropsychology, University of Missouri, Columbia, MO, USA

John E. Mendoza Department of Psychiatry and Neuroscience, Tulane Medical School and SE Louisiana Veterans Healthcare System, New Orleans, LA, USA

Mark Mennemeier Neurobiology and Developmental Sciences, University of Arkansas for Medical Sciences, Little Rock, AR, USA

Randall E. Merchant Department of Anatomy and Neurobiology, Virginia Commonwealth University Medical Center, Richmond, VA, USA

Brad Merker Henry Ford Health Systems, Detroit, MI, USA

Carolyn B. Mervis Department of Psychological and Brain Sciences, University of Louisville, Louisville, KY, USA

Gary B. Mesibov University of North Carolina at Chapel Hill, Chapel Hill, NC, USA

Linda A. Meyer Speech Therapy, Augusta Health, Waynesboro, VA, USA

John E. Meyers Department of Neuropsychology, Comprehensive Medpsych Systems, Sarasota, FL, USA

David Michalec Division of Psychology Ohio State University Nationwide Children's Hospital, Developmental Assessment Program, Columbus, OH, USA

Jackie L. Micklewright Georgia State University, Department of Psychology and the Neuroscience Institute, Atlanta, GA, USA

Christine J. Mihaila Northeast Regional Epilepsy Group, New York, NY, USA

Eric N. Miller Palm Springs, CA, USA

Ana Mills Department of Physical Medicine and Rehabilitation, Virginia Commonwealth University, Richmond, VA, USA

Ginger Mills Graduate Institute of Professional Psychology, University of Hartford, West Hartford, CT, USA

Brenda Atkinson Milner Montreal Neurological Institute and Hospital, Montreal, QC, USA

Kristin Moffett Emory University, Atlanta, GA, USA

Ethan Moitra Department of Psychiatry and Human Behavior, Brown University, Providence, RI, USA

Doris S. Mok Department of Psychology, Faculty of Social Sciences and Humanities University of Macau, Taipa, Macau SAR, China

Ashley Mondragon Department of Psychology, William Paterson University, Wayne, NJ, USA

Anna Bacon Moore Department of Rehabilitation Medicine, Division of Neuropsychology, Emory University School of Medicine, Atlanta, GA, USA

Brittney Moore Department of Educational Psychology, Ball State University, Muncie, IN, USA

Lisa Moran Department of Psychology, Nationwide Children's Hospital, Columbus, OH, USA

Joseph E. Mosley Department of Psychology, William Paterson University, Wayne, NJ, USA

Margaret Moult Olin Neuropsychiatry Research Center, Institute of Living, Hartford, CT, USA

Martin Mrazik Department of Educational Psychology, University of Alberta, Edmonton, AB, Canada

Christine Mullen Emory Health Care, Atlanta, GA, USA

Courtney Murphy Belmont Behavioral Hospital, Philadelphia, PA, USA

Mary Pat Murphy MSN, CRRN, Paoli, PA, USA

Suzanne Musil Rush University Medical Center, Chicago, IL, USA

Charlsie Myers Department of Social Sciences, Coastal College of Georgia, Brunswick, GA, USA

Sylvie Naar-King Detroit, MI, USA

Risa Nakase-Richardson Mental Health and Behavioral Sciences, Department of Medicine, James A. Haley Veterans Hospital, University of South Florida, Defense and Veterans Brain Injury Center, Center of Innovation in Disability and Rehabilitation Research, Tampa, FL, USA

Luba Nakhutina Department of Neurology, SUNY Downstate Medical Center, Brooklyn, NY, USA

Madison Neirmeyer Department of Psychology, The University of Utah, Salt Lake City, UT, USA

Robi L. Nelson Department of Psychiatry and Behavioral Sciences, University of South Florida College of Medicine, Tampa, FL, USA

Department of Pharmacology, Virginia Commonwealth University, Richmond, VA, USA

Aaron P. Nelson Center for Brain Mind Medicine, Brigham and Women's Hospital and Harvard Medical School, Boston, MA, USA

Christina Nessler VA Salt Lake City Health Care System, Salt Lake City, UT, USA

Robert Newby Division of Neurology and Pediatrics, Medical College of Wisconsin, Milwaukee, WI, USA

Paul Newman Department of Medical Psychology and Neuropsychology, Drake Center, Cincinnati, OH, USA

Christine Maguth Nezu Department of Psychology, Drexel University–Hahnemann Campus, Philadelphia, PA, USA

Louisa Ng Department of Rehabilitation Medicine, Royal Melbourne Hospital, Parkville, VIC, Australia

Hien Nguyen Department of Pediatrics, Kaiser Permanente East Bay, Oakland, CA, USA

Jody S. Nicholson Department of Psychology, University of Notre Dame, Notre Dame, IN, USA

Jared A. Nielsen Departments of Psychiatry and Psychology, Harvard University and Massachusetts General Hospital, Cambridge, MA, USA

Janet P. Niemeier Carolinas Rehabilitation, Carolinas Healthcare System, Charlotte, NC, USA

Madison Niermeyer Department of Psychology, Clinical Psychology, The University of Utah, Salt Lake City, UT, USA

Christine Nieves Robert Wood Johnson Medical School, Rutgers University, Piscataway, NJ, USA

C. Michael Nina Department of Psychology, William Paterson University, Wayne, NJ, USA

Ignatius Nip School of Speech, Language, and Hearing Sciences, San Diego State University, San Diego, CA, USA

Nicole R. Nissim Department of Clinical and Health Psychology College of Public Health and Health Professions, Center for Cognitive Aging and Memory, McKnight Brain Institute (Primary), University of Florida, Gainesville, FL, USA
Department of Neuroscience, University of Florida, Gainesville, FL, USA

Natalie O. Nordlund Legal Psychology (Psychology and Law), Neuropsychology, Clinical Psychology, The Chicago School of Professional Psychology, Chicago, IL, USA

David Nordstokke Werklund School of Education, University of Calgary, Calgary, AB, Canada

Virginia A. Norris San Quentin State Prison, San Quentin, CA, USA

Olga Noskin Neurology Group of Bergen County, P.A, Ridgewood, NJ, USA

Thomas A. Novack Department of Physical Medicine and Rehabilitation, University of Alabama at Birmingham, Birmingham, AL, USA

Alicia Nuñez Department of Psychology, University of Nevada, Las Vegas, NV, USA

Meena Nuthi University of Florida, Gainesville, FL, USA

Andrew O'Shea Department of Aging and Geriatric Research, College of Medicine, Institute on Aging, University of Florida, Gainesville, FL, USA

Deirdre M. O'Shea Department of Clinical and Health Psychology, Center for Cognitive Aging and Memory, University of Florida, Gainesville, FL, USA

Kathleen O'Toole Children's Healthcare of Atlanta, Atlanta, GA, USA

Thomas Oakland Department of Educational Psychology, College of Education University of Florida, Gainesville, FL, USA

Thomas Oakland: deceased.

Christa Ochoa Center for Cognitive Aging and Memory, Department of Clinical and Health Psychology, University of Florida, Gainesville, Florida, USA

Natalia Ojeda Department of Methods and Experimental Psychology, Faculty of Psychology and Education, University of Deusto, Bilbao, Spain

Jonathan A. Oler Department of Psychiatry, University of Wisconsin-Madison, Madison, WI, USA

Traci W. Olivier Neuropsychology Section, Department of Psychology, St. Jude Children's Research Hospital, Memphis, TN, USA

Katie Osborn Florida School of Professional Psychology at Argosy University, Tampa, FL, USA

Zachary H. Osborn Behavioural Health Service Line, Harry S. Truman Memorial Veteran's Hospital, Columbia, MO, USA

Celita J. Owens Immaculata University, Immaculata, PA, USA

Matthew J. L. Page Allegheny General Hospital, Pittsburgh, PA, USA
Psychology, Allegheny Health Network, Pittsburgh, PA, USA

Rohan Palmer Institute for Behavioral Genetics, University of Colorado at Boulder, Boulder, CO, USA

Christina A. Palmese Department of Neurology, Mount Sinai Beth Israel, New York, NY, USA

Teresa Palumbo Administration Communications Senior University Relations Specialist, University of Wisconsin-Madison Waisman Center, Madison, WI, USA

Juhi Pandey Department of Psychology, University of Connecticut, Storrs, CT, USA

Carlos Bo Pang Department of Psychology, Faculty of Social Sciences and Humanities, University of Macau, Macao, Macau SAR, China

Aimilia Papazoglou Department of Psychology and the Neuroscience Institute, Georgia State University, Atlanta, GA, USA

Kathryn V. Papp Department of Psychology, The University of Connecticut, Storrs, CT, USA

Rick Parente Department of Psychology, Towson University, Towson, MD, USA

John Parkhurst Psychiatry and Behavioral Medicine, Children's Hospital of Wisconsin, Medical College of Wisconsin, Milwaukee, WI, USA

Matthew R. Parry Neurosurgery, Virginia Commonwealth University, Richmond, VA, USA

Lisa A. Pass Department of Educational Psychology, Ball State University, Muncie, IN, USA

Nicholas Pastorek Rehabilitation and Extended Care Line, Michael E. DeBakey VA Medical Center, Houston, TX, USA

Janet P. Patterson Audiology and Speech-Language Pathology Service, VA Northern California Health Care System, Martinez, CA, USA

Diane Paul Clinical Issues in Speech-Language Pathology, American Speech-Language-Hearing Association, Rockville, MD, USA

Nina Paul Department of Psychology, University of Nevada-Las Vegas, Las Vegas, Nevada, USA

Rebecca Pavlick Department of Psychology, William Paterson University, Wayne, NJ, USA

Shelley Pelletier Board Certified in School Psychology, Shoreline Pediatric Neuropsychology Services, LLC, Old Saybrook, CT, USA

Javier Peña Department of Methods and Experimental Psychology, Faculty of Psychology and Education, University of Deusto, Bilbao, Spain

Suzanne Penna Department of Rehabilitation Medicine, Emory University School of Medicine, Atlanta, GA, USA

Dana L. Penney Department of Neurology, The Lahey Clinic, Burlington, MA, USA

Molly Penzenik Rocky Mountain Mental Illness Research Education and Clinical Center, Denver, CO, USA

University of Colorado, Anschutz Medical Campus, Aurora, CO, USA

Alexandra Perrault University of Cincinnati, Cincinnati, OH, USA

Lexi Perrault University of Cincinnati, Cincinnati, OH, USA

Paul B. Perrin Department of Psychology, Virginia Commonwealth University, Richmond, VA, USA

Kenneth R. Perrine Neurological Surgery, Weill Cornell Medicine, New York, NY, USA

Amy Peterman Department of Psychological Science, University of North Carolina at Charlotte, Charlotte, NC, USA

Maria Petracca Department of Neurology, Icahn School of Medicine at Mount Sinai, New York, NY, USA

Jo Ann Petrie Department of Psychology and the Neuroscience Center, Brigham Young University, Provo, UT, USA

LeAdelle Phelps University at Buffalo, State University of New York, Buffalo, NY, USA

Angela M. Philippus Craig Hospital, Englewood, CO, USA

Linda L. Phillips Anatomy and Neurobiology, Virginia Commonwealth University, Richmond, VA, USA

Jesse J. Piehl Department of Pharmacology, Virginia Commonwealth University, Richmond, VA, USA

Elizabeth I. Pierpont Department of Pediatrics, Division of Clinical Behavioral Neuroscience, University of Minnesota, Minneapolis, MN, USA

Eric E. Pierson Department of Educational Psychology, Ball State University, Muncie, IN, USA

Irene Piryatinsky Butler Hospital and Alpert Medical School of Brown University, Providence, RI, USA

Jenni Pitkanen Product Development at MHS Inc., Toronto, ON, Canada

Kenneth Podell Houston Methodist Hospital, Houston, TX, USA
Henry Ford Health Systems, Detroit, MI, USA

Ben Polakoff Department of Educational Psychology, The University of Utah, Salt Lake City, UT, USA

Elena Polejaeva Department of Clinical and Health Psychology, University of Florida, Gainesville, FL, USA

Donna Polelle Communication Sciences and Disorders, College of Science and Mathematics, University of South Florida Sarasota-Manatee, Sarasota, FL, USA

Eric S. Porges Department of Clinical and Health Psychology, University of Florida, Gainesville, FL, USA
Center for Cognitive Aging and Memory, McKnight Brain Institute, University of Florida, Gainesville, FL, USA
Department of Neurology, University of Florida, Gainesville, FL, USA

Matthew R. Powell Division of Neurocognitive Disorders, Department of Psychiatry and Psychology, Mayo Clinic, Rochester, MN, USA

Tiffany L. Powell Department of Neurosurgery, Virginia Commonwealth University, Richmond, VA, USA

Elizabeth Power Legal Psychology (Psychology and Law), Neuropsychology, Clinical Psychology, Chicago School of Professional Psychology, Chicago, IL, USA
The College of Saint Rose, Albany, NY, USA

Natalia Ojeda Del Pozo Fundamentals and Methods of Psychology, University of Deusto, Bilbao, Spain

Victor R. Preedy Faculty of Life Sciences and Medicine, King's College London, London, UK

Andrew Preston Department of Pediatrics, Chapel Hill Pediatric Psychology, Chapel Hill, NC, USA

Catherine C. Price Department of Clinician and Health Psychology and Dept of Anesthesiology, University of Florida, Florida, USA

George P. Prigatano Department of Clinical Neuropsychology, Barrow Neurological Institute, St. Joseph's Hospital and Medical Center, Phoenix, AZ, USA

Michelle Ann Prosje NeuroBehavioral Specialists of Jacksonville, Inc., Jacksonville, FL, USA

Antonio E. Puente Depatment of Psychology, University of North Carolina Wilmington, Wilmington, NC, USA

Anneliese Radke Department of Neurology, University of California, Davis, CA, USA

Susie Engi Raiford Assessment and Instruction, Pearson, San Antonio, TX, USA

Robert D. Rainer Department of Psychology, University of Florida, Gainesville, FL, USA

Vanessa L. Ramos Scarborough Department of Neuropsychology, Kennedy Krieger Institute, Baltimore, MD, USA

Kate D. Randall Department of Psychology, University of Victoria, Victoria, BC, Canada

Steven Z. Rapcsak Neurology Section, Southern Arizona VA Healthcare System, Tucson, AZ, USA

Department of Neurology, University of Arizona, Tucson, AZ, USA

Sarah A. Raskin Department of Psychology and Neuroscience Program, Trinity College, Hartford, CT, USA

Joseph F. Rath NYU Langone Medical Center, Department of Psychology, Rusk Institute of Rehabilitation Medicine, New York, NY, USA

Holly Rau Department of Psychology, The University of Utah, Salt Lake City, UT, USA

Anastasia Raymer Communication Disorders and Special Education, Old Dominion University, Norfolk, VA, USA

Jennifer Linton Reesman Kennedy Krieger Institute/Johns Hopkins University School of Medicine, Baltimore, MD, USA

Christine Reid Department of Rehabilitation Counseling, Virginia Commonwealth University, Richmond, VA, USA

Stephanie A. Reid-Arndt School of Health Professions – Health Psychology, University of Missouri, Columbia, MO, USA

Sheryl Reminger Psychology Department, University of Illinois at Springfield, Springfield, IL, USA

Kathryn K. Reva University of Northern Colorado, New York, NY, USA

Jose A. Rey College of Pharmacy, Nova Southeastern University, Ft. Lauderdale, FL, USA

Cecil R. Reynolds Texas A&M University, College Station, TX, USA

Jill B. Rich Department of Psychology, York University, Toronto, ON, Canada

Lindsey Richards Department of Clinical and Health Psychology, Center for Cognitive Aging and Memory, University of Florida, Gainesville, FL, USA

Robert Rider Department of Psychology, Drexel University, Philadelphia, PA, USA

Giulia Righi Visual Neuroscience Laboratory, Brown University, Providence, RI, USA

Diana L. Robins AJ Drexel Autism Institute, Drexel University, Philadelphia, PA, USA

Tresa Roebuck-Spencer Jefferson Neurobehavioral Group, Metairie, LA, USA

Daniel E. Rohe Mayo Clinic, Rochester, MN, USA

Cynthia Rolston Department of PM&R, Virginia Commonwealth University-Medical College of Virginia, Richmond, VA, USA

Maryellen Romero Department of Psychiatry and Behavioral Sciences, Tulane University School of Medicine, New Orleans, LA, USA

Katherine A. Roof Department of Psychology, University of North Carolina at Charlotte, Charlotte, NC, USA

Susan Ropacki VA Palo Alto, Polytrauma System of Care, Polytrauma Transitional Rehabilitation Program, VA Palo Alto Health Care System, Palo Alto, California, USA
Neurosurgery, Stanford University, Palo Alto, California, USA

Jon Rose Spinal Cord Injury Clinic, Veterans Affairs Palo Alto Healthcare System, Palo Alto, CA, USA

Carole R. Roth Otolaryngology Clinic, Speech Division, Naval Medical Center, San Diego, CA, USA

Elliot J. Roth Department of Physical Medicine and Rehabilitation, Northwestern University, Feinberg School of Medicine, Chicago, IL, USA

Robert M. Roth Geisel School of Medicine at Dartmouth / DHMC, Lebanon, NH, USA

Linda Rowley Waisman Center Family Village, University of Madison, Madison, WI, USA

Donald R. Royall Deptartment of Psychiatry, The University of Texas Health Center at San Antonio, San Antonio, TX, USA

Shahal Rozenblatt Advanced Psychological Assessment P. C., Smithtown, NY, USA

Alexandra Rudd-Barnard One Neuro, West Los Angeles, California, USA

Ronald Ruff San Francisco Clinical Neurosciences, University of California, San Francisco, CA, USA

Jessica Somerville Ruffolo Department of Psychology, University of Washington, Seattle, Washington, DC, USA

Ruba Rum College of Medicine Psychiatry and Behavioral Neurosciences, University of South Florida, Tampa, FL, USA

Anthony C. Ruocco Department of Psychology, University of Toronto, Toronto, ON, Canada

Beth Rush Psychiatry and Psychology, Mayo Clinic, Jacksonville, FL, USA

Michele Rusin Emory University/Rehabilitation Medicine, Atlanta, GA, USA

Julia Rutenberg Rehabilitation Medicine, Emory University, Atlanta, GA, USA

John P. Ryan Department of Psychiatry, University of Pittsburgh, Pittsburgh, PA, USA

Bruce Rybarczyk Department of Psychology, Virginia Commonwealth University, Richmond, VA, USA

Catherine M. Rydell American Academy of Neurology, Minneapolis, MN, USA

Sara R. Rzepa Clinical, Education, and Public Safety at MHS Inc, Toronto, ON, Canada

Bonnie C. Sachs Parkinson's and Movement Disorders Center, Virginia Commonwealth University, Richmond, VA, USA

Amanda L. Sacks-Zimmerman Department of Neurological Surgery, Weill Cornell Medicine, New York, NY, USA

Donald H. Saklofske Department of Psychology, University of Western Ontario, London, ON, Canada

Christina Salama Kennedy Krieger Institute/Johns Hopkins University School of Medicine, Baltimore, MD, USA

Christine M. Salinas Space Coast Neuropsychology Center, Melbourne, FL, USA

Stephanie L. Salinas Department of Rehabilitation Medicine, The Georgia School of Professional Psychology at Argosy University-Atlanta, Atlanta, GA, USA

Stephen P. Salloway Butler Hospital Alpert Medical School of Brown University, Providence, RI, USA

Jeffery Samuels Inpatient Rehabilitation Unit, North Broward Medical Center, Deerfield Beach, FL, USA

Orlando Sánchez Minneapolis VA Health Care System, Minneapolis, MN, USA

Mark A. Sandberg Neuropsychology, Northport VA Medical Center, Smithtown, NY, USA

Chelsea Sanders Department of Psychology, Utah State University, Logan, UT, USA

R. Sands Legal Psychology (Psychology and Law), Neuropsychology, Clinical Psychology, The Chicago School of Professional Psychology, Chicago, IL, USA

Marla Sanzone Independent Practice, Loyola College of Maryland, Annapolis, MD, USA

Celine A. Saulnier Department of Pediatrics, Emory University School of Medicine, Atlanta, GA, USA

Lynn A. Schaefer Physical Medicine and Rehabilitation, Nassau University Medical Center, East Meadow, NY, USA

Philip Schatz Department of Psychology, Saint Joseph's University, Philadelphia, PA, USA

Mike R. Schoenberg Department of Psychiatry and Behavioral Sciences, University of South Florida College of Medicine, Tampa, FL, USA

Aaron Schrader Applied Psychology and Counselor Education, University of Northern Colorado, Greeley, CO, USA

William A. Schraegle Pediatric Neuropsychology, Dell Children's Medical Center of Central Texas, Austin, TX, USA

Department of Educational Psychology, The University of Texas at Austin, Austin, TX, USA

Jillian Schuh Department of Psychology, University of Connecticut, Storrs, CT, USA

Christian Schutte Henry Ford Allegiance, Jackson, MI, USA

John D. Dingell VA Medical Center, Psychology Section (11MHPS), Detroit, MI, USA

Kerri A. Scorpio Department of Psychology, Queens College of the City University of New York, Flushing, NY, USA

Paige Seegan Clinical Psychology Program, Texas Tech University, Lubbock, TX, USA

Peter W. Seely Department of Pharmacology, Virginia Commonwealth University, Richmond, VA, USA

Daniel L. Segal Department of Psychology, University of Colorado at Colorado Springs, Colorado Springs, CO, USA

Talia R. Seider Department of Clinical and Health Psychology, College of Public Health and Health Professions, University of Florida, Gainesville, FL, USA

Center for Cognitive Aging and Memory, McKnight Brain Institute, University of Florida, Gainesville, FL, USA

Robin Sekerak Waikato District Health Board, Hamilton, New Zealand

Svetlana Serova Department of Rehabilitation Medicine, Mount Sinai School of Medicine, New York, NY, USA

Laura Shank Rehabilitation Psychology and Neuropsychology, Physical Medicine and Rehabilitation University of Michigan, Ann Arbor, MI, USA

Casey R. Shannon University of Northern Colorado, Greeley, CO, USA

Anuj Sharma Virginia Commonwealth University School of Medicine, Richmond, VA, USA

Rhonna Shatz Department of Neurology and Rehabilitation, MED-Neurology, University of Cincinnati, Cincinnati, OH, USA

Bennett A. Shaywitz Department of Pediatrics, Yale University School of Medicine, New Haven, CT, USA

Sally E. Shaywitz Department of Pediatrics, Yale University School of Medicine, New Haven, CT, USA

Victoria Shea University of North Carolina at Chapel Hill, Chapel Hill, NC, USA

Judith A. Shechter Wynnewood, PA, USA

Tamara Goldman Sher Institute of Psychology, Illinois Institute of Technology, Chicago, IL, USA

Elisabeth M. S. Sherman Copeman Healthcare Centre, Calgary, AB, Canada

Cynthia X. Shi Emory College at Emory University, Atlanta, GA, USA

Cheryl L. Shigaki Department of Health Psychology, University of Missouri, Columbia, MO, USA

Lindsay C. Shima Department of Psychology, Neuropsychology Research Group, West Chester University of Pennsylvania, West Chester, PA, USA

Gerald Showalter Department of Psychiatry and Neurobehavioral Sciences, University of Virginia School of Medicine, Charlottesville, VA, USA

Seema Shroff Department of Anatomy and Neurobiology, Virginia Commonwealth University, Richmond, VA, USA

David Ho Keung Shum Griffith University, School of Psychology, Mt Gravatt Campus Griffith University, Brisbane, QLD, Australia

Melissa Shuman-Paretsky Department of Rehabilitation Medicine, Mount Sinai School of Medicine, New York, NY, USA

Linda Shuster Interdisciplinary Health Sciences Ph.D. Program and Department of Speech, Language, and Hearing Sciences, Western Michigan University, Kalamazoo, MI, USA

Kevin Sickinger Chronic Effects of Neurotrauma Consortium (CENC), Virginia Commonwealth University, Richmond, VA, USA

Marc A. Silva Mental Health and Behavioral Sciences Service, James A. Haley Veterans' Hospital, Tampa, FL, USA

Preeti Sinha Department of Clinical and Health Psychology, University of Florida, Gainesville, FL, USA

Sue Ann Sisto School of Health Technology and Management Stony Brook University, Stony Brook, NY, USA

Gill Sitarenios Multi-Health Systems Inc., Toronto, ON, Canada

Ketharini Sivasegaran Whitby Vision Care, Whitby, ON, Canada

Amanda Skierkiewicz School Psychology, The Chicago School of Professional Psychology, Chicago, IL, USA

Beth Slomine Johns Hopkins University School of Medicine, Baltimore, MD, USA

Audrey Smerbeck School and Educational Psychology, University at Buffalo, The State University of New York, Buffalo, NY, USA

Daniel Smith Department of Psychology, Drexel University, Philadelphia, PA, USA
Winship Cancer Institute, Emory University, Atlanta, GA, USA

Kristen Smith Department of Psychology and the Neuroscience Institute, Georgia State University, Atlanta, GA, USA

Marian L. Smith Via Christi Behavioral Health Crossroads Counseling Center, Via Christi Hospital Pittsburg Mt. Carmel, Pittsburg, KS, USA

Nicholas David Smith Educational and Psychological Studies, University of South Florida/TBI Model Systems, James A. Haley VA Hospital, Tampa, FL, USA

Lucia Smith-Wexler Rusk Rehabilitation, New York University Langone Health, New York, NY, USA

Kayle E. Sneed Department of Communication Sciences and Disorders, The University of Oklahoma Health Sciences Center, Oklahoma City, OK, USA

Jill Snyder Behavioral Health Services, Boston Public Schools, Roxbury, MA, USA

McKay Moore Sohlberg Communication Disorders and Sciences, University of Oregon, Eugene, OR, USA

Carney Sotto College of Allied Health Sciences, University of Cincinnati, Cincinnati, OH, USA

Barbara Spacca Anna Meyer Children's Hospital, Florence, Italy

Sara S. Sparrow Yale University Child Study Center, New Haven, CT, USA

Ferrinne Spector Psychology, Edgewood College, Madison, WI, USA

April Spivack Department of Management and Human Resources, University of Wisconsin Oshkosh, Oshkosh, WI, USA

Beth Springate Department of Psychiatry, University of Connecticut Health Center, Farmington, CT, USA

Maria St. Pierre Department of Psychology, Towson University, Towson, MD, USA

Vess Stamenova Rotman Research Institute at Baycrest, Toronto, ON, Canada

Amy J. Starosta Departments of Psychiatry and Physical Medicine and Rehabilitation, University of Colorado Denver, Aurora, CO, USA

Susan Steffani CCC-SLP, Department of Communication Sciences and Disorders, California State University, Chico, Chico, CA, USA

Taryn M. Stejskal Department of Physical Medicine and Rehabilitation, Virginia Commonwealth University Medical Center, Virginia, VA, USA

Jeremy Stevenson Department of Family Medicine, University of Kansas Medical Center, Kansas City, KS, USA

William Stiers Johns Hopkins University School of Medicine, Baltimore, MD, USA

Jordan Stiver UCSF Memory and Aging Center, University California San Francisco, San Francisco, CA, USA

Esther Strauss Department of Psychology, University of Victoria, Victoria, BC, Canada

Anthony Y. Stringer Department of Rehabilitation Medicine, Emory University, Atlanta, GA, USA

Donald T. Stuss University of Toronto, Toronto, ON, Canada

Sunnybrook Health Sciences Centre, Toronto, ON, Canada

Rotman Research Institute of Baycrest, Toronto, ON, Canada

Lauren Stutts Department of Health and Human Values, Davidson College, Davidson, NC, USA

Yana Suchy Department of Psychology, The University of Utah, Salt Lake City, UT, USA

Joyce Suh Kennedy Krieger Institute/Johns Hopkins University School of Medicine, Baltimore, MD, USA

James F. Sumowski Teachers College Columbia University, New York, NY, USA

Dong Sun Department of Aantomy and Neurobiology, School of Medicine, Virginia Commonwealth University Medical Center, Richmond, VA, USA

Uma Suryadevara Department of Psychiatry, University of Florida, Gainesville, FL, USA

Zoë N. Swaine Keele University, Keele, Newcastle ST5 5BG, UK

Joan Swearer Department of Neurology, University of Massachusetts Medical School, Worcester, MA, USA

Lawrence H. Sweet Department of Psychology, University of Georgia, Athens, GA, USA

Rod Swenson Department of Psychiatry and Behavioral Science, University of North Dakota School of Medicine, Fargo, ND, USA

Russell H. Swerdlow University of Kansas School of Medicine, Landon Center on Aging, Kansas City, KS, USA

Sarah M. Szymkowicz Department of Clinical and Health Psychology, College of Public Health and Health Professions, University of Florida, Gainesville, FL, USA

Jing Ee Tan Division of Neurology, University of British Columbia, Vancouver, BC, Canada

Vancouver General Hospital, Vancouver, BC, Canada

Department of Psychology, University of Victoria, Victoria, BC, Canada

Michael J. Tarr Visual Neuroscience Laboratory, Brown University, Providence, RI, USA

David F. Tate Brain Imaging and Behavior Laboratory, Missouri Institute of Mental Health (MIMH), University of Missouri, St. Louis (UMSL), Berkeley, MO, USA

Ella B. Teague Department of Neurorehabilitation, Reykjalundur Rehabilitation Center, Mosfellsbær, Iceland

Richard Temple Clinical Operations, CORE Health Care, Dripping Springs, TX, USA

Claire Thomas-Duckwitz University of Northern Colorado, Greeley, CO, USA

Cynthia K. Thompson Northwestern University, Evanston, IL, USA

Esther Strauss: deceased.

Jacob W. Tickle School of Psychology, The Chicago School of Professional Psychology, Chicago, IL, USA

Jennifer Tinker Department of Neurology, Thomas Jefferson University, Philadelphia, PA, USA

Michelle Marie Tipton-Burton Physical Medicine and Rehabilitation, Santa Clara Valley Medical Center, San Jose, CA, USA

Jeffrey B. Titus Comprehensive Epilepsy Program, Dell Children's Medical Center of Central Texas, Austin, TX, USA

Department of Psychology, The University of Texas at Austin, Austin, TX, USA

Teri A. Todd California State University, Northridge, Northridge, CA, USA

Nam Tran Neurosurgery, Virginia Commonwealth University Medical Center, Richmond, VA, USA

Alexander I. Tröster Department of Clinical Neuropsychology and Center for Neuromodulation, Barrow Neurological Institute, Phoenix, AZ, USA

Daniel Tranel Department of Neurology, The University of Iowa, Iowa City, USA

Angela K. Troyer Neuropsychology and Cognitive Health Program, Baycrest Centre for Geriatric Care, Toronto, ON, Canada

Tina Trudel Northeast Evaluation Specialists, PLLC, Dover, DE, USA

William Tsang Department of Psychology, William Paterson University, Wayne, NJ, USA

Theodore Tsaousides Department of Rehab Medicine Brain Injury Research, Mount Sinai School of Medicine, New York, NY, USA

JoAnn Tschanz Department of Psychology, Utah State University, Logan, UT, USA

Center for Epidemiologic Studies, Utah State University, Logan, UT, USA

Jessica Tsou Department of Psychiatry, University of Kansas Medical Center, Kansas City, KS, USA

Lyn S. Turkstra School of Rehabilitation Science, McMaster University, Hamilton, ON, Canada

Margaret Tuttle Department of Psychiatry, Massachusetts General Hosptial, Boston, MA, USA

Jamie T. Twaite Department of Psychology, Queens College and The Graduate Center of the City University of New York, Flushing, NY, USA

Gary Tye Neurosurgery, Virginia Commonwealth University, Richmond, VA, USA

Katherine Tyson Department of Psychology, University of Connecticut, Storrs, CT, USA

Michelle Uher Marketing Communications, American Academy of Neurology, Minneapolis, MN, USA

Jason Van Allen Clinical Psychology Program, Texas Tech University, Lubbock, TX, USA

Faye van der Fluit Department of Psychology, University of Wisconsin-Milwaukee, Milwaukee, WI, USA

Timothy E. Van Meter Neurosurgery, Virginia Commonwealth University, Richmond, VA, USA

Gertina J. van Schalkwyk Department of Psychology, University of Macau, Taipa, Macao (SAR), China

Emily Vanderbleek Department of Psychology, University of Notre Dame, Notre Dame, IN, USA

Susan Vandermorris Neuropsychology and Cognitive Health Program, Baycrest, Toronto, ON, USA

Kimberly J. Vannest Department of Educational Psychology, Texas A&M University, College Station, TX, USA

Jamie Vannice Applied Psychology and Counselor Education, University of Northern Colorado, Greeley, CO, USA

Laura M. Vasel Department of Educational Psychology, Ball State University, Muncie, IN, USA

Rebecca Vaurio Kennedy Krieger Institute, Baltimore, MD, USA

Jennifer Venegas Department of Educational Psychology, The University of Utah, Salt Lake City, UT, USA

Mieke Verfaellie Memory Disorders Research Center, VA Boston Healthcare System and Boston University School of Medicine, Boston, MA, USA

Elizabeth K. Vernon Department of Psychology, Utah State University, Logan, UT, USA

Jean Vettel US Army Research Laboratory, National Academy of the Sciences, Washington, DC, USA

Clara Vila-Castelar Department of Psychology, Queens College and The Graduate Center, The City University of New York, New York, NY, USA

Michael R. Villanueva Department of Psychology, University of North Carolina at Charlotte, Charlotte, NC, USA

Martin A. Volker School and Educational Psychology, University at Buffalo, The State University of New York, Buffalo, NY, USA

Fred R. Volkmar Child Study Center, Child Psychiatry, Pediatrics and Psychology, Yale University School of Medicine, New Haven, CT, USA

Scott Vota Department of Neurology, Virginia Commonwealth University, Richmond, VA, USA

Christopher Wagner Department of Rehabilitation Counseling, Virginia Commonwealth University, Richmond, VA, USA

George C. Wagner Department of Psychology, Rutgers University, New Brunswick, NJ, USA

Natalie Wahmhoff Department of Educational Psychology, The University of Utah, Salt Lake City, UT, USA

Sarah E. Wallace John G. Rangos Sr. School of Health Sciences, Department of Speech-Language Pathology, Duquesne University, Pittsburgh, PA, USA

Erin Walsh Department of Pharmacology, Virginia Commonwealth University, Richmond, VA, USA

James Walsh School of Psychology, The Chicago School of Professional Psychology, Chicago, IL, USA

Julie L. Wambaugh Veterans Affairs Salt Lake City Healthcare System, University of Utah, Salt Lake City, UT, USA

Yuan Yuan Wang Faculty of Health Sciences, University of Macau, Macao, China

Adam B. Warshowsky Clinical Neuropsychologist, Dual/SCI Unit, Mount Sinai Medical Center, Shepherd Center, Atlanta, GA, USA

Seth Warschausky Department of Physical Medicine and Rehabilitation, University of Michigan, Ann Arbor, MI, USA

David Watson Department of Psychology, 124B Haggar Hall, University of Notre Dame, Notre Dame, IN, USA

Nadia Webb Children's Hospital of New Orleans, New Orleans, LA, USA

Victoria L. Webb Department of Behavioral Sciences, Rush University Medical Center, Chicago, IL, USA

Erica Weber Department of Physical Medicine and Rehabilitation, Kessler Foundation, East Hanover, NJ, USA

Stephen T. Wegener Division of Rehabilitation Psychology and Neuropsychology Department of Physical Medicine and Rehabilitation, The Johns Hopkins School of Medicine, Baltimore, MD, USA

Alan Weintraub Craig Hospital, Rocky Mountain Regional Brain Injury System, Englewood, CO, USA

Devon H. Weir Department of Psychology, University of Florida, Gainesville, FL, USA

Jonathan Wellman St. Luke's Hospital, Kansas City, MO, USA

John D. Westbrook National Center for the Dissemination of Disability Research (NCDDR), SEDL, Austin, TX, USA

Michael Westerveld Medical Psychology Associates, Florida Hospital, Orlando, FL, USA

Holly James Westervelt Memory and Cognitive Assessment Program, Department of Psychiatry, Rhode Island Hospital, Providence, RI, USA

Kristine B. Whigham Department of Neuropsychology, Children's Healthcare of Atlanta, Atlanta, GA, USA

Gale G. Whiteneck Craig Hospital, Englewood, CO, USA

John Whyte Moss Rehabilitation Research Institute, Albert Einstein Healthcare Network, Elkins Park, PA, USA

Robert G. Will University of Edinburgh, Edinburgh, UK

Gavin Williams Epworth Rehabilitation Centre Epworth Hospital, Richmond Melbourne, VIC, Australia

Travis Williams Department of Physical Medicine and Rehabilitation, Indiana University, Indianapolis, IN, USA

Tricia S. Williams Division of Neurology and Department of Psychology, Sick Kids-Centre for Brain and Mental Health, Toronto, ON, Canada

John B. Williamson Department of Neurology, University of Florida College of Medicine, Center for Neurological Studies and the Research Service of the Malcom Randall Veterans Affairs Medical Center, Gainesville, FL, USA

Meredith L. C. Williamson Department of Primary Care Medicine, College of Medicine, Texas A&M Health Science Center, Bryan, TX, USA

Brenda Wilson Department of Communication Disorders and Sciences, Eastern Illinois University, Charleston, IL, USA

Jill Winegardner Oliver Zangwill Centre, Ely, UK

Melissa Wingate Neuropsychology, The Chicago School of Professional Psychology, Chicago, IL, USA

Deborah Witsken University of Minnesota Medical School, Minneapolis, MN, USA

Ericka L. Wodka Center for Autism and Related Disorders, Kennedy Krieger Institute and The Johns Hopkins University School of Medicine, Baltimore, MD, USA

Thomas R. Wodushek School of Medicine, Department of Neurosurgery, University of Colorado, Aurora, CO, USA

Edison Wong Center for Pain and Medical Rehabilitation, Fitchburg, MA, USA

Sarah Woodrow Oak Grove School District, San Jose, CA, USA

Adam J. Woods Department of Clinical and Health Psychology, College of Public Health and Health Professions, University of Florida, Gainesville, FL, USA

Center for Cognitive Aging and Memory, McKnight Brain Institute, University of Florida, Gainesville, FL, USA

Department of Neuroscience, University of Florida, Gainesville, FL, USA

Michael S. Worden Department of Neuroscience, Brown University, Providence, RI, USA

Jerry Wright Rehabilitation Research Center, Santa Clara Valley Medical Center, San Jose, CA, USA

Fan Wu Outcomes Management, The Harris Center for Mental Health and IDD, Houston, TX, USA

Glenn Wylie Neuropsychology and Neuroscience Laboratory, Kessler Medical Rehabilitation Research and Education Center Kessler Foundation, West Orange, NJ, USA

Naohide Yamamoto Queensland University of Technology, Brisbane, Queensland, Australia

Keith Owen Yeates Department of Psychology, University of Calgary, Calgary, AB, Canada

Angela Yi Department of Rehab Medicine, Mount Sinai School of Medicine, New York, NY, USA

Brian Yochim Department of Psychology, University of Colorado at Colorado Springs, Colorado Springs, CO, USA

Sevilay Yumusak Department of Psychology, University of Florida, Gainesville, FL, USA

Michele L. Zaccario Department of Psychology, Pace University, Dyson College of Arts and Sciences, New York, NY, USA

Christina Zafiris Applied Psychology and Counselor Education, University of Northern Colorado, Greeley, CO, USA

Ross Zafonte Department of Physical Medicine and Rehabilitation, Spaulding Rehabilitation Hospital, Massachusetts General Hospital, Brigham and Women's Hospital, Harvard Medical School, Boston, MA, USA

Nathan D. Zasler Concussion Care Centre of Virginia, Ltd., Richmond, VA, USA

Islam Zaydan Neurology, Virginia Commonwealth University, Richmond, VA, USA

Fadel Zeidan Department of Neurobiology and Anatomy, Wake Forest School of Medicine, Winston-Salem, NC, USA

J. Zhou School Psychology, The Chicago School of Professional Psychology, Chicago, IL, USA

Zheng Zhou Department of Psychology, St. John's University, Queens, NY, USA

Miriam Zichlin Health Economics and Outcomes Research, Analysis Group, Inc., Boston, MA, USA

Rosemary Ziemnik Department of Psychology, The University of Utah, Salt Lake City, UT, USA

Molly E. Zimmerman Department of Psychology, Fordham University, Bronx, NY, USA

Davor Zink Neuropsychology Research Program, University of Nevada, Las Vegas, Las Vegas, NV, USA

A

AACN Practice Guidelines

Robert L. Heilbronner
Chicago Neuropsychology Group, Chicago,
IL, USA

Synonyms

Practice development; Practice guidelines

Historical Background

The American Board of Clinical Neuropsychology (ABCN) is a specialty board within the American Board of Professional Psychology (ABPP). For those seeking board certification in clinical neuropsychology, ABCN is the board responsible for overseeing the examination process. The American Academy of Clinical Neuropsychology (AACN) is the organization for those awarded board certification by the ABCN. In 2007, AACN produced the first set of practice guidelines, which were intended to "...facilitate the continued systematic growth of the profession of clinical neuropsychology, and to help assure a high level of professional practice."

Current Knowledge

Given the recent growth of clinical neuropsychology, coupled with the American Psychological Association's focus on evidence-based practice, the AACN established (AACN 2007) guidelines for the practice of neuropsychological assessment and consultation. The guidelines are intended to provide standards for competence and professional conduct within the practice of neuropsychology by describing the "most desirable and highest level of professional conduct" for clinical neuropsychologists providing clinical neuropsychology services. It is important to note that the guidelines are fully compatible with the current APA (2002b) Ethical Principles of Psychologists and Code of Conduct (EPPCC) as well as the Criteria for Practice Guideline Development and Evaluation (2002a) and Determination and Documentation of the Need for Practice Guidelines (2005). The AACN practice guidelines include recommendations for the practice of clinical neuropsychology, and they are not to be regarded as mandatory standards. The guidelines detail consideration of ethical and clinical issues as well as specific methods and procedures for the practice of neuropsychology.

There are several major areas of emphasis in the guidelines. They include (1) definitions, (2) purpose and scope, (3) education and training, (4) work settings, (5) ethical and clinical issues (e.g., informed consent, patient issues in third party assessments, test security; underserved populations/cultural issues, and (6) methods and procedures (e.g., review of records, measurement procedures, test administration and scoring, and interpretation).

© Springer International Publishing AG, part of Springer Nature 2018
J. S. Kreutzer et al. (eds.), Encyclopedia of Clinical Neuropsychology,
https://doi.org/10.1007/978-3-319-57111-9

References and Readings

American Psychological Association. (2002a). Criteria for practice guideline development and evaluation. *American Psychologist, 57*, 1048–1051.

American Psychological Association. (2002b). Ethical principles of psychologists and code of conduct. *American Psychologist, 57*, 1060–1073.

American Psychological Association. (2005). Determination and documentation of the need for practice guidelines. *American Psychologist, 60*, 976–978.

Committee on Ethical Guidelines for Forensic Psychologists. (1991). Specialty guidelines for forensic psychologists. *Law and Human Behavior, 15*, 655–665.

The AACN practice guidelines can be found on the AACN's web site (www.theaacn.org) and are also published in the AACN's journal: *The Clinical Neuropsychologist, 21*, 209–231.

AAMD Adaptive Behavior Scales

Crista A. Hopp[1] and Ida Sue Baron[2]
[1]Connected Pathways Coaching, Herndon, VA, USA
[2]Potomac, MD, USA

Synonyms

AAMD ABS: 2; AAMR ABS-RC: 2; AAMR ABS-S: 2

Description

The American Association for Mental Deficiency Adaptive Behavior Scales (AAMD ABS) is a revised edition (1993) of the original assessments that were published in 1969. The American Association for Mental Retardation (AAMR) (formerly known as the American Association for Mental Deficiency) has changed its name to American Association on Intellectual and Developmental Disabilities (AAIDD). Therefore, *intellectual disabilities* have replaced *mental retardation* as the terminology

of choice. The behavior scales have been published in two versions, the Adaptive Behavior Scales-Residential and Community, 2nd edition (ABS-RC: 2) and the Adaptive Behavior Scales-School, 2nd edition (ABS-S: 2). Current versions are a comprehensive compilation of the past versions. These assessments seek to develop an estimate of adaptive behaviors in two scales defined with personal independence and maladaptive behaviors in individuals with intellectual disabilities. Items are rated with a yes/no response, on a 0–3 scale, or by frequency. Historically, the ABS-RC: 2 was used in institutions, but it is now also used in community settings, whereas the ABS-S: 2 was designed for school settings.

For both the ABS-RC: 2 and the ABS-S: 2, the assessment can be administered by two approaches. The assessment can be completed by a professional or paraprofessional or by someone familiar with the individual. Interpretation of results should be completed by someone formally trained in psychometrics and these scales.

The ABS-S: 2 evaluates an individual's ability to cope with challenges they encounter in their school, and aids in the diagnosis of intellectual disabilities at ages 3–21. There are nine subscales in the first part of the assessment, measuring personal independence and responsibility of daily living: independent functioning, physical development, economic activity, language development, numbers and time, prevocational/vocational activity, self-direction, responsibility, and socialization. Part two of the assessment addresses behavioral domains and consists of seven subscales: social behavior, conformity, trustworthiness, stereotyped and hyperactive behavior, self-abusive behavior, social engagement, and disturbing interpersonal behavior.

The ABS-S: 2 was normed on 2,074 students with intellectual disabilities and 1,254 of their peers without intellectual disabilities. Administration takes place in an interview format with parents or teachers and may vary from 20 min to 2 h. Scoring is completed by hand.

Raw scores are converted into percentiles, standard scores, and age equivalents for each subdomain. Five factors can be derived: personal self-sufficiency, community self-sufficiency, personal social responsibility, social adjustment, and personal adjustment. Percentiles, factor standard scores, and age equivalents are then reported based on factor scores.

The ABS-RC: 2 is also useful for the assessment of personal development and social behavior in individuals with intellectual disabilities, but it has been developed for individuals aged 18–79. Like the ABS-S: 2, the assessment has two parts, but there are more subscales in each part. The first part has ten subscales: independent functioning, physical development, economic activity, language development, numbers and time, domestic activity, prevocational/vocational activity, self-direction, responsibility, and socialization. The second part contains eight subscales: social behavior, conformity, trustworthiness, stereotyped and hyperactive behavior, sexual behavior, self-abusive behavior, social engagement, and disturbing interpersonal behavior. The ABS-RC: 2 was normed on a sample of 4,000 adults with intellectual disabilities, and administration times vary between 15 and 40 min, depending on the informant's knowledge of the individual being assessed. Raw scores are recorded and then converted to standard scores and percentiles. The subscales yield the same five-factor scales as the ABS-S: 2.

Historical Background

The AAMD first published the ABS in 1969 in response to the definition of mental retardation that was amended in 1959 to include adaptive behavior. The ABS-S: 2, first published in 1969 by Nihira, Foster, Shellhaas, and Leland, was revised and standardized in 1974 by Lambert, Windmiller, and Cole and again in 1981 by Lambert and Windmiller. The second and current edition was published in 1993. The ABS-RC:2

was also first published in 1969 by Nihira, Foster, Shellhaas, and Leland. It was revised in 1974, and again in 1993. The goals of the revisions were to improve the reliability of the interviewer in differentiating between individuals with intellectual disabilities who are institutionalized and those living in the community. Previously, these individuals had been classified at different adaptive behavior levels according to the AAIDD.

Psychometric Data

The authors of the ABS-S: 2 report three types of reliability: internal consistency, stability, and interscorer. Internal consistency is reported to range from 0.79 to 0.98, while measures of stability range from 0.82 to 0.97. For Part I, interscorer reliability ranges from 0.95 to 0.98 whereas it is 0.96–0.99 for Part II. Authors report criterion validity in Part 1 moderately correlated with the ABS and the Vineland Adaptive Behavior Scales, although Part II was not significantly related to either (Lyman 2007).

The ABS-RC: 2 reports an internal consistency ranging from 0.81 to 0.97. Concerning discriminant validity, adaptive behavior as measured in Part II was not related to the Vineland Adaptive Behavior Scale and Adaptive Behavior Inventory (ABI), other measures of maladaptive behaviors.

Clinical Uses

The ABS: 2 assesses the status of individuals with intellectual disability, emotional maladjustment, autism, or developmental disability. It enables a professional to evaluate strengths and weaknesses of an individual in adaptive areas, document progress, and measure the effectiveness of intervention/school programs. The manual cautions that the examiner should interview a significant informant or administer the instrument to that significant informant. If an informant is unable to provide needed information, then another informant needs to be interviewed. Whereas the ABS is a standard assessment used in determining adaptive and maladaptive behavior, its psychometric properties are limited, especially compared to other measures such as the Vineland Adaptive Behavior Scales.

Whereas a strength of the ABS-S: 2 is that it was normed on students with and without intellectual disabilities, the ABS-RC: 2's standard scores and percentile ranks were not compared to individuals without intellectual disabilities. Another weakness is that it has not been renormed in two decades.

Therefore, assessment may not meet criteria for a diagnosis of mental retardation according to the AAMR requirements.

Cross-References

▶ Adaptive Behavior Assessment System: Third Edition
▶ Vineland Adaptive Behavior Scales

References and Readings

Aiken, L. (1996). *Assessment of intellectual functioning*. Basel: Burkhauser.

Balboni, G., Tasse, M., Schalock, R., Borthwick-Duffy, S., Spreat, S., Thissen, D., Widaman, K., Zhang, D., & Navas, P. (2014). The diagnostic adaptive behavior scale: Evaluating its diagnostic sensitivity and specificity. *Research in Developmental Disabilities, 35*, 2884–2893.

Bracken, B., & Nagle, R. (2007). *Psychoeducational assessment of preschool children*. New York: Routledge.

Hogg, J., & Langa, A. (2005). *Assessing adults with intellectual disabilities*. Malden: Blackwell.

Lyman, W. C. (2007). Test Review:Lambert, N., Nihira, K., &Lel, H. (1993), AAMR Adaptive Behavior Scales: School (ABS-S:2) *Assessment for Effective Intervention, 33*(1), 55–57.

Reynolds, C., & Fletcher-Janzen, E. (2014). *Encyclopedia of special education, a reference for the education of children, adolescents, and adults with disabilities and other exceptional individuals* (Vol. 3, 4th ed.). Hoboken: Wiley.

Abasia

Douglas I. Katz
Department of Neurology, Boston University School of Medicine, Braintree, MA, USA

Definition

This refers to an inability to walk. Abasia may be caused by a variety of conditions including weakness, spasticity, cerebellar incoordination, and movement disorders of various types.

Cross-References

▶ Ataxia
▶ Spastic Gait

Abbreviated Injury Scale

Edison Wong[1] and Richard Kunz[2]
[1]Center for Pain and Medical Rehabilitation, Fitchburg, MA, USA
[2]Department of Physical Medicine and Rehabilitation, Virginia Commonwealth University, Richmond, VA, USA

Synonyms

Organ injury scale

Definition

The Abbreviated Injury Scale (AIS) is an anatomical scoring system first introduced in 1969. It has been revised and updated against survival data so that it now provides a reasonably accurate way of ranking the severity of injury.

Abbreviated Injury Scale, Table 1 AIS scores and their definition of injury severity

AIS score	Injury
1	Minor
2	Moderate
3	Serious
4	Severe
5	Critical
6	Unsurvivable

Injuries are ranked on a scale of 1–6, with 1 being minor, 5 severe, and 6 representing an unsurvivable injury (Table 1). This represents the "threat to life" associated with an injury and is not meant to represent a comprehensive measure of severity. An additional code of AIS9 is used to indicate an injury for which more detailed coding is not possible due to lack of information. The AIS is not a linear scale, in that the difference between AIS1 and AIS2 is not the same as that between AIS4 and AIS5. Organ Injury Scales of the American Association for the Surgery of Trauma are mapped to the AIS score for calculation of the Injury Severity Score.

Current Knowledge

The latest incarnation of the AIS score is the 2008 update. AIS is monitored by a scaling committee of the Association for the Advancement of Automotive Medicine and has been adopted by the American Association for the Surgery of Trauma since its publication in the *Journal of Trauma* in 1985.

References and Readings

Copes, W. S., Sacco, W. J., Champion, H. R., & Bain, L. W. (1989). Progress in characterizing anatomic injury. In *Proceedings of the 33rd Annual Meeting of the Association for the Advancement of Automotive Medicine* (pp. 205–218), Baltimore, 2–4 Oct 1989.
Gennarelli, T. A., Wodzin, E., & Association for the Advancement of Automotive Medicine. (2008). *The abbreviated injury scale 2005. Update 2008.* Des Plaines: American Association for Automotive Medicine (AAAM).

Greenspan, L., McClellan, B. A., & Greig, H. (1985). Abbreviated injury scale and injury severity score: A scoring chart. *The Journal of Trauma, 25*, 60–64.
Peitzman, A. B., Rhodes, M., Schwab, C. W., Yealy, D. M., & Fabian, T. C. (2002). *The trauma manual* (pp. 29–30). Hagerstown: Lippincott Williams & Wilkins.
Yentis, S. M., Hirsch, N. P., & Smith, G. B. (2004). *Anaesthesia and intensive care A–Z.* New York: Butterworth & Heinemann.

Ablation

Edison Wong[1] and Richard Kunz[2]
[1]Center for Pain and Medical Rehabilitation, Fitchburg, MA, USA
[2]Department of Physical Medicine and Rehabilitation, Virginia Commonwealth University, Richmond, VA, USA

Synonyms

Resection

Definition

Ablation is the removal or destruction of an anatomical structure by means of surgery, disease, or other physical or energetic process. Ablation can be performed on any tissue (e.g., cardiac, neurologic, or endometrium). Ablation is employed as a treatment of various medical conditions and includes recent advances in technology. Surgical ablation of neuronal pathways to the globus pallidus or thalamus has been used historically to treat Parkinsonism. Interventional pain experts use radiofrequency ablation of nerves in the spine to treat chronic back pain. Gamma radiation or "gamma knife surgery" is used to excise brain tumors when traditional surgical ablation is too destructive to neighboring tissues. Even with sophisticated neurosurgical techniques, ablation of any type in the central nervous system may still produce unwanted motor, sensory, or cognitive-behavioral impairments.

Cross-References

► Commissurotomy
► Craniotomy
► Gamma Knife
► Hemispherectomy
► Lobectomy
► Pallidotomy
► Prefrontal Lobotomy
► Radiosurgery, Stereotactic Radiosurgery
► Temporal Lobectomy

References and Readings

Ansari, S. A., Nachanakian, A., & Biary, N. M. (2003). Current surgical treatment of Parkinson's disease. *Neuroscience, 8*(1), 3–7.
Lord, S. M., & Bogduk, N. (2002). Radiofrequency procedures in chronic pain. *Best Practice & Research. Clinical Anaesthesiology, 16*, 597–617.
Lunsford, L. D., Flickinger, J. C., & Steiner, L. (1988). The gamma knife. *JAMA, 259*, 2544.
Shah, R. V., Ericksen, J. J., & Lacerte, M. (2003). Interventions in chronic pain management. 2. New frontiers: Invasive nonsurgical interventions. *Archives of Physical Medicine and Rehabilitation, 84*, S39–S44.

Absence Epilepsy

Jeffrey B. Titus[1,2], Hayley Loblein[3] and Dave Clarke[1,4]
[1]Comprehensive Epilepsy Program, Dell Children's Medical Center of Central Texas, Austin, TX, USA
[2]Department of Psychology, The University of Texas at Austin, Austin, TX, USA
[3]Department of Educational Psychology, The University of Texas at Austin, Austin, TX, USA
[4]Department of Pediatrics, Dell Medical School, The University of Texas at Austin, Austin, TX, USA

Synonyms

Childhood absence epilepsy; Juvenile absence epilepsy; Petit mal epilepsy

Definition

Childhood and juvenile absence epilepsy are forms of idiopathic (genetic) generalized epilepsy that are characterized by seizures that involve sudden arrest in activity, awareness, and responsiveness, and may include some mild motor features. Typical absence seizures usually last less than 20 s and end as abruptly as they start. Patients have no recollection of the event and often return immediately to their previous activity with little or no postictal alterations in functioning. Generalized 3 Hz spike-and-wave discharges on EEG are required for the diagnosis and are strongly correlated with the clinical events.

Categorization

Childhood absence epilepsy (CAE)
Juvenile absence epilepsy (JAE)

Epidemiology

The incidence of CAE is estimated at 6–8% per 100,000 in children younger than 15 years, and the estimated prevalence is 10–12% in children younger than 16 years with epilepsy. The incidence of JAE is less clear, but it is accepted as being less common than CAE. Some estimates suggest that JAE occurs in 10–15% of individuals with epilepsy, though there is likely a pattern of under diagnosis in this condition due to less frequent seizure and the higher rate of other seizure types. CAE is typically considered to be more common in females, but gender differences in JAE have not been reported.

CAE is strongly associated with a family history of seizures, and there is robust concordance among identical twins. Siblings of patients with CAE have about a 10% chance of having seizures, and about one third of patients with CAE have a family member with epilepsy. Heritability of the spike-and-wave trait has been found to peak at the age of 10 years and goes away almost completely by the age of 40. Only about 20% of family members with the spike-and-wave trait develop epilepsy. Multiple genes likely account for transmission, but the causal influences are believed to be multifactorial, depending on both genetic and nongenetic factors. Causal factors in JAE have not been well-studied but may be similar to what is found in CAE.

Natural History, Prognostic Factors, and Outcomes

Typical age of onset in CAE is between 3 and 10 years, with average age of onset of 6 years. Rare cases of onset prior to 3 years of age have been reported. Most cases of JAE are believed to manifest between 10 and 17 years, and average age of onset is 12 or 13 years. Because of variability in onset, there is diagnostic overlap between CAE and JAE, potentially amounting to about 22% of cases with absence seizures. EEG and clinical findings are often useful in differentiating CAE from JAE in older children and younger adolescents, and it is highly unusual for a child with CAE to experience onset of seizures after 11 years of age.

CAE and JAE are both associated with favorable outcomes. Most patients with CAE experience remission of seizures by mid-adolescence, with only a small proportion experiencing absence seizures into adulthood. About 40% of patients with CAE also exhibit generalized tonic-clonic seizures that emerge around the time of puberty, are relatively easy to control, and more commonly persist into adulthood than absence seizures. Generalized tonic-clonic seizures are significantly more common in JAE and occur in about 80% of cases. Some patients with JAE also exhibit myoclonic seizures, but they are typically mild and infrequent. While most patients with CAE become seizure-free by adolescence, seizure outcome in JAE is not well known.

CAE is considered a benign childhood epilepsy because of relatively good seizure and functional outcomes. Seizure control is less common in JAE, but functional outcomes may be similar. Further research is needed to examine this. Tonic-clonic seizures are believed to be a marker for poorer seizure outcome in both CAE and JAE. Functional outcomes in CAE are thought to be most heavily influenced by psychosocial factors, such as family adjustment, support systems, educational attitudes, and stigma toward the condition. Cognitive and/or behavioral side effects from antiepileptic drug (AED) therapy may also limit outcomes.

Neuropsychology and Psychology of Absence Epilepsy

Cognitive functioning in CAE is traditionally considered "benign" because children typically present with normal intelligence and exhibit no significant impairments in functional outcomes. However, more recent research has found evidence that patients with CAE are more prone to having cognitive deficits and psychosocial problems, and they are more likely to receive special education services and display low academic achievement. While patients with poor seizure control exhibit the greatest difficulties, cognitive and behavioral problems are also experienced by patients with good seizure control. While limited information is known about cognitive and psychological functioning in JAE, some reports suggest that about one-third of patients have attention, concentration, or memory problems before their diagnosis of JAE. These cognitive concerns may improve with treatment.

Patients with CAE do not have a characteristic cognitive profile. Cognitive difficulties have been reported in multiple domains, including attention, executive functioning, memory, and visual-spatial processing. A study by Caplan et al. (2008) revealed the presence of subtle cognitive impairments in children with CAE. When compared with controls, they found that children with CAE (ages 6.7–11.2 years) had significantly lower intelligence, as measured by the Wechsler Intelligence Scale for Children – Revised/Third Edition. While, as a group, children with CAE performed in the average range, they were below the performance of a control group. Similar differences were noted on verbally based and visually based intellectual tasks. The difference in performance IQ was less robust, but still significant, between children with CAE and controls. Among their sample of 69 children with CAE, 27% demonstrated overall intelligence at least one standard deviation below the mean. Similar rates were found for VIQ and PIQ. Their spoken language quotient (SLQ), as measured by various versions of the Test of Language Development, was average, but it was also lower than controls. A high percentage of children with CAE performed at least one standard deviation below the mean on language measures.

In the double-blind, randomized controlled clinical trial conducted by the Childhood Absence Epilepsy Study Group, 36% of children with CAE had pretreatment attention problems at a rate estimated to be fourfold that of the general population (Masur et al. 2013). This was despite average intelligence and otherwise normal neurocognitive functioning. Attention problems were disproportionately higher for children being treated with valproic acid. Preferential cognitive deficits in executive functioning have been found in multiple studies affecting problem solving, planning, and fluency.

Caplan et al. (2008) confirmed that children with CAE are at higher risk for emotional and behavioral problems. Among the 69 children with CAE in their sample, 30% had a diagnosis of attention-deficit/hyperactivity disorder (ADHD), with 52% of those children diagnosed as ADHD-inattentive type. Moreover, about 29% of their sample were diagnosed with a form of internalizing psychopathology. Among those children, 75% had a diagnosis of anxiety, 20% had a diagnosis of depression, and 5% had both anxiety and depression. After controlling for IQ and demographic variables, children with CAE were found to have significantly higher ratings on scales of the Child Behavior Checklist (CBCL) that assess attention problems, somatic problems, social problems, withdrawal, and thought problems. The authors discovered that children with lower intelligence had greater social problems, and females in the CAE sample were almost six times more likely to be diagnosed with an anxiety disorder. In addition, children with CAE were more likely to be diagnosed with ADHD or anxiety if they had more frequent seizures or a longer duration of illness. Verrotti et al. (2015) proposed

that it is unclear whether psychological concerns in CAE are a consequence of disease related factors or are part of the epileptic syndrome; however, a recent report by Schwartz and Titus (2015) with the BASC-2 suggested that children with CAE may be more predisposed to depression than other epilepsy syndromes.

Evaluation

Children and adolescents with CAE and JAE typically present with no focal neurological abnormalities on examination. The presence of absence seizures is a defining feature of absence epilepsy, and hyperventilation or light stimulation can be highly effective at eliciting an event. In CAE, absence seizures occur multiple times per day, but, in JAE, seizures are less frequent.

Absence seizures can be either typical or atypical, and discrimination between the two types is typically accomplished through EEG and clinical presentation. While typical absence seizures are characterized by clearly delineated episodes of activity arrest and impaired consciousness for less than 20 s, atypical absence seizures are associated with less abrupt onset and termination, and they may more commonly involve various semiological phenomena. Atypical absence seizures are also frequently observed in epilepsy syndromes that are characterized by more severely impaired neurocognitive functioning, such as Lennox-Gastaut syndrome. Tonic seizures are also frequently present in children with atypical absence seizures.

Typical absence seizures can be subdivided into simple or complex. Simple typical absence seizures constitute about 90% of cases and may involve only minor motor mannerisms (e.g., mild eyelid fluttering) and usually last less than 10 s. Patients with complex typical absence seizures display more involvement of motor features, such as automatisms or decreased or increased muscle tone.

Complex partial seizures can often mimic absence seizures, particularly when their expression is limited. Typical absence seizures can be distinguished from complex partial seizures because they are briefer, more frequent, and have no postictal impairment. EEG characteristics and the presence of various seizure types often distinguish atypical absence seizures from complex partial epilepsy.

When evaluating for the presence of absence seizures, it is important to consider whether the episodes can be accounted for by variations in attention. This is especially important when considering the high rate of attention problems in children with epilepsy. Attempting to determine the degree of responsiveness during the episodes often helps with making the differential diagnosis; however, this can be difficult to determine when episodes are very brief. Moreover, it is not uncommon for patients to have both absence seizures and attention problems. Therefore, a child's ability to respond during an episode cannot be used to rule-out the presence of absence seizures. Sometimes a neuropsychological assessment can be helpful in differentiating between absence seizures and episodes of inattention. If the examiner has experience with absence seizures, the neuropsychological assessment can provide multiple hours of one-on-one observation and interaction that might provide opportunities to observe the episodes and attempt to elicit responses. This can also be helpful if mental fatigue tends to elicit more events.

On EEG, absence seizures are characterized by paroxysmal bursts of high amplitude 2.5–4 Hz spike and slow waves that are superimposed on a normal background. The bursts vary in length (3–20 s), and the clinical absence is time-locked to the burst period. This activity (clinical and electrographic) can be provoked during a routine EEG recording using the hyperventilation activation procedure and, infrequently, from photic stimulation.

Treatment

Response to AED therapy in CAE and JAE is good, and ethosuximide is considered the drug of first choice. Valproic acid or lamotrigine have also been recommended. In rare cases of more difficult to control seizures, polytherapy may be needed. In patients with CAE, a seizure-free period of 2 years is often recommended prior to discontinuation of therapy; however, this should be determined on a case-by-case basis. About 40% of children with CAE develop generalized tonic-clonic seizures. Patients with JAE will require longer treatment and may continue using AEDs indefinitely. In adolescent patients, it is important to educate about the increased risk of seizures with poor medication compliance, alcohol consumption, or sleep deprivation.

See Also

▶ Petit Mal Seizure

Absence Epilepsy – CAE and JAE

EEG signature	Characteristic generalized 3 Hz spike and slow wave (may slow to 2.5 Hz during the absence and may be faster in JAE). Activated by hyperventilation is more common than photic stimulation.
Age of onset	CAE: 3–10 years JAE: 10–17 years
Clinical features	Typical events last 4–20 s. Seizure semiology: (a) Frequent staring spells with abrupt onset and offset without aura (fewer seen in JAE). Occasional automatic mouth or hand movements or subtle myoclonus. (b) Generalized tonic-clonic seizures are more common in JAE. MRI is typically normal.
AED management	Ethosuximide Valproic acid or lamotrigine can be helpful if generalized tonic-clonic seizures manifest.
Response to treatment with AEDs	Good
Seizure freedom	CAE: Expected by adolescence JAE: Less common
Functional outcome	CAE: Good JAE: Unknown

References and Readings

Berkovic, S. F., & Benbadis, S. (2001). Childhood and juvenile absence epilepsy. In E. Wyllie (Ed.), *The treatment of epilepsy: Principles and practice* (3rd ed., pp. 485–490). Philadelphia: Lippincott Williams & Wilkins.

Caplan, R., Siddarth, P., Stahl, L., Lanphier, E., Vona, P., Gurbani, S., et al. (2008). Childhood absence epilepsy: Behavioral, cognitive, and linguistic comorbidities. *Epilepsia, 49*(11), 1838–1846.

Holtkamp, M. (2017). Genetic generalized epilepsies with adolescent onset. In J. M. Pellock, D. R. Nordli Jr., R. Sankar, & J. W. Wheless (Eds.), *Pellock's pediatric epilepsy: Diagnosis and therapy* (4th ed., pp. 337–346).

Masur, D., Shinnar, S., Cnaan, A., Shinnar, R. C., Clark, P., Wang, J., Weiss, E. F., Hirtz, D. G., Glauser, T. A., & Childhood Absence Epilepsy Study Group. (2013). Pretreatment cognitive deficits and treatment effects on attention in childhood absence epilepsy. *Neurology, 81*, 1572–1580.

Pearl, P. L., & Holmes, G. L. (2017). Childhood absence epilepsy. In J. M. Pellock, D. R. Nordli Jr., R. Sankar, & J. W. Wheless (Eds.), Pellock's pediatric epilepsy: Diagnosis and therapy, (4th ed) pp. 309–336).

Schwartz, J. K., & Titus, J. B. (2015). Executive functioning and behavioral profiles in childhood absence epilepsy and juvenile myoclonic epilepsy [Abstract]. *Journal of the International Neuropsychological Society, 21*(s1), 87–88.

Verrotti, A., Matricardi, S., Rinaldi, V. E., Prezioso, G., & Coppola, G. (2015). Neuropsychological impairment in childhood absence epilepsy: Review of the literature. *Journal of the Neurological Sciences, 359*(1–2), 59–66.

Absence Seizure

Kenneth R. Perrine
Neurological Surgery, Weill Cornell Medicine, New York, NY, USA

Synonyms

Petit mal seizure; Psychomotor seizures

Definition

An *absence* (usually pronounced with a French accent as "ab-SAWNS") *seizure* is a type of generalized seizure caused by a large burst of electrical discharges that begins in broad, bilaterally distributed networks simultaneously as opposed to a *complex partial seizure* (focal seizure with altered awareness/responsiveness).[1] During an absence seizure, the patient will lose interaction with the environment, stare blankly ("zone out"), and perhaps blink the eyes (eyelid myoclonia) or have sudden jerks (myoclonic absence). There is no true loss of consciousness or motor functions. The seizure is typically short in duration (only several seconds), and patients often resume their ongoing activity without realizing even that they had a seizure (but will be amnestic for anything occurring during the episode). There are no postictal problems after the end of the seizure. Although no first aid is required, the patient should be protected from doing anything dangerous during the episode (e.g., cooking, crossing the street), but the episodes are often so brief that intervention is difficult.

Current Knowledge

The cause of absence seizures is unknown. Patients with typical absence seizures have no positive neuroimaging findings but usually have bursts of 3-per-second bilaterally synchronous spike/wave epileptiform activity on a routine EEG (even when not having a seizure). Atypical absence seizures can have a slightly different frequency or pattern. Absence seizures can be differentiated clinically from *complex partial seizures* (focal seizures with altered awareness/responsiveness), in which there is a similar disruption of consciousness and "zoning out," by the duration of the episode. Absence seizures last only a few seconds, while *complex partial seizures* usually last 1–1.5 min. Absence seizures typically begin in childhood, respond well to medication, and often remit spontaneously by adulthood. Common medications for absence seizures include divalproex/valproate sodium (Depakote),

---

[1] The International League Against Epilepsy suggested new terminology for seizure types (Berg et al. 2010). These new terms have not yet been fully adopted but are given in parentheses.

ethosuximide (Zarontin), and lamotrigine (Lamictal). Although the frequency of absence seizures can approach dozens per day, only mild (at worst) neuropsychological deficits are typically shown if the absence episodes occur without other seizure types. They do not have a dramatic impact on academic performance. However, absence seizures may occur with other seizure types in serious disorders such as Lennox-Gastaut syndrome, in which case there is considerable cognitive dysfunction and a worse prognosis.

Cross-References

▶ Complex Partial Seizure
▶ Epilepsy
▶ Seizure

References and Readings

Berg, A. T., Berkovic, S. F., Brodie, M. J., Buchhalter, J., Cross, J. H., van Emde, B. W., Engel, J., French, J., Glauser, T. A., Mathern, G. W., Moshe, S. L., Nordli, D., Plouin, P., & Scheffer, I. E. (2010). Revised terminology and concepts for organization of seizures and epilepsies: Report of the ILAE Commission on Classification and Terminology, 2005–2009. *Epilepsia, 51*(4), 676–685.
www.epilepsyfoundation.org
www.ilae.org
Wyllie, E. (Ed.). (2015). *Wyllie's treatment of epilepsy: Principles and practice* (6th ed.). New York: Lippincott Williams & Wilkins.

Absolute Threshold

Mark Mennemeier
Neurobiology and Developmental Sciences, University of Arkansas for Medical Sciences, Little Rock, AR, USA

Synonyms

Stimulus threshold

Definition

The absolute threshold is the smallest amount of stimulus energy necessary to produce a sensation of the stimulus. The idea that a mental event has to exceed some critical amount is central to the concept of a sensory threshold. The absolute threshold refers to the measurement of that critical amount.

See Also

▶ Just Noticeable Difference

References and Readings

Gescheider, G. A. (1997). *Psychophysics: The fundamentals* (3rd ed.). London: Erlbaum, Chapter 1.

Abstract Reasoning

David Hulac
Department of School Psychology, College of Education and Behavioral Sciences, University of Northern Colorado, Greeley, CO, USA

Synonyms

Logical reasoning

Definition

The neuropsychological construct of abstract reasoning refers to an individual's ability to recognize patterns and relationships of theoretical or intangible ideas. Abstract reasoning is contrary to concrete reasoning whereby an individual recognizes patterns in information obtained through the immediate senses. When thinking abstractly, an individual must be able to identify rules and apply those rules to information without the aid of empirical help or personal experience.

Abstract reasoning is most closely related to rational thought as opposed to empirical thought. While using deductive reasoning, a purely rational thinker does not look to determine the accuracy of a premise, but seeks only to understand the relationship between the premises.

An example of deductive reasoning, which requires abstract reasoning, may go like this:

1. Premise 1: Egypt is located in South America.
2. Premise 2: The Sphinx lies in Egypt.
3. Conclusion: The Sphinx is located in South America.

Empirically and concretely, it is obvious that Egypt is not in South America, but in Africa. To complete the syllogism, however, the thinker must ignore the concrete distortion and instead focus on the two premises and understand if the conclusion logically flows.

Common measures of abstract intelligence include the similarities, picture concepts, and matrix reasoning subtests of the Wechsler scales. During a mental status exam, abstract reasoning is measured by asking a subject to describe the meanings of proverbs or to describe word similarities.

Abstract reasoning, most commonly understood as being a function of the frontal lobes of the brain, is a precursor for using and understanding language and mathematics. Individuals who struggle with abstract reasoning benefit when an instructor uses examples to make the concept more concrete or observable. Frequently, children with learning disabilities have difficulty with these abstract concepts, but achieve greater success in courses with more concrete subject matter such as social studies and science.

References and Readings

Goldstein, G. (2004). Abstract reasoning and problem solving in adults. In M. Hersen (Ed.), *Comprehensive handbook of psychological assessment, Intellectual and neuropsychological assessment* (Vol. 1, pp. 293–308). Hoboken: Wiley.

Abulia

Irene Piryatinsky
Butler Hospital and Alpert Medical School of Brown University, Providence, RI, USA

Synonyms

Apathy; Athymia; Loss of psychic self-activation; Psychic akinesia
Also spelled Aboulia

Definition

The term is derived from the Greek "boul" (will). Abulia is manifested by lack of motivation; lack of spontaneity in speech and action; deficiency in initiation, inertia, mental, and motor slowness; poor attention; and easy distractibility. Inactivity comes from an inability to select a course of action, although a wish to participate may be present. Some research indicates that abulia occurs due to malfunction of the brain's dopamine-dependent circuitry. In neurologic diseases, it is associated with bilateral lesions in the medial or orbital frontal lobes. The following criteria have been suggested for the diagnosis of abulia: (i) decreased spontaneity in activity and speech; (ii) prolonged latency in responding to queries, directions, and other stimuli; and (iii) reduced ability to persist with a task.

Further Reading

Berrios, G. E., & Grli, M. (1995). Abulia and impulsiveness revisited: A conceptual history. *Acta Psychiatrica Scandinavica, 92*(3), 161–167.
Caplan, L. R., Schmahmann, J. D., Kase, C. S., Feldmann, E., Baquis, G., Greenberg, J. P., et al. (1990). Caudate infarcts. *Archives of Neurology, 47*(2), 133–143.
Drubach, D. A., Zeilig, G., Perez, J., Peralta, L., & Makley, M. (1995). Treatment of abulia with carbidopa/levadopa. *Journal of Neuroengineering and Rehabilitation, 9*, 151–155.

Egnelborghs, S., Marien, M. A., Pickut, B. A., Verstraeten, M. A., & De Deyn, P. P. (2000). Loss of psychic self-activation after paramedian bithalamic infarction. *Stroke, 31*, 1762–1765.

Forstl, H., & Sahakian, B. A. (1991). A psychiatric presentation of abulia: Three cases of frontal lobe ischaemia and atrophy. *Journal of the Royal Society of Medicine, 84*, 89–91.

Kumral, E., Evyapan, D., & Balkir, K. (1999). Acute caudate vascular lesions. *Stroke, 30*, 100–108.

Laplande, D., Attal, N., Sauron, B., de Billy, A., & Dubois, B. (1992). Lesions of the basal ganglia due to disulfiram neurotoxicity. *Journal of Neurology, Neurosurgery, and Psychiatry, 55*, 925–929.

Liddle, P. F. (1987). The symptoms of chronic schizophrenia. *British Journal of Psychiatry, 151*, 145–151.

Litvan, I., Paulsen, J. S., Mega, M. S., & Cummings, J. L. (1998). Neuropsychiatric assessment of patients with hyperkinetic and hypokinetic movement disorders. *Archives of Neurology, 55*, 1313–1319.

Powell, J. H., Al-Adawi, S., Morgan, J., & Greenwood, R. J. (1996). Motivation deficits after brain injury: Effects of bromocriptine in 11 patients. *Journal of Neurology, Neurosurgery, and Psychiatry, 60*, 416–421.

Abusive Head Trauma

Jennifer Ann Niskala Apps[1] and
Amy Heffelfinger[2]
[1]Department of Psychiatry and Behavioral Medicine, Children's Hospital of Wisconsin/Medical College of Wisconsin, Milwaukee, WI, USA
[2]Medical College of Wisconsin, Milwaukee, WI, USA

Synonyms

Inflicted childhood neurotrauma; Nonaccidental or inflicted traumatic brain injury; Pediatric abusive head trauma; Shaken baby syndrome

Short Description or Definition

Pediatric abusive head trauma (AHT) is a form of inflicted traumatic brain injury in an infant or small child due to blunt trauma, being shaken, or a combination of both. Rapid rotation and movement, acceleration and deceleration changes, of the brain within the cranial vault of a small child result in significant neural trauma. The National Center for Injury Prevention and Control defines pediatric abusive head trauma as "an injury to the skull or intracranial contents of an infant or young child (<5 years of age) due to inflicted blunt impact and/or violent shaking." This definition excludes unintentional injuries and penetrating trauma (Parks et al. 2012).

Categorization

A form of child maltreatment or abuse, AHT occurs as a result of a baby's weak neck muscles in relation to its proportionally large head being unable to compensate for rapid shaking, accelerating and decelerating velocity changes, and/or impact to the head. While the injury itself can present with a wide variety of clinical sequela, the mechanism behind the injury is more extensive force than noted in accidental or neglectful events and different from penetrating injuries. The most common injuries related to AHT include subdural hematomas and retinal hemorrhage, with additional physical injuries such as fractures, signs of impact, and spinal injuries noted (Nadarasa et al. 2014).

Epidemiology

Determination of frequency, morbidity, and mortality is difficult because oftentimes no clear, visible injury occurs. In addition, given the abusive nature of the injury, significant motives to avoid detection often make investigating possible cases of AHT difficult. AHT likely occurs most often in children under 2 years of age, but can occur through 5 years of age. AHT can occur in the context of additional abusive injuries, either current or historical. Among cases of nonaccidental pediatric trauma, more than half of deaths are a result of AHT (Ross and Juarez 2014). Many children had prior additional abusive injuries or nonspecific signs in the past of head trauma such

that those nonfatal, non-life-threatening incidences were not detected. Overall mortality is
estimated to range up to almost 40%, with upward
of 60% of infants who have been shaken dying or
experiencing profound long-term medical and
cognitive consequences (www.dontshake.org).
Incidence, according to research, is estimated to
be as many as 39.8 per 100,000 in children under
1 year of age, with rates decreasing sharply as
children age (Niederkrotenthaler et al. 2013).

Natural History, Prognostic Factors, and Outcomes

In the early 1970s, the term "whiplash shaken
baby syndrome" was used to describe symptoms
consistent with AHT, which had been identified
over two decades prior (Caffey 1974). Over the
last four decades, debate has centered on the
methods for standardizing the diagnosis of
AHT, as well as the implications of various
nomenclature to describe the trauma. Identification of AHT generally includes neurological dysfunction (i.e., apnea), subdural hemorrhage, and
retinal hemorrhage. As there are other possible
causes for this triad that does not include inflicted
trauma, it is difficult to correctly identify and to
convict the suspected perpetrator of committing
abuse. Formal definitions and nomenclature for
AHT have been developed in order to drive diagnostic classifications. The CDC currently defines
pediatric abusive head trauma "as an injury to the
skull or intracranial contents of an infant or young
child (<5 years of age) due to inflicted blunt
impact and/or violent shaking" (Parks et al.
2012). This definition excludes unintentional
injuries, such as from lack of supervision and
any penetrating trauma. Research has indicated
that medical signs such as the presence of intracranial injuries in coordination with a lack of
specific signs of impact assist in differentiating
between inflicted versus accidental trauma
(Vinchon et al. 2009).

Educational campaigns help new parents
expect intense crying, to recognize frustration
that is theorized to lead to abusive shaking, and

to leave the baby in a safe place and walk away.
Unlike other forms of abuse, risk for AHT cuts
across all social classes, races, and gender
although recent studies indicate that it may be
more prevalent for babies in lower socioeconomic
homes. Known risk factors of AHT include male
sex (Keenan et al. 2003), age under 1 year
(Keenan et al. 2003), having a young mother
(Overpeck et al. 1998), having parents with low
socioeconomic status (Christian and Block 2009),
and some studies indicate a higher risk for racial/
ethnic minorities (Bennett et al. 2006; Drake et al.
2011). However, research on prevalence of risk
factors related to race or socioeconomic status is
unclear and extremely variable, with possible
reporting issues related to these same factors.
Therefore, many authors urge caution when
interpreting overall risk factors (Niederkrotenthaler et al. 2013).

Outcomes for children experiencing AHT are
extremely variable and relate to the amount of
damage inflicted and interventions received.
More subtle signs of neurotrauma after injury
can be mistaken for flu-like symptoms or other
common presentations of childhood (i.e., colic),
and in some cases when a child is shaken into a
comatose state, the caretaker may believe that
the child has gone to sleep or finally stopped
crying. Such complicating factors may result in
significant delays before a child is brought for
medical attention and lead to significant mortality rates. Children who survive AHT may experience blindness if they have had retinal
hemorrhaging, as well as significant long-term
neurological conditions such as mental retardation, seizure disorders, muscular spasticity or
cerebral palsy, and structural abnormalities
such as microcephaly, hydrocephaly, cerebral
atrophy, or encephalomalacia as a direct result
of neural trauma.

Neural System Damage and Neuropsychology Outcomes of AHT

Symptoms of AHT vary with the severity of
the inflicted neural trauma. The neural injury

typically includes acceleration injury during shaking and deceleration when the shaking is stopped or the child is slammed or thrown into an object. Recent research indicate differences between AHT and accidental injury on retinal hemorrhages, suggesting AHT causes diffuse, multilayered hemorrhages, and additional research suggests AHT results in increased intracranial pressure, brain swelling, as well as possible rupture of bridging veins, often found in coordination with spinal injuries (Nadarasa et al. 2014). Subdural hemorrhage and subarachnoid hemorrhage are most often bilateral. Further, neuronal injury occurs with resultant cerebral edema. Additional pathology often includes spine and neck injuries, rib fractures, and fractures to the long bones of the infant (particularly, if they have been held by an appendage while shaken). As a result of neurological pathology, immediate observable symptoms can include lethargy, irritability, a high-pitched cry, poor sucking and feeding, problems breathing, a blue or pale pallor, vomiting, and seizures. Literature suggests that apnea and severe retinal hemorrhages are strongest indicators of AHT. Of those who survive, approximately two thirds are either moderately or severely impaired (Narang and Clarke 2014). Long-term outcomes of these injuries are difficult to study and quantify in a rigorous manner. Therefore, most descriptions of AHT are based on the case studies, indicating that children who survive are more severely impaired as they experience more severe injuries, including lacerations of brain tissue, excessively elevated intracranial pressure, infarcts, and hemorrhage. A study of a small number of children with inflicted head trauma that were followed postinjury indicated over half experienced significant cognitive impairments, as well as language delays (Barlow et al. 2005). Limited research indicates that comparisons to children experiencing nonabusive or accidental head trauma indicate far greater incidences of long-term cognitive impairments (Ewing-Cobbs et al. 1998). Those with AHT more likely experienced deeper, more extensive cortical injury, more often resulting in impairments in

cardiorespiratory functioning or consciousness and resulting in more frequent bilateral and ischemic injuries and lower developmental scores post-injury (Hymel et al. 2007).

Evaluation

Diagnosis of AHT requires extensive medical evaluations including radiology studies as well as sociological evaluations of the caregivers. Evidence of additional physical injuries indicative of abuse on the child should be documented. The presence or absence of retinal hemorrhages should be evaluated by a pediatric ophthalmologist or neurologist. Laboratory values can indicate the presence of blood in the cerebral spinal fluid, coagulation changes following cerebral injury, and possible pancreas and liver damage. X-ray can reveal rib injuries. Most significantly, CT scan is the primary method of evaluation for brain injury. Consecutive CT scans can reveal ongoing changes in a recently injured child as well as the evidence of older brain injuries. Utilizing MRI as an adjunct in longer-term diagnosis can reveal more subtle white matter changes related to injury.

Treatment

Treatment of AHT most often involves life-saving measures initially, including neurosurgery to address active bleeding and excessive intracranial pressure. Medical life support may be required for some time while swelling subsides. Long-term treatment of AHT involves addressing the most salient of the resulting neurobiological symptoms. Children with more significant injuries often begin rehabilitation therapies immediately, much like other children who experience accidental brain injuries. Neuropsychological evaluations across development are often useful to detect specific cognitive, functional, or educational impairments, with the most common believed to be attention, executive, and visual perceptual deficits.

Cross-References

► Cerebral Edema
► Subarachnoid Hemorrhage
► Traumatic Brain Injury (TBI)

References and Readings

Barlow, K. M., Thomson, E., Johnson, D., & Minns, R. A. (2005). Late neurologic and cognitive sequelae of inflicted traumatic brain injury in infancy. *Pediatrics, 116*, 174–185.

Caffey, J. (1974). The whiplash-shaken infant syndrome: Manual shaking by the extremities with whiplash-induced intra cranial and intra ocular bleeding, linked with residual permanent damage and mental retardation. *Pediatrics, 54*(4), 396–403.

Ewing-Cobbs, L., Kramer, L., Prasad, M., Canales, D. N., Louis, P. T., Fletcher, J. M., Vollero, H., Landry, S. H., & Cheung, K. (1998). Neuroimaging, physical, and developmental findings after inflicted and noninflicted traumatic brain injury in young children. *Pediatrics, 102*(2), 300–307.

Hymel, K. P., Makoroff, K. L., Laskey, A. L., Conaway, M. R., & Blackman, J. A. (2007). Mechanisms, clinical presentations, injuries, and outcomes from inflicted versus noninflicted head trauma during infancy: Results of a prospective, multicentered, comparative study. *Pediatrics, 119*, 922–929.

Lopes, N. R. L., Eisenstein, E., & Williams, L. C. A. (2013). Abusive head trauma in children: A literature review. *Journal de Pediatria, 89*, 426–433.

Nadarasa, J., Deck, C., Meyer, F., Willinger, R., & Raul, J. S. (2014). Update on injury mechanisms in abusive head trauma – Shaken baby syndrome. *Pediatric Radiology, 44*(Suppl 4), S565–S570.

Narang, S., & Clarke, J. (2014). Abusive head trauma: Past, present, and future. *Journal of Child Neurology, 29*(12), 1747–1756.

National Institutes of Health, National Institute of Neurological Disorder & Stroke NINDS Shaken Baby Syndrome Information page. www.ninds.nih.gov/disorders/shakenbaby

Niederkrotenthaler, T., Xu, L., Parks, S. E., & Sugerman, D. E. (2013). Descriptive factors of abusive head trauma in young children – United States, 2000–2009. *Child Abuse & Neglect, 37*, 446–455.

Parks, S. E., Annest, J. L., Hill, H. A., & Karch, D. L. (2012). *Pediatric abusive head trauma: Recommended definitions for public health surveillance and research*. Atlanta: Centers for Disease Control and Prevention.

Ross, A. H., & Juarez, C. A. (2014). A brief history of fatal child maltreatment and neglect. *Forensic Science, Medicine, and Pathology, 10*, 413–422.

Shaken Baby Association, Inc. www.shakenbaby.net

The National Center on SBS. www.dontshake.org

Academic Competency

Kristy K. Kelly
Educational Psychology, University of Wisconsin-Madison, Madison, WI, USA

Synonyms

Academic ability; Academic performance; Educational productivity

Definition

Academic competency is the multidimensional characteristics of a learner – including skills, attitudes, and behaviors – that factor into their academic success. These characteristics can be separated and considered in one of two primary domains: academic skills or academic enablers (DiPerna and Elliot 2000; Elliot and DiPerna 2002). Academic skills are both the basic and complex skills (e.g., reading, writing, calculating, and critical thinking) needed to access and interact with content-specific knowledge. Academic enablers, however, are the attitudes and behaviors (e.g., interpersonal skills, motivation, study skills, and engagement) that a learner needs in order to take advantage of education.

Research indicates that prior achievement and interpersonal skills influence motivation, thereby impacting study skills and engagement (e.g., time on task), which are skills positively associated with achievement (DiPerna et al. 2002, 2005).

Cross-References

► Academic Skills
► Learning

References and Readings

DiPerna, J. C., & Elliot, S. N. (2000). *The academic competence evaluation scales (ACES college)*. San Antonio: The Psychological Association.

DiPerna, J. C., Volpe, R. J., & Elliott, S. N. (2002). A model of academic enablers and elementary reading/language arts achievement. *School Psychology Review, 31*(3), 298–312.

DiPerna, J. C., Volpe, R. J., & Elliott, S. N. (2005). A model of academic enablers and and mathematics achievement in the elementary grades. *Journal of School Psychology, 43*(5), 379–392.

Edl, H. M., Jones, M. H., & Estell, D. B. (2008). Ethnicity and english proficiency: Teacher perceptions of academic and interpersonal competence in European American and Latino students. *School Psychology Review, 37*(1), 38–45.

Elliot, S. N., & DiPerna, J. C. (2002). Assessing the academic competence of college students: Validation of a self-report measure of skills and enablers. *Journal of Postsecondary Education and Disability, 15*(2), 87–100.

Hutto, L. (2009). *Measuring academic competence in college students: A review of research and instruments.* Saarbrücken: VDM Verlag.

Ma, L., Phelps, E., Lerner, J. V., & Lerner, R. M. (2009). Academic competence for adolescents who bully and who are bullied. *Journal of Early Adolescence, 29*(6), 862–897.

Shapiro, E. S. (2008). From research to practice: Promoting academic competence for underserved students. *School Psychology Review, 37*(1), 46–51.

Academic Skills

Christina Zafiris[1] and Rachel Losoff[2]
[1]Applied Psychology and Counselor Education, University of Northern Colorado, Greeley, CO, USA
[2]School Psychology, The Chicago School of Professional Psychology, Chicago, IL, USA

Definition

Academic skills refer to a student's ability to perform age-appropriate school activities related to reading, writing, and mathematics. **Reading skills** include the five building blocks skills of phonemic awareness, phonics, fluency, vocabulary, and comprehension. These are listed in hierarchical order, as the ultimate goal is comprehending whatever one reads (National Reading Panel 2015). **Writing skills** begin with the basic skill of letter formation and progress to the more advanced skills of fluency (production of simple sentences), syntactic maturity (production of increasingly complex sentences),

semantic maturity or vocabulary use, organization of thought or content, and conventions (including grammar, spelling, and punctuation) (Howell and Nolet 2000). **Math skills** include the general skills of basic fact fluency (i.e., addition, subtraction, multiplication, division), math computation and operations (e.g., multi-digit addition, fractions), and math application/problem-solving. Math skills can further be categorized by the ten common core math standards: counting and cardinality, operations and algebraic thinking, numbers and operations in base 10, numbers and operations-fractions, measurement and data, geometry, ratios and proportional relationships, the number system, expression and equations, functions, and statistics and probability (Common Core Standards Initiative 2016). These three academic skills of reading, writing, and math allow for the acquisition of other content area school subjects. For example, social studies and history require reading and writing, while science and technology require math and reading (and often writing). These academic skills are differentiated from academic enabler skills, which enable the acquisition of academic skills and include motivation, interpersonal skills, engagement, and study skills (DiPerna et al. 2001).

Cross-References

► Academic Competency
► Educational Testing
► Learning
► Reading

References and Readings

Common Core State Standards Initiative. (2016). Common core state standards for mathematics. Retrieved from http://www.corestandards.org/Math/

DiPerna, J. C., Volpe, R. J., & Elliot, S. N. (2001). A model of academic enablers and elementary reading/language art achievement. *School Psychology Review, 31*(3), 298–312.

Howell, K. W., & Nolet, V. (2000). *Curriculum-based evaluation: Teaching and decision making* (3rd ed.). Belmont: Wadsworth.

National Reading Panel. (2015, March 17). National Reading Panel. Retrieved from https://www.nichd.nih.gov/research/supported/Pages/nrp.aspx

Academic Techniques

Ginger Mills
Graduate Institute of Professional Psychology,
University of Hartford, West Hartford, CT, USA

Definition

Academic techniques are a set of rehabilitation strategies that are aimed at facilitating learning. While there are a myriad of techniques available to aid in learning, evidence continues to grow for the effectiveness of specific instructional strategies. These strategies assist individuals with cognitive impairments in learning new information and skills. Various models for improving learning and memory have been developed, some of which include TEACH-M (*T*ask Analysis, *E*rrorless learning, *A*ssessment, *C*umulative review, *H*igh rates of correct practice, *M*etacognitive strategies); PQRST (*P*review, *Q*uestion, *R*ead, *S*tate, and *T*est); and the pediatric neurocognitive intervention (PNI) methods.

Historical Background

Much of the research for academic techniques and strategies stems from the special education field, which utilizes such techniques to teach those with learning disabilities (Sohlberg et al. 2005). Researchers in the neuropsychology field have continued to build upon such literature in order to highlight and develop effective interventions for individuals with neuropsychological impairments. The various models developed from such research have their own unique origin and history, but many have been developed in response to the needs of specific populations. For example, the direct instruction method was developed by Engelmann and Carnine (Sohlberg et al. 2005) as a model for teaching economically disadvantaged children. Other approaches such as the PQRST, stemmed from the notion that individuals with partially intact explicit memory capabilities,

such as those with acquired brain injury, could benefit from strategies that are aimed at improving encoding and retrieval (Wilson 2009). Thus, while academic techniques, and the models that use them, are varied and diverse, they were developed to facilitate learning and in turn improve functioning in individuals with cognitive impairments.

Rationale or Underlying Theory

Acquiring new information and skills is an important part of recovery for individuals with cognitive impairment. It is through learning that individuals are able to remediate and/or compensate for impairments and improve their daily functioning. The underlying theory behind several rehabilitation strategies geared at improving learning and memory is to structure the input of information in a way that aids learning, and in turn memory (Ehlhardt et al. 2008). For some more extensive models, such as the PNI, hierarchal levels are designed so that higher-level skills are built on lower-level skills (Limond and Adlam 2015).

Goals and Objectives

Specific goals vary from technique to technique and within specific models of rehabilitation. Generally, academic techniques are meant to facilitate the learning process for individuals with cognitive impairments. General cognitive rehabilitation objectives include changing target behavior and/or restitution of cognitive abilities (Raskin 2010). Academic techniques can be viewed as targeting both objectives, depending on the technique and model, in that many strategies seek to change the individual's approach to learning (e.g. PQRST) as well as restore certain learning and memory capacities. Academic strategies seek to structure the manner in which information or procedures are taught and practiced so as to facilitate learning (Ehlhardt et al. 2008).

Treatment Participants

Given their variety, academic techniques and strategies can be utilized across settings with different individuals. Specific applications include cognitive rehabilitation and special education instruction. Individuals with cognitive impairment due to developmental disabilities and neurological conditions would benefit from academic techniques and strategies. Additionally, various treatment approaches could be effective across populations with learning and memory impairments, including individuals with learning disabilities, psychiatric disorders such as schizophrenia, and dementia (Sohlberg et al. 2005).

Treatment Procedures

Strategies for learning can be grouped into direction instruction, strategy-based instruction, a combined strategy and direction instruction approach, and nondirect/non-strategy techniques (Sohlberg et al. 2005). Direct instruction includes breaking down instructions into smaller steps, modelling of a skill, and providing frequent feedback. Strategy-based instructions involve teaching individuals to self-monitor, use prompts to foster self-assessment, summarize and elaborate, and outline important themes. A combined approach utilizes both a direct and strategy-based approach (Sohlberg et al. 2005). Examples of techniques include vanishing cues, a technique in which the amount of cuing is reduced over specific number of trials. Errorless learning is another example of a technique used for learning and involves reducing errors during learning by breaking down tasks into discrete steps, providing sufficient examples before the patient is asked to perform the task, and correcting errors immediately (Raskin 2010; Sohlberg et al. 2005).

Several models utilize academic techniques and strategies in their protocols. TEACH-M is an instructional package designed to identify a sequence of strategies that would be helpful in facilitating learning and memory in individuals with memory impairments, specifically related to an acquired brain injury (Ehlhardt et al. 2005). Techniques used include task analysis, errorless learning, assessment of skills, review of new and learned skills, frequent and distributed practice, as well as encouragement of active processing and self-reflection (Sohlberg et al. 2005). The PQRST model encourages individuals to develop questions about the information they are learning, read information carefully while thinking about their questions, summarize the information, and test the knowledge acquired (Wilson 2009). This method allows for a systematic review of information that encourages analysis and organization of information, which is thought to later improve retention. The PNI model consists of various levels that build on previously learned skills. The first level focuses on interventions and techniques designed to aid in learning and memory in addition to other cognitive skills (Limond and Adlam 2015). This model is unique in that in addition to the use of academic techniques and strategies, it also utilizes strategies to increase metacognitive skills and encompasses both compensatory and restorative strategies.

While specific strategies and models can be used with a variety of patients, it is important that individuals working to teach these strategies engage in careful and specific planning for their patients. Specifically for instructional strategies, Ehlhardt et al. (2008) recommend the following: clear specification of intervention targets, constraining errors, sufficient and distributed practice, using multiple examples, promoting effortful processing, and selection of ecologically valid targets.

Efficacy Information

Research on instructional methods suggests that they are effective, although questions regarding what and how specific strategies are implemented for maximum benefit remain to be answered (Glang et al. 2008; Ehlhardt et al. 2008). Several models utilizing academic techniques have been found to be effective in facilitating learning and the retention of information. The PQRST method has been found to be effective for individuals with memory impairments (Wilson 2009) and individuals with memory impairments due to prefrontal cortex lesions (Ciaramelli et al. 2015). The TEACH-M method was also found to be effective in facilitating learning in a group of four individuals, as discussed by Ehlhardt et al. (2005).

Qualifications of Treatment Providers

Those individuals teaching academic strategies or rehabilitation techniques should be individuals trained in special education and cognitive rehabilitation. Some professions include special education teachers, cognitive rehabilitation specialists, clinicians, and speech and language pathologists.

See Also

▶ Cognitive Rehabilitation
▶ Errorless Learning
▶ Evidence-Based Practice
▶ Metacognitive Skills
▶ Method of Vanishing Cues
▶ Mnemonic Techniques

References and Readings

Ciaramelli, E., Neri, F., Marini, L., & Braghittoni, D. (2015). Improving memory following prefrontal cortex damage with the PQRST method. *Frontiers in Behavioral Neuroscience, 9*(211), 1–9. https://doi.org/10.3389/fnbeh.2015.00211.

Ehlhardt, L. A., Sohlberg, M. M., Glang, A., & Albin, R. (2005). TEACH-M: A pilot study evaluating an instructional sequence for persons with impaired memory and executive functions. *Brain Injury, 19*(8), 569–583. https://doi.org/10.1080/02699050400013550.

Ehlhardt, L. A., Sohlberg, M. M., Kennedy, M., Coelho, C., Ylvisaker, M., Turkstra, L., & Yorkston, K. (2008). Evidence-based practice guidelines for instructing individuals with neurogenic memory impairments: What have we learned in the past 20 years? *Neuropsychological Rehabilitation, 18*(3), 300–342. https://doi.org/10.1080/09602010701733190.

Glang, A., Ylvisaker, M., Stein, M., Ehlhardt, L., Todis, B., & Tyler, J. (2008). Validated instructional practices: Application to students with traumatic brain injury. *The Journal of Head Trauma Rehabilitation, 23*(4), 243–251. https://doi.org/10.1097/01.HTR.0000327256.46504.9f.

Limond, J., & Adlam, A. L. (2015). Cognitive interventions for children with brain injury. In J. Reed, K. Byard, & H. Fine(Eds.), *Neuropsychological rehabilitation of childhood brain injury* (pp. 82–105). London: Palgrave Macmillan.

Raskin, S. A. (2010). Current approaches to cognitive rehabilitation. In C. L. Armstrong, L. Morrow, C. L. Armstrong, & L. Morrow (Eds.), *Handbook of medical neuropsychology: Applications of cognitive neuroscience* (pp. 505–517). New York: Springer Science + Business Media. https://doi.org/10.1007/978-1-4419-1364-7_28.

Sohlberg, M. M., Ehlhardt, L., & Kennedy, M. (2005). Instructional techniques in cognitive rehabilitation: A preliminary report. *Seminars in Speech and Language, 26*(4), 268–279. https://doi.org/10.1055/s-2005-922105.

Swanson, H. L. (1999). Instructional components that predict treatment outcomes for students with learning disabilities: Support for a combined strategy and direct instruction model. *Learning Disabilities Research & Practice, 14*(3), 129–140. https://doi.org/10.1207/sldrp1403_1.

Wilson, B. A. (2009). *Memory rehabilitation: Integrating theory and practice.* New York: The Guilford Press.

Acalculia

Kelly Broxterman[1], Natalie Wahmhoff[2], Elaine Clark[2] and Alyssa Beukema[1]
[1]School Psychology, The Chicago School of Professional Psychology, Chicago, IL, USA
[2]Department of Educational Psychology, The University of Utah, Salt Lake City, UT, USA

Synonyms

Mathematics disability

Definition

Acalculia is an acquired impairment in which people have difficulty performing mathematical tasks, such as adding, subtracting, multiplying, and dividing. Acalculia deficits can manifest in a wide variety of number processing and calculation abilities.

Categorization

Generally, authors have agreed on two major distinctions: primary and secondary acalculia (Growth-Marnat 2000). These terms were first described by Berger in 1926 (Boller and Grafman 1983). Primary acalculia refers to a basic defect in computational abilities, not resulting from separate cognitive deficits. It is also known as anarithmetia. Deficits in primary acalculia include poor estimation, number comparison difficulties, and difficulty understanding procedural rules and numerical signs. In primary acalculia, these deficits will exist regardless of whether tasks are presented in an oral or written format (Ardila and Rosselli 2002).

Secondary acalculia refers to calculation defects due to primary deficits in other areas: memory disorders, attention impairments, language defects, spatial deficits, etc. (Berger 1926). The secondary acalculias include aphasic acalculia, alexic acalculia, agraphic acalculia, frontal acalculia, and spatial acalculia.

Aphasic acalculia occurs in patients with Broca's and Wernicke's aphasia. The deficits seen in patients with Broca's aphasia are linguistic in nature, and these individuals often have impairments in the *syntax of calculation*. This includes problems when translating word representations of numbers (three hundred and forty-five) to their numeral form (345). They may also read numbers with morphological errors (15 is read as 50) (Ardila and Rosselli 2002; Basso et al. 2000). When the secondary acalculia stems from Wernicke's aphasia, deficits are more severe. Reading and writing of numbers often have semantic errors, and poor verbal memory often impacts the calculation abilities of these patients (Grafman and Rickart 2000).

Alexic acalculia is the inability to read number and correlations with the inability to read text. People with this type of acalculia may focus only on beginning digits (538 is read as 53). For those with alexic acalculia, mental calculation abilities exceed written calculation abilities (Ardila and Rosselli 2002).

Agraphic acalculia is the inability to write numbers. Like aphasic acalculia, agraphic acalculia correlates with Broca's and Wernicke's aphasia. In Broca's aphasia, acalculia deficits manifest as omissions, substitutions, and order reversal. In Wernicke's aphasia, difficulties are especially evident when required to write quantities when they are orally dictated. Those with Wernicke's aphasia also tend to make paralexias and paragraphias (Ardila and Rosselli 2002; Growth-Marnat 2000).

Frontal acalculia deficits occur in conjunction with attention difficulties, perseveration, and impairment of more complex math concepts (Dehaene et al. 1998). Patients with frontal acalculia often have significant damage to the prefrontal areas of their brain, which can cause trouble with mental operations, operations that need to be carried out successively, backward operations, and numerical problems that require multiple steps. In these individuals, written mathematical problem-solving is easier to do than mental math operations. While complex concepts are difficult for patients with frontal acalculia, more basic math concepts are usually maintained (Ardila and Rosselli 2002).

Spatial acalculia impacts written mathematical tasks more than mental math tasks. A difficulty with writing numbers is quite apparent in these cases and manifests in several ways. Writing on only one side of the page, inability to write numbers in a straight line, and general disorganization are some of the deficits that impact math performance (Basso et al. 2000). Patients with spatial acalculia often forget where to place remainders and carried numbers, despite understanding the basic division and multiplication functions. Math procedure signs are often undetected or switched (add instead of subtract).

Epidemiology

Acalculia can result from stroke, tumors, and trauma. It is also seen in patients with degenerative dementia (Ardila and Rosselli 2002).

Prognostic Factors and Outcomes

There is noted variability in prognosis for acalculia, ranging from no recovery to full recovery. For primary acalculia, improvement is limited. In the case of secondary acalculias, when recovery from the primary deficit, such as aphasia, alexia, and agraphia, occur, the corresponding acalculia deficits tend to improve as well.

Neuropsychology and Psychology of Acalculia

Primary acalculia is associated with left posterior parietal lesions. More specifically, damage to the left angular and supramarginal gyri occurs with primary acalculia (Grafman and Rickart 2000). It is suggested that there are separate neuropathways for rote number knowledge and semantic number knowledge.

Neuroimaging techniques reveal that several brain areas are active when performing calculations and also that the pattern differs according to what type of calculation is done (Dehaene et al. 1998). This occurs to the many abilities that calculation often requires, including verbal, spatial, executive functioning, and memory. The areas most associated with calculation are the upper cortical surface and anterior aspect of the left middle frontal gyrus, the bilateral supramarginal and angular gyrus, the left dorsolateral prefrontal and premotor cortices, Broca's area, inferior parietal and left parietal cortex, and the inferior occipitotemporal regions (Ardila and Rosselli 2002).

It is important to keep in mind that damage to the right hemisphere and the frontal lobes also impact the occurrence of acalculia, especially when it is a secondary acalculia.

Evaluation

The arithmetic section of the Wide Range Achievement Test (WRAT) has often been used to test operational skills. The Key Math, which is designed for children and adolescents, tests most targeted and specific abilities that are suggested for an acalculia assessment (Grafman and Rickart 2000). Many authors have suggested experimental batteries that target specific functions and include error analysis. These batteries often assess skills in the following areas: number recognition, number writing, number transcoding, quantification, magnitude estimation, basic arithmetic operations, calculation fact verification, multicolumn calculations, magnitude comparison, fractions, algebra, and numeric knowledge. When possible, these skills should be assessed in both written and oral forms (Ardila and Rosselli 2002; Grafman and Rickart 2000).

Treatment

Some authors have suggested beginning rehabilitation with an error analysis if it was not completed during the assessment. This will provide explicit areas to target during rehabilitation (Grafman and Rickart 2000). Long-term rehabilitation programs should begin simply and progressively work toward more complex tasks. With secondary acalculia, focusing rehabilitation on the primary deficit may significantly improve the secondary acalculia deficits (Ardila and Rosselli 2002).

Cross-References

▶ Agraphia
▶ Alexia
▶ Aphasia
▶ Gerstmann's Syndrome
▶ Spatial Dyscalculia

References and Readings

Ardila, A., Matute, E., & Inozemtseva, O. (2003). Progressive agraphia, acalculia, and anomia: A single-case report. *Applied Neuropsychology, 10*, 205–214.

Ardila, A., & Rosselli, M. (2002). Acalculia and dyscalculia. *Neuropsychology Review, 12*, 179–231.

Basso, A., Burgio, F., & Caporali, A. (2000). Acalculia, aphasia, and spatial disorders in left and right brain-damaged patient. *Cortex, 36*, 265–280.

Berger, H. (1926). Uber Rechenstorunger bei Herderkraunkunger des Grosshirns. *Arch Psychiatr Nervenkr, 78*, 236–263.

Boller, F., & Grafman, J. (1983). Acalculia: Historical development and current significance. *Brain and Cognition, 2*(3), 205–223.

Dehaene, S., Cohen, L., & Changeux, J. P. (1998). Neuronal network models of acalculia and prefrontal deficits. In R. W. Parks, D. S. Levine, & D. L. Long (Eds.), *Fundamentals of neural network modeling: Neuropsychology and cognitive neuroscience* (pp. 233–255). Cambridge, MA: MIT.

Grafman, J., & Rickart, T. (2000). Acalculia. In M. J. Farah & T. E. Fienberg (Eds.), *Patient based approaches to cognitive neurosciences: Issues in clinical and cognitive neuropsychology.* Cambridge, MA: MIT.

Growth-Marnat, G. (Ed.). (2000). *Neuropsychological assessment in clinical practice.* New York: Wiley.

Scruggs, T. E., & Mastropieri, M. A. (2000). Acalculia. In *Encyclopedia of special education* (Vol. 1, 2nd ed., p. 27). New York: Wiley.

Acceleration Injury

Beth Rush
Psychiatry and Psychology, Mayo Clinic, Jacksonville, FL, USA

Synonyms

Acceleration-deceleration injury

Definition

Traumatic injury to the brain resulting from high-speed acceleration of the brain within the skull cavity in the direction of inertial force.

Current Knowledge

During acceleration injury, movement of the head is unrestricted. One of the most common scenarios resulting in acceleration injury is a high-speed motor vehicle accident. Primary brain injury results from brain tissue and brain structures compressing against one another in the force of inertia. This may result in bruising, hemorrhage, and shearing of the underlying tensile strength of white matter connections deep within the brain. Secondary injury may occur hours or even days after the inciting traumatic event. Secondary effects of injury can include decreased cerebral blood flow, edema, hemorrhage, increased intracranial pressure, and biochemical changes that may cause excitotoxicity and more extensive damage to the surrounding brain structures and their associated connections.

Theoretical models of linear acceleration injury now address the heterogeneity of effects that can result from such biomechanical injuries. Although diffuse brain damage may result from this type of injury, a key factor that predicts the extent of damage following acceleration injury is the area of initial impact. Given that the structure and projection pathways of the brain have varying densities and tensile strengths within different regions of the brain, the point of impact is most likely the key in determining the extent of damage that takes place and the likelihood and course of recovery that is possible following injury.

Patients sustaining acceleration injury may experience headache, photophobia, phonophobia, nausea, and dizziness immediately following injury onset. On neuropsychological evaluation, patients with acceleration injuries are more likely to demonstrate a diffuse, rather than focal, profile of cognitive impairment when cognitive impairment is present. The lateralization of cognitive impairment that is typically observed in focal brain injury is relatively uncommon following acceleration injury. A diffuse profile of cognitive impairment in acceleration injury is due to the disruption of white matter tracts that are responsible for efficiency and coordination of communication between functional brain injuries. As such, a patient with acceleration injury may demonstrate cognitive slowing, executive dysfunction, and problems with simple and complex attention as a consequence of his/her brain injury.

Cross-References

▶ Biomechanics of Injury
▶ Deceleration Injury
▶ Diffuse Axonal Injury

References and Readings

Bayly, P. V., Cohen, T. S., Leister, E. P., Ajo, D., Leuthardt, E. C., & Genin, G. M. (2005). Acceleration-induced deformation of the human brain. *Journal of Neurotrauma, 22*(8), 845–856.

Li, Y., Zhang, L., Kallakuri, S., Zhou, R., & Cavanaugh, J. M. (2011). Quantitative relationship between axonal injury and mechanical response in a rodent head impact acceleration model. *Journal of Neurotrauma, 28*(9), 1767–1782.

Sabet, A. A., Christoforou, E., Zatlin, B., Genin, G. M., & Bayly, P. V. (2008). Deformation of the human brain induced by mild angular head acceleration. *Journal of Biomechanics, 41*, 307–315.

Accessory Cuneate Nucleus

John E. Mendoza
Department of Psychiatry and Neuroscience, Tulane Medical School and SE Louisiana Veterans Healthcare System, New Orleans, LA, USA

Synonyms

Lateral cuneate nucleus

Definition

Nucleus in the dorsolateral portion of the medulla that receives sensory information likely from touch, pressure, and stretch receptors in the upper extremities. It gives rise to the *cuneocerebellar tract* which enters the cerebellum via the inferior cerebellar peduncle. The accessory cuneate nucleus is thought to be the equivalent of the dorsal nucleus of Clarke in the lumbar, thoracic, and lower cervical cord which is the source of the dorsal spinocerebellar tract. These nuclei and tracts provide unconscious (as opposed to "conscious") sensory feedback to the cerebellum in its regulation of individual muscles. Lesions of this nucleus might be expected to produce cerebellar type symptoms of the ipsilateral upper extremity (i.e., ataxia/incoordination of

movement), but it is relatively small and isolated lesions are likely to be extremely rare.

Accommodations

Jacob T. Lutz[1] and David E. McIntosh[2]
[1]Department of Special Education, Ball State University, Muncie, IN, USA
[2]Department of Special Education, Teachers College, Bell State University, Muncie, IN, USA

Synonyms

Reasonable accommodations

Definition

In order to provide students with disabilities the free, appropriate public education mandated by IDEA 2004 and Section 504 of the Rehabilitation Act of 1973, changes typically must be made to a child's educational curriculum or environment. These accommodations include changes in the method of presentation of material, classroom seating location, availability of an interpreter for those with hearing impairment, response format, testing time allowed, setting, or other reasonable steps that do not significantly alter the content of educational material or the validity of tests. To be eligible to receive accommodations, students must be identified as having a disability consistent with the guidelines presented in IDEA 2004 or Section 504 of the Rehabilitation Act of 1973.

Accommodations may also be required in the workplace under the Americans with Disabilities Act. These could include installation of a ramp to permit wheelchair access, flexible working hours, or provision of TTY machines.

Cross-References

▶ Americans with Disabilities Act of 1990

References and Readings

Education, 34 C.F.R. §104.
Individuals with Disabilities Education Improvement Act
    of 2004, 20 U.S.C. § 1400 et seq.
Rehabilitation Act, 29 U.S.C. § 794.

Acetylcholine

JoAnn Tschanz[1,2] and Elizabeth K. Vernon[1]
[1]Department of Psychology, Utah State
University, Logan, UT, USA
[2]Center for Epidemiologic Studies, Utah State
University, Logan, UT, USA

Synonyms

ACh; Cholinergic system

Definition

Acetylcholine has been identified as a neurotransmitter substance since the mid-1920s. It is the neurotransmitter substance present at the neuromuscular junction and also innervates structures of the parasympathetic and sympathetic nervous systems (Feldman et al. 1997; Iversen et al. 2008). In the brain, cholinergic neurons have a wide distribution. Projections emanate from the basal forebrain in the medial septal nucleus and terminate in the hippocampus and limbic cortex. Among other areas receiving cholinergic input are the neocortex, olfactory bulbs, amygdala, neostriatum (caudate nucleus and putamen), the hypothalamus, and various regions in the brain stem (Feldman et al. 1997).

Acetylcholine is synthesized from the precursors Acetyl CoA and choline in a chemical reaction involving the catalytic enzyme, choline acetyltransferase (ChAT). The presence of this enzyme has been used as a marker to locate cholinergic neurons. Acetylcholine degradation (the primary mode of removal from synapses) is accomplished by the activity of a group of enzymes known as cholinesterases. Acetylcholinesterase is the primary enzyme that breaks down acetylcholine in the synapse. Thus, to enhance cholinergic function, a number of substances have been developed that inhibit the activity of this enzyme (Iversen et al. 2008).

Based on differences in the agonists that stimulate cholinergic receptors, two receptor subtypes have been identified, nicotinic and muscarinic. Nicotinic receptors are stimulated by nicotine, are excitatory, and show a rapid response to stimulation. Muscarinic receptors are stimulated by muscarine, have either excitatory or inhibitory effects, and show a slower response to stimulation. Further subtypes exist within the nicotinic and muscarinic classes (Feldman et al. 1997; Iversen et al. 2008).

Acetylcholine is involved in a number of behavioral processes. As a neurotransmitter substance at the neuromuscular junction, it acts on motor neurons of the spinal cord and cranial motor nerve nuclei, playing an important role in the contraction of skeletal muscles. Studies also suggest a role in cortical arousal, REM sleep, and cognitive functions such as attention, learning, and memory. Its presence in cardiac and smooth muscles, organs, and salivary, tear and sweat glands affect autonomic functions (Feldman et al. 1997).

Current Knowledge

Applications
Dysfunction in the cholinergic system has been implicated in a number of clinical conditions including Alzheimer's Disease (AD), Diffuse Lewy Body Dementia (Londos et al. 2003), and Huntington's Disease and Myasthenia Gravis (Iversen et al. 2008). Recent work also suggests a reduction in cholinergic activity in Parkinson's disease that may appear relatively early in the course of the condition (Shimada et al. 2009). Acetylcholinesterase inhibitors are used in the palliative treatment of AD and myasthenia gravis. Cholinergic or anticholinergic compounds are also used as a muscle relaxant for surgery,

treatment of parkinsonism, glaucoma, urinary retention, and in nonclinical applications such as insecticides in agriculture and neurotoxins (and their antidotes) in warfare (Feldman et al. 1997; Iversen et al. 2008). Antagonism of brain cholinergic function has been associated with worse cognitive performance, particularly in older adults. One longitudinal study reported that continuous use of medications with anticholinergic effects was associated with poorer reaction time, attention, delayed nonverbal memory, narrative recall, visuospatial construction, and verbal fluency, but no increase in conversion to dementia after an 8-year follow-up (Ancelin et al. 2006). However, a recent study reported that use of medications with medium or high anticholinergic effects was associated with worse performance in delayed narrative recall and executive functions. Use of anticholinergic medications was also associated with lower cortical volumes and reduced cortical thickness of the temporal lobe as well as greater ventricular volumes. Conversion to Alzheimer's disease was significantly greater in users of anticholinergic medications, and especially among those with evidence of Amyloid Beta deposition on scans or inferred in cerebrospinal fluid (Risacher et al. 2016).

See Also

▶ Alzheimer's Disease
▶ Anticholinesterase Inhibitors
▶ Cholinergic System
▶ Cholinesterase Inhibitors
▶ Donepezil

References and Readings

Ancelin, M. L., Artero, S., Portet, F., Dupuy, A. M., Touchon, J., & Ritchie, K. (2006). Non-degenerative mild cognitive impairment in elderly people and use of anticholinergic drugs: Longitudinal cohort study. *British Medical Journal, 332*, 455–459.

Feldman, R. S., Meyer, J. S., & Quenzer, L. F. (1997). Acetylcholine. In *Principles of neuropsychopharmacology* (pp. 235–276). Sunderland: Sinauer Associates, Inc.

Iversen, L. L., Iversen, S. D., Bloom, F. E., & Roth, R. H. A. (2008). *Introduction to neuropsychopharmacology* (pp. 128–149). New York: Oxford University Press.

Londos, E., Brun, A., Gustafson, L., & Passant, U. (2003). Lewy body dementia. Clinical challenges in diagnosis and management. In K. Iqbal & B. Winblad (Eds.), *Alzheimer's disease and related disorders: Research advances* (pp. 133–142). Bucharest: Ana Asian International Academy of Aging.

Risacher, S. L., McDonald, B. C., Tallman, E. F., West, J. D., Farlow, M. R., Unverzagt, F. W., Gao, S., Boustani, M., Crane, P. K., Petersen, R. C., Jack, C. R., Jr., Jagust, W. J., Aisen, P. S., Weiner, M. W., Saykin, A. J., & Alzheimer's Disease Neuroimaging Initiative. (2016). Association between anticholinergic medication use and cognition, brain metabolism, and brain atrophy in cognitively normal older adults. *JAMA Neurology, 73*, 721–732.

Shimada, H., Hirano, S., Shinotoh, H., Aotsuka, A., Sato, K., Tanaka, N., Ota, T., Asahina, M., Fukushi, K., Kuwabara, S., Hattori, T., Suhara, T., & Irie, T. (2009). Mapping of brain acetylcholinesterase alterations in Lewy body disease by PET. *Neurology, 73*, 273–278.

Achenbach System of Empirically Based Assessment (ASEBA)

Thomas M. Achenbach
Department of Psychiatry, University of Vermont, Burlington, VT, USA

Synonyms

Achenbach System of Empirically Based Assessment (ASEBA)

Description

The Achenbach System of Empirically Based Assessment (ASEBA) comprises a family of forms for rating behavioral/emotional/social problems and adaptive characteristics. For ages 1½ to 90+ years, developmentally appropriate forms are designed to be completed by collaterals who know the person who is being assessed. These forms

Achenbach System of Empirically Based Assessment (ASEBA), Table 1 ASEBA assessment instruments

Instrument	Ages	Completed by	Reference
CBCL/1½–5	1½–5	Parent figures	Achenbach and Rescorla (2000)
C-TRF	1½–5	Daycare providers, preschool teachers	Achenbach and Rescorla (2000)
CBCL/6–18	6–18	Parent figures	Achenbach and Rescorla (2001, 2007a)
TRF	6–18	Teachers	Achenbach and Rescorla (2001, 2007a)
YSR	11–18	Youths	Achenbach and Rescorla (2001, 2007a)
TOF	2–18	Psychological examiner	McConaughy and Achenbach (2004)
DOF	6–11	Observer	McConaughy and Achenbach (2009)
SCICA	6–18	Interviewer	McConaughy and Achenbach (2001)
ASR	18–59	Adults	Achenbach and Rescorla (2003)
ABCL	18–59	Collaterals	Achenbach and Rescorla (2003)
OASR	≥60	Older adults	Achenbach et al. (2004)
OABCL	≥60	Collaterals	Achenbach et al. (2004)

include versions of the Child Behavior Checklist (CBCL), completed by parent figures for 1½- to 5-year-olds and for 6- to 18-year-olds; the Caregiver-Teacher Report Form (C-TRF) for ages 1½–5, completed by daycare providers and preschool teachers; the Teacher's Report Form (TRF) for ages 6–18, completed by teachers and other school personnel; the Adult Behavior Checklist (ABCL) for ages 18–59, completed by spouses, partners, family members, friends, therapists, and other collaterals; and the Older Adult Behavior Checklist (OABCL) for ages 60 and older, completed by caregivers as well as by collaterals.

The ASEBA also includes parallel forms completed by the people being assessed, including the Youth Self-Report (YSR) for ages 11–18, the Adult Self-Report (ASR) for ages 18–59, and the Older Adult Self-Report (OASR) for ages 60 and older. The collateral and self-report forms assess functioning in everyday contexts over periods of 2–6 months.

In addition to the collateral and self-report forms, other ASEBA forms are designed for rating behavior observed in specific situations. These forms include the Direct Observation Form (DOF), which is completed by observers who rate two or more 10-min samples of children's behavior observed in classrooms and other group settings; the Semistructured Clinical Interview for Children and Adolescents (SCICA), which provides an interview protocol and a rating form completed by the interviewer who administers the SCICA to 6- to 18-year-olds, and the Test Observation Form (TOF), which test examiners

use to rate the behavior observed during the administration of individual ability and achievement tests to 2- to 18-year-olds. Table 1 summarizes the ASEBA forms, ages covered, who completes the forms, and references to manuals for each form.

Normed Profiles

Scores obtained from all ASEBA forms are displayed on profiles in relation to norms that are based on distributions of scale scores obtained by large samples of peers. For the collateral and self-report forms for ages 1½ to 90+ years, norms are based on a US national probability sample of people who had not received mental health or substance abuse services in the preceding 12 months. For the CBCL/6–18, TRF, and YSR, norms are provided for many cultures in addition to the USA, as detailed later (Achenbach and Rescorla 2007a, b). Multicultural norms for the CBCL/1½–5 and C-TRF were released in 2010 and for the ASR and ABCL in 2015 (Achenbach and Rescorla 2010, 2015). For the DOF, SCICA, and TOF, norms are based on ratings of children observed in the contexts for which these instruments are designed.

Each profile displays an individual's scale scores in terms of standard scores (T scores) and percentiles based on the normative sample of that individual's peers, as rated by a particular type of informant (e.g., parent, teacher, self). The profiles also display demarcations between the normal range, borderline clinical range, and clinical range on each scale. Figure 1 illustrates a profile

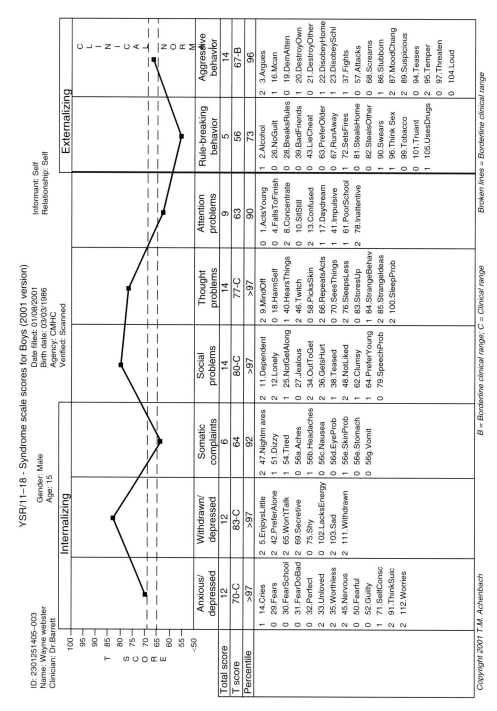

Achenbach System of Empirically Based Assessment (ASEBA), Fig. 1 Syndrome profile scored from the Youth Self-Report completed by 15-year-old Wayne Webster (Copyright Achenbach and Rescorla 2001, p. 33)

of syndrome scales scored from the YSR completed by 15-year-old Wayne Webster (not his real name).

Scales on Which ASEBA Instruments Are Scored

ASEBA problem items are scored on scales for syndromes derived empirically via exploratory factor analyses (EFAs) and confirmatory factor analyses (CFAs). These empirically derived syndromes reflect patterns of problems found to co-occur in ratings by each kind of informant.

In addition to the syndrome scales, each form is scored on DSM-oriented scales constructed by having experts from many cultures select ASEBA problem items that are very consistent with particular diagnostic categories of the American Psychiatric Association's (2013) *Diagnostic and Statistical Manual-Fifth Edition* (DSM-5). Like the syndrome scales, the DSM-oriented scales are displayed on profiles in terms of *T* scores, percentiles, and normal, borderline clinical, and clinical ranges. Most forms are also scored on scales comprising critical items that are of particular concern to clinicians.

The collateral and self-report forms are additionally scored on scales for favorable characteristics, such as competence, adaptive functioning, and personal strengths. The particular items and scales are geared to the developmental level of people being assessed and to the informants' knowledge of people being assessed. For example, parents of 6- to 18-year-olds provide data regarding their children's involvement in sports, nonsports activities, organizations, jobs and chores, friendships, and relationships with parents, siblings, and peers. Teachers provide data on children's academic performance and adaptive characteristics at school. For adults, data are requested regarding friendships, relations with spouse or partner, children, job, and enrolment in educational programs. Only the items relevant to the adult being assessed are scored. For example, adults who lack a spouse or partner, children, job, or enrolment in educational programs are not scored on those items. Adult forms also have normed scales for substance use.

Cross-Informant Comparisons

Meta-analyses have revealed that correlations between parent, teacher, and self-reports of children's problems are typically only low to moderate (Achenbach et al. 1987). Consequently, professionals who work with children recognize the need to obtain reports from multiple informants. Meta-analyses of correlations between collateral and self-reports of adult psychopathology have also revealed only modest correlations that argue for using multi-informant data to assess adults (Achenbach et al. 2005).

Because each informant may provide valid and useful information that differs from what other informants provide, data from multiple informants should be compared. Software for scoring ASEBA forms facilitates cross-informant comparisons by printing scores obtained from parallel forms on parallel profiles. In addition, it prints side-by-side comparisons of ratings by up to ten informants on all problem items that have counterparts on forms completed by different informants. It also prints *Q* correlations that measure the degree of agreement between each pair of informants and compares them with *Q* correlations between pairs of informants in large reference samples.

An especially useful kind of comparison between informants' reports is illustrated in Fig. 2. This is a comparison between syndromes scored from the YSR completed by Wayne Webster, CBCLs completed by Wayne's parents, and TRFs completed by three of Wayne's teachers. For each syndrome, such as the Anxious/Depressed syndrome shown in the upper left-hand corner, the bars reflect the magnitude of standard scores (*T* scores) obtained from ratings by each kind of informant. Because the *T* scores are based on ratings by each kind of informant for a normative sample of children, the height of the bar indicates the level of the problems reported by a particular kind of informant compared to problems reported by that kind of informant for a normative sample of children. For example, the leftmost bars indicate that the Anxious/Depressed syndrome scores obtained from CBCL ratings by Wayne's parents are above the top broken line compared to parents' CBCL ratings of a

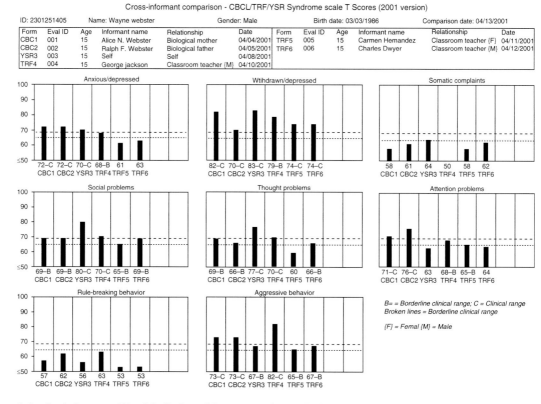

Achenbach System of Empirically Based Assessment (ASEBA), Fig. 2 Cross-informant comparisons of syndrome scores for Wayne Webster (Copyright Achenbach and Rescorla 2001, p. 39)

normative sample of adolescent boys. As scores above the top broken line are in the clinical range, the CBCL bars indicate that Wayne's parents reported more problems of this syndrome than were reported by parents of 97% of boys in the normative sample.

Multicultural Norms

Norms obtained in one society may not be generalizable to other societies. To determine the degree of generalizability across societies, the same assessment instruments must be administered to large representative samples of people in different societies. This has been done with ASEBA instruments in many societies. CFAs of CBCL, TRF, and YSR data from many societies support the generalizability of syndromes that were initially derived from US samples. Comparisons of scale scores show that the distributions of CBCL, TRF, and YSR scores in many societies approximate those obtained in the USA.

However, some societies have substantially lower or higher mean scores. To take account of societal differences in scale scores, separate sets of norms have been constructed for the societies obtaining relatively low scores, societies obtaining intermediate scores, and societies obtaining relatively high scores. Because parent, teacher, and self-ratings often yield different scores, the multicultural CBCL, TRF, and YSR norms were constructed separately. For some societies, problem scores obtained from one kind of informant are relatively low, while scores obtained from another kind of informant are intermediate or high. For example, CBCL and TRF problem scores obtained from Japanese parents and teachers are in the low range, whereas YSR scores obtained from self-ratings by Japanese youths are in the intermediate range.

To enable practitioners and researchers to compare CBCL, TRF, and YSR scores with culturally appropriate norms, the scoring software provides options for displaying problem scale scores in relation to norms for low-scoring, intermediate-scoring, and high-scoring societies. For example, CBCL and TRF scores for a Japanese youth would typically be displayed in relation to norms for low-scoring societies. However, the youth's YSR scores would be displayed in relation to norms for intermediate-scoring societies. If the Japanese youth lived in the USA and attended an American school, the TRF scores would be displayed in relation to US norms for teachers' ratings. If the youth's parents were well accultur-ated to the USA, the CBCL scores could be displayed in relation to US norms and also in relation to Japanese norms to see whether the scores were clinically deviant according to either set of norms.

Historical Background

The ASEBA stems from Achenbach's (1966) factor-analytic derivation of syndromes of child and adolescent psychopathology. Since then, five decades of research and practical experience have produced ASEBA instruments for ages 1½ to 90+

years. Achenbach (2009) documents the historical development of ASEBA research, instruments, theory, and applications, as well as directions in which the ASEBA is now moving. Translations are available in 100 languages. Over 9500 publi-cations by some 15,000 authors report use of the ASEBA in 100 cultural groups and societies (Bérubé and Achenbach 2017). ASEBA instru-ments are available in paper and Internet-based electronic versions in many countries around the world for practical assessment in clinical, educa-tional, forensic, and other services, as well as for research on countless topics, such as genetics, medical conditions, outcome evaluations, epidemiology, development, diagnosis, and mul-ticultural comparisons. Because the ASEBA's conceptual framework is open ended and generative, it continues to advance in multiple directions.

Psychometric Data

Table 2 summarizes psychometric data for all ASEBA instruments in terms of mean alphas, test-retest reliability, and the percentage of

Achenbach System of Empirically Based Assessment (ASEBA), Table 2 Summary of ASEBA psychometric data

Instrument	Alpha[a]		Reliability[b]		Validity[c]	
	Narrow	Broad	Narrow	Broad	Narrow	Broad
CBCL/1½–5	0.76	0.92	0.82	0.89	11	17
C-TRF	0.80	0.94	0.78	0.85	13	20
CBCL/6–18	0.83	0.94	0.88	0.92	24	32
TRF	0.86	0.94	0.84	0.90	15	20
YSR	0.78	0.92	0.78	0.85	10	14
TOF	0.82	0.90	0.76	0.84	9	14
DOF	0.68	0.79	0.51	0.72	7	20
SCICA	0.70	0.84	0.75	0.80	9	16
ASR	0.78	0.93	0.84	0.91	10	14
ABCL	0.80	0.94	0.84	0.88	6	8
OASR	0.80	0.96	0.86	0.95	13	20
OABCL	0.83	0.97	0.94	0.95	19	29

Narrow = mean for syndrome and DSM-oriented scales; broad = mean for internalizing, externalizing, and total problems. Data are from manuals listed in the Further Reading
[a]Cronbach's coefficient *alpha* for the internal consistency of scales
[b]Pearson *r*s for test-retest reliability over 8- to 16-day intervals. SCICA *r*s are between ratings by different interviewers who interviewed children over intervals averaging 12 days
[c]Percentage of variance accounted for by clinical referral status (referred vs. nonreferred) in multiple regressions of referral status on ASEBA scale scores with demographic variables partialed out

variance in ASEBA scale scores accounted for by clinical referral status, after partialing out demographic effects. Many additional psychometric findings – including goodness of fit obtained from CFAs in diverse samples – are reported in ASEBA manuals and in refereed publications listed by Bérubé and Achenbach (2017).

Clinical Uses

ASEBA instruments have numerous clinical uses. Bérubé and Achenbach (2017) list publications reporting use of the ASEBA in relation to over 150 medical conditions. Over 1100 publications report use of the ASEBA for evaluating treatments and outcomes for many kinds of psychopathology and other problems.

ASEBA instruments can be used at many stages of clinical processes, including screening to identify needs for help, documentation of problems and adaptive functioning for use in clinical referrals, and intake assessment on which to base treatment decisions. During the course of treatment, ASEBA instruments are useful for determining whether goals are being met. Following the treatment, ASEBA instruments can be readministered to evaluate outcomes and subsequent functioning. At any point, ASEBA instruments can be used to assess behavioral/emotional/social concomitants of neuropsychological and medical disorders. The availability of similar ASEBA instruments for children and adults facilitates family assessment, as well as close coordination between interventions for parents and their children.

References and Readings

Achenbach, T. M. (1966). The classification of children's psychiatric symptoms: A factor-analytic study. *Psychological Monographs, 80*(7), 1–37. (No. 615).

Achenbach, T. M. (2009). *The Achenbach system of empirically based assessment (ASEBA): Development, findings, theory, and applications*. Burlington: University of Vermont, Research Center for Children, Youth, and Families.

Achenbach, T. M., & Rescorla, L. A. (2000). *Manual for the ASEBA preschool forms & profiles*. Burlington: University of Vermont, Research Center for Children, Youth, and Families.

Achenbach, T. M., & Rescorla, L. A. (2001). *Manual for the ASEBA school-age forms & profiles*. Burlington: University of Vermont, Research Center for Children, Youth, and Families.

Achenbach, T. M., & Rescorla, L. A. (2003). *Manual for the ASEBA adult forms & profiles*. Burlington: University of Vermont, Research Center for Children, Youth, and Families.

Achenbach, T. M., & Rescorla, L. A. (2007a). *Multicultural supplement to the manual for the ASEBA school-age forms & profiles*. Burlington: University of Vermont Research Center for Children, Youth, and Families.

Achenbach, T. M., & Rescorla, L. A. (2007b). *Multicultural understanding of child and adolescent psychopathology: Implications for mental health assessment*. New York: Guilford Press.

Achenbach, T. M., & Rescorla, L. A. (2010). *Multicultural supplement to the manual for the ASEBA preschool forms & profiles*. Burlington: University of Vermont Research Center for Children, Youth, and Families.

Achenbach, T. M., & Rescorla, L. A. (2015). *Multicultural supplement to the manual for the ASEBA adult forms & profiles*. Burlington: University of Vermont Research Center for Children, Youth, and Families.

Achenbach, T. M., McConaughy, S. H., & Howell, C. T. (1987). Child/adolescent behavioral and emotional problems: Implications of cross-informant correlations for situational specificity. *Psychological Bulletin, 101*, 213–232.

Achenbach, T. M., Newhouse, P. A., & Rescorla, L. A. (2004). *Manual for the ASEBA older adult forms & profiles*. Burlington: University of Vermont, Research Center for Children, Youth, and Families.

Achenbach, T. M., Krukowski, R. A., Dumenci, L., & Ivanova, M. Y. (2005). Assessment of adult psychopathology: Meta-analyses and implications of cross-informant correlations. *Psychological Bulletin, 131*, 361–382.

American Psychiatric Association. (2013). *Diagnostic and statistical manual of mental disorders* (5th ed.). Washington, DC: Author.

Bérubé, R. L., & Achenbach, T. M. (2017). *Bibliography of published studies using the Achenbach system of empirically based assessment (ASEBA)*. Burlington: University of Vermont, Research Center for Children, Youth, and Families.

McConaughy, S. H., & Achenbach, T. M. (2001). *Manual for the semistructured clinical interview for children and adolescents* (2nd ed.). Burlington: University of Vermont, Research Center for Children, Youth, and Families.

McConaughy, S. H., & Achenbach, T. M. (2004). *Manual for the test observation form for ages 2–18*. Burlington: University of Vermont, Research Center for Children, Youth, and Families.

McConaughy, S. H., & Achenbach, T. M. (2009). *Manual for the ASEBA direct observation form for ages 6–11*. Burlington: University of Vermont, Research Center for Children, Youth, and Families.

Achromatopsia

Sophie Lebrecht and Michael J. Tarr
Visual Neuroscience Laboratory, Brown University, Providence, RI, USA

Synonyms

Acquired achromatopsia; Color agnosia; Color blindness; Cortical color blindness

Short Description or Definition

Following damage to the ventral medial region of the occipital lobe, known as the "color center" of the brain (Bartels and Zeki 2000), patients lose the ability to perceive color and therefore experience the world as varying shades of gray. This disorder is termed cerebral achromatopsia. The loss of color vision in these patients cannot be explained by the photoreceptors typically damaged or absent in patients with other types of color blindness.

Categorization

Cerebral achromatopsia results from bilateral damage to the V4/V4α region of the color center. If patients experience complete ablation of V4, they lose color vision in their entire visual field. However, if patients experience unilateral damage to V4, hemi-achromatopsia ensues, where patients only lose color vision in the contralateral half of their visual field. In less extreme cases, known as dyschromatopsia, patients lose the ability to perceive selective colors and/or color constancy. These neuropsychological disorders, which are the result of damage to the cerebral cortex, should not be confused with congenital achromatopsia, which occurs as a malfunction of the cone photoreceptors.

Epidemiology

Cerebral achromatopsia arises following brain damage to V4/V4α located in the ventral medial region of the occipital lobe, typically caused by a tumor, a hemorrhage, or some sort of brain trauma. Due to the low incidence rate of cerebral achromatopsia, it is difficult to provide a reliable estimate of its prevalence. However, it seems safe to say that it is extremely rare. A review of the documented cases showed that of the 27 cases reported, 3 patients recovered, 3 partially recovered, and 21 showed no recovery (Bartels and Zeki 2000).

Natural History, Prognostic Factors, and Outcomes

The first cases of cerebral achromatopsia were reported by Verrey (1888). In response to these patients, Verrey introduced the concept of a "color center" in the brain. Continued research confirmed the existence of a cortical region devoted to color processing. Almost a century later, Meadows demonstrated a correlation between the cortical regions sensitive to color and the damaged cortical regions in achromatopsic patients (Meadows 1974).

Neuropsychology and Psychology of Achromatopsia

The region of damage in the visual field of achromotopsic patients, V4/V4α, is organized retinotopically; therefore, damage to a particular region of V4 results in a loss of color vision at the corresponding location in the visual field. For example, if damage to V4 occurs in the *left* hemisphere, the patient will lose color vision in the *right* half of their visual field. Because V4 is located in the vicinity of the fusiform gyrus and the lingual gyrus, known to process faces (Kanwisher et al. 1997), the comorbidity between achromatopsia and prosopagnosia is extremely high (Bouvier and Engel 2006). In addition, patients with achromatopsia also have a higher incidence of spatial and shape deficits. It has been noted that patients with complete achromatopsia cannot even imagine color, which means they cannot dream in color or use color during mental imagery. This absence of color vision often leaves patients with no appetite for foods, which appear gray, and no desire for intimacy, as flesh appears gray. An insightful case study of a color-blind painter describes these experiences in detail (Sacks 1995).

Evaluation

Cerebral achromatopsia can be diagnosed using a range of color vision tests. The simplest test is an explicit color-naming task that requires patients to name the color of individual flash cards. The most common test for color blindness is the Ishihara plate test. These plates contain isoluminant colored dots of varying sizes that together create the perception of a number embedded in noise. In order to perceive the number, patients must be able to distinguish between the different colored dots. Another widely used test is the Farnsworth-Munsell 100-Hue test, in which patients are required to order colored caps based on gradual shifts in hue from light to dark. Patients with color blindness are unable to perform this task. Rarely, a diagnosis is made using a Nagel anomaloscope. This apparatus is typically used to determine whether a patient is a monochromat or a dichromat; however, some experimenters/practitioners use it in the study of cerebral achromatopsia.

Treatment

There is a period of spontaneous recovery for neurovisual lesions, which typically lasts 3 months post-lesion, but can occur for up to a year. With regard to the treatment and diagnosis of cerebral achromatopsia, experimenters report that some patients are not conscious of the absence of color vision. This phenomenon has been explained by the ablation of a color module leaving patients without even the concept of color post-lesion. This symptom of achromatopsia should be noted when addressing patients, because pushing a patient to describe a condition they are not aware of could be distressing for the patient.

Cross-References

▶ Scotoma

References and Readings

Bartels, A., & Zeki, S. (2000). The architecture of the color centre in the human visual brain: New results and a review. *The European Journal of Neuroscience, 12*(1), 172–193.

Bouvier, S. E., & Engel, S. A. (2006). Behavioral deficits and cortical damage loci in cerebral achromatopsia. *Cerebral Cortex (New York, N.Y.: 1991), 16*(2), 183–191.

Kanwisher, N., McDermott, J., & Chun, M. M. (1997). The fusiform face area: A module in human extrastriate cortex specialized for face perception. *Journal of Neuroscience, 17*(11), 4302–4311.

Meadows, J. C. (1974). Disturbed perception of colors associated with localized cerebral lesions. *Brain: A Journal of Neurology, 97*(4), 615–632.

Sacks, O. W. (1995). *An anthropologist on mars: Seven paradoxical tales.* New York: Vintage Books.

Verrey, D. (1888). Hémiachromatopsie Droite Absolue. Conversation Partielle De La Perception Lumineuse Et Des Formes. Ancien Kyste Hémorrhagique De La Partie Inférieure Du Lobe Occipital Gauche. *Archives d'ophtalmologie, 8,* 289–300.

Werner, J. S., & Chalupa, L. M. (2004). *The visual neurosciences.* Cambridge, MA: MIT Press.

Acoustic Neuroma

Ethan Moitra
Department of Psychiatry and Human Behavior,
Brown University, Providence, RI, USA

Synonyms

Neurolemmoma; Vestibular schwannoma

Definition

A benign tumor of the Schwann cells occurring near the cerebellopontine angle of the brain stem. Typically, it arises from the vestibulocochlear or eighth cranial nerve, which connects the brain to the inner ear. It is commonly associated with neurofibromatosis type 2 and often occurs bilaterally. Tumor growth is usually slow and may result in some hearing loss or deafness, tinnitus, vertigo, and vestibular dysfunction. Most acoustic neuromas are diagnosed in patients between the ages 30 and 60. Etiology is possibly related to gene malfunction on chromosome 22. Treatment options include radiosurgery and microsurgical removal (Figs. 1 and 2).

Cross-References

▶ Radiosurgery, Stereotactic Radiosurgery
▶ Radiotherapy

References and Readings

Jørgensen, B. G., & Pedersen, C. B. (1994). Acoustic neuroma. Follow-up of 78 patients. *Clinical Otolaryngology, 19*, 478–484.

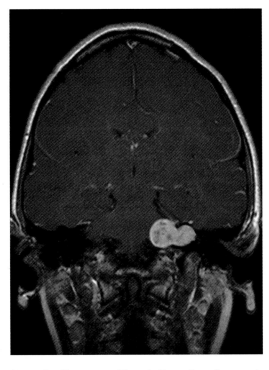

Acoustic Neuroma, Fig. 1 Example of acoustic neuroma

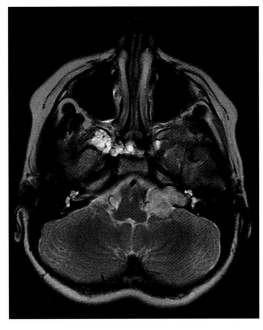

Acoustic Neuroma, Fig. 2 Example of acoustic neuroma

Acquired Immunodeficiency Syndrome (AIDS)

Bruce J. Diamond, William Tsang, Cody Curatolo, Savannah Crippen and C. Michael Nina
Department of Psychology, William Paterson University, Wayne, NJ, USA

Short Description or Definition

Acquired immunodeficiency syndrome (AIDS) is a disease caused by infection with the human immunodeficiency virus (HIV) (Portegies and Berger 2007). HIV is a viral pathogen that targets CD4+ T cells (also called T4 or T helper cells), which are lymphocyte cells with cluster determinant 4 + surface receptor sites, originating in the thymus of the human body's immune system. HIV is known to cause damage to the immune system as well as the central nervous system. The exact cause of this damage is unclear, but explanatory models have been proposed. For example, the "Trojan horse" or neuroinflammation model is thought to involve immune system cells known as macrophages which conceal and convey HIV into the brain, where they can disrupt supportive brain cells such as astrocytes and microglia. In the neuroinflammation model, the body's over-stimulated immune system causes an increased production of CD14+ CD16+ monocytes which flood the brain, causing inflammation and damage to brain cells and structures (Bartlett and Finkbeiner 2006) (Table 1).

Acquired Immunodeficiency Syndrome (AIDS), Table 1 Differentiation between human immunodeficiency virus (HIV) infection and acquired immunodeficiency syndrome (AIDS) in individuals infected with HIV

Symptom	Diagnosis
CD4+ T cell count of 200 or higher per mm^3/blood	HIV infection
CD4+ T cell count below 200 per mm^3/ blood	AIDS
Presence of one or more opportunistic infection	AIDS

AIDS is the name given to the end stage of HIV infection when the body's ability to fight off microorganisms is compromised, resulting in debilitating or fatal diseases, which are known as "opportunistic infections." An individual with HIV infection receives a formal diagnosis of AIDS when the individual has at least one opportunistic infection or when the individual's CD4+ T cell count is below 200 per mm^3 of blood (normal count is typically 500–1500 per mm^3).

In the absence of anti-HIV or antiretroviral drug therapy, progression to AIDS can take an average of 8–12 years for adults and adolescents and 3 years from birth in prenatally infected children. A quarter of a century after the first deaths from AIDS were identified, the AIDS pandemic has killed approximately 25 million people worldwide. UNAIDS, a joint program of the United Nations and the World Health Organization, estimates that globally, in 2014, 36.9 million people lived with HIV, two million became newly infected, and 1.2 million died from AIDS. In Western and Central Europe and North America alone, 2.4 million lived with HIV, 85,000 became newly infected, and 26,000 died from AIDS (UNAIDS 2015).

Categorization

Differentiation between diagnoses of HIV or AIDS depends on CD4+ T cell count and the presence of opportunistic infections.

Etiology/Epidemiology

In 1981, the US Centers for Disease Control and Prevention (CDC) began receiving reports about unusual cases of *Pneumocystis carinii* pneumonia (PCP) and Kaposi's sarcoma in young men who have sex with men (MSM) and PCP in injection drug users. These diseases were uncommon in individuals with healthy immune systems, and in early 1982, similar disease patterns were seen in blood transfusion recipients, hemophiliacs, and female partners of those already infected (Portegies and Berger 2007). In late 1982, the

CDC officially named this disease pattern as acquired immune deficiency syndrome (AIDS). In 1984, a previously unknown human retrovirus was discovered in the blood of individuals with AIDS by teams in the United States and France and in 1986, the retrovirus was officially named human immunodeficiency virus (HIV) by the CDC.

In 1985, a second strain of the virus was discovered, which was designated as HIV-2. The original strain of the virus was designated as HIV-1. HIV-1 is much more common throughout the world, while HIV-2 is more common in certain parts of Africa. HIV-2 appears to be milder than HIV-1, with a slower progression to AIDS. Since its establishment in humans, HIV-1 has undergone mutation of its genome, and there are now three groups of HIV-1.

Globally in 2014, there were approximately 36.9 (34.3–41.4) million people living with HIV (PLHIV), with 2.0 [1.9–2.2] million new infections. Sub-Saharan Africa has the highest global HIV rates, with 25.8 [24.0–28.7] million PLHIV in 2014 (WHO 2015). In recent years, there has been a global increase in prevalence and decrease in incidence attributable to a variety of factors including reduced infectiousness of PLHIV individuals on antiretroviral therapy medications (ART) and expansion of HIV prevention programs focusing on mother-to-child transmission, safer sex, and outreach to high-risk populations. From 2000 to 2015, new HIV infections have decreased by 35% and AIDS-related deaths by 24% (WHO 2015).

HIV transmission varies worldwide depending upon the geographic region. In the United States, the estimated incidence is 50,000 new HIV infections per year. At the end of 2013, 70% of HIV infections were attributed to male-to-male sexual contact, 11% to injection drug use, 10% to heterosexual contact, 7% to male-to-male sexual contact *and* injection drug use (IDU), and 1% to perinatal transmission (CDC 2014). Transmission in women is primarily associated with heterosexual contact and IDU. The HIV incidence rate among women was 20% in 2010, and prevalence rate was 23% in 2011 (CDC 2015). In 2014, males accounted for 81% of all diagnoses of HIV infection among adults and adolescents. Black, Latino, younger White MSM bear the greatest burden of HIV infection, due to higher-risk sexual behavior (CDC 2012).

In Africa, transmission is primarily due to male-to-female sexual contact. Asia has the second greatest rates associated with IDU, paid sex, and MSM. In the Middle East, infection is thought to be associated with commercial sex work and IDU. In Latin America, transmission is primarily due to IDU, paid sex, and MSM. Females constitute a higher proportion of PLHIV (60%) in Latin America and the Caribbean than in any other region. In Eastern Europe, the major vectors are IDU and heterosexual sexual contact. Western Europe and Oceania are similar to North America in HIV transmission from MSM, IDU, and male-to-female sexual contact. The HIV epidemic is most severe in developing countries with inadequate medical and health education resources. Among high-income nations, racial and ethnic minority groups experience higher HIV prevalence compared with the general population (Fettig et al. 2014).

Natural History, Prognostic Factors, and Outcomes

HIV is not transmitted through casual contact, such as touching. It can be transmitted when the bodily fluids of infected individuals – primarily blood, semen, vaginal fluid, or breast milk – comes into contact with the bloodstream or mucosal tissues of uninfected individuals. Transmission can occur through:

1. Unprotected sexual contact (anal, vaginal, or oral) with an individual infected with HIV
2. Sharing needles or syringes with HIV-infected individuals
3. Transfusion of infected blood or other bodily incorporation of infected blood
4. A fetus or infant exposed to HIV before or during birth or through breastfeeding

The natural progression of HIV infection can be divided into three stages: primary infection, clinical latency, and symptomatic disease stage. The symptomatic disease stage is further divided into early and late stages, with AIDS being equated with the late-symptomatic disease stage. After a person is initially infected with HIV, a primary or acute infection stage commences, in which HIV replicates up to ten billion copies of itself daily; high levels of HIV in the blood or viremia is evident. Approximately 2–4 weeks after exposure, nearly 70% of those newly infected will experience an acute illness, which has symptoms similar to influenza or mononucleosis, including fever, fatigue, muscle weakness, headache, ocular pain, sensitivity to light, sore throat, diarrhea, and lymphadenopathy. This illness is due to the temporary reduction of CD4+ T cells; it lasts for approximately 2 weeks and then resolves spontaneously. It is during this stage that the individual typically first begins to produce antibodies to HIV, which is designated as seroconversion.

Serological testing of blood can reliably detect HIV antibodies 2–6 months after seroconversion. Testing typically begins with an enzyme-linked immunosorbent assay (ELISA) or test that looks for antibodies to HIV. A second positive ELISA is needed in order to confirm the result. This would then be followed by the Western blot procedure to confirm the presence of at least two specific HIV antigen groups. A diagnosis of HIV infection is given after a positive Western blot test follows two positive ELISA tests. If HIV is confirmed, additional tests for plasma viral RNA (viral load) and CD4+ T cell counts are then typically completed, in order to assess the state of the immune system and disease prognosis. Higher viral load counts are typically related to faster disease progression. Lower CD4+ T cell counts are typically related to greater clinical vulnerabilities.

After the acute illness disappears, the individual enters the clinical latency stage in which symptoms are typically absent, other than possible chronic lymphadenopathy. This stage lasts an average of 10 years. During the clinical latency stage, HIV continues to replicate and attack CD4+ T cells, which in turn continue to counter attack.

As the immune system becomes progressively compromised, individuals eventually enter the early symptomatic disease stage, when a variety of symptoms begin to manifest, including lymphadenopathy, lack of energy, diarrhea, unintentional weight loss, chronic low-grade fever and sweats, frequent rashes or fungal infections, headaches, or short-term memory loss.

Finally, individuals enter the late stage of the symptomatic disease stage or AIDS when the person has at least one opportunistic infection or when the individual's CD4+ T cell count is below 200 per mm^3 of blood. The most common opportunistic infections are PCP, Kaposi's sarcoma, HIV wasting syndrome, and HIV encephalopathy (also known as dementia due to HIV disease or AIDS dementia complex).

People who benefit from access to ART and lifelong treatment no longer see AIDS-related illnesses as primary threats. Instead, new HIV-related complications have emerged; serious non-AIDS events include cardiovascular disease, cancer, kidney disease, liver disease, osteopenia/osteoporosis, and neurocognitive disease. Additional vulnerabilities include myocardial infarction, hypertension, hyperlipidemia, and diabetes mellitus. There can also be complications from opportunistic infections such as human papillomavirus, Epstein-Barr virus, and hepatitis B and C (Deeks et al. 2013).

Psychological and Neuropsychological Correlates of HIV Infection

As HIV infection progresses, various psychological and neuropsychological complications involving both the central and peripheral nervous systems can arise. During primary infection, reports of headaches and aseptic meningitis are common. During the clinical latency stage, an acute inflammatory demyelinating neuropathy (similar to Guillain-Barre syndrome and characterized by progressive muscle weakness) can occasionally develop. During the early symptomatic disease stage, peripheral neuropathy is common. This is characterized by spontaneous pain (dysesthesia), pain due to light touches or changes in temperature (hyperesthesia), and weakness and wasting in arms/legs (distal atrophy).

Several major neuropsychological complications can develop during the late symptomatic disease stage or AIDS, including:

1. HIV encephalopathy (HIV dementia)
2. Opportunistic infections
   1. Viral (cytomegalovirus, herpes simplex virus I and II, herpes zoster, and JC virus, a polyomavirus or papovavirus which causes PML [progressive multifocal leukoencephalopathy])
   2. Fungal/protozoan (toxoplasmosis, Cryptococcus, Candida, Mycobacterium)
3. Lymphomas
   1. Primary central nervous system lymphomas
   2. Systemic (metastatic) lymphomas (The most common systemic lymphomas are Hodgkin's, immunoblastic; Burkitt's; and non-Hodgkin's, which is particularly prevalent.)

HIV encephalopathy is the term used to describe the pathological features of encephalitis of the brain due to HIV, while HIV dementia (also known as AIDS dementia complex) is used to describe the clinical syndrome. This syndrome is characterized by behavioral, cognitive, and motor declines and difficulties (Table 2). Initial symptoms typically manifest as cognitive difficulties (loss of concentration and mild deficits in memory) with motor and behavioral difficulties

Acquired Immunodeficiency Syndrome (AIDS), Table 2 HIV dementia symptoms

Behavioral difficulties
Depression
Apathy, anhedonia, social withdrawal
Personality changes, including spontaneous, sudden, and strong emotions
Cognitive difficulties
Confusion
Short-term memory lapses
Loss of concentration
Motor difficulties
Lack of muscular coordination
Tremors
Muscle weakness
Loss of balance

frequently occurring. This early stage is often labeled as HIV-associated minor cognitive motor disorder. Later symptoms include partial paralysis, incontinence, and severe cognitive impairment. Death usually occurs within 1–6 months after onset of severe symptoms. Individuals who are co-infected with hepatitis C or were intravenous drug users (IDU) typically display more severe symptoms faster. As HIV-infected individuals now live longer from ART, it is estimated that 47% experience HIV-associated neurocognitive disorders (McGuire et al. 2013).

While HIV can be present in any region of the brain, it is commonly observed in the basal ganglia and central white matter (and to a lesser extent in neocortical gray matter, the brainstem, and the cerebellum) in individuals not receiving highly active antiretroviral therapy (HAART) (see below). In those receiving HAART, there is evidence of greater inflammation in the hippocampus and surrounding entorhinal and temporal cortex which would account for associated memory difficulties.

Peripheral mitochondrial DNA oxidative damage has been found to be associated with reduced hippocampal and subcortical gray matter volumes in chronic stable HIV disease. Oxidative stress-mediated neuroinflammation, caused by dysfunctional reactive oxygen species producing mitochondrial DNA, may contribute to neuronal loss in HIV. Findings have shown that volumes of multiple brain regions (e.g., enlarged lateral ventricles, reduced hippocampal volume) are negatively correlated with mitochondrial DNA in peripheral blood mononuclear cells of HIV-infected individuals (Kallianpur 2016). HIV infection may initiate several potentially inflammatory cascades that cause demyelinating lesions (Lescure et al. 2013).

A therapeutic gap seems to exist between the salutary effects of antiretroviral regimens and the normalization of neurological function in HIV-associated neurocognitive disorders. Despite the advances in antiretroviral therapy, CNS opportunistic infections remain a serious health burden worldwide (Tan et al. 2012). ART regimens differ in their ability to penetrate CNS, and the problem is that most of them do not. The current goal is to develop new medications that can penetrate the CNS and eradicate HIV (Ene et al. 2011).

Treatment

While there is no cure or vaccine for HIV or AIDS at this time, there are currently four different classes of antiretroviral drugs that interfere with the ability of HIV to replicate: reverse transcriptase inhibitors (nucleoside and non-nucleoside types), protease inhibitors, entry/fusion inhibitors, and integrase inhibitors. In 1987, the US Food and Drug Administration (FDA) approved azidothymidine (AZT, also known as zidovudine), the first nucleoside-reverse transcriptase inhibitor (NRTIs). Saquinavir, the first protease inhibitor, was approved in 1995. Nevirapine, the first non-nucleoside-reverse transcriptase inhibitor, was approved in 1996. Enfuvirtide, the first fusion inhibitor, was approved in 2003. Maraviroc, the first entry inhibitor, and raltegravir, the first integrase inhibitor, were approved in 2007.

In 1996, combination drug therapy began and was called "highly active antiretroviral therapy" (HAART) (Portegies and Berger 2007). Three or more drugs are used in combination in order to counter the development of drug resistance by HIV. Strict adherence to medication intake schedules is required. Not only is this schedule difficult to follow for many individuals, HAART often produces unpleasant and toxic side effects, including stomach problems and lipodystrophy. If followed correctly, HAART typically and drastically reduces viral load, often to undetectable levels in the blood, which allows the immune system to rebound. Antiretroviral drug therapy and treatments for opportunistic infections have greatly increased life expectancy of those with HIV infection, but due to the presence of HIV in cells that remain out of reach of antiretroviral drugs, eradication of HIV from the human body is unattainable at this time.

Several recent widespread interventions involve treatment as prevention (TASP), preexposure prophylaxis (PrEP), and postexposure prophylaxis (PEP). In TASP, treatment through adherence to ART reduces likelihood of transmission. In 2011, the World Health Organization found a 96% transmission risk reduction in PLHIV who used ART. PrEP is a preventative combination ART pill regimen (tenofovir and emtricitabine) that has been shown to reduce HIV transmission up to 92% but is significantly less effective if not taken consistently. Lastly, PEP exists as a postexposure ART regimen that must be taken within 72 h (Department of Health and Human Services 2016).

Current treatment investigations are seeking approaches that carry fewer side effects and do not require daily administration and thus increase compliance. Many vaccine trials have taken place with nonsignificant results, but the Thai RV144 trial could lead to improved approaches in vaccines. A major recent development involves the "Berlin patient" and a gene called CCR5. In this case, a patient with HIV and leukemia no longer showed evidence of either disease, after stem cell transplantation from a donor with CCR5 (Levy et al. 2012).

Cross-References

▶ Dementia
▶ Encephalitis (Viral)
▶ Meningitis

References and Readings

Bartlett, J., & Finkbeiner, A. (2006). *The guide to living with HIV infection, developed at the John Hopkins AIDS clinic* (6th ed.). Baltimore: Johns Hopkins University Press.
CDC (2012). *HIV surveillance supplemental report*, Vol. 17, No. 4.
Centers for Disease Control and Prevention. (2014). HIV surveillance report, vol. 26. http://www.cdc.gov/hiv/library/reports/surveillance/. Published November 2015. Accessed 13 April 2016.
Centers for Disease Control and Prevention. (2015). Prevalence of diagnosed and undiagnosed HIV infection — United States, 2008–2012. *MMWR, 64*, 657–662.
Deeks, S. G., Lewin, S. R., & Havlir, D. V. (2013). The end of AIDS: HIV infection as a chronic disease. *The Lancet, 382*(9903), 1525–1533.
Ene, L., Duiculescu, D., & Ruta, S. (2011). How much do antiretroviral drugs penetrate into the central nervous system? *Journal of Medicine and Life, 4*(4), 432–439.
Fettig, J., Swaminathan, M., Murrill, C. S., & Kaplan, J. E. (2014). Global epidemiology of HIV. *Infectious Disease Clinics of North America, 28*(3), 323–337.
Kallianpur, J. K. (2016). oxidative mitochondrial DNA damage in peripheral blood mononuclear cells is associated with reduced volumes of hippocampus and subcortical gray matter in chronically HIV-infected patients. *Mitochondrion, 28*, 8–15.

Lescure, F., Moulignier, A., Savatovsky, J., Amiel, C., Carcelain, G., Molina, J., et al. (2013). CD8 encephalitis in HIV-infected patients receiving cART: A treatable entity. *Clinical Infectious Diseases, 57*(1), 101–108.

Levy, J. A., Autran, B., Coutinho, R. A., & Phair, J. P. (2012). 25 years of AIDS: Recording progress and future challenges. *AIDS, 26*(10), 1187–1189.

McGuire, J. L., Goodkin, K., & Douglas, S. D. (2013). Neuropathogenesis of central nervous system HIV infection. *Psychiatric Annals, 43*(5), 212–216.

Panel on Antiretroviral Guidelines for Adults and Adolescents. (2016). Guidelines for the use of antiretroviral agents in HIV-1-infected adults and adolescents. Department of Health and Human Services. Available at http://www.aidsinfo.nih.gov/ContentFiles/AdultandAdolescentGL.pdf. Accessed 03 April 2016.

Portegies, P., & Berger, J. (Eds.). (2007). *HIV/AIDS and the nervous system: Handbook of clinical neurology.* Amsterdam: Elsevier.

Pratt, R. (2003). *HIV & AIDS: A foundation for nursing and healthcare practice.* London: Arnold Publishers.

Sande, M., & Volberding, P. (Eds.). (1999). *The medical management of AIDS* (6th ed.). Philadelphia: Saunders.

Stine, G. (2005). *AIDS update 2005.* San Francisco: Pearson/Benjamin Cummings.

Tan, I. L., Smith, B. R., von Geldern, G., Mateen, F. J., & McArthur, J. C. (2012). HIV-associated opportunistic infections of the CNS. *The Lancet Neurology, 11*(7), 605–617.

UNAIDS. (2015). UNAIDS annual report 2015: Knowing your epidemic. Retrieved 22 Mar 2016 from www.unaids.org/sites/default/files/media_assest/AIDS_by_the_numbers_2015_en.pdf

Weeks, B. S., & Alcamo, I. E. (2006). *AIDS: The biological basis* (4th ed.). Sudbury: Jones and Bartlett Publishers.

World Health Organization (2015, November). *HIV/AIDS fact sheet.* Retrieved from http://www.who.int/mediacentre/factsheets/fs360/en/

Action Tremor

Anna DePold Hohler[1] and Marcus Ponce de Leon[2]
[1]Boston University Medical Center, Boston, MA, USA
[2]Madigan Army Medical Center, Tacoma, WA, USA

Synonyms

Intention tremors

Definition

Action tremor is a rhythmic, oscillatory, and involuntary movement of the limb that is seen with movement of an extremity. It may be seen in isolation with a cerebellar lesion or associated with other tremor types such as the postural tremor of essential tremor or the rest tremor of Parkinson's disease.

Cross-References

▶ Essential Tremor
▶ Parkinson's Disease

References and Readings

Fahn, S., & Jankovic, J. (Eds.). (2007). Tremors: Diagnosis and treatment. In *Movement disorders* (pp. 451–479). Philadelphia: Churchill Livingstone Elsevier.

Action-Intentional Disorders

Kenneth M. Heilman
Department of Neurology, University of Florida College of Medicine, Center for Neurological Studies and the Research Service of the Malcom Randall Veterans Affairs Medical Center, Gainesville, FL, USA

Synonyms

Abulia; Akinesis; Hypokinesis; Motor impersistence (These terms are not fully synonymous with action-intentional disorders, but comprise important elements of the syndrome and are often used when describing specific these elements.)

Definition

In the absence of weakness, patients can have a disability with initiating (akinesia, hypokinesia, abulia) or sustaining actions (impersistence), inhibiting irrelevant actions (defective response inhibition), and stopping an action when the task has been completed (motor perseveration).

Current Concepts

The motor system allows humans to interact with their environment and alter themselves as well as others. The human corticospinal motor system together with the motor units and muscles can mediate an almost infinite number of movements, and thus the human motor system needs to be guided by at least two major types of programs: *praxic* and *intentional*. The praxic programs provide the corticospinal system with the knowledge of *how* to make skilled movements (spatial and temporal aspects of movements), and the intentional programs provide the corticospinal system with information about *when* to move. In this section, we will discuss disorders of the intentional, or "when," systems. When interacting with environmental stimuli or the self, there are four "when" questions that must be addressed: these are (1) when to move, (2) when to persist at a movement or movements, (3) when to end a movement or a series of movements, and (4) when not to move. The inability to initiate a movement in the absence of a corticospinal or motor unit injury is called *akinesia*. Some patients are able to move after a delay, and we call this *hypokinesia*. *Motor impersistence* is when a patient cannot sustain a movement or a series of movements that are needed to complete a task. The inability to stop a movement or an action program when it is no longer required is called *motor perseveration* and the inability to withhold a response to a sensory stimulus is called *defective response inhibition*.

These motor intentional disorders are parallel to disorders of sensory attention, akinesia being akin to unawareness, impersistence being the motor parallel of decreased vigilance, motor perseveration being parallel to failures of extinction or habituation, and defective response inhibition being similar to distractibility. There are also cognitive defects that mirror four types of intentional

motor disorders mentioned above, but these will not be discussed here.

In the next section, we briefly describe each of these intentional disorders, including subtypes of each category, and in the final section, we briefly discuss the possible pathophysiology.

Clinical Manifestations

Akinesia

An organism might fail to initiate a movement for many reasons, but comprehension, attentional, perceptual, sensory, and motor disorders that lead to a failure of movement initiation should not be termed *akinesia*. In contrast to these disorders, akinesia is caused by a failure of the systems that are responsible for activating the motor system.

There are three methods by which akinesia can be distinguished from extreme weakness. Certain forms of akinesia are present under certain sets of circumstances and absent in others. Thus, using the behavioral method, if it can be demonstrated that a patient makes movements in one set of circumstances (e.g., a motionless left hand is brought over to the right side of the body, and the patient is able to now move this hand) and not in the other, this failure to move is related to an akinesia. If the akinesia is not limited to a set of circumstances then the clinician may have to depend on brain imaging, or physiological techniques such as magnetic stimulation of the motor cortex to demonstrate that the brain lesion did not involve the motor system and thus the failure to move is not caused by weakness.

There are at least three subtypes of akinesia: (1) *body part*: akinesia may involve the eyes, the neck and head, a limb, or the total body; (2) *action space*: akinesia of the limbs, eyes, or head may depend on where in space the body part is moved or in what direction it is moved. The former is called *spatial akinesia* (e.g., a hand that does not move in left hemispace but does move in right body-centered hemispace), and the latter is called *directional akinesia* (e.g., a horizontal gaze palsy where patients cannot move their eyes to the left); (3) *stimulus-response conditions*: some patients, such as those with Parkinson's disease, are impaired in spontaneously initiating a movement, but in response to a stimulus often have no trouble initiating a movement. We call this *endogenously evoked akinesia* (*endo-evoked*). Patients who fail to move to an imperative stimulus but will move spontaneously, we call *exogenously evoked akinesia*. A patient may have both exo-evoked and endo-evoked akinesia, which we term *mixed or global akinesia*.

Hypokinesia

A milder defect in the intentional motor ("when") systems might not induce a total inability to initiate a response (i.e., akinesia), but rather these patients' intentional deficit might be manifested by a delay in initiating a response. We call this delay *hypokinesia*. The hypokinesias may also be subtyped into body part (e.g., limb or eyes) and action space (e.g., directional and hemispatial).

Motor Extinction

Patients with *sensory extinction* are able to detect single stimuli on either side of their body, but when presented with two stimuli one on each side of their body, they remain unaware of contralesional stimuli. *Motor extinction* is a form of akinesia or hypokinesia where a patient who is without sensory extinction is asked to respond by moving the hand (or hands) that was (were) touched. The examiner then delivers stimuli to the right, left, and both hands, and patients with motor extinction are aware that both hands have been touched, but either fail to lift the contralesional hand to simultaneous stimuli or lift it after a delay.

Motor Impersistence

The inability to sustain a motor act or a series of motor acts that are required to complete a goal is called *motor impersistence*. Like akinesia, impersistence can be associated with various *body parts* including the limbs, eyes, neck, eyelids (e.g., keep your eyes closed for until I tell you to open them), jaw, and tongue. Patients can even demonstrate impersistence in activities such as walking. Like akinesia, it may also be *directional* (e.g., inability to maintain leftward gaze) or

hemispatial (inability to maintain dorsiflexion of the wrist in left space with the left arm but able to do so in right space).

Defective Response Inhibition

Not all stimuli require a response, and sometimes a response might interfere with goal-oriented behavior. *Defective response inhibition* is defined as responding when no response of that body part is required. It can be seen in a variety of body parts and might also be directional and perhaps hemispatial.

There are several forms of defective response inhibition. One means of testing for this disorder is to use the *crossed response task*. A blindfolded patient is instructed to raise the hand opposite to that touched. Patients with defective response inhibition will often raise the touched hand first. This type of defective response inhibition may be termed *motor* (*limb* or *eye directional*) *response disinhibition*. These can be either contralesional or bilateral. The eye directional defective response inhibition has also been called a *visual grasp*. There are some patients, however, who have a perceptual disorder and when stimulated on one side (e.g., left hand), feel that they were stimulated on the other (e.g., right hand). This phenomenon is called *allesthesia*, and it should not be confused with defective crossed response inhibition.

Patients with defective response inhibition may also fail on the types of go-no-go tasks described by Luria. For example, the patient may be instructed to put up two fingers when the examiner puts up one finger and to put up no fingers if the examiner puts up two fingers. If the patient mimics the examiner such that when the examiner puts up one finger, the patient puts up one finger and when the examiner puts up two fingers, the patient puts up two fingers, the patient has *echopraxia*.

Motor Perseveration

When a patient incorrectly repeats a prior response or when a patient continues to perform the same act when the goal of the act has been completed, it is called *motor perseveration*. In one type of motor perseveration, when the task requirements have changed, the patient is unable to switch to a different motor program and incorrectly repeats the movements. Luria (1965) calls this *inertia of program action*, and Sandson and Albert (1987) call this *recurrent perseveration*. In the second type, the patient continues to perform movements even though the task is completed. Luria (1965) called this *efferent perseveration*; however, Sandson and Albert (1987) call this *continuous perseveration*.

Pathophysiology of Intentional Disorders

Intentional motor disorders are often associated with bilateral hemispheric lesions, but when these disorders are caused by a unilateral hemispheric lesion, they are more commonly associated with right than left-hemisphere lesions. The intentional disorders that have been reported to be induced by primarily right-hemisphere lesions include akinesia (e.g., left-sided limbs, leftward arm movements, and even left horizontal gaze), hypokinesia (slowed reaction times), motor impersistence of the left-sided limbs, left-sided gaze), and motor (continuous) perseveration. Many of the intentional defects associated with right-hemisphere dysfunction, however, are not just limited to the left limbs. For example, patients with a right-hemisphere lesion are more often abulic, have slowed reaction times of their right hand, and have motor impersistence of eye closure. These clinical studies suggest that the right hemisphere may be dominant for intentional control of the motor systems. Studies with normal subjects provide further evidence for right-hemisphere intentional dominance. The anatomic and physiological basis for this dominance is not entirely understood.

Studies of patients with focal lesions and studies of monkeys suggest that the frontal lobes may play a critical role in mediating intentional activity. The most important areas of the frontal lobes appear to be the medial and lateral frontal lobes. The frontal cortex has strong projections to the striatum. The lateral portion of the frontal lobe projects to the caudate. The premotor cortex projects to the putamen and the cingulate gyrus projects to the ventral striatum. The striatum projects to the pars reticularis of the substantia nigra and the globus pallidus. The globus pallidus projects to specific thalamic nuclei, and these thalamic nuclei project back to the frontal cortex. Just as injury of the frontal lobes can induce intentional deficits, injuries, or diseases that injure the basal ganglia, the substantia nigra (e.g., Parkinson's disease), portions of the thalamus, as well as the white matter connections can also induce intentional deficits.

Future Directions

Disorders of intention have received considerably less neuroscientific study than have disorders of sensory selective attention. There is a need for additional experimental and clinical neuropsychological studies of these disorders. Furthermore, assessment batteries are needed that will facilitate the assessment of the subtypes of motor intention disturbances and which may provide additional quantitative data for experimental analysis and normative comparison between patient groups and healthy individuals.

Cross-References

▶ Attention
▶ Impersistence
▶ Neglect Syndrome

References and Readings

Heilman, K. M. (2004). Intentional neglect. *Frontiers in Bioscience, 9,* 694–705.
Heilman, K. M., Valenstein, E., Rothi, L. J. G., & Watson, R. T. (2004). Intentional motor disorders and apraxia. In W. G. Bradley, R. B. Daroff, G. M. Fenichel, & J. Jankovic (Eds.), *Neurology in clinical practice: Principles of diagnosis and management* (pp. 117–130). Phila Penn: Butterworth Heineman.

Heilman, K. M., Watson, R. T., & Valenstein, E. (2003). Neglect and related disorders. In K. M. Heilman & E. Valenstein (Eds.), *Clinical neuropsychology* (4th ed., pp. 296–346). New York: Oxford University Press.

Luria, A. R. (1965). Two kinds of motor perseveration in massive injury to the frontal lobes. *Brain, 88*, 1–10.

Sandson, J., & Albert, M. L. (1987). Varieties of perseveration. *Neuropsychologia, 22*, 715–732.

Active Limb Activation

Sarah A. Raskin
Department of Psychology and Neuroscience Program, Trinity College, Hartford, CT, USA

Synonyms

Limb activation

Definition

Active limb activation is a rehabilitation technique for individuals with unilateral neglect. In a series of studies, Robertson and North (1992, 1993, 1994) and others (Mattingly et al. 1998) have demonstrated that moving the upper or lower extremity on the affected side can reduce neglect symptoms. The effect is seen only with active movement, as opposed to passive movement, and only when the limb is moved in the effected hemispace. However, the limb need not be observed visually. It should be noted that the effect has not been demonstrated universally (e.g., Brown et al. 1999), and treatment effects may be specific to movements in peripersonal space (Priftis et al. 2013).

Cross-References

▶ Attention Training
▶ Behavioral Inattention Test (BIT)
▶ Cognitive Rehabilitation
▶ Neglect Syndrome

References and Readings

Brown, V., Walker, R., Gray, C., & Findlay, J. (1999). Limb activation and the rehabilitation of unilateral neglect: Evidence of task-specific effects. *Neurocase, 5*, 129–142.

Mattingly, J., Robertson, I., & Driver, J. (1998). Modulation of covert visual attention by hand movement: Evidence from parietal extinction after right hemisphere damage. *Neurocase, 4*, 245–253.

Priftis, K., Passarini, L., Pilosio, C., Meneghello, F., & Pitteri, M. (2013). Visual scanning training, limb activation treatment, and prism adaptation for rehabilitating left neglect: Who is the winner? *Frontiers in Human Neuroscience, 7*, 1–12.

Robertson, I., & North, N. (1992). Spatio-motor cueing in unilateral left neglect: The role of hemispace, hand and motor activation. *Neuropsychologia, 30*, 553–563.

Robertson, I., & North, N. (1993). Active and passive activation of left limbs: Influence on visual and sensory neglect. *Neuropsychologia, 31*, 293–300.

Robertson, I., & North, N. (1994). One hand is better than two: Motor extinction of left hand advantage in unilateral neglect. *Neuropsychologia, 32*, 1–11.

Activities of Daily Living (ADL)

Angela K. Troyer
Neuropsychology and Cognitive Health program, Baycrest Centre for Geriatric Care, Toronto, ON, Canada

Synonyms

Adaptive functions; Functional abilities

Definition

Activities of daily living (ADLs) are self-care activities that are important for health maintenance and independent living. ADLs comprise a broad spectrum of activities, traditionally classified as basic and instrumental ADLs (BADLs and IADLs, respectively). BADLs, also called physical or self-maintenance ADLs, are life-sustaining self-care activities such as feeding, grooming, bathing, dressing, toileting, and ambulation.

IADLs are more complex activities that are necessary for independent living, such as using the telephone, preparing meals, shopping, managing finances, taking medications, arranging appointments, and driving. These activities are important for participating in one's usual work, social, or leisure roles.

Historical Background

The evolution of the concept of ADLs is reflected in the development of instruments to measure these abilities. Measures of BADLs were first developed in the 1940s and 1950s, primarily to determine the required levels of care for institutionalized older adults and those with chronic illnesses. These early measures include the PULSES profile, the Barthel Index, and the Katz Index of ADL, among others. Later, in the 1960s and 1970s, there was increased interest in caring for older and disabled individuals in the community, and this spawned the need for tools to measure IADLs that are important for independent living. Some of the first of these measures were Lawton and Brody's IADL Scale and the Disability Interview Schedule. Recent work has focused on the development of disorder-specific measures that take into account characteristics of the disorder that can systematically impact ADLs, such as changes in motivation, behavior, vision, or motor functioning.

Current Knowledge

ADLs are of interest across various health disciplines. Current knowledge in this area is based on research conducted by psychologists, occupational therapists, nurses, psychiatrists, neurologists, and social workers, among others.

Relevance to Neuropsychology

For the neuropsychologist, an understanding of the patient's level of independence in ADLs, and in particular IADLs, is of interest for several reasons. The diagnosis of a number of cognitive and mental disorders requires an appraisal of the patient's functional ability (American Psychiatric Association 2013). For example, impairment in adaptive or functional ability is a diagnostic criterion for intellectual disability and for schizophrenia. Impaired daily functioning is also required for the diagnosis of dementia and is one of the defining differences between dementia (in which IADLs are impaired) and mild cognitive impairment (in which IADLs are intact or minimally affected).

Increasingly, the evaluation of daily functioning is also used to identify appropriate treatments for cognitive and mental disorders. In particular, an important part of determining the effectiveness of behavioral or pharmacological interventions is measuring the impact of the intervention on the patient's daily functional ability, in addition to cognitive or affective outcomes.

The ability to perform ADLs, and IADLs in particular, is related to sensory, motor, cognitive, and behavioral functioning. Within cognition, the domain most consistently related to IADLs is executive function, although memory, language, visuospatial ability, and attention also play a role (Royall et al. 2007). Thus, neuropsychologists can expect that their clients with executive dysfunction are most likely to experience difficulties with daily functioning.

Assessment of ADLs

Assessment of ADLs can be accomplished in a number of ways. *Real-world observation* of the patient in his or her own home provides relevant, objective information about daily function. However, this method is obviously time and labor intensive, and there are practical limits to the number of behaviors that can be observed within a given time period. An alternative is the use of *performance-based measures*, which require the patient to complete functional tasks – such as preparing a meal, using the telephone, or making personal financial transactions – that are presented in a standardized way in the laboratory or clinic. A number of such instruments have been developed to measure single or multiple functional domains. Tests include the Direct

Assessment of Functional Status, the Independent Living Scales, the Structured Assessment of Independent Living Skills, the Medication Management Abilities Assessment, and many others.

The use of questionnaires administered either on paper or by interview allows the sampling of a large number of behaviors in a short period of time. *Self-report questionnaires* may be appropriate for use with cognitively normal or mildly impaired populations. In the evaluation of dementia and other cognitive disorders, however, self-reported abilities may be difficult to interpret because of disease-related decreases in self-awareness. The use of *informant-based questionnaires* avoids this limitation, although informants can also be biased in their reports and may not always be available. Nevertheless, this is one of the most common methods for measuring IADLs, and a large number of informant-based questionnaires exist, such as the Lawton-Brody IADL Scale, the Bristol ADL Scale, Vineland Adaptive Behavior Scales, and the ADL questionnaire.

The choice of which particular method of assessment to be used will depend, in addition to practical considerations such as time, on the purpose of the assessment. Real-word observations and performance-based measures provide information about what the person is *capable of doing*. Questionnaires, on the other hand, measure what the individual is *actually doing* in his or her day-to-day life.

Future Directions

Although there are a large number of relevant instruments that have been developed to assess ADLs, they vary in terms of how well their psychometric properties have been characterized. Systematic literature reviews (e.g., Floyd et al. 2015; Moore et al. 2007; Sikkes et al. 2009) indicate that, for many of these measures, there is a need for better theoretical justification of the content of the instrument, additional information about test validity and reliability, indication of what constitutes a meaningful change over time, information about the relation between test performance and actual real-world functioning, and the development of comprehensive normative data.

Cross-References

▶ Functional Status
▶ Instrumental Activities of Daily Living
▶ Lawton-Brody Instrumental Activities of Daily Living Scale
▶ Vineland Adaptive Behavior Scales

References and Readings

American Psychiatric Association. (2013). *Diagnostic and statistical manual of mental disorders* (5th ed.). Washington, DC: American Psychiatric Association.

Floyd, R. G., Shands, E. I., Alfonso, V. C., Phillips, J. F., Autry, B. K., Mosteller, J. A., Skinner, M., & Irby, S. (2015). A systematic review and psychometric evaluation of adaptive behavior scales and recommendations for practice. *Journal of Applied School Psychology, 31*, 83–113.

Lawton, M. P., & Brody, E. M. (1969). Assessment of older people: Self-maintaining and instrumental activities of daily living. *Gerontologist, 9*, 179–186.

McDowell, I. (2006). *Measuring health: A guide to rating scales and questionnaires* (3rd ed.). New York: Oxford.

Moore, D. J., Palmer, B. W., Patterson, T. L., & Jeste, D. V. (2007). A review of performance-based measures of functional living skills. *Journal of Psychiatric Research, 41*, 97–118.

Pendleton, H. M., & Schultz-Krohn, W. (Eds.). (2011). *Pedretti's occupational therapy: Practice skills for physical dysfunction* (7th ed.). St. Louis: Mosby.

Royall, D. R., Lauterbach, E. C., Kaufer, D., Malloy, P., Coburn, K. L., & Black, K. J. (2007). The cognitive correlates of functional status: A review from the Committee on Research of the American Neuropsychiatric Association. *The Journal of Neuropsychiatry and Clinical Neurosciences, 19*, 249–265.

Sikkes, S. A. M., de Lange-de Klerk, E. S. M., Pijnenburg, Y. A. L., Scheltens, P., & Uitdehaag, B. M. J. (2009). A systematic review of instrumental activities of daily living scales in dementia: Room for improvement. *Journal of Neurology, Neurosurgery, and Psychiatry, 80*, 7–12.

Activities of Daily Living Questionnaire

Jessica Fish
Medical Research Council Cognition and Brain
Sciences Unit, Cambridge, UK

Synonyms

ADLQ

Description

The activities of daily living questionnaire (ADLQ) was developed to measure the functional abilities of people with dementia. It is an informant-rated questionnaire and should be completed by the patient's primary caregiver. It consists of 28 items covering both basic and instrumental activities of daily living, organized into six subscales: self-care activities, household care, employment and recreation, shopping and money, travel, and communication. The informant rates the subject's competence in each area according to a set of four descriptions of different competence levels; scores range from 0 to 3 where higher scores indicate greater impairment. A fifth response option, "don't know/has never done" is also available, and if this option is selected, the item is excluded from scoring. Scores from individual items are summed (with adjustment for any items marked "don't know/has never done") to form subscale scores and then transformed to a percentage impairment total score. Scores of 0–33% are classified as no/mild impairment, those of 34–66% as moderate impairment, and those of 67–100% as severe impairment.

Historical Background

The first reported use of the ADLQ was in a longitudinal study looking at cognitive test performance and daily functioning in patients with Alzheimer's disease (Locascio et al. 1995). However, the development and psychometric properties of the measure were first reported in Johnson et al. (2004). Since then, a Chinese version has been developed and evaluated (ADLQ-CV; Chu and Chung 2008), and it has been used in several studies involving people with non-Alzheimer's dementia.

Psychometric Data

Johnson et al. (2004) collected ADLQ data from the primary caregivers of 140 people with dementia of various types (Alzheimer's disease, vascular/mixed, and frontotemporal/primary progressive aphasia). The scale was completed twice, with a 1 year interval between completions. Evidence of convergent validity was in the form of correlations with global severity ratings (clinical dementia rating $r = 0.5$ and 0.55 for first/second ratings, respectively; MMSE $r = -0.42$ and -0.38 for first and second ratings, respectively). Further evidence of its validity came from the finding that scores declined significantly over the year-long interval between testings, as would be expected in people with degenerative conditions. A subgroup of 28 participants took part in a test-retest reliability study, with a 2–8 week interval between testings (mean 25.6 days, SD 12.2). Correlations between first and second ratings for the six subscales were high, between 0.86 and 0.92, with the exception of the employment subscale, which correlated at 0.65. Kappa scores for 25% of scale items were 0.42–0.60 (classified as "moderate"), for 54% of scale items were 0.61–0.80 (classified as "good"), and for 21% of scale items 0.81–1.0 (classified as "very good"). The validity of the ADLQ was investigated via correlations between 29 participants' scores on the ADLQ and the record of independent living (RIL), another ADL measure. In line with Johnson et al.'s predictions, there were significant correlations between the ADLQ and the "activities" and "communication" subscales of the RIL but not the "behavior" subscale of the RIL.

Chu and Chung (2008) conducted a study examining the psychometric properties of a Chinese translation of the ADLQ (ADLQ-CV), with 125 caregivers of people with moderate Alzheimer's disease. The ADLQ-CV was shown to have good internal consistency ($\alpha = 0.81$), test-retest reliability at a 2-week interval (intra-class correlation (ICC) = 0.998), and inter-rater reliability (ICC = 0.997, for primary and secondary caregiver ratings). Correlations with the disability assessment for dementia were strong ($r = 0.92$), suggesting that it is a valid measure. A factor analysis also confirmed that the ADLQ-CV has a six-factor structure, following the six proposed subscales.

Clinical Uses

The ADLQ may be used to assist in the diagnosis of dementia, in decision-making regarding necessary intervention and/or assistance, and in monitoring change over time or in response to treatment.

Cross-References

▶ Alzheimer's Disease Cooperative Study ADL Scale
▶ Bristol Activities of Daily Living Scale
▶ Disability Assessment for Dementia
▶ Lawton-Brody Instrumental Activities of Daily Living Scale

References and Readings

Chu, T. K. C., & Chung, J. C. C. (2008). Psychometric evaluation of the Chinese version of the activities of daily living questionnaire (ADLQ-CV). *International Psychogeriatrics, 20*, 1251–1261.
Johnson, N., Barion, A., Rademaker, A., Rehkemper, G., & Weintraub, S. (2004). The activities of daily living questionnaire: A validation study in patients with dementia. *Alzheimer's Disease and Associated Disorders, 18*, 223–230.
Locascio, J. J., Growdon, J. H., & Corkin, S. (1995). Cognitive test performance in detecting, staging, and tracking Alzheimer's disease. *Archives of Neurology, 52*(11), 1087–1099.

Activity Restrictions, Limitations

Brian Yochim
Department of Psychology, University of Colorado at Colorado Springs, Colorado Springs, CO, USA

Definition

This idea refers to restrictions prescribed by clinicians who treat patients with recent strokes, head injuries, or other neurological conditions, after a neurological event has left the patient with deficits in important areas of functioning. Patients are often restricted from driving, cooking, managing finances, or completing other instrumental activities of daily living after a neurological event. The activities of focus must be tailored to the patient and can range from restrictions in playing professional sports to restrictions in managing small amounts of cash.

Current Knowledge

Rehabilitation professionals encounter patients whose injuries have left them with deficits both in physical and cognitive realms. Strokes and traumatic brain injuries can cause physical impairments in walking, swallowing, use of an arm and/or leg, communication, and other important skills. Injuries can also lead to cognitive deficits in memory, executive functioning, social functioning, language, visuospatial skills, attention, and/or processing speed. These basic deficits in turn lead to impaired functioning in everyday life. Rehabilitation professionals must assess patients' abilities to complete these daily activities and often must place restrictions on what activities patients can continue to complete. If patients are deemed to be unable to drive, for example, clinicians must follow appropriate legal and ethical channels to protect the patient and public.

These limitations in activities can lead to difficulties in adjustment for the patient, which can sometimes result in depressed mood and other affective symptoms. This notion is related to the Activity Restriction Model of Depressed Affect (Williamson and Shaffer 2000), which has been studied as one etiology of depressive symptoms among older adults.

Cross-References

▶ Instrumental Activities of Daily Living
▶ Recommendation

References and Readings

Greenwood, R. J., Barnes, M. P., McMillan, T. M., & Ward, C. D. (Eds.). (2003). *Handbook of neurological rehabilitation* (2nd ed.). New York: Psychology Press.

Mills, V. M., Cassidy, J. W., & Katz, D. I. (Eds.). (1997). *Neurologic rehabilitation: A guide to diagnosis, prognosis, and treatment planning*. Malden: Blackwell.

Williamson, G. M., & Shaffer, D. R. (2000). The activity restriction model of depressed affect: Antecedents and consequences of restricted normal activities. In G. M. Williamson, D. R. Shaffer, & P. A. Parmelee (Eds.), *Physical illness and depression in older adults: A handbook of theory, research, and practice*. New York: Kluwer/Plenum Publishers.

Actus Reus

Moira C. Dux
US Department of Veteran Affairs, Baltimore, MD, USA

Definition

Actus reus is Latin for "guilty act." Under most circumstances, a crime consists of at least two factors. The first factor is the physical conduct or act associated with the crime, which is known as the "actus reus." In order for an individual to be convicted of a crime, it must be demonstrated beyond a reasonable doubt that the defendant committed the physical act of the crime or the "actus reus." However, it must concurrently be established that the defendant also possessed "mens rea," which translates to "guilty mind," referring to the mental element of the crime. Thus, a conviction necessitates, beyond reasonable doubt, establishment of an illegal act coupled with a particular mental state (e.g., intent, knowledge, recklessness, or negligence). Description of the actus reus is typically classified into one of three categories: commissions, omissions, and/or commonwealth. Commission refers to an affirmative act; omission refers to a failure to act; and commonwealth refers to a state of affairs or circumstances. Commissions and omissions necessitate causation; commonwealth does not always require voluntariness; and instead the actus reus is viewed in light of the severity of the offense.

Cross-References

▶ Insanity
▶ Insanity Defense
▶ Mens Rea

References and Readings

Melton, G. B., Petrila, J., Poythress, N. G., & Slobogin, C. (1997). *Psychological evaluations for the courts: A handbook for mental health professionals and lawyers*. New York: Guilford.

Acute Lymphoblastic Leukemia

Jacqueline L. Cunningham[1] and
Carol L. Armstrong[2]
[1]Department of Psychology, Children's Hospital of Philadelphia, Philadelphia, PA, USA
[2]Child and Adolescent Psychiatry and Behavioral Sciences, The Children's Hospital of Philadelphia, Philadelphia, PA, USA

Synonyms

ALL

Definition

Acute lymphoblastic leukemia (ALL) is a form of cancer of the white blood cells (leukocytes). ALL is the most common type of childhood leukemia and is distinguished from chronic lymphoblastic leukemia (CLL) and acute myeloid (or myelogenous) leukemia, which are more prevalent in adults.

Current Knowledge

Symptoms

ALL is characterized by the rapid proliferation of immature blood cells (lymphoblasts), which crowd out mature, functional cells. It is associated with the enlargement of lymphoid tissue in areas including the lymph nodes, spleen, bone marrow, and lungs and with increased lymphocytic cells circulating in blood and in various tissues and organs. Persons afflicted will experience weakness and fatigue, anemia, unexplained fever and infections, weight loss, or loss of appetite.

Pathophysiology

Cancer, including ALL, is caused by damage to DNA.

Treatment

The earlier the ALL is detected, the more effective is its treatment. The goal is to induce a lasting remission, considered to be a prevalence of less than 5% of lymphoblasts in bone marrow. Advances made in the ability to match the genetic properties of the blast cells to treatment options, in association with the availability of new drugs and improvements made in bone marrow and stem cell transplantation, have changed the prognosis for ALL from a zero to a 75% survival rate over the past 40 years.

Most (if not all) patients with a childhood history of ALL have brain atrophy. MRI has also demonstrated white matter changes in a minority of children. A large study identified reduced cortical gray and white matter, caudate nucleus, amygdala, and hippocampus in adult survivors in both those who were not treated with cranial irradiation and those who were. Whereas atrophy is associated with treatment-effects of cranial irradiation therapy and intrathecal chemotherapy (usually methotrexate), it can also occur as a result of the condition, itself, rather than as an outcome of treatment, as it appears to cause atrophy of the brain, which is not specific to certain brain tissues (Lucy Rorke, M.D., personal communication); however, few children with ALL are naïve to chemotherapy and radiotherapy, and the effects of time are not controlled in studies so that the developmental effects of damage from the disease and from the treatments both magnify over time. A study to discriminate the effects of treatment versus disease would require studies of children with ALL at diagnosis and prior to treatments. Nonetheless, the strongest detrimental impacts on cognition are attributable to treatment effects and their damaging influence on the biological substrates of core neurocognitive abilities, including executive functions (self-regulation, inhibitory control, cognitive flexibility, problem-solving), memory, verbal skills, and information processing. Such impacts disrupt the secondary abilities, i.e., those that are acquired and knowledge-based. The main approaches to alleviating neurocognitive effects of treatment include cognitive remediation, pharmacology, and ecological alterations in the classroom.

The presentation of survivors in adulthood is highly variable in both IQ and neuropsychological tests, with clinical factors intermediating, including polymorphisms that regulate inflammatory cytokine expression, cumulative dose, intensity of cancer therapy, age at diagnosis, years since diagnosis, and gender. Adult survivors are at heightened risk of neurocognitive disorders.

Cross-References

▶ Acute Myelogenous Leukemia
▶ Leukemia
▶ Neoplasms

References and Readings

Butler, R. W., & Mulhern, R. K. (2005). Neurocognitive interventions for children and adolescents surviving cancer. *Journal of Pediatric Psychology, 30*, 65–78.

Crosley, C. J., Rorke, L. B., Evans, A., & Nigro, M. (1978). Central nervous system lesions in childhood leukemia. *Neurology, 28*, 678–685.

De Oliveira-Gomes, E. R., Leite, D. S., Garcia, D. F., Maranhao, S., & Hazin, I. (2012). Neuropsychological profile of patients with actue lymphoblastic leukemia. *Psychology & Neuroscience, 5*(2), 175–182. https://doi.org/10.3922/j.psns.2012.2.07.

Edelmann, M. N., & Krull, K. R. (2013). Brain volume and cognitive function in adult survivors of childhood acute lymphoblastic leukemia. *Translational Pediatrics, 2*(4), 143–147.

Lofstad, G. E., Reinfjell, T., Hestad, K., & Diseth, T. H. (2009). Cognitive outcome in children and adolescents treated for acute lymphoblastic leukaemia with chemotherapy alone. *Acta Paediatrica, 98*(1), 180–186.

Pääkkö, E., Harila-Saari, A., Vanionpää, L., Himanen, S., Pyhtinen, J., & Lanning, M. (2000). White matter changes on MRI during treatment in children with acute lymphoblastic leukemia: Correlation with neuropsychological findings. *Pediatric Blood & Cancer, 35*(5), 456–461.

Prassopoulos, P., Carouras, D., Golfinopoulos, S., Evlogias, N., Theodoropoulos, V., & Panagiotou, J. (1996). Quantitative assessment of cerebral atrophy during and after treatment in children with acute lymphoblastic leukemia. *Investigational Radiology, 12*, 749–754.

Pui, C.-H. (2003). *Treatment of acute leukemias: New directions for clinical research*. New York: Humana Press.

Zeller, B., Tamnes, C. K., Kanellopoulos, A., Amlien, I. K., Andersson, S., Due-Tønnessen, P., Fjell, A. M., Walhovd, K. B., Westlye, L. T., & Ruud, E. (2013). Reduced neuroanatomic volumes in long-term survivors of childhood acute lymphoblastic leukemia. *Journal of Clinical Oncology, 31*(17), 2078–2085.

Acute Myelogenous Leukemia

Jacqueline L. Cunningham
Department of Psychology, Children's Hospital of Philadelphia, Philadelphia, PA, USA

Synonyms

Acute myeloid leukemia; AML

Definition

Acute myelogenous leukemia (AML) is a form of cancer of the white blood cells (leukocytes). It is a relatively rare cancer that occurs more commonly in adults than in children, with more men affected than women. The median age at diagnosis is 63 years.

Current Knowledge

Symptoms

Acute forms of leukemia are characterized by the rapid proliferation of immature blood cells which rapidly crowd out mature, functional cells. In AML, the cell type is granuloid, whose cancerous change disrupts its normal ability to form red cells, some types of white cells, and platelets. Resulting symptoms are anemia, easy bruising and bleeding, and disruption to the body's ability to resist infection. Impaired cognition and fatigue are also strongly associated with AML. Whereas impairments in these areas have been attributed to effects of chemotherapy, recent research by Meyers, Albitar, and Estey (2005) has identified differing cytokine levels present prior to chemotherapy as also contributing to these symptoms.

Pathophysiology

The malignant cell in AML is the myeloblast, a mutated and immature cell in the granulocytic series, which undergoes combinations with other mutations, to produce a leukemic clone of cells. Because the process contributes to much diversity and heterogeneity in cell differentiation, the diagnosis of AML can be challenging. It remains important, however, since the chromosomal structure of the leukemic cells is the disease's most critical prognostic factor.

Treatment

Treatment in AML consists primarily of chemotherapy, with the goal of achieving remission. Without postremission (consolidation) therapy, almost all patients eventually relapse. Neurocognitive and neuropsychiatric symptoms are highly prevalent in patients with cancer and cause significant impairments in their ability to function. Whereas such impairments are known to be associated with aggressive cancer treatment, they are additionally attributed to biologic mechanisms underlying the cancer itself. Recent research (Meyers et al. 2005) on AML has made linkages between cytokine-immunologic activation and factors including cognitive functioning, significant fatigue, and quality of life in AML patients studied *prior* to the initiation of treatment.

Cross-References

▶ Acute Lymphoblastic Leukemia
▶ Leukemia
▶ Neoplasms

References and Readings

Meyers, C. A., Albitar, M., & Estey, E. (2005). Cognitive impairment, fatigue, and cytokine levels in patients with acute myelogenous leukemia or myelodysplastic syndrome. *Cancer, 104*, 788–793.
Pui, C.-H. (2003). *Treatment of acute leukemias: New directions for clinical research.* New York: Humana Press.

Acute Radiation Somnolence

Jacqueline L. Cunningham
Department of Psychology, Children's Hospital of Philadelphia, Philadelphia, PA, USA

Definition

Acute radiation somnolence is a relatively transient and benign effect of cranial irradiation. It is manifested as sleepiness occurring during irradiation used to treat brain tumors. Multiple variables are associated, including total dose, fraction size, time between fractions, treatment volume, and concurrent chemotherapy. It occurs in both children and adults and usually affects daily functioning during the course of treatment and is a less common acute side effect during radiotherapy than other complications that depend on the specific structures in the pathway of the target of the radiation. Although it is self-limiting, and resolves with medication and with the termination of irradiation, symptoms can be upsetting to patients. Nursing intervention which focuses on preparation through counseling and education serves to alleviate distress. Acute radiation somnolence is usually treated with steroids.

Cross-References

▶ Radiation Oncology
▶ Radiotherapy

References and Readings

Brady, L. W., Heilmann, H. P., Molls, M., & Schlegel, W. (2006). *New techniques in radiation oncology.* New York: Springer.
Walker, A. J., Ruzevick, J., Malayeri, A. A., Rigamonti, D., Lim, M., Redmond, K. J., & Kleinberg, L. (2014). *Future Oncology, 10*(7), 1277–1297.

Acute Respiratory Distress Syndrome

Dona Locke
Psychiatry and Psychology, Mayo Clinic, Scottsdale, AZ, USA

Synonyms

Adult respiratory distress syndrome; Respiratory distress syndrome

Definition

Acute respiratory distress syndrome (ARDS) is the presence of pulmonary edema in the absence of volume overload or depressed left ventricular function and is characterized by the development of sudden breathlessness within hours to days of an inciting event. ARDS is not a specific disease; instead, it is a type of severe, acute lung dysfunction that is associated with a variety of diseases and trauma.

Historical Background

In the past, ARDS signified adult respiratory distress syndrome to separate this from infant respiratory distress syndrome seen in premature infants. However, this type of pulmonary edema can also occur in children, so ARDS has gradually evolved to mean acute rather than adult.

Current Knowledge

ARDS typically develops within 12–48 h after the inciting event, although, in rare instances, it may take up to a few days. Persons developing ARDS are critically ill, often with multisystem organ failure. It is a life-threatening condition; therefore, hospitalization is required for prompt management.

ARDS is associated with severe and diffuse injury to the alveolar-capillary membrane (the air sacs and small blood vessels) of the lungs. Fluid accumulates in some alveoli of the lungs, while some other alveoli collapse. This alveolar damage impedes the exchange of oxygen and carbon dioxide, which leads to a reduced concentration of oxygen in the blood. Low levels of oxygen in the blood cause damage to other vital organs of the body such as the kidneys.

The 1994 American-European Consensus Committee defines ARDS as the acute onset of bilateral infiltrates on chest radiography, a partial pressure of arterial oxygen (PaO_2) to fraction of inspired oxygen (FIO_2) ratio of less than 200 mmHg and a pulmonary artery occlusion pressure of less than 18, or the absence of clinical evidence of left arterial hypertension. Revised definition in 2012 (JAMA) describes criteria for mild, moderate, and severe ARDS based on PaO_2 and FIO_2. Mortality rate is approximately 27% for mild, 32% for moderate, and 45% for severe.

Death usually results from multisystem organ failure rather than lung failure alone.

Causes: A number of clinical conditions are associated with the development of ARDS.

- Sepsis and the systemic inflammatory response syndrome (SIRS) are the most common conditions associated with the development of ARDS.
- Severe traumatic injury (especially multiple fractures), severe head injury, and pulmonary contusion are strongly associated with the development of ARDS. In traumatic injury, factures of the long bones can cause ARDS through fat embolism. In severe brain injury, ARDS is thought to develop owing to a sudden discharge of the sympathetic nervous system, which then leads to acute pulmonary hypertension and injury to the pulmonary capillary bed. In pulmonary contusions, ARDS develops through direct trauma to the lung.
- Multiple blood transfusions are an independent risk factor for ARDS. The risk is independent of the reason for the transfusion or the coexistence of trauma. The incidence of ARDS increases with the number of units of blood transfused. If the patient has preexisting abnormal liver functioning or a coagulation abnormality, the risk is further increased.
- Near drowning can be another cause of ARDS. Development of ARDS is slightly more common with saltwater than with freshwater. Aspiration leads to an osmotic gradient that favors movement of water into air spaces of the lung. Aspiration may be visible with chest radiography, although the chest radiograph may be normal early in the course of the disease.
- Smoke inhalation is another possible cause of ARDS. Smoke inhalation causes lung tissue damage from direct heat, toxic chemicals, and particulate matter carried into the lung. Patients with smoke inhalation initially may be asymptomatic, but patients with airway burns, exposure to toxic fumes, or exposure to carbon monoxide should be monitored closely for the development of ARDS, even if the symptoms are initially absent.

- Overdoses of narcotics, tricyclic antidepressants, and other sedatives have been associated with the development of ARDS. Overdoses of tricyclic antidepressants are the most common. This risk is independent of the risk from concurrent aspiration.

Medical treatment for ARDS:

- People with ARDS require hospitalization and treatment in an intensive care unit.
- There is no specific treatment for ARDS, but, rather, treatment is primarily supportive using a mechanical respirator and supplemental oxygen.
- Diuretics can be given to eliminate fluid from the lungs. However, fluids are often given via IV to provide nutrition and prevent dehydration, but fluids must be carefully monitored to avoid fluid accumulation in the lungs.
- Antibiotic therapy may be administered to treat infection, which is often the underlying cause of ARDS.
- Corticosteroids may sometimes be given late in the process of ARDS or if the patient is in shock. If the patient is in shock, drugs to counteract low blood pressure caused by shock may be administered.
- If the patient is experiencing anxiety, this can be treated with antianxiety medications.

Respiratory therapists may see these patients to provide inhaled drugs to decrease inflammation and provide respiratory comfort.

Because of the acute and medically serious nature of ARDS, it would be unlikely for neuropsychological exam to be requested when a person is acutely ill with ARDS. Mortality with ARDS is 30–40%, and the person would typically be treated in an intensive care unit. If the person survives, outpatient neuropsychological evaluation could be requested, and results may show memory deficits related to the hypoxia as well as neuropsychological deficits related to the underlying medical cause for ARDS (e.g., severe TBI, near drowning, sepsis, medication overdose).

Cross-References

▶ Anoxia

References and Readings

Acute Respiratory Distress Syndrome. (2012). The Berlin definition. *Journal of the American Medical Association, 307*(23), 2526–2533.

Bernard, G. R., Artigas, A., Brigham, K. L., Charlet, J., Falke, K., Hudson, L., Lamy, M., Legall, J. R., Morris, A., & Spragg, R. (1994). Report of the American-European consensus conference on ARDS: Definitions, mechanisms, relevant outcomes and clinical trial coordination. *Intensive Care Medicine, 20*, 225–232.

Acute Stress Disorder

Daniel W. Klyce
Virginia Commonwealth University – School of Medicine, Richmond, VA, USA

Synonyms

Acute stress response; Stress reaction

Short Description or Definition

Acute stress disorder (ASD) is defined in the *Diagnostic and Statistical Manual of Mental Disorders* (5th ed.; *DSM-5*; American Psychiatric Association 2013) by a pattern of symptoms associated with exposure to an actual or threatened trauma or stressor. Exposure may involve (1) direct experience of traumatic events, (2) personally witnessing events, (3) learning of events that occurred to others, and (4) repeated or extreme exposure to details of traumatic events. Symptoms associated with the exposure may include intrusion symptoms (i.e., involuntary memories, distressing dreams, flashbacks, intense responses to triggers), negative mood, dissociative symptoms, avoidance symptoms, and symptoms of physiological arousal (i.e., sleep disturbance, irritability/anger, hypervigilance, poor concentration, and exaggerated startle response). To be diagnosed as ASD, symptoms must persist for at least 3 days and not longer than a month (at which point they might be more representative of posttraumatic stress disorder).

Categorization

The disorder is classified with the trauma- and stressor-related disorders in *DSM-5*.

Current Knowledge

Development and Course
Prevalence rates for ASD tend to vary in association with the nature or severity of the stressor and situational factors following the onset of the stressor (e.g., the persistence of the initial threat). Prevalence rates tend to be higher if the trauma involves interpersonal violence, and these rates have been reported to range from as much as 20% to 50% of such cases. Other common index traumas include motor vehicle accidents, severe burns, work-related or industrial accidents, and traumatic medical events. In a 2011 review of studies reporting incidence of ASD associated with a variety of stressors, Bryant found rates of ASD ranging from 7% to 28%, with a mean incidence rate of 13%. By definition, ASD cannot be diagnosed beyond 1 month from the onset of the stressor or trauma. During this period, symptoms may worsen along with exacerbation of stress. Women appear to be at higher risk for the development of ASD. The risk of ASD also appears to increase among individuals who have a history of other psychological disorders and who perceive the index trauma as more severe.

Associated Disorders and Current Research
Originally, ASD was developed to identify individuals who may eventually develop symptoms of posttraumatic stress disorder (PTSD). Acute stress disorder remains strongly associated with PTSD, with at least half of trauma survivors who have a diagnosis of ASD progressing to PTSD. Among individuals with a diagnosis of PTSD, it is estimated that 48% originally had symptoms of ASD. Acute stress disorder is a narrower form of an acute stress reaction with a prominent anxiety or fear component. The diagnosis of adjustment disorder more appropriately captures the breadth of disruptive psychological reactions to stress or trauma that may be characterized by grief, anger, depression, etc. Acute stress disorder may also be difficult to distinguish from postconcussive symptoms following head trauma. These two disorders share many physiological, cognitive, emotional, and behavioral sequelae (e.g., sensitivity to environmental stimuli, difficulty concentrating, and irritability). Recent research has revealed that individuals exposed to experimentally induced acute psychosocial stressors exhibit impairments in attentional processes and spatial working memory (e.g., Sänger et al., 2014; Olver et al., 2015).

Assessment and Treatment
A diagnosis of ASD should capture an individual's current distress and indicate the importance of facilitating treatment and resources. An essential feature of assessment involves the identification of an index stressor or trauma. Assessment and treatment may be complicated in situations involving persistent threat. Given the temporal proximity to traumatic events associated with a diagnosis of ASD (i.e., as little as 3 days), it may be important to rule out physical or medical conditions associated with trauma or to facilitate medical stabilization and treatment. Acute stress disorder may be assessed with measures such as the Acute Stress Disorder Scale (Bryant et al., 2000) and the National Stressful Events Survey Acute Stress Disorder Short Scale (Kilpatric et al., 2013).

Given the relatively brief course of symptoms associated with ASD, it has been difficult to establish an evidence base for potential interventions. Generally, once ASD has been diagnosed, it is helpful to provide psychoeducation and normalization regarding common psychological reactions to trauma, along with normative expectations for recovery. Given the likelihood that individuals with ASD may go on to develop PTSD, it may be helpful to facilitate case management and referrals for mental health treatment including psychopharmacological or psychotherapeutic treatments for posttraumatic stress.

During the acute phase of recovery from a stressor or trauma, it may also be possible to provide brief interventions for cognitive and physiological symptoms of anxiety. These may include strengths-based coping strategies, behavioral strategies for addressing symptoms of anxious arousal (e.g., relaxation training), and elements of trauma-focused cognitive-behavioral therapies to address common negative or catastrophic thoughts associated with the trauma.

See Also

▶ Adjustment Disorder
▶ Postconcussion Syndrome
▶ Post-traumatic Stress Disorder

References

American Psychiatric Association. (2013). *Diagnostic and statistical manual of mental disorders* (5th ed.). Arlington: American Psychiatric Association Publishing.

Bryant, R. A. (2010). Acute stress disorder as a predictor of posttraumatic stress disorder: A systematic review. *The Journal of Clinical Psychiatry, 72*(2), 233–239.

Bryant, R. A., Moulds, M. L., & Guthrie, R. M. (2000). Acute stress disorder scale: A self-report measure of acute stress disorder. *Psychological Assessment, 12*(1), 61–68.

Bryant, R. A., Friedman, M. J., Spiegel, D., Ursano, R., & Strain, J. (2011). A review of acute stress disorder in DSM-5. *Depression and Anxiety, 28*(9), 802–817.

Kilpatrick, D. G., Resnick, H. S., & Friedman, M. J. (2013). *National stressful events survey ASD short scale (NSESSS-ASD)*. Arlington: American Psychiatric Association.

Olver, J. S., Pinney, M., Maruff, P., & Norman, T. R. (2015). Impairments of spatial working memory and attention following acute psychosocial stress. *Stress and Health, 31*(2), 115–123.

Sänger, J., Bechtold, L., Schoofs, D., Blaszkewicz, M., & Wascher, E. (2014). The influence of acute stress on attention mechanisms and its electrophysiological correlates. *Frontiers in Behavioral Neuroscience, 8*, 353.

Ursano, R. J., Bell, C., Eth, S., Friedman, M., Norwood, A., Pfefferbaum, B., ... & Charles, S. C. (2004). Practice guideline for the treatment of patients with acute stress disorder and posttraumatic stress disorder. *The American Journal of Psychiatry, 161*(Suppl 11), 3–31.

Adaptive Behavior Assessment System: Third Edition

Patti L. Harrison[1] and Thomas Oakland[2]
[1]School Psychology, The University of Alabama, Tuscaloosa, AL, USA
[2]Department of Educational Psychology, College of Education University of Florida, Gainesville, FL, USA

Synonyms

ABAS; ABAS-II; ABAS-3

Description

The Adaptive Behavior Assessment System – Third Edition (ABAS-3; Harrison and Oakland 2015) provides an assessment of adaptive behavior and skills for persons from birth through age 89. Five forms are available: parent/primary caregiver form (for ages 0–5), teacher/day-care provider form (for ages 2–5), parent form (for ages 5–21), teacher form (for ages 5–21), and adult form (for ages 16–89). The ABAS-3 standardization samples are large (4,500) and representative of 2010 US census data with respect to gender, race/ethnicity, and socioeconomic status and included individuals with typical abilities as well as those with disabilities. Forms are available in Spanish in the USA and are being adapted for use in a number of other countries, including in Europe and Asia.

Foundation and Structure

Criteria for a diagnosis of intellectual disability have been identified in policy and legislation for community services and special education. A diagnosis of intellectual disability requires documentation of deficits in both intelligence and

---

Thomas Oakland: deceased.

adaptive behavior. Although supported by its foundation in assessment for intellectual disabilities, adaptive behavior assessment has broader uses for numerous individuals with a variety of disabilities and challenges. Adaptive behavior assessment is conducted routinely to identify strengths and weaknesses and plan supports and services for children and adults with limitations that may interfere with daily functioning.

The ABAS (Harrison and Oakland 2000) and ABAS-II (Harrison and Oakland 2003) preceded the development of the ABAS-3. As with previous editions, the ABAS-3 was developed to be a measure of adaptive behavior consistent with current definitions (e.g., most recently those promulgated by the American Psychiatric Association's (APA 2013) Diagnostic and Statistical Manual of Mental Disorders and the American Association on Intellectual and Developmental Disabilities' (AAIDD 2010) models of adaptive behavior) that underscored the importance of three broad domains of adaptive behavior: conceptual, social, and practical. In addition, the three editions of the ABAS have included measurement of ten specific adaptive skill areas commonly identified in definitions and measure of adaptive behavior: communication, community use, functional academics, health and safety, home or school living, leisure, self-care, self-direction, social, and work skills.

Scaled scores (M = 10, SD = 3) for adaptive skill areas are provided (Table 1). Ten skill area scores combine to produce standard scores (M = 100, SD = 15) in their respective domains: conceptual (communication, functional academics, and self-direction), social (social skills and leisure), and practical (self-care, home or school living, community use, health and safety, and work for adults). Motor skill is an additional adaptive skill area assessed for young children but is not included in a broad domain. A General Adaptive Composite standard score (M = 100, SD = 15) also is derived from the adaptive skill area scores.

Item Rating Data

ABAS-3 items are administered in rating scales completed by respondents (e.g., parents,

caregivers, teachers, other relatives) familiar with the daily functioning of an individual. All items are scored on a four-point scale: 0 (cannot perform the behavior), 1 (can perform the behavior yet does not), 2 (performs the behavior sometimes), and 4 (performs the behavior most or all of the time). This feature is consistent with the World Health Organization's International Classification of Functioning (Mpofu and Oakland 2010) effort to distinguish abilities and performance.

Respondents may indicate that they guessed item scores for behaviors that they have not observed but can estimate based on the person's performance of other skills. Data from adaptive skill areas with four or more guesses should not be used. The ABAS-3's scoring and reporting system informs clinicians of interventions likely to promote the development of selected behaviors associated with critical items.

Psychometric Data

General Adaptive Composite and domain standard scores generally range from 40 to 120. Consistent with all measures of adaptive behavior, the ABAS-3 is more sensitive to the assessment of adaptive behavior and skills at lower to average ranges than at higher ranges. Cut scores are not provided by disability category; instead, reliance is placed on diagnostic standards established by state and national authorities.

The ABAS-3 demonstrates suitable psychometric qualities. Internal consistency is high, with reliability coefficients of 0.85–0.99 for the General Adaptive Composite and three adaptive behavior domains and somewhat lower coefficients for the briefer adaptive skill areas. Test-retest and interrater reliability coefficients generally are in the 0.70s and 0.80s for the General Adaptive Composite, three domains, and skill areas. The ABAS-3 construct validity is strong as displayed through factor analyses. Its concurrent validity with the Vineland Adaptive Behavior Scales – Second Edition – is generally high. The validity of the ABAS-3 also is supported by evidence that its scores distinguish between

Adaptive Behavior Assessment System: Third Edition, Table 1 Adaptive skills and three adaptive domains (Adapted from Harrison and Oakland 2015)

Adaptive skills	
Communication	Speech, language, and listening skills needed for communication with others, including vocabulary, responding to questions, and participating in conversations
Community use	Skills needed for functioning in the community, including use of community services, shopping, and getting around in the neighborhood
Functional academics (functional pre-academics for young children)	Basic reading, writing, math, and other skills needed for daily functioning, including telling time, measurement, writing, and counting money
Home living (school living for teacher forms)	Skills needed for basic care of a home or school setting, including cleaning, straightening, cooking, and completing chores
Health and safety	Skills needed to promote health and safety and respond to illness and injury, including following safety rules, using medication, and staying away from danger
Leisure	Skills needed for participating in leisure and recreational activities, including playing, attending community activities, and following game rules
Self-care	Skills needed for personal care including eating, dressing, bathing, toileting, and grooming
Self-direction	Skills needed for independence, responsibility, and self-control, including completing tasks, keeping schedules, following directions, and making choices
Social	Skills needed to interact socially and get along with others, including having friends, demonstrating emotions, and helping others
Work	Skills needed for successful functioning in a part-time or full-time work setting, including completing tasks, working with supervisors, and following a schedule (completed only for individuals who have a job)
Motor skills[a]	Basic gross and fine motor skills needed for movement and manual manipulation of objects, including sitting, standing, walking, and fine motor control
Three domains and associated skill areas	
Conceptual	Includes communication, functional academics, self-direction,
Practical	Includes social skills and leisure skills
Social	Includes self-care, home/school living, community use, health and safety, and work skills
General adaptive composite: Derived from all adaptive skill areas	

[a]Although fine and gross motor development is not included as one of the ten skills identified by the American Association on Intellectual and Developmental Disabilities, it is included in some scales of adaptive behavior, including the ABAS-3 parent/primary caregiver form (for ages 0-5) and teacher/daycare provider form (for ages 2-5)

individuals with typical functioning and those in clinical groups, such as individuals with intellectual disabilities, autism, and attention disorders.

Clinical Uses

Measures of adaptive behavior have been most important in the assessment of persons with intellectual disabilities The ABAS-3 is useful in this diagnosis as well as in intervention planning and monitoring for this and other disorders. The ABAS-3 also may assist in promoting an understanding of the impact on daily life activities for people with a number of other disorders and limitations, as described in resources about the ABAS-II and applicable to the comparable ABAS-3 (e.g., Ditterline et al. 2008; Harman et al. 2009; Oakland and Harrison 2008; Olley and Cox 2008).

The ABAS-3 provides important information for the assessment and planning services for children with limitations often diagnosed first during infancy or early childhood including autism; disorders of attention, communication, conduct, elimination, feeding and eating, learning, and motor skills; and pervasive developmental disorders. The ABAS-3 is useful with children and adolescents who display disorders including attention deficit hyperactivity, acquired brain injury, auditory or visual impairment, autism, developmental delays, emotional/behavioral disorders, learning disabilities, and physical impairments.

Adults diagnosed with such disorders as anxiety, acute stress, or adjustment disorder, bipolar disorder, depression, mood disorders, psychosis, Parkinson's, postpartum depression, substance abuse, schizophrenia, and sleep disturbance may display impairments in their functional daily living skills. Older adults diagnosed with Alzheimer's type dementia and other cognitive and neuropsychological disorders with late-life onset often display impairments in their functional daily living skills. Although data from the ABAS-3 may not be crucial in the diagnosis of some of these disorders, ABAS-3 data will promote an understanding of their impact on daily living skills. The ABAS-3 is used in the assessment of intellectual disabilities among death row inmates in light of the 2002 US Supreme Court Atkins decision.

Cross-References

▶ Activities of Daily Living (ADL)
▶ Activity Restrictions, Limitations
▶ Intellectual Disability

References

American Association on Intellectual and Developmental Disabilities. (2010). *Intellectual disability: Definition, classification, and systems of support* (11th ed.). Washington, DC: Author.

American Psychiatric Association. (2013). *Diagnostic and statistical manual of mental disorders* (5th ed.). Washington, DC: Author.

Ditterline, J., Banner, D., Oakland, T., & Becton, D. (2008). Adaptive behavior profiles of students with disabilities. *Journal of Applied School Psychology, 24,* 191–208.

Harman, J., Smith-Bonahue, T., & Oakland, T. (2009). Assessment of adaptive behavior development in young children. In E. Mpofu & T. Oakland (Eds.), *Rehabilitation and health assessment: Applying ICF guidelines.* New York: Springer.

Harrison, P., & Oakland, T. (2000). *Adaptive behavior assessment system.* San Antonio: Psychological Corporation.

Harrison, P., & Oakland, T. (2003). *Adaptive behavior assessment system* (2nd ed.). San Antonio: Psychological Corporation.

Harrison, P., & Oakland, T. (2015). *Adaptive behavior assessment system* (3rd ed.). Torrance: Western Psychological Services.

Mpofu, E., & Oakland, T. (2010). *Assessment in rehabilitation and health.* Upper Saddle River: Merrill.

Oakland, T., & Harrison, P. (2008). *Adaptive behavior assessment system-II: Clinical use and interpretation.* New York: Elsevier.

Olley, J. G., & Cox, A. (2008). Assessment of adaptive behavior in adult forensic cases: The use of the ABAS-II. In T. Oakland & P. Harrison (Eds.), *Adaptive behavior assessment system-II: Clinical use and interpretation.* Boston: Elsevier.

Adenoma

Ethan Moitra
Department of Psychiatry and Human Behavior, Brown University, Providence, RI, USA

Definition

A benign tumor of glandular origin. There are three types of adenomas: tubular (most common, tubelike structure), villous (least common, most likely to become cancerous, ruffled structure), and tubulovillous (blend of tubular and villous structures). Adenomas do not metastasize, though they can develop into malignancies known as adenocarcinomas. Most adenomas occur spontaneously. The tumor may occur throughout the endocrine system, including the pituitary gland.

Pituitary adenomas occur at a much higher incidence in adults than in children. Because their invasiveness is local, they are almost always benign and can be difficult to detect. There is the secreting and the nonsecreting type. Clinical symptoms come from the endocrine dysfunction or from mass effect and include headaches, hypopituitarism, and visual loss (caused by compression in the optic chiasm). Treatment of pituitary adenomas includes correction of electrolyte dysfunction, replacement of pituitary hormones, surgical resection, and radiotherapy.

Cross-References

► Pituitary Adenoma

References and Readings

Mazzaferri, E. L., & Saaman, N. A. (Eds.). (1993). *Endocrine tumors*. Boston: Blackwell.

Adjustment Disorder

Daniel W. Klyce
Virginia Commonwealth University – School of Medicine, Richmond, VA, USA

Synonyms

Stress reaction

Short Description or Definition

Adjustment disorders are defined in the *Diagnostic and Statistical Manual of Mental Disorders* (5th ed.; *DSM-5*; American Psychiatric Association 2013) by patterns of clinically significant behavioral or emotional symptoms related to a distinct stressor. The behavioral or emotional response is usually disruptive to everyday functioning, disproportionate to the intensity or severity of the stressor, and must begin within 3 months of the stressor's onset. Symptoms do not last for longer than 6 months from the time the stressor or its consequences have resolved. The adjustment disorder may be characterized by depressed mood, anxiety, mixed anxiety and depressed mood, disturbance of conduct, mixed disturbance of emotions and conduct, or otherwise unspecified. The adjustment disorder is specified to be "acute" if the pattern of response lasts less than 6 months or "persistent" if longer than 6 months. Adjustment disorders are distinguished from normal bereavement or the exacerbation of a preexisting psychological disorder.

Categorization

The disorder is classified with the trauma- and stressor-related disorders in *DSM-5*.

Current Knowledge

Development and Course

An adjustment disorder may develop from a variety of stressors, including single events, recurrent events, ongoing or continuous stressors, and developmental or social milestones (e.g., graduation, marriage, retirement, etc.). The prevalence rate for adjustment disorders as a primary diagnosis in outpatient mental health settings is estimated to range from 5% to 20% (Casey and Bailey 2011; American Psychiatric Association 2013). Adjustment disorders are frequently diagnosed in medical settings and associated with such conditions as cancers, critical illness, traumatic injuries, childhood-onset diabetes, etc. The disorder accounts for as much as 50% of diagnoses encountered by psychiatric consult and liaison services in hospital settings (American Psychiatric Association, 2013). The expected course of an adjustment disorder is that symptoms will remit within 6 months of the resolution of the initial stressor.

Associated Disorders and Current Research

Adjustment disorders are often associated with symptoms of depressed mood, anxiety, grief, and acute or posttraumatic stress. Up to 25% of adolescents and 60% of adults with a diagnosis of an adjustment disorder have been noted to engage in suicidal behavior (Kryzhanovskaya and Canterbury, 2001; Pelkonen et al., 2005; Casey and Bailey, 2011). Suicidal behavior associated with an adjustment disorder tends to occur earlier in the course of the disorder, whereas suicidal behaviors associated with major depression tend to occur later. When compared to major depressive disorder, adjustment disorders tend to be associated with shorter time between communication of suicidal ideation to completion, lower hospital readmission rates, and shorter hospital stays. Common criticisms of the validity of adjustment disorder have been related to the diagnosis being too broad, overused to justify reimbursement, and resulting in overpathologizing reactions to everyday stressors.

Assessment and Treatment

Diagnosis of an adjustment disorder depends upon identifying a distinct stressor and distinguishing normal from pathological psychological responses to the onset of a stressor in the context of factors such as cultural normativity and relative personal circumstances. It may also be challenging to diagnose an adjustment disorder among individuals with neurological injuries or illnesses due to factors such as emotional lability or injury-related sequelae that impact social functioning.

Given the expectation for a relatively brief course of symptoms (i.e., less than 6 months after resolution of the stressor), it is challenging to establish an evidence base for empirically supported interventions. Treatment tends to involve brief interventions with emphasis on problem-solving skills, stress management strategies, and medical management or behavioral health interventions for health-related stressors.

See Also

▶ Acute Stress Disorder
▶ Major Depression
▶ Post-traumatic Stress Disorder
▶ Stress
▶ Stress Management
▶ Trauma- and Stressor-Related Disorders

References

American Psychiatric Association. (2013). *Diagnostic and statistical manual of mental disorders* (5th ed.). Arlington: American Psychiatric Association Publishing.

Arends, I., Bruinvels, D. J., Rebergen, D. S., Nieuwenhuijsen, K., Madan, I., Neumeyer-Gromen, A., Bültmann, U., & Verbeek, J. H. (2012). Interventions to facilitate return to work in adults with adjustment disorders. *Cochrane Database of Systematic Reviews, 12*, CD006389.

Casey, P. (2014). Adjustment disorder: New developments. *Current Psychiatry Reports, 16*(6), 1–8.

Casey, P., & Bailey, S. (2011). Adjustment disorders: The state of the art. *World Psychiatry, 10*(1), 11–18.

Kryzhanovskaya, L., & Canterbury, R. (2001). Suicidal behavior in patients with adjustment disorders. *Crisis: The Journal of Crisis Intervention and Suicide Prevention, 22*(3), 125.

Pelkonen, M., Marttunen, M., Henriksson, M., & Lönnqvist, J. (2005). Suicidality in adjustment disorder. *European Child & Adolescent Psychiatry, 14*(3), 174–180.

Admissibility

Moira C. Dux
US Department of Veteran Affairs, Baltimore, MD, USA

Definition

Admissibility of evidence refers to any testimonial, documentary material, or other form of tangible evidence that can be considered by the trier of fact, most typically a judge or a jury, in the context of a judicial or administrative proceeding. In order for evidence to be admissible, it must be relevant, non-prejudicial, and possess some indicia of reliability. For example, if evidence consists of a witness testimonial, it must be established that the witness is credible and that he/she has knowledge of that which he/she is declaring. For neuropsychologists, a central issue is the admissibility of one's data and opinions. Rules 401, 402, and 702–705 from Article VII of the Federal Rules of Evidence (FRE) relate to "Opinions and Expert Testimony." Perhaps of most relevance to psychologists is rule FRE 702 which states, "If scientific, technical, or other specialized knowledge will assist the trier of fact to understand the evidence or to determine a fact in issue, a witness qualified as an expert by knowledge, skill, experience, training or education, may testify thereto in the form of an opinion or otherwise." In other words, the expert should possess some form of knowledge that a typical judge or juror would not be expected to know or understand. Rule 703 states, "The facts or data in the particular case upon which an expert bases an opinion or inference may be those perceived by or made known to the expert at or before the hearing. If of a type reasonably relied upon by experts in the particular field in forming opinions or inferences upon the subject, the facts or data need not be admissible in evidence in order for the opinion or the inference to be admitted. Facts or data that are otherwise inadmissible shall not be disclosed to the jury by the proponent of the opinion or inference unless the court determines that their probative value in assisting the jury to evaluate the expert's opinion substantially outweighs their prejudicial effect."

Several important cases have addressed the admissibility of scientific testimony. In the case of *Frye v. United States* (1923), the *Frye* standard was established which stated that only scientific methods and concepts with "general acceptance" within a particular field are admissible. In the more recent case of *Daubert v. Merrell Dow* (1993), it was determined that scientific testimony has to abide by two criteria; the testimony must be (a) scientifically valid and (b) relevant to the case at hand.

Cross-References

▶ Daubert v. Merrell Dow Pharmaceuticals (1993)

References and Readings

A complete list of the federal rules of evidence. Available at: http://judiciary.house.gov/media/pdfs/printers/108th/evid2004.pdf

Greiffenstein, M. F. (2009). Basics of forensic neuropsychology. In J. Morgan & J. Ricker (Eds.), *Textbook of clinical neuropsychology*. New York: Taylor & Francis.

Jenkins v. United States, 307 F. 2d 637 (1962).

Kaufmann, P. M. (2008). Admissibility of neuropsychological evidence in criminal cases: Competency, insanity, culpability, and mitigation. In R. Denney & J. Sullivan (Eds.), *Clinical neuropsychology in the criminal forensic setting*. New York: Guilford.

Adoption Studies

Rohan Palmer[1] and Martin Hahn[2]
[1]Institute for Behavioral Genetics, University of Colorado at Boulder, Boulder, CO, USA
[2]Department of Biology, William Paterson University, Wayne, NJ, USA

Definition

Adoption studies typically compare pairs of persons, e.g., adopted child and adoptive mother or adopted child and biological mother to assess genetic and environmental influences on behavior.

Current Knowledge

Design

Familial resemblance of behaviors is due to genetic and/or common familial environmental influences. Adoption studies provide a direct test of the role of both factors. This is possible by drawing comparisons between families that share genetic and environmental influences and families that share only genetic or environmental factors. Adoption creates two types of families. The "genetic family" consists of pairs of genetically related individuals who do not share a common family environment (e.g., biological parent and adopted-away child). The similarity between these pairs of relatives provides a direct estimate of genetic effects on behaviors. The second type family is the "environmental family," which is made up of pairs of individuals who are not genetically related but who share a common family environment (e.g., adoptive parent and adopted child). The similarity between pairs of relatives from an "environmental family" indicates the presence of environmental influences on behavior. Adoption studies utilize either parent-offspring pairs or sibling pairs. Because data on biological parents and siblings of adoptees are sometimes rare, comparison between "genetic-plus-environmental" families (i.e., intact families) and adoptive families also provides evidence of genetic and environmental influences.

Relevance to Neuropsychology

The Colorado Adoption Project has been collecting longitudinal data on biological and adoptive parents and their biological or adopted children for over 30 years (Petrill et al. 2003). In one set of analyses from that project reported by Plomin et al. (1997), parent-offspring correlations were calculated for children aged 3–16 years. The results of the analyses show increasing correlations across those ages between biological parents and their adopted-away children on such special cognitive abilities as verbal skills and perceptual speed. Correlations between adoptive parents and adopted children remained about zero across those ages. The authors interpret the results to indicate that heritability increases for those special cognitive abilities with age and that the role of shared environment is low or nonexistent.

Today, adoption study data are used to assess the genetic and environmental influence on a variety of clinical outcomes that include drug addiction (Young et al. 2006) and age of sexual initiation (Bricker et al. 2006), to name a few.

Cross-References

► Twin Studies

References and Readings

Bricker, J. B., Stallings, M. C., Corley, R. P., Wadsworth, S. J., Bryan, A., Timberlake, D. S., et al. (2006). Genetic and environmental influences on age at sexual initiation in the Colorado adoption project. *Behavior Genetics, 36*, 820–832.

Petrill, S. A., Plomin, R., DeFries, J. C., & Hewitt, J. K. (2003). *Nature, nurture, and the transition to early adolescence.* Oxford: Oxford University Press.

Plomin, R., Fulker, D. W., Corley, R., & DeFries, J. C. (1997). Nature, nurture, and cognitive development from 1 to 16 years: A parent-offspring adoption study. *Psychological Science, 8*, 442–447.

Young, S. E., Rhee, S. H., Stallings, M. C., Corley, R. P., & Hewitt, J. K. (2006). Genetic and environmental vulnerabilities underlying adolescent substance use and problem use: General or specific? *Behavior Genetics, 36*, 603–615.

Adrenocorticotropic Hormone

David J. Libon
Departments of Geriatrics, Gerontology, and Psychology, Rowan University, New Jersey Institute for Successful Aging, School of Osteopathic Medicine, Stratford, NJ, USA

Definition

Adrenocorticotropic hormone (ACTH) is produced by the anterior pituitary gland and is a component of the hypothalamic-pituitary-adrenal axis. The release of ACTH is associated with the biological response to stress. The production of ACTH from the pituitary gland stimulates the adrenal glands to produce cortisol. The ACTH stimulation test is a common procedure used to assess the integrity of the adrenal glands. This test is used to identify a number of medical conditions including adrenal insufficiency, Addison's disease, and related medical conditions (Melmed and Kleinberg 2008).

Cross-References

► Hypothalamus

References and Readings

Melmed, S., & Kleinberg, D. (2008). Anterior pituitary. In H. M. Kronenberg, S. Melmed, K. S. Polonsky, & P. R. Larsen (Eds.), *Williams textbook of endocrinology* (11th ed.). Philadelphia: Saunders Elsevier.

Advanced Progressive Matrices

Victoria M. Leavitt[1] and Erica Weber[2]
[1]Cognitive Neuroscience Division, Columbia University Medical School, New York, NY, USA
[2]Department of Physical Medicine and Rehabilitation, Kessler Foundation, East Hanover, NJ, USA

Synonyms

APM

Description

First developed in the 1940s as an additional form of the Raven's progressive matrices, the advanced progressive matrices (APM) were developed to test intellectual efficiency in people with greater than average intellectual ability and to differentiate clearly between people of superior ability. A nonverbal test of inductive reasoning, the APM contains 48 items, presented as one set of 12 (Set I) and another of 36 (Set II). As in the standard version of the test (SPM), items are presented in black ink on a white background and become increasingly difficult as progress is made through each set. Although it is an untimed task, some clinicians administer the APM under time constraints. Set II can be used without a time limit to assess the examinee's total reasoning capacity. In this case, the examinee would first be shown the problems of Set I as examples to explain the principles of the test and would then be given approximately 1 h to complete the task. Alternately, Set I can be given as a short practice test followed by Set II as a speed test. In this case, 40 min is the time limit most commonly given for Set II.

Historical Background

The APM was designed in the 1940s to assess nonverbal abstract conceptualization skills of individuals for whom the standard version was too easy, that is, those achieving a raw score of 50 or above on the SPM. For children over 10 years of age with high intellectual functioning, the APM may be the appropriate version to ensure an adequate ceiling (Mills et al. 1993). For additional information about the historical background of the original test, please refer to the entry for Raven's Progressive Matrices.

Psychometric Data

Norms for adolescents (ages 12–16.5) and adults (18–68+; Sets I and II) for untimed (ages 12–70+) and timed (ages 17–28) versions are provided for North America (Raven et al. 1998). The reliability of the test is considered good, with high internal consistency of APM Set II, and split-half reliability coefficients varying between 0.83 and 0.87 (Strauss et al. 2006). Set I, as it has only 12 items, yields lower figures. Reliability of the original 48-item version was found to be high for adults and children aged 11.5 years + (>0.80); for younger children, it was only reasonably reliable (0.76). Overall, Set II scores increased by three points on retest (Raven et al. 1998).

Clinical Uses

The SPM and CPM have been found to be sensitive to a variety of neurological and neuropsychiatric conditions (Raven's Progressive Matrices). The APM, designed for use with higher functioning individuals, may be more appropriately employed for assessing an individual's capacity for decision-making or strategic planning at the management level in the workplace or in a higher education setting. However, clinical utility for the APM has been more recently realized, in that discrepancy between expected (via regression-based prediction models using NART scores; Freeman and Godfrey 2000) and observed APM scores has been used to detect intellectual decline in older adults (van den Berg et al. 2013). Additionally, the first set of items of the APM has been validated for use as a short form of Raven's SPM to assess fluid intelligence (Chieri et al. 2012).

Cross-References

▶ Colored Progressive Matrices
▶ Raven's Progressive Matrices
▶ Standard Progressive Matrices

References and Readings

Chiesi, F., Ciancaleoni, M., Galli, S., & Primi, C. (2012). Using the advanced progressive matrices (set I) to assess fluid ability in a short time frame: An item response theory-based analysis. *Psychological Assessment, 24*, 892–900.

Freeman, J., & Godfrey, H. (2000). The validity of the NART-RSPM index in detecting intellectual decline following traumatic brain injury: A controlled study. *British Journal of Clinical Psychology, 39*, 95–103.

Mills, C. J., Ablard, K. E., & Brody, L. E. (1993). The Raven's progressive matrices: Its usefulness for identifying gifted/talented students. *Roeper Review, 15*, 183–186.

Raven, J. C. (1965, 1994). Advanced progressive matrices sets I and II. Oxford: Oxford Psychologists Press.

Raven, J., Raven, J. C., & Court, J. H. (1996). *Progressive matrices: A perceptual test of intelligence. Individual form.* Oxford: Oxford Psychologists Press. (Original work published 1938).

Raven, J., Raven, J. C., & Court, J. H. (1998). *Raven manual: Section 4. Advanced progressive matrices.* Oxford: Oxford Psychologists Press Ltd..

Raven, J., Raven, J. C., & Court, J. H. (2003). *Manual for Raven's progressive matrices and vocabulary scales. Section 1: General overview.* San Antonio: Harcourt Assessment.

Strauss, E., Sherman, E. M. S., & Spreen, O. (2006). *A compendium of neuropsychological tests* (3rd ed.). NY: Oxford University Press.

van den Berg, E., Nys, G. M. S., Brands, A. M. A., Ruis, C., van Zandvoort, M. J. E., & Kessels, R. P. C. (2013). Exploration of the Raven APM – National Adult Reading Test discrepancy as a measure of intellectual decline in older adults. *Applied Neuropsychology: Adult, 20*, 7–14.

Advocacy

Amy J. Armstrong
Department of Rehabilitation Counseling, Virginia Commonwealth University, Richmond, VA, USA

The process of supporting or acting on behalf of a cause, facilitating equal community access and participation of individuals or groups that have typically been socially and/or economically marginalized. There are several types of advocacy to include:

Systems advocacy: the process in which any system (public, private, community based) is made more responsive to the needs of the individual served by the system. This process may include increasing awareness of services and resources available within a community, identifying unmet needs of individuals, identifying existing barriers that impede access to community services and resources, and developing strategies to eliminate legislative, regulatory, social and economic barriers that may impede access to one's community supports and resources.

Individual advocacy: the process of increasing awareness of unmet needs and procuring rights or benefits on behalf of another individual or group of individuals.

Self-advocacy: the process of empowering an individual to rely upon him or herself to make his/her own choices and decisions in order to direct the course of his/her life.

The People First movement of the 1970s was a progenitor of self-advocacy as a civil rights movement. The independent living movement engaged in systems advocacy and also fostered self-advocacy, providing a foundation for self-advocacy activism in which people with significant disabilities had a right to live in an accessible community of their choice. A core service of Centers of Independent Living is individual and systems advocacy, including providing opportunities for skill development in self-advocacy. The Protection and Advocacy (P&A) System protects the rights of people with disabilities by providing legal representation and other advocacy services associated with state and federal laws. P&A Offices exist in each state.

Cross-References

▶ Americans with Disabilities Act of 1990
▶ Independent Living Centers

References and Readings

Dell Orto, A. E., & Marinelli, R. P. (Eds.). (1995). *Encyclopedia of disability and rehabilitation*. New York: MacMillian Publishing.
Test, D., Fowler, C. H., Wood, W. M., Brewer, D. M., & Eddy, S. (2005). Conceptual framework of self-advocacy for students with disabilities. *Remedial and Special Education, 26*, 43–54.
Wehmeyer, M. L. (2004). Self-determination and the empowerment of people with disabilities. *American Rehabilitation, 28*, 22–29.

Adynamia

Irene Piryatinsky
Butler Hospital and Alpert Medical School of Brown University, Providence, RI, USA

Synonyms

Asthenia

Definition

Adynamia refers to a general weakness and lack of energy evident through lack of verbal or overt behavior due to a disease or neurological conditions. It can manifest as lethargy, loss of strength, weakness in extremities, and difficulty initiating activities or completing tasks. Adynamia can be observed after trauma to the frontal lobes, multiple sclerosis, and other conditions. In language, verbal adynamia (lack of spontaneity of speech) is seen with lesions of the medial frontal lobes and refers to difficulty in initiation and maintenance of language output.

Cross-References

▶ Abulia
▶ Apathy
▶ Transcortical Motor Aphasia

References and Readings

Berrios, G. E. (2008). Classic text no. 76: 'Asthenia' by A. Dechambre (1865). *History of Psychiatry, 19*(4), 490–501.
Caplan, D. (1987). *Neurolinguistics and linguistic aphasiology: An introduction*. New York: Cambridge University Press.

Affect

Joel W. Hughes
Department of Psychology, Kent State University, Kent, OH, USA

Synonyms

Affect display

Definition

Affect is the displaying and experiencing of emotion. It includes positive dimensions such as joy, interest, and contentment, as well as negative dimensions of emotion such as disgust, fear, and anger. Affect is a very rapid response to internal (e.g., thoughts, memory) or external stimuli (e.g., other people). It is different from mood, in that it is more momentary and observable by others, whereas mood is longer lasting and constitutes a symptom that patients may report (e.g., depression). Affect can be observed from facial expression, gestures, posture, and speech (e.g., word choice, tone, rate).

Cross-References

▶ Affective Disorder
▶ Emotionality
▶ Mood Disorder
▶ Pseudobulbar Palsy

References and Readings

Batson, C. D., Shaw, L. L., & Oleson, K. C. (1992). *Differentiating affect, mood and emotion: Toward functionally-based conceptual distinctions. Emotion.* Newbury Park: Sage.
Blechman, E. A. (1990). *Moods, affect, and emotions.* Hillsdale: Lawrence Erlbaum Associates.
Ekman, P. (1993). An argument for basic emotion. *Cognition and Emotion, 6,* 169–200.

Affective Disorder

Joel W. Hughes
Department of Psychology, Kent State University, Kent, OH, USA

Synonyms

Emotional disorder; Mood disorder

Short Description or Definition

An affective disorder is a mental disorder predominantly characterized by altered mood characterized by feelings of emptiness, irritability, or sadness for a prolonged period that results in a significant impairment in social, occupational, or another important area of functioning. Affective disorders include depressive disorders such as major depressive disorder and dysthymia, as well as manic disorders such as bipolar disorder and cyclothymic disorder. Affective disorders may be primary or caused by medical conditions or substances.

Categorization

Mania and depression seem to anchor the ends of an emotional and behavioral continuum, an observation that dates from ancient times. In Hippocrates' humoral theory, mania resulted from an excess of yellow bile and depression to an excess of black bile. In the early twentieth century, German psychiatrist Emil Kraepelin described affective disorders as belonging to a manic-depressive form of psychosis, which he differentiated from *dementia praecox*. The term "manic depression" was replaced by more contemporary language, including major depressive disorder and bipolar disorder in the twentieth century, and for example, major depressive disorder was first incorporated into the third edition of the Diagnostic and Statistical Manual (DSM-III).

Depressive disorders include major depressive disorder and persistent depressive disorder. Diagnosis of major depressive disorder is made by symptoms, as there is no physiological test that reliably diagnoses depression. Major depressive disorder requires at least 2 weeks of depressed mood and loss of interest in usually pleasurable activities (anhedonia). In addition, at least four of the following seven symptoms must also be present: significant weight gain or loss or appetite changes, sleep disturbance (e.g., early morning awakening with difficulty returning to sleep), observable disturbances in psychomotor speed (increased or diminished), loss of energy or excessive fatigue, feelings of low self-worth or inappropriate guilt, cognitive changes such as the subjective experience of difficulty concentrating, and thinking about or planning suicide.

Persistent depressive disorder is similar to major depressive disorder, although the depression must be chronic (i.e., 2 or more years of depressed mood), and during the first 2 years of dysthymia, there must not have been an episode of major depression or a period of longer than 2 months with no symptoms.

Bipolar disorder is diagnosed when there is a "manic" mood disturbance characterized by markedly expansive, elevated, or irritable mood, lasting at least 1 week. The mood disturbance must be accompanied by additional symptoms such as grandiosity, excessive risky behavior such as sexual behavior or irresponsible spending, and decreased need for sleep. A "mixed" episode denotes mood disturbances that are characterized by both manic and depressive symptoms. A "hypomanic" episode is a less pronounced elevation of mood that would not qualify as a true manic episode. Bipolar disorders follow a course in which periods of elevated mood alternate with periods of depression and are categorized according to the nature of these episodes. For example, bipolar I involves alternating manic and depressive episodes; in bipolar II, there are alternating hypomanic and depressive episodes; cyclothymic disorder involves alternating hypomanic and depressive episodes that do not meet full criteria for major depression.

Epidemiology

Affective disorders are very common. At any one time, approximately 10% of the adult population, or nearly 20 million Americans, have a depressive illness. Rates of depression are even higher in patients with comorbid medical conditions, and for example, about 30% of patients with cardiac disease have clinically significant depression. Bipolar disorder is much less common than unipolar depression, occurring in between 2% and 4% of the population (including bipolar I, bipolar II, and cyclothymic disorder). While depression is twice as common among women as men, bipolar is equally common in men and women.

Natural History, Prognostic Factors, and Outcomes

Affective disorders often start in adolescence. For example, the onset of bipolar disorder is typically 15–24 years of age. However, the most likely ages for a first major depressive episode are 30–40 years of age. Depressive disorders often remit spontaneously, but recurrence is common, and about 15% of individuals experiencing an initial major depressive episode will develop chronic recurrent depression. The bipolar disorders are highly heritable, and research continues to determine genetic risk markers for bipolar disorder. Brain imaging studies also suggest that a broad risk for unstable moods may underlie bipolar disorder, but more research is warranted. The causes of depression are not fully understood, but appear to involve the interaction of genetic and environmental factors such as stress and disruptions in interpersonal relationships. Thus, in addition to female gender, risk factors for depression include severe life stress such as traumatic events and loss of significant relationships. Depression is associated with shorter life expectancy from suicide and other causes of death. For example, depression increases the risk of cardiac disease, as well as the risk of mortality among individuals with cardiac disease.

Neuropsychology and Psychology of Affective Disorder

Depression is common in neurological conditions such as stroke and traumatic brain injury (Robinson 2006; Rosenthal et al. 1998). Even without an obvious neurologic insult, individuals with alterations in executive control, memory, and emotion regulation are at increased risk for depression. Furthermore, individuals with depression often show neuropsychological deficits in the absence of neurological conditions. The neuropsychological deficits specified in the diagnostic criteria for depression include difficulty concentrating and making decisions. Thus, depressed patients often exhibit deficits in executive control, memory, and processing speed. For bipolar disorder, distractibility is typically present, as well as impaired decision-making reflected in the criterion relating to distractibility of excessive involvement in activities that present a significant risk of negative consequences. Current neuropsychological theories of depression emphasize the frontal lobes and basal ganglia, including abnormalities in neural circuitry involving the prefrontal cortex, mesiotemporal cortex, striatum, amygdala, and thalamus (Chamberlain and Sahakain 2006). These areas may also be implicated in bipolar disorder, as they appear to underlie mood symptoms and treatment effects.

Evaluation

Assessment of affective disorders focuses on self-report instruments and clinical interviews. Neuropsychological testing may reveal deficits in executive function, attention psychomotor slowing, and biases in the processing of emotional stimuli. Specifically, depressed individuals have exaggerated responses to negative feedback, including rumination. Neuropsychological evaluations in depression and bipolar disorder are frequently used in research, as tests with broad clinical utility in the context of assessing or treating affective disorders have not been widely disseminated.

Treatment

Depression is often treated with medication and psychotherapy. A large number of medications are available to treat depression, including selective serotonin reuptake inhibitors, which typically have relatively milder side effects and lower risks than older drugs such as monoamine oxidase inhibitors. Treatment of bipolar disorders requires pharmacotherapy. In contrast to major depressive disorder, bipolar cannot be successfully treated by psychotherapy alone.

Cross-References

▶ Depressive Disorder

References and Readings

Allen, L. B., McHugh, R. K., & Barlow, D. H. (2008). Emotional disorders: A unified protocol. In D. H. Barlow (Ed.), *Clinical handbook of psychological disorders: A step-by-step treatment manual* (4th ed., pp. 216–249). New York: Guilford Press.

American Psychiatric Association. (2013). *Diagnostic and statistical manual of mental disorders (DSM-5®).* Arlington: American Psychiatric Association.

Chamberlain, S. R., & Sahakain, B. J. (2006). The neuropsychology of mood disorders. *Current Psychiatry Reports, 8,* 458–463.

Clark, L., Chamberlain, S. R., & Sahakian, B. J. (2009). Neurocognitive mechanisms in depression: Implications for treatment. *Annual Review of Neuroscience, 32,* 57–74.

Robinson, R. (2006). *The neuropsychiatry of stroke* (2nd ed.). New York: Cambridge University Press.

Rosenthal, M., Christensen, B., & Ross, T. (1998). Depression following traumatic brain injury. *Archives of Physical Medicine and Rehabilitation, 79,* 90–103.

Afferent

John Bigbee
Anatomy and Neurobiology, Virginia Commonwealth University, Richmond, VA, USA

Synonyms

Sensory

Definition

Afferent is an anatomical term that indicates functional directionality. In nervous tissue, afferent is often used synonymously with sensory information when it refers to nerves carrying impulses from peripheral receptors toward the central nervous system. Afferent can also be used in general to refer to any connection coming into a structure within the nervous system. The opposite direction of conduction is efferent.

See Also

► Efferent

Further Reading

Purves, D., et al. (Eds.). (2012). *Neuroscience* (5th ed.).
    Sunderland: Sinauer Associates.

Afferent Paresis

Maryellen Romero
Department of Psychiatry and Behavioral
Sciences, Tulane University School of Medicine,
New Orleans, LA, USA

Definition

A deficit in the ability to perform voluntary movements due to loss of kinesthetic feedback. The primary and secondary motor cortices have extensive inputs from the somatosensory areas in the parietal lobes. Following lesions to this latter area, particularly the post-central gyrus or to the lemniscal system which provides proprioceptive information to it, motor difficulties may be observed either in the limbs or in speech production. Although the muscles involved in such activities are not weak *per se*, the loss of sensory information results in a disruption of motor control and an imprecise excitation of muscle groups required to execute specific, voluntary fine-motor responses.

References and Readings

Luria, A. L. (1976). *The working brain: An introduction
    to neuropsychology*. New York: Perseus Books
    Group.

Age Decrements

Michael Franzen
Allegheny General Hospital, Pittsburgh, PA, USA

Synonyms

Age-associated cognitive decline

Definition

The concept of age decrements in neuropsychology refers to a decline in cognitive performance due to normal aging rather than due to an extraneous or internal event that is known to negatively affect cognitive performance, such as a traumatic brain injury, stroke, psychiatric condition, or extensive drug use history.

Current Knowledge

Variability in the performance of aging individuals adds complexity to the determination of specific age decrements on neuropsychological tests. It is generally thought that individuals are more likely to retain "crystallized" knowledge (e.g., that which is practiced, overlearned, and skill-based) than "fluid" knowledge (e.g., problem-solving). As there are factors that heighten the risk for age decrements, protective factors may counteract the risk. For instance, higher levels of education and positive health status may slow down the rate of cognitive decline that would otherwise occur with increasing age.

One concept that illustrates age decrements is age-associated memory impairment (AAMI), which pertains to age-related decline in performance specifically in terms of memory.

Cross-References

► Cognitive Reserve
► Memory Impairment

References and Readings

Lezak, M., Howieson, D. B., Bigler, E. D., & Tranel, D. (2012). *Neuropsychological assessment* (5th ed.). New York: Oxford University Press.

Agenesis of Corpus Callosum

John E. Mendoza
Department of Psychiatry and Neuroscience, Tulane Medical School and SE Louisiana Veterans Healthcare System, New Orleans, LA, USA

Definition

A developmental defect in which either all or part of the corpus callosum fails to develop.

Current Knowledge

Agenesis can result from various etiologies, including genetic predisposition, chromosomal abnormalities, or intrauterine trauma, such as infection. When present, this condition is commonly associated with other neuroanatomical anomalies, metabolic disturbances, and/or neurobehavioral deficits. The latter might include mental retardation, seizures, motor deficits, and psychiatric disturbances. However, some patients may be relatively asymptomatic, the callosal defect being discovered only serendipitously late in life. The latter is more likely to occur when the agenesis is not accompanied by other neurological or metabolic defects. Whereas "disconnection syndromes" are routinely present following surgical commissurotomy for intractable epilepsy, they are generally not present with agenesis.

References and Readings

Aicardi, J., Chevrie, J.-J., & Baraton, J. (1987). Agenesis of the corpus callosum. In P. J. Vinken, G. W. Bruyn, & H. L. Klawans (Eds.), *Handbook of clinical neurology* (Vol. 50, pp. 149–173). New York: Elsevier.

Marszal, E., Jamroz, E., Pilch, J., Kluczewska, E., Jablecka, H., & Krawczyk, R. (2000). Agenesis of the corpus callosum: Clinical description and etiology. *Journal of Child Neurology, 15*, 401–405.

Zaidel, E., & Iacoboni, M. (2003). *The parallel brain: The cognitive neuroscience of the corpus callosum*. Cambridge, MA: MIT Press.

Agent Orange

Ben Dodsworth
PM&R, University of South Florida, Tampa, FL, USA

Synonyms

None

Definition

A tactical herbicide and defoliant (chemical used to remove leaves from trees and plants) employed by the US military during the Vietnam War during "Operation Ranch Hand." It was sprayed from aircraft with the purpose of depriving the enemies of food and removing dense tropical foliage that provided enemy cover. The name was derived from the orange stripe that identified the large drums in which it was stored. It was composed of two active ingredients: 2,4-dichlorophenoxyacetic acid (2,4-D) and 2,4,5-trichlorophenoxyacetic acid (2,4,5-T). Studies involving US military personnel have linked exposure to these chemicals with higher incidence of various cancers, diabetes, heart disease, Parkinson's disease, and other medical issues (US Department of Veterans Affairs).

See Also

▶ Parkinson's Disease

References and Readings

US Department of Veterans Affairs. Facts About Herbicides. Retrieved January 24, 2017, from http://www.publichealth.va.gov/exposures/agentorange/basics.asp.

Ageusia

Maryellen Romero
Department of Psychiatry and Behavioral Sciences, Tulane University School of Medicine, New Orleans, LA, USA

Definition

Ageusia is the loss of the sense of taste. The disorder should be distinguished from a disruption in the ability to perceive *flavor*, which requires a combination of olfactory, gustatory, and somatosensory functions. Frequently, complaints of ageusia are often explained by olfactory dysfunction rather than a disruption in taste perception, *per se*. The majority of taste receptors (buds) are located on the tongue and this information is carried by the VIIth (anterior two thirds) and IXth (posterior third) cranial nerves, with other taste receptors (cranial nerve X) located in other regions of the mouth and throat. These taste fibers enter the solitary nucleus (rostral portion) in the upper medulla and from there second-order neurons travel to the ventral posterior medial nuclei of the thalamus. Thalamic projections carrying this gustatory information then project to the postcentral gyrus in the region of the parietal operculum and to the underlying insular cortex where the sensation of taste is likely experienced.

Lesions of the VIIth nerve can result in loss of taste in the ipsilateral anterior two thirds of the tongue which is more readily assessable to clinical testing than lesions of the IXth or Xth nerve. However, total loss of taste (ageusia) is seldom seen as a result of structural lesions because of the multiple and bilateral pathways involved. Ageusia (or hypogeusia) is more likely to result from more systemic problems such as treatments for cancer (radiation, chemotherapy), certain types of influenza, diabetes, or certain medications. Taste acuity (hypogeusia) can decline with age and may contribute to the anorexia and weight loss often seen in elderly persons. The prognosis in acquired ageusia is often correlated directly with the expected course of the illness or injury causing the dysfunction.

Cross-References

▶ Taste

References and Readings

Cerf-Ducastel, B., Van de Moortele, P. F., MacLeod, P., Le Bihan, D., & Faurion, A. (2001). Interaction of gustatory and lingual somatosensory perceptions at the cortical level in the human: A functional magnetic resonance imaging study. *Chemical Senses, 26*(4), 371–383.

Doty, R. L., & Kimmelman, C. P. (1992). Lesser20R.-P. Smell and taste and their disorders. In A. K. Asbury, G. M. McKhann, & W. I. McDonald (Eds.), *Diseases of the nervous system* (2nd ed., pp. 390–403). Philadelphia: W.B. Saunders.

Wilson-Pauwek, L., Akesson, E., & Stewart, P. (1988). *Cranial nerves: Anatomy and clinical comments.* Philadelphia: B.C. Decker.

Aggravating Factors

Robert L. Heilbronner
Chicago Neuropsychology Group, Chicago, IL, USA

Definition

Refers to any relevant circumstances in correspondence with the evidence presented during the trial that, from the perspective of the jurors, makes the harshest penalty appropriate. By contrast, mitigating factors refer to evidence regarding the defendant's character or circumstances related to the crime that would provide foundation for a juror to vote for a lesser sentence.

Historical Background

In 1972, the US Supreme Court considered the death penalty to be a cruel and an unusual punishment because the manner in which capital sentences were decided in Georgia was capricious (*Furman v. Georgia* 1972). This decision discontinued death penalty litigation in the USA at that time because none of the states had a system that was substantially different. In 1976 (*Gregg v. Georgia*), the Court accepted as constitutional Georgia's rewrite of their statute which included a capital sentencing process that required presentation before a judge or jury of aggravating and mitigating factors. It required at least one or ten specified aggravating circumstances to be established beyond reasonable doubt to impose the death penalty. Some examples include whether the crime (murder) was particularly cruel and atrocious, if more than one victim was murdered, whether the murder occurred during the commission of a felony, etc.

Current Knowledge

Laws regarding how aggravating or mitigating factors should be weighed by jurors vary based on state laws. Neuropsychological assessments in death penalty cases typically focus on mitigating factors, such as neuropsychological or neurobehavioral impairments, as there is an increased body of evidence demonstrating a preponderance of neurocognitive deficits in violent criminals. Neuropsychological assessment with respect to aggravating factors is less common and typically addresses increased risk of future dangerousness.

Cross-References

▶ Mitigating Factors

References and Readings

Denney, R. L. (2005). Criminal responsibility and other criminal forensic issues. In G. Larrabee (Ed.), *Forensic neuropsychology: A scientific approach*. New York: Oxford University Press.

Furman v. Georgia, 408 U.S. 238 (1972).

Gregg v. Georgia, 49 L.Ed.2d. 859 (1976).

Melton, G. B., Petrila, J., Poythress, N. G., & Slobogin, C. (2007). *Psychological evaluations for the courts: A handbook for mental health professionals and lawyers* (3rd ed.). New York: Guilford Press.

Agitated Behavior Scale

Megan Becker and Daniel N. Allen
Department of Psychology, University of Nevada, Las Vegas, NV, USA

Synonyms

ABS

Description

The agitated behavior scale (ABS) was designed to evaluate agitation and other problematic behaviors that commonly occur during the acute recovery phase following traumatic brain injury (Corrigan 1989). The ABS is composed of 14 items that represent a number of commonly occurring problematic behaviors such as short attention span, impulsivity, uncooperativeness, violence, and angry outbursts. Information that assists in ABS scoring is available from the author (Corrigan) and includes descriptions of item ratings and other examples. Each item on the ABS is rated on a 1–4-point scale based on the intensity or frequency of the behavior's occurrence. Additionally, when assigning ratings, the degree to which the behavior interferes with functional behavior is also considered. If the behavior is absent, a rating of 1 is assigned. When the behavior is present, a rating of 2 or greater is assigned, with a rating of 4 indicating the presence of a behavior to an extreme degree.

A total score is derived through a summary of all 14 items (range 14–56) and interpreted as normal range (<22), mild agitation (22–28), moderate agitation (29–35), or severe agitation (35–56). Subscale scores can also be calculated for disinhibition, aggression, and lability although it appears that ABS primarily measures a single construct (Bogner et al. 2000), so interpretation of the total score may be most appropriate.

Current Knowledge

The ABS is often used to perform serial assessments and track changes in agitation that occur as a natural part of the recovery process and as a result of treatment. Although designed for assessment of traumatic brain injury, the ABS has also been used to assess agitation in other populations, such as patients with progressive dementia (Corrigan et al. 1996; Tabloski et al. 1995). No differences have been found between males and females with brain injury on the total score or the subscale scores (Kadyan et al. 2004). Internal consistency estimates range from 0.74 to 0.92 (Bogner et al. 1999; Corrigan 1989), with interrater reliability of 0.92 for the total score and with comparable reliabilities of 0.90, 0.91, and 0.73 for the disinhibition, aggression, and lability scores, respectively. Subscale to total score correlations range from 0.43 to 0.55. The construct validity of the ABS has been supported by factor-analytic studies that demonstrated the presence of three factors: disinhibition, aggression, and lability (Corrigan and Bogner 1994). ABS scores account for a substantial portion of the variance (from 36% to 62%) in independent observations of agitation (Corrigan 1989) and are able to predict changes in cognition (Corrigan and Mysiw 1988), which provide additional support for its validity. The ABS was also translated into German (ABS-G) and Danish, and both translations demonstrated interrater reliability in individuals with traumatic brain injury (0.85 and 0.75–0.91, respectively) with an internal consistency of 0.66 in the ABS-G (Hellweg and Schuster-Amft 2016;

Wolffbrandt et al. 2013). Thus, there is evidence for the clinical utility of the ABS, a highly practical measure with sound psychometric properties that allow for assessment of agitation in populations with brain injury (Amato et al. 2012).

Cross-References

▶ Post-Traumatic Confusional State
▶ Traumatic Brain Injury (TBI)

References and Readings

Amato, S., Resan, M., & Mion, L. (2012). The feasibility, reliability, and clinical utility of the agitated behavior scale in brain-injured rehabilitation patients. *Rehabilitation Nursing, 37*, 19–24.

Bogner, J. A., Corrigan, J. D., Stange, M., & Rabold, D. (1999). Reliability of the agitated behavior scale. *The Journal of Head Trauma Rehabilitation, 14*, 91–96.

Bogner, J. A., Corrigan, J. D., Bode, R. K., & Heinemann, A. W. (2000). Rating scale analysis of the agitated behavior scale. *The Journal of Head Trauma Rehabilitation, 15*, 656–659.

Corrigan, J. D. (1989). Development of a scale for assessment of agitation following traumatic brain injury. *Journal of Clinical and Experimental Neuropsychology, 11*, 261–277.

Corrigan, J. D., & Bogner, J. A. (1994). Factor structure of the agitated behavior scale. *Journal of Clinical and Experimental Neuropsychology, 16*, 386–392.

Corrigan, J. D., & Mysiw, W. J. (1988). Agitation following traumatic head injury: Equivocal evidence for a discrete stage of cognitive recovery. *Archives of Physical Medicine and Rehabilitation, 69*, 487–492.

Hellweg, S., & Schuster-Amft, C. (2016). German version, inter- and intrarater reliability and internal consistency of the "Agitated Behavior Scale" (ABS-G) in patients with moderate to severe traumatic brain injury. *Health and Quality of Life Outcomes, 14*(106), 1–8.

Kadyan, V., Mysiw, W. J., Bogner, J. A., Corrigan, J. D., Fugate, L. P., & Clinchot, D. M. (2004). Gender differences in agitation after traumatic brain injury. *American Journal of Physical Medicine & Rehabilitation, 83*, 747–752.

Wolffbrandt, M. M., Poulsen, I., Engberg, A. W., & Hornnes, N. (2013). Occurrence and severity of agitated behavior after severe traumatic brain injury. *Rehabilitation Nursing, 38*, 133–141.

Agitation

Paul Newman
Department of Medical Psychology and
Neuropsychology, Drake Center, Cincinnati,
OH, USA

Synonyms

Posttraumatic agitation

Definition

Agitation is an *excess* of one or more behaviors that occur during the course of delirium when cognition is impaired. The behaviors most often in excess during agitation include aggression, akathisia, disinhibition, and/or emotional lability. Specific examples of agitated behavior may include pacing, hand wringing, pulling at tubes or restraints, inappropriate verbalizations, excessive crying or laughter, etc.

Agitation is often conceptualized to result from an inability to cope with overstimulation. Stimulation may be internal (e.g., pain or hallucinations) or external (e.g., noise, light, or conversation). One's ability to cope with stimulation may be viewed as a threshold. Adverse changes to the brain's typical functioning have the potential to lower this threshold. Thus, individuals with traumatic brain injury or dementia may become agitated at lower levels of stimulation than noninjured individuals.

Current Knowledge

There was no consensus on the definition of agitation within the greater health-care profession for many years. Clinicians in neuro-rehabilitation were using the term in the early 1980s to describe a pattern of behavior observed during recovery from traumatic brain injury. The development of the Agitated Behavior Scale by Corrigan and associates in the late 1980s to measure this brain-injury-related behavior led to a more refined definition of the term. The term is not limited to just traumatic brain injury

as agitation can manifest in any setting in which an individual experiences delirium and impaired cognition (e.g., dementia).

The importance of the concept of agitation and its measurement was vital to the establishment of the now accepted viewpoint that recovery from agitation is preceded by improvement in cognition. Or conversely, interventions that decrease arousal and/or cognition can lead to a worsening of agitation.

Cross-References

▶ Agitated Behavior Scale
▶ Behavior Management
▶ De-escalation
▶ Dementia
▶ Frustration Tolerance
▶ Post-traumatic Confusional State
▶ Traumatic Brain Injury (TBI)

References and Readings

Corrigan, J. D. (1989). Development of a scale for assessment of agitation following traumatic brain injury. *Journal of Clinical and Experimental Neuropsychology, 69*, 261–277.

Sandel, M. E., & Bysiw, W. J. (1996). The agitated brain injured patient. Part 1: Definitions, differential diagnosis, and assessment. *Archives of Physical Medicine and Rehabilitation, 77*, 617–623.

Smith, M., Gardner, L. A., Hall, G. R., & Buckwalter, K. C. (2004). History, development, and future of the progressively lowered stress threshold: A conceptual model for dementia care. *Journal of the American Geriatric Society, 52*, 1755–1760.

Agnosia

Anastasia Raymer
Communication Disorders and Special Education,
Old Dominion University, Norfolk, VA, USA

Definition

Agnosia is a failure to recognize a sensory stimulus that is not attributable to dysfunction of peripheral sensory mechanisms or to other cognitive impairments associated with brain damage (Bauer 2012). Agnosia is often described as a percept that is "stripped of its meaning" (Teuber 1968). The individual can respond to the presence of the stimulus but has difficulty processing the perceptual information in sufficient detail to make sense of and meaningfully recognize the stimulus. The difficulty is modality specific (e.g., visual), so the stimulus can be recognized through other sensory modalities (e.g., tactile or auditory).

Current Knowledge

Different forms of agnosia have been described that depend upon the detail with which the incoming stimulus is processed and the sensory modality and type of materials that pose difficulty. Lissauer (1890) used the terms apperceptive and associative, to classify the agnosias, terms that continue to guide descriptions of agnosia (Farah 2004). Agnosia is also described with respect to the sensory modality affected (e.g., auditory agnosia, tactile agnosia), although it is most commonly reported to affect the visual modality (Farah 2004). Rarely, multimodality forms of agnosia also have been described (Feinberg et al. 1986). Finally, agnosia is discussed in the context of the material to be perceived, for example, objects, sounds, or faces (i.e., prosopagnosia, Gainotti 2014). Lesions that lead to agnosia vary across sensory modalities, usually affecting bilateral post-Rolandic cortical sensory regions or disconnecting incoming pathways from one hemisphere to the other (Bauer 2012).

Apperceptive agnosia is associated with disruption at early stages of perceptual processing beyond primary sensory appreciation of a stimulus. For example, in the visual modality, the person can see the percept but has difficulty copying or matching an incoming percept to a like stimulus and may make perceptual confusions, yet when asked can conjure up some visual information from memory or answer questions about visual attributes of a named stimulus in visual imagery tasks (e.g., What number does a peanut look like in its shell? 8). In contrast, Lissauer's associative agnosia refers to a pattern in which the person can perform elementary perceptual tasks, such as copying or matching, but is not able to conjure up information about perceptual characteristics of a stimulus from memory and also has difficulty interpreting the meaning of a percept, its category, context, associated objects, and actions, despite the ability to perform those interpretations through alternative sensory modalities (e.g., failure to sort pictures by category and retained ability to identify the category for the same spoken words). Accurate diagnosis of agnosia depends upon careful examination across modalities to rule out alternative cognitive and linguistic bases for processing failure (Bauer 2012).

Cross-References

▶ Apperceptive Visual Agnosia
▶ Associative Visual Agnosia
▶ Auditory Agnosia
▶ Prosopagnosia
▶ Pure Word Deafness
▶ Tactile Agnosia
▶ Visual Object Agnosia

References and Readings

Bauer, R. M. (2012). Agnosia. In K. M. Heilman & E. Valenstein (Eds.), *Clinical neuropsychology* (5th ed., pp. 238–295). New York: Oxford University Press.

Farah, M. J. (2004). *Visual agnosia* (2nd ed.). Cambridge, MA: MIT Press.

Feinberg, T. E., Rothi, L. J. G., & Heilman, K. M. (1986). Multimodal agnosia after unilateral left hemisphere lesion. *Neurology, 36*, 864–867.

Gainotti, G. (2014). Familiar people recognition disorders: An introductory review. *Frontiers in Bioscience, S6*, 58–64.

Lissauer, H. (1890). Ein fall von seelenblindheit nebst einem beitrage zur theorie derselben. *Archiv für Psychiatrie und Nervenkrankheiten, 21*, 222–270.

Teuber, H. L. (1968). Alteration of perception and memory in man. In L. Weiskrantz (Ed.), *Analysis of behavioral change*. New York: Harper & Row.

Agrammatism

Lyn S. Turkstra[1] and Cynthia K. Thompson[2]
[1]School of Rehabilitation Science, McMaster University, Hamilton, ON, Canada
[2]Northwestern University, Evanston, IL, USA

Synonyms

Agrammatic aphasia

Definition

Agrammatism refers to language production that is lacking in grammatical structures. The basic signs of agrammatism are short phrase length, simplified syntax, errors and omissions of main verbs, and omission or substitution of grammatical morphemes such as plural markers or functors (Saffran et al. 1989). There may also be errors in tense, number, and gender, and difficulty in producing sentences with movement of grammatical elements, such as passive sentences, Wh- questions, and complex sentences (Benedet et al. 1998; Caplan and Hanna 1998; Goodglass 1997; Faroqi-Shah and Thompson 2004). Spoken and written production typically shows similar error patterns. Typically, individuals with agrammatic aphasia also show impaired comprehension of grammatical structures, particularly noncanonical semantically reversible sentences (e.g., "the boy was kicked by the horse"; Berndt et al. 1996; Caramazza and Zurif 1976).

Historical Background

Historically, agrammatism was thought of as a syndrome typically associated with nonfluent aphasia (Goodglass 1997). More recent studies (e.g., Dick et al. 2001) have shown that features of agrammatism are present in the production of many individuals with various forms of aphasia, as well as in normal speakers under stressful conditions, and agrammatism is not attributable to any single site of lesion.

Current Knowledge

The underlying mechanisms of agrammatism have been debated in the literature over the past several decades. Some authors have argued that agrammatism reflects an *underlying impairment* in language representation and/or processing (Grodzinsky 1986, 1990, 1995; Zurif et al. 1993), while others contend that they represent the speaker's *strategic adaptation* to an underlying language processing impairment that is not specific to grammar (Kolk and Heeschen 1990; also see discussion in Beeke et al. 2007). Consistent with the processing deficit view, individuals with agrammatic aphasia show problems computing syntactic structures in real time (Dickey et al. 2007; Swinney et al. 2000; but see Blumstein et al. 1998); and may have deficits that impact both production and comprehension, although not always the same structures (Dickey et al. 2008); and their performance is influenced by contextual factors such as elicitation task (Faroqi-Shah and Friedman 2015). Also, the structures that typically are impaired in agrammatic aphasia are similar across many languages. In support of the adaptation view, there is evidence that the grammatical structures used by individuals with agrammatic aphasia vary as a function of the task. For example, individuals with agrammatic aphasia may produce more complex sentences on standardized language tests, in which grammatical completeness is the focus, than in conversational interactions, in which the message and interaction are the focus and the communication partners are coconstructing a dialog (Beeke et al. 2008).

There is evidence of treatment efficacy for interventions aimed improvement of underlying representation/processing impairments and deficits in adaptation. Verb as Core (Loverso et al. 1986), Mapping Therapy (Schwartz et al. 1994), and Treatment of Underlying Forms (TUF; Thompson et al. 2003; Thompson et al. 2010) focus treatment on verbs and verb argument structure, training patients to map form to meaning in both simple and complex sentences. Notably, TUF results in strong generalization from complex to simple structures by controlling the lexical and syntactic variables of sentences trained (see Thompson and Shapiro 2007, for review). Various approaches to treatment of grammatical morphology, such as deficits in verb tense and agreement, also have been shown to be efficacious (Faroqi-Shah 2008; Friedmann et al. 2000; Mitchum and Berndt 1994; Weinrich et al. 1999).

Cross-References

▶ Aphasia
▶ Grammar
▶ Nonfluent Aphasia
▶ Paragrammatism
▶ Syntax
▶ Telegraphic Speech

References

Beeke, S., Maxim, J., & Wilkinson, R. (2008). Rethinking agrammatism: Factors affecting the form of language elicited via clinical test procedures. *Clinical Linguistics & Phonetics, 22*(4-5), 317–323.

Beeke, S., Wilkinson, R., & Maxim, J. (2007). Individual variation in agrammatism: A single case study of the influence of interaction. *International Journal of Language and Communication Disorders, 42*(6), 629–647.

Benedet, M. J., Christiansen, J. A., & Goodglass, H. (1998). A cross-linguistic study of grammatical morphology in Spanish- and English-speaking agrammatic patients. *Cortex, 34*(3), 309–336.

Berndt, R. S., Mitchum, C. C., & Haendiges, A. N. (1996). Comprehension of reversible sentences in "agrammatism": A meta-analysis. *Cognition, 58*(3), 289–308.

Blumstein, S. E., Byma, G., Kurowski, K., Hourihan, J., Brown, T., & Hutchinson, A. (1998). On-line processing of filler-gap construction in aphasia. *Brain and Language, 61*, 149–168.

Caplan, D., & Hanna, J. E. (1998). Sentence production by aphasic patients in a constrained task. *Brain and Language, 63*(2), 184–218.

Caramazza, A., & Zurif, E. B. (1976). Dissociation of algorithmic and heuristic processes in language comprehension: Evidence from aphasia. *Brain and Language, 3*(4), 572–582.

Dick, F., Bates, E., Wulfeck, B., Utman, J. A., Dronkers, N., & Gernsbacher, M. A. (2001). Language deficits, localization, and grammar: Evidence for a distributive

model of language breakdown in aphasic patients and neurologically intact individuals. *Psychological Review, 108*(4), 759–788.

Dickey, M. W., Choy, J., & Thompson, C. K. (2007). Real-time comprehension of wh-movement in aphasia: Evidence from eyetracking while listening. *Brain and Language, 100*, 1–22.

Dickey, M. W., Milman, L. H., & Thompson, C. K. (2008). Judgment of functional morphology in agrammatic aphasia. *Journal of Neurolinguistics, 21*(1), 35–65.

Faroqi-Shah, Y., & Thompson, C. K. (2004). Semantic, lexical, and phonological influences on the production of verb inflections in agrammatic aphasia. *Brain and Language, 89*(3), 484–498.

Faroqi-Shah, Y. (2008). A comparison of two theoretically-driven treatments of verb inflections in agrammatic aphasia. *Neuropsychologia, 46*, 3088–3100.

Faroqi-Shah, Y., & Friedman, L. (2015). Production of verb tense in agrammatic aphasia: A meta-analysis and further data. *Behavioural Neurology, 2015*, 983870.

Friedmann, N., Wenkert-Olenik, D., & Gil, M. (2000). From theory to practice: Treatment of agrammatic production in hebrew based on the tree pruning hypothesis. *Journal of Neurolinguistics, 13*, 250–254.

Grodzinsky, Y. (1986). Language deficits and syntactic theory. *Brain and Language, 27*, 135–159.

Grodzinsky, Y. (1990). *Theoretical perspectives on language deficits.* Cambridge, MA: MIT Press.

Grodzinsky, Y. (1995). A restrictive theory of agrammatic comprehension. *Brain and Language, 50*, 27–51.

Goodglass, H. (1997). Agrammatism in aphasiology. *Clinical Neuroscience, 4*(2), 51–56.

Kolk, H. H. J., & Heeschen, C. (1990). Adaptation symptoms and impairment symptoms in Broca's aphasia. *Aphasiology, 4*, 221–231.

Loverso, F. L., Prescott, T. E., & Selinger, M. (1986). Cuing verbs: A treatment strategy for aphasic adults. *Journal of Rehabilitation Research, 25*, 47–60.

Mitchum, C., & Berndt, R. (1994). Verb retrieval and sentence construction: Effects of targeted intervention. In M. J. Riddoch & G. Humphreys (Eds.), *Cognitive neuropsychology and cognitive rehabilitation.* Hove: Erlbaum.

Saffran, E. M., Berndt, R. S., & Schwartz, M. F. (1989). The quantitative analysis of agrammatic production: Procedure and data. *Brain and Language, 37*(3), 440–479.

Schwartz, M. F., Saffran, E. M., Fink, R. B., & Myers, J. L. (1994). Mapping therapy: A treatment programme for agrammatism. *Aphasiology, 8*, 19–54.

Swinney, D., Prather, P., & Love, T. (2000). The time course of lexical access and the role of context: Converging evidence from normal and aphasic processing. In Y. Grodzinsky, L. P. Shapiro, & D. Swinney (Eds.), *Language and the brain: Representation and processing.* New York: Academic.

Thompson, C. K., & Shapiro, L. P. (2007). Complexity in treatment of syntactic deficits. *American Journal of Speech-Language Pathology, 16*, 30–42.

A

Thompson, C. K., Shapiro, L. P., Kiran, S., & Sobecks, J. (2003). The role of syntactic complexity in treatment of sentence deficits in agrammatic aphasia: The complexity account of treatment efficacy (CATE). *Journal of Speech, Language, and Hearing Research, 42,* 690–707.

Thompson, C. K., Choy, J.J., Holland, A., Cole, R. (2010). Sentactics®: Computer-Automated Treatment of Underlying Forms. *Aphasiology, 24*(10), 1242–1266.

Weinrich, M., Boser, K. I., & McCall, D. (1999). Representation of linguistic rules in the brain: Evidence from training an aphasic patient to produce past tense verb morphology. *Brain and Language, 70,* 144–158.

Zurif, E., Swinney, D., Prather, P., Solomon, J., & Bushell, C. (1993). On-line analysis of syntactic processing in Broca's and Wernicke's aphasia. *Brain and Language, 45,* 448-464.

Agraphia

Pélagie M. Beeson[1], Steven Z. Rapcsak[2] and Angel Ball[3]
[1]Department of Speech, Language, and Hearing Sciences, The University of Arizona, Tucson, AZ, USA
[2]Neurology Section, Southern Arizona VA Healthcare System, Tucson, AZ, USA
[3]Department of Clinical Health Sciences, Texas A&M University – Kingsville, Kingsville, TX, USA

Synonyms

Dysgraphia; Written language disorders

Short Description or Definition

Agraphias are acquired disorders of spelling or writing caused by neurological damage in individuals with normal premorbid literacy skills. There are several different agraphia profiles that variously result from impairments of spelling knowledge, sound-to-letter correspondences, letter-shape information, or motor control for handwriting. Although agraphia can occur in relative isolation (*pure agraphia*), more often agraphia co-occurs with acquired impairments of reading (alexia) and spoken language (aphasia).

Categorization

Historically, the term *agraphia* was introduced in 1867 by Ogle with a description of two types: *amnemonic* and *atactic* (Lorch 2013). As researchers have developed models of writing processes, these types have become termed *central* and *peripheral* syndromes, each with subcategories. Generally speaking, several distinct forms of acquired agraphia occur that reflect specific combinations of impaired and preserved spelling and writing abilities following damage to certain brain regions.

Central agraphia produces one of five types of word spelling difficulties, each associated with damage to a part of the linguistic processing model and having specific distinctive features and characteristic errors (Rapszak and Beeson 2000). Agraphia may result from damage to multiple areas of linguistic processing; therefore, multiple subtypes may occur concurrently.

Some central agraphia syndromes:

- *Phonological agraphia* refers to an impaired ability to manipulate the sound system of the language (phonology) which manifests as a disproportionate difficulty with the spelling of nonwords (e.g., *flig, merber*) compared with real words.
- *Deep agraphia* is characterized by a marked impairment of spelling ability for nonwords, as seen in phonological agraphia, but with the additional hallmark feature of semantic errors (e.g., *car* for *vehicle*).
- *Surface agraphia* (also called *lexical agraphia*) is characterized by relatively preserved ability to spell nonwords and regularly spelled words in the face of marked impairment of spelling words with irregular sound-to-letter correspondences, such as *choir*.

Peripheral agraphias have been described as disorders of writing based on the final stage of production; they often spare oral spelling. The disorder occurs in the *peripheral* processing components that guide the selection and production of appropriate letter shapes. Individuals can display both central and peripheral type agraphias if, for example, there is coexisting motor dysfunction.

Some peripheral agraphia syndromes:

- *Allographic agraphia* is an impairment of written spelling due to errors in letter selection.
- *Apraxic agraphia* is an impairment of the selection and implementation of graphic motor programs necessary to move the hand to form letter shapes.
- *Nonapraxic disorders of motor execution*, due to motor system control of movements. This subcategory includes *micrographia,* which is the production of abnormally small letters due to defective control of the force, speed, and amplitude of handwriting movements.

Writing disorders also occur at the sentence and narrative levels. These are behaviors that occur when the left language dominant hemisphere is affected. Disorders of syntax include written agrammatism, with limited or misuse of low content or function words (e.g., articles, prepositions), and decrease in clausal complexity, as in fragmented clauses, restarts, and abandoned sentences (as seen in cases of dementia). Perseverative letters and words are also observed in dementia-type written language, occurring along with decline in meaning.

Individuals with both left and right hemisphere damage can also demonstrate written disorders related to visuoperceptual deficits (e.g., hemispatial neglect), characterized by avoiding one side of the page, slanted writing, overwriting letters, etc. The reader is encouraged to seek entry on hemispatial neglect.

Epidemiology

Agraphia is commonly observed following damage to the language-dominant hemisphere and can follow any kind of focal damage to the brain regions critical for implementing the various cognitive operations necessary for normal spelling and writing. One primary cause is a stroke with the agraphia being worse immediately following or in the acute stages post stroke. Agraphia post stroke often occurs concurrently with aphasia, motor apraxia, or dysarthria (when affecting the writing limb), but specific prevalence data are not available. Agraphia is also observed in individuals with neurodegenerative disorders including (but not limited to) those with primary progressive aphasia, amyotrophic lateral sclerosis, multiple sclerosis, or Alzheimer's disease. Detection of deterioration in writing is easily done when comparison is made to premorbid samples. Sampling of written narratives over time provides information about communicative and cognitive declines as seen in Alzheimer's disease (Neils-Strunjas et al. 2006; Kemper et al. 2001).

Natural History, Prognostic Factors, and Outcomes

The prognosis for recovery from agraphia depends on the etiology of the lesion and the extent of the underlying brain damage. Agraphia following stroke or traumatic brain injury tends to show some spontaneous recovery in the first months after damage occurs, but residual impairments often persist. Additional improvements may be achieved with behavioral treatment directed toward strengthening the weakened cognitive processes that support spelling, syntax, and morphology, or motor control for writing. In individuals with neurodegenerative disorders, progressive worsening of the spelling impairment is observed along with the gradual deterioration of other language and cognitive functions.

Neuropsychology and Psychology of Agraphia

Neuroimaging of normal functioning individuals provides knowledge of brain pathways involved in writing, which aids in describing the impaired neurologic processing of writing. A recent meta-

Agraphia, Fig. 1 A
cognitive model indicating
the component processes
involved in spelling and
writing

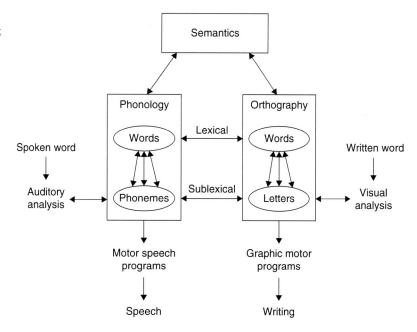

analysis of 18 neuroimaging studies during hand-writing provides a template for cortical and sub-cortical involvement, with support for superior parietal involvement in the language dominant hemisphere that could function to interface between linguistic and motor systems (Planton et al. 2013). Meanwhile, research that identifies regions of brain damage associated with various types of agraphia continues to help us understand the disorder and its subtypes. Nonetheless, researchers have not entirely unraveled specific brain regions for each step of the process (Lorch 2013).

Written words are typically produced in response to activation of a concept in the seman-tic system. The motivation to write a word may be driven by the desire to convey a message or in response to an auditory stimulus, as in the con-text of writing a word to dictation. As depicted in the cognitive model of single-word processing in Fig. 1, the word meaning (semantics) and the phonological word form (phonology) both provide access to spelling knowledge (orthography). In literate adults, the spellings of familiar words are easily recalled as whole words from one's spelling vocabulary (i.e., orthographic lexicon). In contrast to this *lexical* approach, spellings can be assembled on the basis of the knowledge of sound-to-letter corre-spondences using a *sublexical* processing strat-egy as depicted in Fig. 1. A sublexical approach is often employed when one is unsure about the spelling of a word, or when required to spell an unfamiliar word or a nonword, such as *glope*. Spelling via sound-to-letter correspondences is likely to yield correct responses for regularly spelled words, such as *drive*, but overreliance on the sublexical route will result in phonologi-cally plausible errors for irregularly spelled words, such as *kwire* for *choir*. Thus, according to a dual-route model as depicted in Fig. 1, only the lexical route can deliver correct spellings for irregularly spelled words. The final stages of writing require translation of abstract spelling knowledge into letter shapes and selection and implementation of the graphic motor programs for the appropriate handwriting movements. The various agraphia syndromes reflect specific impairments to these component processes nec-essary for spelling and writing.

Phonological/Deep Agraphia

Phonological agraphia is characterized by diffi-culty in the generation of spellings on the basis of sound-to-letter correspondences. This problem is particularly evident during clinical evaluation when an individual is asked to generate plausible spellings for nonwords. The disproportionate difficulty in spelling nonwords compared to familiar words gives rise to an exaggerated *lexicality effect* (Henry et al. 2007; Rapcsak et al. 2009). According to a dual-route model (Fig. 1), poor nonword spelling in phonological agraphia is attributable to damage to the sublexical route, while the better preserved real-word spelling by these patients reflects the residual functional capacity of the lexical and semantic routes. There is evidence to suggest that phonological agraphia reflects a central impairment of phonological processing ability that is also apparent on reading tasks; however, the spelling impairment is typically of greater severity due to the fact that spelling is a harder task than reading (Rapcsak et al. 2009). Although spelling accuracy for words (both regular and irregular) is better preserved than spelling of nonwords, performance is often degraded to some extent relative to premorbid performance. Due to the reliance on lexical processing with limited sublexical input, real-word spelling is typically influenced by lexical-semantic variables such as word frequency (high > low), imageability (concrete > abstract), and grammatical class (nouns > verbs > functors). Deep agraphia

includes all of the characteristic features of phonological agraphia, but it is distinguished from the latter by the production of semantic errors (e.g., *husband* written as *wife*). In essence, deep agraphia can be considered a more severe form of phonological agraphia.

Like phonological/deep alexia, phonological/deep agraphia is typically encountered in patients with aphasia syndromes characterized by phonological impairment including Broca's, conduction, and Wernicke's aphasia. In such cases, there is damage to a network of *perisylvian* cortical regions involved in speech production/perception and phonological processing including Broca's area, precentral gyrus, insula, Wernicke's area, and supramarginal gyrus (Fig. 2). The contribution of these regions to phonological processing skills is evident from both lesion studies and also in functional imaging studies of healthy individuals performing a variety of written and spoken language tasks requiring phonological processing (Jobard et al. 2003; Vigneau et al. 2006; Rapcsak et al. 2009). In individuals with deep agraphia, the left hemisphere damage tends to be more extensive than that associated with phonological agraphia, and it has been hypothesized that the right hemisphere may be responsible for the characteristic deep agraphia profile (Rapcsak et al. 1991).

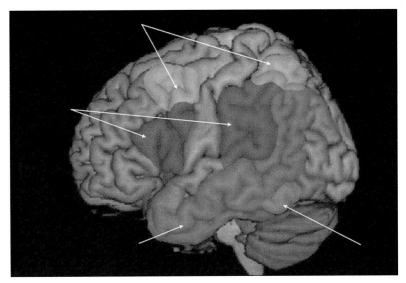

Agraphia, Fig. 2 Cortical regions involved in spelling and writing

Surface Agraphia

Surface agraphia is characterized by difficulty in spelling irregular words – i.e., those that contain atypical sound-to-letter correspondences. Regular words are spelled with significantly better accuracy, thus yielding a *regularity effect*. Nonword spelling is relatively preserved. In a manner analogous to surface alexia, a dual-route theory attributes surface agraphia to dysfunction of the lexical spelling route (Fig. 1). Specifically, it has been suggested that the spelling disorder results from damage to the orthographic lexicon (Rapcsak and Beeson 2004). The loss of word-specific orthographic knowledge prompts reliance on a sublexical phoneme-grapheme conversion strategy that produces phonologically plausible regularization errors on irregular words, a finding that is most pronounced for low-frequency items (e.g., *yot* for *yacht*). A functional MRI study with normal right-handed adults recently identified cluster of brain regions more activated with irregular spelling: specifically involving the "left posterior IFG (pars, triangularis/opercularis) and adjacent insula, left mid-posterior superior temporal sulcus (STS) and the anterior cingulate/supplementary motor area (SMA)" and suggesting a network of cortical processing engaging orthographic and phonological systems (De Marco et al. 2017, p. 121).

Surface agraphia may also result from damage to central semantic representations as observed in individuals with semantic dementia (Graham et al. 2000). The reduction in the ability to process lexical-semantic information in such individuals results in overreliance on sublexical spelling procedures and regularization errors. As expected, it is not uncommon to observe co-occurrence of surface alexia and agraphia in individuals with semantic dementia (Graham et al. 2000).

Surface agraphia, like surface alexia, is typically associated with *extrasylvian* brain pathology (Fig. 2). Focal lesions that give rise to surface agraphia have been documented in the left inferior occipito-temporal cortex (Rapcsak and Beeson 2004). This region includes a portion of the fusiform gyrus known as the visual word form area that has been shown to be engaged in healthy adults during reading (Cohen et al. 2002) and

spelling tasks (Beeson et al. 2003) and may represent the neural substrate of the orthographic lexicon. Surface agraphia has also been described following focal damage to posterior middle/inferior temporal gyrus and angular gyrus (Rapcsak and Beeson 2004) and in patients with left anterior temporal lobe atrophy (Graham et al. 2000). In these cases, the spelling deficit may reflect damage to a distributed extrasylvian cortical network involved in semantic processing (Fig. 2).

Allographic Agraphia

Allographic agraphia refers to a disturbance of the ability to activate or select appropriate letter shapes for the abstract orthographic representations generated by central spelling routes. This impairment of handwriting is characterized by letter selection errors that often include the substitution of physically similar letter forms (e.g., *b* for *h*). The allographic difficulty may be specific to letter case (upper vs. lower) or style (print vs. cursive). When allographic agraphia occurs in isolation, oral spelling is preserved, as well as the ability to correctly arrange component letters that make up a word (i.e., anagram spelling) and typing. Allographic agraphia is often associated with damage to left temporo-parieto-occipital regions.

Apraxic Agraphia

Apraxic agraphia is characterized by poor letter formation in handwriting that is not attributable to allographic disorder or sensorimotor, cerebellar, or basal ganglia dysfunction. The difficulty arises at the level of motor programming for the skilled movements of the hand so that the spatiotemporal aspects of writing are disturbed. Individual letters are often difficult to recognize and may simply appear to be meaningless scrawls. Lesions associated with apraxic agraphia have been noted in the hemisphere contralateral to the dominant hand. Thus, in right-handed individuals, the damage typically involves the left superior parietal lobe in the region of the intraparietal sulcus, the dorsolateral premotor cortex just anterior to primary motor cortex for the hand, or the supplementary motor area. More recently, cases of thalamic damage have also demonstrated disturbances of the graphomotor process (Vandenborre et al. 2015).

Nonapraxic Disorders of Motor Execution

In addition to apraxic agraphia, there are several additional disorders of motor execution that affect the ability to form legible letter shapes. These writing difficulties include disturbances of the regulation of movement force, speech, and amplitude. Micrographia (the production of small letters with reduced legibility) is a common example that is associated with the basal ganglia pathology in Parkinson disease. Cerebellar pathology can also result in poor handwriting due to irregular and disjointed hand movements. Handwriting difficulty is also associated with damage to primary sensorimotor cortex and/or associated corticospinal tracts that cause hemiparesis of the dominant hand. When the hemiparesis is marked, individuals typically shift to writing with the nondominant hand. Improvement in graphomotor control of the non-dominant hand is apparent with practice and often provides a fully functional substitute; however, the automaticity of motor movements is rarely comparable to the premorbidly dominant hand.

Evaluation

The evaluation of writing in individuals with neurological impairments is often part of a broader language and cognitive assessment. No current modality-specific formal test tool is available for acquired agraphia. An evaluation of adult writing must first include information regarding educational level, premorbid reading level, visual ability (e.g., access to glasses if needed), and observations of any dominant hand paresis/paralysis/praxis. If the evaluation is proceeding with an unimpaired dominant limb, then the focus can be primarily on linguistic features. However, if either an impaired dominant limb or use of unimpaired nondominant limb is used, then consideration must be given for slow productions, poor legibility, and possible apraxic-type errors. In some cases, keyboard writing can be assessed particularly if the individual used a keyboard premorbidly. In addition, access to premorbid handwriting samples is beneficial for identification of change in ability via comparisons (Papathanasiou and Cséfalvay (2013).

To evaluate word level spelling and determine the agraphia subcategory type(s), several tasks should be included: spelling aloud, written spelling of regular and irregular words, comparing word class (content vs functor), and word length. Input stimuli to test routes of processing include written picture naming (pictorial visual), writing to dictation (auditory), and manipulation of letters (graphemic visual). The Johns Hopkins University Dyslexia and Dysgraphia Batteries (JHU Battery: Goodmann and Caramaaza 1986b, published in Chapey 2008) is a word-only tool that includes data on word frequency, word length, regular vs. irregular spelling, and nonwords, but is primarily dictated task.

To evaluate sentence level writing acquired disorders, the tasks of writing to dictated sentences or picture description are used in formal tests. Researchers are also finding valuable diagnostic information from narrative discourse samples, using picture description, story retell, story scripts from sequential picture, or generated essays (e.g., Groves-Wright et al. 2004; Mitzner and Kemper 2003; Neils et al. 1989; Pennebaker and Stone 2003, Nippold et al. 2005). Discourse samples will provide information on ability to express content (information units) and demonstrate syntactic and morphological forms and clausal complexity and measures of semantic usage (number of words, and type token ratio -TTR).

Standardized tests with writing subtests include:

- *Boston Diagnostic Aphasia Examination-3* (Goodglass et al. 2001) – writing subtests include person's name, dictated letters and numbers, abbreviations, one copied sentence, the alphabet, dictated primer words, regular and irregular spelling words, nonsense words of irregular spelling, written picture naming of objects and actions, functor words, morphological endings, functor loaded sentences, and picture description of the Cookie Theft line drawing.

- *Examining for Aphasia-4* (EFA-4; LaPointe and Eisenson 2008) – writing subtests include dictated letters, numbers, words, and short sentences (six to eight words in length) and a written narrative (either self-generated or story-retell) based on a Beach scene line drawing.
- *Multilingual Aphasia Examination* 3rd Ed (MAE-3; Benton et al. 1978) – writing subtest includes word level only for oral spelling, dictated words, and manipulation of tactile letters.
- *Psycholinguistic Assessment of Language Processing in Aphasia* (PALPA: Kay et al. 1992) – writing subtests include writing at word level for word length, imageability and frequency of words, grammatical class, morphological endings, regularity, nonwords, and homophones and option of written picture naming.
- *Western Aphasia Battery-R* (WAB-R; Kertesz 2007) – writing subtests include dictated letters and numbers, dictated words of increasing length, irregular words and nonwords, one dictated sentence, name and address, and written description of a Picnic scene line drawing.

Treatment

Several behavioral treatment approaches have shown positive outcomes in the rehabilitation of agraphia (for reviews see Beeson and Henry 2008; Murray and Clark 2015; Papathanasiou and Cséfalvay 2013; Peach and Shapiro 2012). In general, treatment is directed toward strengthening impaired processes and training the use of compensatory strategies necessary to bypass the functional deficit. Most evidenced-based practice researches on clinical application of spelling intervention are case studies. For example, one approach involves phoneme-to-grapheme correspondence learning (e.g., Beeson et al. 2010; Tsapkini and Hillis 2013).

Treatment programs also include hierarchical cueing, with the intention of providing cues to trigger accessing at the graphemic, phonologic, or semantic level (e.g., cue to the grapheme,

visual shape of word, or provide letter anagrams) (Murray and Clark 2015). To address peripheral dysgraphia or visual perceptual difficulties, clinicians can employ techniques such as using prompts (e.g., lined paper), encouraging print or typing in lieu of handwriting, verbal cues to attend to left visual field, or writing prosthesis. Facilitated writing with technology also provides functional abilities for use with computer or tablets. Software and apps with word prediction and cued choices (auditory and visual) are growing in use, but research is needed to demonstrate efficacy in the adult populations (Dietz et al. Griffith 2011).

Cross-References

- ► Alexia
- ► Aphasia
- ► Hemispatial Neglect
- ► Phonological Disorder
- ► Visual Neglect

References and Readings

Beeson, P. M., & Henry, M. L. (2008). Comprehension and production of written language. In R. Chapey (Ed.), *Language intervention strategies in adult aphasia* (5th ed., pp. 654–688). Baltimore: Wolters Kluwer/ Lippincott, Williams & Wilkins.

Beeson, P. M., & Rapcsak, S. Z. (2002). Clinical diagnosis and treatment of spelling disorders. In A. E. Hillis (Ed.), *Handbook on adult language disorders: Integrating cognitive neuropsychology, neurology, and rehabilitation* (pp. 101–120). Philadelphia: Psychology Press.

Beeson, P. M., & Rapcsak, S. Z. (2006). Treatment of alexia and agraphia. In J. H. Noseworthy (Ed.), *Neurological therapeutics: Principles and practice* (2nd ed., pp. 3045–3060). London: Martin Dunitz.

Beeson, P. M., Rapcsak, S. Z., Plante, E., Chargualaf, J., Chung, A., Johnson, S. C., et al. (2003). The neural substrates of writing: A functional magnetic resonance imaging study. *Aphasiology, 17*, 647–665.

Beeson, P. M., Rising, K., Kim, E. S., & Rapcsak, S. Z. (2010). A treatment sequence for phonological alexia/ agraphia. *Journal of Speech, Language, and Hearing Research, 53*(2), 450–468.

Benton, A. L., deS Hamsher, K., & Sivan, A. B. (1978). *Multilingual aphasia examination 3rd Ed (MAE-3)*. Lutz: Psychological Assessment Resources.

Cohen, L., Lehéricy, S., Chochon, F., Lemer, C., Rivaud, S., & Dehaene, S. (2002). Language-specific tuning of visual cortex? Functional properties of the visual word form area. *Brain, 125*, 1054–1069.

DeMarco, A. T., Wilson, S. M., Rising, K., Rapcsak, S. Z., & Beeson, P. M. (2017). Neural substrates of sublexical processing for spelling. *Brain and Language, 164*, 118–128.

Dietz, A., Ball, A., & Griffith. (2011). Reading and writing with aphasia in the 21st century: Internet applications of supported reading comprehension and written expression. *Topics in Stroke Rehabilitation, 18*(6), 758–769.

Goodglass, H., Kaplan, E., & Barresi, B. (2001). *The Boston diagnostic aphasia examination* (3rd ed.). Baltimore: Lippincott Williams & Wilkins.

Goodman & Caramazza (1986) In R. Chapey (Ed.). (2008). *Language intervention strategies in aphasia and related neurogenic communication disorders* (5th ed., Appendix 25-1, pp. 596–603). Philadelphia: Wolters Kluwer Health/Lippincott Williams & Wilkins.

Graham, N. L., Patterson, K., & Hodges, J. R. (2000). The impact of semantic memory impairment on spelling: Evidence from semantic dementia. *Neuropsychologia, 38*, 143–163.

Groves-Wright, K., Neils-Strunjas, J., Burnett, R., & O'Neill, M. J. (2004). A comparison of verbal and written language in Alzheimer's disease. *Journal of Communication Disorders, 37*, 109–130.

Henry, M. L., Beeson, P. M., Stark, A. J., & Rapcsak, S. Z. (2007). The role of left perisylvian cortical regions in spelling. *Brain and Language, 100*, 44–52.

Jobard, G., Crivello, F., & Tzourio-Mazoyer, N. (2003). Evaluation of the dual route theory of reading: A metaanalysis of 35 neuroimaging studies. *NeuroImage, 20*, 693–712.

Kay, J., Lesser, R., & Coltheart, M. (1992). *Psycholinguistic assessments of language processing in aphasia (PALPA)*. East Sussex: Lawrence Erlbaum Associates.

Kemper, S., Greiner, L. H., Marquis, J. G., Prenovost, K., & Mitzner, T. L. (2001). Language decline across the life span: Findings from the Nun study. *Psychology and Aging, 169*(2), 227–239.

Kertesz, A. (2007). *Western aphasia battery – Revised (WAB-R)*. San Antonio: PsychCorp.

LaPointe, L. L., & Eisenson, J. (2008). *Examining for aphasia: Assessment of aphasia and related communication disorders-4th Ed. (EFA-4)*. Austin: Pro-Ed.

Lorch, M. (2013). Written language production disorders: Historical and recent perspectives. *Current Neurology and Neuroscience Reviews, 13*(7), 1–6.

McNeil, M. R., & Tseng, C.-H. (2005). Acquired neurogenic agraphias: Writing problems. In L. L. LaPointe (Ed.), *Aphasia and related neurogenic language disorders* (3rd ed., pp. 97–116). New York: Thieme.

Mitzner, T. L., & Kemper, S. (2003). Oral and written language in late adulthood: Findings from the Nun study. *Experimental Aging Research, 29*, 457–474.

Murray, L. L., & Clark, H. M. (2015). *Neurogenic disorders of language and cognition: Evidence-based clinical practice* (2nd ed.). Clifton Park: Thomson Delmar Learning.

Neils, J., Boller, F., Gerdeman, B., & Cole, M. (1989). Descriptive writing abilities in Alzheimer's disease. *Journal of Clinical and Experimental Neuropsychology, 11*(5), 692–698.

Neils-Strunjas, J., Groves-Wright, K., Mashima, P., & Harnish, S. (2006). Dysgraphia in Alzheimer's disease: A review for clinical and research purposes. *Journal of Speech, Language, and Hearing Research, 49*, 1313–1330.

Nippold, M. A., Ward-Lonergan, J. M., & Fanning, J. L. (2005). Persuasive writing in children, adolescents and adults: A study of syntactic, semantic and pragmatic development. *Language, Speech, and Hearing Services in Schools, 36*, 125–138.

Papathanasiou, I., & Cséfalvay, Z. (2013). Written language and its impairments. In I. Papathanasiou, P. Coppens, & C. Potagas (Eds.), *Aphasia and related neurogenic communication disorders* (pp. 173 195). Burlington: Jones & Bartlett Learning.

Peach, R. K., & Shapiro, L. P. (2012). *Cognition and acquired language disorders*. St. Louis: Elsevier Mosby.

Pennebaker, J. W., & Stone, L. D. (2003). Words of wisdom: Language use over the life span. *Journal of Personality and Social Psychology, 85*(2), 291–301.

Planton, S., Jucla, M., Roux, F.-E., & Démonet, J.-F. (2013). The "handwriting brain": A meta-analysis of neuroimaging studies of motor versus orthographic processes. *Cortex, 49*, 2772–2787.

Rapcsak, S. Z., & Beeson, P. M. (2000). Agraphia. In L. J. G. Rothi, B. Crosson, & S. Nadeau (Eds.), *Aphasia and language: Theory and practice* (pp. 184–220). New York: Guilford.

Rapcsak, S. Z., & Beeson, P. M. (2004). The role of left posterior inferior temporal cortex in spelling. *Neurology, 62*, 2221–2229.

Rapcsak, S. Z., Beeson, P. M., & Rubens, A. B. (1991). Writing with the right hemisphere. *Brain and Language, 41*, 510–530.

Rapcsak, S. Z., Beeson, P. M., Henry, M. L., Leyden, A., Kim, E. S., Rising, K., et al. (2009). Phonological dyslexia and dysgraphia: Cognitive mechanisms and neural substrates. *Cortex, 45*(5), 575–591.

Tainturier, M.-J., & Rapp, B. (2001). The spelling process. In B. Rapp (Ed.), *The handbook of cognitive neuropsychology* (pp. 233–262). Philadelphia: Psychology Press.

Tsapkini, K., & Hillis, A. E. (2013). Spelling intervention in post-stroke aphasia and primary progressive aphasia. *Behavioural Neurology, 26*, 55–66.

Vandenborre, D., van Dun, K., Engelborghs, S., & Mariën, P. (2015). Apraxic agraphia following thalamic damage: Three new cases. *Brain and Language, 150*, 153–165.

Vigneau, M., Beaucousin, V., Hervé, P. Y., Duffau, H., Crivello, F., Houdé, O., et al. (2006). Meta-analyzing left hemisphere language areas: Phonology, semantics, and sentence processing. *NeuroImage, 30*, 1414–1432.

Ahylognosia

John E. Mendoza
Department of Psychiatry and Neuroscience, Tulane Medical School and SE Louisiana Veterans Healthcare System, New Orleans, LA, USA

Definition

Inability to determine by touch alone certain physical properties of an object such as its texture, density (weight), or resistance to pressure, with difficulties in perceiving size or shape is referred to as amorphognosia. While perhaps seeming a bit artificial, according to Bauer and Demery (2003), the distinction between ahylognosia and amorphognosia apparently traces back to 1935 when a French neurologist, Delay, divided astereognosis into two subtypes of deficits: amorphognosia, which was defined as a difficulty in recognizing the size or shape of an object by touch, and ahylognosia, which was described as a failure to differentiate the "molecular qualities" of an object, such as its density, weight, thermal conductivity, or roughness. Delay also defined a third type of astereognosis, tactile asymboly, which was characterized as the inability to identify an object by touch in the absence of amorphognosia and ahylognosia. These same distinctions were followed by Critchley (1969) and continue to be used by more recent authors (Bauer and Demery 2003). Hecaen and Albert (1978) in their book, *Human Neuropsychology*, attempted to explain these distinctions by suggesting that ahylognosia was "the loss of the capacity to differentiate structural components of objects, resulted from impairment of intensity analyzers." By contrast, amorphognosia, was thought to reflect "the loss of the capacity to differentiate forms, resulted from impairment of the analyzers of extent." Because determining any of these qualities requires discriminatory judgments, in the absence of more elementary tactual defects, such disturbances suggest pathology involving the somatosensory areas of the parietal lobe.

Cross-References

▶ Amorphognosis
▶ Astereognosis
▶ Tactile Agnosia

References and Readings

Bauer, R. M., & Demery, J. A. (2003). Agnosia. In K. Heilman & E. Valenstein (Eds.), *Clinical Neuropsychology* (4th ed., pp. 236–295). New York: Oxford University Press.

Critchley, M. (1969). *The parietal lobes*. New York: Hafner Publishing Co.

Delay, J. (1935). *Les astereognosis. Pathologie due Toucher, Clinque, Physiologie, Topographie*. Paris: Masson.

Hecaen, H., & Albert, M. L. (1978). Chapter 6, Disorders of somesthesis and somatognosis. In *Human neuropsychology*. New York: Wiley.

Akathisia

Anna DePold Hohler[1] and Marcus Ponce de Leon[2]
[1]Boston University Medical Center, Boston, MA, USA
[2]Madigan Army Medical Center, Tacoma, WA, USA

Synonyms

Restlessness

Definition

Akathisia is a syndrome characterized by unpleasant sensations of inner restlessness that manifests itself with an inability to sit still or remain motionless.

Current Knowledge

It is most often seen as a side effect of medications, mainly neuroleptic antipsychotics. Patients may have difficulty describing their symptoms, leading to a misdiagnosis of anxiety and worsening of the condition upon treatment with neuroleptic antipsychotic agents. Several medications have been used to treat the condition, including benztropine and beta-blocking agents. Withdrawal of the offending agent is often most effective. It may be seen with Parkinson's disease.

Cross-References

▶ Parkinson's Disease
▶ Tardive Dyskinesia

References and Readings

Kumar, A., & Calne, D. (2004). Approach to the patient with a movement disorder and overview of movement disorders. In R. L. Watts & W. C. Koller (Eds.), *Movement disorders* (2nd ed., p. 9). New York: McGraw-Hill.

Akelaitis, Andrew John Edward ("A.J.") (1904–1955)

Michael J. Larson and Joseph E. Fair
Brigham Young University, Provo, UT, USA

Major Appointments

- Dr. A.J. Akelaitis began his career as an assistant professor in the Department of Medicine, Division of Psychiatry, at the University of Rochester School of Medicine and Dentistry. At the same time, he also held appointments at the clinics of the Strong Memorial and Rochester Municipal Hospitals in Rochester, New York. He left these appointments to serve in the Navy during World War II. Following his service in the war, Dr. Akelaitis worked as an Assistant Professor of Neurology at the New York Medical College and Assistant Professor of Clinical Medicine in Neurology at Cornell University Medical College. He also served as the attending neuropsychiatrist at Mount Vernon (New York) Hospital and on the staff of the Bellevue Hospital and the New York Hospital.

Major Honors and Awards

- Dr. Akelaitis was a Fellow of the American Psychiatric Association. He was specialty certified by the American Board of Psychiatry and Neurology and held membership appointments in the American Medical Association, the New York State Medical Society, the New York Society for Clinical Psychiatry, and the New York Neurological Society.

Landmark Clinical, Scientific, and Professional Contributions

- Dr. A.J. Akelaitis is best known for his observations of patients who underwent sectioning of the corpus callosum (i.e., "split-brain" patients). Beginning in the late 1930s, the neurosurgeon Dr. William P. van Wagenen pioneered surgical sectioning of the corpus callosum for the treatment of intractable epilepsy (Mathews et al. 2008). Dr. Akelaitis worked closely with Dr. van Wagenen and performed pre and postoperative tests of cognitive and neurological functioning on many of these individuals. According to Akelaitis' reports, patients who underwent callosotomy surgery largely did not show lasting changes in cognitive, intellectual, or motor functioning, although their seizure activity was consistently alleviated. For nearly two decades, Akelaitis' reports of largely normal functioning after callosotomy perpetuated the generally accepted belief that sectioning the corpus callosum did not impact cognitive or motor functioning in humans.

- Despite his reports of few neurological changes following callosotomy, Akelaitis noted periodic cases with hemiplegia and praxic disturbances. He was slow, however, to include the sectioning of the corpus callosum in his explanations for these changes; rather, he attributed the symptoms to unintended operative damage to adjacent cortical areas. In some cases, postoperative symptoms were seen as exacerbations of pre-callosotomy characteristics or were attributed to preexisting and/or postoperative psychological or behavioral factors. Further, many of the symptoms observed by Akelaitis were transient and consequently not considered to be conclusively linked with callosal sectioning (Sauerwein and Lassonde 1996).

- Several factors most likely influenced Akelaitis' reports of minimal neurological changes following callosotomy surgery. First, the majority of patients Akelaitis observed did not have complete callosotomies, nor were neurosurgical procedures well standardized at the time. Of the 28 patients he studied, only one third were reported to have undergone "complete" callosal sectioning, with the remainder "nearly complete" or "partial" sectioning (Bogen 1995). The patients with only partially sectioned callosal fibers undoubtedly continued to have interhemispheric transmission, thereby contributing to Akelaitis' findings of generally intact functioning. Next, emerging research at the time reported no cognitive changes following sectioning of the corpus callosum. For example, Walter Dandy stated in 1936 that when "the corpus callosum is split longitudinally... no symptoms follow its division. This simple experiment at once disposes of the extravagant claims to the functions of the corpus callosum" (see Zaidel et al. 2003). Finally, Akelaitis lacked the technologies, such as the tachistoscope used by his successors, to present stimuli to one visual field. Such technology would possibly have given him insight into the specialization of the two hemispheres and interhemispheric transfer of information via the corpus callosum (Mathews et al. 2008).

- Despite his contributions as one of the first individuals to study neurological functioning following callosotomy, Akelaitis has been criticized for employing insensitive or inadequate testing procedures. However, reviews of his cases have confirmed that his patients did exhibit what are now considered typical symptoms, although his explanations for these manifestations, while consistent with much of the research of the time, were often inadequate (Sauerwein and Lassonde 1996). In the 1950s and 1960s, researchers including Roger Sperry, Michael Gazzaniga, Norman Geschwind, Edith Kaplan, and Joseph Bogen began to publish articles involving callosotomies in animals and humans, which contradicted many of Akelaitis' findings. This sparked renewed interest in the function of the corpus callosum and eventually earned Sperry the Nobel Prize in 1981.

- Through the course of his short career, Dr. Akelaitis made significant contributions toward research on the corpus callosum and advanced the treatment of intractable epilepsy. He also published articles regarding the psychiatric aspects of myxedema (severe hypothyroidism), hereditary and vascular cerebral atrophy, lead encephalopathy, acute demyelinating processes (multiple sclerosis), and Pick's disease.

Short Biography

Andrew John ("A.J.") Akelaitis was born in Baltimore, Maryland, on July 11, 1904. He studied medicine at Johns Hopkins University and received his M.D. in 1929. In the early 1930s, he practiced clinical neurology in Rochester, New York. He subsequently became an Assistant Professor of Medicine at the University of Rochester School of Medicine and Dentistry. Dr. Akelaitis joined the Navy during World War II where he served with distinction at the rank of Commander. He married the former Victoria Chesno. The couple had one son, Andrew, and a daughter, Lillian. Akelaitis died at the New York Hospital on November 24, 1955 at the young age of 51.

Cross-References

▶ Corpus Callosum
▶ Epilepsy
▶ Split-Brain

References and Readings

Akelaitis, A. J. (1941a). Psychobiological studies following section of the corpus callosum: A preliminary report. *American Journal of Psychiatry, 97*, 1147–1157.
Akelaitis, A. J. (1941b). Studies on the corpus callosum. II. The higher visual functions in each homonymous field following complete section of the corpus callosum. *Archives of Neurology and Psychiatry, 45*, 788–796.
Akelaitis, A. J., Risteen, W. A., Herren, R. Y., & Van Wagenen, W. P. (1942). Studies on the corpus callosum. III. A contribution to the study of dyspraxia and apraxia following partial and complete section of the corpus callosum. *Archives of Neurology and Psychiatry, 47*, 971–1008.
Akelaitis, A. J. (1944a). Studies on the corpus callosum. IV. Diagonistic dyspraxia in epileptics following partial and complete section of the corpus callosum. *American Journal of Psychiatry, 101*, 594–599.
Akelaitis, A. J. (1944b). Study on gnosis, praxis, and language following section of corpus callosum and anterior commisure. *Journal of Neurosurgery, 1*, 94–102.
Bogen, J. (1995). Some historical aspects of callosotomy for epilepsy. In A. G. Reeves & D. W. Roberts (Eds.), *Epilepsy and the corpus callosum 2* (pp. 107–121). New York: Plenum Press.
Gazzaniga, M. S. (1995). Principles of human brain organization derived from split brain studies. *Neuron, 14*, 217–228.
Gazzaniga, M. S. (2005). Forty-five years of split-brain research and still going strong. *Nature Reviews: Neuroscience, 6*, 653–659.
Mathews, S., Linskey, M., & Binder, D. (2008). William P. van Wagenen and the first corpus callosotomies for epilepsy. *Journal of Neurosurgery, 108*, 608–613.
Sauerwein, H. C., & Lassonde, M. (1996). Akelaitis' investigations of the first split-brain patients. In C. Code, C.-W. Wallesh, Y. Joanette, & A. R. Lecours (Eds.), *Classic cases in neuropsychology* (pp. 305–317). Hove: Psychology Press.
Zaidel, E., Iacoboni, M., Zaidel, D., & Bogen, J. (2003). The callosal syndromes. In K. M. Heilman & E. Valenstein (Eds.), *Clinical neuropsychology* (pp. 347–403). New York: Oxford University Press.

Akinesis

Douglas I. Katz
Department of Neurology, Boston University School of Medicine, Braintree, MA, USA

Synonyms

Akinesia; Akinetic

Definition

Akinesis is an absence or paucity of movement, resulting from an abnormal motor control. It is a problem that may occur in Parkinson's disease when patients develop freezing or inability to initiate movement. It may also occur as a result of a paralyzed muscle, such as with an anesthetic nerve block.

Cross-References

▶ Action-Intentional Disorders
▶ Akinetic Mutism
▶ Bradykinesia
▶ Parkinson's Disease

Akinetic Mutism

Michael S. Mega
Center for Cognitive Health, Portland, OR, USA

Synonyms

A spectrum of motivational impairment has abulia at one end and akinetic mutism at the other. Coma vigil is not akinetic mutism; it arises when a comatose patient regains the sleep-wake cycle, eyes open during the day and closed during sleep at night, usually after 2 weeks of a brain lesion that produces irreversible coma. Coma vigil is also referred to as a persistent vegetative state. When brain lesions disconnect all descending motor output but preserve conscious awareness the patient is said to be *locked in*. In akinetic mutism, patients still respond to their internal and external environment – and thus are not in coma, and they are not locked in since they can accomplish motor output, given sufficient motivation.

Short Description or Definition

The fully formed akinetic mute state usually results from bilateral anterior cingulate lesions (Fig. 1). Patients are profoundly apathetic, incontinent, and akinetic. They do not initiate eating or drinking and if speech occurs, it is restricted to terse responses. They seem awake, visually tracking objects, but displaying no emotions – even during painful circumstances, they remain indifferent. The akinetic mute state also results from bilateral subcortical paramedian diencephalic and midbrain lesions possibly affecting the ascending reticular core, medial forebrain bundles, and isolated bilateral globus pallidus lesions.

Categorization

When anterior cingulate lesions are bilateral, limbic, cognitive, and motor activation is disrupted producing profound akinetic mutism. Loss of ascending input from the reticular core, due to bilateral lesions of the medial forebrain bundle, may also produce akinetic mutism. Rarely are complete bilateral lesions seen in humans, more frequently partial circuit disruption results in a graded loss in motivation depending upon which circuit is damaged.

Five frontal-subcortical circuits have been named according to their function or cortical site of origin: the motor circuit, originating in the supplementary motor area, and the oculomotor circuit, originating in the frontal eye fields, are dedicated to motor function. The dorsolateral prefrontal, lateral orbitofrontal, and anterior cingulate circuits support executive cognitive functions, personality, and motivation, respectively (Mega and Cummings 1994). Each of the five circuits has the same member structures: the frontal lobe, striatum, globus pallidus, substantia nigra, and thalamus. There is a progressive spatial compaction of the circuits as they travel through the basal ganglia. A lesion anywhere along the path of a circuit will produce the same clinical result but only in the globus pallidus interna are all the frontal-subcortical circuits in such

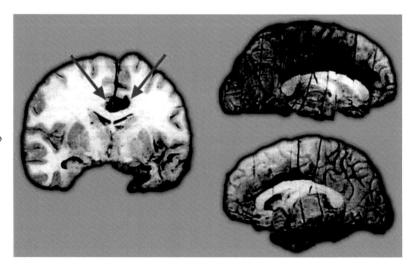

Akinetic Mutism,
Fig. 1 *Arrows* show the left greater than right anterior cingulate lesions due to bilateral anterior cerebral artery (*ACA*) ischemic stroke. Bilateral ACA lesions usually result in death due to loss of all limbic motivational input to prefrontal cortex

a compact spatial volume that a relatively small lesion can have profound effects.

Epidemiology

Akinetic mutism is exceedingly rare when permanent, since a bilateral lesion is necessary and usually results in death. Unilateral anterior cerebral artery (ACA) strokes are the usual cause of transient akinetic mutism, but ACA strokes only make up 1% of all cerebral vascular lesions.

Natural History, Prognostic Factors, and Outcomes

The natural history of akinetic mutism, when it arises from a unilateral lesion, is usually a 2-week period of gradual improvement from the fully formed syndrome to near-complete recovery presumably enabled by contralateral limbic activation gaining access to deafferented networks. The outcome from bilateral lesions is usually death, given no ability for cross-hemispheric motivation. Thus, prognosis will rely upon neuroimaging documenting the extent of the lesion.

Neuropsychology and Psychology

Extracingulate connections support a segregation of the cingulate into functional subregions (for a complete discussion of these circuits, *Cingulate Gyrus*). Paralleling the general distinction between posterior granular sensory cortices and anterior agranular executive cortices, the anterior cingulate can be considered an executive region for affective motivation and cognition, while the posterior cingulate, with its prominent granular layer IV receiving sensory input, is engaged in visuospatial and memory processing. The interconnections between the anterior and posterior cingulate allow for regulatory control by the anterior executive effector regions over posterior sensory processing and reciprocal modulation of that regulatory input by the posterior cingulate.

Three anterior effector regions include a *visceral effector region* inferior to the genu of the corpus callosum encompassing area 25, the anterior subcallosal portions of 24a-b, and 32; a *cognitive effector region* that includes most of the supracallosal area 24, and areas 24a′-b′ and 32′; and a *skeletomotor effector region* within the depths of the cingulate sulcus, that includes areas 24c′/23c on the ventral bank, with 24c′g and 6c on the dorsal bank. These three cingulate effector regions integrate ascending input concerning the internal milieu of the organism with visceral motor systems, cognitive-attentional networks, and skeletomotor centers to produce the affective motivation necessary for the organism's engagement in the environment.

Circumscribed lesions in humans are rarely confined to one region of the cingulate. With an anterior lesion, the cognitive, skeletomotor, and visceral effector regions are often affected. Bilateral lesions result in an akinetic mute state. The loss of spontaneous motor activity results when the lesion involves the supplementary motor area and the skeletomotor effector region. When these two motor regions are spared, motor activity will be normal but the patient will demonstrate profound indifference, docility, and the loss of motivation to engage in a task. They can be led by the examiner to engage in a task but will fail to self-generate sustained directed attention. They lack cognitive motivation.

The role of the anterior cingulate as a cognitive effector is appreciated within the realm of language. Language, a cognitive function, is distinguished from the motor function of speech. Transcortical motor aphasia (TCMA) is the usual result of left anterior medial or anterior dorsolateral prefrontal lesions. The classic syndrome of TCMA is initial mutism that resolves in days to weeks, yielding a syndrome featuring delayed initiation of brief utterances without impaired articulation, excellent repetition, inappropriate word selection, agrammatism, and poor comprehension of complex syntax. Activation of dorsolateral prefrontal cortices enabling language and speech arises from two sources: the anterior cingulate and the supplementary motor area (with the cingulate skeletomotor region). When the executive prefrontal cortex (areas 9, 10, and 46) is disrupted, cognitive language deficits are prominent (TCMA, type I); when motor neurons in area 4, devoted to the speech apparatus, are disconnected from their activation, speech hesitancy and impoverished output ensues (TCMA, type II). These two functional realms are separable and can be disconnected anywhere along two pathways. Direct damage to the supplementary motor area or its outflow to the motor cortex traveling in the anterior superior paraventricular white matter will produce TCMA type II. Direct damage to the anterior cingulate, its outflow to areas 9, 10, and 46, or to the caudate – via the subcallosal fasciculus, just inferior to the frontal horn of the lateral ventricle – will disrupt frontal-subcortical circuits involved in motivation and executive cognitive function. The initial muteness has been described by a patient after recovery from an anterior cingulate/supplementary motor infarction as a loss of the "will" to reply to her examiners, because she had "nothing to say," her "mind was empty," and "nothing mattered" (Damasio and Van Hoesen 1983).

The loss of will to initiate a motor function results from supplementary motor or cingulate skeletomotor region damage, while poor initiation of a cognitive process results from lesions in supracallosal cingulate areas. Loss of emotional vigilance ranging from flattened affect to neglect can be produced by surgery in this region. Anterior cingulate lesions in monkeys – difficult subjects in which to evaluate subtle behavioral changes – produce either no observable change or result in a transient stupor with ensuing lethargy, tameness, disturbed intraspecies social behavior, and decreased pain sensitivity (Pribram and Fulton 1954). Removal of the anterior cingulate (areas 24 and 32) in humans (cingulectomy) has been employed as a treatment for epilepsy, psychiatric, and pain disorders.

The cingulum bundle has also been the site of surgical lesions (cingulumotomy when only the bundle is transected, or cingulotomy when cingulate cortex is also removed) to treat psychiatric and pain disorders. The cingulum contains the efferents and afferents of the cingulate to the hippocampus, basal forebrain, amygdala, and all cortical areas, as well as fibers of passage between hippocampus and prefrontal cortex, and from the median raphe to the dorsal hippocampus. Surgical ablation of the anterior portion (sparing fibers relevant to memory function) is most successful when treating aggression, extreme anxiety, obsessive-compulsive behaviors, and severe pain. Psychotic symptoms show only a temporary response. The only prospective long-term follow-up of patients undergoing supracallosal anterior cingulotomy for the treatment of medically refractory obsessive-compulsive disorder revealed a clear response in 28% and a partial response in 17% (Baer et al. 1995). Including the subcallosal anterior cingulate/medial orbital cortex may provide the best result in treating the refractory obsessive-compulsive patient (Hay et al. 1993) due to the elimination of the visceromotor aspects of the disorder. Postsurgical personality changes are subtle after the acute attentional disorder resolves. Although formal cognitive testing is unaltered, affect is flattened. Motivation for previous enjoyments, such as reading, hobbies, and even spectator sports, is lost (Tow and Whitty 1953) subtle changes that reflect the loss of higher *cognitive* motivation. The three anterior cingulate regions, by virtue of the distinct functional systems they coordinate, are the conduits through which limbic motivation can activate feeling, thought, and movement – partial lesions produce partial aspects of the akinetic mute state depending upon their location.

Subcortical lesions can also produce the fully formed syndrome. Carbon monoxide poisoning with resultant apathy and placidity was described in a patient with a ventral pallidal lesion who also had hypoperfusion on single photon emission computed tomography (SPECT) predominately in the cingulate bilaterally (Mori et al. 1996). Hypometabolism on ^{18}F-fluorodeoxyglucose positron emission tomography (FDG-PET) in frontal cortex has also resulted from pallidal lesions (Laplane et al. 1989) disconnecting their cortical targets. Yet, when pallidal lesions result from carbon monoxide poisoning, microscopic cortical lesions may contribute to the functional imaging abnormalities. Ventral extension of a pallidal lesion appears to disconnect the anterior cingulate circuit, in nonhuman primates and humans (Mega and Cohenour 1997), from limbic drive. Bilateral paramedian or anterior thalamic lesions (Nagaratnam et al. 2004) caudate (Grunsfeld and Login 2006) or putamen (Ure et al. 1998) lesions will also disrupt the anterior cingulate frontal-subcortical circuit.

Evaluation

Evaluation of the patient suspected of suffering from akinetic mutism is to first rule out other causes of possible unresponsiveness. Documenting the response to first verbal stimuli, and then sensory stimuli, will provide evidence for or against coma. Patients in coma will not respond to internal (e.g., hunger) or external (e.g., pain) stimuli. All patients who survive the myriad of insults producing coma will regain the sleep-wake cycle and will eventually open their eyes spontaneously. They are then described as being in a persistent vegetative state. The locked-in patient will blink to command and can be taught to use blinking as a form of communication. The patient with akinetic mutism will respond to stimuli but will not initiate an unprovoked response. When any patient with limited response is encountered, a brain imaging study is required in their evaluation.

Treatment

Time is the best treatment for unilateral lesions producing akinetic mutism since after the acute phase of the lesion (4–6 weeks) the patients usually recover limbic activation from unaffected regions. When subcortical lesions destroy ascending dopaminergic fibers in the medial forebrain bundle, patients may respond to dopaminergic agonist (Psarros et al. 2003), or paradoxically antagonists of the D2 receptor (Brefel-Courbon et al. 2007) and GABA activation (Spiegel et al. 2008), perhaps due to blocking feedback-loop inhibition.

Cross-References

► Abulia
► Apathy
► Cingulate Gyrus
► Motivation

References and Readings

Baer, L., Rauch, S. L., Ballantine, H. T., Martuza, R., Cosgrove, R., Cassem, E., et al. (1995). Cingulotomy for intractable obsessive-compulsive disorder: Prospective long-term follow-up of 18 patients. *Archives of General Psychiatry, 52*, 384–392.

Brefel-Courbon, C., Payoux, P., Ory, F., Sommet, A., Slaoui, T., Raboyeau, G., et al. (2007). Clinical and imaging evidence of zolpidem effect in hypoxic encephalopathy. *Annals of Neurology, 62*(1), 102–105.

Damasio, A. R., & Van Hoesen, G. W. (1983). Focal lesions of the limbic frontal lobe. In K. M. Heilman & P. Satz (Eds.), *Neuropsychology of human emotion* (pp. 85–110). New York: Guilford.

Grunsfeld, A. A., & Login, I. S. (2006). Abulia following penetrating brain injury during endoscopic sinus surgery with disruption of the anterior cingulate circuit: Case report. *BMC Neurology, 6*, 4.

Hay, P., Sachdev, P., Cumming, S., Smith, J. S., Lee, T., Kitchener, P., et al. (1993). Treatment of obsessive-compulsive disorder by psychosurgery. *Acta Psychiatrica Scandinavica, 87*, 197–207.

Laplane, D., Levasseur, M., Pillon, B., Dubois, B., Baulac, M., Mazoyer, B., et al. (1989). Obsessive-compulsive and other behavioural changes with bilateral basal ganglia lesions. *Brain: A Journal of Neurology, 112*, 699–725.

Mega, M. S., & Cohenour, R. C. (1997). Akinetic mutism: A disconnection of frontal-subcortical circuits. *Neurology, Neuropsychology, and Behavioral Neurology, 10*, 254–259.

Mega, M. S., & Cummings, J. L. (1994). Frontal subcortical circuits and neuropsychiatric disorders. *Journal of Neuropsychiatry and Clinical Neurosciences, 6*, 358–370.

Mori, E., Yamashita, H., Takauchi, S., & Kondo, K. (1996). Isolated athymhormia following hypoxic bilateral pallidal lesions. *Behavioral Neurology, 9*, 17–23.

Nagaratnam, N., Nagaratnam, K., Ng, K., & Diu, P. (2004). Akinetic mutism following stroke. *Journal of Clinical Neuroscience: Official Journal of the Neurosurgical Society of Australasia, 11*(1), 25–30.

Pribram, K. H., & Fulton, J. F. (1954). An experimental critique of the effects of anterior cingulate ablations in monkey. *Brain: A Journal of Neurology, 77*, 34–44.

Psarros, T., Zouros, A., & Coimbra, C. (2003). Bromocriptine-responsive akinetic mutism following endoscopy for ventricular neurocysticercosis. Case report and review of the literature. *Journal of Neurosurgery, 99* (2), 397–401.

Spiegel, D. R., Casella, D. P., Callender, D. M., & Dhadwal, N. (2008). Treatment of akinetic mutism with intramuscular olanzapine: A case series. *Journal of Neuropsychiatry and Clinical Neurosciences, 20*(1), 93–95.

Tow, P. M., & Whitty, C. W. M. (1953). Personality changes after operations of the cingulate gyrus in man. *Journal of Neurology, Neurosurgery, and Psychiatry, 16*, 186–193.

Ure, J., Faccio, E., Videla, H., Caccuri, R., Giudice, F., Ollari, J., et al. (1998). Akinetic mutism: A report of three cases. *Acta Neurologica Scandinavica, 98*(6), 439–444.

Alcohol Abuse

Nathan Ewigman
Mental Health Service Line, San Francisco VA
Health Care System, San Francisco, CA, USA

Synonyms

Alcoholism; Binge drinking; Excessive alcohol use

Short Description or Definition

Alcohol abuse refers to a "maladaptive pattern of alcohol [use] leading to clinically significant impairment or distress." The DSM-5 criteria for substance use disorders as applied to alcohol abuse are presented below.

DSM-5 Criteria for Alcohol Use Disorder

1. A minimum of 2–3 criteria is required for a mild substance use disorder diagnosis, while 4–5 is moderate and 6–7 is severe (APA 2013):
   - Taking alcohol in larger amounts and for longer than intended
   - Wanting to cut down or quit but not being able to do it
   - Spending a lot of time obtaining alcohol
   - Craving or a strong desire to use alcohol
   - Repeatedly unable to carry out major obligations at work, school, or home due to alcohol use
   - Continued use despite persistent or recurring social or interpersonal problems caused or made worse by alcohol use
   - Stopping or reducing important social, occupational, or recreational activities due to alcohol use
   - Recurrent use of alcohol in physically hazardous situations
   - Consistent use of alcohol despite acknowledgment of persistent or recurrent physical or psychological difficulties from using alcohol
   - Tolerance as defined by either a need for markedly increased amounts to achieve intoxication or desired effect or markedly diminished effect with continued use of the same amount
   - Withdrawal manifesting as either characteristic syndrome or alcohol is used to avoid withdrawal

Although alcohol abuse is diagnosed primarily by observed or reported impairment and distress related to alcohol use, the *Dietary Guidelines for Americans* recommends no more than one drink per day for women and two drinks per day for men (USDA 2005).

Categorization

In the DSM-5, alcohol abuse and dependence are combined into alcohol use disorder (AUD) with a severity specifier from mild to severe (DSM-5 2013). Individuals with AUD may continue to drink despite awareness of the potential negative physical, social, and legal consequences.

Epidemiology

Alcohol abuse is associated with diseases of the liver, hypertension, neurological damage, and cardiac diseases such as heart failure. In 2000, alcohol abuse was responsible for 85,000 deaths in the USA. National data suggest that the prevalence of DSM-IV-TR alcohol abuse (not including alcohol dependence) was 4.65% in 2001–2002 (Grant et al. 2004). More recent data on 12-month and lifetime prevalence on AUD (which combines abuse and dependence diagnoses) was 13.9% and 29.1%, respectively. Being male, white, Native American, younger, low income, and having a disability has been associated with AUD prevalence. Approximately one out of five individuals with AUD has ever been treated (Grant et al. 2015). It appears that alcohol abuse is generally more severe with earlier onset in age of alcohol use (Grant et al. 2001). Results from a national survey suggest that close to one fifth of adolescents and adults engaged in binge drinking one or more times within the last 30 days (US DHHS 2002).

Natural History, Prognostic Factors, and Outcomes

In *The Natural History of Alcoholism Revisited*, George Vaillant (1995) described alcohol dependence as a condition of gradual onset over 5–15 years of continuous alcohol abuse. He found that the average age of onset was 29 years among a cohort of delinquent youth and 41 among a higher-educated group. In the cohorts that Vaillant (1995) studied, the prevalence of alcoholism increased until age 40 and then declined at a rate of 2–3% per year thereafter.

Potential risk factors for alcohol abuse in adolescence and early adulthood include being in areas of high availability and accessibility, early alcohol use (DeWit et al. 2014), sensation seeking and low harm-avoidance in youth, family history of alcohol abuse, liberal family attitude toward alcohol use, lack of family closeness, and early behavioral problems (Hawkins et al. 1992). Another risk factor appears to be comorbid mental disorders. Epidemiological data suggest that 37% of people who have an alcohol disorder also have another mental disorder (Regier et al. 1990), emphasizing the importance of mental and behavior health screening.

In Vaillant (1995) delinquent youth cohort, by age 70, 54% had already died, 32% were abstinent, 12% were still abusing alcohol, and 1% were controlled drinkers (i.e., drinking but not abusing).

In terms of prognostic factors, Vaillant (1995) suggests that those who achieve "long-term sobriety usually [are characterized by] (1) a less harmful, substitute dependency; (2) new relationships; (3) sources of inspiration and hope; and (4) experiencing negative consequences of drinking." From a neurobiological perspective, a pattern of long-term structural damage with region-specific recovery is observable in alcoholics who have achieved long-term abstinence (O'Neill et al. 2001). Neuropsychologically, early gains from abstinence include improved short-term memory and visuospatial, attentional, and balance abilities (Sullivan et al. 2000).

Neuropsychology and Psychology of Alcohol Abuse

In a review of the literature of neuropsychological deficits in chronic alcohol abusers, Chelune and Parker (1981) found patterns of neurological damage such as cerebral atrophy, ventricular enlargement, and decreased cerebral blood flow. Approximately 10% of chronic alcohol abusers have neurocognitive deficits commensurate with diagnoses of alcohol-related amnesia or dementia. A large portion of those without diagnosable neurocognitive deficits still evince disturbed neuropsychological performance (Rourke and Grant 2009). Alcoholics generally function in the average to above average range on IQ tests with consistently lower performance IQ (PIQ) scores relative to verbal IQ (VIQ). Their PIQ scores are similar to those of persons with brain damage, whereas VIQ scores are comparable with those of normal controls (Chelune and Parker 1981; Rourke and Grant 2009). However, this discrepancy is not diagnostic of alcoholism. Within the Wechsler subtests, Block Design appears to be the most frequently impaired relative to normal controls in all studies reviewed. Block Design impairment has been cited as an effective discriminator between alcoholics and nonalcoholics. Object Assembly and Digit Symbol were also impaired relative to normal controls in more than 3/4 of the studies. Other tests that have revealed impairment in alcoholics include the Category Test, Wisconsin Card Sorting Test, Raven's Progressive Matrices, Shipley-Hartford Abstract Age, and other tests of abstract thinking. Alcoholics also generally perform poorly on Part B of the Trail Making Test relative to matched control groups (Chelune and Parker 1981).

Overall, the most consistently impaired neuropsychological domains include verbal and nonverbal learning and perceptual motor skills. More broadly, most reviews conclude that abstraction-executive abilities are impaired among alcohol abusers (Rourke and Grant 2009). Despite the consistency of these neuropsychological findings, many of the samples from these studies are recently detoxified adults. Grant and Adams (2009) point out that neuropsychological recovery typically occurs following the first year – and perhaps more – of detoxification.

Although the exact mechanisms of these neuropsychological deficits are not known, some of the major hypotheses attempting to explain these deficits have been (Chelune and Parker 1981):

1. Chronic alcohol abuse results in premature aging of the brain.
2. Chronic alcohol abuse leads to global generalized CNS dysfunction.
3. Chronic alcohol abuse differentially disrupts the right hemisphere of the brain.
4. Chronic alcohol abuse exerts its detrimental effect *on the* anterior-basal regions of the brain.
5. Chronic alcohol abuse produces a generalized CNS impairment that is particularly disruptive of the frontoparietal association areas of the brain.

More recent neural hypotheses of the mechanisms of neuropsychological deficits include reduced regional blood flow to the frontal lobes, reduction in metabolites (e.g., NAA) that indicate lack of neuronal integrity, and frontal-striatal and cerebellar dysfunction manifesting as loss of dendritic arbor (Rourke and Grant 2009). Grant and Adams (2009) note that molecular mechanisms of the influence of chronic alcohol abuse on neuropsychological functioning are largely unknown.

Evaluation

A common screening tool for alcohol abuse is the CAGE questionnaire (Ewing 1984; see An even briefer CAGE Questionnaire, Table B). The CAGE is highly effective at identifying problem drinkers among adults (Bernadt 1982). Two "yes" responses on the CAGE indicate that the respondent should be investigated further. The questionnaire asks the following questions:

- Have you ever felt you needed to *C*ut down on your drinking?
- Have people *A*nnoyed you by criticizing your drinking?
- Have you ever felt *G*uilty about drinking?
- Have you ever felt you needed a drink first thing in the morning (*E*ye-opener) to steady your nerves or to get rid of a hangover?

Other brief assessments for alcohol abuse include the POSIT and CRAFFT for adolescents (Knight et al. 2003), the Michigan Alcoholism Screen Test (MAST) for adults (Magruder-Habib et al. 1993), and the AUDIT-C for both adults and adolescents (Bush et al. 1998). According to Fiellin et al. (2000), the CAGE and the AUDIT are the superior screening instruments in primary care settings compared with other alcohol abuse screeners and other clinical methods. The CAGE is superior at detecting diagnosable abuse and dependence, and the AUDIT is superior at detecting at-risk and harmful drinking (Fiellin et al. 2000). AUDIT-C has been shown to be effective in screening for alcohol use disorder in DSM-5 (Dawson et al. 2012).

Treatment

Treatment ranges from support groups to rehabilitation centers. Treatments of alcohol abuse appear to be largely psychosocial. In a systematic review, brief psychosocial interventions among primary care patients were found to be effective at reducing alcohol consumption (Kaner et al. 2007). Although well-known support groups such as Alcoholics Anonymous (AA) have been helpful to many people and likely constitute the most accessible form of treatment, evidence has not supported AA's effectiveness at reducing alcohol problems (Ferri et al. 2006). Medical treatments of alcohol abuse focus on reducing craving. Naltrexone (Chick et al. 2000) and acamprosate (Garbutt et al. 1999) have been found to be effective at reducing craving. However, most medications are aimed at dependence, not abuse symptoms. A common framework called SBIRT (screening, brief intervention, and referral to treatment) has shown promising outcomes toward a population-based management approach of AUD (Babor et al. 2007). Secondary effects of alcohol abuse, such as Wernicke-Korsakoff syndrome, can be treated through monitoring and infusion to correct for vitamin deficiency (Isenberg-Grzeda et al. 2012); however, longer-term neurocognitive consequences can only be managed and can lead to placement in long-term care facilities (Bommersbach et al. 2015).

Cross-References

▶ Alcoholic Brain Syndrome
▶ Alcohol Dependence
▶ Blood Alcohol Level
▶ Fetal Alcohol Spectrum Disorder
▶ Michigan Alcoholism Screen Test
▶ Substance Abuse
▶ Wernicke-Korsakoff Syndrome

References and Readings

American Psychiatric Association. (2013). *Diagnostic and statistical manual of mental disorders: DSM-5*. Washington, DC: American Psychiatric Association.

Babor, T. F., et al. (2007). Screening, brief intervention, and referral to treatment (SBIRT) toward a public health approach to the management of substance abuse. *Substance Abuse, 28*(3), 7–30.

Bernadt, M. W. (1982). Comparison of questionnaire and laboratory tests in the detection of excessive drinking and alcoholism. *Lancet, 6*, 325–328.

Bommersbach, T. J., et al. (2015). Geriatric alcohol use disorder: A review for primary care physicians. *Mayo Clinic Proceedings, 90*(5), 659–666. Elsevier.

Bush, K., et al. (1998). The AUDIT alcohol consumption questions (AUDIT-C): an effective brief screening test for problem drinking. *Archives of internal medicine, 158*(16), 1789–1795.

Chelune, G. J., & Parker, J. B. (1981). Neuropsychological deficits associated with chronic alcohol abuse. *Clinical Psychology Review, 1*, 181–195.

Chick, J., Anton, R., Checinski, K., Croop, R., Drummond, D. C., Farmer, R., et al. (2000). A multicentre, randomized, double-blind, placebo-controlled trial of naltrexone in the treatment of alcohol dependence or abuse. *Alcohol, 35*, 587–593.

Dawson, D. A., et al. (2012). Comparative performance of the AUDIT-C in screening for DSM-IV and DSM-5 alcohol use disorders. *Drug and Alcohol Dependence, 126*(3), 384–388.

DeWit, D. J., et al. (2014). Age at first alcohol use: a risk factor for the development of alcohol disorders. *American Journal of Psychiatry, 157*(5), 745–750.

Ewing, J. A. (1984). Detecting alcoholism: The CAGE questionnaire. *JAMA, 252*, 1905–1907.

Ferri, M. M. F., Amato, L., & Davoli, M. (2006). Alcoholics anonymous and other 12-step programmes for alcohol dependence. *Cochrane Database of Systematic Reviews, 19*(3), CD005032. https://doi.org/10.1002/14651858.CD005032.pub2.

Fiellin, D. A., Reid, M. C., & O'Connor, P. G. (2000). Screening for alcohol problems in primary care: A systematic review. *Archives of Internal Medicine, 160*(13), 1977–1989.

Garbutt, J. C., West, S. L., Carey, T. S., Lohr, K. N., & Crews, F. T. (1999). Pharmacological treatment of alcohol dependence: A review of the evidence. *JAMA, 281*, 1318–1325.

Grant, I., & Adams, K. M. (Eds.). (2009). *Neuropsychological assessment of neuropsychiatric disorders* (3rd ed.pp. 127–158). New York: Oxford University Press.

Grant, B. F., Stinson, F. S., & Harford, T. C. (2001). Age at onset of alcohol use and DSM-IV alcohol abuse and dependence: A 12-year follow-up. *Journal of Substance Abuse, 13*, 493–504.

Grant, B. F., Dawson, D. A., Stinson, F. S., Chou, S. P., Dufour, M. C., & Pickering, R. P. (2004). The 12-month prevalence and trends in DSM-IV alcohol abuse and dependence: United States, 1991–1992 and 2001–2002. *Drug and Alcohol Dependence, 74*, 223–234.

Grant, B. F., et al. (2015). Epidemiology of DSM-5 alcohol use disorder: Results from the national epidemiologic survey on alcohol and related conditions III. *JAMA Psychiatry, 72*(8), 757–766.

Hasin, D. S., Van Rossem, R., McCloud, S., & Endicott, J. (1997). Alcohol dependence and abuse diagnoses: Validity in a community sample of heavy drinkers. *Alcoholism, Clinical and Experimental Research, 21*, 213–219.

Hawkins, J. D., Catalano, R. F., & Miller, J. Y. (1992). Risk and protective factors for alcohol and other drug problems in adolescence and early adulthood: Implications for substance abuse prevention. *Psychological Bulletin, 112*, 64–105.

Isenberg-Grzeda, E., Kutner, H. E., & Nicolson, S. E. (2012). Wernicke-Korsakoff-syndrome: Under-recognized and under-treated. *Psychosomatics, 53*(6), 507–516.

Kaner, Eileen F. S., et al. (2007). Effectiveness of brief alcohol interventions in primary care populations. The Cochrane Library.

Knight, J. R., Sherritt, L., Harris, S. K., Gates, E. C., & Chang, G. (2003). Validity of brief alcohol screening tests among adolescents: A comparison of the AUDIT, POSIT, CAGE, and CRAFFT. *Alcoholism, Clinical and Experimental Research, 27*, 67–73.

Magruder-Habib, K., Stevens, H. A., & Alling, W. C. (1993). Relative performance of the MAST, VAST, and CAGE versus DSM-III-R criteria for alcohol dependence. *Journal of Clinical Epidemiology, 46*, 435–441.

O'Neill, J., Cardenas, V. A., & Meyerhoff, D. J. (2001). Effects of abstinence on the brain: Quantitative magnetic resonance imaging and magnetic resonance spectroscopic imaging in chronic alcohol abuse. *Alcoholism: Clinical and Experimental Research, 25*(11), 1673–1682.

Regier, D. A., Farmer, M. E., Rae, D. S., Locke, B. Z., Keith, S. J., Judd, L. L., et al. (1990). Comorbidity of mental disorders with alcohol and other drug abuse. Results from the epidemiologic catchment area (ECA) study. *JAMA, 264*, 2511–2518.

Rourke, S. B., & Grant, I. (2009). The neurobehavioral correlates of alcoholism. In I. Grant & K. M. Adams (Eds.), *Neuropsychological assessment of neuropsychiatric and neuromedical disorders* (3rd ed., pp. 398–454). New York: Oxford University Press.

Sullivan, E. V., et al. (2000). Longitudinal changes in cognition, gait, and balance in abstinent and relapsed alcoholic men: Relationships to changes in brain structure. *Neuropsychology, 14*(2), 178.

U.S. Department of Health and Human Services. Substance Abuse and Mental Health Services Administration(US DHHS). (2002). *Results from the 2001 national household survey on drug abuse: Volume I. Summary of national findings (Office of Applied Studies, NHSDA Series H-17 ed.) (BKD461, SMA 02-3758)*. Washington, DC: U.S. Government Printing Office. Retrieved 14 Mar 2009, from the World Wide Web: http://www.oas.samhsa.gov/nhsda/2k1nhsda/vol1/Chapter3.htm.

United States Department of Agriculture and United States Department of Health and Human Services (USDA).
(2005). *Dietary guidelines for Americans: Chap. 9 – Alcoholic beverages* (pp. 43–46). Washington, DC: US Government Printing Office.

Vaillant, G. E. (1995). *The natural history of alcoholism revisited*. Cambridge, MA: Harvard University Press.

Alcohol Dependence

Glenn S. Ashkanazi
Department of Clinical and Health Psychology, Clinical and Health Psychology Clinic, College of Public Health and Health Professions, University of Florida, Gainesville, FL, USA

Synonyms

Alcoholism

Definition

This diagnosis no longer exists and has been replaced by "Alcohol Use Disorder" in DSM-5

As described in DSM-IV, alcohol dependence is a set of symptoms encompassing dysfunction in cognitive, behavioral, and physiological domains caused by continued alcohol use. A pattern of repeated alcohol ingestion exists, resulting in increasing amounts consumed in order to obtain the desired effect (i.e., tolerance) and characteristic symptoms if use is suddenly suspended (i.e., withdrawal). There is a perceived loss of control over drinking, exhibited by repeated failed attempts to decrease or quit drinking. Individuals may spend increasing amounts of time in drinking-related behaviors without being able to stop, despite being aware that drinking is causing, or exacerbating, psychological or medical problems. Cognitive consequences can include memory loss, difficulty performing familiar tasks, poor or impaired judgment, and problems with language.

Cross-References

▶ Alcohol Abuse

► Alcoholic Brain Syndrome
► Substance Abuse
► Substance Use Disorders
► Wernicke-Korsakoff Syndrome

References and Readings

American Psychiatric Association. (1994). *Diagnostic and statistical manual of mental disorders* (4th ed.). Washington, DC: American Psychiatric Association.

Alcohol Use Disorders Indentification Test (AUDIT), The

Matthew P. Martens
University of Missouri, Columbia, MO, USA

Synonyms

AUDIT; AUDIT Alcohol Consumption Questions (AUDIT-C)

Description

The Alcohol Use Disorders Identification Test (AUDIT: Saunders et al. 1993) consists of ten questions that assess quantity/frequency of alcohol consumption (e.g., number of drinks typically consumed when drinking alcohol), symptoms of a potential alcohol use disorder (e.g., frequency of not engaging in expected activities due to alcohol use), and specific problems associated with alcohol use (e.g., injuring someone else). It is not a formal diagnostic measure but is used to identify individuals who may be engaging in harmful alcohol use. Scores on each item range from 0 to 4, with higher scores indicating more problematic alcohol use. Scores of 8+ on the measure have generally been used to identify individuals engaging in potentially hazardous or harmful alcohol use. The developers of the measure recommend that those who exceed the screening threshold should be advised to consider cutting down on their alcohol use and/or receive further in-depth assessment (e.g., a structured diagnostic interview).

Researchers and clinicians sometimes use a shortened measure of the AUDIT that assesses only alcohol consumption, the AUDIT-C (AUDIT Alcohol Consumption Questions; Bush et al. 1998). The AUDIT-C consists of the first three items of the full measure, which assess frequency of alcohol use, typical number of drinks consumed on a drinking day, and number of days engaging in heavy drinking (6+ drinks). The brevity of the AUDIT-C makes it appealing as an alcohol use screener in very busy clinical settings. For example, the Veterans Administration uses the AUDIT-C for annual routine alcohol screening (Bradley et al. 2006), and those who exceed the screening threshold (4+ for men, 3+ for women) are required to receive a brief alcohol counseling session from their provider.

Historical Background

The Alcohol Use Disorders Identification Test (AUDIT) is one of the most commonly used measures to screen for at-risk alcohol use and is available for public use. It was originally developed as part of a World Health Organization initiative (Saunders et al. 1993), and has been used extensively by researchers and clinicians throughout the world. The original article detailing its development has been cited in the Web of Science Core Collection database over 3,000 times and in Google Scholar over 5,000 times. The primary rationale for developing the AUDIT was the need for a screening measure that identified problematic alcohol consumption at the lower end of a severity continuum. Measures that existed at the time, such as the Michigan Alcoholism Screening Test (MAST) or the CAGE, were reasonably effective at identifying individuals with the most severe alcohol-related problems. However, they were considerably less effective at identifying those experiencing milder alcohol-related problems that might be in an emerging phase. Without an effective screening measure for less-severe alcohol-related problems, it would be impossible to provide early intervention services that could inhibit the development of a formal alcohol use disorder. Researchers subsequently examined an even shorter version of the AUDIT, the AUDIT-C, due in part to logistical concerns about the willingness of physicians and others in primary care settings to administer a ten-item screening instrument (Bush et al. 1998).

Psychometric Data

A vast array of research studies have examined reliability and validity of scores on both the full AUDIT and the AUDIT-C. Scores on the AUDIT are consistently associated in the expected direction with other alcohol-related constructs, such as alcohol cravings and drinking motives. Considering that the measure is designed to classify individuals into potential at-risk drinking categories, it is particularly important to assess the accuracy of cutoff scores on the measures. In general, research has shown that both the AUDIT and AUDIT-C have relatively high sensitivity (i.e., accurately identifying those with an alcohol use disorder and/or who are engaging in high-risk drinking) and specificity (i.e., accurately identifying those without an alcohol use disorder and/or who engage in low-risk drinking). For example, in a national study of over 40,000 adults, a cutoff score of 4+ on the AUDIT-C yielded sensitivity values of 91.2 for alcohol dependence and 92.6 for at-risk drinking, with corresponding specificity values of 80.2 and 92.0 (Dawson et al. 2005). Similar findings have been reported for the full AUDIT with specific at-risk subgroups, such as young adults.

Clinical Uses

The AUDIT and its shortened version are excellent measures to screen for at-risk alcohol consumption and related problems in a variety of settings, including those where individuals may be experiencing neuropsychological problems. The AUDIT or AUDIT-C has been used as a screening measure when neuropsychological researchers were interested in recruiting participants experiencing alcohol-related problems (e.g., Houben et al. 2011), or when researchers were interested in association between harmful alcohol consumption and cognitive abilities (e.g., following a brain injury, see Ponsford et al. 2007, 2013). The full ten-item version can be used in research settings and in clinical settings where patients have more time to complete assessment measures, and the three-item AUDIT-C can be completed in less than a minute and provide an accurate picture of an individual's drinking risk. Cutoff scores on the AUDIT can be easily adjusted to meet the needs of a specific setting (e.g., using a lower cutoff score to increase sensitivity and/or identify individuals experiencing even mild alcohol-related problems).

See Also

▶ Alcohol Abuse
▶ Alcohol Dependence
▶ Michigan Alcoholism Screen Test

References and Readings

Bradley, K. A., Williams, E. C., Achtmeyer, C. E., Volpp, B., Collins, B. J., & Kivlahan, D. R. (2006). Implementation of evidence-based alcohol screening in the Veterans Health Administration. *American Journal of Managed Care, 12*, 597–606.

Bush, K., Kivlahan, D. R., McDonell, M. B., Fihn, S. D., & Bradley, K. A. (1998). The AUDIT alcohol consumption questions (AUDIT-C): An effective brief screening test for problem drinking. *Archives of Internal Medicine, 158*, 1789–1795.

Dawson, D. A., Grant, B. F., Stinson, F. S., & Zhou, Y. (2005). Effectiveness of the derived Alcohol Use Disorders Identification Test (AUDIT-C) in screening for alcohol use disorders and risk drinking in the US general population. *Alcoholism: Clinical and Experimental Research, 29*, 844–854.

Houben, K., Wiers, R. W., & Jansen, A. (2011). Getting a grip on drinking behavior: Training working memory to reduce alcohol use. *Psychological Science, 22*, 968–875.

Ponsford, J., Whelan-Goodinson, R., & Bahar-Fuchs, A. (2007). Alcohol and drug use following traumatic brain injury: A prospective study. *Brain Injury, 21*, 1385–1392.

Ponsford, J., Tweedly, L., & Taffe, J. (2013). The relationship between alcohol and cognitive functioning following traumatic brain injury. *Journal of Clinical and Experimental Neuropsychology, 35*, 103–112.

Saunders, J. B., Aasland, O. G., Babor, T. F., De La Fuente, J. R., & Grant, M. (1993). Development of the Alcohol Use Disorders Identification Test (AUDIT): WHO collaborative project on early detection of persons with harmful alcohol consumption-II. *Addiction, 88*, 791–804.

Alcoholic Brain Syndrome

Glenn S. Ashkanazi
Department of Clinical and Health Psychology, Clinical and Health Psychology Clinic, College of Public Health and Health Professions, University of Florida, Gainesville, FL, USA

Synonyms

Alcoholic dementia; Alcoholic hallucinosis; Delirium tremens; Korsakoff's syndrome; Wernicke-Korsakoff syndrome

Short Description or Definition

"Alcoholic brain syndrome" is a collection of several syndromes associated with the acute or chronic use of alcohol, resulting in significant impairment on normal brain functioning (APA Dictionary of Psychology 2007), also referred to as alcohol-related dementia (ARD).

Categorization

As mentioned in the definition, alcoholic brain syndrome encompasses several syndromes (newly named "major neurocognitive disorder (NCD)-substance/medication induced" in DSM-5):

1. *Alcohol withdrawal delirium (ICD-9)*: A reversible condition that develops after cessation of chronic, extreme alcohol intake. Symptoms include disturbed consciousness (e.g., disruption in attention/concentration) and disruption in memory, orientation, and language beyond what would be expected from typical alcohol withdrawal.

2. *Alcohol-induced persisting dementia (ICD-9)*: A chronic condition that includes multiple cognitive deficits as a result of prolonged alcohol abuse. Cognitive areas generally impaired include memory, speech, motor/sensory functions, and executive functions. Global impairment in intellectual functioning evolves gradually over time.

3. *Alcohol-induced persisting amnestic disorder (ICD-10)*: A persistent disturbance in memory functioning caused by chronic alcohol abuse. Memory impairment is severe enough to cause significant disturbance in occupational or social functioning.

4. *Wernicke's encephalopathy (WE) (ICD-10)*: A syndrome resulting from chronic alcoholism leading to nutritional deficiency (i.e., vitamin B1 [thiamine]) and characterized by acute confusion, ataxia, sluggish pupillary reflexes, nystagmus, and memory deficits. The syndrome can result in coma or death. Lesions are centered in the midbrain, cerebellum, and diencephalon.

5. *Korsakoff's syndrome (ICD-10)*: This condition often follows episodes of WE. Thiamine deficiency, as a result of chronic, severe alcohol abuse, leads to a dense anterograde and retrograde amnesia. Patients with Korsakoff's syndrome can store information for only a few seconds before they forget it. The resulting amnesia is thought to be due to damage in the mammillary bodies and anterior or dorsomedial nuclei (or both) of the thalamus. Another common feature is confabulation, in which the patient recounts detailed and convincing memories for events that have never happened.

6. *Alcohol-induced psychotic disorder (ICD-10)*: A condition involving the presence of delusions and/or hallucinations due to the physiological effects of alcohol.

Epidemiology

Up to two million alcoholics have developed permanent and debilitating conditions that require lifetime custodial care. A number of factors influence how and to what extent alcohol affects the brain. These include the age at which the person started drinking, duration of drinking, amount of alcohol consumed, drinking style/pattern, patient's age, education, genetic background, family history of alcoholism, neuropsychiatric risk factors (e.g., prenatal alcohol exposure), and general health status. Studies comparing men and women's sensitivity to alcohol-induced brain damage have not been conclusive. Of all cases of dementia, ARD accounts between 4% and 20%.

Poor nutrition has been a major contributor to the development of alcohol-induced brain damage. Up to 80% of alcoholics have a deficiency in thiamine (i.e., vitamin B1). This vitamin is an essential nutrient required by all tissues including the brain. Some of these people will progress to WE. Approximately 80–90% of alcoholics with Wernicke's develop Korsakoff's psychosis, which is more prevalent in men aged 45–65. Women who develop this condition tend to do so at a younger age (i.e., 35–55).

Natural History, Prognostic Factors, and Outcomes

Wernicke 's encephalopathy is a medical emergency and requires immediate treatment, as it can lead to death in approximately 20% of untreated cases. Symptoms can develop within hours and can be easily missed as many mimic intoxication. If treatment is given in time, usually through the administration of thiamine, progression of symptoms can be slowed or stopped. Ocular abnormalities usually recover within a few days to a few weeks, but ataxia takes 1–2 months longer to resolve. The acute confusion/delirium usually improves within 1–2 days after the treatment but may take 1–3 months to completely clear.

If treatment is not provided, then irreversible brain damage, or even death, is possible. Of those who survive, approximately 85% develop Korsakoff's syndrome. However, not every person who develops Korsakoff's syndrome has a previous episode of Wernicke's. Some will develop Korsakoff's gradually with either no known history or brief episodes of Wernicke's. Some patients are initially comatose or semiconscious and only when the acute disorder has resolved is the underlying Korsakoff's syndrome manifests. These patients are still susceptible to developing Wernicke's, especially if drinking were to continue.

Loss of some cognitive functions including memory in Korsakoff's syndrome may be permanent. Once the patient has developed Korsakoff's, the treatment strategies are not clear. However, it is important for patients to remain abstinent from alcohol. Depending on the degree of memory and executive function impairment, and availability of family support, patients with Korsakoff's may require long-term custodial care.

Neuropsychology and Psychology of Alcoholic Brain Syndrome

The classic symptom in Korsakoff's syndrome is the inability to form new memories (i.e., anterograde amnesia). However, patients also demonstrate significant deficits in their ability to recall incidents or events from their own past as well (i.e., episodic memory). Memory for facts, concepts, and language (i.e., semantic memory) is variable, while perceptual-motor memory is thought to be preserved.

The inability to recall previously learned information (i.e., retrograde amnesia) can often extend back 20–30 years in a person's life with Korsakoff's patients. Generally, a temporal gradient exists such that memories from the more distant past are recalled better than the more recent ones. The basis of this extensive retrograde amnesia is still a matter of great controversy.

These patients are typically younger than most patients presenting to dementia services, and because they often present as initially confused, with concomitant frontal lobe pathology, they are more likely to demonstrate aggressive, agitated behaviors and anxiety. Those with irreversible brain damage are unlikely to be able to live alone but also typically lack available social services. These patients often have a difficult time maintaining social and familial relationships and live isolated lives.

The classic triad of symptoms for Wernicke's encephalopathy is:

- Encephalopathy – demonstrative of damage to the frontal lobes, mammillary bodies, thalamus, and cerebellum
- Ataxic gait
- Some variant of oculomotor dysfunction

Evaluation

For patients who meet the ICD-10 criteria for Wernicke 's encephalopathy or Korsakoff's syndrome, neuropsychological assessment is useful for documenting functions that are impaired, the severity of impairment, and the prognostic factors involved in determining the patient's ability to manage daily life either independently or with assistance. However, it is preferable for the neuropsychological assessment to occur when the patient has been abstinent from alcohol for a long enough period of time to insure that the acute symptoms of alcohol withdrawal have subsided. Cognitive dysfunction includes aphasia, apraxia, agnosia, memory impairment, and decreased executive functions. Neuroimaging evidence of cerebellar atrophy/shrinkage also supports the diagnosis.

Treatment

The primary treatment option for patients experiencing alcoholic brain syndrome is to stop drinking and remain abstinent. Without additional alcohol exposure, the recovery from the delirium caused by alcohol is usually good. This is obviously the first treatment to be utilized. As mentioned above, thiamine deficiency is an important contributor to alcohol-related brain damage;

therefore, vitamin B1 supplementation is necessary. Initially, the vitamins can be given intravenously or intramuscularly followed by oral administration. Wernicke 's encephalopathy responds well to high-dose vitamins, and such treatment can prevent the occurrence of severe, chronic Korsakoff's syndrome. Secondarily, nutritional counseling to promote a vitamin-rich and balanced diet is also part of this initial treatment protocol, especially for longer-term recovery and prevention.

Cross-References

- ► Alcoholism
- ► Amnesia
- ► Anterograde Amnesia
- ► Dementia
- ► Encephalopathy
- ► Episodic Memory
- ► Korsakoff's Syndrome
- ► Organic Brain Syndrome
- ► Retrograde Amnesia
- ► Semantic Memory
- ► Substance Abuse

References and Readings

Horton, L., Duffy, T., & Martin, C. (2014). Comprehensive assessment of alcohol-related brain damage (ARBD): Gap or chasm in the evidence? *Journal of Psychiatric and Mental Health Nursing, 22*(1), 3–14.

Kopelman, M., Thomson, A., Guerrini, I., & Marshall, E. (2009). The Korsakoff syndrome: Clinical aspects, psychology and treatment. *Alcohol & Alcoholism, 44*(2), 148–154.

Martin, P., Singleton, C., & Hiller-Sturmhofel, S. (2003). The role of thiamine deficiency in alcoholic brain disease. *Alcohol Research & Health, 27*(2), 134–142.

Moriyama, Y., Mimura, M., Kato, M., & Kashima, H. (2006). Primary alcoholic dementia and alcohol-related dementia. *Psychogeriatrics, 6*(3), 114–118.

Oscar-Berman, M., & Marinkovic, K. (2003). Alcoholism and the brain: An overview. *Alcohol Research & Health, 27*(2), 125–133.

Parsons, O. (1996). Alcohol abuse and alcoholism. In R. Adams, O. Parsons, J. Culbertson, & S. Nixon (Eds.), *Neuropsychology for clinical practice: Etiology, assessment, and treatment of common neurological disorders*. Washington, DC: American Psychological Association.

Ridley, N., & Draper, B. (2015). Alcohol-related dementia and brain damage. In J. Svanberg, A. Withall, B. Draper, & S. Bowden (Eds.), *Alcohol and the adult brain*. New York: Psychology Press.

Ridley, N., Draper, B., & Withall, A. (2013). Alcohol-related dementia: An update of the evidence. *Alzheimer's Research & Therapy, 5*, 3.

Rourke, S., & Grant, I. (2009). The neurobehavioral correlates of alcoholism. In I. Grant & K. M. Adams (Eds.), *Neuropsychological assessment of neuropsychiatric and neuromedical disorders* (3rd ed.). New York: Oxford University Press.

Sachdev, P., Blacker, D., Blazer, D., Ganguli, M., Jeste, D., Paulsen, J., & Petersen, R. (2014). Classifying neurocognitive disorders: The DSM-5 approach. *Nature, 10*, 634–642.

White, A. (2003). What happened? Alcohol, memory blackouts, and the brain. *Alcohol Research & Health, 27*(2), 186–196.

Alcoholism

Glenn S. Ashkanazi
Department of Clinical and Health Psychology, Clinical and Health Psychology Clinic, College of Public Health and Health Professions, University of Florida, Gainesville, FL, USA

Synonyms

Alcohol abuse; Alcohol addiction; Alcohol dependence; Problem drinking; Substance abuse

Definition

The term "alcoholism" has a variety of definitions. For some, it is a disease that makes a person dependent on alcohol and causes an obsession with alcohol and inability to control how much they drink even though their drinking causes serious problems in their relationships, health, work, and finances. Others do not define it as a "disease" per se but rather a "condition," behavioral in nature, which results in continued consumption of alcohol despite health problems and negative social consequences. For some, the definition

must include the concepts of addiction and physiological withdrawal mechanisms, while for others, these are consequences of drinking.

It is common for laypeople to equate any kind of excessive drinking with alcoholism. Those in the mental health fields see that disorders related to alcohol use lie along a continuum of severity that *may* include physical dependency/withdrawal (i.e., alcohol dependence) or may involve impaired drinking habits that lead to health or social problems/consequences but without dependency/withdrawal (i.e., alcohol abuse). According to the *APA Dictionary of Psychology*, alcoholism is the popular term for "alcohol dependence." "Alcoholism" is not an official diagnostic term. The DSM-5 term for alcohol-related problems is alcohol use disorder.

Historical Background

The term "alcoholism" was first used in 1849 by a physician, Magus Haas, to describe the systematic adverse effects of alcohol overconsumption. In the USA, it became a popular term in the 1930s as a result of the growth of Alcoholics Anonymous (AA). Previously, society viewed those who drank to excess as immoral, weak of character, and irresponsible. Society's response was punishment and removal of over-consumers from sober society to protect the community. With the rise of AA, and their publication (i.e., the "Big Book"), the view of alcoholism changed from character flaw to medical disease. AA viewed alcoholism as a physical allergy to alcohol accompanied by an obsession with drinking. This organization began to dispel the previously held beliefs that alcoholics were unemployable, destitute, and isolated individuals by demonstrating that some highly respected people who had been alcohol dependent had eventually overcome their disorder and went on to lead productive lives.

Epidemiology

The epidemiology of alcoholism can be confusing and contradictory, depending on the definition being utilized and the measurement tool. The generally accepted overall rate of occurrence of alcoholism in the USA is 10%. The US National Longitudinal Alcohol Epidemiologic Study concluded that alcoholism is prevalent in 20% of adult hospital inpatients and in 17% of community-based primary care practices. A 1985 US National Hospital Survey found that 528,000 patients were discharged from hospitals with a primary diagnosis of substance abuse, and for 81% (428,000), alcohol was the abused substance.

According to a 2001 survey conducted by the National Institute on Alcohol Abuse and Alcoholism (NIAAA) in the USA, approximately 48% of adults (aged 12 or older) are reported being current drinkers of alcohol (approximately 109 million). That number drops to 44% when the age is 18 or older. A 2014 survey found that 87.6% of people over age 18 reported they drank alcohol at some point in their lifetime and 56.9% within the last month. Approximately 20% of persons aged 12 or older participated in binge drinking at least once in 30 days prior to the 2001 survey. In the 2014 survey, that number was 24.7%.

"Heavy drinking" was reported by 5.7% of the 12 or older population (12.9 million). The highest prevalence for both binge and heavy drinking was for those in the 18–25 age groups with the peak rate occurring at age 21. Studies have found those who begin drinking at an earlier age are at higher risk to develop dependency. Those Americans who wait till age 21 are four times less likely to become dependent than those who begin drinking before the age of 15 (i.e., 40% who start before age 15 develop dependency on alcohol at some point in their lives). The risk for developing dependency declines with age, as the prevalence rate for alcoholism in those persons greater than 65 years old is 3%.

There are other nonage risk factors as well. Those with lower education and lower socioeconomic status are also at higher risk. There are also gender differences as men are at minimum 2.5 times more likely to be defined as "alcoholic" as women; however, the proportion of female alcoholics is increasing. White, non-Hispanic individuals are more likely to develop alcoholism than African-Americans. The risk for Hispanics is generally the same as Whites.

Alcoholism is estimated to be the third leading cause of preventable death in the USA (after smoking and obesity). In the USA, 85,000 deaths are attributable to alcohol each year at a cost of $185 billion. The NIAAA estimates that intoxication is present in 30–60% of homicides, 22% of suicides, 33–50% of automobile accidents, 67% of drownings, and 70–80% of fire-related deaths. More than 50% of American adults have a close family member who has or has had alcoholism. Approximately one in four children younger than 18 in the USA is exposed to alcohol abuse or alcohol dependence in their family.

Internationally, the World Health Organization estimates that there are 140 million people worldwide that are alcohol dependent and they account for 3.5% of the total cases of disease worldwide, which is a higher rate than tobacco or illicit drugs. They estimated that 5.9% of all global deaths were attributable to alcohol consumption.

Current Knowledge

Causes

There is no identifiable single cause of alcoholism. Scientists believe that a myriad of factors play a role in the development of alcoholism:

1. *Genetics*: Previous twin and adoption studies have demonstrated that genes play an important role in the development of alcoholism. Researchers found that identical twins (i.e., identical genes) have a higher concordance rate for drinking behavior than fraternal twins. Other studies have cast some doubt on these twin studies by suggesting the environment of identical twins is more alike than fraternal twins, thus suggesting a weakening of the argument in favor of genes. In the adoption studies, researchers found that whether reared by biologic or adoptive parents, the sons of males with alcohol problems are four times more likely to have alcohol problems than sons of persons who are not. In either case, epidemiologic studies indicate that alcoholism

tends to run in families. Alcoholics are six times more likely than nonalcoholics to have blood relatives who are alcohol dependent. In summary, a person's genetic makeup can predispose them to alcoholism or not.

2. *Peer influence*: Social networks that include heavy drinkers and alcohol abusers increase an individual's risk for alcoholism.

3. *Cultural influence*: Cultures that include well-established taboos against drunkenness and rules regarding drinking have lower alcoholism rates than those who do not.

4. *Psychiatric conditions*: Certain psychiatric diagnoses increase the risk of alcoholism. These include ADHD, panic disorder, schizophrenia, and antisocial personality disorder.

Screening

There are a variety of measures for alcoholism including the following:

1. CAGE: The CAGE is named for the four questions asked of a patient before any questions regarding quantities drank are asked.
   1. Have you ever felt the need to **C**ut down on your drinking?
   2. Have people **A**nnoyed you by criticizing your drinking?
   3. Have you ever felt **G**uilty about drinking?
   4. Have you ever felt you needed a drink in the morning to steady your nerves or get rid of a hangover? (**E**ye-opener)

   The CAGE has been extensively validated. Those who answer "YES" to two or more questions are seven times more likely to be alcohol dependent. It is not an adequate measure by itself but can alert a health-care provider to probe further. Another weakness is that it tends to be less reliable with populations with lower alcoholism rates (e.g., elderly) and does not identify "hazardous drinking."

2. Alcohol Use Disorders Identification Test (AUDIT): The AUDIT can detect both hazardous drinking and alcohol abuse. It does not need to be administered face to face like the CAGE. It was developed by the World Health Organization and yields scores for consumption, dependency, and alcohol-related problems.

3. Short Alcohol Dependence Data Questionnaire (SADD): More sensitive than the CAGE and can distinguish abuse versus dependence.

Diagnosis

Alcoholism is not a diagnosable term. The current term to describe "problem drinking" is alcohol use disorder found in the *Diagnostic Statistical Manual of the Mental Disorders, Fifth Edition* (DSM-V). The diagnosis requires:

1. A problematic pattern of alcohol use leading to clinically significant impairment or distress as manifested by at least two of the below occurring in the same 12-month period.
   (a) Tolerance (as defined by either of the following).
      (i) A need for markedly increased amounts of alcohol to achieve intoxication or desired effect
      (ii) A markedly diminished effect with continued use of the same amount of alcohol
   (b) Withdrawal (as manifested by either of the following).
      (i) The characteristic withdrawal syndrome for alcohol.
      (ii) Alcohol (or benzodiazepines) is taken to relieve or avoid withdrawal syndrome.
   (c) Alcohol is often taken over longer period of time or in larger amounts than intended.
   (d) Persistent desire to drink or unsuccessful efforts to cut down or control use.
   (e) Great deal of time spent in acquiring/using alcohol or recovering from its effects.
   (f) Important social, occupational, or recreational activities given up or reduced because of alcohol.
   (g) Drinking continues despite knowledge of persistent or recurrent physiological or psychological problems caused or exacerbated by drinking.
   (h) Craving, or strong desire or urge to use alcohol.

Treatment

There are several well-accepted avenues of treatment:

1. *Psychosocial*: Studies have shown that simple, brief interventions can be effective in those not severely alcohol dependent. One of those getting an extensive trial has been "motivation interviewing" based on Prochaska's five stages of change model. A summary of the treatment approach is as follows:

   - *Precontemplation* – Patient expresses no interest or need for change. The healthcare professional's options are limited. They can point to discrepancies between the patient's goals and behavior and recommend 2 weeks of abstinence.
   - *Contemplation* – Patient expresses ambivalence or skepticism about change. The provider should work to influence them in direction of change, provide information about the dangers of alcohol abuse, and recommend an abstinence trial.
   - *Preparation* – Patient accepts need for change and makes plans to accomplish changed drinking goal.
   - *Action* – Patient recognizes problem in drinking behavior and takes observable steps to decrease alcohol use. Professional reinforces decision for change and may introduce self-help groups and/or medications.
   - *Maintenance* – Patient and professional work together to maintain change and prevent relapse.
2. *Medications*: The most common medications in the treatment of alcoholism are:
   - *Disulfiram (Antabuse)* – Prevents the elimination of acetaldehyde, which is a by-product of alcohol metabolism. Results in unpleasant side effects in persons still drinking including nausea, dizziness, headache, flushing, vomiting, heart palpitations, and sudden drop in blood pressure. Disulfiram needs to be taken daily to be effective. However, in at least one large clinical trial, it did not increase abstinence.

   - *Naltrexone (ReVia)* – May work by blocking the positive effects felt from drinking by blocking opiate receptors in the brain thereby decreasing craving for alcohol. Clinical studies have found a modest decrease in relapse (12–20%). This drug has an unknown cause of action.
   - *Acamprosate (Campral)* – Used to maintain abstinence once alcoholics have stopped drinking. Thought to work by stabilizing the chemical balance in the brain. In clinical trials, the 1-year abstinence rates have been 18% and 12% at 2 years.
3. *Self-help groups*: Perhaps the best-known organization involving alcoholism is AA. Until the mid-1930s in the USA, alcohol-dependent persons who could not afford a private hospital or private psychiatrist could only find help in state hospitals, jails, or churches. AA was the first self-directed approach toward treatment. The AA treatment model includes self-help groups, utilizing psychological principles organized in small local community groups. The "12 steps" of AA encourage confrontation of denial and admission of powerlessness over alcohol and strives for people to atone for harm caused by their behavior while drinking. It encourages its members to live ethically with a reliance on a "higher power." It is this sense of AA as a "religion" that has led to nonreligious self-help groups including rational recovery, LifeRing, and SOS.

Future Directions

The following are areas needing continued study:

1. *Genetic research* – Current and future studies are looking at individuals with a family history of alcoholism to pinpoint the location of genes that influence vulnerability to alcoholism. This line of study will assist in the early identification of individuals at risk and of new, gene-based treatment approaches.
2. *Treatment approaches* – The NIAAA has been funding a study called "Project MATCH"

whose goal is to identify variables important in predicting outcome based on patient characteristics and treatment design.

3. *Medications* – Naltrexone was the first drug approved by the FDA in 45 years to help alcoholics stay sober following detoxification. More research is needed.

Cross-References

► Alcoholic Brain Syndrome
► Fetal Alcohol Spectrum Disorder
► Korsakoff's Syndrome
► Michigan Alcoholism Screen Test
► Motivational Interviewing
► Substance Use Disorders
► Twin Studies
► Wernicke-Korsakoff Syndrome

References and Readings

Borsari, B., & Carey, K. (2001). Peer influences on college drinking: A review of the research. *Journal of Substance Abuse, 13*(4), 391–424.

Cavanaugh, S. (2014). Alcoholism and mental illness: Overlapping diseases requiring a renewed focus. *Mental Health and Substance Abuse, 7*(4), 487–496.

Davidson, R., & Raistrick, D. (1986). The validity of the Short Alcohol Dependence Data Questionnaire (SADD): A short self-report questionnaire for the assessment of alcohol dependence. *British Journal of Addiction, 81*(2), 217–222.

Dhalla, S., & Kopec, J. (2007). The CAGE questionnaire for alcohol misuse: A review of reliability and validity studies. *Clinical and Investigative Medicine, 30*(1), 33–41.

Ducci, F., & Goldman, D. (2012). The genetic basis of addictive disorders. *Psychiatric Clinics of North America, 35*(2), 495–519.

National Institute on Alcohol Abuse and Alcoholism. (2005). *Helping patients who drink too much: A clinician's guide, updated 2005 edition.* http://www.niaaa.nih.gov/Publications/EducationTrainingMaterials/guide.htm.

National Institute on Alcohol Abuse and Alcoholism. *Etiology and natural history of alcoholism.* http://pubs.niaaa.nih.gov/publications/social/module2etiology&naturalhistory/module2.html.

Prochaska, J., DiClemente, C., & Norcross, J. (1992). In search of how people change: Applications to addictive behaviors. *American Psychologist, 47*(9), 1102–1114.

Reinert, D., & Allen, J. (2007). The alcohol use disorders identification test: An update of research findings. *Alcoholism Clinical & Experimental Research, 31*(2), 185–199.

Room, R., & Makela, K. (2000). Typologies of the cultural position of drinking. *Journal of Studies on Alcohol and Drugs, 61*(3), 475–483.

Schuckit, M. (2000). *Drug and alcohol abuse: A clinical guide to diagnosis and treatment.* New York: Kluwer/Plenum Publishers.

U.S. Department of Health and Human Services and SAMHSAs National Clearinghouse for Alcohol and Drug Information. http://ncadistore.samhsa.gov/catalog/facts.aspx?topic=3.

Alertness

Chris Loftis
National Council for Community Behavioral Healthcare, Alexandria, VA, USA

Synonyms

Awareness; Consciousness; Vigilance; Watchfulness

Definition

A state of being mentally perceptive and responsive to external stimuli. A "readiness to respond" that can be detected by electroencephalography (EEG). Alertness is susceptible to fatigue; maintaining a constant level of alertness is difficult, particularly for monotonous tasks demanding continuous attention. Stimulants such as nicotine, caffeine, and amphetamines can temporally boost alertness. Diminished alertness is often associated with the physiological response of yawning, which may boost the alertness of the brain. Impaired alertness is a common symptom of a number of conditions, including narcolepsy, attention deficit disorder, traumatic brain injury, chronic fatigue syndrome, depression, Addison's disease, and sleep deprivation. Although a broad neurological network modulates alertness, the basal forebrain and a distinct group of neurons located in the periventricular areas of the midbrain, pons, and medulla, referred to as the reticular activating system (RAS), appear to be most directly responsible for modulating alertness and sleep.

Cross-References

▶ Attention
▶ Attention Deficit Hyperactivity Disorder
▶ Basal Forebrain
▶ Coma
▶ Consciousness
▶ Hindbrain
▶ Reticular Activating System
▶ Severe Brain Injury
▶ Vigilance

Alexia

Angel Ball
Department of Clinical Health Sciences,
Texas A&M University-Kingsville, Kingsville,
TX, USA

Synonyms

Acquired reading disorder

Short Description or Definition

The term alexia is applied to acquired disorders of reading produced by neurological injury in individuals with normal premorbid literacy skills. We differentiate here from developmental dyslexia which reflects a failure to attain normal reading skills. Clinically, patients with alexia have difficulty in recognizing, pronouncing, or comprehending written words. Although alexia can occur in relative isolation, it is more frequently encountered in the context of spoken language dysfunction or aphasia. Most individuals with alexia have concomitant spelling impairment, suggesting that reading and spelling rely on shared cognitive representations and neural substrates.

Categorization

Alexia is not a single clinical entity. Instead, there are several distinct forms of alexia characterized by specific combinations of impaired and preserved reading abilities and associated with unique lesion profiles. The three most common alexia syndromes include pure alexia/letter-by-letter reading, phonological/deep alexia, and surface alexia. Some individuals may also have a coexisting visual field deficit, which causes errors in reading. Clinicians should attempt to differentiate the linguistic processing aspect from the visual deficit. In order to understand the neuropsychological mechanisms underlying different subtypes of alexia, it is important to briefly review the cognitive processes involved in normal reading.

Reading is a complex cognitive skill that requires rapid visual discrimination of letters and words, as well as the ability to link information about visual word forms (orthography) with knowledge about word sounds (phonology) and word meanings (semantics). According to an influential dual-route model of reading (Coltheart et al. 2001), perceptual processing of written words begins with visual feature analysis and letter shape detection (Fig. 1). Following the letter identification stage, the model postulates two distinct procedures or processing routes for deriving phonology from print. The lexical route requires the activation of memory representations of written word forms stored in the orthographic lexicon, followed by the retrieval of the corresponding spoken word forms from the phonological lexicon. The lexical route is normally used to read familiar words and can support the processing of both regular words that have predictable spelling-sound relationships (e.g., spring)

Alexia, Fig. 1 A cognitive model indicating the component processes involved in reading

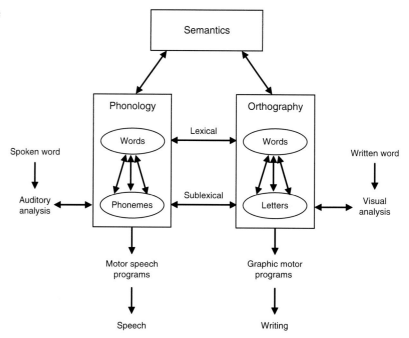

and irregular words that contain atypical letter-sound or grapheme-phoneme mappings (e.g., choir). By contrast, the sublexical route operates on units smaller than the whole word and is thought to rely on the serial conversion of individual graphemes to the corresponding phonemes. The sublexical route is essential for accurate reading of unfamiliar words or nonwords (e.g., nace) because these novel items, by definition, do not have preexisting representations in the orthographic or phonological lexicon. The sublexical route can also be used to generate plausible pronunciations for regular words that strictly obey spelling-sound conversion rules. However, processing irregular words by the sublexical procedure results in regularization errors (e.g., *have* read to rhyme with *save*). Thus, according to dual-route theory, only the lexical reading route can deliver a correct response to irregular words. Note that the model depicted in Fig. 1 also includes an indirect route from orthography to phonology via the semantic system. The activation of word meanings by this semantic reading route is critical for written word comprehension. However, whether semantic mediation is also normally required for accurate oral reading of familiar words is a topic of controversy (Coltheart et al. 2001; Plaut et al. 1996;

Woollams et al. 2007). In summary, skilled reading depends on interactions among visual/orthographic processing, phonology, and semantics. Damage to these functional domains or the disruption of the transfer of information between the cognitive/brain systems that support these operations results in alexia.

Epidemiology

Alexia is commonly observed following damage to the language-dominant hemisphere. Although it is most frequently caused by stroke, alexia can follow any kind of focal injury (e.g., trauma, tumor) to the brain regions critical for implementing the various cognitive operations necessary for normal reading. Data on stroke prevalence in the USA, Canada, and worldwide can be accessed via the Internet Stroke Center (n.d.); however, data on prevalence with alexia as an outcome is not well known. Alexia is also often seen in the setting of neurodegenerative disorders, especially in patients with primary progressive aphasia/semantic dementia or Alzheimer's disease. In general, the specific alexia profile is determined not so much by the etiology of the brain damage as by the location of the responsible lesions.

Natural History, Prognostic Factors, and Outcomes

The prognosis for recovery from alexia depends both on the etiology of the lesion and the extent of the underlying brain damage. Alexia following stroke tends to show some spontaneous recovery over time, but patients with extensive brain damage may never regain useful reading function and typically stop reading for pleasure. In individuals with neurodegenerative disorders, progressive worsening of the reading impairment is observed along with the gradual deterioration of other language and cognitive functions.

Neuropsychology and Psychology of Alexia

Pure Alexia/Letter-by-Letter Reading

In pure alexia, the rapid visual identification of familiar words that characterizes normal skilled reading is disrupted. Reading is slow and laborious, often relying on a serial letter-naming strategy known as "letter-by-letter" reading. Typically, there is a monotonic increase in reading latencies as a function of the number of letters in the word, giving rise to an abnormal *word length effect* that is considered the hallmark feature of the syndrome. Varying degrees of letter identification difficulty are present, and visual reading errors are common (e.g., chain – charm). Collectively, these behavioral observations suggest that visual processing impairment plays a critical role in the pathogenesis of pure alexia (Behrmann et al. 1998). Although the reading disorder may be unaccompanied by significant aphasia or agraphia, many patients with pure alexia demonstrate concomitant anomia and spelling impairment (Rapcsak and Beeson 2004). Furthermore, patients often perform poorly on non-reading tasks that require fine-grained visual discrimination, suggesting that the reading impairment is part of a more general visual

processing deficit (Behrmann et al. 1998). Within the framework of the cognitive model depicted in Fig. 1, pure alexia is attributable to dysfunction at the visual feature analysis and/or letter identification stages of reading, or it may be produced by damage to the orthographic lexicon. Damage to any of these visual processing components would be expected to interfere with the rapid perceptual identification of familiar orthographic word forms and result in an abnormal word length effect in oral reading.

Pure alexia/letter-by-letter reading is most commonly seen following left inferior occipito-temporal damage caused by posterior cerebral artery strokes. It has been proposed that the critical lesions degrade or disrupt visual input to the visual word form area (VWFA) or directly damage the VWFA itself (Cohen et al. 2003; Epelbaum et al. 2008). The VWFA is consistently activated in functional imaging studies of reading in normal individuals and has been localized to the mid-lateral portions of the left fusiform gyrus (BA37) (Cohen et al. 2002; Jobard et al. 2003) (Fig. 2). The VWFA receives converging input from bilateral posterior occipital areas (BA17,18/ 19) involved in visual feature analysis and letter shape detection, and it integrates this information into larger perceptual units corresponding to whole words (Fig. 2). Activation of the VWFA is sensitive to the orthographic familiarity of the letter string, consistent with the notion that this cortical region may constitute the neural substrate of the orthographic lexicon. The orthographic codes computed by the VWFA are subsequently transmitted to cortical systems involved in the phonological and semantic components of reading (Fig. 3). Importantly, it has been shown that spelling familiar words also activates the VWFA (Beeson et al. 2003). These observations confirm the central role for the VWFA in orthographic processing and support the view that the same orthographic lexical representations mediate reading and spelling. Consistent with this hypothesis, patients with damage to the VWFA are likely to show evidence of reading and spelling impairment attributable to the loss of word-specific orthographic representations (Rapcsak and Beeson 2004).

Phonological/Deep Alexia

Phonological alexia is characterized by a dispro-portionate difficulty in processing nonwords compared with familiar words, giving rise to an exaggerated *lexicality effect* in reading (Crisp and

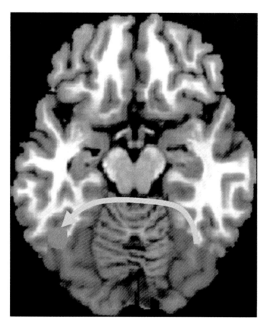

Alexia, Fig. 2 Location of the visual word form area (VWFA) (indicated by green circle) as determined by functional neuroimaging studies of reading. This region receives input from bilateral posterior occipital visual areas (shown in purple). Arrow indicates callosal transfer of information initially processed by right visual cortex

Lambon Ralph 2006; Patterson and Lambon Ralph 1999; Rapcsak et al. 2009). Attempts to read nonwords often result in real word responses known as lexicalization errors (e.g., nace – name). Although in phonological alexia reading of familiar words (both regular and irregular) is relatively preserved, performance is typically influenced by lexical-semantic variables including word frequency (high > low), imageability (concrete > abstract), and grammatical class (nouns > verbs > functors). Deep alexia includes all the characteristic features of phonological alexia, but it is distinguished from the latter by the production of prominent semantic reading errors (e.g., boy – son) (Coltheart et al. 1980). Although phonological and deep alexia were originally considered separate entities, there is now much evidence to suggest that the difference between these syndromes is quantitative rather than qualitative. Thus, phonological and deep alexia are more appropriately considered as points along a continuum, with the latter representing a more severe version of the former (Crisp and Lambon Ralph 2006; Rapcsak et al. 2009).

Phonological alexia is typically encountered in patients with aphasia syndromes characterized by phonological impairment (i.e., Broca's, conduction, Wernicke's). Furthermore, it has been shown that most patients with phonological alexia demonstrate prominent deficits and increased

Alexia, Fig. 3 Cortical regions involved in reading

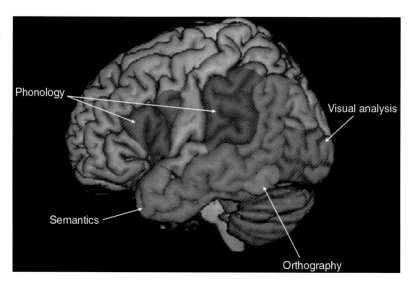

lexicality effects in spoken language tasks that require the manipulation and maintenance of sub-lexical phonological information (e.g., repetition, rhyme judgments, phoneme segmentation, and blending) and also that such non-orthographic measures of phonological ability correlate with and are predictive of reading performance (Crisp and Lambon Ralph 2006; Rapcsak et al. 2009). These observations suggest that the written and spoken language impairments in phonological alexia have a common origin and are merely dif-ferent manifestations of a central or modality-independent phonological deficit (Crisp and Lambon Ralph 2006; Patterson and Lambon Ralph 1999; Rapcsak et al. 2009). Consistent with this view, the reading disorder in phonolog-ical alexia is usually accompanied by a qualita-tively similar spelling impairment (phonological agraphia) (Rapcsak et al. 2009). According to dual-route models (Fig. 1), poor nonword reading in phonological alexia is attributable to damage to the sublexical route, while the relatively preserved real word reading performance of these patients reflects the residual functional capacity of the lexical and semantic routes. The general phono-logical impairment observed in the vast majority of patients suggests that the most common site of damage may be at the level of the phoneme units (with additional damage to the phonological lex-icon in more severe cases), as these phonological processing components are shared between writ-ten and spoken language tasks.

Phonological alexia is most often associated with damage to a network of *perisylvian* cortical regions involved in speech production/perception and phonological processing in general. Compo-nents of this distributed phonological system include posterior-inferior frontal gyrus/Broca's area (BA44/45), precentral gyrus (BA4/6), insula, superior temporal gyrus/Wernicke's area (BA22), and supramarginal gyrus (BA40) (Rapcsak et al. 2009). Consistent with the phonological deficit hypothesis, there is an excellent neuroanatomical correspondence between the location of the lesions that produce phonological alexia and the location of the perisylvian cortical areas that show activation in normal individuals during a variety of written and spoken language tasks requiring

phonological processing (Jobard et al. 2003; Rapcsak et al. 2009; Vigneau et al. 2006). As predicted by the continuum model, there is con-siderable overlap between the perisylvian lesion profiles of patients with phonological and deep alexia, although the damage in deep alexia tends to be more extensive. In fact, the massive destruc-tion of left-hemisphere language areas in deep alexia has led to the hypothesis that reading per-formance in these patients may be mediated by the intact right hemisphere (Coltheart et al. 1980).

Surface Alexia

In surface alexia, the main difficulty involves reading irregular words, especially when these items are of low frequency. Regular words of comparable frequency are processed more effi-ciently, and the discrepancy in performance between words with predictable versus atypical spelling-sound relationships is reflected by an increased *regularity effect* in reading. Nonword reading is typically preserved. According to dual-route theory, surface alexia is attributable to dysfunction of the lexical reading route (Fig. 1). Specifically, it has been suggested that the reading disorder in some cases may result from damage to the orthographic lexicon (Coltheart et al. 2001; Patterson et al. 1985). Due to the loss of word-specific orthographic knowledge, patients with this type of deficit will be forced to rely on a sublexical grapheme-phoneme conversion strategy that pro-duces phonologically plausible regularization errors on irregular words. Low-frequency irregular words are especially vulnerable because the acti-vation of representations in the orthographic lexi-con is normally modulated by word frequency, and the relative refractoriness of low-frequency items may be further exaggerated by the brain damage. Consistent with the notion that reading and spell-ing rely on shared orthographic representations, patients with surface alexia following damage to the orthographic lexicon show similar difficulty in spelling irregular words (surface agraphia) (Patterson et al. 1985; Rapcsak and Beeson 2004). Alternatively, surface alexia may result from damage to central semantic representations (Woollams et al. 2007). Specifically, it has been proposed that accurate oral reading of low-frequency irregular words normally requires additional support from the semantic reading route and cannot be mediated efficiently by pathways that rely on direct transcoding between orthographic and phonological representations (Plaut et al. 1996). With the degradation of semantic knowledge, the relative inadequacy of non-semantic reading routes is revealed and manifests itself as surface alexia. Consistent with the semantic deficit hypothesis, many patients with surface alexia perform poorly on verbal and nonverbal cognitive tasks requiring semantic processing (e.g., picture naming, verbal fluency, spoken word, and picture comprehension). Furthermore, the severity of the semantic impairment on these nonreading tasks has been shown to correlate with reading accuracy for low-frequency irregular words (Woollams et al. 2007). The proposed central semantic deficit may also explain the frequent co-occurrence of surface alexia and surface agraphia (Graham et al. 2000).

In contrast to the strong association between perisylvian damage and phonological alexia, surface alexia is typically encountered in the setting of *extrasylvian* brain pathology. Although uncommon in patients with stroke, surface alexia has been described in individuals with left temporoparietal lesions centered on posterior middle/inferior temporal gyrus and angular gyrus (BA20/21,37/39), and also following inferior occipitotemporal lesions that involved the VWFA (Rapcsak and Beeson 2004; Vanier and Caplan 1985). As expected, patients with surface alexia following VWFA damage also showed evidence of visual processing impairment and features of pure alexia/letter-by-letter reading (Rapcsak and Beeson 2004). A particularly dramatic and pure form of surface alexia is consistently observed in patients with semantic dementia (SD) (Woollams et al. 2007). SD is a subtype of primary progressive aphasia/ frontotemporal dementia in which the neurodegenerative process has a predilection for left anterior and inferolateral temporal cortex, including the temporal pole, middle/inferior temporal gyri, and anterior fusiform gyrus

(BA38,20/21) (Galton et al. 2001; Mummery et al. 2000). Surface alexia has also been described in patients with Alzheimer's disease (Patterson et al. 1994) and is likely to reflect the frequent involvement of left temporoparietal cortex by the disease process. Although distributed over a large anatomical area, the disparate extrasylvian lesion sites in surface alexia seem to have in common the potential for disrupting either lexical orthographic or semantic processing. Specifically, in patients with VWFA involvement, the reading disorder may reflect damage to the orthographic lexicon resulting in the loss of word-specific orthographic knowledge. By contrast, in patients with anterior temporal lobe lesions, and possibly also in patients with posterior temporoparietal damage, surface alexia may be attributable to the degradation of central semantic representations. The latter hypothesis is supported by functional imaging studies of semantic processing in normal individuals that have shown activation of a large-scale left-hemisphere extrasylvian cortical network that included both anterior temporal lobe and posterior temporoparietal sites (Vigneau et al. 2006; Binder et al. 2009) (Fig. 3).

Evaluation

In evaluating adults with alexia, it is important to assess the status of all the relevant component processes involved in reading (Fig. 1). A comprehensive battery should include tests of letter and word recognition, as well as measures of oral reading and reading comprehension. The evaluation should allow the clinician to identify the nature of the functional impairment and to locate the level of breakdown with reference to a cognitive model of normal reading. It is equally important to document relatively spared reading abilities and the use of compensatory strategies by the patient, as this information may be helpful in planning treatment.

As reading inherently is a visual task, the examiner must inquire as to any visual limitations with or without corrective lenses. One compensation may be to change font size or spacing, which if successful, will help distinguish a reading disorder from a visual limitation. In addition, the examiner should consider the age-level readability of the material, in comparison to the premorbid reading level of the client.

Silent reading is an internal event which may be processed differently depending on the type of reading. Stories and books for pleasure are often read with a mental image of the story with no effort to memorize or learn material. Reading texts or articles for learning requires acquisition of knowledge, and readers vary in their style. Most formal test does not prepare the examiner for these differences. Test measurement has traditionally required a technique to judge the internal comprehension. Usually this is done by asking questions on content information in a series of yes/no questions or multiple choice with visual choices or matching word or sentence to a picture.

Oral reading accuracy can be monitored by the examiner during the event. This task will help to reveal visual spatial or attention errors, such as skipped words or lost place. Recording the oral words per minute provides information on word fluency.

The only reading modality-specific commercially available reading test is the *Reading Comprehension Battery for Aphasia-2 (RCBA-2;* LaPointe and Horner 1998)*, which includes oral and silent reading at word, sentence, paragraph levels, and functional reading tasks (i.e., calendar).

Standardized tests with reading subtests include:

- *Boston Diagnostic Aphasia Examination-3* (Goodglass et al. 2001) – reading subtests include symbol letter and number recognition, word identification given choice of 4 words with visually and semantically similar foils, lexical decision of real word from nonwords, homophone matching, nonword to homophone matching, matching written to spoken target

(including bound morphemes, derivational morphemes(suffixes), word and sentence (4–14 words) oral reading, and sentence and paragraph comprehension with word and phrase choices.

- *Examining for Aphasia-4* (EFA-4; LaPointe and Eisenson 2008) – reading subtests include silent reading interrogative sentences (five to seven words) with semantic matching from set of four words, silent paragraph reading with interrogative sentence to test comprehension from set of four sentence choices, and oral paragraph reading with interrogative sentences to test comprehension given set of four short phrases or sentences.
- *Multilingual Aphasia Examination* 3rd Ed (MAE-3; Benton et al. 1978) – provides a picture matching words and two to four word phrases to picture choices of four items.
- *Psycholinguistic Assessment of Language Processing in Aphasia* (PALPA English Ed: Kay et al. 1992) – reading subtests include letter discrimination (mirror reversal, upper and lower case matching), spoken letter to written letters, recognition of non- and real words, homophones, oral reading tasks for letter and syllable length, word frequency and grammatical class, regularity of spelling, and sentence-level oral reading (five to seven words), and defining with reading word tasks.

Treatment

A variety of behavioral treatment approaches have shown positive outcomes in the rehabilitation of alexia. In general, treatment is directed toward strengthening the impaired reading procedure/route or it encourages the use of compensatory strategies to bypass the functional deficit (for a review, see Beeson and Rapcsak 2006; Murray and Clark 2015; Riley and Kendall 2013; Peach and Shapiro 2012). Treatment approaches often align with the underlying problem, e.g., syntactic, visual-attention, memory.

Material choices have extended beyond traditional text and into using supported technology such as highlighted text, read-aloud technology (text to speech), and electronic access to dictionary (Deitz et al. 2011; Helm-Estabrooks et al. 2014). The number of software programs and apps designed for stimulation and practice are ever increasing (e.g., Lingraphica TalkPath, Bungalow software). Readers are encouraged to view the online tables for evidence-based treatment for individuals with aphasia (Beeson, n.d.) for a list of reading treatments.

See Also

▶ Aphasia
▶ Boston Diagnostic Aphasia Examination
▶ Multilingual Aphasia Examination
▶ Reading Comprehension Battery for Aphasia-2
▶ Western Aphasia Battery

References and Readings

Beeson, P. M. (n.d). Aphasia treatment evidence tables: Written language-reading. The University of Arizona-Academy of Neurologic Communication Disorders and Sciences Retrieved 15 Oct 2015 from http://aphasiatx. arizona.edu/written_reading?order=field_data_year_ value&sort=asc&page=2

Beeson, P. M., & Rapcsak, S. Z. (2006). Treatment of alexia and agraphia. In J. H. Noseworthy (Ed.), *Neurological therapeutics: Principles and practice* (2nd ed., pp. 3045–3060). London: Martin Dunitz.

Beeson, P. M., Rapcsak, S. Z., Plante, E., Chargualaf, J., Chung, A., Johnson, S. C., et al. (2003). The neural substrates of writing: A functional magnetic resonance imaging study. *Aphasiology, 17*, 647–665.

Behrmann, M., Plaut, D. C., & Nelson, J. (1998). A literature review and new data supporting an interactive account of letter-by-letter reading. *Cognitive Neuropsychology, 15*, 7–51.

Benton, A. L., Hamsher, K. d S., & Sivan, A. B. (1978). *Multilingual aphasia examination* (3rd ed.). Lutz: Psychological Assessment Resources.

Binder, J. R., Desai, R. H., Graves, W. W., & Conant, L. L. (2009). Where is the semantic system? A critical review and meta-analysis of 120 functional neuroimaging studies. *Cerebral Cortex, 19*, 2767–2796.

Cohen, L., Lehéricy, S., Chochon, F., Lemer, C., Rivaud, S., & Dehaene, S. (2002). Language-specific tuning of

visual cortex? Functional properties of the visual word form area. *Brain, 125*, 1054–1069.

Cohen, L., Martinaud, O., Lemer, C., Lehéricy, S., Samson, Y., Obadia, M., et al. (2003). Visual word recognition in the left and right hemispheres: Anatomical and functional correlates of peripheral alexias. *Cerebral Cortex, 13*, 1313–1333.

Coltheart, M., Patterson, K., & Marshall, J. C. (1980). *Deep dyslexia*. London: Routledge & Kegan Paul.

Coltheart, M., Rastle, K., Perry, C., Langdon, R., & Ziegler, J. (2001). DRC: A dual route cascaded model of visual word recognition and reading aloud. *Psychological Review, 108*, 204–256.

Crisp, J., & Lambon Ralph, M. A. (2006). Unlocking the nature of the phonological-deep dyslexia continuum: The keys to reading aloud are in phonology ad semantics. *Journal of Cognitive Neuroscience, 18*, 348–362.

Epelbaum, S., Pinel, P., Gaillard, R., Delmaire, C., Perrin, M., Dupont, S., et al. (2008). Pure alexia as a disconnection syndrome: New diffusion imaging evidence for an old concept. *Cortex, 44*, 962–974.

Galton, C. J., Patterson, K., Graham, K., Lambon Ralph, M. A., Williams, G., Antoun, N., et al. (2001). Differing patterns of temporal atrophy in Alzheimer's disease and semantic dementia. *Neurology, 57*, 216–223.

Goodglass, H., Kaplan, E., & Barresi, B. (2001). *The Boston diagnostic aphasia examination* (3rd ed.). Baltimore: Lippincott Williams & Wilkins.

Graham, N. L., Patterson, K., & Hodges, J. R. (2000). The impact of semantic memory impairment on spelling: Evidence from semantic dementia. *Neuropsychologia, 38*, 143–163.

Greenwald, M. (2000). The acquired dyslexias. In S. E. Nadeau, L. J. Gonzelez Rothi, & B. Crosson (Eds.), *Aphasia and language* (pp. 159–183). New York: The Guilford Press.

Helm-Estabrooks, N., Albert, M. L., & Nicholas, M. (2014). *Manual of aphasia and aphasia therapy* (3rd ed.). Austin: Pro-Ed.

Internet Stroke Center. (n.d.). Stroke statistics Retrieved 15 Oct 2015 from http://www.strokecenter.org/ patients/about-stroke/stroke-statistics/

Jobard, G., Crivello, F., & Tzourio-Mazoyer, N. (2003). Evaluation of the dual route theory of reading: A metanalysis of 35 neuroimaging studies. *NeuroImage, 20*, 693–712.

Kay, J., Lesser, R., & Coltheart, M. (1992). *Psycholinguistic assessments of language processing in aphasia (PALPA)*. East Sussex: Lawrence Erlbaum Associates.

Kertesz, A. (2007). *Western aphasia battery – revised (WAB-R)*. San Antonio: PsychCorp.

LaPointe, L. L. (2005). *Aphasia and related neurogenic language disorders* (3rd ed.). New York: Thieme Medical Publishers.

LaPointe, L. L., & Eisenson, J. (2008). *Examining for aphasia: Assessment of aphasia and related communication disorders (EFA-4)* (4th ed.). Austin: Pro-Ed.

LaPointe, L. L., & Horner, J. (1998). *Reading comprehension battery for aphasia (RCBA-2)* (2nd ed.). Austin: Pro-Ed.

Mummery, C. J., Patterson, K., Price, C. J., Ashburner, J., Frackowiak, R. S. J., & Hodges, J. R. (2000). A voxel-based morphometry study of semantic dementia: Relationship between temporal lobe atrophy and semantic memory. *Annals of Neurology, 47*, 36–45.

Murray, L. L., & Clark, H. M. (2015). *Neurogenic disorders of language and cognition: Evidence-based clinical practice* (2nd ed.). Austin: Pro-Ed.

Patterson, K., Graham, N., & Hodges, J. R. (1994). Reading in dementia of the Alzheimer type: A preserved ability? *Neuropsychology, 8*, 835–407.

Patterson, K., & Lambon Ralph, M. A. (1999). Selective disorders of reading? *Current Opinion in Neurobiology, 9*, 235–239.

Patterson, K. E., Marshall, J. C., & Coltheart, M. (1985). *Surface dyslexia: Neuropsychological and cognitive studies of phonological reading*. London: Lawrence Erlbaum.

Peach, R. K., & Shapiro, L. P. (2012). *Cognition and acquired language disorders*. St. Louis: Elsevier Mosby.

Plaut, D. C., McClelland, J. L., Seidenberg, M. S., & Patterson, K. (1996). Understanding normal and impaired word reading: Computational principles in quasi-regular domains. *Psychological Review, 103*, 56–115.

Rapcsak, S. Z., & Beeson, P. M. (2000). Agraphia. In S. E. Nadeau, L. J. Gonzelez Rothi, & B. Crosson (Eds.), *Aphasia and language* (pp. 184–220). New York: The Guilford Press.

Rapcsak, S. Z., & Beeson, P. M. (2004). The role of left posterior inferior temporal cortex in spelling. *Neurology, 62*, 2221–2229.

Rapcsak, S. Z., Beeson, P. M., Henry, M. L., Leyden, A., Kim, E. S., Rising, K., et al. (2009). Phonological dyslexia and dysgraphia: Cognitive mechanisms and neural substrates. *Cortex, 45*(5), 575–591.

Riley, E. A., & Kendall, D. L. (2013). The acquired disorders of reading. In I. Papathanasiou, P. Coppens, & C. Potagas (Eds.), *Aphasia and related neurogenic communication disorders* (pp. 157–172). Burlington: Jones & Bartlett Learning.

Sampson, G. (1985). *Writing systems*. Stanford: Stanford University Press.

Vanier, M., & Caplan, D. (1985). CT correlates of surface dyslexia. In K. E. Patterson, J. C. Marshall, & M. Coltheart (Eds.), *Surface dyslexia: Neuropsychological and cognitive studies of phonological reading* (pp. 511–525). London: Lawrence Erlbaum.

Vigneau, M., Beaucousin, V., Hervé, P. Y., Duffau, H., Crivello, F., Houdé, O., et al. (2006). Meta-analyzing left hemisphere language areas: Phonology, semantics, and sentence processing. *NeuroImage, 30*, 1414–1432.

Woollams, A., Lambon Ralph, M. A., Plaut, D. C., & Patterson, K. (2007). SD-squared: On the association between semantic dementia and surface dyslexia. *Psychological Review, 114*, 316–339.

Alexithymia

Joel W. Hughes
Department of Psychology, Kent State University, Kent, OH, USA

Definition

A deficit in apprehending, experiencing, and describing emotions, including difficulty perceiving and understanding the feelings of others. In particular, difficulty distinguishing between emotions and bodily sensations that indicate emotional arousal.

Current Knowledge

The term "alexithymia" was coined by the late psychiatrist Peter Sifneos to describe patients who could not find the appropriate words to describe their emotional states. Literally meaning "without words for emotions" in Sifneos' native Greek, alexithymia is a trait that overlaps with a number of medical and psychiatric disorders. Alexithymia is associated with somatic complaints such as headaches, lower back pain, irritable bowel syndrome, and fibromyalgia. It is also associated with psychiatric conditions such as anorexia nervosa, autism spectrum disorders including Asperger's, major depressive disorder, panic disorder, post-traumatic stress disorder, and substance abuse.

See Also

▶ Emotional Intelligence

Further Reading

Sifneos, P. E. Alexithymia: Past and present. *The American Journal of Psychiatry*, *153*, 137–142.

Taylor, G. J., & Taylor, H. S. (1997). Alexithymia. In M. McCallum & W. E. Piper (Eds.), *Psychological mindedness: A contemporary understanding*. Munich: Lawrence Erlbaum Associates.

Taylor, G. J., Bagby, R. M., & Parker, J. D. A. (1997). *Disorders of affect regulation: Alexithymia in medical and psychiatric illness*. Cambridge: Cambridge University Press. ISBN 052145610X.

Alien Hand Syndrome

Gary Goldberg[1] and Matthew E. Goodwin[2]
[1]Hunter Holmes McGuire Veterans Administration Medical Center, Department of Physical Medicine and Rehabilitation, Virginia Commonwealth University School of Medicine/Medical College of Virginia, Richmond, VA, USA
[2]Central Arkansas Veterans Healthcare System, Little Rock, AR, USA

Synonyms

Alien limb phenomenon; Anarchic hand; Callosal apraxia; Diagnostic dyspraxia; Dr. Strangelove syndrome; Intermanual conflict; Magnetic apraxia; Wayward hand

Short Description or Definition

Alien hand syndrome (AHS) is a relatively rare manifestation of damage to specific brain regions involved in purposive voluntary movement. It is postulated to be an impairment of the "sense of agency" or, alternatively, an impairment of intentionality. The core observation is the patient report that one of his/her hands is displaying purposeful, coordinated, and goal-directed behavior over which the patient feels he/she has no direct voluntary control. The patient fails to recognize the action of one of

their hands as their own. The hand, effectively, appears to manifest a "will of its own." This unique involuntary movement disorder is characterized by coordinated, well-organized, and clearly goal-directed limb movements that would otherwise be indistinguishable from normal voluntary movement. This definition excludes disordered, non-purposeful, and dyskinetic movements associated with other involuntary movement disorders such as chorea, athetosis, hemiballism, and myoclonus.

The alien hand can be engaged in performing a specific goal-directed task or the purposeful use of an external object. Distinguishing this condition from asomatognosia, there is typically normal awareness and recognition of the limb reported by the patient. However, the patient perceives a lack of self-agency ("I am not doing that. . .") with regard to the observed behavior of the limb but displays an intact "sense of ownership" (". . .even though I know this is my hand"). While the original description of this condition occurred in patients with well-defined focal lesions of cerebral cortex, with the majority of cases due to cerebral infarction, it has since been described in a variety of different clinical conditions including corticobasal syndrome, progressive supranuclear palsy, Alzheimer's disease, and Creutzfeldt-Jakob disease. Furthermore, while the alien limb is typically and most often noted in an upper extremity, it has been described in the lower extremity as well.

This suggests that the alien hand syndrome reflects a phenomenon that may result from impaired function at a variety of different points in a widely distributed brain system involved in the intentional preparation and generation of purposeful voluntary movement. This system would be expected to include both specifically defined motor and premotor regions of the cerebral cortex as well as related interconnected subcortical regions such as the basal ganglia. The different clinical variants of AHS associated with circumscribed cortical damage which will be reviewed below may reflect varying clusters of clinical manifestations resulting from disrupted functions at different points and levels within this distributed brain system. As noted, this distributed brain system would be expected to involve a variety of both cortical and associated subcortical regions engaged together in the emerging brain process linked to voluntary movement generation, with the common pathophysiologic manifestation being a dissociation between self-perceived will and action.

One of the significant difficulties in conceptualizing and studying AHS in the context of a conventional scientific paradigm is that a mechanistic explanation alone cannot adequately account for the process linked to intentionality and the teleological aspect of goal-directed behavior. The emerging field of "biosemiotics" that recognizes the process of semiosis through which meaning and action-associated intentionality emerge in the behavior of living organisms promises to provide a new perspective and, in the process, provide potential insights into this disorder.

Categorization

Two major forms of AHS can be distinguished. One form is related to focal cortical and intercortical white matter damage and the other is associated with more diffusely distributed cortical/subcortical damage (e.g., as seen in corticobasal syndrome). Three variants of the focal cortical form of AHS have been described, each with unique behavioral manifestations and neuroanatomical correlations. These variants include the frontal, callosal, and posterior forms.

Cortical Form

Frontal Variant

Neuroanatomy The most common variant is the "frontal" form. It is typically associated with damage to the medial surface of the cerebral hemisphere in the frontal region. This variant has been described in cerebral infarction in the territory of the anterior cerebral artery, with tumors involving the medial surface of the cerebral hemisphere, and in other conditions affecting the function of the medial frontal lobe region. When the region of

injury extends posteriorly to involve the medial aspect of the prefrontal gyrus associated with the primary motor cortex (PMC), the patient may present with crural hemiparesis, with greater weakness in the leg as compared to the arm. This presentation corresponds to the topographical organization of the PMC with control of lower limb movement located more medially than the areas on the exterior lateral surface that control the upper limb and face. The frontal variant is seen with involvement of the medial aspect of the premotor cortex anterior to PMC including the pre-supplementary (pre-SMA) and supplementary motor area (SMA), and anterior cingulate cortex (ACC), as well as connections to the posterior cingulate cortex (PCC). In functional activation studies, the medial frontal cortex has also been found to activate spontaneously with complex purposeful movements and with internal imaging of voluntary movement, suggesting that it may serve as a higher-level system that modulates the activation of PMC in accordance with volitional features of the performance. The readiness potential, or Bereitschaftspotential, a slowly developing surface-negative shift that precedes an overt voluntary movement by over 1200 ms, arises through activation of the anteromedial frontal cortex, suggesting that excitation of this system precedes the appearance of the overt movement and activation of the PMC. Activation of the ACC is involved in intentional suppression of prepotent responses as tested with the Stroop test. These areas may serve as a higher-level system modulating the activation of PMC in accordance with the volitional self-referenced aspects of the performance. Alternatively, they may be part of a feed-forward system that generates an efference copy of the generated motor command that is transmitted to sensory cortex as a means of distinguishing active self-generated limb movement with its associated sensory re-afference, from passive movement produced by external forces associated with sensory ex-afference.

Clinical Presentation Behaviors seen frequently with the frontal variant include involuntary, visually driven reaching and grasping onto objects, an inability to voluntarily release these objects, and utilization behavior in which the presence of a frequently encountered object used in daily activities such as a comb or a toothbrush elicits behavior in which the object may be put to use independent of the general interpersonal context. A grasp reflex to tactile stimulation is often present in the affected hand. The patient may wake themselves up from sleep by grasping onto and pulling at their own body parts. Patients may show a prepotent tendency to be drawn toward external objects. They also may demonstrate alien-associated sexual self-stimulation or involuntary fondling of another's body, a great source of public embarrassment (Ong Hai and Odderson 2000). Interestingly, while the patient clearly manifests purposeful involuntary coordinated behaviors in the affected limb that appear to flow effortlessly, attempts to willfully move the limb are effortful and arduous. Voluntary movement in the affected limb is often hypokinetic and hypometric with greater activation of the axial and proximal limb muscles compared to the distal muscles controlling the wrist and fingers, even though these muscles are fully and dexterously activated in the alien movements. Generally, these alien behaviors appear in the hand contralateral to the damaged hemisphere regardless of hemispheric dominance. When the dominant hemisphere is damaged, in addition to alien hand behavior in the dominant hand, they may experience difficulty with the initiation of spontaneous speech while still being able to follow verbal commands and repeat phrases without difficulty. These findings are consistent with a transcortical motor aphasia that affects spontaneous verbalization and production of propositional speech more than repetition and generally responsive language output. Alternatively, this has been interpreted as a partial mutism manifesting as an inability to initiate spontaneous propositional verbal output.

Callosal Variant

Neuroanatomy The "callosal" variant is seen with an isolated lesion of the corpus callosum.

The voluntary motor systems of the two hemispheres are isolated from each other due to lost interhemispheric communication resulting in impaired intermanual coordination. This variant has been described most frequently as a transient condition following callosotomy in the treatment of intractable seizures. It may also be seen following infarction or tumors selectively involving the corpus callosum.

Clinical Presentation In the "callosal" variant of AHS, the appearance of "intermanual conflict" or "self-oppositional" behaviors is the predominant feature. Grasping behaviors and externally driven reaching movements seen in the frontal variant are notably less prominent. When there is a major disconnection between the two hemispheres resulting from callosal injury, the language-linked dominant hemispheric agent that maintains its primary control over the contralateral dominant limb effectively loses its direct and linked control over the separate "agent" based in the nondominant hemisphere (and, thus, the nondominant limb), which had been previously responsive and "obedient" to the dominant agent. The possibility of purposeful action in the nondominant limb occurring outside of the realm of influence of the dominant agent thus can occur. In the callosal variant, the problematic alien hand is consistently the nondominant hand, while the dominant hand is the identified "good" normally controlled hand. The patient may express frustration and bewilderment at the conflicting and disruptive behavior of the alien hand whose motivations remain inaccessible to consciousness. There may be an attentional component that modulates the appearance of these episodes of self-oppositional behavior since intermanual conflict is observed more frequently when the patient is fatigued, stressed, or is engaged in effortful multitasking and divided-attention activity. Occasionally, rather than acting in a contradictory manner, the two hands are observed to be engaged in two different and entirely unrelated activities as if being guided by completely separate and independent intentions.

In a dramatic example of this behavior, one patient was observed to initiate smoking a cigarette by pulling the cigarette out of the package and placing it in her mouth with the controlled dominant hand followed by the alien non-dominant hand, rather than beginning to light the cigarette, suddenly reaching up, pulling it out of her mouth, and throwing it across the room. Astonished, the patient reasoned that perhaps the alien hand was not in favor of her smoking!

The callosal and frontal variants are often seen in combination with a corresponding overlap of observed behaviors. For example, following cerebral infarction in the territory of the anterior cerebral artery, there may be ischemic injury to both the medial frontal lobe and the corpus callosum. In this circumstance, there may be both visually directed reaching and grasping alien behaviors in the limb contralateral to the area of injury as well as episodes of intermanual conflict. However, a clear differentiation between apparent intermanual conflict due to attempts to restrain alien behaviors associated with the frontal variant (e.g., as in the case of "self-grasping" described below), and true intermanual conflict, in which the two hands are directed toward independently contradictory purposes, may be difficult to differentiate.

Posterior or "Sensory" Variant

Neuroanatomy The third identified variant of AHS is the "posterior" or "sensory" form, which appears most often with a parietal or parieto-occipital focus of circumscribed damage. As in the frontal variant, the alien behavior appears in the hand contralateral to the damaged hemisphere.

Clinical Presentation In the patient with the posterior variant, the movement of the affected alien limb is typically less organized and often has an ataxic instability particularly with visually guided reaching. The limb also may show proprioceptive sensory impairment with hypesthesia, so that kinesthetic impairment limits the monitoring of limb position. Visual field deficits as well as hemi-inattention may be seen on the same side as the alien hand. In this variant, the limb may be observed to lift up off of support surfaces involuntarily and "levitate" in the air seemingly to

avoid contact between the palmar surface of the affected hand and support surfaces. It may also be seen to withdraw from objects approaching the hand in distinct contrast to the reaching and grasping behaviors that are seen in the frontal variant. The alien hand may assume a characteristic posture of fully extended digits with the palmar surface retreating from environmental objects, and support surfaces an observation that has been labeled an "instinctive avoidance reaction" by Denny-Brown and has also been referred to as a "parietal hand." At times, grasping behaviors can also be observed with the posterior variant.

Alien hand behavior has also been reported in association with focal subcortical thalamic infarction.

Distributed Cortical/Subcortical Form
In addition to having been observed in the context of stroke, tumors, and callosotomy, alien hand behavior has been described in a second general form linked to degenerative neurological conditions that tend to affect cortical and subcortical regions together. The progressive neurodegenerative disorders associated with this form of AHS include corticobasal syndrome, progressive supranuclear palsy, multiple sclerosis, spongiform encephalopathy, and Alzheimer's disease. When AHS appears with these progressive encephalopathies, it is usually accompanied by various forms of motor apraxia, along with multiple additional cognitive and motor disturbances characteristic of the particular condition.

Epidemiology

While there are no epidemiologic studies of the occurrence of AHS variants in association with acquired brain damage, it can be assumed that this is a relatively rare but striking manifestation of neurologic pathology.

Pathophysiology and Prognosis

Adapting the concept developed by Derek Denny-Brown regarding positive and negative cortical tropisms based in the parietal lobe and frontal lobes (Denny-Brown 1956, 1966), respectively, a heuristic model has been proposed. In this model, there are two separable but interactive components of an intrahemispheric premotor intentional system that modulate the output of the PMC of the hemisphere and its direct influence via the corticospinal tract over the spinal motor nuclei innervating the distal muscles of the contralateral limbs (Goldberg and Bloom 1990).

The first component is a posterolateral premotor system (PLPS) based in the posterior parietal region that is involved in generating movements of the contralateral arm and hand, as well as the lower limb, that are perceptually driven toward external objects and are responsive to externally sensed, contextually relevant, ecological contingencies. The second component is an anteromedial premotor system (AMPS) based in the medial frontal region including medial prefrontal, pre-SMA, SMA, and ACC that is involved in generating movements in the contralateral upper limb that are guided by an outwardly directed intentional action plan and driven by an anticipatory internally based model of projected future contingencies. It presumably is also involved in activating withdrawal movements that pull the limb back and away from external stimuli. It also functions to withhold action directly responsive to surrounding objects through inhibitory influence over the PLPS. These two systems are proposed to be in a metastable balance through mutually inhibitory influence. Together, these two hemispheric agency systems form an integrated intrahemispheric agency system. Furthermore, each intrahemispheric agency system has the capability of acting autonomously in its control over the contralateral limb, although overall unitary control by a singular conscious agent is maintained through interhemispheric communication between these systems via the corpus callosum at the cortical level and other interhemispheric commissures linking the two cerebral hemispheres at the subcortical level. Thus, conscious human agency can be thought of as emerging through the linked and coordinated action of at least four major premotor

systems, two in each hemisphere. The overall general configuration of this postulated heuristic model is shown in Fig. 1.

It is proposed that AHS, in its different variants described above, appears due to damage either to the corpus callosum in the callosal variant (Fig. 2), the AMPS of either hemisphere in the frontal variant (Figs. 3 and 4), or to the PLPS of either hemisphere in the posterior variant (Figs. 5 and 6).

The common factor in these anomalous conditions is the relative sparing of the PMC region controlling the contralesional alien hand, while the premotor regions involved in the intentional selection of action and the inhibition of automatic behaviors in response to external factors are impaired. A recent fMRI study of cortical activation patterns associated with alien and non-alien movement has demonstrated that alien movement is in fact characterized by isolated activation of PMC without concomitant activation of intrahemispheric premotor regions, while voluntary behavior includes the activation of PMC in concert with activation of intrahemispheric premotor regions (Assal et al. 2007).

Neuropsychology and Psychology of AHS

The presence of AHS can cause the patient significant psychological distress as the hand seems to possess the capability for acting autonomously, independent of their conscious voluntary control. The patient may become fearful that they will be held accountable for consequences of an action of the alien hand over which they do not feel control. The patient may display "autocriticism" complaining that the alien hand is not doing what it has been "told to do" and is therefore characterized as disobedient, wayward, or "evil." The hand is felt to be under the control of an external unknown agent to whose narrative and intentions the patient is not privy. They may even physically strike the alien hand with the controlled hand as a "punishment" intended to discourage its wayward behavior, or restrain the movement of the alien hand by grasping tightly onto it with the controlled hand ("self-grasping"). They may

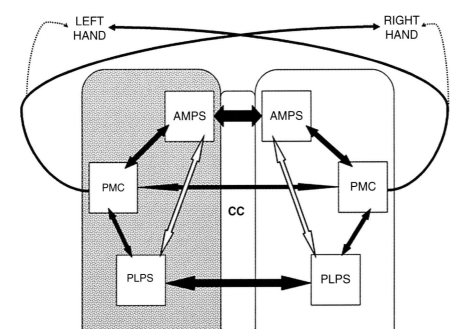

Alien Hand Syndrome, Fig. 1 Heuristic Model for Understanding Alien Hand Syndrome (AHS). Abbreviations: *RH* right hemisphere, *LH* left hemisphere, *CC* corpus callosum, *PMC* primary motor cortex, *AMPS* anteromedial premotor system, *PLPS* posterolateral premotor system. This view is shown looking down from above the vertex with the face located at the *top* of the drawing and the *back* of the head noted at the *bottom* of the drawing, the *left side to the left* and the *right side to the right* of the diagram. The *open bidirectional arrow* between the AMPS and the PLPS indicates an interaction characterized by mutually interactive inhibition creating a complementary metastable control of the contralateral hand. *Solid arrows* indicate facilitatory connections or connections that maintain synchrony and coherence between the connected structures. Output from PMC is directed primarily to the distal contralateral limb with some less potent ipsilateral projections to primarily axial postural muscles illustrated by a *dotted line*. See text for further detail. Note that the left hemisphere is stippled in the diagram designating this as the dominant hemisphere for most individuals in correspondence with a dominant right hand

verbally address and instruct the hand as if it were an unruly child acting autonomously and in need of disciplinary intervention. Conversely, they may respond to these contrary actions with amusement.

Given the predicament created, the patient may develop depersonalization and dissociate themselves from the unintended actions of the hand. They often choose to identify an external "alien" source for the voluntary control of the hand, or assign a distinct personality to the hand as a way of seeking a satisfactory narrative to explain this perplexing and disturbing situation.

From a psychological perspective, it is helpful to counsel the patient regarding the organic basis of their problem and provide assurance that there is a rational explanation for their concerns and that there is evidence that these problems can be treated and are likely to gradually improve over time.

In AHS, different regions of the brain are able to command purposeful limb movements, without generating the conscious feeling of self-control over these movements. There is thus a dissociation between the actual execution of the physical movements of the limb and the process that produces an internal sense of voluntary control over the movements. This latter process, impaired in AHS, normally produces the conscious sense of agency that conveys that the movement is being internally initiated and produced by an active self. Presumably, this process differentiates reliably between "re-afference" (i.e., the return of

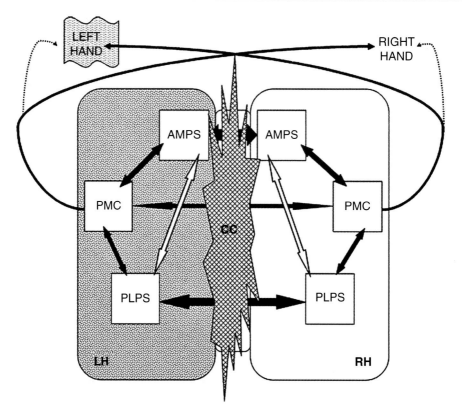

Alien Hand Syndrome, Fig. 2 The Callosal Variant of AHS. Theoretical explanatory model for the alien behaviors observed in callosal damage. In this instance, there are findings consistent with callosal apraxia in addition to intermanual conflict associated with the complete separation of the two intrahemispheric premotor intentional control systems. The limbs appear to be operated by two relatively autonomous hemispheric control systems that function as two distinct agents. The intentional premotor system in the dominant hemisphere is linked to the language system while that of the nondominant hemisphere is separated from it. The dominant hand is understood as connected to the language-mediated narrative "self," while the nondominant hand is not directly accessible to this narrative self. The alien hand in this variant is the nondominant hand that operates outside of the dominant narrative. This is indicated by the stippled overlay in the diagram on the left nondominant hand

kinesthetic sensation from the self-generated "active" limb movement) and "ex-afference" (i.e., kinesthetic sensation generated from an externally produced "passive" limb movement). It may do this by giving rise to a parallel output signal from motor regions, a so-called efference copy. The efference copy is then translated into a corollary discharge, which conveys the expected re-afferent sensory response from the commanded movement. The corollary discharge can then be used in somatosensory cortex as a referent to distinguish re-afference from ex-afference and thus differentiate a self-produced active movement from a passive movement resulting from external forces. AHS may thus involve impaired production and transmission of either an efference copy or a corollary discharge signal.

Evaluation

Evaluation of the patient with AHS involves careful observation of limb movement in various naturalistic contexts, along with reports from the patient regarding their sense of control over these movements. The relative dependence of movement on external context should be evaluated through assessment for utilization behaviors elicited by the

Alien Hand Syndrome, Fig. 3 The Non-dominant Frontal Variant of AHS. Theoretical explanatory model for the alien behaviors observed in the frontal variant associated with damage to the AMPS of the nondominant hemisphere. In this case, the contralesional nondominant hand develops alien hand findings due to the release by disinhibition of the reaching and grasping behaviors driven from the nondominant PLPS

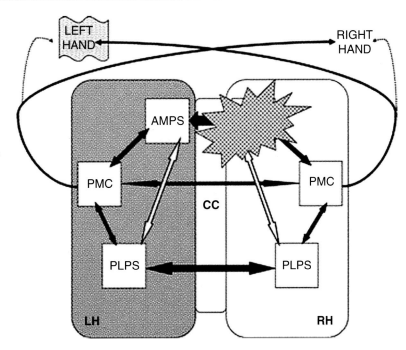

Alien Hand Syndrome, Fig. 4 The Dominant Frontal Variant of AHS. Theoretical explanatory model for the alien behaviors observed in the frontal variant associated with damage to the AMPS of the dominant hemisphere. In this case, the contralesional dominant hand develops alien hand findings due to the release by disinhibition of the reaching and grasping behaviors driven from the dominant PLPS. In addition, spontaneous expressive language initiation is impaired due to the role of the AMPS of the dominant hemisphere in the initiation of propositional verbal output

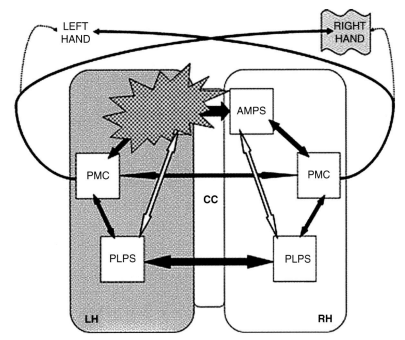

presentation of external objects commonly encountered in daily activities. A phenomenological approach to assessing and documenting the motor behavior and linking it to introspective first-person report of the patient's own experience is essential. Not only should the verbal reports of the patient be noted but also the associated affect. The limb should be evaluated for evidence of a grasp reflex with both tactile and visual stimulation. The ability to release objects that have been grasped should

**Alien Hand Syndrome,
Fig. 5** The Non-dominant
Posterior Variant of AHS.
Theoretical explanatory
model for the alien
behaviors observed in the
posterior variant associated
with damage to the PLPS of
the nondominant
hemisphere. In this case, the
contralesional nondominant
hand develops alien hand
findings due to the release
by disinhibition of
behaviors driven from the
nondominant AMPS

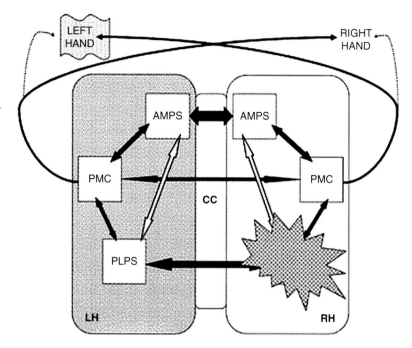

**Alien Hand Syndrome,
Fig. 6** The Dominant
Posterior Variant of AHS.
Theoretical explanatory
model for the alien
behaviors observed in the
posterior variant associated
with damage to the PLPS of
the dominant hemisphere.
In this case, the
contralesional dominant
hand develops alien hand
findings due to the release
by disinhibition of
behaviors driven from the
dominant AMPS

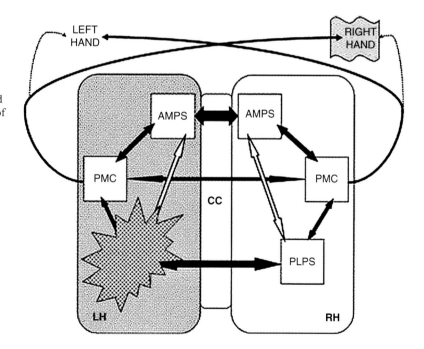

also be assessed. Evaluation for callosal apraxia and impairment of interhemispheric transfer of information should be included. When the posterior variant of AHS is suspected, a visual field assessment and careful sensory examination of the affected limb should be completed as well as assessment for hemi-inattention. Evidence of an avoidant tendency to withdraw the limb from tactile and visual stimulation should also be elicited and noted when present.

Treatment

There is no definitive specific treatment for AHS but a number of different rehabilitative approaches have been described. Furthermore, in the presence of unilateral damage within a single cerebral hemisphere, there is often a gradual reduction in the frequency of alien behaviors observed over time and a gradual restoration of normal voluntary control over the affected hand. This suggests that neuroplasticity in the bihemispheric and subcortical brain systems involved in voluntary movement production can serve to reestablish functional connection between the executive production process and the internal self-generation and volitional registration process. Exactly how this may occur is not well understood but could involve a reorganization within residual elements of the intrahemispheric premotor systems both at the cortical and subcortical levels. In addition, some degree of expanded participation of the intact ipsilateral hemisphere may be involved in the recovery process by extending ipsilateral motor projections and influence.

Different strategies can be used to reduce the interference of the alien hand behavior in the ongoing coherent controlled functional actions of everyday life being performed by the patient. In the frontal variant, an object such as a cane can be placed in the grip of the alien hand so that it does not reach out to grasp onto other objects, thus impeding the patient's forward progress during walking. In another approach, voluntary control of the limb is developed by training the patient to perform a specific task with the alien limb, such as moving the alien hand to contact a specific object or a highly salient environmental target. Through training to enhance volitional control, the patient can effectively override the alien behavior when it occurs. Recognizing that alien behaviors in the frontal variant are often sustained by tactile input, another approach involves simultaneously "muffling" the actions of the alien hand and limiting sensory feedback by placing it in a restrictive "cloak" such as a specialized soft foam hand orthosis or, alternatively, an everyday oven mitt. Of course, this then limits the degree to which the hand can engage in functional tasks. It may also be possible to develop improved participation of ipsilateral hemispheric premotor mechanisms by engaging the patient in coordinated bimanual activities that necessitate cooperative coherent coordinative mechanisms within residual intact components of the motor control systems in both hemispheres.

Cross-References

▶ Anterior Cingulate Cortex
▶ Apraxia
▶ Corpus Callosum
▶ Environmental Dependency
▶ Movement Disorders
▶ Utilization Behavior

References and Readings

Assal, F., Schwartz, S., & Vuilleumier, P. (2007). Moving with or without will: Functional neural correlates of alien hand syndrome. *Annals of Neurology, 62*, 301–306.

Bakheit, A. M., Brennan, A., Gan, P., Green, H., & Roberts, S. (n.d.). Anarchic hand syndrome following resection of a frontal lobe tumor. *Neurocase, 19*, 36–40.

Biran, I., & Chatterjee, A. (2004). Alien hand syndrome. *Archives of Neurology, 61*, 292–294.

Brugger, F., Galovic, M., Weder, B. J., & Kägi, G. (2015). Supplementary motor complex and disturbed motor control. A retrospective clinical and lesion analysis of patients after anterior cerebral artery syndrome. *Frontiers in Neurology.* https://doi.org/10.3389/fneur.2015.00209. Available online at: http://journal.frontiersin.org/article/10.3389/fneur.2015.00209/full.

Denny-Brown, D. (1956). Positive and negative aspects of cerebral cortical functions. *North Carolina Medical Journal, 17*, 295–303.

Denny-Brown, D. (1966). *The cerebral control of movement.* Liverpool: Liverpool University Press.

Fried, I., Mukamel, R., & Kreiman, G. (2011). Internally generated preactivation of single neurons in human medial frontal cortex predicts volition. *Neuron, 69*, 548–562.

Frith, C. D., Blakemore, S.-J., & Wolpert, D. M. (2000). Abnormalities in the awareness and control of action. *Philosophical Transactions of the Royal Society of London, 355*, 1771–1788.

Giovanetti, T., Buxbaum, L. J., Biran, I., & Chatterjee, A. (2005). Reduced endogenous control in alien hand syndrome: Evidence from naturalistic action. *Neuropsychologia, 43*, 75–88.

Goldberg, G. (1992). Premotor systems, attention to action and behavioural choice. In J. Kien, C. McCrohan, & W. Winlow (Eds.), *Neurobiology of motor programme selection. New approaches to mechanisms of behavioural choice* (pp. 225–249). Oxford: Pergamon.

Goldberg, G., & Bloom, K. K. (1990). The alien hand sign. Localization, lateralization, and recovery. *American Journal of Physical Medicine and Rehabilitation, 69*, 228–238.

Graff-Radford, J., Rubin, M. J., Jones, D. T., Aksamit, A. J., Ahlskog, J. E., Knopman, D. S., Peterson, R. C., Boeve, B. F., & Josephs, K. A. (2013). The alien limb phenomenon. *Journal of Neurology, 260*, 1880–1888.

Hoffmeyer, J. (2011). The natural history of intentionality. A biosemiotic approach. In T. Schilhab, F. Stjernfelt, & T. Deacon (Eds.), *Biosemiotics vol. 6: The symbolic species evolved* (pp. 97–116). New York: Springer.

Hu, W. T., Josephs, K. A., Ahlskog, J. E., Shin, C., Boeve, B. F., & Witte, R. J. (2005). MRI correlates of alien leg-like phenomenon in corticobasal degeneration. *Movement Disorders, 20*, 870–873.

Kalckert, A., & Ehrsson, H. H. (2012). Moving a rubber hand that feels like your own. A dissociation of ownership and agency. *Frontiers in Human Neuroscience, 6*, Article 40. https://doi.org/10.3389/fnhum.2012.00040.

McBride, J., Sumner, P., Jackson, S. R., Bajaj, N., & Husain, M. (2013). Exaggerated object affordance and absent automatic inhibition in alien hand syndrome. *Cortex, 49*, 2040–2054.

Nowak, D. A., Bösl, K., Lüdemann-Podubecka, J., Gdynia, H. J., & Ponfick, M. (2014). Recovery and outcome of frontal alien hand syndrome after anterior cerebral artery stroke. *Journal of the Neurological Sciences, 338*, 203–206.

Ong Hai, B. G., & Odderson, I. R. (2000). Involuntary masturbation as a manifestation of stroke-related alien hand syndrome. *Archives of Physical Medicine and Rehabilitation, 79*, 395–398.

Pack, B. C., Stewart, K. J., Diamond, P. T., & Gate, S. D. (2002). Posterior-variant alien hand syndrome: Clinical features and response to rehabilitation. *Disability and Rehabilitation, 24*, 817–818.

Pynn, L. K., & DeSouza, J. E. X. (2013). The function of efference copy signals: Implications for symptoms of schizophrenia. *Vision Research, 76*, 124–133.

Romano, D., Sedda, A., Dell'aquila, R., Dalla Costa, D., Beretta, G., Maravita, A., & Bottini, G. (2014). Controlling the alien hand through the mirror box. *Neurocase, 20*, 307–316.

Sarva, H., Deik, A., & Severt, W. L. (2014). Pathophysiology and treatment of alien hand syndrome. *Tremor and Other Hyperkinetic Movements, 4*, 241. https://doi.org/10.7916/D8VX0F48. Available online at: http://www.tremorjournal.org/index.php/tremor/article/view/241

Scepkowski, L. A., & Cronin-Golomb, A. (2003). The alien hand: Cases, categorizations, and anatomical correlates. *Behavioral and Cognitive Neuroscience Reviews, 2*, 261–277.

Schaefer, M., Heinze, H. J., & Galazky, I. (2010). Alien hand syndrome: Neural correlates of movements without conscious will. *PLoS ONE, 5*(12), e15010. https://doi.org/10.1371/journal.pone.0015010.

Schaefer, M., Heinze, H. J., & Galazky, I. (2013). Waking up the alien hand: Rubber hand illusion interacts with alien hand syndrome. *Neurocase, 19*, 371–376.

Sumner, P., & Husain, M. (2008). At the edge of consciousness: Automatic motor activation and voluntary control. *The Neuroscientist, 14*, 474–486.

Synofzik, M., Vosgerau, G., & Newen, A. (n.d.). I move, therefore I am: A new theoretical framework to investigate agency and ownership. *Consciousness and Cognition, 17*, 411–424.

Wolfe, N., Moore, J. W., Rae, C. L., Rittman, T., Altena, E., Haggard, P., & Rowe, J. B. (2013). The medial frontal-prefrontal network for altered awareness and control of action in corticobasal syndrome. *Brain, 137*, 208–220.

Zénon, A., Sidibé, M., & Olivier, E. (2015). Disrupting the supplementary motor area makes physical effort appear less effortful. *Journal of Neuroscience, 35*, 8737–8744.

Allele

John DeLuca
Research Department, Kessler Foundation, West Orange, NJ, USA

Definition

Allele is an alternate form of a gene, which is the basic unit of inheritance. A gene is located at a particular site on the chromosome and can have several alleles for that locus. For example, A, B, and O are different alleles for the ABO blood-type marker locus of a gene. Alleles greatly influence the expression of physical and behavioral phenotypes or traits such as eye color. For instance, the apolipoprotein E (APoE) gene is a well-known risk factor for developing Alzheimer's disease. The APoE gene has three common alleles: epsilon

2, epsilon 3, and epsilon 4. There is some evidence that carriers of the APoE epsilon 4 allele are at a greater risk for the development of Alzheimer's disease. In contrast, the APoE epsilon 3 allele has been suggested as a "protective" factor in the development of Alzheimer's disease (Plomin et al. 2003).

Cross-References

► Alzheimer's Disease
► Apolipoprotein E
► Chromosome
► Deoxyribonucleic Acid (DNA)
► Gene
► Phenotype

References and Readings

Plomin, R., Defries, J. C., Craig, W., & McGuffin, P. (2003). *Behavioral genetics in the postgenomic era.* Washington, DC: American Psychological Association.

Allesthesia

John E. Mendoza
Department of Psychiatry and Neuroscience, Tulane Medical School and SE Louisiana Veterans Healthcare System, New Orleans, LA, USA

Definition

Misperception of the location of a stimulus. Although it can occur in other modalities, it is most commonly elicited by tactile stimulation and is often seen in the presence of other symptoms of unilateral asomatognosia. If a tactual stimulus is applied to the side of the body contralateral to a hemispheric lesion, the allesthetic patient may perceive the nature of the stimulus correctly but identify it as being applied to the comparable area on the opposite (unaffected) side of the body. In some instances the stimulus may be perceived as being on the same side of the body to which it was applied, but displaced significantly from the point of the actual stimulation (usually toward the midline). When present, this phenomenon likely results from post-rolandic (parietal) lesions of the right rather than the left hemisphere. More rarely it has been associated with brainstem lesions.

Cross-References

► Asomatognosia

Allokinesia

Douglas I. Katz
Department of Neurology, Boston University School of Medicine, Braintree, MA, USA

Definition

This phenomenon refers to a motor response in the wrong limb, contralateral to the requested side, sometimes opposite to the direction requested. It can include nonvoluntary, mirror movements.

Current Knowledge

Allokinesia is often associated with neglect syndromes, usually involving damage to the right hemisphere. It is the motor counterpart of allesthesia. Typically, a patient moves the right limb in response to a request to move the left limb or moves toward the right, away from the neglected side, when asked to move toward the neglected side. In animal models, the phenomena has been associated with frontal, arcuate gyrus lesions (Heilman et al. 1995) and disconnections of frontal and posterior parietal cortices (Burcham et al. 1997).

Cross-References

▶ Allesthesia
▶ Neglect Syndrome

References and Readings

Burcham, K. J., Corwin, J. V., Stoll, M. L., & Reep, R. L. (1997). Disconnection of medial agranular and posterior parietal cortex produces multimodal neglect in rats. *Behavioural Brain Research, 86*(1), 41–47.

Heilman, K. M., Valenstein, E., Day, A., & Watson, R. (1995). Frontal lobe neglect in monkeys. *Neurology, 45*(6), 1205–1210.

Alpha Rhythm

Cindy B. Ivanhoe[1] and Ana Durand Sanchez[2]
[1]Neurorehabilitation Specialists Baylor College of Medicine, The Institute for Rehabilitation and Research, Houston, TX, USA
[2]Physical Medicine and Rehabilitation, Baylor College of Medicine, Houston, TX, USA

Synonyms

Alpha waves; Berger's waves

Definition

Normal electromagnetic oscillations produced by the brain when in a state of relaxation. They are in the frequency range of 8–12 Hz and arise from synchronous and coherent electrical activity of the thalamic pacemaker cells in the human brain. Also called Berger's waves.

Current Knowledge

Alpha waves are believed to arise from the white matter of the occipital lobes. They increase during periods of relaxation with eyes closed. Alpha waves are thought to represent activity in the visual cortex and are associated with feelings of calmness and relaxation. Alpha waves increase when eyes are closed and during meditation and are associated with creativity and mental coordination.

After sustained wakefulness and during the transition from waking to sleeping when the ability to respond to external stimuli ceases, upper alpha power decreases, whereas theta increases.

It is suggested that the encoding of new information is reflected by theta oscillations in hippocampo-cortical feedback loops, whereas search and retrieval processes in (semantic) long-term memory are reflected by upper alpha oscillations in thalamocortical feedback loops.

The neuronal currents resulting from spontaneous alpha wave activity have been shown to generate the largest extracranial magnetic fields. An important application of this knowledge is the use of eye closure as a way to modulate alpha wave reactivity. There is technology that allows paralyzed individuals to operate hand-free controls with the use of eye closure.

See Also

▶ Electroencephalography

References and Readings

Bragatti, J. A., De Moura Cordova, N., Rossato, R., & Bianchin, M. M. (2007). Alpha coma and locked-in syndrome. *Journal of Clinical Neurophysiology, 24*(3), 308.

Craig, A., McIsaac, P., Tran, Y., Kirkup, L., & Searle, A. (1999). Alpha wave reactivity following eye closure: A potential method of remote hands free control for the disabled. *Technology and Disability, 10*(3), 187–194.

Klimesch, W. (1999). EEG alpha and theta oscillations reflect cognitive and memory performance: A review and analysis. *Brain Research Reviews, 29*(2–3), 169–195.

Konn, D., Leach, S., Gowland, P., & Bowtell, R. (2004). Initial attempts at directly detecting alpha wave activity in the brain using MRI. *Magnetic Resonance Imaging, 22*(10), 1413–1427.

Min, B. K., Busch, N. A., Debener, S., Kranczioch, C., Hansimayr, S., Engel, A. K., et al. (2007). The best of both worlds: Phase reset of human EEG alpha activity and additive power contribute to ERP generation. *International Journal of Psychophysiology, 65*(1), 58–68.

Alprazolam

John C. Courtney[1] and Efrain Antonio Gonzalez[2,3]
[1]Socorro Mental Health, Presbyterian Medical Services, Socorro, NM, USA
[2]College of Psychology, Nova Southeastern University, Fort Lauderdale, FL, USA
[3]Utah State University, Logan, UT, USA

Generic Name

Alprazolam

Brand Name

Xanax, Xanax XR, Niravam

Class

Antianxiety agents, anxiolytics, benzodiazepines

Proposed Mechanism(s) of Action

Binds to benzodiazepine receptors at the GABA-A ligand-gated channel, thus allowing for neuronal hyperpolarization. Benzodiazepines enhance the inhibitory action of GABA via boosted chloride conductance.

Indication

Generalized anxiety and panic disorder

Off-Label Use

Other anxiety disorders, irritable bowel syndrome, insomnia, adjunctive treatment in mania and psychosis, premenstrual dysphoric disorder.

Side Effects

Serious

Respiratory depression, hepatic dysfunction (rare), renal dysfunction and blood dyscrasias, grand mal seizures

Common

Sedation, fatigue, depression, dizziness, memory problems, disinhibition, confusion, ataxia, slurred speech

References and Readings

Physicians' Desk Reference (71st ed.). (2017). Montvale: Thomson PDR.
Stahl, S. M. (2007). *Essential psychopharmacology: The prescriber's guide* (2nd ed.). New York: Cambridge University Press.

Additional Information

Drug Interaction Effects: http://www.drugs.com/drug_interactions.html
Drug Molecule Images: http://www.worldofmolecules.com/drugs/
Free Drug Online and PDA Software.: www.medscape.com
Free Drug Online and PDA Software: www.epocrates.com
Gene-Based Estimate of Drug interactions: http://mhc.daytondcs.com:8080/cgibin/ddiD4?ver=4&task=getDrugList
Pill Identification.: http://www.drugs.com/pill_identification.html

Alternate Test Forms

Grant L. Iverson[1] and Kyle E. Ferguson[2]
[1]Department of Psychiatry, British Columbia Mental Health and Addictions, University of British Columbia, Vancouver, BC, Canada
[2]University of British Columbia, Vancouver, BC, Canada

Synonyms

Equivalent forms; Parallel forms

Definition

Alternate test forms are designed to avoid or reduce *content-* or *item-specific* practice effects that are associated with repeated administrations of the same neuropsychological test(s) (Fastenau et al. 2002). Examination of the manuals for many intellectual and neuropsychological tests illustrates that practice effects are common, especially over brief retest intervals (e.g., days or weeks). Regarding test construction, alternate test forms should include the same number of items, and the items should be of equivalent difficulty. Moreover, the test instructions, time limits, examples, and format should be identical to the original instrument developed during standardization, to reduce measurement error (Jackson 2009). Of course, measurement error can never be eliminated. For example, content-sampling error and time-sampling error – inherent in all test-retest paradigms – are always concerns in developing alternate test forms (Strauss et al. 2006). Additionally, alternate test forms cannot control other factors such as positive carry-over effect (i.e., developing better test-taking strategies), familiarity with the testing context (i.e., novelty effects), performance anxiety, and regression to the mean, among others (Busch et al. 2006; Salinsky et al. 2001). This might, to some extent, explain why some studies show that alternate test forms reduce or eliminate practice effects, whereas other studies do not.

Current Knowledge

Alternate test forms are developed by administering an equivalent test – comprising items of similar difficulty – to the same group of examinees or normative sample, shortly before or after being administered the original test form. Scores from the two forms are then correlated (This is called alternate form reliability, or equivalent or parallel form reliability), which yields a reliability coefficient – otherwise known as the coefficient of equivalence. If the original and alternate test forms are truly equivalent, then there would be (theoretically) a one-to-one correspondence between the two sets of scores (Petersen 2008). Moreover, their means and variances would also be very similar. Therefore, the coefficient of equivalence should be high (i.e., >0.80; Sattler 2001). Of course, though they appear similar, the two forms are often not of equivalent difficulty, or otherwise parallel. Thus, in the absence of employing special empirical procedures like test equating, which "fine-tune the test construction process" (Petersen 2008, p. 99), the two forms cannot be used interchangeably.

Test equating refers to a class of statistical concepts and procedures that adjust for differences in difficulty level on alternate test forms (please note that these procedures adjust for differences in test difficulty, not differences in content (see Kolen and Brennan 2004)), so that the forms can be used interchangeably (see Kolen and Brennan 2004, pp. 2–3, for a discussion of this procedure; White and Stern 2003). Test equating establishes, empirically, "a relationship between raw scores on two test forms that can then be used to express the scores on one form in terms of the scores on the other form" (Petersen et al. 1989, p. 242; see also Dorans and Holland 2000; Petersen 2008). Common types of test equating are Item Response Theory (IRT), linear, and equipercentile (Ormea et al. 2001).

The Neuropsychological Assessment Battery (Stern and White 2003), Hopkins Verbal Learning Test-Revised (Brandt and Benedict 2001), Brief Visuospatial Memory Test-Revised (Benedict 2001), and Wide Range Achievement Test-Fourth Edition (Wilkinson and Robertson 2006) are several examples of tests (or test batteries) that provide alternate test forms. With the above caveats in mind, alternate test forms can be useful in serial neuropsychological evaluations.

Cross-References

▶ Item Response Theory
▶ Reliable Change Index
▶ Test Construction
▶ Test Reliability

References and Readings

Benedict, R. H. B. (2001). *Brief visuospatial memory test – Revised*. Odessa: Psychological Assessment Resources.

Brandt, J., & Benedict, R. H. B. (2001). *Hopkins verbal learning test-revised*. Odessa: Psychological Assessment Resources.

Busch, R. M., Chelune, G. J., & Suchy, Y. (2006). Using norms in neuropsychological assessment. In D. K. Attix & K. A. Welsh-Bohmer (Eds.), *Geriatric neuropsychology: Assessment and intervention* (pp. 133–157). New York: Guilford.

Dorans, N. J., & Holland, P. W. (2000). Population invariance and equitability of tests: Basic theory and the linear case. *Journal of Educational Measurement, 37*, 281–306.

Fastenau, P. S., Hankins, W. T., McGinnis, C. M., Moy, T., & Richard, M. (2002). Effects of alternate forms on retest effects in clinical testing. *Journal of International Neuropsychological Society, 7*(2), 151.

Jackson, S. L. (2009). *Research methods and statistics: A critical thinking approach* (3rd ed.). Belmont: Wadsworth Cengage Learning.

Kolen, M. J., & Brennan, R. L. (2004). *Test equating, scaling, and linking: Methods and practices* (2nd ed.). New York: Springer.

Ormea, D., Reeb, M. J., & Riouxc, P. (2001). Premorbid IQ estimates from a multiple aptitude test battery: Regression vs. equating. *Archives of Clinical Neuropsychology, 16*, 679–688.

Petersen, N. S. (2008). A discussion of population invariance of equating. *Applied Psychological Measurement, 32*, 98–101.

Petersen, N. S., Kolen, M. J., & Hoover, H. D. (1989). Scaling, norming, and equating. In R. L. Linn (Ed.), *Educational measurement* (3rd ed., pp. 221–262). New York: Macmillan.

Salinsky, M. C., Storzbach, D., Dodrill, C. B., & Binder, L. M. (2001). Test-retest bias, reliability, and regression equations for neuropsychological measures repeated over a 12–16-week period. *Journal of the International Neuropsychological Society, 7*(5), 597–605.

Sattler, J. M. (2001). *Assessment of children: Cognitive applications* (4th ed.). San Diego: Jerome M. Sattler.

Stern, R. A., & White, T. (2003). *Neuropsychological assessment battery*. Lutz: Psychological Assessment Resources.

Strauss, E., Sherman, E. M. S., & Spreen, O. (2006). *A compendium of neuropsychological tests: Administration, norms, and commentary* (3rd ed.). New York: Oxford University Press.

White, T., & Stern, R. A. (2003). *Neuropsychological assessment battery: Psychometric and technical manual*. Lutz: Psychological Assessment Resources.

Wilkinson, G. S., & Robertson, G. J. (2006). *Wide range achievement test* (4th ed.). Lutz: Psychological Assessment Resources.

Alzheimer, Alois (1864–1915)

Katherine S. McClellan[1] and Anna Bacon Moore[2]
[1]Rehabilitation Research and Development Center, Atlanta Veterans Affairs Medical Center, Decatur, GA, USA
[2]Department of Rehabilitation Medicine, Division of Neuropsychology, Emory University School of Medicine, Atlanta, GA, USA

Major Appointments

- Intern – Mental Asylum at Frankfurt am Main, 1888–1895
- Senior Physician – Mental Asylum at Frankfurt am Main, 1895–1903
- Researcher – Royal Psychiatric Clinic and District Mental Asylum, Munich, 1903–1912
- Assistant Professor – Ludwig-Maximilian University, Munich, 1904–1912
- Chief Physician – Royal Psychiatric Clinic and District Mental Asylum, Munich, 1906–1909
- Professor of Psychiatry – Psychiatry Clinic of Silesian Friedrich-Wilhelm University, Breslau, 1912–1915

Major Honors and Awards

- Extraordinary Professor, Ludwig-Maximilian University (1909)
- *Geheimer Ministerialrat* (Cabinet Councillor) (1915)

Landmark Clinical, Scientific, and Professional Contributions

- Alois Alzheimer was both an excellent clinician and a notable researcher. He is best remembered for being the first to definitively describe the symptoms and cerebral lesions of the disease now known as Alzheimer's disease. Nonetheless, his contributions to science and medicine did not begin, nor do they end, there. He was one of the leaders of the movement to implement the nonrestraint principle (explained more fully below) in asylums. His neurohistological work advanced the idea that psychiatric diseases were biological in origin. And, through his roles as both doctor and scientist, he contributed to our understanding of a variety of conditions such as cerebral atherosclerosis, alcoholism, and general paresis.

Short Biography

In the German municipality Marktbreit, Alois Alzheimer was born on June 14, 1864, to Eduard and Theresia Alzheimer. Eduard, a Royal Notary, provided his family with a comfortable upbringing. Although Alois had only an older brother when he was born, six more siblings followed him. Alois spent the first 4 years of his education at Catholic school in Marktbreit, until his family left the area to find a new home with superior educational opportunities for the children. The family's chosen residence was in Aschaffenburg, and in 1874, Alois moved there in order to study at the Royal Humanistic Gymnasium. Alois completed his high school degree in 1883 with excellent grades. He then decided to study medicine because of his aptitude and fondness for the natural sciences, as well as a sense of duty to mankind.

He enrolled at the Royal Friedrich-Wilhelm University in Berlin for the 1883–1884 winter semester. In his psychiatry lecture there, he learned of John Conolly's nonrestraint principle. Also called open treatment, the nonrestraint principle proposed the novel view that the mentally ill should be treated with a minimal amount of physical constraint. Although Berlin was the medical capital of Germany, Alois disliked Berlin and its distance from his family. Therefore, he was transferred to the University of Würzburg (Lower Franconia, Germany), where his older brother was studying. As an aside, due to the influence of his older brother, Alois joined and later held several officer positions in the Franconian Corps. His histology professor, Alfred von Kölliker, gave him his first experience with microscopes and staining techniques, which lead to his passion for forensic psychiatry. In

the fall of the following year, Alois left to spend his winter semester at the Eberhard Karls University of Tübingen. He returned in 1887 to the Würzburg Anatomical Institute's department of microscopy to write his doctoral thesis, "On the Earwax Glands." The intricate figures he presented in the paper, as in all his papers, were proof of how scrupulously he conducted his research and clinical work. With the completion of his thesis, Alois Alzheimer received his doctor of medicine degree. He passed the state medical examination and was awarded a license to practice medicine in 1888.

Shortly thereafter, he became a personal physician to a mentally ill woman and traveled with her for 5 months. Emil Sioli, the director of the Municipal Asylum for the Insane and Epileptic in Frankfurt am Main had advertized for an intern, specifically hoping for a competent doctor who was also adept with a microscope. Upon his return, the 24-year-old Dr. Alzheimer was hired immediately. Dr. Franz Nissl also was hired as senior physician for the asylum. Nissl not only became one of Alzheimer's closest friends but also taught him a powerful staining technique for highlighting neuronal cell bodies (the Nissl stain), which helped Alzheimer achieve success in his histological studies. Sioli's main goal for the asylum was to fully employ the nonrestraint principle. Alzheimer was particularly skilled at gaining the trust of patients through conversation, and he often documented these conversations. The dialogues often were central to diagnosing a patient and even more so to research. His talent in clinical interviewing was such that clinicians who later read his notes had sufficient information to evaluate his opinions and to make their own diagnoses. Alzheimer drew on his microscopy and forensic psychiatry training, to do histological investigations into the physical origins of psychiatric disorder. In Frankfurt, his topics of study included epilepsy, senile dementia, criminal minds, and a variety of psychoses. He established himself as a well-rounded physician by publishing papers on a wide variety of topics. Aside from his duties as a physician and researcher, he also appeared as an expert before courts and presented at many scientific meetings. While at Frankfurt,

Alzheimer became an expert on general paresis, which later became the subject of his postdoctoral thesis.

In Algeria, a personal physician who had been traveling with a man suffering from general paresis sent a telegram to Alzheimer in 1892 to request that he treat the worsening patient. Alzheimer obliged and went to North Africa. He intended to bring the patient back to his hospital in Germany, but the patient died before reaching Germany, leaving his wife, Cecilie, a widow. Alzheimer and Cecilie became close friends, and eventually the widow asked him to marry her. They were married in April 1894 in the registry office of Frankfurt. Because Cecilie was Jewish, she had to convert to Catholicism before the two could be married by the church in February 1895. On March 10, 1895, their first child, Gertrud, was born, and Dr. Nissl was chosen to be her godfather. But Nissl soon moved to work with Emil Kraepelin in Heidelberg. Nissl's departure created room for Alzheimer to be promoted to senior physician within Sioli's asylum. Also that year, to lessen the overcrowding of the main hospital, a new branch asylum opened. With this addition, Sioli and Alzheimer furthered their goal of fully implementing the nonrestraint principle by instituting duration baths rather than isolation. The asylum became known as a revolutionary clinic, and it elevated the reputations of all its doctors. But above all, in 1901, Alzheimer met the patient who would immortalize his name: Auguste D. Auguste had been admitted to the asylum because of delusional and excessively forgetful behavior. Although at admission she was disoriented, anxious, and suspicious, over time she became unruly and disruptive. Alzheimer was particularly intrigued by her case for the duration of her stay in the hospital.

Alzheimer's second child, Hans, was born in 1896, and his third, Maria, was born in 1900. However, the lavish lifestyle he had lived with Cecilie ended when she died in February 1901. Alzheimer's sister, Elisabeth, took over his household. Though she was strict, she became an integral part of the family. Without Cecilie, Alzheimer no longer had a reason to stay in Frankfurt. After his application to be director of a regional asylum was rejected, he joined Nissl in Heidelberg in 1903 and went to work for Emil Kraepelin. The group he joined there was an international team of researchers. Later that same year, Kraepelin was named director of the Royal Psychiatric Clinic and the District Mental Asylum in Munich. Alzheimer followed him, but was not paid in Munich due to the lack of a position for him and also his desire to manage his own time. Despite his absence from Frankfurt, Alzheimer still received updates on Auguste D.

By this point, Alzheimer's thesis on general paresis was finished, but because he moved twice in such a short time, he had not yet turned it in. Alzheimer submitted his postdoctoral thesis to the Ludwig-Maximilian University in Munich with the hopes of gaining associate professorship. In it, he published not only his clinical dialogues but also his postmortem histological findings. With this paper, he asserted that histological examinations could definitively show the presence of general paresis. Until then, few doctors suspected that syphilis was a cause of general paresis, but shortly thereafter the link between the two was found. His work was surpassed by the discovery of a way to diagnose syphilis, without resorting to autopsies. In August 1904, he joined the university's medical faculty.

Because of his experience at remodeling the Frankfurt clinic, Alzheimer was fundamental in finishing the plans for the new Munich clinic. He furnished his anatomic laboratory with the best equipment and the brightest students – many of whom went on to make great contributions to science, including Ugo Cerletti, electrical shocks to generate convulsions; Hans Gerhard Creutzfeldt and Alfons Jakob, Creutzfeldt-Jakob disease; Frederic Lewy, Lewy bodies; and others. Alzheimer was made chief physician in 1906, a paid position, but also one that took away much of his time in the laboratory.

Two topics that consumed Alzheimer in Munich were psychiatric symptoms resulting from pathological anatomy and classification of mental illnesses by etiology. The latter faced much opposition from the scientific community. Yet, the most opposition he ever faced was his presentation of the Auguste D. case. Auguste

D. had always fascinated Alzheimer. He had paid special attention to her, taking copious notes about their conversations. When he moved away, he still received updates about her condition, which worsened progressively until her death. When Auguste D. died in 1906, her files, brain, and spinal cord were sent to Munich. Alzheimer, along with his student Gaetano Perusini, immediately began examining the case. In Tübingen, Alzheimer presented her case in a lecture entitled "On a Peculiar Severe Disease Process of the Cerebral Cortex," in which he described the lesions (now known to be neurofibullary tangles) that he believed caused Auguste's symptoms. Based on records from the time, his peers did not bother to ask questions, nor were there any comments about the lecture in the minutes. He later published the entire lecture, but still it received little attention. He then tasked Perusini to find more patients, similar to Auguste D. in the clinic. Perusini found four cases and published an article entitled "On Clinically and Histologically Peculiar Mental Illnesses in Advanced Age." Another student of Alzheimer's, Francesco Bonfiglio, found another case of presenile dementia and also published on the disease. Spurred by Bonfiglio's paper, Kraepelin included a section on "Alzheimer's Disease," in the 1910 edition of his textbook *Clinical Psychiatry*. This publication is acknowledged as the origin of the term. Alzheimer himself never referred to it as "Alzheimer's disease," though he had later publications on the disease. Alzheimer decided to resign his post as chief physician in order to devote more time to research, specifically traveling to study epilepsy. Although he was no longer employed by Kraepelin, Alzheimer undertook the responsibilities of coeditor of Kraepelin's *Journal of Complete Neurology and Psychiatry*.

Recognition for Alzheimer and the disease carrying his name began to spread. In 1912, the Silesian Friedrich-Wilhelm University in Breslau asked him to join their faculty as a full professor of psychiatry. During the move to Breslau, Alzheimer fell ill, but nevertheless assumed his duties with vivacity. His patients and coworkers, including Georg Stertz, Ottfried Förster, and Ludwig Mann, took

notice of his kind, yet authoritative presence. In 1913, his health forced him to visit a private clinic. Though he returned to work, his health had not improved. This did not impede his ability to make significant contributions to science: in 1913 he found the syphilis pathogen in the central nervous system of a patient with general paresis.

After a long illness, Alois Alzheimer died on December 19, 1915, from a heart condition and kidney failure. Though no one immediately took over his pursuit of an understanding of Alzheimer's disease, people recommenced research on Alzheimer's disease cases in the 1950s. Studies of the disease began in earnest after Martin Roth's assertion in the 1960s that Alzheimer's disease was the most common cause of senile dementia. In the 1970s, Robert Katzman further propelled the surge of interest in Alzheimer's disease by stating that it was one of the most widespread diseases. Since then, the amount of research on Alzheimer's disease has increased exponentially, resulting in multiple foundations and centers devoted solely to the disease that Alois Alzheimer's colleagues considered trivial.

Cross-References

▶ Alzheimer's Dementia
▶ Alzheimer's Disease
▶ Paresis

References and Readings

Alzheimer, A. (1906). Über einen eigenartigen schweren Erkrankungsprozeß der Hirnrincle. *Neurol Central, 25,* 1134. (On a peculiarly difficult malady/pathology of the cerebral cortex).
Engstrom, E. (2007). Researching dementia in imperial Germany: Alois Alzheimer and the economies of psychiatric practice. *Culture, Medicine and Psychiatry, 31,* 405–413.
Graeber, M., Kösel, S., Egensperger, R., Banati, R., Müller, U., Bise, K., et al. (1997). Rediscovery of the case described by Alois Alzheimer in 1911: Historical and molecular genetic analysis. *Neurogenetics, 1*(73), 80.
Lage, J. (2006). 100 years of Alzheimer's disease (1906–2006). *Journal of Alzheimer's Disease, 9,* 15–26.

Maurer, K., & Maurer, U. (1998). *Alzheimer: The life of a physician and the career of a disease.* New York: Columbia University Press.

Morris, R., & Salmon, D. (2007). The centennial of Alzheimer's disease and the publication of "Über eine eigenartige Erkankung der Hirnrinde" by Alöis Alzheimer. *Cortex, 43*, 821–825.

Small, D., & Cappai, R. (2006). Alois Alzheimer and Alzheimer's disease: A centennial perspective. *Journal of Neurochemistry, 99*, 708–710.

Snyder, P., & Pearn, A. (2007). Historical note on Darwin's consideration of early-onset dementia in older persons, thirty-six years before Alzheimer's initial case report. *Alzheimer's & Dementia, 3*, 137–142.

Zilka, N., & Novak, M. (2006). The tangled story of Alois Alzheimer. *Bratislavské Lekárske Listy, 107*, 343–345.

Alzheimer's Dementia

Chelsea Sanders[1], Joshua M. Matyi[1],
JoAnn Tschanz[1,2] and Aaron Andersen[3]
[1]Department of Psychology, Utah State University, Logan, UT, USA
[2]Center for Epidemiologic Studies, Utah State University, Logan, UT, USA
[3]Utah State University, Logan, UT, USA

Synonyms

Alzheimer's disease; Early-onset Alzheimer's disease; Familial Alzheimer's disease; Late-onset Alzheimer's disease; Senile dementia of the Alzheimer's type

Short Description or Definition

One of the leading causes of dementia in late life, Alzheimer's dementia (AD) is a progressive neurodegenerative disorder characterized by a gradual onset and progressive course, affecting memory and other cognitive domains. Traditionally, a diagnosis of AD is made if the cognitive impairments do not occur exclusively in the context of other conditions that affect cognitive status (e.g., delirium, depression, medication side effects, thyroid malfunction, or certain vitamin deficiencies) and are of sufficient severity to cause impairment in social or occupational functioning. Recent changes to the *Diagnostic and Statistical Manual of Mental Disorders, Fifth Edition* (DSM-V), allow a diagnosis of AD under either major or mild neurocognitive disorder. The criteria for major neurocognitive disorder state that cognitive decline must be significant and interfere with daily activities (e.g., paying bills, managing household chores, or shopping), whereas mild neurocognitive disorder represents "modest" decline that does not necessarily interfere with accomplishing daily tasks. A diagnosis of mild neurocognitive disorder due to Alzheimer's disease can be made if the condition has not yet progressed to interfere with daily functioning (American Psychiatric Association 2013). Diagnoses of AD are based on the history and presentation of clinical symptoms, evidence of cognitive impairment, and the exclusion of other causes of dementia such as stroke, metabolic disorders, or other conditions that may account for the cognitive impairment. A diagnosis of definite AD is based upon postmortem neuropathological analysis and is made when there are sufficient numbers of senile plaques and neurofibrillary tangles in specific brain regions.

Categorization

AD may be categorized according to onset age, family history, or presenting clinical features. Age categories distinguish between early (occurring before age 65) and late (occurring at age 65 and older) onset. Classifications based on family history (familial AD vs. sporadic AD) distinguish AD forms that show high heritability. Familial AD is rare, generally of early onset, and has been associated with mutations in the APP gene on chromosome 21, presenilin 1 gene on chromosome 14, and presenilin 2 gene on chromosome 1 (Hardy 2003). Its transmission resembles an autosomal dominant pattern (Morris and Nagy 2004).

AD has also been classified according to the clinical presentation of symptoms. Its most common presentation involves early and significant memory impairment. Variants to this presentation have been reported in the literature and include a visual (posterior) form with significant impairment in higher-level processing of visual stimuli, an aphasic form with significant language involvement, and a frontal form with prominent impairment of executive functions. At autopsy, these variants usually exhibit AD neuropathology in brain regions typically involved in the specific neuropsychological domain (Grabowski and Damasio 2004).

Epidemiology

AD is the most common cause of dementia in late life, accounting for 60–80% of all cases ("2015 Alzheimer's" 2015). Current estimates suggest 5.3 million individuals suffer from AD in the United States, and projections based on population trends suggest an increase to 13.8 million by 2050, including approximately seven million individuals aged 85 and older (Hebert et al. 2013). The overall prevalence of AD is about 11% in individuals age 65 years or older in America and increases with age to include 32% of persons aged 85 and older (Hebert et al. 2013). Incidence rates also exhibit an age-related increase. For example, of the 473,000 individuals that are projected to develop AD in 2015, just 61,000 new cases represent those aged 65 to 74, while 172,000 new cases are among those age 75 to 84, and the final 240,000 cases are among individuals aged 85 and older (the "oldest-old") ("2015 Alzheimer's" 2015; Hebert et al. 2013). Studies report differing patterns of AD prevalence and incidence at the upper end of the life span, with some reporting a plateau at very old ages (age 90 or 100; Mendez and Cummings 2003). Additionally, research demonstrates racial differences in the prevalence of dementia with higher rates among Black and Latino populations. Some of these differences are attributed to differences in cardiovascular risk ("2015 Alzheimer's" 2015).

Risk Factors

Increasing age is among the strongest risk factor for AD. Other risk factors include the e4 allele of the apolipoprotein E (APOE) gene, positive family history (also in sporadic AD), low education (possibly due to less neural reserve), female sex (even after accounting for differential survival), history of head trauma, and cardiovascular factors ("2015 Alzheimer's" 2015; Tschanz et al. 2013). Well-established vascular risk factors include hypertension, high cholesterol, and diabetes (Tschanz et al. 2013). Some of these risk factors affect AD risk when occurring earlier in the life span. For example, studies suggest that high blood pressure, high serum cholesterol, and obesity in *midlife* increase the risk of AD later in life ("2015 Alzheimer's" 2015; Kivipelto et al. 2005). Although inconsistent, some studies report treatment with antihypertensive medications or cholesterol-lowering agents reduces risk for AD (Soininen et al. 2003). Among potential "protective" factors, data from epidemiological studies suggest a *lower* risk of AD among women receiving hormone replacement therapy (Zandi et al. 2002b; Kawas et al. 1997). However, a large randomized clinical trial of estrogen and estrogen-+progesterone in elderly women suggested an *increase* in all-cause dementia in those receiving the combination hormone treatment. Thus hormone therapy is not recommended for cognitive health (Malaspina et al. 2008). Other modifiable risk factors that have shown potential benefits for cognitive health and reduced risk for dementia include diet, nutrients, and nutrient supplements such as antioxidant vitamins, omega-3 fatty acid, medications such as nonsteroidal anti-inflammatory agents, and lifestyle practices such as physical activity and cognitive and social engagement (Scarmeas et al. 2009; Zandi et al. 2002a; Wengreen et al. 2009; Morris 2012; Engelhart et al. 2002; Norton et al. 2012; Wang et al. 2012).

Natural History, Prognostic Factors, Outcomes

The clinical course of AD is usually one of the gradual onset of symptoms with progressive decline. Many scientists believe the disease process starts in the brain decades before overt symptoms emerge. A preclinical phase, characterized primarily by episodic memory deficits, heralds the onset of symptoms. This stage, also referred to as mild cognitive impairment (MCI), lasts approximately 1–3 years. Progression to dementia is characterized by increasing severity of cognitive impairment with severe memory deficits, visuospatial impairment, and other perceptual disturbances. Language impairment begins with mild naming difficulties and circumlocutory speech but progresses to include comprehension deficits. Apraxia (difficulty performing learned motor tasks in the absence of impairment in primary motor or sensory functions) and impaired executive functions and computational ability are also apparent. Behavioral changes are common with indifference, irritability, and sadness, progressing to delusions and, in some individuals, more severe psychiatric disturbances such as hallucinations and agitation. In end stages, there is severe deterioration of all cognitive functions, speech is generally unintelligible, and motor rigidity and urinary and fecal incontinence are present. Death may occur as the result of other causes such as pneumonia or infections (Mendez and Cummings 2003). On postmortem exam, the brain is characterized by generalized atrophy and sulcal and ventricular enlargement. Figure 1a and b display gross atrophy of an AD brain compared with a brain from a cognitively normal elderly individual. Figure 2 displays a coronal section of an AD brain at the level of the hippocampus.

Alzheimer's Dementia, Fig. 1 (**a** and **b**) Displays the brains from a cognitively normal elderly individual and an individual who suffered from advanced AD, respectively. Note the severe atrophy apparent in the AD brain (Photo courtesy of Christine Hulette, M.D., Bryan Alzheimer Disease Research Center, Duke University. Used by permission of Elsevier Limited)

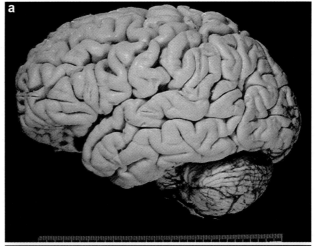

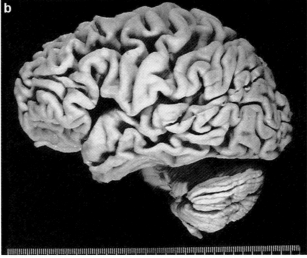

Alzheimer's Dementia,
Fig. 2 Displays atrophy in
AD in this coronal section
including the hippocampi.
Note dilated lateral
ventricles and loss of
inferior temporal mass are
present bilaterally (Photo
courtesy of Steven S. Chin,
M.D., Ph.D., University of
Utah Health Sciences
Center)

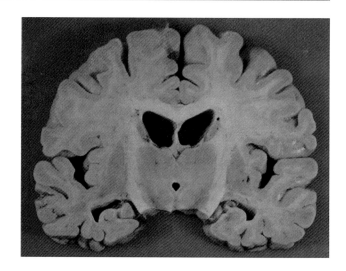

The duration of the entire disease course from MCI to death is highly variable. Mean survival estimates from symptom onset range from 4 to 8 years, but some studies have reported considerably longer duration of 20 years ("2015 Alzheimer's" 2015). Regardless of duration, one study suggests that individuals will spend the majority of their total years with AD in the most severe stage (Arrighi et al. 2010). More rapid rate of disease progression has been associated with early, prominent language impairment, frontal features, and extrapyramidal signs (Mendez and Cummings 2003). Studies examining risk factors of progression after AD onset indicate more rapid decline of cognitive and functional deficits for females, those with earlier onset ages, and those with comorbid vascular risk factors. Alternatively, use of various vascular treatments and cholinesterase inhibitors has been associated with *slower* rates of decline (Tschanz et al. 2013).

Neuropsychology and Psychology of Alzheimer's Dementia

Neuropsychological Deficits

The neuropsychology of AD follows the clinical progression. In early stages, memory is almost always involved, with specific deficit in learning new information. Remote memory such as memory for autobiographical or other knowledge-based systems (semantic memory) is relatively unaffected. In early stages, standardized testing with word lists may reveal relative preservation of immediate or working memory but impairment in delayed (free) recall. There is usually some benefit from cuing or recognition procedures. With progression, cuing is no longer helpful, and remote recall is affected. Implicit memory may be relatively spared as patients show evidence of learning on priming or procedural motor tasks. Orientation to time and place is also affected in AD (Knopman and Selnes 2003).

Language impairments progress from mild anomia and word finding difficulties in early stages to include impairment in comprehension and writing. Errors in speech (paraphasias) become more common, and word substitutions become progressively less related to the target words. Repetition of speech may be relatively unaffected until late in the disease course (Mendez and Cummings 2003; Knopman and Selnes 2003). Sensitive to changes in language are tests of verbal fluency and confrontation naming. Visuospatial disturbances may be subtle or nonexistent in the earliest stages of AD. In moderate and severe stages, impairment may be evident on figure copying tasks or judgment of line orientation (Knopman and Selnes 2003). Figure 3 displays characteristic examples of visuoconstructional impairment in four representative patients with AD.

Impaired abstract reasoning, sustained attention, planning, judgment, and problem-solving

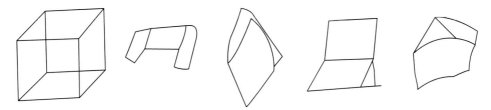

A

Alzheimer's Dementia, Fig. 3 Displays visuocon-structional impairments in the drawings of four individuals with possible or probable AD. The stimulus is the left-most figure (Photographs courtesy of Norman L. Foster, M.D., and Angela Y. Wang, Ph.D., Center for Alzheimer's Care, Imaging and Research, University of Utah)

may characterize impairment in executive functions. Deficits in executive functions may be demonstrated on tests of verbal fluency, trailmaking, and set shifting. Tests such as the Rey complex figure and clock drawing may also elicit impairment in executive functions with poor planning and execution of the tasks. Deficits in working memory may be evident on tasks requiring mental manipulation or divided attention (Knopman and Selnes 2003).

Other neurocognitive aspects of AD include apraxia and anosognosia. In mild AD, deficits in praxis are not common but emerge later in the disease course. Assessment of apraxia may involve pantomiming the execution of a task. Anosognosia or an unawareness of disability is extremely common (Knopman and Selnes 2003). Standardized assessment approaches are few. Some approaches rely on clinical observation, noting a discrepancy between self-report of cognitive impairment and test performance or a discrepancy between caregiver and patient report of impairment.

Behavioral Symptoms

Behavioral changes are extremely common in AD, with nearly all individuals exhibiting at least one symptom at some point over the disease course. Among the most common of these changes is apathy, characterized by a lack of interest and indifference. Anxiety, irritability, and depression are also common, as are delusions. Some patients may exhibit hallucinations, and particularly challenging for caregivers and family are disruptive behaviors such as agitation and aggression. The course of behavioral symptoms is variable, with severe episodes alternating with

milder ones, raising questions about environmental triggers. Noting the co-occurrence of several behaviors, some scientists believe these symptoms are better conceptualized as behavioral *syndromes*, with implications for underlying brain pathology. Several questionnaires are available for assessing behavioral symptoms, ranging from a single symptom questionnaire to a large inventory of symptoms. Assessment of behavioral symptoms is particularly important in an AD evaluation as their presence may suggest other causes for dementia.

Evaluation

A thorough dementia work-up is important for diagnosing AD or determining the etiology of dementia. Critical elements of an evaluation include a detailed clinical history, mental status and physical exam, and, due to potential inaccuracies in patient reporting, an interview with a reliable informant. Neuropsychological testing, laboratory, and neuroimaging are important to exclude other causes of dementia.

Neuropsychological testing is especially important in determining severity of cognitive decline and developing a differential diagnosis between dementia and cognitive deficits due to other conditions. Neuropsychologists may administer a battery of standardized assessments of memory, visuospatial functioning, language, and executive functions and estimate a discrepancy between current and premorbid functioning based on normative data associated with those tests. Alternatively, many neuropsychologists may administer several follow-up examinations to identify patterns of cognitive change over time in establishing a diagnosis. Psychometric properties of these assessments as well as reliable change methods should be considered when determining the validity and reliability of results. While practice effects are generally considered problematic, recent research has elucidated the utility of practice effects for prognosis and differential diagnosis (Chelune and Duff 2013).

Laboratory testing may include a blood count, routine chemistries, thyroid function, and B12 levels. Neuroimaging with MRI or CT may reveal generalized cerebral atrophy with associated sulcal widening and ventricular enlargement. In early stages of the disorder, the brain may appear normal on MRI/CT. PET imaging is a more sensitive technique for detecting changes in brain function in early stages. Reduced glucose metabolism, usually in the temporoparietal regions, is a

consistent pattern in early AD. Figures 4, 5, and 6 display the pattern of glucose hypometabolism in MCI and AD compared with a cognitively normal elderly individual. Additional examination of biomarkers, such as sampling cerebrospinal fluid for tau and amyloid-B42 assays, may be helpful as supplemental procedures for complex cases (Mendez and Cummings 2003).

All acquired data are used in differential diagnosis under the DSM-V and National Institute of Neurological and Communicative Disorders and Stroke and the Alzheimer's Disease and Related Disorders Association (NINCDS-ADRDA) criteria (American Psychiatric Association 2013; McKhann et al. 1984). In 2011 the National Institute on Aging (NIA) and Alzheimer's Association workgroup proposed updated criteria to increase diagnostic range and specificity, including a preclinical stage of AD before symptom onset and

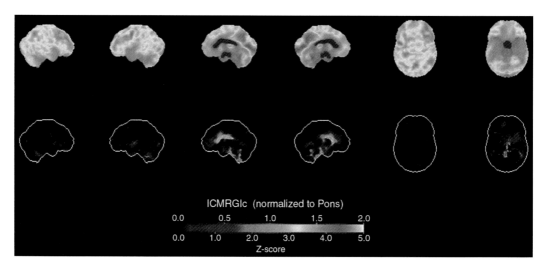

Alzheimer's Dementia, Fig. 4 These images are processed FDG-PET images obtained from elderly subjects. The images have been processed using Neurostat stereotactic surface projections to illustrate the changes of the brain in Alzheimer's disease. Subject scans are shown in two rows in each figure, depicting projections onto six surfaces: R-lateral, L-lateral, R-medial, L-medial, superior, and inferior. The top row in each figure displays regional glucose metabolism with "cooler" colors (purple, blue) reflecting areas of hypometabolism. The bottom row in each figure displays relative glucose metabolism for each participant as compared with a normative sample of 27 cognitively normal elderly individuals. In this bottom series, the images display the statistical significance, expressed as Z-scores, of the hypometabolism when compared to those of the normative sample. The brighter colors (red, white) represent areas of significant hypometabolism, and the cooler colors of blues and purples represent relatively normal brain metabolism. 74-year-old control subject with normal cognition. The top row shows normal brain metabolic activity, and the lower row shows very few regions of hypometabolism. The areas of significant hypometabolism indicated in the medial views are due to this individual having enlarged lateral ventricles relative to normative subjects (Photographs courtesy of Norman L. Foster, M.D., and Angela Y. Wang, Ph.D., Center for Alzheimer's Care, Imaging and Research, University of Utah)

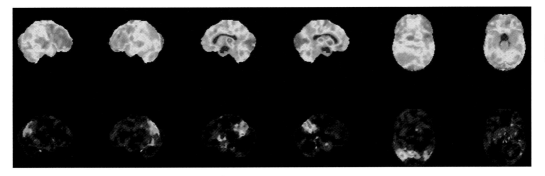

A

Alzheimer's Dementia, Fig. 5 These images are processed FDG-PET images obtained from elderly subjects. The images have been processed using Neurostat stereotactic surface projections to illustrate the changes of the brain in Alzheimer's disease. Subject scans are shown in two rows in each figure, depicting projections onto six surfaces: R-lateral, L-lateral, R-medial, L-medial, superior, and inferior. The top row in each figure displays regional glucose metabolism with "cooler" colors (purple, blue) reflecting areas of hypometabolism. The bottom row in each figure displays relative glucose metabolism for each participant as compared with a normative sample of 27 cognitively normal elderly individuals. In this bottom series, the images display the statistical significance, expressed as Z-scores, of the hypometabolism when compared to those of the normative sample. The brighter colors (red, white) represent areas of significant hypometabolism, and the cooler colors of blues and purples represent relatively normal brain metabolism. 60-year-old subject clinically diagnosed with MCI. The top row shows symmetric decreases in metabolic activity in both hemispheres of the brain. Abnormalities are primarily in the parietal lobe (shown in the R-lateral and L-lateral views) and the posterior cingulate cortex (shown in the R-medial and L-medial views), as seen in the green regions. The bottom row confirms that these regions (green, yellow, and red areas) are indeed significantly (Z-scores $> = 2.5$) hypometabolic. This pattern is a distinguishing feature of AD seen in FDG-PET studies (Photographs courtesy of Norman L. Foster, M.D., and Angela Y. Wang, Ph.D., Center for Alzheimer's Care, Imaging and Research, University of Utah)

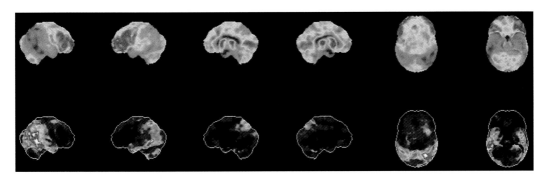

Alzheimer's Dementia, Fig. 6 These images are processed FDG-PET images obtained from elderly subjects. The images have been processed using Neurostat stereotactic surface projections to illustrate the changes of the brain in Alzheimer's disease. Subject scans are shown in two rows in each figure, depicting projections onto six surfaces: R-lateral, L-lateral, R-medial, L-medial, superior, and inferior. The top row in each figure displays regional glucose metabolism with "cooler" colors (purple, blue) reflecting areas of hypometabolism. The bottom row in each figure displays relative glucose metabolism for each participant as compared with a normative sample of 27 cognitively normal elderly individuals. In this bottom series, the images display the statistical significance, expressed as Z-scores, of the hypometabolism when compared to those of the normative sample. The brighter colors (red, white) represent areas of significant hypometabolism, and the cooler colors of blues and purples represent relatively normal brain metabolism. 72-year-old subject clinically diagnosed with AD. This subject shows an even greater and more widely distributed decrease in glucose metabolism. Parietal and temporal lobes and posterior cingulate cortex (green and blue regions in the top row) are affected. The statistically significant changes in metabolic pattern (red and white regions in the lower row) are much greater than the MCI case (Photographs courtesy of Norman L. Foster, M.D., and Angela Y. Wang, Ph.D., Center for Alzheimer's Care, Imaging and Research, University of Utah)

incorporation of diagnostic biomarkers (McKhann et al. 2011). These criteria are gaining supporting scientific evidence toward their validity although further evaluation is required before they are adopted in clinical settings ("2015 Alzheimer's" 2015).

Treatment

Treatment for AD is palliative, with medications and therapies for symptom management. Medications most commonly used are cholinesterase inhibitors that functionally address the cholinergic deficit of AD by blocking the activity of the acetylcholine-degrading enzyme, acetylcholinesterase (see ► "Cholinesterase Inhibitors"). These medications are modestly effective, and patients and family may note an improvement in some cognitive and behavioral symptoms. However, the medications do not modify the trajectory of disease progression. In general, cholinesterase inhibitors are well-tolerated. The use of the first FDA-approved drug of this class, tacrine, however, is rarely administered now due to risk of liver toxicity. Other medications include donepezil, rivastigmine, and galantamine. Side effects include gastrointestinal symptoms such as diarrhea, nausea, and vomiting (Orgogozo 2003). Memantine, an NMDA glutamate receptor blocker, has been approved for use in moderate and severe AD with the mechanism of action presumably reducing neuronal excitotoxicity. Additionally, a sixth drug combining donepezil and memantine was approved in 2014 for use in moderate and severe AD ("2015 Alzheimer's" 2015). Other treatments include the use of psychotropic medications (such as antidepressant and antipsychotic medications) to address the behavioral symptoms. Cognitive rehabilitation may be attempted early in the disease course while patients are still able to participate, and personalized psychosocial interventions such as reminiscence therapy and music therapy have gathered support (Cotelli et al. 2012). Furthermore, psychoeducation, behavioral techniques, and caregiver support and interventions are also important elements of clinical care.

See Also

► Cholinesterase Inhibitors
► Neurofibrillary Tangles
► Senile Dementia
► Senile Plaques

References and Readings

2015 Alzheimer's. (2015). 2015 Alzheimer's disease facts and figures. *Alzheimer's & Dementia: The Journal of the Alzheimer's Association, 11*(3), 332–384. https://doi.org/10.1016/j.jalz.2015.02.003

American Psychiatric Association. (2013). *Diagnostic and statistical manual of mental disorders: DSM-5.* Washington, DC: American Psychiatric Association.

Arrighi, H. M., Neumann, P. J., Lieberburg, I. M., & Townsend, R. J. (2010). Lethality of Alzheimer disease and its impact on nursing home placement. *Alzheimer Disease and Associated Disorders, 24*(1), 90–95. https://doi.org/10.1097/WAD.0b013e31819fe7d1

Chelune, G. J., & Duff, K. (2013). The assessment of change: Serial assessments in dementia evaluations. In L. D. Ravdin, H. L. Katzen, L. D. Ravdin, & H. L. Katzen (Eds.), *Handbook on the neuropsychology of aging and dementia* (pp. 43–57). New York: Springer Science + Business Media. https://doi.org/10.1007/978-1-4614-3106-0_4

Cotelli, M., Manenti, R., & Zanetti, O. (2012). Reminiscence therapy in dementia: A review. *Maturitas, 72*(3), 203–205.

Engelhart, M. J., Geerlings, M. I., Ruitenberg, A., Van Swieten, J. C., Hofman, A., Witteman, J. C., & Breteler, M. M. (2002). Dietary intake of antioxidants and risk of Alzheimer disease [abstract]. *JAMA, 287*(24), 3223–3229. PubMed PMID: 12076218.

Grabowski, T. J., & Damasio, A. R. (2004). Definition, clinical features and neuroanatomical basis of dementia. In M. M. Esiri, V. M.-Y. Lee, & J. Q. Trojanowski (Eds.), *The neuropathology of dementia* (2nd ed., pp. 1–33). Cambridge, UK: Cambridge University Press.

Hardy, J. (2003). The genetics of Alzheimer's disease. In K. Iqbal & B. Winblad (Eds.), *Alzheimer's disease and related disorders: Research advances* (pp. 151–153). Bucharest: Ana Asian Intl. Acad. of Aging.

Hebert, L. E., Weuve, J., Scherr, P. A., & Evans, D. A. (2013). Alzheimer disease in the United States (2010–2050) estimated using the 2010 census. *Neurology, 80*(19), 1778–1783. https://doi.org/10.1212/WNL.0b013e31828726f5

Kawas, C., Resnick, S., Morrison, A., Brookmeyer, R., Corrada, M., Zonderman, A., ..., & Metter, E. (1997). A prospective study of estrogen replacement therapy and the risk of developing Alzheimer's disease: The

Baltimore Longitudinal Study of Aging. *Neurology, 48* (6), 1517–1521.

Kivipelto, M., Ngandu, T., Fratiglioni, L., Viitanen, M., Kåreholt, I., Winblad, B., ..., & Nissinen, A. (2005). Obesity and vascular risk factors at midlife and the risk of dementia and Alzheimer disease. *Archives of Neurology, 62*(10), 1556–1560. https://doi.org/10.1001/archneur.62.10.1556

Knopman, D., & Selnes, O. (2003). Neuropsychology of dementia. In K. M. Heilman & E. Valenstein's (Eds.), *Clinical neuropsychology* (4th ed., pp. 574–616). New York: Oxford University Press.

Malaspina D., Corcoran C., Schobel, S., Hamilton, S.P. (2008). Epidemiological and genetic aspects of neuropsychiatric disorders. In S.C. Yudofsky and R.E. Hales' Neuropsychiatry and behavioral neurosciences (5th ed) (pp. 301–362). Washington, DC: American Psychiatric Association Press.

McKhann, G., Drachman, D., Folstein, M., Katzman, R., Price, D., & Stadlan, E. M. (1984). Clinical diagnosis of Alzheimer's disease: Report of the NINCDS–ADRDA work group under the auspices of Department of Health and Human Services Task Force on Alzheimer's disease. *Neurology, 34*, 939–944.

McKhann, G. M., Knopman, D. S., Chertkow, H., Hyman, B. T., Jack, C. R., Kawas, C. H., ... & Phelps, C. H. (2011). The diagnosis of dementia due to Alzheimer's disease: Recommendations from the National Institute on Aging-Alzheimer's Association workgroups on diagnostic guidelines for Alzheimer's disease. *Alzheimer's & Dementia, 7*(3), 263–269.

Mendez, M. F., & Cummings, J. L. (2003). *Dementia a clinical approach* (3rd ed.). Philadelphia: Butterworth.

Morris, M. C. (2012). Nutritional determinants of cognitive aging and dementia. *Proceedings of the Nutrition Society, 71*, 1–13. https://doi.org/10.1017/S0029665111003296

Morris, J. H., & Nagy, Z. (2004). Alzheimer's disease. In M. M. Esiri, V. M.-Y. Lee, & J. Q. Trojanowski (Eds.), *The neuropathology of dementia* (2nd ed., pp. 161–206). Cambridge, UK: Cambridge University Press.

Norton, M. C., Dew, J., Smith, H., Fauth, E., Piercy, K. W., Breitner, J. S., ..., & Welsh-Bohmer, K. (2012). Lifestyle behavior pattern is associated with different levels of risk for incident dementia and alzheimer's disease: The Cache County Study. *Journal of The American Geriatrics Society, 60*(3), 405–412. https://doi.org/10.1111/j.1532-5415.2011.03860.x

Orgogozo, J.-M. (2003). Treatment of Alzheimer's disease with cholinesterase inhibitors. An update on currently used drugs. In K. Iqbal & B. Winblad (Eds.), *Alzheimer's disease and related disorders: Research advances* (pp. 663–675). Bucharest: Ana Asian Intl. Acad. of Aging.

Scarmeas, N., Luchsinger, J. A., Schupf, N., Brickman, A. M., Cosentino, S., Tang, M. X., & Stern, Y. (2009). Physical activity, diet, and risk of Alzheimer disease. *JAMA: Journal of The American Medical Association, 302*(6), 627–637. https://doi.org/10.1001/jama.2009.1144

Soininen, H., Kivipelto, M., Laakso, M., & Hiltunen, M. (2003). Genetics, molecular epidemiology and cardiovascular risk factors of Alzheimer's disease. In K. Iqbal & B. Winblad (Eds.), *Alzheimer's disease and related disorders: Research advances* (pp. 53–62). Bucharest: Ana Asian Intl. Acad. of Aging.

Tschanz, J. T., Norton, M. C., Zandi, P. P., & Lyketsos, C. G. (2013). The cache county study on memory in aging: Factors affecting risk of Alzheimer's disease and its progression after onset. *International Review of Psychiatry, 25*(6), 673–685. https://doi.org/10.3109/09540261.2013.849663

Wang, H. X., Xu, W., & Pei, J. J. (2012). Leisure activities, cognition and dementia. *Biochimica et Biophysica Acta, 1822*(3), 482–491.

Wengreen, H. J., Neilson, C., Munger, R., & Corcoran, C. (2009). Diet quality is associated with cognitive test performance among aging men and women. *Journal of Nutrition, 139*, 1944–1949.

Zandi, P. P., Anthony, J. C., Hayden, K. M., Mehta, K., Mayer, L., & Breitner, J. S. (2002a). Reduced incidence of AD with NSAID but not H2 receptor antagonists: The cache county study. *Neurology, 59*(6), 880–886.

Zandi, P. P., Carlson, M. C., Plassman, B. L., Welsh-Bohmer, K. A., Mayer, L. S., Steffens, D. C., & Breitner, J. S. (2002b). Hormone replacement therapy and incidence of Alzheimer disease in older women: The cache county study. *JAMA: Journal of The American Medical Association, 288*(17), 2123–2129. https://doi.org/10.1001/jama.288.17.2123

Alzheimer's Disease

Russell H. Swerdlow[1], Heather Anderson[2] and Jeffrey M. Burns[2]
[1]University of Kansas School of Medicine, Landon Center on Aging, Kansas City, KS, USA
[2]Department of Neurology, University of Kansas School of Medicine, Kansas City, KS, USA

Definition

A neurodegenerative disease of the brain characterized clinically by insidious, chronic, and progressive cognitive decline and histologically by cerebral accumulations of the proteins beta amyloid (plaques) and tau (tangles).

Historical Background

In 1902, a woman called Auguste D. came under the care of Dr. Alois Alzheimer and then at the University of Frankfurt. The patient manifested changes in behavior and cognition. Her clinical course was characterized by progressive paranoia, delusional thinking, disorientation, and poor memory. She was institutionalized for the last 3 years of her life. Upon her death, Alzheimer analyzed her brain using a silver stain and described both extracellular and intracellular protein accumulations. The extracellular protein accumulations were termed plaques, and the intraneuronal protein accumulations were called tangles. Alzheimer presented the results of this autopsy in 1906. Several other similar cases of relatively "presenile" (i.e., arbitrarily defined as an onset prior to age 55–65) clinical dementia associated with plaques and tangles were noted by Alzheimer and others over the next 4 years. In 1910, Alzheimer's departmental chair, Emil Kraepelin, published a textbook covering the fields of neurology and psychiatry and referred to patients with presenile dementia, plaques, and tangles as having "Alzheimer's disease."

Concurrently, other investigators, such as Oscar Fischer, also reported plaque presence in elderly demented individuals. These individuals were older than those with "presenile" dementia (i.e., generally older than age 55–65). As the commonality of progressive dementia in the elderly was well recognized, the presence of plaques in elderly demented individuals was felt to represent a normal phenomenon. Such individuals were not diagnosed with Alzheimer's disease. Instead, cognitive decline in elderly adults was attributed to normal aging or other poorly described conditions, such as "hardening of the arteries." As a result, Alzheimer's disease remained relatively uncommon for a number of subsequent decades.

In the 1960s, investigators began comparing elderly demented subjects to those diagnosed with "presenile" Alzheimer's disease. Notable similarities were observed regarding the clinical course (chronic and progressive), the clinical features (cognitive decline that featured evolution of an amnestic state, followed by behavioral changes), and histopathology (plaques and tangles). By the 1970s, the number of demented elderly was growing fast as demographic shifts in the aging population combined with increased recognition of the syndrome. At this point, the original definition of Alzheimer's disease (as described by Alzheimer and named by Kraepelin) was expanded to account for all dementing individuals with plaques and tangles, although some separation of these groups was envisioned. Those meeting the original criteria of plaque and tangle dementia in presenile adults were designated as having dementia of the Alzheimer type (DAT), while the previously unconsidered elderly cases were designated as having senile dementia of the Alzheimer type (SDAT). With increasing recognition of the problem, Alzheimer's disease very quickly became incredibly common, as well as a Western civilization health priority.

In the USA, the 1980s saw the establishment of federally funded Alzheimer's disease research centers, which began to systematically study the clinical course of this progressive dementia, mostly in the common SDAT form. Academic research began to unravel the chemical makeup of plaques and tangles. Investigations into patterns and causes of neurodegeneration were performed. This advancing knowledge enhanced the ability of clinicians to diagnose Alzheimer's disease at increasingly subtle stages, as well as the ability to pharmacologically intervene to achieve partial, temporary symptomatic benefits in at least some individuals.

Current Knowledge

Scientific Perspective

The plaques seen in persons with Alzheimer's disease contain several aggregated proteins. The major constituent is a protein called amyloid beta (Aβ). "Beta" is a chemical term that specifies a certain pattern of protein folding. "Amyloid" is a general term that refers to proteins that give a particular appearance when exposed to a particular type of stain, Congo red. The beta amyloid, or Aβ, found in the brains of Alzheimer's disease patients derives from a particular protein called the amyloid precursor protein (APP).

In the human brain, the APP is 695 amino acids long. It is a transmembrane protein. One end (the carboxyl end) is found inside neurons, in the cytoplasm. The other end (the amino end) extends outside the cell. In between the cytoplasmic and extracellular portions is a stretch that runs through the membrane. The normal function of APP is not well known. APP is digested by different enzymes, which cut the protein at different points. An enzyme complex called the beta secretase (BACE) cuts APP in its extracellular portion. An enzyme or group of enzymes referred to as the alpha secretase cuts APP in its intramembrane segment. The gamma secretase cuts APP twice, both times in its intramembrane segment. Both of the gamma secretase cuts occur closer to the carboxyl end of the APP than the alpha secretase cut.

Different cutting combinations generate various APP by-products. Cutting of an APP by beta and gamma secretases generates a 38–43 amino acid stretch, and this stretch tends to assume a beta folding conformation and has the features of an amyloid protein (i.e., birefringence under the microscope when stained with Congo red). The 40 and 42 amino acid-long variants of Aβ predominate in plaques and are often designated Aβ40 and Aβ42. Aβ42 seems to be particularly important to the formation of the amyloid plaques of Alzheimer's disease, probably because this version of the protein is quite insoluble. When Aβ accumulations begin to form in brain, they are not associated with disrupted cell elements and are called "diffuse plaques." Another type of more evolved plaque can also be found in Alzheimer's disease patients, in which Aβ becomes condensed at the center of the plaque, and the vicinity of the plaque is associated with disrupted cell elements such as degenerating axons and dendrites. As axons and dendrites are collectively called "neurites," this type of plaque is called a "neuritic plaque."

The tangles of Alzheimer's disease are found primarily in neurons. Under the microscope tangles have a fibrous quality to them, and hence tangles in Alzheimer's disease are referred to as "neurofibrillary tangles." Neurofibrillary tangles consist of a protein called tau. Normally, tau is found in association with microtubules, which act as a skeleton, or "cytoskeleton" supporting the cellular structure. The function of tau appears to be the stabilization of these microtubules. Like many proteins, after its production tau is modified by the addition and subtraction of phosphate groups on certain amino acids, especially serine and threonine. During embryonic development, tau is heavily phosphorylated, but during youth and early adulthood, this heavily phosphorylated pattern is rare if at all seen. In Alzheimer's disease, though, tau again takes on a heavily phosphorylated pattern, which is felt to reflect an abnormal physiologic event and is referred to as tau "hyperphosphorylation." Hyperphosphorylated tau molecules begin to pair off, a process called "dimerization." Hyperphosphorylated tau dimers, also called "paired helical filaments," are quite insoluble and begin to aggregate with each other. This aggregation, typically visible extending from cell bodies into axons, comprises the neurofibrillary tangle.

As impressive as this advancing understanding of plaque and tangle composition is, recognizing what constitutes these aggregations does not address why they form. In this regard, genetic studies of DAT subjects who inherit the disorder in an autosomal-dominant fashion have had a large impact. Several hundred such families have been documented. In these families the disease affects about 50% of each generation, with typical onset occurring in the third, fourth, fifth, or sixth decades. A small number of these families have demonstrable mutations in the gene that encodes the APP. This gene is located on chromosome 21, the same chromosome that is present in excess in Down's syndrome. Down's syndrome patients invariably accumulate Aβ plaques in their fifth decade. A somewhat larger number of these families have mutations in the gene that encodes a protein called presenilin 1. This gene is found in chromosome 14. Presenilin 1 protein constitutes part of the gamma secretase complex. A smaller number of families have mutation of a related gene on chromosome 1, which encodes a related protein, presenilin 2. Presenilin 2 can also participate in formation of the gamma secretase. Mutations in the genes that encode APP, presenilin 1, and presenilin 2 all enhance the production of Aβ42. This has lent support to the "amyloid cascade hypothesis," which posits as Aβ42 is generated it begins to interfere with neuronal function, kill neurons, and generate the other histologic features seen in Alzheimer's disease. While the logic underlying this hypothesis is obvious, it is important to keep in mind it assumes the very small subset of early-onset, autosomal-dominant Alzheimer's disease (which accounts for far less than 1% of those affected) have a similar if not identical etiology to the common sporadic, late-onset cases that constitute the vast majority. In those subjects, what initiates Aβ42 production remains an open area of debate. Conceivably, population diversity in genes that contribute to APP production or processing could cause Aβ42 to appear. Environmental factors could lead to Aβ42 formation. Also, a variety of age-related factors promote Aβ42 formation.

Other factors are recognized to play a role in Alzheimer's disease, and where these factors fit into or what they tell us about the etiologic hierarchy of the disease is unclear. One factor relates to the *APOE* gene on chromosome 19. The *APOE* gene shows population variability due to the presence of two polymorphic positions. The common *APOE* variants are the ε2, ε3, and ε4 forms. The *APOE* ε4 form is over represented in those with Alzheimer's disease, where it seems to move up the age of presentation in those destined to develop the disorder. Mitochondrial function is also altered in Alzheimer's disease, and these alterations are not limited to the brain.

Diagnostic Perspective

Dementia is defined as a cognitive decline that has advanced to that point it interferes with activities of daily living. While dementia has many different etiologies, Alzheimer's disease is the most common cause of dementia, accounting for 50–60% of dementia verified by neuropathological examination of the brain at autopsy. The clinical diagnosis (i.e., diagnosis in life) of Alzheimer's disease is made in patients who have progressive dementia with no other systemic or brain diseases that could account for the progressive cognitive decline. A diagnosis of "definite Alzheimer's disease" is

traditionally diagnosed at autopsy by the presence of plaques and tangles (although in some older schemas tangles are not requisite) in an individual with a clinical history suggestive of dementia. The presence of plaques and tangles in typical brain regions (mesial temporal, parietal, and inferior frontal structures) is quite common in elderly persons with the clinical syndrome of Alzheimer's disease. As a result of the high prevalence of Alzheimer's disease with advancing age (at least one commonly quoted study estimates approximately half of those over the age of 85 have it), the specificity of the clinical diagnosis is high. Recognition of how common Alzheimer's disease is in later life has also served to enhance clinician awareness, thus improving sensitivity of the diagnosis. In the hands of an experienced physician, clinical diagnostic accuracy is excellent.

Criteria originally designed to facilitate identification of subjects for clinical trials have helped to standardize clinical diagnostic approaches. These criteria, such as those proposed by the National Institute of Neurologic, Communicative Disorders, and Stroke (NINCDS) and the Alzheimer's Disease and Related Disorders Association (ADRDA) in the 1980s emphasize the importance of establishing that a progressive dementia exists in a patient. Two basic approaches are commonly used toward this end. One is to demonstrate a pattern of cognitive domain strengths and weaknesses that reliably suggest decline from a previous level of cognitive function has emerged. For example, defective memory retention in the presence of another defective cognitive domain (language, executive function, visuospatial function, and praxis) in an elderly patient with cognitive complaints and an otherwise unremarkable physical exam is strongly suggestive of Alzheimer's disease. The other approach focuses more on defining the degree and nature of emerging declines in daily living activities. This latter technique focuses extensively on collateral history obtained from family members or friends of the patient.

The diagnosis is made primarily through clinical impression, although that impression is influenced by a small set of recommended laboratory and imaging tests. These tests are serologic (vitamin B12 level, thyroid function tests, electrolytes with renal and hepatic indices, and a blood cell count) and structural (brain imaging by either computed tomography or magnetic resonance imaging) in nature. As currently used, they mostly serve to rule out the presence of concomitant pathologies that can interfere with cognition. Although this has contributed to the view that the Alzheimer's disease diagnosis is one of exclusion, it should be noted that certain patterns of cognitive decline elicited by clinical history or demonstrable by neuropsychological testing are so typical of Alzheimer's disease they can be used to support a diagnosis of inclusion. It is important to note, though, that while fluorodeoxyglucose PET and *APOE* genotyping are occasionally used to address specific questions, such as whether the presence of Alzheimer's disease versus a frontotemporal dementia is more likely in a patient, these tests are not routinely used in the diagnosis of Alzheimer's disease and cannot by themselves establish a diagnosis of Alzheimer's disease.

Another PET application is also now available, which reveals the presence of brain fibrillary Aβ deposition (in essence, the presence of amyloid plaques). At the time of this writing amyloid plaque scanning, which is expensive and not covered by third-party payers, is not routinely used to diagnose Alzheimer's disease although the utility of this test is under study and this may change in the future. Spinal fluid measurements of Aβ and tau protein levels yield similar information to that which is obtained through an amyloid scan, but this test is currently used more in research settings than it is in the clinic setting.

An increasing emphasis on Alzheimer's disease biomarker measurements is apparent in new Alzheimer's disease diagnostic research criteria that were formulated in 2011. In addition to essentially continuing recognition of existing Alzheimer's disease criteria, two new largely biomarker-driven Alzheimer's disease categories were proposed. One new category, "prodromal Alzheimer's disease," captures individuals with a mild cognitive impairment (MCI) syndrome and evidence of fibrillary brain amyloid plaque deposition. "Preclinical Alzheimer's disease" is defined as intact cognitive function in an individual with evidence of fibrillary brain amyloid plaque deposition.

Treatment Perspective

Although Alzheimer's disease is currently neither reversible nor curable, it is possible to treat its symptoms. The first approved treatment for Alzheimer's disease was tacrine, a cholinesterase inhibitor. This drug increased levels of brain acetylcholine by antagonizing its synaptic degradation. Increasing brain cholinergic tone was identified as a pharmacologic target because Alzheimer's disease patients show a profound loss of acetylcholine due to degeneration of cholinergic neurons in the basal forebrain. Safer cholinesterase inhibitors (donepezil, rivastigmine, and galantamine) have since superseded tacrine. In addition to inhibiting acetylcholinesterase, rivastigmine also inhibits butyrylcholinesterases that also hydrolyze acetylcholine, and galantamine is an allosteric modulator of acetylcholine nicotinic receptors. Each agent shows a similar overall degree of efficacy, although the individual with Alzheimer's disease may respond to or tolerate one drug better than the other. Treatment cohorts followed for 12 weeks to 3 years indicate that as a group, those started on cholinesterase inhibitors tend to perform and appear slightly improved compared to their immediate pretreatment baseline. This improvement appears detectable for 6–12 months. By 12 months, though, treatment groups return to their pretreatment performance as ascertained by cognitive testing, clinical impression, and caregiver impression. Beyond 12 months, patients continuously decline below their pretreatment baseline, although for at least the next several years, patients appear to perform better on cognitive testing than would otherwise be expected. The clinical meaningfulness of this sustained benefit has fueled considerable debate. Benefits have been observed on measures of cognitive ability, functional ability, behavior, and caregiver stress.

At the time of this writing, memantine is the only non-cholinesterase inhibitor specifically approved for the treatment of Alzheimer's disease. Under in vitro conditions, memantine blocks a cation channel associated with the NMDA type of glutamate-activated ionotropic receptors. Whether or not this is its primary mechanism of action in Alzheimer's disease has been questioned. In any case, cohorts of patients with moderate or severe Alzheimer's disease, when randomized to memantine, perform better on measures of cognitive and functional performance than do concurrent placebo treatment groups. In severe Alzheimer's disease, the magnitude of observed benefit is similar to that obtained with donepezil. Memantine and donepezil have been studied in combination with each other. Subjects with mini-mental state exam scores of 5–14, who were already on donepezil, did better as a group when memantine was added to their treatment regimen than when placebo was added. Demonstrable benefits in mild Alzheimer's disease are lacking, and thus the role of memantine in the mild stages of Alzheimer's disease is not clear.

Two studies concluded high-dose vitamin E (2000 IU each day) might slightly slow decline in Alzheimer's disease patients. Other studies, though, suggest taking more than 400 IU of vitamin E on a daily basis increases overall mortality. The marginality of any vitamin E benefit, in conjunction with safety concerns, has reduced enthusiasm for the use of vitamin E in Alzheimer's disease. Although a variety of other prescription medications (estrogens, statins), nonprescription medications (nonsteroidal anti-inflammatories), and nutraceuticals (gingko biloba) have been considered for the treatment of Alzheimer's disease, published data to date on all other treatment options has been at worst negative and at best insufficient to earn regulatory approval.

Other drug categories are commonly used to treat targeted symptoms associated with Alzheimer's disease. For instance, antipsychotic medications are often used to treat agitated behavior. Some studies do show efficacy in this regard, although other studies have argued the limited behavioral benefits antipsychotics may confer is canceled out by increased morbidity.

Future Directions

Scientific Perspective

In the short term, considerable effort will be directed at additional studies of Aβ dynamics and homeostasis. Research will focus on the toxicities of different degrees of Aβ aggregation (especially oligomers, defined as short, soluble polymers of amyloid), cellular mechanisms of Aβ disposal, and tissue-level mechanisms of Aβ disposal.

Research over the longer term will need to address the fact that the predominant etiologic hypothesis, the amyloid cascade hypothesis, cannot yet explain why Aβ homeostasis changes in most of those affected or how Aβ might give rise to other aspects of Alzheimer's disease pathology. It is possible the amyloid cascade hypothesis will prove valid in those with early-onset, autosomal-dominant Alzheimer's disease caused by mutations of the genes encoding APP, presenilin 1, and presenilin 2 proteins, but not the late-onset cases (the vast majority). Disproving the amyloid cascade hypothesis in the late-onset cases will likely require two events. First, interventions that attempt to treat Alzheimer's disease by targeting Aβ will need to show absent or limited efficacy. Second, other hypotheses better able to explain the overall Alzheimer's clinical, and pathological big picture will need to demonstrate viability and durability.

Diagnostic Perspective

Because it may prove easier in the future to prevent neurodegeneration rather than reverse it, the ability to render an early, accurate diagnosis is crucial. Also, the ability to treat the disease (either symptomatically or disease modifying) increases the importance of early diagnosis. This has led the field to recently define prodromal and preclinical Alzheimer's disease categories. A key question is how these new categories, which were proposed for research purposes, should extrapolate to the clinical setting. The use of biomarkers to define how close an asymptomatic or very mildly impaired individual is to clinical Alzheimer's disease outside of the research setting requires, and is receiving, careful consideration.

Treatment Perspective

None of the treatments approved for use in Alzheimer's disease are approved for use in MCI/prodromal Alzheimer's disease, although available data argue cholinesterase inhibition (at least with donepezil) may provide a marginal benefit. Such a benefit would not be surprising, especially if MCI represents very early Alzheimer's disease in most people.

Over a decade of experience with symptomatic treatment has made it abundantly clear that disease-modifying treatments are required. Most current approaches toward disease modification are targeted to Aβ homeostasis. Inhibition of its production (gamma secretase inhibitors and modifiers), its targeted removal (active and passive immunization approaches), prevention of its aggregation, and enhancement of enzymatic degradation are all under active pursuit. To date, a phase II Aβ vaccination trial (AN1792) was halted when several of the subjects developed encephalitis. Other data obtained through this trial suggest the approach was successful in reducing cerebral amyloid plaques. However, the most extensive published clinical data from AN1792 indicate that 1 year after vaccination, the rate of cognitive decline was similar to (unchanged from or only very slightly reduced from) the rate of decline shown by the placebo group of that trial. Other anti Aβ trials have featured drugs designed to prevent generation of Aβ from APP, drugs designed to prevent the collection of Aβ monomers into oligomers, and the administration of antibodies to Aβ that are intended to remove Aβ from the brain. To date a number of trials of these agents have not succeeded in reaching their primary end point, while other trials are still underway. It is worth noting that anti-Aβ trial design increasingly is focusing on subjects whose brains show Aβ deposition, but who are clinically asymptomatic or only mildly affected from a clinical perspective. The proposed but unproven rationale for this is that if it turns out to be the case that Aβ does initiate neurodegeneration in Alzheimer's disease, once the neurodegeneration proceeds to a certain point, it may continue to advance whether or not Aβ is present.

If attacking Aβ fails to meaningfully benefit Alzheimer's disease patients, the validity of the amyloid cascade hypothesis in late-onset, sporadic Alzheimer's disease will be called into question. If this happens, new models for drug design will be needed. Currently, mice expressing a mutant APP transgene, sometimes in conjunction with other mutant human transgenes, serve as the gold standard for preclinical testing of potential Alzheimer's disease treatments.

Cross-References

► Alzheimer's Dementia
► Memory Impairment
► Mental Status Examination
► Mini-Mental State Exam
► Senile Dementia

References and Readings

Albert, M. S., DeKosky, S. T., Dickson, D., Dubois, B., Feldman, H. H., et al. (2011). The diagnosis of mild cognitive impairment due to Alzheimer's disease: Recommendations from the National Institute on Aging-Alzheimer's Association workgroups on diagnostic guidelines for Alzheimer's disease. *Alzheimers Dement, 7*, 270–279.

Amaducci, L. A., Rocca, W. A., & Schoenberg, B. S. (1986). Origin of the distinction between Alzheimer's disease and senile dementia: How history can clarify nosology. *Neurology, 36*, 1497–1499.

Blacker, D., & Tanzi, R. E. (1998). The genetics of Alzheimer disease: Current status and future prospects. *Archives of Neurology, 55*, 294–296.

Blessed, G., Tomlinson, B., & Roth, M. (1968). The association between quantitative measures of dementia and of senile change in the cerebral grey matter of elderly subjects. *The British Journal of Psychiatry, 114*, 797–811.

Campion, D., Dumanchin, C., Hannequin, D., Dubois, B., Belliard, S., Puel, M., et al. (1999). Early-onset autosomal dominant Alzheimer disease: Prevalence, genetic heterogeneity, and mutation spectrum. *The American Journal of Human Genetics, 65*, 664–670.

Corder, E. H., Saunders, A. M., Strittmatter, W. J., Schmechel, D. E., Gaskell, P. C., Small, G. W., et al. (1993). Gene dose of apolipoprotein E type 4 allele and the risk of Alzheimer's disease in late onset families. *Science, 261*, 921–923.

De Leon, M. J., & Klunk, W. (2005). Biomarkers for the early diagnosis of Alzheimer's disease. *Lancet Neurology, 5*, 198–199.

Evans, D. A., Funkenstein, H. H., Albert, M. S., Scherr, P. A., Cook, N. R., Chown, M. J., et al. (1989). Prevalence of Alzheimer's disease in a community population of older persons. Higher than previously reported. *JAMA, 262*, 2551–2556.

Gearing, M., Mirra, S. S., Hedreen, J. C., Sumi, S. M., Hansen, L. A., & Heyman, A. (1995). The consortium to establish a registry for Alzheimer's disease (CERAD). Part X. Neuropathology confirmation of the clinical diagnosis of Alzheimer's disease. *Neurology, 45*, 461–466.

Gilman, S., Koller, M., Black, R. S., Jenkins, L., Griffith, S. G., Fox, N. C., et al. (2005). Clinical effects of Abeta immunization (AN1792) in patients with AD in an interrupted trial. *Neurology, 64*, 1553–1562.

Hardy, J., & Allsop, D. (1991). Amyloid deposition as the central event in the aetiology of Alzheimer's disease. *Trends in Pharmacological Sciences, 12,* 383–388.

Hardy, J. A., & Higgins, G. A. (1992). Alzheimer's disease: The amyloid cascade hypothesis. *Science, 256,* 184–185.

Jack Jr., C. R., Knopman, D. S., Jagust, W. J., Shaw, L. M., Aisen, P. S., et al. (2010). Hypothetical model of dynamic biomarkers of the Alzheimer's pathological cascade. *Lancet Neurology, 9,* 119–128.

Katzman, R. (1976). The prevalence and malignancy of Alzheimer's disease: A major killer. *Archives of Neurology, 33,* 217–218.

Khachaturian, Z. S. (1985). Diagnosis of Alzheimer's disease. *Archives of Neurology, 42,* 1097–1106.

Klunk, W. E., Engler, H., Nordberg, A., Wang, Y., Blomqvist, G., Holt, D. P., et al. (2004). Imaging brain amyloid in Alzheimer's disease with Pittsburgh compound-B. *Annals of Neurology, 55,* 306–319.

Mayeux, R., Saunders, A. M., Shea, S., Mirra, S., Evans, D., Roses, A. D., et al. (1998). Utility of the apolipoprotein E genotype in the diagnosis of Alzheimer's disease. Alzheimer's Disease Centers Consortium on Apolipoprotein E and Alzheimer's Disease. *The New England Journal of Medicine, 338,* 506–511.

McKhann, G., Drachman, D., Folstein, M., Katzman, R., Price, D., & Stadlan, E. M. (1984). Clinical diagnosis of Alzheimer's disease: Report of the NINCDS-ADRDA Work Group under the auspices of Department of Health and Human Services Task Force on Alzheimer's Disease. *Neurology, 34,* 939–944.

McKhann, G. M., Knopman, D. S., Chertkow, H., Hyman, B. T., Jack Jr., C. R., et al. (2011). The diagnosis of dementia due to Alzheimer's disease: Recommendations from the National Institute on Aging-Alzheimer's Association workgroups on diagnostic guidelines for Alzheimer's disease. *Alzheimers Dement, 7,* 263–269.

Morris, J. C. (2006). Mild cognitive impairment is early-stage Alzheimer disease: Time to revise diagnostic criteria. *Archives of Neurology, 63,* 15–16.

Mosconi, L., De Santi, S., Li, J., Tsui, W. H., Li, Y., Boppana, M., et al. (2007). Hippocampal hypometabolism predicts cognitive decline from normal aging. *Neurobiology of Aging.* https://doi.org/10.1016/j.neurobiolaging.2006.12.008.

National Institute on Aging, and Reagan Institute Working Group on Diagnostic Criteria for the Neuropathological Assessment of Alzheimer's Disease. (1997). Consensus recommendations for the postmortem diagnosis of Alzheimer's disease. *Neurobiology of Aging, 18* (4 Suppl), S1–S2.

Petersen, R. C., Smith, G. E., Waring, S. C., Ivnik, R. J., Tangalos, E. G., & Kokmen, E. (1999). Mild cognitive impairment: Clinical characterization and outcome. *Archives of Neurology, 56,* 303–308.

Petersen, R. C., Thomas, R. G., Grundman, M., Bennett, D., Doody, R., Ferris, S., et al. (2005). Vitamin E and donepezil for the treatment of mild cognitive impairment. *The New England Journal of Medicine, 352,* 2379–2388.

Ronald and Nancy Reagan Research Institute of the Alzheimer's Association and the National Institute on Aging Work Group. (1998). Consensus report of the work group on: Molecular and biochemical markers of Alzheimer's disease. *Neurobiology of Aging, 19,* 109–116.

Sano, M., Ernesto, C., Thomas, R. G., Klauber, M. R., Schafer, K., Grundman, M., et al. (1997). A controlled trial of selegiline, alpha-tocopherol, or both as treatment for Alzheimer's disease. The Alzheimer's Disease Cooperative Study. *The New England Journal of Medicine, 336,* 1216–1222.

Scheuner, D., Eckman, C., Jensen, M., Song, X., Citron, M., Suzuki, N., et al. (1996). Secreted amyloid beta-protein similar to that in the senile plaques of Alzheimer's disease is increased in vivo by the presenilin 1 and 2 and APP mutations linked to familial Alzheimer's disease. *Nature Medicine, 2,* 864–870.

Schneider, L. S., Tariot, P. N., Dagerman, K. S., Davis, S. M., Hsiao, J. K., et al. (2006). Effectiveness of atypical antipsychotic drugs in patients with Alzheimer's disease. *The New England Journal of Medicine, 355,* 1525–1538.

Snowdon, D. A., Kemper, S. J., Mortimer, J. A., Greiner, L. H., Wekstein, D. R., & Markesbery, W. R. (1996). Linguistic ability in early life and cognitive function and Alzheimer's disease in late life. Findings from the Nun Study. *JAMA, 275,* 528–532.

Sperling, R. A., Aisen, P. S., Beckett, L. A., Bennett, D. A., Craft, S., et al. (2011). Toward defining the preclinical stages of Alzheimer's disease: Recommendations from the National Institute on Aging-Alzheimer's Association workgroups on diagnostic guidelines for Alzheimer's disease. *Alzheimers Dement, 7,* 280–292.

Swerdlow, R. H. (2007). Is aging part of Alzheimer's disease, or is Alzheimer's disease part of aging? *Neurobiology of Aging, 28,* 1465–1480.

Alzheimer's Disease Cooperative Study ADL Scale

Jessica Fish
Medical Research Council Cognition and Brain Sciences Unit, Cambridge, UK

Synonyms

Alzheimer's disease cooperative study ADL scale for mild cognitive impairment (ADCS-ADL-MCI); Alzheimer's disease cooperative study ADL scale for severe impairment (ADCS-ADL-sev)

Description

The ADCS-ADL assesses the competence of patients with Alzheimer's disease (AD) in basic and instrumental activities of daily living (ADLs). It can be completed by a caregiver in questionnaire format or administered by a clinician/researcher as a structured interview with a caregiver. All responses should relate to the 4 weeks prior to the time of rating. The six basic ADL items each take an ADL (e.g., eating) and provide descriptions of level of competence, with the rater selecting the most appropriate option (e.g., ate without physical help and used a knife, used a fork or spoon but not a knife, used fingers to eat, was usually fed by someone else). The 16 instrumental ADL items follow the format "In the past 4 weeks, did s/he *use the telephone*," with the response options of yes/no/don't know. If the response is "yes," a rating is then made regarding his/her competence according to a set of descriptions tailored to that activity (e.g., for the telephone item, whether the person looked up phone numbers and made calls, made calls only to well-known numbers without referring to a directory, made calls only to well-known numbers using a telephone directory, answered the phone but did not make calls, or only spoke when put on the line). Adapted versions of the scale suitable for people with MCI (ADCS-MCI-ADL) and moderate–severe AD (ADCS-ADL-sev) have also been developed. Scores on the 24-item ADCS-ADL range from 0 to 78, those on the 18-item ADCS-MCI-ADL range from 0 to 57, and on the 19-item ADCS-ADL-sev from 0 to 54, where higher scores reflect greater competence (see section "Psychometric Data" for further details). The entire instrument takes 15–30 min to administer.

Historical Background

The ADCS is a US-based initiative that aims to conduct research informing the prevention and treatment of AD, as well as developing measures for use in people with AD, particularly in clinical trials. The ADCS-ADL was the first ADL scale to be developed for use specifically in clinical trials with people with AD across the range of severity. The 24 items in the standard version were selected from a pool of 45 items based upon a stringent set of psychometric criteria (see section "Psychometric Data"). Using the same criteria, Galasko et al. (2005) developed a version of the ADCS-ADL for more severely impaired participants, which is known as the ADCS-ADL-sev, and a version for people with MCI has also been developed (ADCS-MCI-ADL, Perneczky et al. 2006). The ADCS-ADL has been used in a variety of clinical trials.

Psychometric Data

Galasko et al. (1997) selected the items for the ADCS-ADL from a pool of 45 items thought to be relevant to the target population on the basis of existing scales and clinical experience. To determine which ADLs were most suitable for inclusion, the 45-item version was administered at baseline, 6 months and 12 months later to 64 elderly controls and 242 people with AD, stratified by MMSE score at baseline assessment. Half of participants were additionally assessed at 1 and 2 months post-baseline. An item was included in the final measure if it fits the criteria that it was performed either premorbidly or at baseline by >90% of participants (showing it was applicable to the target group), had a kappa agreement statistic at 1–2 months of >0.4 (indicating good test-retest reliability), had a significant correlation with MMSE score (indicating appropriate scaling and validity), and showed decline over 12 months in at least 20% of participants (indicating validity and sensitivity to change).

Galasko et al. (2005) used the same criteria in the development of the ADCS-ADL-sev, based on longitudinal data of 145 patients with Mini-Mental State Examination (MMSE) scores between 0 and 15. Galasko et al. reported good test-retest reliability (baseline-1 month $r = 0.94$, baseline-2 months $r = 0.89$, month1–month2 $r = 0.94$), and there was evidence of convergent validity based upon the strong correlation between ADCS-ADL-sev and other global impairment measures (ADCS-ADL-sev – MMSE $r = 0.64$; ADCS-ADL-sev – severe Impairment Battery $r = 0.71$). The mean score on the first test was 25.4 (SD 12.7, maximum obtainable 54), with a mean decline of 5.6 points (SD 7.5) over 6 months and 10.3 points (SD 10.3) over 12 months.

Perneczky et al. (2006) have found that the ADCS-MCI-ADL scale can discriminate people with MCI from control participants (a cutoff score of 52 gives sensitivity of 0.89 and specificity of 0.97). Further the scale has been shown to have high discriminatory power to distinguish between MCI and AD (a cutoff score of 37/38 has a sensitivity of 85% and specificity of 87%) (Pedrosa et al. 2010).

Clinical Uses

The ADCS-ADL and its variants are the only ADL scales designed with AD specifically in mind and can provide a fairly detailed assessment of competence in a variety of ADLs. Galasko et al. (2005) state that the measure takes too long to administer for it to be widely adopted in clinical practice, but it would be useful in intervention studies, and the ADL-sev in particular where the severity of the disorder may render measures such as the MMSE unsuitable due to floor effects. The careful selection of items for the ADCS-ADL suggests that they are eminently suitable for use in clinical trials. Perneczky et al. (2006) found that even patients with a diagnosis of mild cognitive impairment exhibit deficits in instrumental ADLs on the ADCS-ADL-MCI and that scores can successfully discriminate patients with MCI from healthy controls; as such, results from this scale may be useful in forming an MCI diagnosis.

Cross-References

▶ Activities of Daily Living Questionnaire
▶ Bristol Activities of Daily Living Scale
▶ Disability Assessment for Dementia
▶ Lawton-Brody Instrumental Activities of Daily Living Scale

References and Readings

Galasko, D., Bennett, D., Sano, M., Ernesto, C., Thomas, R., Grundman, M., et al. (1997). An inventory to assess activities of daily living for clinical trials in Alzheimer's disease. The Alzheimer's disease cooperative study. *Alzheimer's Disease and Associated Disorders, 11*(S2), S33–S39.

Galasko, D., Schmitt, F., Thomas, R., Jin, S., Bennett, D., & Ferris, S. (2005). Detailed assessment of activities of daily living in moderate to severe Alzheimer's disease. *Journal of the International Neuropsychological Society, 11*, 446–453.

Pedrosa, H., De Sa, A., Guerreiro, M., Maroco, J., Simoes, M. R., Galasko, D., & de Mendonca, A. (2010). Functional evaluation distinguishes MCI patients from healthy elderly people – The ADCS/MCI/ADL scale. *The Journal of Nutrition, Health & Aging, 14*, 703–709.

Perneczky, R., Pohl, C., Sorg, C., Hartmann, J., Komossa, K., Alexopoulos, P., et al. (2006). Complex activities of daily living in mild cognitive impairment: Conceptual and diagnostic issues. *Age and Ageing, 35*, 240–245.

Ambidexterity

John E. Mendoza
Department of Psychiatry and Neuroscience, Tulane Medical School and SE Louisiana Veterans Healthcare System, New Orleans, LA, USA

Definition

Ambidexterity is the tendency for one to be more or less equally proficient in carrying out complex or skilled motor tasks with either the right or the left hand. While complete ambidexterity is relatively rare, mixed proficiencies or preferences are not uncommon, with men more frequently demonstrating such mixed preferences than women. Tan (1988) found that approximately 66% of the population was noted to express a strong right-handed preference, while a little more than 3%

were predominately left handed. The remaining 30% evidenced mixed hand preferences. As noted elsewhere in this volume, handedness is a common, but not the only measure of what is referred to as "cerebral dominance." Another of the more frequent indices of dominance is language, which is typically organized primarily in the left hemisphere. While in the majority of non-brain-injured individuals, the control of both complex motor skills and language functions rest within the left hemisphere, this may not always be the case, particularly for those who are either left handed or ambidextrous. It has been shown that while right hemisphere dominance for language is quite rare in right-handers, it could approach 30% in strong left-handers. Individuals who are ambidextrous or whose parents are left handed tend to fall somewhere in between these two groups with regard to the hemispheric localization of language. Furthermore, the localization of language may not be an all-or-none phenomena. While one hemisphere may be more predominant, language functions may be mediated to some extent by both hemispheres. Individuals with mixed or anomalous dominance, including those who were ambidextrous, tend to have a greater incidence of at least some degree of bilateral representation of language. In the event of unilateral strokes, such individuals may evidence less severe residual aphasic deficits when compared to patients with strongly lateralized language when that hemisphere is affected.

Cross-References

▶ Anomalous Dominance
▶ Dominance (Cerebral)

References and Readings

Benson, D. F., & Geschwind, N. (1985). Aphasia and related disorders: A clinical approach. In M. Mesulam (Ed.), *Principles of behavioral neurology* (pp. 193–238). Philadelphia: F.A. Davis Co..
Knecht, S., Drager, B., Deppe, M., Bode, L., Lohmann, H., Floel, A., et al. (2000). Handedness and hemispheric language dominance in healthy humans. *Brain, 123*, 2512–2518.
Pieniadz, J. M., Naeser, M. A., Koff, E., & Levine, H. L. (1983). CT scan hemispheric asymmetry measurements in stroke cases with global aphasia: Atypical asymmetries associated with improved recovery. *Cortex, 19*, 371–391.
Pujol, J., Deus, J., Losilla, J. M., & Capdevila, A. (1999). Cerebral lateralization of language in normal left-handed people studied by functional MRI. *Neurology, 52*, 1038–1043.
Tan, Ü. (1988). The distribution of hand preference in normal men and women. *International Journal of Neuroscience, 41*, 35–55.

American Academy of Clinical Neuropsychology (AACN)

Rebecca McCartney
Department of Behavioral Health,
Kaiser Permenante, Atlanta, GA, USA

Membership

American Academy of Clinical Neuropsychology (AACN) is an organization for psychologists who have achieved board certification in the specialty of clinical neuropsychology, under the American Board of Clinical Neuropsychology (ABCN). Membership in the Academy consists of three classes: active, senior, and affiliate. Active members are elected from among psychologists who have been certified in clinical neuropsychology by the ABCN in affiliation with the American Board of Professional Psychology (ABPP). Senior members are elected from among active members who have been academy members, for a period of no less than the five preceding years, are age 65 or older or disabled, and are fully retired from the active practice of clinical neuropsychology. They continue to be listed in the membership directory of the academy, and they continue to receive any newsletters distributed to academy members. Senior members have no financial obligations to the academy and are allowed to continue to subscribe to any journal available through the academy. At the time of this publication, there were 1045 members listed in the online directory.

Affiliate members are elected from among all others who are intellectually interested in the purposes of the academy and wish to participate in its nonvoting activities. All members are provided with a subscription to *The Clinical Neuropsychologist*, access to the AACN Clinical Discussion Email List, and discounted fees to meetings and workshops.

Presidents of the Academy include Byron P. Rourke, (1995–1996), Wilfred van Gorp (1996–2002), Catherine A. Mateer (2002–2004), Robert L. Mapou (2004–2006), Jerry J. Sweet (2006–2008), Gregory J. Lamberty (2008–2010), Michael A. McCrea (2010–2012), Aaron Nelson (2012–2014), E. Mark Mahone, (2014–2016), and Karen Postal (2016–2018).

Major Areas or Mission Statement

AACN's stated mission is to advance the profession of clinical neuropsychology through its advocacy of outstanding educational and public policy initiatives. The academy holds the following objectives:

1. To promote board certification by the ABCN as the standard for competence in the practice of clinical neuropsychology
2. Support for those principles, policies, and practices that seek the attainment of the best in clinical neuropsychological patient care
3. The pursuit of excellence in psychological education, especially as it concerns the clinical neuropsychological sciences
4. The pursuit of high standards in the practice of clinical neuropsychology and support of the credentialing activities of the ABCN
5. Support for the quest of scientific knowledge by support for research in neuropsychology and related fields
6. The communication of scientific and scholarly information through continuing education, scientific meetings, and publications
7. Provision for communication with other groups and representation for clinical neuropsychological opinion to best achieve and preserve the purposes of the academy

Landmark Contributions

AACN was founded in 1996. The first appointed president was Byron Rouke, Ph.D., and the first elected president was Wilfred Van Gorp, Ph.D. AACN cosponsored the Houston Conference on Specialty Education and Training in Clinical Neuropsychology in 1997. This conference was a national consensus conference of neuropsychological organizations held with the purpose of establishing training guidelines for clinical neuropsychology. The Houston Conference guidelines have since become the model for most programs offering formal training in clinical neuropsychology. AACN held its first annual conference in 2003. During that same year, *The Clinical Neuropsychologist* became AACN's official journal. In 2007, AACN began online continuing education (CE) programs. In 2009, the American Academy of Clinical Neuropsychology Foundation (AACNF) was established to help fund outcome-oriented research for neuropsychological services. The first AACNF outcome grant was awarded in 2011. During that same year, *Child Neuropsychology* became the official journal of AACN's Pediatric Special Interest Group.

Major Activities

AACN hosts one conference each year. This conference is open to both members and nonmembers. The official journal published by AACN is *The Clinical Neuropsychologist.*

Cross-References

▶ American Board of Clinical Neuropsychology (ABCN)
▶ International Neuropsychological Society
▶ National Academy of Neuropsychology (NAN)

References and Readings

Boake, C. (2008). Clinical neuropsychology. *Professional Psychology: Research and Practice, 39*(2), 234–239.
Boake, C., & Bieliauskas, L. A. (2007). Development of clinical neuropsychology as a psychological specialty: A timeline of major events. *The ABPP Specialist, 26*, 42–43.

Lucas, J. A., Mahone, E. M., Westerveld, M., Bieliauskas, L., & Baron, I. S. (2014). The American Board of Clinical Neuropsychology and American Academy of Clinical Neuropsychology: Updated milestones 2005–2014. *The Clinical Neuropsychologist, 28*(6), 889–906.

Yeates, K. O., & Bieliauskas, L. A. (2004). The American Board of Clinical Neuropsychology and American Academy of Clinical Neuropsychology: Milestones past and present. *The Clinical Neuropsychologist, 18*, 489–493.

American Academy of Neurology (AAN)

Catherine M. Rydell[1] and Michelle Uher[2]
[1]American Academy of Neurology, Minneapolis, MN, USA
[2]Marketing Communications, American Academy of Neurology, Minneapolis, MN, USA

Address (and URL)

American Academy of Neurology

201 Chicago Avenue
Minneapolis, Minnesota 55415
www.aan.com
(800) 879–1960 (US)
(612) 928–6000 (International)
(612) 454–2746 (fax)

Membership

The American Academy of Neurology (AAN) is the world's largest professional association of neurologists and the leading online resource for neurologists across the world.

Founded in 1948, the AAN now represents 33,000 members and is dedicated to promoting the highest quality patient-centered care and enhancing member career satisfaction.

Major Areas or Mission Statement

The vision of the AAN is to be indispensable to its members by providing guidance and inspiration through education, information, policy development, and advocacy for our members and their patients while maintaining the highest ethical and professional standards.

The mission of the AAN is to promote the highest-quality patient-centered neurologic care and enhance member career satisfaction.

Landmark Contributions

The AAN was founded in 1948 by A. B. Baker, M. D., chair of the neurology department of the University of Minnesota, in response to the difficulties of one of his residents, Joseph Resch, M.D., in finding a society that he could join to continue his education and network with fellow neurologists. Baker was aided by Adolph L. Sahs, M.D., of the University of Iowa; Francis M. Forster, of Jefferson Medical Hospital in Philadelphia; and Russell DeJong, M.D., of the University of Michigan. Baker served as the first academy president, and Forster and Sahs later had terms as president. DeJong was the founding editor in chief of the journal *Neurology*®, which began publication in 1951.

The AAN had 52 founding members. The establishment of the academy, coupled with the increased need for neurologists due to World War II, helped elevate the status of neurology as a practice distinct from psychiatry. In 1947, there were between 300 and 325 physicians in the USA who designated themselves as primary neurologists, and there were 32 residency positions available nationwide. By 1970, there were 2,727 primary neurologists and some 700 residents in training. By the end of 2007, there were more than 16,000 neurologists in the USA. In 2016, the AAN has over 33,000 members worldwide.

Major Activities

Physician Education and Lifelong Learning
The AAN Annual Meeting is one of the largest gatherings of neurology professionals in the world. Held each spring, the event attracts over 14,000 clinicians, academicians, researchers, exhibitors, and media representatives to share

the latest in neurology science and education. The AAN also offers members a yearly 3-day regional Educational Fall Conference, The Sports Concussion Conference in the summer and a Breakthroughs in Neurology science conference in the winter. Education activities and programs are structured to support the ongoing development of neurology professionals from medical students to accomplished clinicians and scientists.

Science and Research

The annual meeting is a leading forum for sharing the latest developments in science and research, as is the weekly peer-reviewed *Neurology*® journal along with its spoke journals *Neurology*® *Neuroinflammation & Neuroimmunology* and *Neurology*® *Genetics*. AAN scientific awards, presented at the annual meeting, honor outstanding achievements in neurology, from aspiring medical students to veteran researchers. The American Academy of Neurology Institute provides support to young researchers through clinical research training fellowships, enabling them to pursue research initiatives and helping them to secure academic appointments and future fundings.

Clinical Practice

The AAN develops evidence-based clinical practice guidelines to assist its members in clinical decision making related to the prevention, diagnosis, treatment, and prognosis of neurologic disorders. Each guideline makes specific practice recommendations based upon a rigorous and comprehensive evaluation of all available scientific data. The AAN develops position statements on a variety of ethical issues to help guide neurologists and others in decision making. Members also rely on the AAN for the latest information on coding, reimbursement, quality initiatives, patient safety, and practice management issues.

Advocacy

To help foster changes in health care that will benefit patients and enhance the practice of neurology, the AAN presents advocacy training opportunities for members through the Donald M. Palatucci Advocacy Leadership Forum. Members also participate in the annual Neurology on the Hill visits to the Capitol in Washington, DC. The Brain PAC political action committee also is instrumental in representing neurology's interests on the federal level and supporting federal legislators who support the profession and patients with neurologic disorders.

Publishing

The AAN has several highly successful publications published by Lippincott Williams and Wilkins.

- The weekly scientific journal *Neurology*® is the most widely read peer-reviewed neurology journal in North America.
- *Neurology*® *Clinical Practice*, published bimonthly, is the first "spoke" journal in the *Neurology* family of publications.
- *Neurology*® *Neuroinflammation & Neuroimmunology* is the first open-access online journal in the *Neurology* portfolio of publications.
- *Neurology*® *Genetics*, launched in 2015, is the academy's latest open-access online journal.
- *Neurology Today*®, published biweekly, leads all other neurology tabloids in readership.
- *Neurology Now*®, a bimonthly patient-oriented magazine available to patients and caregivers currently, has a readership of 1.6 million.
- *Continuum: Lifelong Learning in Neurology*®, the AAN's bimonthly continuing education monograph, is recognized by the American Board of Psychiatry and Neurology as a key tool for maintenance of certification.
- The AAN also publishes the monthly member magazine *AANnews*®, which focuses on AAN activities, events, and services; a book series for patient and their families on treating and living with neurologic disorders; and textbooks geared toward professionals.

Cross-References

▶ Neuropsychiatry

References and Readings

Visit the AAN at American Academy of Neurology (AAN)

American Board of Clinical Neuropsychology (ABCN)

John A. Lucas[1] and Michael Westerveld[2]
[1]Department of Psychiatry and Psychology, Mayo Clinic, Jacksonville, FL, USA
[2]Medical Psychology Associates, Florida Hospital, Orlando, FL, USA

Address (and URL)

The American Board of Clinical Neuropsychology (ABCN) is the specialty board of the American Board of Professional Psychology (ABPP) that is responsible for the development and administration of examinations of competence for independent practice of Clinical Neuropsychology. Information about ABCN can found at the following websites:

American Board of Clinical Neuropsychology
 (www.theabcn.org)
American Board of Professional Psychology
 (www.abpp.org)
American Academy of Clinical Neuropsychology
 (www.theaacn.org)

Mail correspondence can be directed to ABCN at the following street address:
 Department of Psychiatry (F6248, MCHC-6)
 University of Michigan Health System
 1500 East Medical Center Drive, SPC 5295
 Ann Arbor, MI 48109-5295

Membership

As of June 2017, ABCN/ABPP has awarded specialty certification in clinical neuropsychology to 1201 specialists practicing across the United States and Canada. Of these, 91 have been awarded subspecialty certification in the practice of pediatric clinical neuropsychology. Neuropsychologists certified through ABCN demonstrate their scientific knowledge and clinical expertise through a staged examination process that includes (1) review of training credentials, (2) written examination, (3) review of case materials from the candidate's clinical practice, and (4) oral examination.

Candidates who pass all stages of the ABCN examination process are awarded specialty certification in clinical neuropsychology and are eligible for membership in the American Academy of Clinical Neuropsychology (AACN). All board-certified specialists in good standing may vote in elections for the ABCN Board of Directors (BOD), which is comprised of 15 members each elected to 5-year terms. Officers of the ABCN BOD include the president, vice president, secretary, treasurer, the ABCN representative to the ABPP board of trustees, and other agents as may be directed by the board.

Neuropsychologists who possess subspecialty education, training, and clinical expertise in pediatric clinical neuropsychology may pursue subspecialty certification after passing all stages of the ABCN specialty examination process. Subspecialty candidates must resubmit credentials for review of education and training specific to the science and practice of pediatric neuropsychology. Once subspecialty credentials are approved, candidates may take a subspecialty written examination and, when passed, may submit a case sample from their pediatric neuropsychology practice for peer review.

Mission Statement

The mission of ABCN is to (1) develop and conduct examinations to determine the qualifications of individuals who apply for board certifications, (2) award certification in clinical neuropsychology and its subspecialties to candidates who pass all stages of the examination process, and (3) evaluate compliance of certified specialists with maintenance of certification requirements.

Landmark Contributions

Origins of ABCN. In June 1981, a joint task force of the International Neuropsychological Society and Division 40 of the American Psychological Association met to discuss education, credentialing, and accreditation in the specialty of clinical neuropsychology. The task force concluded that training as a neuropsychologist was poorly standardized and that many professionals claimed expertise in clinical neuropsychology without proper training or skill sets. During the meeting, several members of the task force discussed the need to develop a formal credentialing process to assist the public in identifying professionals capable of providing competent neuropsychological services (Report of the Division 40/INS Joint Task Force on Education, Accreditation, and Credentialing 1984; Reports of the INS – Division 40 Task Force on Education, Accreditation, and Credentialing 1987). A small planning group was subsequently formed to create a peer-review mechanism for this purpose, and in August 1981, the American Board of Clinical Neuropsychology was incorporated in the state of Minnesota as an independent credentialing body.

The ABCN planning group included Linas Bieliauskas, Louis Costa, Edith Kaplan, Muriel Lezak, Charles Matthews, Steven Mattis, Manfred Meier, and Paul Satz, who together developed a three-stage board certification process. At its inception, the ABCN examination process included (1) review of training credentials, (2) submission of case materials reflecting the candidate's practice of clinical neuropsychology, and (3) an oral examination of, but not limited to, clinical and scientific knowledge, assessment practices, and ethical/legal issues. Prominent neuropsychologists of national reputation were chosen by consensus of the planning group to serve as the first board of directors of ABCN. The inaugural board examined each other and, in 1983, conducted the first formal set of board examinations in clinical neuropsychology. Following the first formal exams, ABCN affiliated with ABPP, the unifying governing body for specialty examining boards in psychology. The first official ABPP/ABCN certifications in the specialty of clinical neuropsychology were awarded in 1984. Twenty years later, in 2004, ABCN awarded its 500th certification (Yeates and Bieliauskas 2004), demonstrating continued interest among clinical neuropsychologists in the peer-review process. In 2014, ABCN awarded board certification to its 1000th specialist, doubling the previous milestone in half the time (Lucas et al. 2014).

Enhancements to the Board Certification Process. Bieliauskas and Matthews provided detailed facts and data regarding the development and enhancement of ABCN policies and procedures in updates published in 1987, 1990, and 1996 (Bieliauskas and Matthews 1990, 1997, 1987). In 1997, representatives from each professional neuropsychology organization were invited to meet in Houston to review current training models and propose universal standards for education and training in the specialty. The proceedings and consensus statement of the Hou*ston Conference on Specialty Education and Training in Clinical Neuropsychology* were published the following year (Hannay et al. 1998). Although largely aspirational at the time of publication, by 2002 the ABCN Board determined that a sufficient number of neuropsychology training programs had successfully incorporated the Houston Conference (HC) model and voted to include HC training and education guidelines as criteria for passing credential review. In recognition of earlier training models and to allow enough time for transition, the board allowed that only those applicants earning their doctoral degree on or after January 1, 2005, would be held to HC criteria. Others continued to be held to the eligibility criteria that were in place at the time they earned their doctoral degree (or completed respecialization in clinical neuropsychology). A survey conducted in 2012 by Sweet and colleagues (2012) indicated that HC guidelines have become widely adopted by training programs in clinical neuropsychology and that professionals who complete training in HC-adherent programs report being well prepared to engage independently in key professional activities.

In 1988, ABCN partnered with Psychological Examination Services to develop a 100-item written examination whereby candidates could objectively demonstrate the scientific knowledge acquired during their training and years of practice. The written examination was implemented in 1993 as the second stage of the certification process and must be passed before a candidate may submit practice samples. The content and psychometric properties of the written examination are reviewed and updated on an ongoing basis. In 2012 ABCN transitioned the written examination from a paper-and-pencil test administered at national meetings to a computer-based test administered on an electronic platform during 2-week examination windows, four times per year. Candidates who are eligible to sit for the written examination may do so locally at any of nearly 300 PSI testing sites across the United States and Canada. In 2015 a set of 25 beta-test items were added to the core 100 test items to provide psychometric data for informed item selection of subsequent versions of the exam. Only the 100 core test items contribute to candidate's final exam score. In late 2015, the ABCN Board of Directors contracted with Alpine Testing Solutions, Inc. to develop and implement the next revision of the written exam.

ABCN partnered with Thomson-Reuters in 2012 to create an electronic portal in the ScholarOne online manuscript management system to allow candidates to upload electronic copies of their practice sample case materials rather than mailing paper copies, as had been the prior practice. Additionally, the ABCN Practice Sample Committee engaged in a multifaceted approach to enhance both the standardization and turnaround time of reviews. The committee recruited a cohort of dedicated specialists and provided standardized guidelines and training for practice sample reviews, thus allowing candidates to move more efficiently through the board certification pipeline.

Subspecialty Certification. In 2006, the ABPP Board of Trustees requested that ABCN form a work group to consider issues regarding the emerging interest of subspecialty practices within psychological specialties (Baron et al. 2011). After careful deliberation, the work group proposed a model whereby subspecialties reflect the normal evolution of psychological specialty practice, emerging naturally as the core knowledge base of a specialty grows and begins to be applied or tailored to unique populations, settings, or methods. The work group proposed that

subspecialty development begins with the aggregation of board-certified specialists into a "special interest group" (SIG) representing shared expertise and interests in a component of the specialty. This model was endorsed by the ABPP BOT in December 2008 and incorporated into the formal policies and procedures of the ABPP Affiliations and Standards Committee.

In 2009, a group of pediatric clinical neuropsychologists formed the first official SIG within ABPP. The pediatric SIG (P-SIG) met over subsequent years to vet the interest, feasibility, and viability of developing a subspecialty of pediatric clinical neuropsychology within ABCN. Simultaneously, the ABCN BOD tasked its committee on subspecialization to consider and recommend a model of requirements and procedures by which specialists might attain certification in a subspecialty area of neuropsychology practice. The committee reasoned that subspecialty candidates have already demonstrated competencies required for neuropsychology practice by virtue of their board certification through ABCN. Thus, certification in a subspecialty of clinical neuropsychology should require only (1) clear demonstration of subspecialty-specific education, training, and practice requirements as determined by the ABCN Board in consultation with the subspecialty SIG, (2) a written examination of subspecialty knowledge and clinical application, and (3) demonstration of competent, evidence-based clinical practice in the subspecialty as determined by review of a single representative assessment case. In October 2013 ABCN submitted this proposal to ABPP and in December 2013 pediatric clinical neuropsychology was approved as the first official subspecialty within ABPP. In January 2014, all ABCN specialists with expertise in pediatric clinical neuropsychology were invited to submit applications for subspecialty credential review. Those who demonstrated the required education and training were subsequently invited to sit for a calibration administration of an objective written examination. The data from the calibration examination was used to create two parallel 30-item subspecialty written examinations which were fielded in June 2015. The subspecialty written examination is currently

A

administered once per year. As of June 2017, 91 ABCN specialists had passed the practice sample peer-review stage and successfully earned ABPP/ABCN subspecialty certification in pediatric clinical neuropsychology.

Maintenance of Certification. ABCN has always recognized that competence in any field of medical practice is dynamic and that specialists must continuously maintain and update their competencies through ongoing professional education and engagement. In 2010, the ABCN Board endorsed a plan proposed by ABPP to require specialists to formally document the ways in which they maintain the competencies required of ongoing specialty practice. In 2013, ABCN created a maintenance of certification (MOC) committee to develop and implement procedures, materials, and criteria to allow neuropsychology specialists and subspecialists the formal means of demonstrating MOC. This process adapts the core requirements expected across all ABPP specialties in a way that is relevant to the functional competencies specific to ABCN. The MOC policy and procedures developed by ABCN were approved by the ABPP Standards Committee in 2014 and implemented on January 1, 2015.

The American Academy of Clinical Neuropsychology (AACN). ABCN expanded its mission from being a board certification body to being a membership organization of board-certified specialists in 1983. The reason for this transition was to collect dues to fund the development of the written examination. In 1996, ABPP legal counsel advised examining boards against having a dual role of being both a certifying body and membership organization. In response, the ABCN BOD voted to incorporate its membership organization as a separate academy, with an independent board of directors and separate mission statement. The AACN took on the important task of promoting board certification, advocating for standards of training and education in clinical neuropsychology, and disseminating information about the field of neuropsychology to the general public, forensic settings, schools, healthcare professionals, and clinical training programs. The AACN provides mentorship and study support for candidates seeking board certification through ABCN (Armstrong et al. 2008).

Although AACN began as an organization restricted only to board-certified neuropsychology specialists, membership opportunities at this time also extend to students, individuals who are in the midst of the board certification process, and non-neuropsychology professionals (Table 1).

Major Activities

As noted above, ABCN focuses its primary activities on developing, maintaining, reviewing, revising, and implementing the board certification examinations in clinical neuropsychology and its subspecialties. As of 2015, ABCN also conducts reviews of documentation from specialists who wish to demonstrate maintenance of certification.

The ABCN Specialty Certification Examination. A comprehensive overview of the ABCN examination process was published in 2008 (Armstrong et al. 2008) and can also be found within the Candidate's Manual on the ABCN website (www.theabcn.org). Briefly, the specialty examination process consists of four distinct and sequential steps. First, the education and training experiences of the applicant are reviewed by ABPP for appropriate graduate training, internship, and licensure status in psychology. Applications that pass the ABPP general review are then forwarded to ABCN for review of advanced specialty credentials. Applicants who completed their doctoral training on or after January 1, 2005, must demonstrate training consistent with the *Houston Conference on Specialty Education and Training in Clinical Neuropsychology*, including required coursework and completion of a formal 2-year postdoctoral residency program in clinical neuropsychology. Policies and exceptions regarding candidates who received their training before implementation of the Houston Conference criteria respecialized in neuropsychology after obtaining a doctoral degree in another specialty or received training in Canada are detailed on the ABCN website (www.theabcn.org).

Once an applicant's credentials are approved, they may sit for the written examination. The exam consists of 125 multiple-choice questions that cover a range of topics in neuropsychology.

Only 100 items contribute to the candidate's final score. The other 25 items are included to gather psychometric data to determine the item's suitability as a future exam question. The written examination tests the candidate's breadth of knowledge and assures that they have the scientific foundation necessary for competent practice in clinical neuropsychology. Since 2012, the written examination has been administered electronically. It is currently offered in 2-week windows, four times per year through PSI testing centers across the United States and Canada.

Candidates who pass the written examination may submit a practice sample consisting of two typical cases from their neuropsychology practice. The practice samples are peer-reviewed by at least three independent, board-certified neuropsychologists. Reviewers follow a standardized rubric to determine whether the candidate's clinical practices, conclusions, and recommendations as demonstrated in the sample would be defensible upon oral examination.

If the practice sample is approved by at least two reviewers, the candidate is invited to participate in an oral examination of their specialty competencies. The oral examination consists of three 1-h exercises that cover (1) defense of the practice sample, (2) fact-finding, and (3) ethics and professional development. During the practice sample exercise, the candidate is given opportunities to discuss their clinical practice as applied to the specific cases they submitted. The cases also serve as a starting point leading to more in-depth discussion and evaluation of competencies such as assessment, intervention, consultation, and scientific knowledge. The fact-finding exercise presents a brief description of a case that is new to the candidate. The candidate must then gather appropriate information from the clinical history, test data, and medical record to generate an appropriate case conceptualization and differential diagnosis. The ethics and professional development exercise allows candidates to demonstrate knowledge of important ethical considerations as presented in a brief vignette. Candidates are evaluated not only on their ability to identify the ethical issues in the vignette but also on their

ability to demonstrate understanding of why the issues are problematic. During this portion of the exercise, candidates are also invited to discuss their own contributions to research, teaching, practice administration, patient advocacy, or other activities that contribute to their professional development. Currently, oral examinations are conducted twice annually in Chicago, Illinois, hosted by the Neuropsychiatric Institute of the University of Illinois at Chicago.

The ABCN Subspecialty Examination in Pediatric Clinical Neuropsychology. ABCN specialists who wish to become certified in the subspecialty of pediatric clinical neuropsychology may submit their credentials for review. Applicants who have been engaged in an active pediatric neuropsychology practice within the 2 years prior to submission of their application and document a minimum of 4000 h of postdoctoral experience within pediatric neuropsychology meet criteria to pass subspecialty credential review. Applicants who completed doctoral training or respecialization in clinical neuropsychology on or after January 1, 2005, must meet the additional requirement that at least 1000 of their 4000 h of postdoctoral clinical practice was obtained under the direct supervision of a pediatric neuropsychologist. Two letters of reference must verify that the above criteria were met. Candidates who pass the credential review process may take the 30-item subspecialty written examination containing questions related to neurodevelopment, functional neuroanatomy, pediatric clinical syndromes, specialized neuropsychological assessment techniques, developmental psychology, and the ethical and legal issues of pediatric neuropsychological practice. Candidates who pass the written examination may submit a single pediatric neuropsychological case evaluation of a patient age 16 or under that clearly demonstrates independent practice at the subspecialist level of competence. The subspecialty review process differs in important ways from that of the ABCN specialty review process because the specialty review is intended to determine whether a candidate's practice would be defensible at oral examination. In contrast, the subspecialty review process must determine if the

A

American Board of Clinical Neuropsychology (ABCN), Table 1 Timeline for major ABCN milestones

1981	ABCN incorporated in Minnesota
1983	Inaugural ABCN examinations completed and formal affiliation between ABCN and ABPP established
1984	First ABPP/ABCN certifications awarded
1988	Bylaws revised to create membership organization of board-certified neuropsychologists
1988	ABCN partners with professional examinations services to develop a specialty written examination
1993	Written examination implemented as the second stage of ABCN certification process
1996	The American Academy of Clinical Neuropsychology (AACN) becomes independently incorporated as the membership organization of ABCN specialists
2002	ABCN endorses the *Houston Conference on Specialty Education and Training in Clinical Neuropsychology*
2004	500th ABCN certification awarded
2005	Houston Conference guidelines implemented as criteria for ABCN credential review process
2006	ABCN Committee on Innovations and Technology established to transition examination components to electronic platforms
2007	Committee on subspecialization formed
2008	ABCN introduces fast-track credential review for applicants completing postdoctoral training in APPCN member programs and APA-accredited specialty training programs
2009	First meeting of the ABCN Pediatric Special Interest Group (P-SIG)
2010	ABCN endorses the ABPP model for maintenance of certification
2011	P-SIG activities transfer from ABCN to AACN
2012	Written examination transitions to computer-based administration through Prometric
2012	Online ScholarOne portal implemented for electronic submission of practice sample materials
2013	Oral examinations move from Rush Presbyterian Hospital to University of Illinois, Chicago, Neuropsychiatric Institute to accommodate growth of exams
2013	ABPP Board of Trustees approves ABCN subspecialty in pediatric clinical neuropsychology
2014	ABPP Standards Committee approves ABCN MOC procedures
2014	Specialty written examination expands from 100 to 125 items
2014	Implementation of the ABCN Practice Sample review cadre
2014	ABCN awards 1000th board certification.
2015	Credential reviews for the pediatric clinical neuropsychology subspecialty commence
2015	Written examination for the pediatric clinical neuropsychology subspecialty developed and implemented
2015	ABCN contracts with Alpine Testing Solutions and PSI Exams Online to manage and administer the specialty written examination.
2016	Implementation of maintenance of certification policies

case sample *on its own* sufficiently demonstrates competent practice in the subspecialty.

Maintenance of Certification. Maintenance of certification (MOC) is a process of self-examination of a specialist's professional development since his or her initial board certification or last MOC review. The ABPP MOC model asserts that competence for independent specialty practice is established at the time of initial board certification and can be continuously maintained thereafter through lifelong learning, ongoing participation in professional activities, and self-evaluation related to core competencies. In accordance with ABPP policy, MOC is required of all ABCN specialists awarded with board certification on or after January 1, 2015. Specialists who completed board certification prior to that date may "opt in" to the process but are not required by ABPP to do so.

In the course of self-examination, specialists survey their professional activities during the 2 years prior to MOC submission and report/describe the means by which those activities served to maintain the ABCN-defined competencies required for independent practice in clinical neuropsychology. Five broad categories of professional activities support the maintenance of specialty competencies. These include (1) collaborative clinical consultation; (2) teaching and training; (3) ongoing education; (4) research, methodologies, and programs; and (5) professional leadership. Numerous activities fall within each of these categories and specialists must indicate how the activities in which they engaged served to support the competencies defined by ABPP and ABCN as essential to neuropsychological practice. Those with subspecialty certification must further ensure that MOC activities support competencies required for subspecialty practice.

Beyond engagement in professional activities, all ABCN specialists must also demonstrate appropriate self-evaluation by describing their practice, approaches to ethical or diversity issues, and the means by which they evaluate their clinical efficacy (e.g., ongoing peer review, performance evaluations, patient satisfaction data, etc.). Members of the ABCN MOC Committee review all submissions against established ABCN standards to determine if criteria for passing MOC review have been met.

Conclusion

With over 1200 certifications in clinical neuropsychology now awarded, ABCN specialists can be found across a multitude of practice settings, geographic locations, advocacy efforts, training programs, and research endeavors involving pediatric, adult, and older adult populations. Board certification through ABCN reflects validation of competence by one's peers and assures the public that the neuropsychologist has successfully completed the education, training, and experience requirements of the specialty, including examinations designed to assess the competencies required to provide quality services in clinical neuropsychology.

References and Readings

Armstrong, K., Beebe, D. W., Hilsabeck, R. C., & Kirkwood, M. W. (2008). *Board certification in clinical neuropsychology: A guide to becoming ABPP/ABCN certified without sacrificing your sanity.* New York: Oxford Press.
Baron, I. S., Wills, K., Rey-Casserly, C., Armstrong, K., & Westerveld, M. (2011). Pediatric neuropsychology:

Toward subspecialty designation. *The Clinical Neuropsychologist, 25,* 1075–1086. https://doi.org/10.1080/13854046.2011.594455.
Bieliauskas, L. A., & Matthews, C. G. (1987). American Board of Clinical Neuropsychology: Policies and procedures. *The Clinical Neuropsychologist, 1,* 21–28.
Bieliauskas, L. A., & Matthews, C. G. (1990). American Board of Clinical Neuropsychology update, 1990. *The Clinical Neuropsychologist, 4,* 337–343.
Bieliauskas, L. A., & Matthews, C. G. (1997). The American Board of Clinical Neuropsychology, 1996 update: Facts, data, and information for potential candidates. *The Clinical Neuropsychologist, 11,* 222–225.
Hannay, H. J., Bieliauskas, L., Crosson, B. A., Hammeke, T. A., Hamsher K de, S., & Koffler, S. (1998). Proceedings of the Houston Conference on specialty education and training in clinical neuorpsychology. *Archives of Clinical Neuropsychology, 13,* 157–250.
Lucas, J. A., Mahone, M., Westerveld, M., Bieliauskas, L., & Baron, I. S. (2014). The American Board of Clinical Neuropsychology and American Academy of Clinical Neuropsychology: Updated milestones 2005–2014. *The Clinical Neuropsychologist, 28,* 889–906. https://doi.org/10.1080/13854046.2014.935484.
Report of the Division 40/INS Joint Task Force on Education, Accreditation, and Credentialing. (1984). *Division 40 Newsletter, 2*(2), 3–8.
Reports of the INS – Division 40 Task Force on Education, Accreditation, and Credentialing. (1987). *The Clinical Neuropsychologist, 1*(1), 29–34.
Sweet, J. J., Perry, W., Ruff, R. M., Shear, P. K., & Guidotti Breting, L. M. (2012). The Inter-Organizational Summit on Education and Training (ISET) 2010 survey on the influence of the Houston Conference training guidelines. *The Clinical Neuropsychologist, 26*(7), 1055–1076. https://doi.org/10.1080/13854046.2012.705565.
Yeates, K. O., & Bieliauskas, L. A. (2004). The American Board of Clinical Neuropsychology and American Academy of Clinical Neuropsychology: Milestones past and present. *The Clinical Neuropsychologist, 18,* 489–493.

American Board of Pediatric Neuropsychology

Peter Dodzik
Fort Wayne Neurological Center, Fort Wayne, IN, USA

Membership as of (January 2015)

The American Board of Pediatric Neuropsychology (ABPdN) was developed in 1996 by a coalition of clinical practitioners representing institutions hiring pediatric neuropsychologists. The original group conceived the board to advance their belief that a unique interplay exists between neurodevelopmental issues and neuropsychological assessment that requires special sets of expertise not readily assessed by then existing boarding entities. Following discussion with colleagues who were members of medical practice and psychology boards, the coalition elected to establish an independent certifying authority. The examination process evolved into a comprehensive and multi-level process that includes a written application including clinical case vignettes used to determine decision-making strategies of the applicant, scope of practice and a thorough assessment of organized training in pediatric neuropsychology (from graduate school to continuing education), written examination, a practice sample submission, and an oral examination. The ABPdN does not have a "grand fathering" policy and thus all existing board members were required to complete all new phases of the examination process to ensure equality of standards among boarded members.

As of early 2015, one hundred and eighty seven (187) neuropsychologists have submitted applications to ABPdN, and one hundred and thirty (130) members have passed the ABPdN examination process. At present, there are ninety-three (93) active and five (5) emeritus members of the board from 28 states, Canada, and Puerto Rico.

Major Areas or Mission Statement

Board certification in pediatric neuropsychology serves to assist consumers by offering supportive evidence of the competence of the pediatric neuropsychologists. The ABPdN is the only board certification organization with the sole purpose of examining and certifying competence in pediatric neuropsychology.

Landmark Contributions

Members of ABPdN practice in a variety of settings include universities, teaching hospitals, general hospitals, hospital trauma centers, private practices, rehabilitation facilities, stroke centers, memory disorders centers, group practices, and child development centers. Current members hold academic affiliations at over 40 colleges and universities including Ivy League institutions and several university medical centers. Publications from members of ABPdN include over 5000 edited books, book chapters, and scholarly articles. Several members have developed tests commonly used in the practice of pediatric and general neuropsychology. Member accomplishments include:

Professional Contributions

- Two past presidents of APA Division 40
- Past president of APA Division 2, 5 and 16
- Current and past presidents of eight state psychology boards
- Three past presidents of the National Academy of Neuropsychology
- Two past editors of *Archives of Clinical Neuropsychology*
- Current editor of *Archives of Clinical Neuropsychology*
- Current editor, *Psychological Assessment*
- Current editor, *Journal of Attention Disorders*
- Current editor, *Journal of Pediatric Neuropsychology*
- Past editor, *Journal of School Psychology*
- Past editor, *Applied Neuropsychology*
- Eight prescribing psychologists

Major Activities

The American Board of Pediatric Neuropsychology is the board-certifying arm of the American Academy of Pediatric Neuropsychology (AAPN), which is devoted to training and promotion of the field of pediatric neuropsychology. The AAPN holds an annual conference each spring with topics related to the field of pediatric neuropsychology.

The primary activity of ABPdN is conduct of the Board certification process. Board examination through the ABPdN involves several stages. The format of the ABPdN's examination processes has been constant since the examinations held in 2004, but the procedures continue to be reviewed and amended. The purpose of the ABPdN examination process is to ensure that the examinee has demonstrated competency to practice pediatric neuropsychology. The specific stages are discussed below and more detail can be obtained from the ABPdN Web site (Beljan et al. 2006). The overall pass rate for each stage of the examination process is between 73% and 81%.

Credential Review

Minimum training and education standards include completion of a doctoral degree from a regionally accredited program in applied psychology that was, at the time the degree was granted, accredited by the APA and CPA or was listed in the publication *Doctoral Psychology Programs Meeting Designation Criteria* (*"ASPPB National Register designation committee"*, 2008). Membership in the National Register of Health Service Providers in Psychology, the Canadian Register of Health Service Providers, or those holding the Certificate of Professional Qualification qualify as meeting the doctoral requirements for membership. Licensure or certification at the independent practice level as a psychologist in the state, province, or territory in which the psychologist actively practices is also required. The applicant must be practicing as a pediatric neuropsychologist and must have completed an APPIC or APA accredited internship that included a documented rotation or concentration in neuropsychology, and 2 years of postdoctoral supervised experience in neuropsychology, at least 50% of that being pediatric-oriented. In addition, each applicant reviewed by the Board must provide the following:

(A) Education
- (I) Undergraduate degree transcript
- (II) Graduate degree transcript
- (III) Internship verification contact information
- (IV) Postdoctoral residency verification contact information
- (V) Postdoctoral fellowship verification contact information (if applicable)
- (VI) Detailed description of training in pediatric neuropsychology (narrative)

(B) Continuing Education
- (I) Verification of CEUs in pediatric neuropsychology for past 3 years

(C) Clinical Work
- (I) Clinical appointment verification contact information
- (II) Breakdown of clinical practice by age, disorders, and ethnic background
- (III) Completion of clinical vignettes

(D) Educational Appointment (if applicable)
- (I) Academic institution verification contact information

The application is first reviewed by the examination chair for completion and accuracy of documents and licensure status. The application is then reviewed by a panel of three reviewers. A passing score by two of the three reviewers is required to move to the next stage of the examination. Each reviewer evaluates the application for consistent and thorough training in pediatric neuropsychology at multiple levels of training.

Practice Sample

The purpose of the practice sample is determined by the applicant's clinical knowledge. While the written examination was designed to assess content-specific knowledge with regard to pediatric neuropsychology, the practice sample allows the board to evaluate the day-to-day skills of the applicant. To that end, the sample should reflect a typical patient seen in the applicant's clinical practice. Practice samples may include assessment or intervention techniques. After an application is reviewed and the candidate is determined to be board-eligible, they will then be invited to provide a practice sample that reflects their typical work in pediatric neuropsychology. Prior to taking the objective and oral examination, the candidate must prepare and tender one written sample of an original pediatric neuropsychological examination performed solely by the candidate. Appropriate samples may include case analysis/interventions and supervision sessions.

Written Examination

The third step is the written exam, a 100-question, multiple-choice instrument designed and constructed by other pediatric neuropsychologists whose purpose is to assess the candidate's breadth of knowledge in pediatric neuropsychology. The questions were first assessed for face validity, clustered for content area, rank ordered, deleted or refined, reanalyzed, debated, approved, and then compiled into a larger item pool for random selection by domain each year. A passing score of 70% is required. Each exam includes the following basic core areas:

- Psychometrics
- Pediatric Neurosciences
- Psychological and Neurological Development
- Neuropsychological and Neurological Diagnostics
- Ethics and Legal Issues
- Research Design Review for Clinical Application
- Intervention Techniques
- Consultation and Supervisory Practices

Oral Examination

This part of the examination process is comprised of a review of the candidate's practice sample, the nature and application of neuropsychological knowledge to their current practice, appreciation for ethical issues and obligations, and a review of the candidate's views and philosophy on pediatric neuropsychology. The oral examination also includes a mock case review, in which the candidate is given information about a fictional case, and they develop and articulate their working hypothesis. The oral examination is intended to be a collegial opportunity for the reviewers to validate the candidate's ability to "think on their feet" and discern their preparation and readiness for board certification.

The first portion of the oral examination permits the examination team to consider the scope of the candidate's body of training and how they practice pediatric neuropsychology (e.g., acute care, rehabilitation, outpatient, assessment, and/or treatment) so that the fact-finding and practice sample review can be conducted in the most relevant fashion. This section is broken into two parts:

Part I: The examinee will explain their background.
- The examinee will provide a history of their educational and professional background. Special consideration should be given to their pediatric neuropsychological training and background.
- The examinee will explain their current role as a pediatric neuropsychologist and the issues their typical clientele present.

Part II: The examinee will demonstrate pertinent knowledge of practical pediatric neuropsychology.

Part III: Review of the practice sample.

This segment of the oral examination allows the candidate to present the material in their practice sample and to provide an overview of the history, evaluation process, and outcome of the case. The examiners evaluate their ability to articulate the major findings and their rationale. Candidates discuss their rationale in such areas as:

1. Test selection (if applicable)
   Psychometric properties, test validity/reliability, limitations for use, and exclusion of all competing diagnoses
2. Test interpretation (if applicable)
   Alternate interpretations of findings, conflict resolution within the data, discussion of strengths and weaknesses, and environmental and cultural factors
3. Diagnostic conclusions
   Alternate diagnosis, ultimate understanding of neuropathology, prognosis, progression, lateralizing/localizing effects, pathognomonic signs, causality, environmental conditions, and effects on neural development
4. Recommendations and treatment planning
   Best practices for treatment, availability, prognosis, funding, delivery options,

cost/benefit analysis, iatrogenic outcomes, parental compliance/agreement, and ethical issues

5. Consultation and supervision (if applicable)
   Best practices for communication of data, delivery options, supervisee needs/relationships, and rapport/therapeutic relationship
      This process is intended to be collegial and the examiners endeavor to be sensitive to the different and yet equally viable approaches within pediatric neuropsychology. The purpose is to ascertain the candidate's logic and thought processes and to allow them to demonstrate these skills.

Part IV: Fact finding.

The purpose of the fact finding portion of the oral examination is to provide the candidate with the opportunity to review a clinical case vignette including history, medical reports, and test data and to generate diagnoses and recommendations for treatment based on that information. The candidate is expected to use relevant information to generate hypotheses regarding the underlying pathology. Candidates will thoughtfully weigh ethical and clinical considerations in the light of the APA ethics principles, professional practice standards, and relevant statutes.

See Also

▶ American Psychological Association (APA), Division 40
▶ National Academy of Neuropsychology (NAN)

References and Readings

ASPPB National Register Designation Committee. (2008). Retrieved 1 Oct 2009 from http://www.nationalregister.org/designate_stsearch.html

Beljan, P., Bos, J., Courtney, J., & Dodzik, P. (2006). Preparation guide for examination and certification by the American board of pediatric neuropsychology. Retrieved from http://abpdn.org/docs/studyguide.pdf

American Board of Professional Neuropsychology (ABN)

John E. Meyers
Department of Neuropsychology, Comprehensive Medpsych Systems, Sarasota, FL, USA

Address (and URL)

Geoffrey Kanter, Ph.D., ABN
  Executive Director
  1090 S Tamiami Trail
  Sarasota, FL 34236
  (941) 363-0878
  http://www.abn-board.com/

Membership

The American Board of Professional Neuropsychology (ABN) is comprised of over 400 neuropsychologists who have doctoral degrees, are licensed as psychologists, and have completed the ABN diplomate examination process.

ABN was established in 1982 by a group of clinical neuropsychologists, all of whom were diplomates of the American Board of Professional Psychology (ABPP), to provide peer regulation of the practice of professional neuropsychology. The process of obtaining the ABN diplomate is a dynamic one which has changed over the years and is expected to continue to evolve as the field of neuropsychology evolves. Initially, in addition to obtaining a doctoral degree, acquiring licensure as a psychologist, and completing a number of years of postdoctoral experience in neuropsychology, early applicants were required to show evidence of specialized training in neuropsychology and to provide supervisory evaluations of their competency in clinical neuropsychology.

Between 1982 and 1985, following a review of credentials and supervisory evaluations, work samples were required. These were evaluated by multiple examiners on a pass/fail basis. Individuals who passed this final step were awarded a diplomate. Individuals who did not pass the evaluation were allowed to apply for a "Certificate in Professional Neuropsychology," indicating that they had some training in neuropsychology but not sufficient enough to be awarded diplomate status. This was initially intended as an interim credential as part of the process of obtaining a diplomate. After 1985, this process was abandoned as increasing numbers of neuropsychology training programs became available.

In February of 1989, the ABN was reorganized and the bylaws were modified. An annual dues structure was instituted and ABN became a membership organization whose only credential is a diplomate. This newly established organization mandated continuing education for active membership. It was required that all those who had a "Certificate in Professional Neuropsychology" complete the diplomate process to maintain membership. At this time, an oral examination and essay examination were added to the case study reviews, and all previous members were allowed the opportunity to undergo the expanded examination process. Those who successfully completed the process, including the new oral examination, were given full diplomate status in ABN.

After 1991, those who did not successfully complete the additional oral examination were no longer listed as diplomates through ABN. The examination process included the essay examination, and three 1 h oral examinations covering ethics, the work sample, and general knowledge. ABN no longer required letters of competency from supervisors but instead required letters of recommendation from other neuropsychologists.

In 2004, the diplomate evaluation process was again reevaluated and work began on substituting a multiple-choice general knowledge examination for the oral examination on the same subject. This process took several years to complete, and as of January 1, 2009, all applicants were required to complete the multiple-choice written examination; the essay examination was dropped in favor of the multiple-choice exam. The continuing education requirement was expanded to a

Maintenance of Certification requirement. ABN prefers an APA approved education program and internship and for those who graduated after 2005 requires a 2-year postdoctoral fellowship. ABN's application criteria are designed around the Houston Conference Guidelines for postdoctoral training in neuropsychology, though some flexibility is allowed in meeting the internship and postdoctoral requirement, and graduated training requirements are in place tied to era of graduation, to accommodate those who trained prior to 2005. In 2008, the original acronym for ABN was changed from ABPN to ABN to avoid confusion with the American Board of Psychiatry and Neurology. In January 2014 ABN created an affiliate organization the Academy of the American Board of Professional Neuropsychology (AABN), which is a postdoctoral fellowship organization.

The current examination procedure includes:

1. Review of credentials and letters of recommendation
2. A 100-question multiple-choice examination
3. Case study/work samples review
4. A 1 hour ethics oral examination and
5. A 1 hour work style oral examination

The multiple-choice written examination covers areas of general knowledge based on the recommended guidelines of the Houston Conference. The ethics examination addresses ethical situations and current ethical dilemmas, and the work style examination covers clinical vignettes and clinical decision-making.

Major Areas or Mission Statement

ABN recognizes and encourages the pursuit of excellence in the practice of clinical neuropsychology. ABN's primary objective is the establishment of professional standards of expertise for the practice of clinical neuropsychology. Through its credentialing and examination processes and its continuing education requirement, the ABN offers to the medical community, the public, and to individuals who have a need for applied neuropsychological services, a process whereby competent clinical neuropsychologists can be identified.

To achieve the standards set forth by the ABN for competent professional practice of neuropsychology, the following outcome objectives have been developed:

- Validate the skills of clinical practitioners
- Identify competent practitioners
- Provide public information about clinical neuropsychology
- Document the maintenance of competence of professional neuropsychology practitioners with continuing education requirements
- Provide individuals, organizations, and agencies who use neuropsychology services with a referral directory of ABN diplomates

Recognition by ABN signifies to the public and to other health professionals a high level of competency in applied neuropsychology. The ABN does not ascribe to any specific theoretical framework. While recognizing the importance and contribution of a graduate education in neuropsychology and subsequent specialty training, the ABN believes that the critical element in the practice of professional neuropsychology is the application of that training to client issues and needs.

Landmark Contributions

Applied Neuropsychology: Adult, a peer-reviewed edited journal, is an official journal of the ABN.

Applied Neuropsychology: Child, a peer-reviewed edited journal, is an official journal of the ABN.

The Academy of ABN (AABN) is a postdoctoral training site recognition organization. The AABN uses a standard didactic curriculum to ensure that all sites can meet the Houston Conference Training Guidelines.

ABN actively participates in national and international neuropsychological specialty initiatives and interorganizational activities supporting the development of neuropsychology.

Major Activities

ABN holds an annual board of directors meeting at the National Academy of Neuropsychology (NAN) conference. Associated with ABN is the American College of Professional Neuropsychology (ACPN) whose purpose is to provide continuing education programs in neuropsychology.

ABN holds monthly meetings of the board of directors and committee chairs to organize ABN's professional activities. ABN candidate examinations and examiner training workshops are typically held a minimum of twice a year at locations throughout the country. A workshop on the ABN examination process is held at least once a year. Individual candidate mentoring is offered throughout the year.

ACPN is approved by the American Psychological Association to sponsor continuing education for psychologists. ACPN typically holds at least one general meeting each year, covering various subjects, offering continuing education credits to attendees.

References and Readings

Bennett, T. L., Horton Jr., A. M., & Elliott, R. W. (1999). American Board of Professional Neuropsychology (ABPN). *Bulletin of the National Academy of Neuropsychology, 14*, 7–9.

Elliott, R. W., & Horton Jr., A. M. (1994). Philosophy of the American Board of Professional Neuropsychology. *Bulletin of the National Academy of Neuropsychology, 11*, 14–15.

Elliott, R. W., & Horton Jr., A. M. (1995). History and current status of the American Board of Professional Neuropsychology. *The Independent Practitioner, 15*, 175–177.

Goldstein, G. (2001). Board certification in clinical neuropsychology: Some history, facts and opinions. *Journal of Forensic Neuropsychology, 2*, 57–65.

Horton Jr., A. M., Crown, B. M., & Reynolds, C. R. (2001). American Board of Professional Neuropsychology: An update-2001. *Journal of Forensic Neuropsychology, 2*, 67–78.

http://www.abn-board.org/

American Board of Professional Psychology (ABPP)

Christine Maguth Nezu
Department of Psychology, Drexel
University–Hahnemann Campus, Philadelphia,
PA, USA

Membership

The American Board of Professional Psychology (ABPP) has over 3100 currently active board-certified specialists in membership. As a national-in-scope credentialing organization in professional psychology, its membership is comprised doctoral-level psychologists who provide professional services and consultation and are licensed to practice psychology in the jurisdiction in which they practice. Completion of a doctoral degree, completion of a qualified internship, relevant postdoctoral experience, and relevant jurisdictional licensure as a psychologist are the minimum prerequisites for approval to take an ABPP board certification exam. However, through its Early Entry Option, ABPP permits psychology graduate students, interns, and residents to begin the application process at a reduced fee, submitting credentials as they are completed until full eligibility criteria are met for the selected specialty area.

Major Areas or Mission Statement

The American Board of Professional Psychology (ABPP) is a national-in-scope credentialing organization that has been awarding board certification in professional psychology specialties for over 60 years (Bent et al. 1999; Finch et al. 2006; Packard and Reyes 2003). ABPP describes the value of its credential as one that "provides peer and public recognition of demonstrated competence in an approved specialty area in professional psychology" (American Board of Professional

Psychology 2008). Moreover, ABPP board certification is increasingly associated with greater opportunities for career growth, including employment opportunities, practice mobility between jurisdictions, and financial compensation (American Board of Professional Psychology; Sweet et al. 2006).

ABPP is currently a unique and unitary umbrella organization with multiple specialty boards that include Clinical Child and Adolescent Psychology, Clinical Health Psychology, Clinical Neuropsychology, Clinical Psychology, Cognitive and Behavioral Psychology, Counseling Psychology, Couple and Family Psychology, Forensic Psychology, Geropsychology, Group Psychology, Organizational and Business Consulting Psychology, Police and Public Safety Psychology, Psychoanalysis in Psychology, Rehabilitation Psychology, and School Psychology. Many professional psychologists seek dual certifications that reflect the full scope of their specialties. Examples of these might include clinical and cognitive behavioral, clinical neuropsychology and rehabilitation, or counseling and group. Uniquely, the Clinical Neuropsychology board also offers a subspecialty in pediatric neuropsychology, though, as of this writing, other subspecialties are being considered by other ABPP boards.

For a licensed psychologist to be "board eligible," each of the 15 boards requires that he or she meets both generic and specialty eligibility criteria concerning education, professional training, and licensure in the jurisdiction where professional services are provided. Once an individual's credentials are reviewed and approved, the individual seeking board certification moves to the next phase of their candidacy process. In clinical neuropsychology and forensic specialties, this necessitates passing a written examination. In all other specialties, the candidates are not required to take a written exam and may move directly to the final phases in the process. For all specialties, this includes first submitting a professional practice sample. After the practice sample is approved, the oral examination (final phase) is typically scheduled. Specialty boards may also provide a "senior option" regarding practice samples submitted by candidates with at least 15 years of experience post licensure who may submit samples of their professional work such as publications, treatment manuals, program manuals, or a comprehensive summary of their professional practice, to satisfy the requirements of a professional practice sample.

With regard to both practice samples and oral exams, the candidate's competency is assessed across various domains. These competency domains may be *functional* in nature and include the day-to-day activities of specialty practice, such as assessment, intervention, and/or consultation that are informed by a scientific literature base. They also include foundational competencies, such as ethics, individual and cultural diversity, and interpersonal competence, which cut across all of a specialist's other activities. The competency model upon which ABPP board certification is based draws from several important sources such as the APA-sponsored Competencies Conference in 2002 and resulting Task Force on Assessment of Competence in Professional Psychology (Kaslow et al. 2007), and a review of competency assessment models developed both within (e.g., Assessment of Competence Workgroup from Competencies Conference – Roberts et al. 2005; Leigh et al. 2007) and outside (e.g., American Council for Graduate Medical Education and American Board of Medical Specialties 2000) of the profession of psychology.

There is a strong consensus among many professional psychologists that the American Board of Professional Psychology represents a high degree of integrity regarding specialty board certification and serves as a gold standard for demonstration of specialty competency in professional psychology. In recent years, ABPP has turned its attention to maintenance of professional competency over the specialist's career. From 2006 to 2014, ABPP encouraged specialists to periodically review their performance to maintain quality of professional care and to serve and protect consumers of psychological services. ABPP has recently adopted formal Maintenance of Certification (MOC) procedures to standardize this process across specialty boards. Specialists certified after January 1, 2015, must successfully demonstrate maintenance of competency every 10 years to maintain their ABPP board-certified status. This requires detailed reporting of continuing education and other professional competency-related activities, appropriate for the certifying specialty board. Specialists certified before January 1, 2015, may participate in formal MOC but also have the option of waiving this requirement.

Landmark Contributions

The origins of ABPP can be traced back to its establishment in 1947 as the American Board of Professional Examiners in Psychology (Bent et al. 1999). The intention of the original board was to ensure that individuals were qualified to perform the professional service activities associated with clinical and counseling psychology. However, as professional psychology expanded its scope and depth, the organization changed its name to the American Board of Professional Psychology to reflect the expansion of specialization activities that were emerging for professional psychologists. As a result, the number of its affiliated specialty boards and associated academies has grown from 3 to 13, reflecting this professional expansion and the breadth of specialties that have emerged in recent decades (Finch et al. 2006; Packard and Reyes 2003).

Major Activities

Each of the psychology specialty boards under the ABPP umbrella has an elected trustee who participates as a member of the ABPP Board of Trustees as the overall governance group of the ABPP. Each specialty board assumes the responsibility for developing and carrying out the ABPP specialty examinations. The ABPP central office, under the management of a full-time executive officer, executes important day-to-day functions for all of the 13 specialty boards. These include generic candidacy verification of applicants, budget maintenance and accounting responsibilities, record keeping, development and maintenance of an ABPP Directory, development and editing responsibility for the ABPP website, monitoring the organization relative to ethical/legal issues, planning of conference and governance activities, and general administrative support. The primary publication of the organization, *The Specialist*, is published twice annually and available to all members in both electronic and printed format. The organization website (www.ABPP.org) contains important information regarding the mission, governance, and organizational documents. For the public, the website contains listings of board-certified specialists across specialties and practice jurisdictions. For interested applicants, it contains application instructions as well as other helpful information. The organization published its first book, *Becoming Board Certified by the American Board of Professional Psychology (ABPP)*, in 2009. This has been followed by publication of separate guides to become board certified by many individual specialties.

Cross-References

▶ American Academy of Clinical Neuropsychology (AACN)
▶ American Board of Clinical Neuropsychology (ABCN)
▶ American Board of Rehabilitation Psychology

References and Readings

American Board of Professional Psychology. (2008). Retrieved June 25, 2008, from http://www.abpp.org
American Council for Graduate Medical Education and American Board of Medical Specialties. (2000). *Toolbox of assessment methods*. Chicago: American Council for Graduate Medical Education and American Board of Medical Specialties.
Bent, R. J., Packard, R. E., & Goldberg, R. W. (1999). The American board of professional psychology. *Professional Psychology: Research and Practice, 30*, 65–73.
Datillio, F. M. (2002). Board certification in psychology: Is it really necessary? *Professional Psychology: Research and Practice, 33*, 54–57.

Finch, A. J., Simon, N. P., & Nezu, C. M. (2006). The future of clinical psychology: Board certification. *Clinical Psychology: Science and Practice, 13*, 254–257.
Kaslow, N. J., Rubin, N. J., Bebeau, M. J., Leigh, I. W., Lichtenberg, J. W., Nelson, P. D., Portnoy, S. M., & Smith, I. L. (2007). Guiding principles and recommendations for the assessment of competence. *Professional Psychology: Research and Practice, 38*, 441–451.
Leigh, I. W., Smith, I. L., Bebeau, M. J., Lichtenberg, J. W., Nelson, P. D., Portnoy, S., Rubin, N. J., & Kaslow, N. J. (2007). Competency assessment models. *Professional Psychology: Research and Practice, 38*, 463–473.
Nezu, C. M., Finch, A. J., & Simon, N. P. (Eds.). (2009). *Becoming board certified by the American board of professional psychology (ABPP)*. New York: Oxford University Press.
Packard, T., & Reyes, C. J. (2003). Specialty certification in professional psychology. In M. J. Prinstein & M. D. Patterson (Eds.), *The portable mentor: Expert guide to a successful career in psychology* (pp. 191–208). New York: Plenum.
Roberts, M. C., Borden, K. A., Christiansen, M. D., & Lopez, S. J. (2005). Fostering a culture shift: Assessment of competence in the education and careers of professional psychologists. *Professional Psychology: Research and Practice, 36*, 355–361.
Sweet, J. J., Nelson, N. W., & Moberg, P. J. (2006). The TCN/AACN 2005 "salary survey": Professional practices, beliefs, and incomes of U.S. neurophysiologists. *The Clinical Neuropsychologist, 20*, 325–364.

American Board of Rehabilitation Psychology

Daniel E. Rohe
Mayo Clinic, Rochester, MN, USA

Membership

The American Board of Rehabilitation Psychology (ABRP) is 1 of 15-member boards of the American Board of Professional Psychology (ABPP). The ABRP has certified 186 (as of 2017) doctoral-level psychologists who are engaged in provision of rehabilitation psychology services to individuals and their families affected by a wide range of disabilities and chronic health conditions including brain injury, spinal cord injury, amputations, chronic pain, multiple sclerosis, cancer, and sensory impairment such as blindness and deafness. In addition to clinical services, the majority of the board certified rehabilitation psychologists also engage in research, teaching, and administration of rehabilitation programs. Rehabilitation psychologists are also involved in interdisciplinary teamwork with other medical and rehabilitation providers. Rehabilitation psychologists who are boarded in the specialty reside in 30 states and 1 Canadian province.

Major Areas or Mission Statement

The mission of the ABRP is to protect the public and enhance the quality of health care by certifying rehabilitation psychologists who demonstrate the knowledge, skills, and attitudes essential to maximize quality of life for individuals with disabilities and chronic illness. The vision of the ABRP is that all psychologists practicing in rehabilitation will be boarded in the specialty. Psychologists who become board certified in Rehabilitation Psychology must meet the generic requirements for specialty certification by the ABPP that include a doctoral degree in psychology from an accredited degree program and licensure as a psychologist for independent practice in the USA or Canada. The ABRP-specific eligibility requirements include completion of a recognized internship program and 2 years of supervised practice in Rehabilitation Psychology. Given the diverse training experiences of rehabilitation psychologists, the credential review relies on the ratings of supervisors (two required) and the endorsement of colleagues and peers (two required). The candidate then submits a two-part practice sample (typically two case reports) that is evaluated by three ABRP examiners. Finally, the candidate completes an oral examination on two clinical vignettes, their clinical practice sample, and ethics. The entire examination process is designed to ensure that each candidate demonstrates the foundational and the functional competencies required of a psychologist who is board certified in Rehabilitation Psychology. The foundational competencies fall in four domains:

interpersonal interactions, individual and cultural diversity, ethical and legal foundations, and professional identification. The functional competencies encompass science base and application, assessment, intervention, consultation, and consumer protection.

Landmark Contributions

The primary contribution of ABRP is providing the opportunity for psychologists, dedicated to the health and psychological welfare of individuals with a wide range of disabilities and chronic health conditions, to unite and be boarded in a single specialty. The ABRP began as a credentials committee within the Division of Rehabilitation Psychology of the American Psychological Association in 1993. This committee incorporated as the American Board of Rehabilitation Psychology in 1995. On December 4, 1994 they established bylaws and elected officers: Richard Cox (president, 1994–2000), Bernard Brucker (vice president), Mitchell Rosenthal (secretary), and Daniel Rohe (treasurer). The initial members at large were Bruce Caplan, David Cox, Harry Parker, Anthony Ricci, James Whelan, and Mary Willmuth. Subsequent board presidents have included Mitchell Rosenthal (2000–2003), Bernard Brucker (2004–2007), Daniel Rohe (2008–2011), Lester Butt (2012–2013), and Michele Rusin (2014–present). The second major contribution is crafting an organizational structure that reflects the values of Rehabilitation Psychologists. The ABRP designed an innovative examination process that is user-friendly, collegial, inclusive, competency-based, and affirming of the candidate. The ABRP was the first ABPP board to devise a proactive mentoring program that has a credentialed colleague guide the applicant through the process. The ABRP examination and mentoring process has been emulated by other ABPP boards. The third major contribution is cosponsorship of the Rehabilitation Psychology Annual Conference with the Division of Rehabilitation Psychology from 1999 to the present. The annual meeting has become an institutionalized opportunity for rehabilitation psychologists to meet, present research, and promote the specialty to students.

Major Activities

The primary activity of ABRP is examination of psychologists entering the field of Rehabilitation Psychology. The second major activity is providing mentoring in the boarding process by the members of the board. The third major activity of ABRP has been cosponsoring the Rehabilitation Psychology Annual Conference. This conference typically occurs the last weekend of February and provides the opportunity to earn continuing education credits specific to Rehabilitation Psychology. The conference provides ABRP sponsored educational sessions that explain the process of attaining board certification in Rehabilitation Psychology to interested candidates. The conference features nationally recognized leaders in the field of Rehabilitation Psychology. The ABRP board works in concert with the newly created Academy of Rehabilitation Psychology (ARP). The ARP is a separate organization that is assuming the role of providing logistical support for the Rehabilitation Psychology Annual Conference.

Cross-References

▶ American Board of Professional Psychology (ABPP)
▶ American Psychological Association (APA), Division 22
▶ Rehabilitation Psychology

References and Readings

Cox, D., Cox, R., & Caplan, B. (2013). *Specialty competencies in rehabilitation psychology*. New York: Oxford University Press.
Frank, R., Rosenthal, M., & Caplan, B. (Eds.). (2009). *Handbook of rehabilitation psychology* (2nd ed.). Washington, DC: American Psychological Association.
Kennedy, P. (Ed.). (2012). *Oxford handbook of rehabilitation psychology*. New York: Oxford University Press.

American College of Professional Neuropsychology (ACPN)

John E. Meyers
Department of Neuropsychology, Comprehensive Medpsych Systems, Sarasota, FL, USA

Membership

The American College of Professional Neuropsychology (ACPN) is a membership organization formed on September 1, 1995, that is composed of over 400 neuropsychologists who have doctoral degrees, are licensed as psychologists, and have completed the Diplomate examination process of the American Board of Professional Neuropsychology as well as 122 Affiliate members.

Major Areas or Mission Statement

ACPN is the academic arm of the American Board of Professional Neuropsychology (ABN). The mission of the ACPN is to promote and provide the highest levels of services related to professional neuropsychology for the benefit of the public and the profession.

Landmark Contributions

In addition to the continuing education benefit, ACPN also has two official quarterly journals – Applied Neuropsychology: Adult and Applied Neuropsychology: Child, which are dedicated to the presentation of practitioner-based scholarly research.

Diplomates of the ABN who are in good standing are automatically Fellows of ACPN and may use the acronym FACPN on their signature line. Members of other neuropsychological organizations may also join the ACPN as Affiliate members and receive a subscription to the Applied Neuropsychology Journals and can participate in ACPN continuing education programs.

Major Activities

ACPN is approved by the American Psychological Association to sponsor continuing education for psychologists. ACPN typically holds at least one general meeting each year, covering various subjects, and offering continuing education credits to attendees.

Cross-References

▶ American Board of Professional Neuropsychology (ABN)

American Congress of Rehabilitation Medicine

Marcel P. J. M. Dijkers
American Congress of Rehabilitation Medicine, Reston, VA, USA
Department of Rehabilitation Medicine, Icahn School of Medicine at Mount Sinai, New York, NY, USA

Membership as of December 2016

Membership is about 2,300, consisting of clinicians and nonclinicians with an interest in medical rehabilitation (rehabilitation medicine, physical medicine and rehabilitation) research, and training in medicine, (neuro)psychology, occupational and physical therapy, nursing, speech and language pathology, vocational counseling, rehabilitation engineering, medical sociology, etc. Medical rehabilitation concerns restoration of function for individuals who as a result of stroke, traumatic brain injury, spinal cord injury, amputation, cancer, neurodegenerative diseases and other disorders have impairments and activity limitations that are primarily physical in nature but often also include cognitive and behavioral deficits; it is to be distinguished from psychiatric rehabilitation, addiction rehabilitation, etc., although there is an overlap in methods and sometimes clientele. ACRM members share an interest in rehabilitation research, and the translation of research-based knowledge into formats that are of use to medical rehabilitation clinicians. Within the organizations that employ them, ACRM members may play one or more roles: rehabilitation practitioner, rehabilitation researcher, knowledge broker, research funder staff, clinical administrator, teacher, etc. About 550 members are located outside the United States in over 50 countries.

Mission Statement

The slogan currently used by the organization expresses its mission: "Improving lives through interdisciplinary rehabilitation research." This is further clarified by "We enhance the lives of people living with disabilities through a multi-disciplinary approach to rehabilitation. As leaders in the physical medicine and rehabilitation field, we promote innovative research, new technologies, and sharing information, and encourage evidence-based practices in clinical settings" (About ACRM 2015). The interdisciplinary character and research focus of the organization are further expressed by another slogan: "Excellence in the science of rehabilitation medicine through interdisciplinary collaboration" (About ACRM 2015). ACRM supports research that promotes health, independence, productivity, and quality of life and meets the needs of rehabilitation clinicians and people with disabilities. In order to enhance current and future research and knowledge translation, the organization:

- Assists researchers in improving their investigations and dissemination of findings
- Shares this information via education meetings and its journal, *Archives of Physical Medicine and Rehabilitation*
- Encourages leaders in rehabilitation to identify current best practices at all levels of care
- Serves as a forum for creating and discussing new treatment paradigms to achieve optimal functional outcomes for people with chronic disease and disabilities

- Educates providers to deliver best practices
- Advocates for funding of future rehabilitation research

Landmark Contributions

The American Congress of Rehabilitation Medicine was established in 1923 as the American College of Radiology and Physiotherapy, a professional organization of physicians who had a clinical interest in diagnostic and therapeutic radiology, as well as the therapeutic application of electricity and other physical therapies (Dijkers 2009). Reflecting the ongoing differentiation between radiologists and what (much later) would be called physiatrists, the name was changed to American Congress of Physical Therapy in 1925. To emphasize its link to medicine rather than allied health, the organization renamed itself American Congress of Physical Medicine in 1944.

While World War I had given rise to the development of rehabilitation, the involvement of physicians had been limited – rehabilitation was centered on the vocational rehabilitation of discharged servicemen. During World War II, however, a number of military physicians became specialists in rehabilitation; after the war they started to apply the methods they had developed with injured servicemen to the treatment of civilians with amputations, spinal cord injury, stroke, and developmental disabilities such as cerebral palsy. To avoid the creation of a separate organization involving physicians with very similar interests and therapeutic regimens, a "shotgun marriage" between physiatrists and these rehabilitation physicians was acknowledged in 1952 with the expansion of the name of the organization to American Congress of Physical Medicine and Rehabilitation (Zeiter 1954).

In the 1960s, the Congress opened its membership to nonphysician rehabilitation professionals, first only those holding a doctoral degree (1965) and then also to nurses and therapists with a (earned) master's degree (Anonymous 1998). To acknowledge the diminishing emphasis on physical medicine, the Congress changed its name again, to American Congress of Rehabilitation Medicine, in 1966. ACRM accepted rehabilitation professionals with a bachelor's degree as members starting in 1986. The first nonphysician to become president of the organization took office in 1977; neuropsychologists who have served as president include Leonard Diller, Mitchell Rosenthal, and Wayne Gordon.

In recent years, ACRM has redefined itself as an organization focusing on rehabilitation science, with strong interest in both generating knowledge through research and knowledge translation to bring research results to clinical practice in a format that practitioners can use (Hart 1997; Heinemann 2006; Wilkerson 2004). It is now primarily a group of creators, transmitters, and users of research-based rehabilitation knowledge, both those with clinical training (physicians, occupational and physical therapists, psychologists, etc.) and those without (engineers, social scientists, etc.), bound by the conviction that the collaboration of disciplines is the best way to solve the problems inherent in disablement and the rehabilitation of persons with impairment, activity limitations, and participation restrictions.

The seal of the organization until very recently still reflected ACRM's roots in physical medicine, including the traditional symbols for medicine and for the four elements: water, earth, fire, and air. In 2013 a new logo was unveiled, showing the overlapping petals of a lotus flower, to visually communicate the interdisciplinary culture of the organization.

Major Activities

ACRM communicates with its members through its scientific journal (the *Archives of Physical Medicine and Rehabilitation – APM&R*), a newsletter (*Rehabilitation Outlook*), electronic newsletters for various special interest groups, and the weekly E-news, an electronic digest of time-sensitive news. An annual scientific meeting of 3–4 days, often held jointly with other scientific and professional organizations, brings together members and nonmembers to discuss research findings, research methods, and issues relevant to the funding, implementation, and dissemination of rehabilitation research. A midyear meeting brings together members of task forces across the many special interest groups to further their multiple ongoing projects.

A number of standing committees offer members an opportunity to work on issues of special interest. Current committees include the International Committee (focusing on the communications between US and foreign rehabilitation research specialists), the Evidence and Practice Committee (dealing with issues of evidence-based rehabilitation and related matters), and the Health Policy Networking Group. The Early Career Committee aims to assist individuals new to rehabilitation research in mastering the scientific, administrative, and personal aspects of a career in rehabilitation research.

Over the years, a number of interdisciplinary special interest groups (ISIGs) have existed under the aegis of ACRM; current groups include ISIGs focused on pain, spinal cord injury, stroke, measurement, pediatric rehabilitation, geriatric rehabilitation, cancer, and traumatic brain injury.

The Brain Injury ISIG (BI-ISIG) grew out of the ACRM Head Injury Task Force, first called together in 1979. The BI-ISIG, which attracts large numbers of psychologists and especially neuropsychologists, has played a crucial role in the development of services for individuals with traumatic brain injury (TBI) in the United States. A definition of mild TBI often used in the literature emerged from the work of this group (ACRM Head Injury Interdisciplinary Special Interest Group 1993). The *Journal of Head Trauma Rehabilitation* (*JHTR*) was founded by a physician (Sheldon Berrol) and a psychologist (Mitchell Rosenthal) who were active in the BI-ISIG, as well as involved with the fledgling National Head Trauma Foundation, now the Brain Injury Association of America. There is significant overlap between the BI-ISIG membership and both the Editorial Board of JHTR and the leadership of the TBI Model Systems of Care, demonstration, and research grant programs supported by the National Institute on Disability, Independent Living and Rehabilitation Research since 1987 (Dijkers et al. 2010). There also is considerable overlap between the membership of the BI-ISIG and Divisions 22 (Rehabilitation Psychology) and

40 (Clinical Neuropsychology) of the American Psychological Association. Intense collaboration in research and clinical care occurs among the BI-ISIG members, who have their own task forces; communicate through the BI-ISIG newsletter, *Moving Ahead*; and come together at the ACRM midyear meeting.

APM&R began in 1920 as the *Journal of Radiology* and changed its name to the *Archives of Physical Therapy, X-ray, Radium*, in 1926. Later changes in its name paralleled those in the name of its owner: *Archives of Physical Therapy* in 1938 and the *Archives of Physical Medicine* in 1945. In 1953, the journal became the *Archives of Physical Medicine and Rehabilitation*, the name it still has (Nelson 1969). However, the content has shifted gradually from emphasis on physical medicine, with a fairly low research basis, to an accent on rehabilitation as carried out by all disciplines that play a role in medical rehabilitation. It is now almost exclusively a research journal, with non-US contributions constituting over half the contents. It has a respectable impact factor (3.3) ranking it fifth in the "rehabilitation" category, but because of the large number of papers published each year, it has more influence than higher-ranked journals. In fact, the annual number of citations is about is larger than those of the four higher-ranked publications together.

The journal probably gives the best indication of the role of neuropsychology in rehabilitation settings and of neuropsychologists in ACRM. The first paper with neuropsychology in its title or abstract was distributed in 1975. About 300 have been published since, but they did not become an annual presence until 1984. The number now averages over 15 a year. In scanning the contributions of neuropsychologists to *APM&R*, a number of characteristics of neuropsychology in rehabilitation stand out:

- Many of these papers are coauthored with representatives of other disciplines, especially physicians.
- Several straddle neuropsychology and rehabilitation psychology, reflecting the fact that in many rehabilitation programs, psychologists need to wear multiple hats.

- The focus, especially in recent years, is as much on treatment as on diagnosis, with cognitive rehabilitation for TBI and other diagnostic groups most prominent.
- A great variety of diagnostic groups have been studied, including peripheral vascular disease amputations, post-polio fatigue, multiple sclerosis, sickle-cell disease, progressive supranuclear palsy, myotonic muscular dystrophy, and spinal cord injury.
- However, over the years and especially recently, stroke and TBI have been the etiologies of disability that rehabilitation neuropsychologists have most often been concerned with.

While the American Congress of Rehabilitation Medicine is not an organization of psychologists, let alone neuropsychologists, it is safe to say that it has played a key role in the development of neuropsychology for medical rehabilitation patients in the United States. In the foreseeable future, it probably will continue to be the forum in which these specialists, especially those who are interested in research, interact with nurses, speech/language pathologists, neuroscientists, and other specialists who contribute to rehabilitation and its evidence base.

References and Readings

About ACRM. (2015). Retrieved 4 Aug 2015, from http://www.acrm.org/about/

American-Congress-of-Rehabilitation-Medicine.-Head-Injury-Interdisciplinary-Special-Interest-Group. (1993). Definition of mild traumatic brain injury. *The Journal of Head Trauma Rehabilitation, 8*(3), 86–87.

Anonymous. (1998). Development of the American Congress of Rehabilitation Medicine into a multidisciplinary professional society: Final report of the Professional Development Committee, 1969–1972. *Archives of Physical Medicine and Rehabilitation, 79* (12 Suppl. 2), 4–12.

Dijkers, M. P. (2009). International collaboration and communication in rehabilitation research. *Archives of Physical Medicine and Rehabilitation, 90*(5), 711–716.

Dijkers, M. P., Harrison-Felix, C., & Marwitz, J. H. (2010). The traumatic brain injury model systems: History and contributions to clinical service and research. *The Journal of Head Trauma Rehabilitation, 25*(2), 81–91.

Hart, K. A. (1997). Rehabilitation research: The new focus of the American Congress of Rehabilitation Medicine.

Archives of Physical Medicine and Rehabilitation, 78 (12), 1287–1289.

Heinemann, A. W. (2006). ACRM's evolving mission: Opportunities to promote rehabilitation research. *Archives of Physical Medicine and Rehabilitation, 87* (2), 157–159.

Kottke, F. J., & Knapp, M. E. (1988). The development of physiatry before 1950. *Archives of Physical Medicine and Rehabilitation, 69*. Spec No, 4–14.

Krusen, F. H. (1969). Historical development in physical medicine and rehabilitation during the last forty years. Walter J. Zeiter lecture. *Archives of Physical Medicine and Rehabilitation, 50*(1), 1–5.

Nelson, P. A. (1969). History of the archives – a journal of ideas and ideals. *Archives of Physical Medicine and Rehabilitation, 50*(7), 367–405. passim.

Rusk, H. A. (1969). The growth and development of rehabilitation medicine. *Archives of Physical Medicine and Rehabilitation, 50*(8), 463–466.

Wilkerson, D. L. (2004). Individual, science, and society: ACRM's mission and the body politic. *Archives of Physical Medicine and Rehabilitation, 85*(4), 527–530.

Zeiter, W. J. (1954). The history of the American Congress of Physical Medicine and Rehabilitation. *Archives of Physical Medicine and Rehabilitation, 35*(11), 683–688.

American Psychological Association (APA)

Nadine J. Kaslow[1] and Jennifer M. Doran[2]
[1]Department of Psychiatry and Behavioral Sciences, Emory University School of Medicine, APA, Atlanta, GA, USA
[2]VA Connecticut Healthcare System, Yale School of Medicine, Newington, CT, USA

Membership

As of 2017, the American Psychological Association (APA) had a total of 115,492 members (76,174 full members and 39,318 affiliate members, including 31,560 students).

Mission Statement

APA is the leading scientific and professional organization representing psychology in the United States. Its mission is to "advance the creation, communication, and application of psychological knowledge to benefit society and improve people's lives." APA achieves this mission through four interrelated directorates, which focus on education, science, practice, and the public interest. APA's current strategic plan has three primary goals: (1) maximize organizational effectiveness, (2) expand psychology's role in advancing health, and (3) increase recognition of psychology as a science.

History

The APA was founded in 1892 at Clark University by a small group of scholars interested in the "new psychology" (Fernberger 1932). G. Stanley Hall was elected as the inaugural president. The organization's first meeting occurred in December 1892 at the University of Pennsylvania. APA's founding at this time can best be understood in the context of myriad changes occurring in the United States, including the emergence of the modern university system; a broad reorganization of American knowledge production; the formation of several now-standard academic disciplines, including psychology; and mounting societal demands for individuals with advanced degrees to serve in new professional niches. The "new psychology" grew and prospered as it responded to the changing needs of modern American society and contributed to the management of an increasingly complex and diversified world (Benjamin 2009).

Psychology expanded even further after World War II, and funding from various governmental offices began influencing psychology research, training, and practice (Pickren and Schneider 2005). This expansion was largely due to the increased prominence of the applied areas of psychology. Realizing that the growth of applied psychology represented a potential threat to its preeminence, APA's leaders responded via a reorganization plan in which APA merged with other psychological organizations. It was at this time that APA began creating divisions that represented specialized fields of interest (Dewsbury 1997). Seventeen divisions were initially created, with the two most populated being clinical and personnel (now counseling). Growth in the number of divisions was slow until the 1960s in part because there was resistance among APA leaders to increasing the number of divisions. The trajectory with regard to the addition of divisions since the 1960s has been slow but steady, with many of the newer divisions reflecting the growth of particular practice areas (e.g., addictions). Currently, there are 54 divisions, with the most recent division being approved in 2006 (trauma psychology). This divisional structure has resulted in a more broad-based and inclusive organization. In conjunction with APA's four directorates, the organization's scope includes supporting professional practice, promoting human welfare, advancing psychological science, and fostering psychology education and training.

Over the years, concerns mounted among some of the scientists in the organization that APA was no longer providing an adequate home for them and was drifting away from a primary focus on scientific psychology. As a result, in the 1950s, a group of experimental psychologists formed the Psychonomic Society with the aim of fostering psychology as a science. A more serious division occurred in the mid- to late 1980s, as tensions escalated between those who wanted APA to remain a primarily scientific organization and those who sought a greater emphasis on professional practice issues. After a proposed reorganization plan was defeated by a vote of the membership, a group of dissident psychological scientists, including several former APA presidents, left the APA to form what is now the Association for Psychological Science (Evans et al. 1992). Today, all three of these organizations are strong, stable representatives of psychology, with many psychologists belonging to two or more of these associations.

There are multiple smaller organizations that represent various areas of psychology, as well as a growing number of interdisciplinary and interprofessional organizations in which psychology plays a major role. In addition, there are separate organizations for psychologists with various ethnic and racial identities, most notably the Asian American Psychological Association, Association of Black Psychologists, National Latina/o Psychological Association, and Society of Indian Psychologists. These four ethnic minority psychological associations have partnered with the APA to form the Alliance of National Psychological Associations for Racial and Ethnic Equity.

The APA is a nonprofit 501 (c)(3) organization that has a companion 501 (c)(6) organization for practitioners and educators of practitioners, the APA Practice Organization (APAPO). The APAPO is tasked with advancing and protecting the profession of psychology and the economic interests of practicing psychologists. The APAPO focuses on legislative advocacy and mental health policy, as well as serving as a resource for members' professional needs.

Over the past few years, APA has undergone periods of tension and conflict. These have been in response to myriad internal and external challenges, such as those related to the organizational critiques launched in the Independent Review (IR) Relating to APA Ethics Guidelines, National Security Interrogations, and Torture (a.k.a. Hoffman Report); efforts at organizational restructuring; concerns about the lack of prioritization of social justice in the organization's strategic plan; the alienation of marginalized groups; the lack of clarity with regard to the functions of the 501 (c)(3) (i.e., APA) versus the 501(c)(6) (i.e., APAPO); the APA Assessment Fee Litigation (i.e., class action settlement) that impacted both the (c)(3) and (c)(6); and the sharp membership decline of the APAPO.

Despite these challenges, APA remains the largest scientific and professional organization representing psychology in the United States. Its members are scientists, educators, practitioners, and psychologists working for the public interest, as well as students in psychology. It is also the most prominent national organization that advocates at the federal level for psychology. Further, APA is a major publisher of professional books, children's books, journals, magazines and newsletters, the *Publication Manual of the American Psychological Association*, reports and brochures, videos, and data bases. It takes seriously its responsibility to not only communicate with its members but also to inform the general public and the media about the breadth and depth of psychology and its relevance to societal issues. For example, it hosts on its website the Psychology Help Center, which is an online resource for consumers that offers information regarding psychological factors that impact emotional and physical well-being. Moreover, it continues to create, disseminate, and evaluate innovative and state-of-the-art programs designed to enhance psychology education, science, public interest, and practice.

Organizational Structure

At the time the organization was founded, its basic governance structure consisted of a small council that was overseen by an executive committee. This structure remained in effect until the reorganization of APA during World War II. While the APA has undergone a number of reorganizations since this time, its governance structure continues to include a Board of Directors, which includes the Chair of the American Psychological Association of Graduate Students (APAGS), and a large Council of Representatives. Over the years this council has expanded to include more diverse constituent-based representation. For example, in 2017, this Council of Representatives has 177 members, with individual representing the 54 divisions of the APA, the State, Provincial, and Territorial Psychological Associations, and APAGS.

This large governing body creates an inherent tension between representation and a cumbersome and somewhat unwieldy structure that has been criticized. The most recent attempt at structural reorganization has occurred under the auspices of the Good Governance Project (GGP), which had as its aim the enhancement of APA's organizational effectiveness. Recommendations were made regarding distinguishing and clarifying the roles of the Board of Directors and the Council of Representatives, increasing APA's operational efficiency, and becoming a more inclusive organization with a pipeline of diverse and well-trained leaders. While some of the recommended changes have been instituted already, many others have been challenging to implement and/or require a vote of the membership. One of the most controversial sets of recommendations, tabled at the present time, is the reduction of the overall size of the council along with a reconsideration of how membership in this body would be determined. The size of the Council and the issues of representation and loss of voice continue to be debated among governance members. A related challenge has pertained to who should have a seat on the Council, and there have been three failed votes by the members with regard to the inclusion of representatives from the four major ethnic minority psychological associations. Challenges related to the inclusion of diverse psychologists within psychology and APA have a long history (Guthrie 2004).

There also are a significant number of standing boards and committees that help to advance APA's mission, support policy initiatives, and focus on content specific to the discipline. In response to a recent vote by the Council of Representatives, each of these boards and committees is now expected to include at least one Early Career Psychologist (ECP) member in an effort to acknowledge their contributions and to expand the pipeline of emerging leaders.

Membership

Membership growth has fluctuated over time. Growth was modest over the first 50 years of APA's existence; by 1940 there were only 664 members. In 1926, a new class of nonvoting membership was formed, deemed *associate members* (now *affiliate members*). Membership growth reflected the increased interest in the profession following World War II, with rapid growth occurring between 1945 and 1970. During this time, membership increased 630%. Membership continued to boom through the early 2000s, with the peak of membership occurring in 2010, when the association had a robust 155,138 full and affiliate members. The upward trend began to reverse beginning in 2011, when membership dropped 11.6%. Membership has continued to decline at a slow but steady rate since this time, which is consistent with broader trends in association management (Yohn 2016). This decline may also reflect specific sociopolitical factors within the discipline, the profession, and the organization. To alter this membership trajectory, improve the member value proposition and strengthen membership recruitment, retention, and engagement, APA named its first executive director for membership in 2015. Member benefits include, but are not limited to, access to a directory of members, an attendance discount at the annual convention, a subscription to the *American Psychologist* and the *Monitor on Psychology*, access to continuing professional development programs, and discounts on both non-APA- and APA-produced products (e.g., books, journals, apps, videos).

Major Activities

For detailed descriptions of APA's major activities, the reader is referred to the APA website. This section highlights some of the key activities across the organization and is meant to be illustrative rather than inclusive.

APA's Central Office includes the Executive Office, which is responsible for overseeing and managing the association's key functions and implementing APA policies. Associated with the Central Office is APA's Center for Psychology and Health, a cross-directorate center that collaborates with the APAPO in order to provide coordinated activities designed to secure and expand psychology's central role in improving health and healthcare in the United States. Another center that bridges APA's component parts is the recently launched Center for Organizational Excellence, which aims to enhance employee well-being and strengthen organizational performance. Also associated with the Executive Office is APA's Ethics Office, which oversees the development and implementation of the APA's Ethical Principles of Psychologists and Code of Conduct (APA 2002), educates members and the public about ethics throughout the field of psychology, provides ethics consultations, and supports the Ethics Committee's efforts to adjudicate ethics complaints against APA members.

The Central Office also includes the Office of the General Counsel, which is responsible for all aspects of legal counsel and representation of APA. The Office of the General Counsel has often spearheaded the development of amicus briefs, documents used to educate courts on issues relevant to legal cases that include supporting scientific research. These briefs have focused on diverse topics such as abortion, affirmative action, family law, the insanity defense, scientific research, and sexual orientation (discrimination).

Reflecting a life cycle perspective, the Education Directorate focuses on Pre-K to 12, undergraduate, graduate and postgraduate, and continuing education efforts. Through the Education Government Relations Office, it leads federal advocacy efforts relevant to policies and funding for psychology education and training. The Directorate offers tools for teaching psychology, engages in activities that enable APA to be a leader in ensuring that education and training are competency-based, provides information and programs for trainers and trainees about the education and training pipeline and the range of employment opportunities, and collects and disseminates data about the profession of psychology through its Center for Workforce Studies. To support the accreditation of doctoral, internship, and postdoctoral programs, it houses the Office of Program Consultation and Accreditation and the APA Commission on Accreditation. Staff and governance members collaboratively address critical issues facing the field and impacting high-quality education and training, such as the internship imbalance (i.e., more trainees seeking accredited internships than available positions). For example, they were instrumental in APA's 2012 Internship Stimulus Package, in which APA committed $3 million to increase the number of accredited internship positions. Finally, APA sponsors continuing education programs that support psychologists' professional development.

The Science Directorate aims to advance psychological science, address the needs of psychological scientists, promote the integration of psychological science with other core science disciplines, and advocate for psychological science at the federal level (Science Government Relations Office). The Directorate offers a broad array of services, including a Psychology: Science in Action program that underscores how science benefits society and enhances people's lives, guidelines on pertinent topics (e.g., Ethical Conduct in the Care and Use of Nonhuman Animals in Research), and a toolkit for science advocacy. It shares with its constituents information about research funding, analytic tools and methods, and publications. The Directorate houses the Science Student Council to promote trainees in the leadership pipeline and offers fellowships for burgeoning and Early Career Psychologists (e.g., the Summer Science Fellowship, the APA Executive Branch Science Fellowship Program). The Science Directorate is also committed to ensuring that psychological science is translated in meaningful ways to the public.

APA's Public Interest Directorate aims to apply psychological science to the fundamental problems of human welfare and social justice and to promote equitable and just treatment for all individuals through education, training, and policy. It supports offices, programs, governance activities, and the creation of guidelines related to aging; HIV/AIDS; children, youth, and families; disabilities; ethnic minority affairs; lesbian, gay, bisexual, and transgender concerns; socioeconomic status; violence prevention; women; and work, stress, and health. It has a strong Government Relations Office that takes an active role in advocacy related to the aforementioned issues as well as other human rights and social justice concerns, such as health disparities. The Directorate also houses APA's Minority Fellowship Program, which provides funding support to racial and ethnic minority graduate students during their education and training, as one mechanism for increasing the diversity of the profession.

APA's Practice Directorate has as its mission the promotion of the practice of psychology and the availability of behavioral health services through advocacy, public education and outreach, and research. It participates actively in crafting policies and practice guidelines for specific areas of psychological practice and service delivery. It oversees a major Public Education Campaign designed to educate the public about the value of psychology. This campaign has addressed school violence, the mind/body health connection, and the promotion of psychologically healthy workplaces. The Disaster Response Network also falls within the auspices of the Practice Directorate. In collaboration with the American Red Cross, this program involves licensed psychologist volunteers who help individuals and communities cope with and heal from disasters. The Directorate creates and disseminates a range of resources for practitioners, such as information on transitioning to electronic medical records, evidence-based practice in psychology, and documents on self-care and colleague assistance.

Through its Office of International Affairs, APA is very invested in its relations with international psychology organizations. As one example of this, APA engaged in an agreement with the International Union of Psychological Science to provide technical assistance to the World Health Organization (WHO) with regard to the revision of the WHO's International Statistical Classification of Diseases and Related Health Problems (ICD-10; World Health Organisation 1992) "Mental and Behavioural Disorders" chapter.

Concluding Comments

APA continues to adapt and redefine itself in light of a changing healthcare climate, the ongoing implementation of the GGP's recommended structural reorganization, and declining membership trends and in the context of recent controversies and conflict. APA remains the world's largest membership organization of psychologists. It has a fascinating past, marked by growth, conflict, and increasing diversification. Its response to current challenges will likely have long-standing impacts on the association and profession of psychology as a whole. The present moment appears to be a pivotal one in APA's history; how so, only time will tell.

References and Readings

American Psychological Association. (2002). Ethical principles of psychologists and code of conduct. Retrieved from: http://www.apa.org/ethics/code/

American Psychological Association. (2016). About APA. Retrieved from: http://www.apa.org/about/index.aspx

Benjamin, L. T., Jr. (2009). *A history of psychology: Original sources and contemporary research* (3rd ed.). Malden: Blackwell Publishing.

Dewsbury, D. A. (1997). On the evolution of divisions. *American Psychologist, 52*, 733–741. https://doi.org/10.1037/0003-066X.52.7.733.

Evans, R. B., Sexton, V. S., & Cadwallader, T. C. (Eds.). (1992). *The American Psychological Association: A historical perspective*. Washington, DC: American Psychological Association.

Fernberger, S. W. (1932). The American Psychological Association: A historical summary, 1892–1930. *Psychological Bulletin, 29*, 1–89. https://doi.org/10.1037/h0075733.

Guthrie, R. V. (2004). *Even the rat was white: A historical view of psychology*. Boston: Allyn and Bacon.

Pickren, W. E., & Schneider, S. F. (Eds.). (2005). *Psychology and the National Institute of Mental Health: A historical analysis of science, practice, and policy*. Washington, DC: APA Books.

World Health Organisation. (1992). *International statistical classification of diseases and related health problems, 10th revision (ICD-10)*. Geneva: WHO.

Yohn, D. L. (January 2016). To stay relevant, professional associations must rebrand. Harvard Business Review. Retrieved from: https://hbr.org/2016/01/to-stay-relevant-professional-associations-must-rebrand

American Psychological Association (APA), Division 22

William Stiers
Johns Hopkins University School of Medicine, Baltimore, MD, USA

Membership

The American Psychological Association (APA) Division 22 – Rehabilitation Psychology is composed of 1164 psychologists (as of December, 2017) who provide health services, teach, manage rehabilitation programs, conduct research, and perform other professional activities. They work in hospitals and clinics, in independent practice, in other human service settings, and in universities and colleges.

Major Areas or Mission Statement

The Division of Rehabilitation Psychology works to unite psychologists and others interested in the prevention and rehabilitation of disability and chronic illness. Rehabilitation Psychology practice is a specialty within the domain of professional healthcare psychology, which applies psychological knowledge and skills on behalf of individuals with disabilities and chronic health conditions in order to maximize their health and welfare, independence and choice, functional abilities, and social role participation. Such disabilities include spinal cord injury, brain injury, stroke, amputations, burns, work-related injuries, multiple traumatic injuries, chronic pain, cancer, heart disease, multiple sclerosis, neuromuscular disorders, AIDS, developmental disorders, psychiatric impairment, substance abuse, impairments in sensory functioning, and other physical, mental, and/or emotional impairments. The broad field of Rehabilitation Psychology also includes rehabilitation program development and administration, research, teaching, public education and development of policies for injury prevention and health promotion, and advocacy for persons with disabilities and chronic health conditions.

APA Division 22 – Rehabilitation Psychology participates in the Rehabilitation Psychology Specialty Council. In accordance with the policy of the Council of Specialties in Professional Psychology (CoS – https://www.cospp.org/), this Rehabilitation Psychology Specialty Council consists of the professional groups and organizations that represent the major educational, training, and professional constituencies and stakeholders relevant to Rehabilitation Psychology, that is, APA Division 22, the American Board of Rehabilitation Psychology, The Foundation for Rehabilitation Psychology, the Academy of Rehabilitation Psychology, and the Council of Rehabilitation Psychology Postdoctoral Training Programs. The Rehabilitation Psychology Specialty Council selects one of its members to serve as the specialty's representative to CoS, and this representative serves as a voting member on CoS.

Landmarks

- Rehabilitation psychologists have worked in medical settings as part of teams of healthcare professionals for more than 70 years, long before psychologists were regularly involved in other healthcare settings.
- Division 22 was established in 1958, one of the earlier divisions in APA.
- Division 22 members conducted the initial research on individual, interpersonal, and social changes related to changes in appearance and physical capacity, as well as the social psychology of stereotyping and prejudice faced by persons with disability.
- Division 22 members were among the pioneers helping psychology understand the world of work, how work can be affected by impairment and disability, and issues about vocational rehabilitation.
- Rehabilitation psychologists have developed the principles of cognitive rehabilitation and have served as leaders in the federal model systems programs for traumatic brain injury, spinal cord injury, and burns.
- Board Certification in Rehabilitation Psychology was established in 1997.
- Rehabilitation Psychology is recognized by the Commission for the Recognition of Specialties and Proficiencies in Professional Psychology since 2015.

Major Activities

- The journal *Rehabilitation Psychology* is published quarterly by the APA http://www.apa.org/pubs/journals/rep/.

- Division 22, in conjunction with the American Board of Rehabilitation Psychology, holds an annual conference in the early spring of each year.

Resources

- American Psychological Association (APA) – http://www.apa.org
  - General information about psychology and about the divisions or sections within APA
- Rehabilitation Psychology – http://www.div22.org/
  - Specific information about the specialty of Rehabilitation Psychology

Cross-References

▶ American Board of Professional Psychology (ABPP)
▶ American Board of Rehabilitation Psychology
▶ American Psychological Association (APA)
▶ Rehabilitation Psychology

References and Readings

American Psychological Association. (2008). A closer look at Division 22: A growing field meets the challenges of war. *Monitor on Psychology, 38*(8), 54–55.
Frank, R., Rosenthal, M., & Caplan, B. (Eds.). (2009). *Handbook of rehabilitation psychology* (2nd ed.). Washington, DC: American Psychological Association.
Larson, P., & Sachs, P. (2000). A history of Division 22. In D. A. Dewsbury (Ed.), *Unification through division: Histories of the divisions of the American Psychological Association* (Vol. 5, pp. 33–58). Washington, DC: American Psychological Association.

Division Sections
Pediatric Rehabilitation
Women in Rehabilitation Psychology

Special Interest Groups
Assistive Technology
Psychologists with Disabilities
Deafness
Early Career Psychologists

American Psychological Association (APA), Division 40

A

William B. Barr
NYU Langone Medical Center, Comprehensive Epilepsy Center, New York, NY, USA

Membership

The Society for Clinical Neuropsychology (SCN), Division 40 of the American Psychological Association (APA) is one of 56 specialty divisions recognized by the APA. Since its inception, it has become one of APA's most visible and active divisions. In its nearly 40 years, membership has grown from 433 psychologists to its current (based on 2016 statistics) membership of 3,423, which currently makes it the largest of all APA divisions. The division's representation to the APA council has grown over the years from its initial one representative to the current allotment of four seats. This trend coincides with SCN's increasing influence within APA and increasing recognition of neuropsychology as a clinical specialty.

The division voted to change its name to SCN in 2013 as part of a branding and public relations effort to enable greater flexibility in communications and greater clarity for the public. Eligibility for division membership was previously based on membership in APA. That criterion is no longer required. Any psychologist, trainee, or individual with an interest in clinical neuropsychology is encouraged to join SCN. All members are provided access to SCN's Internet LISTERVs and publications. All members of the division who are APA members have additional rights and privileges to hold office and serve on division committees and vote in APA elections. Information for joining SCN can be obtained on the division's website at http://www.scn40.org/mc.html.

APA statistics indicate that the majority of SCN members are women by a slight majority (49.9%). Ethnic minority members constitute 8% of the membership, consistent with larger APA trends. Approximately, 80% of the division memberships have a Ph.D. in clinical psychology or a related field. Based on the previous statistics, nearly half of the members work in independent settings. Most other members work in medical schools, hospitals, and university settings. Many combine their work in institutional and private practice settings. Prior membership surveys have indicated that psychologists in SCN spend a substantially larger amount of time (>40%) in assessment activities than other APA members (<15%). Approximately, one third of the members are actively involved in research activities. Approximately, 40% are involved in clinical training.

Major Areas or Mission Statement

Division 40 was formed in 1980 with the mission of enhancing the understanding of brain-behavior relationships and the application of such knowledge to human problems. Activities of the division encompass the areas of science (e.g., presentations at the annual meeting of APA, awards for outstanding scientific contributions), practice (e.g., Current Procedural Terminology, "CPT," billing codes, educational brochures for patients), education and training (e.g., neuropsychology graduate student organization), and specialty public interest groups (e.g., women, minorities, geriatrics, rural, etc.).

The division upholds APA bylaws and enacted its own divisional bylaws in 1980, which were subsequently revised to their current form in 2005. Over the years, SCN has provided published guidelines on many aspects of neuropsychological practice and training while also fostering continued development of the science of neuropsychology through activity of its committees. The division advances scientific knowledge in the field of neuropsychology through its support of publication and presentation of scientific papers at professional conferences, including the APA's annual convention.

Landmark Contributions

Psychologists interested in the developing field of neuropsychology began participating on a regular basis at APA meetings during the 1960s. The origins of SCN can be traced back to the development of the International Neuropsychological Society (INS), which is known as the field of neuropsychology's first formal organization. Informal meetings of psychologists interested in neuropsychological issues were held at the annual APA meeting dating back to 1965. The INS was formally organized in 1967 as an outgrowth of these meetings with the goal of serving as a scientific and educational organization. The need for formal representation in APA became increasingly apparent as professional issues regarding practice, education, and training in neuropsychology began to emerge. Leaders in the field, including Arthur Benton, Louis Costa, and Manfred Meier, saw the need for the development of an organization to promote the growing specialty of clinical neuropsychology that was independent of INS and APA's Division of Clinical Psychology (Division 12). The application to establish a Division of Clinical Neuropsychology was submitted to APA and approved by its Council of Representatives in September 1979. The formation of Division 40 was made effective in January 1980, consistent with APA procedures. The division's first President was Dr. Harold Goodglass with Dr. Gerald Goldstein serving as both the Secretary and Treasurer. The presidents of the division include many of the most prominent names in the field of neuropsychology (Table 1).

One of the division's earliest activities included working with the INS Task Force on Education, Accreditation, and Credentialing (TFEAC) in establishing guidelines for doctoral, internship, and postdoctoral training in clinical neuropsychology. Recommendations provided by that group, calling for a combination of training experiences in psychology and the neurosciences, continue as the field's dominant model of training. The INS Task Force was eventually discontinued as it became increasingly evident that professional issues were becoming the domain of Division 40. A listing of early

American Psychological Association (APA), Division 40, Table 1 The Society for Clinical Neuropsychology (SCN), Division 40 of the American Psychological Association (APA). Presidents of division, 1979–2017

1980s	1990s	2000s	2010s
1979–1980 Harold Goodglass	1989–1990 Charles G. Matthews	1999–2000 Gordon J. Chelune	2009–2010 Celiane M. Rey-Casserly
1980–1981 Harold Goodglass	1990–1991 Raymond S. Dean	2000–2001 Jason Brandt	2010–2011 H. Gerry Taylor
1981–1982 Louis Costa	1991–1992 Steven Mattis	2001–2002 Allan F. Mirsky	2011–2012 William B. Barr
1982–1983 Nelson M. Butters	1992–1993 Oscar Parsons	2002–2003 Antonio Puente	2012–2013 Munro Cullum
1983–1984 Thomas J. Boll	1993–1994 Robert K. Heaton	2003–2004 Kathleen J. Haaland	2013–2014 Paula K. Shear
1984–1985 Lawrence C. Hartledge	1994–1995 Carl Dodrill	2004–2005 Robert J. Ivnik	2014–2015 Neil Pliskin
1985–1986 Manfred J. Meier	1995–1996 Kenneth M. Adams	2005–2006 Russell M. Bauer	2015–2016 Jennifer Vasterling
1986–1987 Edith F. Kaplan	1996–1997 Eileen B. Fennell	2006–2007 Keith O. Yeates	2016–2017 Mark Bondi
1987–1988 Byron P. Rourke	1997–1998 Linas A. Bieliauskas	2007–2008 Thomas A. Hammeke	
1988–1989 Gerald Goldstein	1998–1999 Cecil R. Reynolds	2008–2009 Glenn E. Smith	

American Psychological Association (APA), Division 40, Table 2 Published guidelines and online toolkits from Division 40 committees and task forces

Year	Activity
1987	Guidelines for Doctoral Training Programs in Clinical Neuropsychology
1987	Task Force Report on Computer-Assisted Neuropsychological Evaluation
1988	Guidelines of Continuing Education in Clinical Neuropsychology
1989	Definition of a Clinical Neuropsychologist
1989	Guidelines Regarding the Use of Nondoctoral Personnel in Clinical Neuropsychological Assessment
1991	Recommendations for Education and Training of Nondoctoral Personnel in Clinical Neuropsychology
1991	Guidelines for Computer-Assisted Neuropsychological Rehabilitation and Cognitive Remediation
2013	Webkit for Interdisciplinary Health Service Psychology Trainees (www.wihpt.com)
2013	Health Care Reform and Neuropsychology Toolkit (https://iopc.online/practice-tools/)
2015	The Concussion Toolkit for Psychologists (www.ucdenver.edu/academics/colleges/medicalschool/departments/pmr/documents/concussion_toolkit/index.htm)

publications of other professional guidelines, statements, and online toolkits developed by Division 40 committees and task forces is provided in Table 2. The purpose of these guidelines was to facilitate an adherence to standards for professionals in the field of clinical neuropsychology with the ultimate goal of ensuring the quality of services provided to consumers.

There has been a more recent trend to publish online WebKits and toolboxes with other APA divisions and neuropsychology organizations. The division has also continued to publish position statements on a variety of topics in association with other neuropsychological organizations, including the National Academy of Neuropsychology (NAN) and the American Academy of Clinical Neuropsychology (AACN). The division, in collaboration with these organizations, became a member of the Inter Organizational Practice Committee (IOPC), which was developed in 2013 to coordinate advocacy efforts and improve the practice climate for neuropsychology as a profession.

During the 1990s, a task force from SCN led by Manfred Meier successfully submitted a petition for clinical neuropsychology to become the first psychological specialty recognized by the APA's Commission on Recognition of Specialties and Proficiencies in Professional Psychology (CRSPP). Recognition of clinical neuropsychology as a specialty became official in 1997. This was followed by a set of activities, working in conjunction with NAN, AACN, American Board of Clinical Neuropsychology, and the Association of Postdoctoral Programs in Clinical Neuropsychology (APPCN) in developing an integrated model for specialty training in clinical neuropsychology. Representatives from these organizations and various training programs across the USA met in 1997 for what was termed the Houston Conference on Specialty Training in Clinical Neuropsychology. The conference led to the development and publication of a document describing an integrated model of education and training. Interactions between SCN and these other groups continued through an organization called the Clinical Neuropsychology Synarchy (CNS). In 2013, the division joined other organizations in forming the Inter Organizational Practice Committee (IOPC), with the goal of joining forces to increase the breadth and reach of grassroots' advocacy for issues having local and national implications. The group published its 360 Degree Advocacy model in TCN and a Neuropsychology Toolkit for Healthcare Reform on its website (http://neuropsychologytoolkit.com).

Major Activities

Officers of SCN include President, President-Elect, Past President, Secretary, and Treasurer. These positions are elected by the general membership with the term of President lasting 1 year and the roles of Secretary and Treasurer lasting 3 years. The officers serve on an Executive Committee (EC) joined by various Division Committee Chairs, Divisional Representatives to APA Council, and three Members-at-Large. Meetings of the EC are held twice yearly, with one of the meetings held at the North American meeting of the INS in midwinter and the other coinciding with the APA convention in the summer. Presidents of the division preside at meetings and serve as the Chairperson of the EC. Terms of office begin and end at the completion of the annual business meeting held during the summer.

The division has four standing committees including Membership, Fellowship, Elections, and Program Committees and four continuing committees consisting of the Science Advisory, Education Advisory, Practice Advisory, and Public Interest Advisory Committees. Special Committees, including Task Force Committees, can also be established by vote of the Executive Committee, when the need arises. The Committee on APA Relations and the Publications and Communications Committee are examples of these. The President, in consultation with the EC, appoints chairs of all divisional committees and task forces. Summaries of divisional activities, minutes of executive committee meetings, and committee

reports are published biannually in *Newsletter 40*, the official division newsletter. Additional communications are provided electronically through the *SCN News*, *SCN NeuroBlog*, and the division's five LISTERVs.

Continued commitments to training and entry level members have been demonstrated by the formation of the Association for Neuropsychology Students in Training (ANST) and the establishment of an Early Career Psychologists committee. Committees and mentoring programs have been established for women entering the field and for ethnic minority members. Brochures describing an introduction to clinical neuropsychology are available through the division's Public Interest Advisory Committee (PIAC). The Practice Advisory Committee (PAC) provides monitoring of legislative activities and both local and national activities affecting the practice of clinical neuropsychology. This committee is also responsible for interactions with government agencies such as the Centers for Medicare and Medicaid Services (CMS). The PAC worked with other organizations in establishing a new set of CPT testing codes aimed at optimizing reimbursement for neuropsychological services. These codes were officially implemented in 2006.

The division has maintained its goal of integrating science and practice. The Science Advisory Committee (SAC) continues in its role of producing scientific programs for the APA's annual convention. Studies on neurologic syndromes, assessment, and developmental issues are among the topics most commonly presented in the SCN program at the annual APA meeting. The SAC also provides a number of awards for students and early career psychologists establishing careers in neuropsychological research. More recent SAC activities include integration of neuropsychology's scientific activities with APA and government agencies such as the National Institutes of Health (NIH).

SCN does not publish or provide an official journal. However, over the years, the division has maintained a close relationship with *The Clinical Neuropsychologist (TCN)*, a journal focusing on clinical issues relevant to neuropsychologists. The journal has published a number of statements and guidelines prepared by SCN task forces relevant to the practice of neuropsychology and abstracts from SCN's scientific program at APA. In 1989, *TCN* also began to publish regular listings of training programs in neuropsychology. In 2006, a user-interactive revision of the list was developed by the Education Advisory Committee (EAC) and transferred to the SCN website. The listing currently includes 40 doctoral training programs, 59 internships, and 114 sites offering postdoctoral residencies for specialty training in clinical neuropsychology. The website also includes descriptions of other divisional activities and links to the division's archival material.

Cross-References

▶ American Academy of Clinical Neuropsychology (AACN)
▶ American Board of Clinical Neuropsychology (ABCN)
▶ American Psychological Association (APA)
▶ Association for Postdoctoral Programs in Clinical Neuropsychology (APPCN)
▶ Houston Conference
▶ International Neuropsychological Society
▶ National Academy of Neuropsychology (NAN)

References and Readings

Adams, K. M., & Rourke, B. P. (Eds.). (1992). *The TCN guide to professional practice in clinical neuropsychology*. Berwyn: Swets & Zeitlinger.

Costa, L. (1998). Professionalization in neuropsychology: The early years. *The Clinical Neuropsychologist, 12*, 1–7.

Meier, M. J. (1992). Modern clinical neuropsychology in historical perspective. *American Psychologist, 47*, 550–558.

Meier, M. J. (2002). In search of knowledge and competence. In A. Y. Stringer, E. L. Cooley, & A.-L. Christensen (Eds.), *Pathways to prominence in neuropsychology: Reflections of twentieth century pioneers*. New York: Psychology Press.

Puente, A. E., & Marcotte, A. C. (2000). A history of Division 40 (clinical neuropsychology). In D. A. Dewsbury (Ed.), *Unification through division: Histories of the divisions of the American Psychological Association* (Vol. V). Washington, DC: American Psychological Association Press.

American Speech-Language-Hearing Association (ASHA)

Lemmietta McNeilly
Speech-Language Pathology, American Speech-Language-Hearing Association, Rockville, MD, USA

Membership

The American Speech-Language-Hearing Association is the national professional, scientific, and credentialing association for 191,500 members and affiliates who are audiologists, speech-language pathologists, and speech, language, and hearing scientists, audiology and speech-language pathology support personnel, and students.

Vision

Vision: Making effective communication, a human right, accessible and achievable for all.

Mission

Empowering and supporting audiologists, speech-language pathologists, and speech, language, and hearing scientists through:

- Advancing science
- Setting standards
- Fostering excellence in professional practice
- Advocating for members and those they serve

Landmark Contributions

ASHA has had several names during its more than 90-year history. The first was the American Academy of Speech Correction (1925). The current name, the American Speech-Language-Hearing Association (ASHA), was adopted in 1978.

ASHA is the nation's leading professional, credentialing, and scientific organization for speech-language pathologists, audiologists, and speech/language/hearing scientists. ASHA has been the guardian of these professions for over 85 years, initiating the development of national standards for each discipline and certifying professionals since 1952.

ASHA began in 1925 at an informal meeting of the National Association of Teachers of Speech (NATS) in Iowa City, IA, an organization of people working in the areas of rhetoric, debate, and theater. Robert W. West was the first president of the association from 1925 to 1928. Its members were becoming increasingly interested in speech correction and wanted to establish an organization to promote "scientific, organized work in the field of speech correction." Accordingly, in December of that year, the American Academy of Speech Correction – ASHA's original predecessor – was born.

ASHA has grown exponentially since its inception – from 25 members in 1925 to 191,500 in 2016. ASHA opened its first national office on January 1, 1958, in Washington, DC. The association subsequently moved four times, most recently settling in its current location in Rockville, MD, in 2008. ASHA's new national office is a LEED certified green building – the first nonprofit company's building of that distinction in Maryland.

Major Activities

Publications: *The ASHA Leader*; *American Journal of Audiology*; *American Journal of Speech-Language Pathology*; *Journal of Speech, Language, and Hearing Research*; *Language, Speech, and Hearing Services in Schools*; and *SIG Perspectives*.

Conferences: Annual convention and niche conferences addressing topics in healthcare and schools, as well as several web events annually.

References and Readings

American Speech-Language-Hearing Association. (2016). *Scope of practice in speech-language pathology* [Scope of practice]. Available from www.asha.org/policy/

American Speech-Language-Hearing Association. www.asha.org

American Speech-Language-Hearing Association Functional Assessment of Communication Skills for Adults

Diane Paul
Clinical Issues in Speech-Language Pathology, American Speech-Language-Hearing Association, Rockville, MD, USA

Synonyms

ASHA FACS

Description

The American Speech-Language-Hearing Association *Functional Assessment of Communication Skills for Adults* (ASHA FACS) was designed as a quick and easily administered measure of functional communication behaviors at the level of disability in adults with speech, language, and cognitive-communication impairments (Frattali et al. 1995; Frattali et al. 2017). The ASHA FACS uses the following definition of functional communication: "the ability to receive or to convey a message, regardless of the mode, to communicate effectively and independently in a given [natural] environment" (ASHA 1990, p. 2). The World Health Organization (WHO 2001) International Classification of Functioning, Disability and Health (ICF) provides the framework for functional assessment. The ICF consists of two components: functioning and disability (body functions/structures and activity/participation) and contextual factors (environmental and personal). The ASHA FACS assesses communication in the context of daily life activities. The ASHA FACS is based on direct observations by speech-language pathologists or significant others who are familiar with the client's typical communication performance across four assessment domains: social communication; communication of basic needs; reading, writing, and number concepts; and daily planning. Within each domain, specific functional behaviors are rated on a seven-point Scale of Communication Independence, which ranges from "does" the activity independently, through five levels of "does with" varying degrees of assistance, to "does not" perform the activity. A second scoring system, the Scale of Qualitative Dimensions of Communication, uses a five-point scale to rate adequacy, appropriateness, promptness, and communication sharing.

Assessment Domains

Table 1 shows the behaviors that are included within the four assessment domains. The measure yields domain and dimension mean scores,

American Speech-Language-Hearing Association Functional Assessment of Communication Skills for Adults, Table 1 ASHA FACS conceptual framework

Qualitative dimensions			
Adequacy	**Appropriateness**	**Promptness**	**Communication sharing**
Definitions			
Frequency with which client understands gist of message and gets point across	Frequency with which client's communication is relevant and done under the right circumstances	Frequency with which client responds without delay and in an efficient manner	Extent to which a client's communication poses a burden to the communication partner
Assessment domains			
Social communication	**Communication of basic needs**	**Readings/writing/ number concepts**	**Daily planning**
Behaviors			
Uses names of familiar people Expresses agreement/disagreement Explains how to do something Requests information Exchanges information on the telephone Answers yes/no questions Follows directions Understands facial expressions/tone of voice Understands nonliteral meaning and intent Understands conversations in noisy surroundings Understands TV/radio Participates in conversations Recognizes/corrects communication errors	Recognizes familiar faces/voices Makes strong likes/dislikes known Expresses feelings Requests help Makes needs/wants known Responds in an emergency	Understands simple signs Uses references materials Follows written directions Understands printed material Prints/writes/types name Completes forms Writes messages Understands signs with numbers Makes money transactions Understands units of measurement	Tells time Dials telephone numbers Keeps scheduled appointments Uses a calendar Follows a map

overall scores, and profiles of both communication independence and qualitative dimensions.

The ASHA FACS includes:

A revised manual (Frattali et al. 2017) detailing the project rationale, review of functional communication measures, description and validation data, and administration and scoring procedures

A score summary and profile forms

A case example

A pull-out rating key with the Scale of Communication Independence and the Scale of Qualitative Dimensions of Communication

Historical Background

The ASHA FACS evolved from the wave of healthcare accountability and the widespread need for an effective instrument to measure the functional communication of adults who have speech, language, or cognitive impairments for purposes of justifying payment, defining service eligibility, and judging the value of care. Developed in 1995 by ASHA, it reflects the collaborative effort of more than 70 individuals, both ASHA members and related professionals. The ASHA FACS was supported in part by the U.S. Department of Education/National Institute on Disability and Rehabilitation Research (NIDRR) and the U.S. Department of Veterans Affairs. The Psychological Corporation provided expert advice and data analysis.

The ASHA FACS originally was validated on adults with aphasia following left hemisphere stroke and adults with traumatic brain injury (TBI). The original validation study was conducted primarily with African American and White adults with these communication impairments. ASHA conducted further validation testing from 1998 to 2003 with other racial/ethnic groups and patient populations and created an addendum to the ASHA FACS (Paul et al. 2004a). The research was supported in part by NIDRR. A revised manual includes the validation data from the addendum (Frattali et al. 2017).

Psychometric Data

The usability, sensitivity, reliability, and validity of the ASHA FACS were demonstrated through two separate pilot tests and one field test. The first version was piloted to determine the measure's usability, resulting in the development of a seven-point observational rating scale. A second pilot test confirmed the usability of the revised version, and acceptable levels of reliability and validity were found. A more sensitive scoring system for capturing qualitative information about the nature of a client's functional communication led to the addition of a second scoring feature, a five-point rating scale of qualitative dimensions.

To establish interrater reliability during the field test, the ASHA FACS was completed independently for 35 subjects by two examiners within a 48-h period after a minimum of three subject-examiner contacts. Interrater reliability correlations on the four assessment domain scores ranged from 0.88 to 0.92. Overall communication independence scores had high interrater agreement (mean correlation = 0.95). Interrater consistencies of the four qualitative dimension mean scores ranged from 0.72 to 0.84. The interrater reliability of overall qualitative dimension mean scores was 0.88. Intrarater reliability (38 subjects) for communication independence mean scores by assessment domain ranged from 0.95 to 0.99 and intrarater reliability of overall communication independence scores was 0.99. Intrarater reliability of qualitative dimension mean scores ranged from 0.94 to 0.99 and 0.99 for the overall qualitative dimension scores.

The ASHA FACS was moderately correlated with other measures of language and cognitive function as demonstrated by external criterion measures used with subjects with aphasia and cognitive-communication impairments from TBI. For subjects with aphasia, a correlation of 0.73 was obtained between the Western Aphasia Battery (WAB) Aphasia Quotient (AQ) (Kertesz 1982), and the ASHA FACS overall communication independence score. Correlations were obtained between ASHA FACS domain scores and WAB subtest scores, with a range of .038 to

0.81. Correlations between the ASHA FACS domain score and overall score and each of the Functional Independence Measure (FIM) scales (FIM 4.0; SUNY at Buffalo Research Foundation 1993) ranged from 0.61 to 0.83. For the subjects with aphasia, correlations also were computed between ASHA FACS qualitative ratings and external criterion measures, the WAB and the FIM. These results indicated moderate correlations. External validation data for the subjects with cognitive-communication impairments ranged from 0.66 to 0.78 between the Scales of Cognitive Ability for Traumatic Brain Injury (SCATBI) (Adamovich and Henderson 1992) severity scores and the ASHA FACS domain scores and a 0.78 correlation between the ASHA FACS overall domain score with the SCATBI severity scores. Correlations ranging from 0.72 to 0.86 were found between ASHA FACS overall mean communication independence scores and FIM scores for subjects with cognitive-communication impairments. Moderate correlations also were found between ASHA FACS qualitative ratings and the SCATBI and the FIM for this subject group.

High internal consistency and social validity were reported. Internal consistency indicated that most item scores covered the full seven-point communication independence rating scale, showed high inter-item correlations between items within assessment domains, were internally consistent with respect to assessment domain, and that all items were measuring the same underlying construct. The data indicated that all domain scores correlated with overall ASHA FACS scores. Evaluation of social validity was accomplished by correlating overall ASHA FACS scores with measures scored by family members or friends of subjects. These measures included the Communicative Effectiveness Index (CETI; Lomas et al. 1989) and a rating of overall communication effectiveness, a single overall index of each subjects' communication effectiveness rated on a scale from 1 (lowest) to 7 (highest). These data indicated high positive correlations between ASHA FACS overall scores and ratings of overall communication effectiveness by clinicians (i.e., $r = 0.81$). The ASHA FACS overall

scores did not correlate well with family members' or friends' ratings of overall communication effectiveness or CETI scores. CETI ratings were consistently higher than those measured using the ASHA FACS.

Clinical Uses

The ASHA FACS was designed for clinicians to rate functional communication behaviors of adults with speech, language, and cognitive-communication impairments resulting from left hemisphere stroke and from TBI. In a review of the evidence leading to recommended best practices for assessment of individuals with cognitive-communication impairments after TBI, the ASHA FACS was one of a few standardized, norm-referenced tests that met most established criteria for validity and reliability for use with this clinical population (Turkstra et al. 2005). It was one of only four of the 31 tests reviewed that evaluated performance outside clinical settings. It was unique in that it was based on research about daily communication needs in the target population and incorporated consumer feedback about ecological validity into the design. The research is rich in the many clinical benefits of the ASHA FACS. For example, this instrument has been used to measure communication disability relative to quality of life in adults with chronic aphasia (Ross and Wertz 2002; Davidson et al. 2003), to evaluate the effectiveness of functionally based communication therapy (Worrall and Yiu 2000), and to evaluate real-life outcomes of aphasia interventions (Kagan et al. 2008). Using Rasch analysis of the ASHA FACS Social Communication Subtest (SCS), Donovan et al. (2006) demonstrated that caregivers were reliable respondents who could use the SCS to rate therapy progress and functional outcomes.

Additional research (Paul et al. 2004a) demonstrated that the ASHA FACS is a reliable and valid measure of functional communication for African American, Hispanic, and White adults with cognitive-communication impairments resulting from right hemisphere stroke or dementia. Validity could not be determined for Asian Americans and Native Americans due to the small sample size. Further research is needed to determine the validity of the ASHA FACS for adults with dysarthria.

ASHA established an international advisory group to determine the validity, reliability, and usability of the ASHA FACS in other English-speaking countries (Australia, Canada, Ireland, New Zealand, South Africa, England, and Scotland). Generally, the ASHA FACS was considered to be appropriate for use in these other countries with adults with aphasia or TBI. Certain test items were not relevant across groups, and there were difficulties in administration in countries where multiple primary languages are used. A Portuguese version was found to be valid and reliable for adults with mild or moderate Alzheimer's disease (de Carvalho and Mansur 2008). There continues to be broad interest in functional communication assessment for populations with communication impairments.

The ASHA FACS should be used as part of a comprehensive communication assessment, in conjunction with measures of impairment and quality of life. Treatment decisions should not be made on the basis of a single instrument. The ASHA Quality of Communication Life Scale (QCL) may be used to assess the impact of communication impairment on an adult's participation in social, leisure, work, and education activities (Paul et al. 2004b).

References

Adamovich, B., & Henderson, J. (1992). *Scales of cognitive ability for traumatic brain injury*. Chicago: Riverside.

American Speech-Language-Hearing Association. (1990). *Advisory report, functional communication measures project*. Rockville: Author.

de Carvalho, I. A. M., & Mansur, L. L. (2008). Validation of ASHA FACS-functional assessment of communication skills for Alzheimer disease population. *Alzheimer Disease & Associated Disorders, 22*(4), 375–381.

Davidson, B., Worrall, L., & Hickson, L. (2003). Identifying the communication activities of older people with aphasia: Evidence from naturalistic observation. *Aphasiology, 17*(3), 243–264.

Donovan, N. J., Rosenbek, J. C., Ketterson, T. U., & Velozo, C. A. (2006). Adding meaning to measurement: Initial Rasch analysis of the ASHA FACS social communication subtest. *Aphasiology, 20*(2–4), 362–373.

Frattali, C. M., Thompson, C. K., Holland, A. L., Wohl, C. B., & Ferketic, M. M. (1995). *American Speech-Language-Hearing Association Functional Assessment of Communication Skills for adults (ASHA FACS)*. Rockville: ASHA.

Frattali, C. M., Thompson, C. K., Holland, A. L., Wohl, C. B., Wenck, C. J., Slater, S. C., & Paul, D. (2017). *American Speech-Language-Hearing Association Functional Assessment of Communication Skills for adults (ASHA FACS)*. Rockville: ASHA.

Kagan, A., Simmons-Mackie, N., Rowland, A., Huijbregts, M., Shumway, E., McEwen, S., Threats, T., & Sharp, S. (2008). Counting what counts: A framework for capturing real-life outcomes of aphasia intervention. *Aphasiology, 22*(3), 258–280.

Kertesz, A. (1982). *Western aphasia battery*. New York: Grune & Stratton.

Lomas, J., Pickard, L., Bester, S., Elbard, H., Finlayson, A., & Zoghaib, C. (1989). The communicative effectiveness index: Development and psychometric evaluation of a functional communication measure for adults. *Journal of Speech and Hearing Disorders, 54*, 113–124.

Paul, D., Frattali, C. M., Holland, A. L., Thompson, C. K., & Slater, S. C. (2004a). *American Speech-Language-Hearing Association Functional Assessment of Communication Skills for adults: Addendum*. Rockville: ASHA.

Paul, D., Frattali, C. M., Holland, A. L., Thompson, C. K., Caperton, C. J., & Slater, S. C. (2004b). *Quality of communication life scale*. Rockville: ASHA.

Ross, K. B., & Wertz, R. T. (2002). Relationships between language-based disability and quality of life in chronically aphasic adults. *Aphasiology, 16*(8), 791–800.

State University of New York at Buffalo Research Foundation. (1993). *Guide for use of the uniform data set for medical rehabilitation: Functional Independence Measure*. Buffalo: Author.

Turkstra, L. S., Coelho, C., & Ylvisaker, M. (2005). The use of standardized tests for individuals with cognitive-communication disorders. *Seminars in Speech and Language, 26*(4), 215–222.

World Health Organization. (2001). *International classification of functioning, disability and health*. Geneva: Author.

Worrall, L., & Yiu, E. (2000). Effectiveness of functional communication therapy by volunteers for people with aphasia following stroke. *Aphasiology, 14*(9), 911–924.

Readings

American Speech-Language-Hearing Association. (n.d.). *National outcomes measurement system (NOMS)*. Available from www.asha.org/NOMS

Davidson, B., & Worrall, L. (2000). The assessment of activity limitation in functional communication: Challenges and choices. In L. E. Worrall & C. M. Frattali (Eds.), *Neurogenic communication disorders: A functional approach* (pp. 19–34). New York: Thieme.

Golper, L. C., & Frattali, C. M. (2012). *Outcomes in speech-language pathology: Contemporary theories, models, and practices* (2nd ed.). New York: Thieme.

Worrall, L., McCooey, R., Davidson, B., Larkins, B., & Hickson, L. (2002). The validity of functional assessments of communication and the activity/participation components of the ICIDH-2: Do they reflect what really happens in real-life? *Journal of Communication Disorders, 35*(2), 107–137.

Americans with Disabilities Act of 1990

Robert L. Heilbronner
Chicago Neuropsychology Group, Chicago, IL, USA

Historical Background

The Americans with Disabilities Act (ADA) was signed by President George Bush in 1990 and went into effect in 1992. It is regarded by many as the most sweeping civil rights legislation since the Civil Rights Act of 1964, with its intent to assist people with disabilities to obtain jobs and achieve the goal of full functioning in the workplace. The ADA contains provisions that outlaw discrimination against people with disabilities (including those with learning disabilities and mental disorders) in hiring, training, compensation, and benefits (Bell 1997) and mandates that employers provide "reasonable accommodations" for disabled workers who could qualify for jobs if such assistance is provided. It also protects individuals against retaliation for filing charges or otherwise being involved in an Equal Employment Opportunity Commission (EEOC)-related action. The act requires that people with disabilities be treated like nondisabled persons, unless it is determined that a certain individual's disability produces significant hindrances to one's involvement in a particular endeavor. It was established due to Congress's recognition of a large number of Americans with one or more disabilities and the discrimination experienced by such individuals with respect to employment and access to services.

Current Knowledge

The ADA includes several sections that cover different types of activities, most notably, employment (Title I), public services (Title II), public accommodations and services operated by private entities (Title III), access to telecommunications (Title IV), and miscellaneous provisions (Title V). Psychologists often conduct evaluations of disabled individuals to determine "reasonable accommodations" in accordance with the ADA. The most common referral involves Title 1, employment issues. The ADA requires that an evaluator assesses four distinct areas: (a) disability, (b) qualifications to perform an essential function of the job, (c) reasonable accommodations, and (d) threats to others. The "reasonable accommodations" are typically broken down by short-term accommodations as well as long-term accommodations.

References and Readings

Americans with Disabilities Act of 1990, 42 U.S.C. 12101–12213 et seq.

Bell, C. (1997). The Americans with Disabilities Act, mental disability and work. In R. Bonnie & J. Monahan (Eds.), *Mental disorder, mental disability and the law.* Chicago: University of Chicago Press.

Foote, W. M. (2003). Forensic evaluation in Americans with disabilities act cases. In A. Goldstein (Ed.), *Handbook of psychology (Vol. 11). Forensic psychology.* Hoboken: Wiley.

Melton, G. B., Petrila, J., Poythress, N. G., & Slobogin, C. (1997). *Psychological evaluations for the courts: A handbook for mental health professionals and lawyers.* New York: Guilford.

More detailed information regarding the Americans with Disabilities Act of 1990 can be found at www.ada.gov

Amitriptyline

Efrain Antonio Gonzalez
College of Psychology, Nova Southeastern
University, Fort Lauderdale, FL, USA
Utah State University, Logan, UT, USA

Generic Name

Amitriptyline

Brand Name

Elavil, Levate

Class

Tricyclic antidepressant

Proposed Mechanism(s) of Action

Increases available norepinephrine and serotonin, blocks serotonin reuptake, and may desensitize both serotonins 1A and beta adrenergic receptors.

Indication

Depression

Off-Label Use

Postherpetic neuralgia, neuropathic pain, fibromyalgia, headache, eating disorder, and insomnia.

Side Effects

Serious
Paralytic ileus, hyperthermia, lowered seizure threshold, sudden death, cardiac arrhythmias, tachycardia, QTc prolongation, hepatic failure, mania, and potential for activation of suicidal ideation.

Common
Blurred vision, constipation, urinary retention, increased appetite, dry mouth, diarrhea, heartburn, weight gain, fatigue, weakness, dizziness, anxiety, sexual dysfunction, sweating, rash, and itching.

References and Readings

Physicians' Desk Reference, (71st ed.). (2017). Montvale: Thomson PDR.
Stahl, S. M. (2007). *Essential psychopharmacology: The prescriber's guide* (2nd ed.). New York: Cambridge University Press.

Additional Information
Drug Interaction Effects. http://www.drugs.com/drug_interactions.html.
Drug Molecule Images. http://www.worldofmolecules.com/drugs/.
Free Drug Online and PDA Software. www.epocrates.com.
Free Drug Online and PDA Software. www.medscape.com.
Gene-Based Estimate of Drug interactions. http://mhc.daytondcs.com:8080/cgi   bin/ddiD4?ver=4&task=getDrugList.
Pill Identification. http://www.drugs.com/pill_identification.html.

Amnesia

Ginette Lafleche and Mieke Verfaellie
VA Boston Healthcare System, Memory
Disorders Research Center, Boston University
School of Medicine, Boston, MA, USA

Definition

Amnesia refers to the loss of ability to recall facts, events, or concepts encountered prior to the onset of illness (retrograde amnesia) or to the loss of the ability to form new memories (anterograde amnesia), or both. Although anterograde and retrograde amnesia can each occur in isolation, they frequently appear together following a single cause. The cause is commonly an organic neurologic insult or illness, but it can also be psychogenic. Although in most organic cases the memory loss is permanent, it can also be temporary, as for example in transient global amnesia.

Cross-References

► Anterograde Amnesia
► Memory Impairment
► Retrograde Amnesia
► Transient Global Amnesia

References and Readings

Baddeley, A. D., Kopelman, M. D., & Wilson, A. W. (2002). *The handbook of memory disorders*. Chichester: Wiley.

Amnestic Disorder

Beth Springate
Department of Psychiatry, University of Connecticut Health Center, Farmington, CT, USA

Short Description or Definition

Amnestic disorders are defined by a decline in explicit memory in the absence of other significant cognitive impairments and represent a deterioration from previous levels of function. The hallmark feature of classic amnestic disorders is anterograde amnesia (impairment in the ability to form new explicit memories), although retrograde amnesia (inability to remember previously learned information) can be seen, usually in a temporal gradient with recent memories affected more than earlier ones. This entry focuses on persistent, nonprogressive etiologies of amnestic disorders, excluding etiologies such as transient global amnesia, neurodegenerative conditions (e.g., Alzheimer's disease), and psychogenic amnesias.

Categorization

Amnestic disorders can result from a variety of causes, including hypoxic/anoxic events, infections, nutritional deficiencies, and lesions such as those occurring following stroke or surgical ablation, and are associated with damage to several brain regions. Two subtypes of amnestic disorders have received the most attention: bitemporal amnesia and diencephalic amnesia (e.g., Korsakoff's syndrome and patients with discrete thalamic or mammillary body lesions). A third subtype, basal forebrain amnesia, is viewed as clinically distinctive (Bauer et al. 2003).

Epidemiology

Amnestic disorders can be observed in several classes of patients, including following viral infections (e.g., herpes encephalitis), anoxic/hypoxic events (e.g., after heart attack or near-drowning, carbon monoxide exposure), nutritional impairments (e.g., Korsakoff's syndrome), bilateral temporal lobectomies, traumatic brain injury, and cerebrovascular events; epidemiological data are available by specific etiology, although pure global amnestic syndromes themselves are relatively rare. For example, herpes simplex encephalitis carries a 70% mortality rate without treatment. The cognitive impairments in survivors are ranging, and in one study of long-term survivors, 19 of 22 participants experienced some form of memory impairment, although only five subjects had memory difficulties that were categorized as severe (Utley et al.

1997). In a review of studies of cerebral anoxia, Caine and Watson (2000) concluded that while 54% of case studies describe memory impairments, only 19% report memory deficits in isolation.

Natural History, Prognostic Factors, and Outcomes

The amnestic disorder is exemplified by the case study of H.M., a patient who underwent a radical, experimental surgery in which the medial temporal lobes were removed bilaterally in an attempt to treat intractable epilepsy. His resection included the hippocampal formation and adjacent structures including most of the amygdala and parahippocampal gyrus, including the entorhinal cortex. Following surgery, H.M. developed severe anterograde amnesia which manifested as impaired episodic memory. In addition, he developed partial retrograde amnesia for events within 19 months before his surgery. However, earlier memories were unaffected, and his working memory and procedural memory (skill learning) also remained intact (Corkin 2002; Scoville and Milner 1957).

Course: Onset is often acute due to the nature of the pathological processes that cause amnestic disorders (e.g., cerebrovascular events, anoxic/hypoxic events, surgical ablation, and infections such as herpes encephalitis). Although some degree of improvement may occur in some patients, for example during the immediate period of natural recovery which occurs following cerebrovascular infarcts or traumatic injuries, deficits typically are persistent. Barring any additional injury, worsening of memory over time would not be anticipated.

General neuropsychological profile: Patients exhibit deficits in explicit memory marked by significant anterograde amnesia. They may also exhibit retrograde amnesia, although this is typically less severe and exhibits a temporal gradient with older memories less likely to be disturbed. Attention, working memory, procedural memory,

implicit learning, and general cognition remain largely intact.

Amnestic disorders resulting from bitemporal or diencephalic insults are the most frequently studied and similar in their neuropsychological profiles. Although early studies suggested that individuals with bitemporal amnesias have a more rapid forgetting rate, McKee and Squire (1992) found equivalent forgetting curves for pictures when severity of amnesia was controlled. Both subtypes of amnesia display a degree of retrograde amnesia (Kopelman et al. 1999). Bauer et al. (2003) argue that despite these similarities, some deficits are unique to patients with diencephalic amnestic disorders; although some studies suggest patients with Korsakoff's syndrome display a unique deficit in memory for temporal order (e.g., Squire 1982; Kopelman et al. 1999), others fail to support this finding (Downes et al. 2002).

Basal forebrain amnesia typically results from vascular lesions or aneurysm surgery in the region of the anterior communicating artery. After basal forebrain damage, patients may demonstrate extensive anterograde amnesia (Bottger et al. 1998; Tidswell et al. 1995). Confabulation is common and may relate to the extent of orbitofrontal involvement (Hashimoto et al. 2000), but it often subsides following the acute phase, while the amnestic state remains. There is evidence that patients with basal forebrain amnesia benefit from the presentation of cues to enhance recall (Osimani et al. 2006).

Evaluation

As amnestic disorders are defined by deficits in new learning, memory is the cognitive domain that should be emphasized within a comprehensive neuropsychological evaluation that also includes assessment of other areas of cognitive function such as orientation, attention, language, executive functions, visuospatial skills, and psychological functioning. Patients fitting the classic amnestic disorder profile will exhibit deficits in memory with generally intact cognition within other domains.

It is important to establish the specific nature of patients' memory impairments. Immediate memory span (typically assessed through tests such as Digit and Spatial Span from the Wechsler Memory Scales) should be within the normal range. Anterograde learning may be assessed with measures such as list learning, story learning, or figure memory. While patients will be able to retain items and repeat them back as long as they can keep them in memory, learning curves are typically flat, and an intervening distractor task will typically cause items to be lost completely. It is important to examine free recall vs. cued/recognition formats, as patients with frontally medicated amnestic disorders may show some benefit (typically no benefit seen for patients with bitemporal or diencephalic etiologies). Some degree of laterality to memory profiles may be expected depending on the nature of injury (e.g., left hemisphere damage leading to verbal memory impairments, right hemisphere damage impacting visual memory).

In addition, retrograde amnesia and memory for remote events can be examined in a qualitative manner by inquiring about autobiographical events or memories that one can assume to be present in most people from a given society (e.g., pictures of famous individuals, questions regarding salient historical events). The aspects of memory that remain intact in classic amnestic disorder patients (such as semantic memory and motor skill learning) could also be assessed.

The main differential diagnoses to consider include delirium and neurodegenerative dementias (e.g., Alzheimer's disease). Delirium is defined by a disturbance in attention and consciousness, both of which are intact in amnestic disorders. Although neurodegenerative dementias present similarly to amnestic disorders in that patients often present with memory impairments, cognitive decline (rather than stability) occurs and impairments in other cognitive domains such as language or executive functions are present.

Treatment

Treatment of amnestic disorders is nonspecific and focused primarily on compensation for memory impairments. Cognitive rehabilitation and memory training programs often emphasize the teaching of mnemonic strategies or the use of external memory aids such as note-taking or audiotaping in order to enhance patients' functioning in daily life, although patients would consciously need to recall learning these strategies and to utilize them. Implicit training procedures, such as those involving errorless learning strategies, can be helpful, as are environmental supports (e.g., electronic reminders) and assistance from family, friends, and/or caregivers.

The use of pharmacologic agents to treat amnestic disorders is not well studied, and large randomized controlled trials are lacking. In an open-label pilot study, Benke et al. (2005) administered donepezil, a cholinesterase inhibitor, to patients with a chronic amnestic syndrome from a ruptured and repaired aneurysm of the anterior communicating, anterior cerebral, or pericallosal artery. Some measures of performance on a list-learning task improved significantly during the 12-week medication administration period, suggesting future double-blind controlled studies would be useful to more thoroughly examine the potential utility of cholinergic medications. Studies have also examined the use of cholinesterase inhibitors following traumatic brain injury; a recent review (Bengtsson and Godbolt 2016) found only three studies meeting somewhat relaxed inclusion criteria (no studies located using their initial inclusion criteria). One study found no effect of treatment, and two studies showed limited effects. Given that included studies had several methodological limitations, further studies are needed to examine whether acetylcholinesterase inhibitors may be beneficial in this population.

In addition, due to their memory impairment, patients are likely to experience impairments in their social and vocational activities and may also require supervision and/or support in their living environment and a guardian or conservator to assist with legal and medical concerns in more severe cases.

Cross-References

▶ Amnesia
▶ Amnestic Syndromes
▶ Dissociative Amnesia
▶ Korsakoff's Syndrome
▶ Temporal Lobectomy

References and Readings

Bauer, R. M., Grande, L., & Valenstein, E. (2003). Amnesic disorders. In K. M. Heilman & E. Valenstein (Eds.), *Clinical neuropsychology* (pp. 495–573). New York: Oxford University Press.

Bengtsson, M., & Godbolt, A. K. (2016). Effects of acetylcholinesterase inhibitors on cognitive function in patients with chronic traumatic brain injury: A systematic review. *Journal of Rehabilitation Medicine, 5,* 1–5.

Benke, T., Köylü, B., Delazer, M., Trinka, E., & Kemmler, G. (2005). Cholinergic treatment of amnesia following basal forebrain lesion due to aneurysm rupture – An open-label pilot study. *European Journal of Neurology, 12,* 791–796.

Bottger, S., Prosiegel, M., Steiger, H., & Yassouridis, A. (1998). Neurobehavioral disturbances, rehabilitation outcome, and lesion site in patients after rupture and repair of anterior communicating artery aneurysm. *Journal of Neurology, Neurosurgery, and Psychiatry, 65,* 93–102.

Caine, D., & Watson, J. D. G. (2000). Neuropsychological and neuropathological sequelae of cerebral anoxia: A critical review. *Journal of the International Neuropsychological Society, 6,* 86–99.

Corkin, S. (2002). What's new with the amnesic patient H. M.? *Nature Reviews: Neuroscience, 3,* 153–160.

Downes, J. J., Mayes, A. R., MacDonald, C., & Hunkin, N. M. (2002). Temporal order memory in patients with Korsakoff's syndrome and medial temporal amnesia. *Neuropsychologia, 40,* 853–861.

Hashimoto, R., Tanaka, Y., & Nakano, I. (2000). Amnesic confabulatory syndrome after focal basal forebrain damage. *Neurology, 54,* 978–980.

Kopelman, M. D., Stanhope, N., & Kingsley, D. (1999). Retrograde amnesia in patients with diencephalic, temporal lobe or frontal lesions. *Neuropsychologia, 37,* 939–958.

McKee, R. D., & Squire, L. R. (1992). Both hippocampal and diencephalic amnesia result in normal forgetting

for complex visual material. *Journal of Clinical and Experimental Neuropsychology, 14,* 103.

Osimani, A., Vakil, E., Blinder, G., Sobel, R., & Abarbanel, J. M. (2006). Basal forebrain amnesia: A case study. *Cognitive and Behavioral Neurology, 19,* 65–70.

Scoville, W. B., & Milner, B. (1957). Loss of recent memory after bilateral hippocampal lesions. *Journal of Neurology, Neurosurgery, and Psychiatry, 20,* 11–21.

Squire, L. R. (1982). Comparisons between forms of amnesia: Some deficits are unique to Korsakoff's syndrome. *Journal of Experimental Psychology: Learning, Memory, and Cogntion, 8,* 560–571.

Tidswell, P., Dias, P. S., Sagar, H. J., Mayes, A. R., & Battersby, R. D. E. (1995). Cognitive outcome after aneurysm rupture: Relationship to aneurysm site and perioperative complications. *Neurology, 45,* 875–882.

Utley, T. F. M., Ogden, J. A., Gibb, A., McGrath, N., & Anderson, N. E. (1997). The long-term neuropsychological outcome of herpes simplex encephalitis in a series of unselected survivors. *Neuropsychiatry, Neuropsychology, and Behavioral Neurology, 10,* 180–189.

Amnestic Syndromes

Ginette Lafleche and Mieke Verfaellie
Memory Disorders Research Center, VA Boston Healthcare System and Boston University School of Medicine, Boston, MA, USA

Short Description or Definition

The amnestic syndromes are a group of neurologic disorders characterized by a dense global amnesia. This amnesia is comprised of an inability to form new memories (anterograde amnesia) and an inability to retrieve old memories (retrograde amnesia) (Anterograde Amnesia and Retrograde Amnesia). A unique feature of these disorders is that the dense memory loss occurs within the context of relatively preserved intelligence, language, attention, and perceptual abilities.

Categorization

The amnestic syndromes can be classified according to cause or site of damage. Possible etiologies include herpes simplex encephalitis, anoxia, Wernicke-Korsakoff syndrome, cerebrovascular accidents, anterior communicating artery aneurysm (ACoA), and tumors. These disorders can give rise to amnesia by damaging any of an array of structures, such as the medial temporal lobes (including the hippocampus), the midline diencephalic nuclei, and the basal forebrain, or by disrupting some of their interconnections such as the fornix. In such cases, the resulting amnestic syndrome tends to be permanent because the structural damage to the brain is irreversible. However, amnesia can also be transient when it is due to a functional disruption of these brain structures (see Transient Global Amnesia) or psychogenic causes.

Neuropsychology of the Amnestic Syndromes

Herpes Simplex Encephalitis (HSE)

HSE is a viral infection of the brain that begins as a flu-like illness with headaches and fever, followed by lethargy, confusion, and disorientation. If treatment is delayed, severe neurological deficits, including amnesia, agnosia (loss of the ability to recognize sensory impressions such as objects, people, and sounds), and aphasia (loss of aspects of speech production or reception) can develop. Recovery varies even with treatment, and many are left with a broad range of cognitive deficits. For a few, an isolated amnestic syndrome persists. Their presentation is similar to that of the well-known amnesic patient HM who became unable to form new memories after undergoing a neurosurgical operation in which a large portion of the medial temporal lobe of his brain was removed bilaterally.

Neuropathologically, the virus preferentially affects limbic regions in the temporal lobe, including the hippocampus and adjacent medial temporal lobe regions, as well as the amygdala and polar limbic cortices. Damage often extends to the lateral aspect of the temporal lobe, affecting the anterolateral aspect, the inferior aspect, or both. Anterior extension of damage into ventromedial areas of the brain, such as the insular cortex and the basal forebrain, has also been documented.

The severity of memory impairment following HSE shows substantial variation that is directly proportional to the extent of medial temporal lobe damage (Stefanacci et al. 2000). Lesions are often asymmetrical, and this will define the clinical presentation. If damage to the left medial temporal region is greater, verbal memory problems dominate, whereas if right medial temporal damage is greater, nonverbal aspects of memory, such as memory for faces and designs, are predominantly impaired.

In addition to an inability to acquire new information (anterograde amnesia), patients also have difficulty remembering events that occurred prior to their illness (retrograde amnesia). Retrograde amnesia can vary considerably in severity but is particularly marked when lesions extend into lateral temporal regions. Impairments in episodic memory, which is memory for specific events of your life, for example, remembering your college graduation, are the primary complaint. Semantic memory, which is memory for non-personal facts, such as remembering that Paris is the capital of France, may be more or less affected depending on the damage. Damage primarily to right anterior temporal regions is more likely to result in extensive loss of personal (i.e., episodic) memories (O'Connor et al. 1992) while damage to the left temporal cortex is associated with the loss of general world knowledge (i.e., semantic memory) (DeRenzi et al. 1987). Unusual selective impairments can also occur, such as the ability to identify inanimate objects but not living things or foods and the ability to comprehend concrete but not abstract words (Warrington and Shallice 1984).

Anoxia

Anoxic brain injury can result from any of a number of diverse etiologies including cardiac arrest, respiratory distress, carbon monoxide poisoning, and drug overdose. These conditions all diminish or cut off the supply of oxygen to the brain, either through reduced blood flow or reduced blood oxygen saturation. The physiological consequences of such anoxic events are complex. Brain areas particularly vulnerable to anoxic injury include the hippocampus, the basal ganglia, and other areas where the distributions of the cerebral arteries overlap in the cerebral cortex. The clinical manifestations of anoxia are highly variable, but memory impairment is a common symptom. A review of 58 studies of cerebral anoxia showed that while damage to hippocampal structures was common, damage restricted to the hippocampus was seen in only 18% of patients (Caine and Watson 2000). Accordingly, in a majority of patients, memory impairment occurs in the context of more diffuse cognitive deficits with executive problems and motor dysfunction being particularly common (Alexander et al. 2011). In a minority of patients, the anoxic injury leads to an isolated amnesia, that is, a memory disorder in the absence of other neuropsychological impairments. In these cases, bilateral hippocampal damage is thought to underlie the amnesic syndrome (Di Paola et al. 2008). As with other forms of amnesia, the severity of the amnesia is proportional to the damage to the hippocampal formation (Zola-Morgan et al. 1986; Rempel-Clower et al. 1996). While anterograde memory impairment is typically accompanied by some degree of retrograde impairment, anterograde amnesia can occur in the absence of retrograde amnesia as evidenced by patient R.B. who exhibited bilateral damage that was limited to the hippocampus (Zola-Morgan et al. 1986).

Relatively selective amnesia has been documented in children and adolescents who experienced a hypoxic-ischemic event at birth or shortly after birth (i.e., developmental amnesia: Vargha-Khadem et al. 1997). Gadian et al. (2000) reported on five cases, all of whom exhibited bilateral damage that was limited to the hippocampus. All had a profound inability to form new episodic memories, but strikingly, they were able to acquire a considerable amount of new factual knowledge, which allowed them to attend mainstream schools and maintain a relatively higher level of functioning compared to adult onset cases of amnesia described above. The relative preservation of semantic learning in these children has been ascribed to the integrity of medial temporal areas outside of the hippocampus. Research on developmental amnesia has provided additional support for the notion that the hippocampus itself is critical for episodic memory but not semantic memory.

Wernicke-Korsakoff Syndrome

See ► Wernicke-Korsakoff Syndrome entry.

Cerebrovascular Accidents

Bilateral posterior cerebral artery (PCA) infarction is a well-recognized cause of amnesia. Because the left and right PCA arise from the bifurcation of a common source, strokes that occur upstream from the bifurcation can affect the medial temporal lobes bilaterally, causing a dense amnesia with dysfunction in both anterograde and retrograde memory. Neuroanatomical studies of patients with PCA infarction have revealed that lesions in the posterior parahippocampus or the collateral isthmus (a pathway connecting the posterior parahippocampus to association cortex) are critical for the development of memory impairment (Von Cramon et al. 1988). When damage extends posteriorly to include occipitotemporal cortices, deficits beyond amnesia are often seen.

Early in their clinical course, patients with PCA infarction exhibit a confusional state that eventually resolves into an amnestic syndrome with or without additional neuropsychological symptoms involving primarily the processing of visual information. The memory disturbance is characterized by a classic profile of consolidation deficits in the context of normal short-term memory and normal intelligence. There may or may not be associated retrograde amnesia. Memory problems have also been described with unilateral, usually left, PCA infarction. In such cases, the memory impairment can be transient or permanent and is typically limited to verbal material. Memory deficits in patients with right PCA infarction have been less well studied, in part because such examination is complicated by the perceptual problems that frequently accompany right PCA infarction.

Thalamic strokes can also lead to significant memory problems. Because the relevant thalamic centers are small and adjacent to one another, it is difficult to establish associations between site of damage and clinical deficits. A review by Van der

Werf et al. (2000) led to the conclusion that damage to the mammillothalamic tract (MTT) invariably causes anterograde amnesia and that no amnesia occurs in the absence of damage to the MTT. Medial dorsal thalamic lesions cause a memory disturbance that is mild in comparison to the severe amnesia that arises when the lesion extends to the MTT. Patients with thalamic amnesia exhibit executive dysfunction, increased sensitivity to interference, and variability in the persistence and extent of retrograde amnesia.

ACoA Aneurysm

Rupture of the ACoA can result in a memory disorder that ranges from mild to severe. The ACoA provides blood supply to the basal forebrain, the anterior cingulate, the anterior hypothalamus, the anterior columns of the fornix (an important neural pathway leading to and from the hippocampus), the anterior commissure, and the genu of the corpus callosum. The pathological consequences of a ruptured aneurysm may be a result of infarction directly, or secondary to subarachnoid hemorrhage, vasospasm, or hematoma formation. Because of the various neuropathological consequences, the clinical profiles associated with ACoA aneurysm are more variable than those seen with diencephalic or medial temporal lobe injuries, and the impairments are often more diffuse in nature (see DeLuca and Diamond 1995 *for review*).

The acute phase of recovery following rupture and repair of ACoA aneurysm is characterized by a severe confusional state and a marked attentional disorder. As the confusion resolves, memory problems become more apparent. These can vary from mild impairments to severe amnesia and can include a retrograde amnesia. Other symptoms, including executive dysfunction, confabulation, and poor insight, are likely to be part of the resulting clinical syndrome if the lesion extends to the medial frontal lobes. The clinical outcome of patients with more extensive lesions is typically worse than that of patients with lesions limited to the basal forebrain (Alexander et al. 1984).

The amnesia associated with ACoA aneurysm has a marked frontal dysexecutive component. Performance on recognition tests of memory is often better preserved than performance on recall tests, particularly following a delay with interference. This reflects a disruption of strategic retrieval processes that allow access to information stored in memory. Deficient strategic memory processes also contribute to poor encoding, and the use of organizational strategies during the learning phase can enhance patients' performance. A failure to monitor whether the outcome of a memory search led to the sought after information can lead to a high number of false alarms in recognition tests. In extreme cases, this can lead to impairment in recognition memory that exceeds that seen in recall. Other features linked to frontal dysfunction include impaired source memory, which refers to when, where, and how information was learned.

Evaluation

Although a primary focus of the assessment in amnesia is on memory function, it is important to assess other cognitive domains as well, including general intelligence, attention, executive functions, language, and visuospatial skills. This comprehensive approach is required to establish whether a patient presents with a pure amnestic syndrome or with memory impairment in the context of more pervasive cognitive difficulty. New learning abilities should be assessed using measures that include free recall (unassisted by the examiner), cued recall (with some guidance from the examiner), and recognition (deciding whether an item was or was not part of a learned list of items). Assessments should examine both immediate and delayed retention. Information derived from specific aspects of performance, such as the shape of the learning curve, the comparison of recall and recognition performance, and the impact of delay, all provide important pointers to the nature of the memory breakdown and will serve to inform remediation.

A variety of standardized tests are available to assess memory function, and the reader is referred to Lezak et al. (2004) for specific examples. The most commonly used standardized memory test is the Wechsler Memory Scale-III or IV, which consists of a series of subtests that probe various aspects of verbal and nonverbal memory in different formats. The assessment of retrograde memory should cover knowledge of public events and people, personal facts, and autobiographical events. With respect to public knowledge, areas of assessment include the knowledge of famous names and faces, public news events, and new vocabulary that has recently entered the language. The assessment of personal facts and events can be challenging, because there are few standardized measures available, and corroboration from a caregiver may be needed to establish the accuracy of reported personal memories.

Treatment

There is no pharmacological or cognitive treatment that can restore memory in organic amnesia. However, cognitive rehabilitation approaches have been developed that aim to foster routines and habits that will increase independence, productivity, and quality of life. The choice of rehabilitation approach should be informed by both cognitive and psychosocial/emotional factors. Cognitive factors include premorbid skills and abilities and current neuropsychological functioning. A clear delineation of impaired and preserved aspects of memory is critical to guide rehabilitation efforts, as is the identification of other areas of cognitive impairment that might hamper therapeutic efforts. Of the psychosocial/emotional factors, insight and motivation are perhaps the two most influential predictors of rehabilitation success. Patients need to have some awareness of their deficits and have some degree of internal drive to understand the value of, and engage in, the rehabilitation process.

Several approaches have been developed to help patients with severe memory impairment learn new information. These approaches take advantage of preserved non-declarative (i.e., implicit) memory abilities to help amnesic patients acquire new information or skills. One approach that capitalizes on preserved implicit perceptual memory is the vanishing cues technique (Glisky et al. 1986). Patients are guided to provide the correct information in response to

perceptual cues, through the use of implicit memory. Once successful, cues are gradually reduced, eventually leading to the spontaneous generation of the to-be-learned information. This technique has proven successful for learning new vocabulary and concepts. A caveat, however, is that such learning is a slow and laborious, and the information learned is typically inflexible and only accessible in the exact form in which it was learned. An important consideration in the use of implicit memory techniques is the avoidance of errors, as patients have no recollection of their mistakes, and consequently, errors, just like correct responses, can be strengthened. Other methods capitalize on preserved procedural learning and use repetition to teach skills and habits that support activities of daily living. Examples of external compensatory aids that rely on procedural memory are the use of notebooks, diaries, and alarm clocks. Electronic devices such as computers, smartphones, and paging systems have great flexibility as compensatory aids, but training in the use of such technology requires very lengthy practice sessions, and transfer of learning outside of the training sessions can be difficult. Such training is therefore more appropriate for individuals who have had premorbid experience with such devices and are highly motivated to use them.

For individuals with milder memory impairments, it may also be possible to directly focus on enhancing impaired forms of memory through the use of internal strategies. The choice of strategy will be dependent on the nature of the memory process that appears defective. Examples of such techniques include enhanced organization of the to-be-learned information through chunking (i.e., breaking down or grouping information in short-term memory to make it more manageable) or through categorization and elaboration of the material, whether through verbal associations or the creation of visual images. Such strategies fall under the category of internal memory aids.

There are no specific methods of treatment available to restore memories from the past. Information and pictures about one's life, such as places where one has resided, can be reintroduced and incorporated into the selected treatment approach. However, emotionally laden facts, such as the death of a family member, can trigger repeated emotional responses that can interfere with adjustment and are best avoided in the early stage of treatment. By nature, relearned personal information about one's life will be recalled without the emotional texture of the original event; however, it can play an important role in helping patients fill in the narrative of their own life.

Cross-References

► Anterograde Amnesia
► Retrograde Amnesia
► Transient Global Amnesia

References and Readings

Alexander, M. P., & Freedman, M. (1984). Amnesia after anterior communicating artery aneurysm rupture. *Neurology, 34*(6), 5–11.

Alexander, M. P., Lafleche, G., Schnyer, D., Lim, C., & Verfaellie, M. (2011). Cognitive and functional recovery after out of hospital cardiac arrest. *Journal of the International Neuropsychological Society, 17*, 1–5.

Caine, D., & Watson, J. D. G. (2000). Neurospsychological and neuropathological sequelae of cerebral anoxia: A critical review. *Journal of the International Neuropsychological Society, 6*, 86–99.

DeLuca, J., & Diamond, B. J. (1995). Aneurysm of the anterior communicating artery: A review of neuroanatomical and neuropsychological sequelae. *Journal of Clinical and Experimental Neuropsychology, 17*, 100–121.

DeRenzi, E., Liotti, M., & Nichelli, P. (1987). Semantic amnesia with preservation of autobiographical memory: A case report. *Cortex, 23*, 578–597.

Di Paola, M., Caltagirone, C., Fadda, L., Sabatini, U., Serra, L., & Carlesimo, G. A. (2008). Hippocampal atrophy is the critical brain change in patients with hypoxic amnesia. *Hippocampus, 18*(7), 719–728.

Gadian, D. G., Aiardi, J., Watkins, K. E., Porter, D. A., Mishkin, M., & Vargha-Khadem, F. (2000). Developmental amnesia associated with early hypoxic-ischaemic injury. *Brain, 123*, 499–507.

Glisky, E. L., Schacter, D. L., & Tulving, E. (1986). Learning and retention of computer-related vocabulary in memory-induced patients: Method of vanishing cues. *Journal of Clinic Journal of Clinical and Experimental Neuropsychology, 8*, 292–312.

Lezak, M. D., Howieson, D. B., & Loring, D. W. (2004). *Neuropsychological assessment*. New York: Oxford University Press.

O'Connor, M. G., Butters, N., Miliotis, P., Eslinger, P., & Cermak, L. S. (1992). The dissociation of anterograde and retrograde amnesia in a patient with herpes simplex encephalitis. *Journal of Clinical and Experimental Neuropsychology, 14*, 159–178.

Rempel-Clower, N. L., Zola, S. M., Squire, L. R., & Amaral, D. (1996). Three cases of enduring memory impairment after damage limited to the hippocampal formation. *The Journal of Neuroscience, 16*(16), 5233–5255.

Stefanacci, L., Buffalo, E. A., Schmolck, H., & Squire, L. R. (2000). Profound amnesia after damage to the medial temporal lobe: A neuroanatomical and neuropsychological profile of patient EP. *The Journal of Neuroscience, 20*, 7024–7036.

Van der Werf, Y. D., Witter, M. P., Uylings, H. B., & Jolles, J. (2000). Neuropsychology of infarctions in the thalamus: A review. *Neuropsychologia, 38*, 613–627.

Vargha-Khadem, F., Gadian, D. G., & Mishkin, M. (2001). Dissociations in cognitive memory: The syndrome of developmental amnesia. *Philosophical Transactions of the Royal Society of London B, 356*, 1435–1440.

Von Cramon, D., Hebel, N., & Schuri, U. (1988). Verbal memory and learning in unilateral posterior cerebral infarction. *Brain, 111*, 1061–1077.

Warrington, E. K., & Shallice, T. (1984). Category specific semantic impairments. *Brain, 107*, 829–854.

Zola-Morgan, S., Squire, L. R., & Amaral, D. G. (1986). Human amnesia and the medial temporal region: Enduring memory impairment following a bilateral lesion limited to field CA 1 of the hippocampus. *The Journal of Neuroscience, 6*(10), 2950–2967.

Amorphognosis

John E. Mendoza
Department of Psychiatry and Neuroscience, Tulane Medical School and SE Louisiana Veterans Healthcare System, New Orleans, LA, USA

Definition

Amorphognosis is that aspect of tactile agnosia which refers specifically to deficits in the ability to appreciate (identify) the external form of an object such as its shape, size, or other contour features by tactual manipulation alone. In the absence of more elementary somatosensory disturbances resulting from either peripheral nerve or the dorsal column system, such deficits suggest lesions in the contralateral postcentral gyrus of the parietal lobe or in its adjacent association cortices.

Cross-References

► Ahylognosia
► Astereognosis
► Tactile Agnosia

References and Readings

Bauer, R. M., & Demery, J. A. (2003). Agnosia. In K. Heilman & E. Valenstein (Eds.), *Clinical neuropsychology* (4th ed., pp. 236–295). New York: Oxford University Press.
Hecaen, H., & Albert, M. L. (1978). Chapter 6. Disorders of somesthesis and somatognosis. In *Human neuropsychology*. New York: Wiley.

Amoxapine

Efrain Antonio Gonzalez
College of Psychology, Nova Southeastern University, Fort Lauderdale, FL, USA
Utah State University, Logan, UT, USA

Generic Name

Amoxapine

Brand Name

Ascendin

Class

Tetracyclic antidepressant

Proposed Mechanism(s) of Action

Amoxapine inhibits reuptake of norepinephrine and noradrenaline. It is also known to antagonize serotonin 2A receptors, thus increasing presynaptic release of amines. Mild dopamine 2 blockade.

Indication

Depression, reactive depressive disorder, psychotic depression, and depression accompanied by anxiety or agitation.

Off-Label Use

Depressive phase of a bipolar disorder, anxiety, insomnia, neuropathic pain, and treatment-resistant depression.

Side Effects

Serious
Paralytic ileus, hyperthermia, lowered seizure threshold, sudden death, cardiac arrhythmias, tachycardia, QTc prolongation, hepatic failure, intraocular pressure, mania, and potential for activation of suicidal ideation.

Common
Blurred vision, constipation, urinary retention, increased appetite, dry mouth, diarrhea, heartburn, weight gain, fatigue, weakness, dizziness, anxiety, sexual dysfunction, sweating, rash, and itching. Can cause extrapyramidal symptoms such as akathisia and potentially tardive dyskinesia.

References and Readings

Physicians' Desk Reference (71st ed.). (2017). Montvale: Thomson PDR.
Stahl, S. M. (2007). *Essential psychopharmacology: The prescriber's guide* (2nd ed.). New York: Cambridge University Press.

Additional Information
Drug Interaction Effects. http://www.drugs.com/drug_interactions.html.
Drug Molecule Images. http://www.worldofmolecules.com/drugs/.
Free Drug Online and PDA Software. www.epocrates.com.
Free Drug Online and PDA Software. www.medscape.com.
Gene-Based Estimate of Drug interactions. http://mhc.daytondcs.com: 8080/cgi bin/ddiD4?ver=4&task=getDrugList.
Pill Identification. http://www.drugs.com/pill_identification.html.

Amphetamine

Elizabeth K. Vernon[1] and JoAnn Tschanz[1,2]
[1]Department of Psychology, Utah State
University, Logan, UT, USA
[2]Center for Epidemiologic Studies, Utah State
University, Logan, UT, USA

Synonyms

Dexedrine; Dextro-amphetamine; d-amphetamine

Definition

Amphetamine refers to a group of synthetic chemicals with psychoactive stimulant effects. Amphetamines are similar in molecular structure to the catecholamine neurotransmitters, norepinephrine and dopamine. They compete with the endogenous monoamine (norepinephrine, dopamine, and serotonin) transporters to be transported into the nerve. Once inside the presynaptic terminal, amphetamine displaces the monoamines from the cytosolic pool, which reverses the direction of the reuptake transporter and thereby increases synaptic concentrations of monoamine neurotransmitters (Heal et al. 2014). There are two forms, dextro-amphetamine (d-amphetamine) and levo-amphetamine (l-amphetamine), of which d-amphetamine is the more active form. Chemical modifications to the basic structure have led to derivatives with even more potent psychoactive properties. For example, addition of a second methyl group to the chemical structure creates methamphetamine, a highly addictive drug. Modification of the benzene ring of the amphetamine structure creates methylenedioxymethamphetamine (MDMA) or ecstacy, another drug with high addiction and abuse potential (Iversen et al. 2009).

The behavioral effects of lower doses of amphetamine include increased alertness, confidence, euphoria, and well-being (Freberg 2014). The drug also reduces fatigue and enhances performance on cognitive tasks, possibly by increasing attention and working memory. However, cognition is reportedly enhanced only among those with poor baseline working memory ability, and even detrimental to those with high baseline ability (Iversen et al. 2009). At higher doses, the drugs produce symptoms similar to schizophrenia (hallucinations, thought disorder, flat affect, and anhedonia) (Freberg 2014). In animals, there is a dose-dependent effect of increasing activity such as locomotion or at higher doses, stereotyped motor behaviors. Amphetamine's reinforcing properties have been demonstrated in operant conditioning studies. The drug also increases both systolic and diastolic blood pressure and increases respiration and heart rate, among other sympathetic effects (Feldman et al. 1997). Amphetamine or its derivatives have been used for clinical purposes (see "Historical Background and Clinical Relevance"). However, its clinical use has been limited due to its abuse potential and dangerous sympathetic effects (Iversen et al. 2009).

At high doses, the drug also inhibits the metabolism of catecholamines by the enzyme monoamine oxidase. Chronic use has been associated with damage to selective dopamine neurons and receptors (Feldman et al. 1997). The derivative methamphetamine is also a potent neurotoxin, although unlike amphetamine, this drug predominantly affects the serotonergic system (Feldman et al. 1997). The reinforcing properties of amphetamine are hypothesized to reflect increased dopamine neurotransmission in the subcortical structure, the nucleus accumbens.

Historical Background and Clinical Relevance

First commercially introduced in 1930s as a nasal or bronchial decongestant, amphetamine was sought after for its psychoactive effects and as an appetite suppressant. One of amphetamines' first clinical uses was for the treatment of narcolepsy. By 1946 there were more than 30 uses for amphetamine, including schizophrenia, opiate addiction, infantile cerebral palsy, seasickness, radiation sickness, and persistent hiccups. At the beginning of the Spanish Civil War, amphetamine was used to promote military alertness (Sulzer et al. 2005). Amphetamine was then used in subsequent wars to enhance attention and fight the effects of sleep deprivation (Iversen et al. 2009; Meyer and Quenzer 2005). Early efforts to synthesize amphetamine on the basis of structure and function have resulted in trimethoxyamphetamine (TMA), which led to nearly 200 potentially hallucinogenic substituted amphetamines (Sulzer et al. 2005). Amphetamine and its derivatives have been used for the treatment of narcolepsy, attentional problems, and as a stimulant to combat fatigue and the need for sleep (Meyer and Quenzer 2005). In the 1930s, amphetamine was discovered to have beneficial effects for treating children with attention deficit/hyperactivity disorder (ADHD). Stimulants (e.g., methylphenidate) persist to this day as one of the most effective drugs available for treating the condition (Heal et al. 2013).

Over time, the addictive properties of amphetamine were realized, particularly of its potent derivatives. The acute effects of the drug could be enhanced by using a rapid route of administration such as an intravenous injection. Following the short-term "rush," however, is a period of restless agitation, depression, irritability, and other symptoms. Repeated, continuous administrations will ultimately lead to a let down, with a prolonged period of sleep. This alternating cycle is often repeated, resulting in a physical toll on the body. As with other drugs of abuse, dependence and tolerance can develop with chronic use, resulting in the administration of increasing doses to achieve the desired effects. With sustained chronic use, negative effects may emerge consisting of repetitive, stereotyped behaviors as well as a psychotic syndrome consisting of hallucinations and paranoid delusions. This syndrome, referred to as "amphetamine psychosis," was notably similar to the symptoms of paranoid schizophrenia and provided some support for the dopamine hypothesis of schizophrenia. However, qualitative differences between the two conditions were also noted (e.g., greater tendency for visual hallucinations in amphetamine psychosis

vs. schizophrenia; Iversen et al. 2009). Other negative effects of chronic amphetamine abuse include possible neurotoxic damage to the dopamine system with reduced numbers of transporters and receptors. Impairments in attention and memory have been reported with abuse, but their long-term persistence, particularly with abstinence, is unknown (Iversen et al. 2009).

Future Directions

Research into the psychoactive and behavioral effects of amphetamine has helped advance knowledge of the psychological role of several monoamine neurotransmitters and their relevance to several clinical conditions such as addiction and schizophrenia and the neurochemistry underlying some cognitive processes such as attention and working memory. Future research will undoubtedly utilize advances in technology to build on past research such as elucidating the neural structures and pathways associated with reward circuits, examining the neuroplasticity of the nervous system after chronic substance abuse, and clarifying the moderating role of genetics in the behavioral response to amphetamine and other compounds (Iversen et al. 2009).

References and Readings

Feldman, R. S., Meyer, J. S., & Quenzer, L. F. (1997). Stimulants: Amphetamine and Cocaine. In *Principles of neuropsychoparhmacology* (pp. 549–568). Sunderland: Sinauer Associates, Inc.

Freberg, L. (2014). *Discovering behavioral neuroscience* (pp. 107–108). Boston: Cenage Learning.

Heal, D. J., Smith, S. L., Gosden, J., & Nutt, D. J. (2013). Amphetamine, past and present – A pharmacological and clinical perspective. *Journal of Psychopharmacology (Oxford, England), 27*(6), 479–496. https://doi.org/10.1177/0269881113482532.

Iversen, L. L., Iversen, S. D., Bloom, F. E., & Roth, R. H. (2009). Psychostimulants. In *Introduction to Neuropsychopharmacology* (pp. 447–472). New York: Oxford University Press.

Meyer, J. S., & Quenzer, L. F. (2005). Psychomotor stimulants: Cocaine and the amphetamines. In *Psychopharmacoogy. Drugs, the brain and behavior* (pp. 292–300). Sunderland: Sinauer Associates, Inc.

Sulzer, D., Sonders, M. S., Poulsen, N. W., & Galli, A. (2005). Mechanisms of neurotransmitter release by amphetamines: A review. *Progress in Neurobiology, 75*(6), 406–433. https://doi.org/10.1016/j.pneurobio.2005.04.003.

Amusia

John E. Mendoza
Department of Psychiatry and Neuroscience, Tulane Medical School and SE Louisiana Veterans Healthcare System, New Orleans, LA, USA

Current Knowledge

"Music" involves both complex qualities such as familiar melodies, rhythm, or tempo, and more elementary aspects such as discrimination of timbre, pitch, or tone. While lesions of the temporal lobes are fairly consistently implicated, the hemispheric localization of lesions responsible for specific deficits has been more controversial. Music, like language, is composed of individual, temporally sequenced stimuli (musical notes, melodies, tunes), each capable of being analyzed with regard to particular features such as pitch and timbre, functions that would appear to be more in keeping with the suspected operations of the left hemisphere. By contrast, melodies may also be perceived as a gestalt, which is more characteristic of right hemisphere functions. There is evidence that well-trained musicians come to rely more heavily on the left hemisphere for processing certain aspects of music when compared with non-musicians. However, the right hemisphere evidences superiority for both the perception and expression of music in studies of non-musicians. Thus, the strategies by which various musical elements are approached, as well as the leading hemisphere in appreciating those elements, are most likely determined in part by one's prior musical experience or training. In summary, while both the right and left hemispheres are apparently involved in the expression and perception or appreciation of music, the specific contributions of each are still somewhat of a mystery.

Amygdala

Rory McQuiston
Anatomy and Neurobiology, Virginia Commonwealth University, Richmond, VA, USA

Synonyms

Amygdaloid body; Amygdaloid nucleus

Historical Background

The amygdala was originally described by Burdach in the late nineteenth century as an almond-shaped structure situated deep in the anterior temporal lobe of the central nervous system. The amygdala was subsequently shown to be important for the appropriate processing of emotional information in nonhuman primates by Kluver and Bucy in the 1930s. This permitted McLean to include the amygdala in the group of brain structures that make up the limbic system thought to be involved in processing of emotional information. Since then, progress has continued toward understanding the role that the amygdala plays in processing and encoding emotional information in the mammalian central nervous system.

Current Knowledge

The amygdala is an almond-shaped structure located in the medial temporal lobe of mammals. However, the first description of this almond-shaped structure only referred to a portion of the amygdala called the basal nucleus. Currently, the amygdala is described as a collection of different subnuclei or subareas, one of which is the basal nucleus. The nuclei have been grouped together based on their phylogenetic similarities or similarities in their neuronal elements. Older phylogenetic nuclei include the olfactory areas (i.e., cortical nucleus and nucleus of the olfactory tract) and the central and medial nuclei. More recent phylogenetic structures include areas similar to the neocortex such as the lateral, basal, and accessory basal nuclei, which are collectively referred to as the basolateral region or complex. Based on similarities in their neuronal components, various nuclei of the amygdala have been defined as neocortical-like nuclei (such as the basolateral complex) that consist of glutamatergic pyramidal-like neurons or striatal-like nuclei (such as the central and medial nuclei) that consist of GABAergic medium spiny neurons.

In humans, the amygdala is located under the uncus of the limbic lobe at the anterior end of the hippocampus. It also merges with the peri-amygdaloid cortex and abuts the putamen and tail of caudate nucleus. As a whole, the amygdala receives diverse inputs from throughout the central nervous system. The basolateral complex receives inputs encoding somatosensory, visual, auditory, gustatory, olfactory, and visceral information from the dorsal thalamus, prefrontal cortex, cingulate, parahippocampal gyrus, insular cortex, and sensory associational areas. The central and medial nuclei receive inputs from olfactory centers, hypothalamus (ventromedial and lateral), dorsomedial and medial nuclei of the thalamus, and visceral inputs from the parabrachial nuclei, solitary nucleus, and periaqueductal gray of the brainstem. Outputs from the amygdala are equally diverse. They leave via two predominant pathways. The central nucleus contributes to the stria terminalis where its efferents make connections with the hypothalamus (preoptic nuclei, ventromedial nucleus, anterior nucleus, and lateral hypothalamic areas), nucleus accumbens, septal nuclei, and rostral portions of the caudate and putamen. However, the primary output of the amygdala is the ventral amygdalofugal pathway. Through this pathway, the basolateral complex sends inputs to the hypothalamus, septal nuclei, substantia innominata, prefrontal, cingulate, insular, and inferior temporal cortices. Through the same pathway, the central nucleus projects diffusely in the brainstem innervating the dorsal vagus, raphe, locus coeruleus, parabrachial nuclei, and the periaqueductal gray. It is the interplay between the diverse afferents projecting to the amygdala, processing within the amygdala, and

the effect of the amygdala on its targets that contribute to the emotional assessment of incoming sensory information and coordinated behavioral responses.

Most of what is known about human amygdala function comes from studies of patients with damage to the amygdala. However, most damage in humans is not restricted to the amygdala alone, and patients with damage to larger areas of the medial temporal lobe have more profound deficits. Nonetheless, patients with temporal lobe damage including the amygdala display a number of emotional and inappropriate behavioral deficits. These include impaired fear responses, hypersexuality, hyperorality, and hyperattention. These behaviors were originally described by Kluver and Bucy in nonhuman primates.

Much of what is known about functional circuitry within the amygdala and how it relates to encoding of emotion has been gleaned from studies in rodents. The amygdala can be divided into many subareas based on functional circuitry. Lateral to the amygdala is the piriform cortex, which encodes olfactory information. Olfactory information from the piriform cortex, and other olfactory structures, projects to the most ventral and lateral portion of the amygdala, the cortical nuclei. The cortical nuclei in turn project medially to the ventrally located medial nuclei, which is a major output for olfactory information from the amygdala. However, less is known about the ventrally located olfactory-associated amygdala nuclei compared to the more dorsal multisensory nuclei. The more dorsal nuclei receive information from all sensory modalities. The major inputs to the amygdala innervate the lateral nuclei. The lateral nuclei are the most dorsally located within the amygdala, medial to the piriform cortex, and underneath the striatum. The lateral nuclei receive associational inputs encoding a single sensation (somatosensory, visual, auditory, gustatory, olfactory, or visceral). This is the first stage where sensory input is assigned emotional value and also where some emotional memories may be stored (however, the amygdala as a site for storing emotional memories remains a contentious issue). Although the lateral nuclei project to multiple areas within and outside the amygdala, a major output is the basal nuclei (located ventral to the lateral nuclei) where the initial sensory processing of the lateral nuclei is integrated with inputs from highly processed areas including polymodal sensory areas and areas involved in memory formation like the hippocampus. The lateral and basal nuclei project medially to the central nucleus either directly or indirectly through intercalated cells (intercalated cells separate the basolateral complex from the central and medial nuclei). The central nuclei send much of the processed emotional content from the amygdala to the rest of the brain. Thus, the central nucleus is seen as the output region of the amygdala. The central nucleus produces emotional responses through its effects on its various targets throughout the central nervous system. For example, the central nucleus produces arousal through its innervation of modulatory systems in the brain stem that release norepinephrine, dopamine, serotonin, and acetylcholine. Its input to the periaqueductal gray produces freezing, startle, analgesia, and cardiovascular changes associated with fear. It also innervates the parabrachial nucleus where it affects pain processing. Its inputs to the dorsal motor vagal nucleus controls parasympathetic nervous system function, and it also affects vagal nerve function through its projection to the solitary nucleus. Finally, the central nuclei projects to the hypothalamus where it controls the release of hormones and activates the sympathetic nervous system.

In summary, the amygdala is a complex group of nuclei that receive diverse inputs from various regions of the central nervous system to assess emotional value. Similarly, after extensive processing, its outputs innervate a diverse group of regions in the central nervous system to exert its effect. The result is that the amygdala is involved in encoding fear, reward, aggression, and sexual, maternal, and ingestive behaviors. This results in effects on cognition, attention, perception, and memory formation. Therefore, it is not surprising that amygdala dysfunction has been associated with anxiety disorders such as posttraumatic stress disorder, phobias and panic attacks, depression, and schizophrenia.

Future Directions

Most of what is known about emotional information processing performed by the amygdala has been gleaned from studies of fear conditioning. However, the amygdala also likely plays a role in the encoding of positive emotions associated with rewarding stimuli. Currently, efforts are being made toward understanding the different types of emotional values encoded in the amygdala. Also, it remains somewhat contentious whether emotional memory is actually stored by the amygdala. It is of great interest to determine where emotional memories are stored in the amygdala (possibly the lateral nuclei) and precisely what types of memories are being stored by the amygdala, that is, whether these memories are of conscious declarative forms or more procedural reflexive forms. Understanding how the amygdala contributes to the formation of different forms of emotional memory will likely provide insights for the treatment of several psychiatric illnesses such as posttraumatic stress disorder, phobias, anxiety, and depression.

Cross-References

▶ Efferent
▶ Insular Lobe
▶ Limbic System
▶ Locus Ceruleus
▶ Midbrain Raphe
▶ Neocortex
▶ Striatum
▶ Temporal Lobe

References and Readings

Ledoux, J. E. (2000). Emotion circuits in the brain. *Annual Review of Neuroscience, 23*, 155–184.
Ledoux, J. (2007). The amygdala. *Current Biology, 17*, 868–874.
Phelps, E. A., & Ledoux, J. E. (2005). Contributions of the amygdala to emotion processing: From animal models to human behavior. *Neuron, 48*, 175–187.
Sah, P., Faber, E. S., Lopez De Armentia, M., & Power, J. (2003). The Amygdaloid complex: Anatomy and physiology. *Physiological Reviews, 83*, 803–834.

Amyloid Plaques

Elizabeth K. Vernon[1] and JoAnn Tschanz[1,2]
[1]Department of Psychology, Utah State
University, Logan, UT, USA
[2]Center for Epidemiologic Studies, Utah State
University, Logan, UT, USA

Synonyms

Diffuse plaques; Neuritic plaques; Senile plaques

Definition

An aggregation of beta-amyloid protein found in the extracellular space between neurons in the brain. Amyloid plaques may be of diffuse, pre-amyloid type or neuritic, mature senile type. The latter is recognized as one of the neuropathological hallmarks of Alzheimer's disease (AD). Mature amyloid plaques are spherical in shape and consist of a central beta-amyloid core, fibrillary outward extensions, and surrounding dystrophic neurites (elements of degenerating neurons). Unlike the mature, senile plaques, diffuse plaques have an amorphous, irregular shape

and lack the surrounding neurites (Serrano-Pozo et al. 2011).

Current Knowledge

It is unknown if the diffuse plaques later form into senile plaques. Both plaque types contain the amyloid β protein (Aβ), a portion of a larger neuronal transmembrane protein of unknown function. Other differences between senile and diffuse plaques include the constituent Aβ protein and their regional distribution in the brain. Diffuse plaques are common in the basal ganglia structures of the caudate nucleus and putamen as well as the cerebellum, where neuritic plaques are rare. In AD, neuritic plaques are more commonly found in the neocortex (Morris and Nagy 2004).

Distribution of amyloid plaques over the course of AD. In AD, amyloid plaque deposition is less predictive than neurofibrillary tangles but can be characterized by using staging system of Braak and Braak. Braak and Braak suggest three stages of progression of amyloid deposition: Stage A is characterized by amyloid deposition in the basal regions of the temporal, frontal, and occipital lobes; Stage B is characterized by involvement of isocortical areas with mild deposition in the hippocampus; and Stage C is characterized by deposition in primary isocortical areas (sensory and motor regions) and less

Amyloid Plaques,
Fig. 1 Amyloid plaques
stained with a modified
Bielschowsky silver stain
(Photo courtesy of Steven S.
Chin, M.D., Ph.D.,
University of Utah Health
Sciences Center)

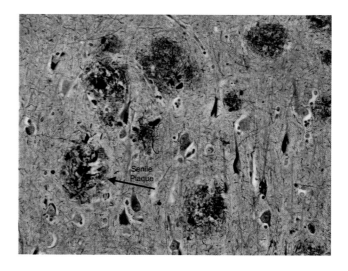

commonly, but in some cases, involving the cerebellum and the striatum, thalamus, hypothalamus, and other subcortical nuclei (Braak & Braak 1991). Other researchers have posited five proposed stages in the progression of amyloid deposition in AD: Stage I, isocortical; Stage II, allocortical deposition (e.g., entorhinal cortex, hippocampal formation, amygdala, insula, and cingulate cortex); Stage III, subcortical nuclei (e.g., striatum, cholinergic nuclei in the basal forebrain, thalamus, and hypothalamus) and white matter; Stage IV, involvement of brainstem structures (e.g., red nucleus, substantia nigra, portions of the medulla oblongata, and superior and inferior colliculi); and Stage V, additional deposition in pontine structures (reticular formation, raphe nuclei, locus ceruleus) (Thal et al. 2002). Recent studies have reported that amyloid burden does not correlate with the severity or duration of dementia, but early amyloid deposition has been correlated with the preclinical stage of AD, where there is Aβ accumulation but no apparent clinical symptoms of the disorder (Serrano-Pozo et al. 2011) (see also Alzheimer's Disease) (Fig. 1).

See Also

▶ Senile Plaques

References and Readings

Braak, H., & Braak, E. (1991). Acta H ' pathologica Neuropathological stageing of Alzheimer-related changes, 239–259.

Morris, J. H., & Nagy, Z. (2004). Alzheimer's disease. In M. M. Esiri, V. M.-Y. Lee, & J. Q. Trojanowski (Eds.), *The neuropathology of dementia* (2nd ed., pp. 161–206). Cambridge: Cambridge University Press.

Serrano-Pozo, A., Frosch, M. P., Masliah, E., & Hyman, B. T. (2011). Neuropathological alterations in Alzheimer disease. *Cold Spring Harbor Perspectives in Medicine, 1*(1), a006189. https://doi.org/10.1101/cshperspect.a006189

Thal, D. R., Rüb, U., Orantes, M., & Braak, H. (2002). Phases of Aβ-deposition in the human brain and its relevance for the development of AD. Neurology, 58 (12), 1791 LP – 1800. Retrieved from http://n.neurology.org/content/58/12/1791

Amyotrophic Lateral Sclerosis

A

Alexander I. Tröster
Department of Clinical Neuropsychology and Center for Neuromodulation, Barrow Neurological Institute, Phoenix, AZ, USA

Synonyms

Lou Gehrig's disease

Short Description or Definition

The features of amyotrophic lateral sclerosis (ALS) were first described by Charcot in the nineteenth century. ALS is a progressive, fatal neurodegenerative disease affecting upper and lower motor neurons, although increasingly ALS is recognized as a multisystem disorder whose manifestations may also include cognitive and behavioral changes. Most patients present with motor neuron symptoms at disease onset, and as the disease progresses, persons with ALS demonstrate impairments in speech, swallowing, breathing, and use of upper and lower limbs, with eventual paralysis. The prevalence of cognitive changes, which is not well studied, is estimated to range from about 20% to 50% and most often involve executive dysfunction. Deficits in visuospatial, language, and memory functions are more inconsistently observed. When dementia is seen, it resembles a frontotemporal lobar degeneration or frontotemporal dementia characterized by personality change, irritability, diminution of insight, poverty of planning, abstraction and initiation, and obsessiveness.

Categorization

Categorizations can be based on genetics, neurological levels inferred from symptoms, severity defined by number of neurological levels involved, and need for gastrostomy or noninvasive ventilation (King's stages) and diagnostic probability (El Escorial criteria). At least eight familial variants of ALS (ALS 1–8) have been identified, though the vast number of cases (about 90%) is sporadic. Of these eight, six forms are inherited in autosomal dominant manner and two in autosomal recessive manner. A large expansion of a hexanucleotide repeat in an intron of the gene *C9orf72* (a gene also implicated in frontotemporal dementia) is responsible for about 30–60% of familial ALS cases. Mutations in the superoxide dismutase 1 gene (*SOD1*) account for about another 20% of familial cases.

Three neurological levels are most often identified in the expression of ALS symptoms: bulbar, cervical, and lumbar. A fourth (thoracic) level is rarely encountered clinically. Persons with bulbar onset demonstrate problems with speech (dysarthria) and/or swallowing (dysphagia), and may have disease that affects lower or upper motor neurons (or both), showing features of bulbar palsy (facial weakness, limited palatal movement and lingual atrophy, weakness, and fasciculation) and/or pseudobulbar palsy (emotional lability, dysarthria, and brisk jaw jerk). Persons with cervical onset can also show upper and or lower motor neuron involvement and have upper limb signs. Such signs may include proximal weakness (shoulder abduction as required in toothbrushing or combing) or distal weakness (carrying out pincer grip movements). Lumbar onset patients have involvement of lower motor neurons and proximal weakness (e.g., difficulty in climbing stairs) or foot drop (resulting in tripping).

The most widely accepted clinical diagnostic criteria (the El Escorial criteria) define definite ALS by the presence of both upper and lower motor neuron signs in three regions, probable ALS by signs in two regions, possible ALS by signs in one region, and suspected ALS by *only* lower *or* upper motor neuron signs in one or more regions. The *suspected ALS* category may be the most controversial, and some consider the presence of only upper motor neuron signs to represent primary lateral sclerosis, while the presence of only lower motor neuron signs represents spinal muscular atrophy. The King's stages of severity are related to the El Escorial criteria. There are four clinical stages (the fifth stage is death), and the first three stages are identified by the involvement of either one, two, or three neurological levels. The fourth stage is identified by the need for either noninvasive ventilation or gastrostomy.

The notion that FTD and ALS may be part of the same spectrum of disorders has become less controversial with the implication of the *C9orf72* gene in both conditions and the observations that persons with ALS may develop FTD and persons with FTD or primary progressive aphasia (PPA) may develop ALS as well as by pathologic (ubiquitin-positive, tau-negative, and synuclein-negative neuronal inclusions in some forms of ALS and FTD). Nonetheless, some propose a categorization of ALS dependent upon the presence or absence of cognitive and behavioral features, namely, ALS, ALS with cognitive impairment, ALS with behavioral impairment, and ALS with FTD. This categorization apparently failed to consider that about 25% of patients may have both cognitive and behavioral abnormalities. Revised consensus criteria for the diagnosis of frontotemporal spectrum disorders in ALS were published in 2017 and these criteria do recognize a group of persons with ALS having both cognitive and behavioral impairment. Additionally, the criteria list both ALS-Frontotemporal dementia and ALS-Parkinsonism-dementia complex, thus highlighting further the neuropsychological heterogeneity of ALS.

Epidemiology

The incidence of ALS is about 1.5–2.5 per 100,000 per year and a prevalence of about 6 per 100,000. Prevalence and incidence of cognitive impairment are not well studied in ALS. Although one study in a specialty clinic indicated a prevalence of FTD features in about 40% of patients with ALS, this might represent an overestimate, given sampling bias, and the figure may be as low as 5%. Generally it has been estimated that dementia may occur at rates of 6–15% and milder cognitive impairment in 20–51% of patients. Other behavioral abnormalities (e.g., disinhibition, apathy) may occur in 14–40% of patients.

Natural History, Prognostic Factors, and Outcomes

Incidence of ALS peaks in the 1960s and drops rapidly thereafter. A broad estimate of mortality is that 50% of patients do not survive beyond 3 years from symptom onset but that some may survive 10 years or more. Three epidemiologic studies provide fairly consistent survival data using time of diagnosis as the reference point (though diagnostic confirmation may lag onset by 13–18 months): 78% at 1 year, 56% at 2 years, and 32% at 4 years. Several factors are associated with poorer prognosis: low-forced vital capacity, bulbar onset (often less tolerant of forced ventilation), older age at onset, and shorter interval between first symptom and presentation. Patients attending tertiary and specialized ALS clinics tend to show longer survival, and treatment with *riluzole*, on average, extends life by 3 months. Longer survival is seen in persons with only upper or lower motor neuron disease, though as noted, it is controversial whether variants such as primary lateral sclerosis are ALS.

Neuropsychology and Psychology of Amyotrophic Lateral Sclerosis

Most common among cognitive declines in ALS is executive dysfunction. A recent meta-analysis has revealed that ALS produces impairments in cognitive domains (without bias due to motor impairment) of medium effect size in verbal fluency, language, and social cognition and of small effect sizes in verbal memory and executive functions. Individual tests, within a domain do, however, reveal impairments of varying magnitude. Card-sorting tasks demanding of conceptualization and cognitive flexibility are less sensitive to executive deficits in ALS than are verbal fluency tasks demanding initiation and deployment of efficient word retrieval strategies. Retrieval of verbs, putatively more dependent upon frontal lobe integrity than upon phonemic or semantic fluency tasks (requiring word retrieval by initial sound or membership in semantic categories, respectively), may be the

most susceptible to ALS. Verbal fluency decrements are observed even if one controls for motor and speech impairments. Another task sensitive to deficits in ALS, and particularly to pseudobulbar ALS, are Tower tasks that place a premium on spatial working memory and planning. Similarly, another test of working memory (digit span backward, requiring examinees to repeat increasingly long series of digits in reverse order of presentation) has also been shown to be sensitive to ALS.

Language (unlike motor speech) is less likely disrupted by ALS, although language task impairments are observed in patients with ALS and dementia. Despite performing well on nonverbal semantic knowledge and grammar tasks, patients with ALS and dementia perform poorly on verbal tasks, making semantic paraphasic errors on naming tests. Some studies have observed tendencies toward echolalia, stereotypy of expression, and perseveration in ALS.

When deficits in memory are observed in ALS, they are more likely to be evident on immediate than delayed recall tasks. Some take this to implicate poorer executive control over encoding processes, whereas others might invoke slowed information processing as an explanation. The finding that patients can benefit disproportionately from the provision of recognition cues relative to free recall formats suggests that retrieval deficits might also be implicated or that shallow levels of encoding are sufficient to support recognition but not recall.

Recent interest has focused on social cognition and especially on theory of mind (the ability to infer another's thoughts, beliefs, intentions, and emotions). Patients with ALS seem to show significant impairments in both the cognitive and affective components of theory of mind.

Concerning behavioral changes, rating scales have revealed that as many as two thirds of persons with ALS show one or more of irritability, disinhibition, inflexibility, restlessness, and apathy. Apathy and questionable or poor social judgment are more likely to be observed in patients with bulbar onset ALS. Surprisingly, although reactive depressive reactions may occur after diagnosis, major depression is quite rare among

ALS patients (about 10%). Symptoms of depression are common, occurring in about half of patients. Persons with ALS may in particular experience hopelessness and end-of-life concerns. Pathological laughing or crying, as seen in pseudobulbar syndromes, should not be confused with depression.

Evaluation

Although consensus guidelines for assessment of cognition in ALS are expected in the future, currently only older suggestions are available. Experimental modifications of tests to eliminate timing and minimize motor requirements, while facilitating patient performance, have unknown sensitivity. Persons with hypophonic speech might be provided an amplifier. Computers as augmentative communication devices, while not practical in traditional neuropsychological assessment, can be helpful in interviewing the patient. Yes-no or forced-choice recognition paradigms might allow patients to demonstrate knowledge of memoranda.

Verbal fluency tests are likely to be helpful in determining which patients might require fuller evaluations because traditional screening instruments, such as the Mini-Mental State Exam, are not sensitive to cognitive impairment in ALS. In addition to measures of executive function, naming, and memory, it is important to include in assessments self- or informant rating scales capturing behavioral changes such as apathy, irritability, depression, disinhibition, etc. Such measures are helpful in identifying those persons with behavioral changes or the behavioral variant of FTD.

Treatment

There are no curative treatments for ALS. The only drug approved for ALS is *riluzole*, a glutamate release inhibitor that shows moderate benefit and extends life on an average of 3 months. Palliative care (symptomatic control and quality-of-life optimization in the absence of a cure) is recommended from the outset, and numerous ameliorative therapies, often multidisciplinary, are available. Cramps and spasticity can be treated with a variety of medications including, for example, *carbamazepine, quinine, baclofen,* and *tizanidine*. Drooling can be treated with anticholinergics such as *scopolamine*, although there is a risk of confusion and memory problems in older patients, and *amitriptyline*, which may also alleviate depression and pathological laughing and crying, may be preferable. Speech therapy is helpful both for swallowing problems and dysarthria, although ultimately, severe swallowing problems necessitate change in diet and choking may necessitate percutaneous endoscopic gastrostomy (PEG) placement. When communication becomes too difficult due to speech problems or difficulty breathing, computers can be used to facilitate communication, in some cases even when paralysis is present. Because breathing difficulty and shortness of breath can be distressing to the patient, a benzodiazepine or *morphine* use is recommended. Respiratory insufficiency can be alleviated with noninvasive ventilation and later invasive ventilation. Mood disturbances and family bereavement issues can be dealt with by counseling and social work intervention. Physical and occupational therapy may also be helpful to facilitate mobility and, perhaps to lesser extent, strength and range of motion.

Cross-References

► Assistive Technology
► Cortical Motor Pathways
► Frontal Lobe
► Frontal Temporal Dementia
► Frontotemporal Lobar Degenerations
► Speech

References and Readings

Averill, A. J., Kasarskis, E. J., & Segerstrom, S. C. (2007). Psychological health in patients with amyotrophic lateral sclerosis. *Amyotrophic Lateral Sclerosis, 8*, 243–254.

Beeldman, E., Raaphorst, J., Twennaar, M. K., de Visser, M., Schmand, B. A., & de Haan, R. J. (2015). The cognitive profile of ALS: A systematic review and meta-analysis update. *Journal of Neurology, Neurosurgery, and Psychiatry.* https://doi.org/10.1136/jnnp-2015-310734. online first, 17 Aug 2015.

Brownlee, A., & Palovcak, M. (2007). The role of augmentative communication devices in the medical management of ALS. *NeuroRehabilitation, 22*, 445–450.

Kiernan, M. C. (2015). Palliative care in amyotrophic lateral sclerosis. *Lancet Neurology, 14*, 347–348.

Lewis, M., & Rushanan, S. (2007). The role of physical therapy and occupational therapy in the treatment of amyotrophic lateral sclerosis. *NeuroRehabilitation, 22*, 451–461.

Logroscino, G., Traynor, B. J., Hardiman, O., Chio, A., Couratier, P., Mitchell, J. D., et al. (2008). Descriptive epidemiology of amyotrophic lateral sclerosis: New evidence and unsolved issues. *Journal of Neurology, Neurosurgery and Psychiatry, 79*, 6–11.

McCluskey, L. (2007). Palliative rehabilitation and amyotrophic lateral sclerosis: A perfect match. *NeuroRehabilitation, 22*, 407–408.

Murphy, J., et al. (2016). Cognitive-behavioral screening reveals prevalent impairment in a large multicenter ALS cohort. *Neurology, 86*, 813–820.

Phukan, J., Pender, N. P., & Hardiman, O. (2007). Cognitive impairment in amyotrophic lateral sclerosis. *Lancet Neurology, 6*, 994–1003.

Radunovic, A., Mitsumoto, H., & Leigh, P. N. (2007). Clinical care of patients with amyotrophic lateral sclerosis. *Lancet Neurology, 6*, 913–925.

Strong, M. J., Grace, G. M., Orange, J. B., & Leeper, H. A. (1996). Cognition, language, and speech in amyotrophic lateral sclerosis: A review. *Journal of Clinical and Experimental Neuropsychology, 18*, 291–303.

Trojsi, F., Santangelo, G., Caiazzo, G., Siciliano, M., Ferrantino, T., Piccirillo, G., Femiano, C., Cristillo, V., Monsurro, M., Espositio, F., & Tedeschi, G. (2016). Neuropsychological assessment at different King's clinical stages of amyotrophic lateral sclerosis. *Amyotrophic Lateral Sclerosis and Frontotemporal Degeneration, 17*, 1–7.

Van der Hulst, E.-J., Bak, T. H., & Abrahams, S. (2015). Impaired affective and cognitive theory of mind and behavioural change in amyotrophic lateral sclerosis. *Journal of Neurology, Neurosurgery, and Psychiatry, 86*, 1208–1215.

Woolley, S. C., & Rush, B. K. (2017). Considerations for clinical neuropsychoplogical evaluation in amyotrophic lateral sclerosis. *Archives of Clinical Neuropsychology, 32*, 906–916.

Amyotrophic Lateral Sclerosis Functional Rating Scale

A

Michelle Marie Tipton-Burton
Physical Medicine and Rehabilitation, Santa Clara Valley Medical Center, San Jose, CA, USA

Synonyms

ALSFRS; ALSFRS-R

Description

The Amyotrophic Lateral Sclerosis Functional Rating Scale (ALSFRS) is a validated instrument designed to assess the functional status and the disease progression in patients with amyotrophic lateral sclerosis (ALS). It is a tool that can be used to monitor functional change in a patient over time. The ALSFRS is a ten-item functional inventory which was devised for use in therapeutic trials in ALS. Each item is rated on a 0–4 scale, (with 0 being severely impaired and 4 being normal) by the patient and/or caregiver, yielding a maximum score of 40 points. The ALSFRS assesses the patients' levels of self-sufficiency in areas of self-feeding, grooming, ambulation, and communication and swallowing. Versions are available in Spanish, Dutch, and German.

Historical Background

The ALSFRS was developed because clinimetric scales being utilized at the time were contaminated with impairment measurements, did not measure the broad range of disabilities that result from ALS, and did not lend themselves to subscore analysis that was based entirely on disability components (Feinstein 1987; Streiner and Norman 1989).

The ALSFRS is a validated rating instrument for monitoring the progression of disability in patients with ALS. One weakness of the ALSFRS, as it was originally designed, was that it granted disproportionate weighting to the limb and bulbar, as compared to respiratory dysfunction. Some patients with ALS are able to live for several years past the lowest measurable level of function on the Amyotrophic Lateral Sclerosis Functional Rating Scale-Revised (ALSFRS-R), a widely used end point in ALS assessment. The ALSFRS-R is also validated and incorporates additional assessments of dyspnea, orthopnea, and the need for ventilator support. The ALSFRS-R retains the properties of the original scale and shows strong internal consistency and construct validity. The ALSFRS extension offers improved sensitivity at lower levels of physical function.

Psychometric Data

The ALSFRS was developed as an internally consistent, reliable, and valid measure of disability in ALS patients as part of the Amyotrophic Lateral Sclerosis Ciliary Neurotrophic Factor (ALS CNTF) Treatment Study (ACTS Phase 1–11 Study Group 1996). The ability of the ALSFRS to be responsive to change in the clinical status of ALS patients was evaluated cross sectionally and prospectively over time in phase 1 and phase 2 studies of CNTF in ALS.

The ALSFRS has been validated both cross sectionally and longitudinally against muscle strength, the Schwab and England ADL rating scale, the Clinical Global Impression of Change (CGIC) scale, and independent assessments of patient's functional status (Cedarbaum and Stambler 1997).

Clinical Uses

The ALSFRS is a straightforward instrument that can be utilized across disciplines to assess the functional status of an individual diagnosed with ALS. The tool has also been utilized to evaluate the disease progression and predict hospital length of stay and survival time in ALS patients treated with tracheostomy-intermittent positive-pressure ventilation. Through observation and interview, the evaluator assesses the following measures: speech, salivation, swallowing, handwriting, cutting food/handling utensils, turning in bed and adjusting bed clothes, walking, climbing stairs, and breathing.

Cross-References

▶ Amyotrophic Lateral Sclerosis

Further Reading

ALS CNTF Treatment Study (ACTS) Phase 1-11 Study Group. (1996). The amyotrophic lateral sclerosis functional rating scale. Assessment of activities of daily living in patients with amyotrophic lateral sclerosis. *Archives of Neurology, 53*, 141–147.

Campos, T. S., Rodriquez-Santos, F., Esteban, J., Vasquez, P. C., Mora Paradivia, J. S., & Carmona, A. C. (2010). Spanish adaption of the revised amyotrophic lateral sclerosis functional rating scale (ALSFRS-R). *Amyotrophic Lateral Sclerosis, 11*(5), 475–477.

Cedarbaum, J. M., & Stambler, N. (1997). Performance of the amyotrophic lateral sclerosis functional rating scale (ALSFRS) in multicenter clinical trials. *Journal of the Neurological Sciences, 152*(Suppl 1), S1–S9.

Feinstein, A. R. (1987) Clinimetric perspectives. *Journal of Chronic Diseases, 40*(6), 635–40.

Herndon, R. M. (2006). *Handbook of neurologic rating scales* (p. 96). New York: Demos Medical Publishing, LLC.

Lo Coco, D., Marchese, S., La Bella, V., Piccoli, T., & Lo Coco, A. (2007). The amyotrophic lateral sclerosis functional rating scale predicts survival time in amyotrophic lateral sclerosis patients on invasive mechanical ventilation. *Chest, 132*(1), 64–69.

Streiner, D. L. & Norman, G. R. (1989). A Review of: "Health Measurement Scales: A Practical Guide to Their Development and Use, Fourth Edition" New York: Oxford University Press, 2008, ISBM 978-0-19-923188-1, xvii + 431 pp

Wicks, P., Massagli, M. P., Wolf, C., & Heywood, J. (2009). Measuring function in Advaced ALS: Validation of ALSFRS-Ex extension items. *European Journal of Neurology, 16*(3), 353–359. https://doi.org/10.1111/j.1468-1331.2008.02434.x.

Analysis of Variance

Matthew J. L. Page
Allegheny General Hospital, Pittsburgh, PA, USA
Psychology, Allegheny Health Network,
Pittsburgh, PA, USA

Synonyms

ANOVA, *F*-test

Definition

Analysis of variance (ANOVA) is a statistical test that identifies whether two or more group means are statistically different. ANOVA evaluates the null hypothesis that the means of each group are equal, and, by implication, that each group represents the same population. The alternative hypothesis is that at least one pair of group means is different, suggesting that these groups reflect different populations and that the independent variable (IV) has a significant effect on the dependent variable (DV). ANOVA uses a statistic referred to as *F*, which is defined as the ratio between the between-group (explained) variance and the within-group (unexplained) variance. A one-way ANOVA analyzes the difference between the means of multiple levels of one independent variable. A factorial ANOVA incorporates multiple independent variables (factors). For example, in a two-way ANOVA, the main effect of both IVs is examined. The interaction effect is also analyzed, which examines whether the effect of one variable changes at different levels of the other variable.

Like a *t*-test, ANOVA is appropriate for categorical IVs and continuous DVs with interval or ratio data. However, *t*-tests are limited in that they can evaluate the significance of the difference between only two group means; thus, multiple *t*-tests are required to examine more than two means. Doing so is problematic because conducting an increasing number of tests increases the probability of making a type I error. ANOVA can identify the presence of a significant difference between any pair of means using a single test. If the *F*-test produces a significant result, the next step is to identify which pairs of means are statistically significantly different using post-hoc analyses, such as Tukey's honest significant difference test.

Current Knowledge

When using ANOVA, observations must be randomly sampled and independent of each other. Additionally, the use of ANOVA requires that the populations under examination are normally distributed, although the *F*-test is fairly robust against violations of this rule with large sample sizes and symmetrical population distributions. Another assumption of ANOVA is that the variances of the group populations are equal, and hence an important step in ANOVA is to test this assumption using the group sample variances (for example, using Levene's test or Bartlett's test).

See Also

▶ False Positive
▶ Multivariate Analysis of Variance
▶ Statistical Significance

Further Reading

Gueorguieva, R., & Krystal, J. H. (2004). Move over ANOVA: Progress in analyzing repeated-measures data and its reflection in papers published in the *Archives of General Psychiatry*. *Archives of General Psychiatry, 61*, 310–317. https://doi.org/10.1001/archpsyc.61.3.310.

Iverson, G. R., & Norpoth, H. (1987). *Analysis of variance*. Newbury Park: Sage.

Watson, P. (2009). Review of analysis of variance and covariance: How to choose and construct models for the life sciences. *Psychological Medicine, 39*, 695–696.

Anarthria

Ignatius Nip[1] and Carole R. Roth[2]
[1]School of Speech, Language, and Hearing
Sciences, San Diego State University, San Diego,
CA, USA
[2]Otolaryngology Clinic, Speech Division, Naval
Medical Center, San Diego, CA, USA

Synonyms

Speechlessness

Definition

Anarthria is speechlessness due to a severe loss of
neuromuscular control over the speech muscula-
ture and is the most severe form of dysarthria.
Language and cognition may be intact, but the
neuromuscular disorder prevents speech.
Anarthric patients are motivated to speak but are
unable.

Some patients with anarthria can produce some
oral movements and/or undifferentiated vocaliza-
tions when attempting to speak. Occasionally,
there is no concomitant limb movement disorder,
but there is almost always a nonspeech oromotor
impairment. Frequent causes include brainstem
stroke, multiple strokes, closed head injury, and
degenerative diseases, including amyotrophic lateral sclerosis (ALS).

Cross-References

▶ Dysarthria

References and Readings

Duffy, J. R. (2013). *Motor speech disorders: Substrates,
    differential diagnosis, and management* (3rd ed.).
    St. Louis: Elsevier Mosby.

ANCOVA/MANCOVA

Michael Franzen
Allegheny General Hospital, Pittsburgh, PA, USA

Synonyms

Analysis of covariance

Definition

ANCOVA or analysis of covariance is a variant
of the ANOVA model in which the statistical
effect of a nuisance variable is removed mathe-
matically from the analysis in order to clarify the
relations between the independent and the
dependent variables (Belin and Normand
2009). The optimal situation would be if the
independent variable levels or groups were not
related to the nuisance variable. However, if the
nuisance variable is related to the dependent
variable and if the nuisance variable is systematically represented among the independent variables, ANCOVA may be used to partial out the
statistical effect of the nuisance variable or
covariate. This is not a substitute for removing
the effect through experimental design. For
example, level of education may be statistically
related to performance on a memory test. If two
groups of depressed and nondepressed individuals differ systematically on the basis of their
level of education, any difference found with
regard to performance on a memory test might
be due to the different level of education. By
employing ANCOVA and using education level
as the covariate, the researcher may have a
clearer understanding of the relation between
the presence of depression and performance on
the memory test by statistically partialling out or
removing the variance associated with the nuisance variable of education.

For example, Airaksinen et al. (2005) were
interested in differences on neuropsychological

tests among groups of individuals with different anxiety disorders. Unfortunately, their experimental groups differed in age, a variable which is known to influence neuropsychological test performance. Therefore age was used as a covariate in their analysis.

Although there are different mathematical methods for conducting an ANCOVA including the use of multiple regression (which see), ANCOVA under the general linear model provides a useful conceptualization of the underlying idea. We can think of calculating the regression between the covariate and the dependent variable and then residualizing the influence of the covariate. Then an ANOVA can be conducted on the residual values. In order to use ANCOVA, the data must satisfy a few basic assumptions. There must be a linear relation between the covariate and the dependent variable. The slope of the regression for each group or level of the independent variable must be the same. The error term should be normally distributed with a mean of zero. The covariate should not be affected by the independent variable (Wildt and Ahtola 1978).

Cross-References

► Analysis of Variance

References

Airaksinen, E., Larsson, M., & Fosell, Y. (2005). Neuropsychological functions in anxiety disorders in population-based samples: Evidence of episodic memory dysfunction. *Journal of Psychiatry Research, 39*, 207–214.

Belin, T. R., & Normand, S.-L. T. (2009). The role of ANCOVA in analyzing experimental data. *Psychiatric Annals, 39*, 753–759.

Watson, P. (2009). Review of analysis of variance and covariance: How to choose and construct models for the life sciences. *Psychological Medicine, 39*, 695–696.

Wildt, A. R., & Ahtola, O. T. (1978). *Analysis of covariance*. Beverly Hills: Sage.

Anencephaly

Erin D. Bigler and Jo Ann Petrie
Department of Psychology and the Neuroscience Center, Brigham Young University, Provo, UT, USA

Synonyms

Amnion rupture; Brain stem; Congenital defects; Exencephaly; Forebrain; Lack of neural tube closure; Magnetic resonance imaging; MRI; Neural tube defects; NTD

Definition

Using "*an*" in front of an anatomical descriptor signifies *absence*. *Cephalic* is Greek for *head* with *encephalon* specifically referring to the brain. Therefore, the term *anencephaly* is used to denote a congenital defect in the development of the head, including the meninges, the cranium, and the scalp and, in particular, abnormal brain growth, with an almost completely diminished *prosencephalon* (*telencephalon* + *diencephalon*) or *forebrain* and only rudimentary development of the *brain stem*.

Categorization

Anencephaly neural tube defects (NTD) result from the failure of closure of the headend of the neural tube in early fetal/embryolic development (first 3–4 weeks); including lack of formation of the brain, skull, and scalp (Greene and Copp 2014; Puvirajesinghe and Borg 2015; Yamaguchi and Miura 2013). Loss of the forebrain includes loss of the two cerebral hemispheres, the connecting corpus callosum, neocortex, thalamus, hypothalamus, and other structures of the limbic system – the amygdala, hippocampus, caudate nucleus, ventricles, etc., and all of their connections (Kandel et al. 2013; Kolb and Whishaw 2008). These structures comprise the majority of human brain tissue and are required for almost all sensation perception and basic physiological functions including body temperature control, eating, sleeping, and motor function, and cognition, language, memory, emotion, thought processing, inhibition, decision making, and/or reasoning (see also Lezack et al. 2012).

Epidemiology

Anencephaly results from NTD (Cohen 2002; Detrait et al. 2005; Mitchell 2005; Yamaguchi and Miura 2013) in approximately three pregnancies for every 10,000 births in the USA and 300,000 births per year worldwide (Flores et al. 2014). Such severe NTDs may be associated with genetics, nutrition, environment, or a combination of all three (Centers for Disease Control and Prevention (CDC) 2015). There is a known higher prevalence of females born with anencephaly NTD as compared to males (James 1980). Over the past several decades, worldwide research has found an association between prenatal folic acid (synthetic vitamin B) deficits leading to folate (natural vitamin B) deficiencies (National Institute of Neurological Disorders and Stroke (NINDS) 2015; National Institutes of Health (NIH): Office of Dietary Supplements 2016) and NTD (Calvo and Biglieri 2008; Kondo et al. 2009; Wolff et al. 2009; Yila et al. 2016). While all the causes of open NTD are not known, research indicates that daily consumption of 4 mg/day of folic acid by women before and during pregnancy brings about a 70% reduction in NTD (Centers for Disease Control and Prevention (CDC) 2015; Cornel and Erickson 1997; MRC Vitamin Study Research Group 1991; National Institutes of Health (NIH): Office of Dietary Supplements 2016). Since 1996 more than 50 countries worldwide have taken the critical step to mandate fortification of staple grain food products with folic acid to prevent NTD such as anencephaly and spina bifida and have been highly successful – especially those with low and middle income populations (Castillo-Lancellotti et al. 2013;

Rampersaud et al. 2016; Wang et al. 2016; Zaganjor et al. 2016). However, since natural folate is also readily available in other staple foods (e.g., dried beans, lentils, and leafy green vegetables) recent research also raises concerns for those areas with folic acid supplementation to watch for *excess* folate consumption which may also adversely *increase* growth in undetected cancer cells (see Castillo-Lancellotti et al. 2013; Herrmann and Obeid 2011; Strickland et al. 2013) or increased malaria infection in those areas at high risk for the disease (Nzila et al. 2016).

Natural History, Prognostic Factors, and Outcomes

With the major portion of an infant's brain being undeveloped, particularly the cerebrum, and coupled with the brain often being exposed in utero, the anencephalic infant is frequently stillborn (Creasy et al. 2014). An infant born alive with anencephaly is, as a rule, blind, deaf, unconscious, and may only reflexively respond. With only a basic brain stem and a nonfunctioning cerebrum, prognosis is poor; anencephalic infants will never gain consciousness and will only have minimal reflex actions such as breathing. There may be intermittent sound or touch responses; however, no further progress can be expected (see National Institute of Neurological Disorders and Stroke 2015).

Neuropsychology and Psychology of Anencephaly

There is essentially no assessment that neuropsychological testing can offer given the absence of cortical development in the anencephalic infant who does survive. Such children have reflexive function only (i.e., breathing and some responses to sound or touch can manifest) and will rarely survive longer than a few hours or days. Neuropsychologists should have an empathetic awareness of this condition and be prepared to consult with parents and families about the nature of the

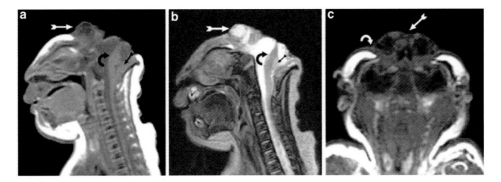

A

Anencephaly, Fig. 1 Magnetic resonance imaging (MRI) findings of the head and neck 8 h after birth. (**a**) Sagittal T1-weighted, (**b**) sagittal T2-weighted, and (**c**) coronal T1-weighted images show cranial schisis. The normal skin stops at the skull base and encircles abnormally developed cerebral structures, the so-called area cerebrovasculosa (*white arrows*). Along the border of the skull defect the skin seems to be in continuity with the superficial layer of the area cerebrovasculosa, probably the pia mater (*curved white arrow*). The posterior fossa is funnel-shaped. A rudimentary brain stem (*curved black arrows*) and primordium of cerebellum (small *black arrows*) are present. The cervical spine is normal (From Calzolari et al. 2004, with permission).

infants' deficits and the poor prognosis (Ashwal 2005; Creasy et al. 2014).

Evaluation

Although the pathogenesis of anencephaly is still not fully understood, several studies suggest that *exencephaly* or the lack of skull growth or separation following NTD allows the cerebral tissue to be exposed in utero causing damage from the amniotic fluid (Calzolari et al. 2004; Sharif and Zhou 2016). As can be seen in Fig. 1, even though there are other anomalies of physical development associated with the presence of anencephaly, the most dramatic is a failure of brain development.

Treatment

Ultimately, mortality rate is 100% with anencephaly. Some anencephalic children do survive from hours to days but rarely longer and in a persistent vegetative state (Payne and Taylor 1997); thus, treatment is purely supportive. The presence of a surviving infant with anencephaly raises numerous ethical questions about care, treatment, and maintenance (Batavia 2002; Castillo-Lancellotti et al. 2013; Cook et al. 2008; Obeidi et al. 2010; Rampersaud et al. 2016; Yila et al. 2016; Zhang et al. 2016), including the importance of continued research to guide worldwide policy making for better ways to prevent and treat neurological birth defects.

References and Readings

Ashwal, S. (2005). Recovery of consciousness and life expectancy of children in a vegetative state. *Neuropsychological Rehabilitation, 15*(3–4), 190–197.

Batavia, A. I. (2002). Disability versus futility in rationing health care services: Defining medical futility based on permanent unconsciousness – PVS, coma, and anencephaly. *Behavioral Sciences & the Law, 20*(3), 219–233. https://doi.org/10.1002/bsl.483.

Calvo, E. B., & Biglieri, A. (2008). Impact of folic acid fortification on women's nutritional status and on the prevalence of neural tube defects. *Archives of Argentina Pediatrics, 106*(6), 492–498. https://doi.org/10.1590/S0325-00752008000600004. S0325-00752008000600004 [pii].

Calzolari, F., Gambi, B., Garani, G., & Tamisari, L. (2004). Anencephaly: MRI findings and pathogenetic theories. *Pediatric Radiology, 34*(12), 1012–1016. https://doi.org/10.1007/s00247-004-1259-8.

Castillo-Lancellotti, C., Tur, J. A., & Uauy, R. (2013). Impact of folic acid fortification of flour on neural tube defects: A systematic review. *Public Health Nutrition, 16*(5), 901–911. 10.1017/S1368980012003576.

Centers for Disease Control and Prevention (CDC). (2015). Facts about anencephaly. Retrieved from http://www.cdc.gov/ncbddd/birthdefects/anencephaly.html

Cohen, M. M., Jr. (2002). Malformations of the craniofacial region: Evolutionary, embryonic, genetic, and clinical perspectives. *American Journal of Medical*

Genetics, 115(4), 245–268. https://doi.org/10.1002/ajmg.10982.

Cook, R. J., Erdman, J. N., Hevia, M., & Dickens, B. M. (2008). Prenatal management of anencephaly. *International Journal of Obstetrics & Gynaecology, 102*(3), 304–308. https://doi.org/10.1016/j.ijgo.2008.05.002. S0020-7292(08)00210-5 [pii].

Cornel, M. C., & Erickson, J. D. (1997). Comparison of national policies on periconceptional use of folic acid to prevent spina bifida and anencephaly (SBA). *Teratology, 55*(2), 134–137. https://doi.org/10.1002/(SICI)1096-9926(199702)55:2<134::AID-TERA3>3.0.CO;2-3.

Creasy, R. K., Resnik, R., Iams, J. D., Lockwood, C. J., Moore, T. R., & Greene, M. F. (Eds.). (2014). *Creasy and Resnik's maternal-fetal medicine: Principles and practice* (7th ed.). Philidelphia: Elsevier Saunders.

Detrait, E. R., George, T. M., Etchevers, H. C., Gilbert, J. R., Vekemans, M., & Speer, M. C. (2005). Human neural tube defects: Developmental biology, epidemiology, and genetics. *Neurotoxicology and Teratology, 27*(3), 515–524. https://doi.org/10.1016/j.ntt.2004.12.007. S0892-0362(04)00156-4 [pii].

Flores, A. L., Vellozzi, C., Valencia, D., & Sniezek, J. (2014). Global burden of neural tube defects, risk factors, and prevention. *Indian Journal of Community Health, 26*(Suppl 1), 3–5.

Greene, N. D., & Copp, A. J. (2014). Neural tube defects. *Annual Review of Neuroscience, 37*, 221–242. https://doi.org/10.1146/annurev-neuro-062012-170354.

Herrmann, W., & Obeid, R. (2011). The mandatory fortification of staple foods with folic acid: A current controversy in Germany. *Deutsches Arzteblatt International, 108*(15), 249–254. https://doi.org/10.3238/arztebl.2011.0249.

James, W. H. (1980). The sex ratios of anencephalics born to anencephalic-prone women. *Developmental Medicine and Child Neurology, 22*, 618–622.

Kandel, E. R., Schwartz, J. H., Jessell, T. M., Siegelbaum, S. A., & Hudspeth, A. J. (Eds.). (2013). *Principles of neural science*. New York: The McGraw-Hill Companies.

Kolb, B., & Whishaw, I. Q. (2008). *Fundamentals of human neuropsychology* (6th ed.). New York: Worth Publishers.

Kondo, A., Kamihira, O., & Ozawa, H. (2009). Neural tube defects: Prevalence, etiology and prevention. *International Journal of Urology, 16*(1), 49–57. https://doi.org/10.1111/j.1442-2042.2008.02163.x.

Lezack, M. D., Howieson, D. B., Bigler, E. D., & Tranel, D. (2012). *Neuropsychological assessment* (5th ed.). New York: Oxford University Press.

Mitchell, L. E. (2005). Epidemiology of neural tube defects. *American Journal of Medical Genetics. Part C. Seminars in Medical Genetics, 135C*(1), 88–94. https://doi.org/10.1002/ajmg.c.30057.

MRC Vitamin Study Research Group. (1991). Prevention of neural tube defects: Results of the Medical Research Council vitamin study. *Lancet, 338*(8760), 131–137.

National Institute of Neurological Disorders and Stroke. (2015). NINDS Anencephaly Information Page. *National institutes of health: Reducing the burden of neurological disease.* Retrieved from http://www.ninds.nih.gov/disorders/anencephaly/anencephaly.htm

National Institutes of Health (NIH): Office of Dietary Supplements. (2016). Health information: Folate, dietary supplement fact sheet: *Strengthening knowledge and understanding of dietary supplements.* Retrieved from https://ods.od.nih.gov/factsheets/Folate-HealthProfessional/#h2

Nzila, A., Okombo, J., & Hyde, J. (2016). Malaria in the era of food fortification with folic acid. *Food and Nutrition Bulletin*, 1–11. https://doi.org/10.1177/0379572116634511.

Obeidi, N., Russell, N., Higgins, J. R., & O'Donoghue, K. (2010). The natural history of anencephaly. *Prenatal Diagnosis, 30*, 357–360. https://doi.org/10.1002/pd.2490.

Payne, S. K., & Taylor, R. M. (1997). The persistent vegetative state and anencephaly: Problematic paradigms for discussing futility and rationing. *Seminars in Neurology, 17*(3), 257–263.

Puvirajesinghe, T. M., & Borg, J. P. (2015). Neural tube defects: From a proteomic standpoint. *Metabolites, 5*(1), 164–183. https://doi.org/10.3390/metabo5010164.

Rampersaud, G. C., Sokolow, A., Gruspe, A., Colee, J. C., & Kauwell, G. P. (2016). Folate/folic acid knowledge, intake, and self-efficacy of college-age women: Impact of text messaging and availability of a folic acid-containing supplement. *Journal of American College Health.* https://doi.org/10.1080/07448481.2016.1179196.

Sharif, A., & Zhou, Y. (2016). Fetal MRI characteristics of exencephaly: A case report and literature review. *Case Reports in Radiology, 2016*, 9801267. https://doi.org/10.1155/2016/9801267.

Strickland, K. C., Krupenko, N. I., & Krupenko, S. A. (2013). Molecular mechanisms underlying the potentially adverse effects of folate. *Clinical Chemistry and Laboratory Medicine, 51*(3), 607–616. https://doi.org/10.1515/cclm-2012-0561.

Wang, H., De Steur, H., Chen, G., Zhang, X., Pei, L., Gellynck, X., & Zheng, X. (2016). Effectiveness of folic acid fortified flour for prevention of neural tubed in a high risk region. *Nutrients, 8*(3). https://doi.org/10.3390/nu8030152.

Wolff, T., Witkop, C. T., Miller, T., & Syed, S. B. (2009). Folic acid supplementation for the prevention of neural tube defects: An update of the evidence for the U.S. preventive services task force. *Annals of Internal Medicine, 150*(9), 632–639. https://doi.org/150/9/632 [pii].

Yamaguchi, Y., & Miura, M. (2013). How to form and close the brain: Insight into the mechanism of cranial neural tube closure in mammals. *Cellular and Molecular Life Sciences, 70*(17), 3171–3186. https://doi.org/10.1007/s00018-012-1227-7.

Yila, T. A., Araki, A., Sasaki, S., Miyashita, C., Itoh, K., Ikeno, T., et al. (2016). Predictors of folate status among pregnant Japanese women: The Hokkaido study on environment and Children's health,

2002–2012. *British Journal of Nutrition*, 1–9. https://doi.org/10.1017/S0007114516001628.

Zaganjor, I., Sekkarie, A., Tsang, B. L., Williams, J., Razzaghi, H., Mulinare, J., ··· & Rosenthal, J. (2016). Describing the prevalence of neural tube defects worldwide: A systematic literature review. *PloS One, 11*(4), e0151586. https://doi.org/10.1371/journal.pone.0151586.

Zhang, R., Wu, K., Zhan, C., Liu, X., & Gong, Z. (2016). Folic acid supplementation reduces the mutagenicity and genotoxicity caused by benzo(a)pyrene. *Journal of Nutritional Science and Vitaminology (Tokyo), 62*(1), 26–31. https://doi.org/10.3177/jnsv.62.26.

Aneurysm

Bruce J. Diamond
Department of Psychology, William Paterson University, Wayne, NJ, USA

Synonyms

Blood-filled dilatation

Short Description or Definition

An aneurysm is an abnormal blood-filled dilatation of a blood vessel that can occur in vascular innervated areas (Webster 2006). Cerebral aneurysms are generally located at arterial curvatures and bifurcations that are exposed to major hemodynamic forces (Kulcsár et al. 2011). Aneurysms generally develop due to trauma, infections, congenital defects, or degenerative diseases (Parkin and Leng 1993). Blood from a ruptured brain aneurysm can leak into the brain (i.e., hemorrhagic stroke). If blood leaks into the space between the brain and the thin tissues covering the brain, this type of hemorrhagic stroke is classified as a subarachnoid hemorrhage (Mayo Clinic Staff 2015). An aneurysm can also dissect, which is a split in one or more layers of the artery wall that causes bleeding into and along the layers of the artery wall (NIH 2011). The size and rate of growth of an unruptured cerebral aneurysm will affect signs and symptoms, and, therefore, a patient with a static aneurysm may be asymptomatic. However, a larger aneurysm with a steady growth pattern may produce a variety of symptoms (e.g., headache, numbness, loss of feeling in the face, or problems with the eyes) (NINDS 2015).

Categorization

Intracranial aneurysms are commonly classified as saccular, mycotic, traumatic, arteriosclerotic, dissecting, or neoplasmic. Giant aneurysms greater than 2.5 cm in diameter are believed to be congenital anomalies. They are generally located on the anterior and middle cerebral, carotid and basilar arteries (Ropper et al. 2005).

Etiology

The combination of high wall shear stress (WSS) and high positive spatial wall shear stress gradient (SWSSG) focused on a small segment of the arterial wall may mediate aneurysm formation (Kulcsár et al. 2011). Additionally, the proximity of the distal anterior cerebral artery (dACA) to the falx has been recently implicated in the pathogenesis of dACA aneurysms with fibrous adhesions between the falx and the dACA observed in patients with this type of aneurysm (Scholtes et al. 2015).

Epidemiological Factors

Ruptured aneurysms, specifically the saccular type, are the most common cause of subarachnoid hemorrhage (SAH) after 20 years of age. This type of aneurysm accounts for about 80% of nontraumatic aneurysms. Cerebral aneurysms can occur throughout the lifespan but tend to be more common in adults than in children. They are also slightly more common in women than in men (NINDS 2015). It has been hypothesized that women may experience more ruptured aneurysms due to their higher proportion of superthin tissue at the dome of their aneurysm in comparison to men. This superthin tissue is more vulnerable to external forces and consequently more susceptible to rupture (Kadasi et al. 2013). Inflammation accompanying cigarette smoke exposure may also be an important pathway underlying the development, progression, and rupture of cerebral aneurysms (Chalouhi et al. 2012).

Natural History, Prognostic Factors, and Outcomes

Unruptured aneurysms may be symptomatic and manifested as cranial nerve palsies. Moreover, unruptured aneurysms of sufficient size can compress cerebral tissue and manifest as various neurological signs (Ko and Kim 2011; Penn et al. 2011). Ruptured cerebral aneurysms can be associated with states of consciousness ranging from lethargy to coma with outcome based on location and severity of bleeding. A sudden loss of consciousness is a presenting feature in about 20% of cases. Commonly observed systemic complications and sequelae are vasospasms, rebleeding, hydrocephalus, herniation, seizures, cardiac dysrhythmias, and respiratory depression (Bonner and Bonner 1991).

Neuropsychological and Medical Outcomes

Symptoms and signs can include retinal hemorrhage, papilledema, and meningeal signs with seizure activity commonly observed. Focal signs are prominent within the first 24 h (e.g., parenchymal dissection, hyperfusion distal to the aneurysm site, cerebral edema). Vasospasm may be the cause of focal signs within the 48–72 h window. Cognitive, psychiatric, and behavioral impairments associated with ruptured and unruptured aneurysms depend on the site and extent of damage, secondary sequelae, complications, and premorbid health (see Table 1).

Aneurysm, Table 1 Symptoms that may be associated with ruptured and unruptured cerebral aneurysms (From Bonner and Bonner 1991; NINDS 2015; Walsh 2014)

Ruptured aneurysms	Unruptured aneurysms
Parenchymal dissection	Headache, neck rigidity
Hyperfusion	Neurologic deficit
Cerebral edema	Drowsiness, confusion, focal neurologic deficit
Cognitive impairments, confusion	Decerebrate rigidity/ vegetative disturbance possible
Disturbances in personality	Deep coma
Eye changes (drooping, blurred vision, light sensitivity)	Dilated pupil
Seizure	Pain above/behind eye, drooping eyelid
Severe headache	Double vision

Assessment and Treatment

The Hunt-Hess grading scale is used for prognosis and for timing of surgical interventions. Diagnostic evaluations commonly include CT scans, angiography, and MR angiography. Surgical treatment consists of clipping and endovascular embolization of the aneurysm or implanting a Woven endobridge device to provide flow disruption at the aneurysm neck–parent artery interface (Klisch et al. 2011). Pharmacologic interventions may include calcium channel blockers (e.g., nimodipine) in order to reduce the severity of vasospasm (Bonner and Bonner 1991). Patients taking Aspirin three times weekly to daily had significantly lower odds of hemorrhage compared with controls, and thus, Aspirin may reduce the risk of intracranial aneurysm rupture. However, additional research is needed using both animal and clinical models in order to verify safety, dosage, and efficacy (Hasan et al. 2011). The putative linkage between cigarette smoke, inflammation and aneurysm formation, progression, and rupture may suggest new targeted interventions to treat aneurysms.

Current research is examining DNA sequences in order to identify families at increased risk for certain types of aneurysm and possibly identify aneurysm-related genetic markers (NINDS 2015). Research on the advantages and disadvantages of microsurgical clipping and endovascular surgery for the treatment of both ruptured and unruptured aneurysms is also underway (Kohyama et al. 2014; Furuichi et al. 2015; Kamensky 2015; NINDS 2015; Suzuki et al. 2015).

Cross-References

▶ Anterior Cerebral Artery
▶ Anterior Communicating Artery
▶ Herniation Syndromes
▶ Hydrocephalus

References and Readings

Bonner, J. S., & Bonner, J. J. (1991). *The little black book of neurology: A manual for neurologic house officers* (2nd ed.). St Louis: Mosby-Year Book.

Chalouhi, N., Ali, M. S., Starke, R. M., Jabbour, P. M., Tjoumakaris, S. I., Gonzalez, L. F., ..., & Dumont, A. S. (2012). Cigarette smoke and inflammation: Role in cerebral aneurysm formation and rupture. *Mediators of Inflammation, 2012*, 271582.

Furuichi, M., Shimoda, K., Kano, T., Satoh, S., & Yoshino, A. (2015). A case of brainstem hemorrhage following embolization of a large basilar aneurysm with hydrogel-coated coils. *No Shinkei Geka. Neurological Surgery, 43(9)*, 835–842.

Hasan, D. M., Mahaney, K. B., Brown, R. D., Meissner, I., Piepgras, D. G., Huston, J., ..., & International Study of Unruptured Intracranial Aneurysms Investigators. (2011). Aspirin as a promising agent for decreasing incidence of cerebral aneurysm rupture. *Stroke, 42(11)*, 3156–3162.

Kadasi, L. M., Dent, W. C., & Malek, A. M. (2013). Cerebral aneurysm wall thickness analysis using intraoperative microscopy: Effect of size and gender on thin translucent regions. *Journal of Neurointerventional Surgery, 5(3)*, 201–206.

Kamensky, J. (2015). Neurosurgical versus endovascular treatment of subarachnoid haemorrhage caused by ruptured cerebral aneurysm: Comparison of patient outcomes. *Journal of Perioperative Practice, 25(3)*, 53–57.

Klisch, J., Sychra, V., Strasilla, C., Liebig, T., & Fiorella, D. (2011). The Woven EndoBridge cerebral aneurysm embolization device (WEB II): Initial clinical experience. *Neuroradiology, 53(8)*, 599–607.

Ko, J. H., & Kim, Y. J. (2011). Oculomotor nerve palsy caused by posterior communicating artery aneurysm: Evaluation of symptoms after endovascular treatment. *Interventional Neuroradiology, 17(4)*, 415–419.

Kohyama, S., Kakehi, Y., Yamane, F., Ooigawa, H., Kurita, H., & Ishihara, S. (2014). Subdural and intracerebral hemorrhage caused by spontaneous bleeding in the middle meningeal artery after coil embolization of a cerebral aneurysm. *Journal of Stroke and Cerebrovascular Diseases, 23(9)*, e433–e435.

Kulcsár, Z., Ugron, A., Marosfőia, M., Berenteia, Z., Paálc, G., & Szikoraa, I. (2011). Hemodynamics of cerebral aneurysm initiation: The role of wall shear stress and spatial wall shear stress gradient. *American Journal of Neuroradiology, 32*, 587–594.

Mayo Clinic Staff. (2015). Brain aneurysm information page. Rochester: Mayo Clinic. http://www.mayoclinic.org/diseases-conditions/brain-aneurysm/basics/definition/con-20028457. Updated 1 Sept 2015.

NIH. (2011). National Heart Lung and Blood Institute aneurysm information page. Bethesda: NIH. https://www.nhlbi.nih.gov/health/health-topics/topics/arm. Updated Oct 2015.

NINDS. (2015). NINDS cerebral aneurysm information page. National Institute of Neurologic Disorders and Stroke website. http://www.ninds.nih.gov/disorders/aneurysm/aneurysm.htm. Updated 23 Feb 2015; accessed 5 Mar 2016.

Parkin, A., & Leng, R. C. (1993). *Neuropsychology of the amnestic syndrome*. Hove: Lawrence Erlbaum.

Penn, D. L., Komotar, R. J., & Connolly, E. S. (2011). Hemodynamic mechanisms underlying cerebral aneurysm pathogenesis. *Journal of Clinical Neuroscience, 18(11)*, 1435–1438.

Ropper, A. H., Brown, R. H., Adams, R. D., & Victor, M. (2005). *Adams & Victor's principles of neurology*. New York: McGraw-Hill.

Scholtes, F., Henroteaux, A., Otto, B., & Martin, D. (2015). Head trauma and distal anterior cerebral artery aneurysm: Potential role of an adhesion to the falx. *Journal of Neurological Surgery. Part A, Central European Neurosurgery, 76(1)*, 72–75.

Suzuki, M., Yoneda, H., Ishihara, H., Shirao, S., Nomura, S., Koizumi, H., ..., & Inoue, T. (2015). Adverse events after unruptured cerebral aneurysm treatment: A single-center experience with clipping/coil embolization combined units. *Journal of Stroke and Cerebrovascular Diseases, 24(1)*, 223–231.

Walsh, M. E. (2014). The nose knows: An unusual presentation of a cerebral aneurysm. *Journal of Emergency Medicine, 47(5)*, e113–e115.

Webster. (2006). *Webster's new explorer medical dictionary* (2nd ed.). Springfield: Merriam-Webster.

Angelman Syndrome

Kristen Smith[1] and Bonita P. "Bonnie" Klein-Tasman[2]
[1]Department of Psychology and the Neuroscience Institute, Georgia State University, Atlanta, GA, USA
[2]Department of Psychology, University of Wisconsin-Milwaukee, Milwaukee, WI, USA

Definition

Angelman syndrome is a neurodevelopmental disorder caused by one of several genetic mechanisms involving maternal chromosome 15, specifically the region 15q11.2-13 (Dagli et al. 2015). Common features include microcephaly, seizure disorder, impaired motor skills, and developmental delays. Absent or extremely limited expressive language skills are also commonly observed. Behaviorally, individuals with Angelman syndrome are known for a happy temperament, frequent laughter, inattention/hyperactivity, and stereotyped behaviors; these features have been identified as the most consistent features within this population (Clayton-Smith and Laan 2003).

Categorization

Deletion or mutation of genetic material on chromosome 15q11-13 can result in one of two distinct neurodevelopmental disorders, depending upon whether the genetic material is from the maternal or paternal chromosome. This parent of origin effect is known as "imprinting." Note that the 15q11-13 region is differently imprinted in maternal and paternal chromosomes, and both imprintings are needed for normal development. If a maternal deletion occurs, the result is Angelman syndrome; if a paternal deletion occurs, then the result is Prader-Willi syndrome. Therefore, Angelman and Prader-Willi have been termed "sister syndromes" or "sister disorders" (e.g., Cassidy et al. 2000).

There are four main classes of Angelman syndrome, based upon four primary genetic mechanisms by which it occurs (Clayton-Smith and Laan 2003). In the general population, UBE3A is expressed only from the maternal chromosome in particular regions of the brain, and the UBE3A gene on the paternal chromosome is inactive. In Angelman syndrome, as a result of the deletion, only about 10% of UBE3A is expressed (Williams 2005).

Epidemiology

Exact prevalence rates of Angelman syndrome are unknown but have been estimated between 1/12,000 and 1/24,000 (Dagli et al. 2015). See Table 1 for estimates by subtype.

Natural History, Prognostic Factors, and Outcomes

Angelman syndrome was first described by Dr. Harry Angelman in 1965. He observed several pediatric patients whom he referred to as "puppet children," in light of their happy expressions and "jerky" movements (Angelman 1965). This term was later abandoned, and the disorder instead came

Angelman Syndrome, Table 1 Sample caption

Genetic mechanism	Incidence	Definition
De novo deletion	75%	Deletion on maternal chromosome region 15q11-13
Uniparental disomy	1–2%	Both copies of chromosome 15 are inherited from the father, rather than one from each parent
Imprinting defect	3%	Genes become inactivated as a result of a disruption in genes controlling the imprinting process itself, or the imprinting center
UBE3A mutation	11%	
Unknown	10%	

Buiting et al. (2015); Dagli et al. (2015)

to be known as Angelman syndrome. Diagnostic clinical criteria were developed by Williams and colleagues in 1995 and revised in 2006. These criteria include severe developmental delay, movement or balance disorder, unique behavior, and severe speech impairment (Williams et al. 2006).

The prenatal and perinatal history of children with Angelman syndrome is typically unremarkable, and developmental delays first become evident around 6–12 months of age (Cassidy et al. 2000). Head circumference is typically normal at birth but growth is then delayed, resulting in microcephaly by age 2 years (Dagli et al. 2015). Puberty usually occurs on time. There is generally no evidence of reduced life span, although the severity of associated medical conditions (e.g., seizures) certainly impacts health and the overall quality of life. Additionally, the long-standing motor difficulties in this population often translate into mobility issues later in life (Clayton-Smith and Laan 2003) (Fig. 1).

Epilepsy is common in Angelman syndrome, reported in at least 80% of cases (Dagli et al. 2015; Williams et al. 2006). A variety of seizure types has been reported, including both generalized and complex-partial types (Thibert et al. 2009). Seizures usually appear in early childhood, with some indication of improvement during late childhood/adolescence, followed by recurrence in some adults with Angelman syndrome (Clayton-Smith 2001). EEGs are typically abnormal and often include large-amplitude spike-and-slow wave discharges (Dagli et al. 2015).

Variability is evident in the phenotypic expression of Angelman syndrome depending upon the specific genetic mechanism by which it occurs. Those with Angelman syndrome due to a de novo deletion appear have the most severe medical/neurological effects, as well as greater motor and language deficits (e.g., Clayton-Smith and Laan 2003; Levitas et al. 2007). In contrast, those with uniparental disomy have lower rates of seizures and less severe language impairments, as well as fewer dysmorphic facial features. Individuals with an imprinting center defect also appear to have milder clinical presentations. Finally, those with UBE3A mutations have been found to have the more severe medical and physical problems seen in individuals with de novo deletions but fewer difficulties with motor and language skills than these individuals (Clayton-Smith and Laan 2003) (Fig. 2).

Neuropsychology and Psychology of Angelman Syndrome

Findings from neuroimaging studies have included smaller gray matter volume in several cortical and subcortical brain regions, as well as abnormal patterns of myelination and white matter abnormalities (Aghakhanyan et al. 2016; Harting et al. 2009; Peters et al. 2011). Cognitive development is severely delayed (Gentile et al. 2010). Adaptive functioning is also delayed, with a relative strength evident in social skills (Peters et al. 2004). As mentioned above, a primary feature of Angelman syndrome is limited expressive language, which typically ranges from no language to very few single words. There are relative strengths in receptive language (Gentile et al. 2010). Marked deficits occur in fine motor skills.

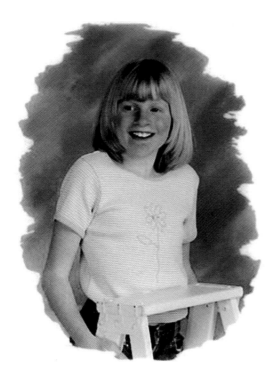

Angelman Syndrome, Fig. 1

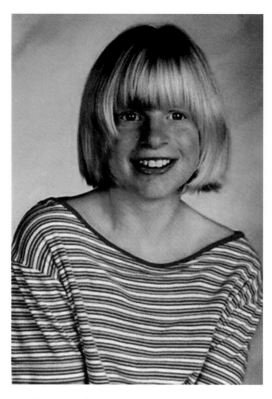

Angelman Syndrome, Fig. 2

A "happy" temperament has been reported among individuals with Angelman syndrome, characterized by frequent smiling and laughter, which persists across the life span (e.g., Clayton-Smith and Laan 2003). A variety of other behavioral concerns have also been reported, most commonly inattention and hyperactivity (Clarke and Marston 2000; Summers et al. 1995). However, there is some indication that these behavioral difficulties improve with age (Clayton-Smith and Laan 2003). Stereotyped motor behaviors, such as hand flapping, have frequently been observed (Williams et al. 2006). Elevated risk of autism spectrum disorder has often been suggested; however, this may be overdiagnosed due to the severity of intellectual disability and especially communication problems and motor abnormalities, whereas social reciprocity is typically relatively intact (Moss and Howlin 2009). Social smiling may appear as early as 1 to 3 months of age, and a strong preference for

social interactions has been described, although the nature of these interactions differs depending upon overall intellectual abilities (Williams 2010). Those with larger deletions have been demonstrated to show more impaired social affect and more repetitive behaviors than those with smaller deletions, when controlling for cognitive and adaptive abilities (Peters et al. 2012). Incidence of parental stress is high and differs by subtype, with those parents of children with imprinting defects reporting the highest stress levels (Miodrag and Peters 2015). Sleep and feeding problems have been identified as associated features of Angelman syndrome (Williams et al. 2006).

Evaluation

Angelman syndrome is confirmed through genetic testing (Dagli et al. 2015). Fluorescence in situ hybridization (FISH) testing is typically employed to identify genetic deletions; chromosomal microarray is utilized in some specific instances. DNA-methylation testing can be used to detect uniparental disomy or imprinting defects.

Treatment

There is no "cure" for Angelman syndrome itself. Given the high incidence of seizure disorder, management and follow-up by a neurologist is usually necessary. Anticonvulsant medications have been used to manage seizures in this population, most often clonazepam, valproic acid, topiramate, lamotrigine, and ethosuximide (Thibert et al. 2009). Sleep difficulties have successfully been addressed through behavioral intervention and with melatonin (Allen et al. 2013; Braam et al. 2008).

Involvement in interventions such as occupational, physical, and speech/language therapy is typically recommended to address language and motor deficits. In addition to speech/language therapy, alternative communication methods typically need to be explored. Special education programming is indicated in light of cognitive deficits. Very few behavioral intervention studies have been conducted for individuals with Angelman syndrome. Behavioral training has been used in an effort to address problematic social behaviors (Fichtner and Tiger 2015; Heald et al. 2013).

Cross-References

▶ Ataxia
▶ Developmental Delay
▶ Epilepsy
▶ Intellectual Disability
▶ Microcephaly
▶ Prader-Willi Syndrome
▶ Seizure
▶ Syndrome

References and Readings

Aghakhanyan, G., Bonanni, P., Randazzo, G., Nappi, S., Tessarotto, F., De Martin, L., et al. (2016). From cortical and subcortical Grey matter abnormalities to neurobehavioral phenotype of Angelman syndrome: A voxel-based Morphometry study. *PloS One, 11*(9), e0162817. https://doi.org/10.1371/journal.pone.0162817.

Allen, K. D., Kuhn, B. R., DeHaai, K. A., & Wallace, D. P. (2013). Evaluation of a behavioral treatment package to reduce sleep problems in children with Angelman syndrome. *Research in Developmental Disabilities, 34*(1), 676–686.

Angelman, H. (1965). 'Puppet' children: A report on three cases. *Developmental Medicine & Child Neurology, 7*, 681–688.

Braam, W., Didden, R., Smits, M. G., & Curfs, L. M. (2008). Melatonin for chronic insomnia in Angelman syndrome: A randomized placebo-controlled trial. *Journal of Child Neurology, 23*, 649–654.

Buiting, K., Clayton-Smith, J., Driscol, D. J., Gillessen-Kaesbach, G., Kanber, D., Schwinger, E., et al. (2015). Clinical utility card for: Angelman syndrome. European journal of human genetics, 23, online.

Cassidy, S. B., Dykens, E., & Williams, C. A. (2000). Prader-Willi and Angelman syndromes: Sister imprinted disorders. *American Journal of Medical Genetics, 97*, 136–146.

Clarke, D. J., & Marston, G. (2000). Problem behaviors associated with 15q- Angelman syndrome. *American Journal on Mental Retardation, 105*, 25–31.

Clayton-Smith, J. (2001). Angelman syndrome: Evolution of the phenotype in adolescents and adults. *Developmental Medicine & Child Neurology, 43*, 476–480.

Clayton-Smith, J., & Laan, L. (2003). Angelman syndrome: A review of the clinical and genetic aspects. *Journal of Medical Genetics, 40*, 87–95.

Dagli, A. I., Mueller, J., & Williams, C. A. (2015). Angelman Syndrome. In: Pagon R. A., Adam, M. P., Ardinger, H. H., Wallace, S. E., Amemiya, A., Bean, L. J. H., . . . & Stephens, K. (Eds.). *GeneReviews*® [Internet]. Seattle: University of Washington, Seattle; 1993–2015. Available from: https://www.ncbi.nlm.nih.gov/books/NBK1144/

Fichtner, C. S., & Tiger, J. H. (2015). Teaching discriminated social approaches to individuals with Angelman syndrome. *Journal of Applied Behavior Analysis, 48*, 734–748.

Gentile, J. K., Tan, W.-H., Horowitz, L. T., Bacino, C. A., Skinner, S. A., Barbieri-Welge, R., et al. (2010). A neurodevelopmental survey of Angelman syndrome with genotype-phenotype correlations. *Journal of Developmental and Behavioral Pediatrics, 31*(7), 592–601.

Harting, I., Seitz, A., Rating, D., Sartor, K., Zschocke, J., Janssen, B., et al. (2009). Abnormal myelination in Angelman syndrome. *European Journal of Pediatric Neurology, 13*(3), 271–275.

Heald, M., Allen, D., Villa, D., & Oliver, C. (2013). Discrimination training reduces high rate social approach behaviors in Angelman syndrome: Proof of principle. *Research in Developmental Disabilities, 34*, 1794–1803.

Levitas, A., Dykens, E., Finucane, B., & Kates, W. (2007). Behavioral phenotype of genetic disorders. In R. Fletcher, E. Loschen, C. Stavrakaki, & M. First (Eds.), *Diagnostic manual - intellectual disability: A textbook of diagnoses of mental disorders in persons with intellectual disability*. Kingston: NADD Press.

Miodrag, N., & Peters, S. (2015). Parent stress across molecular subtypes of children with Angelman syndrome. *Journal of Intellectual Disability Research, 59*, 816–826.

Moss, J., & Howlin, P. (2009). Autism spectrum disorders in genetic syndromes: Implications for diagnosis, intervention and understanding the wider autism spectrum disorder population. *Journal of Intellectual Disabilities Research, 53*, 852–873.

Peters, S. U., Goddard-Finegold, J., Beaudet, A. L., Madduri, N., Turcich, M., & Bacino, C. A. (2004). Cognitive and adaptive behavior profiles of children with Angelman syndrome. *American Journal of Medical Genetics, 128*, 110–113.

Peters, S. U., Horowitz, L., Barbieri-Welge, R., Lounds Taylor, J., & Hundley, R. J. (2012). Longitudinal follow-up of autism spectrum features and sensory behaviors in Angelman syndrome by deletion class. *Journal of Child Psychology and Psychiatry, 53*(2), 152–159.

Peters, S. U., Kaufmann, W. E., Bacino, C. A., Angerson, A. W., Adapa, P., Chu, Z., . . . & Wilde, E. A., (2011). Alterations in white matter pathways in Angelman syndrome. Developmental Medicine & Child Neurology, 53, 361–367.

Summers, J. A., Allison, D. B., Lynch, P. S., & Sandler, L. (1995). Behaviour problems in Angelman syndrome. *Journal of Intellectual Disability Research, 39*, 97–106.

Summers, J. A., & Feldman, M. A. (1999). Distinctive pattern of behavioral functioning in Angelman syndrome. *American Journal on Mental Retardation, 104*, 376–384.

Thibert, R. L., Conant, K. D., Braun, E. K., Bruno, P., Said, R. R., Nespeca, M. P., & Thiele, E. A. (2009). Epilepsy in Angelman syndrome: A questionnaire-based assessment of the natural history and current treatment options. *Epilepsia, 50*, 2369–2376.

Williams, C. A. (2005). Neurological aspects of the Angelman syndrome. *Brain & Development, 27*, 88–94.

Williams, C. A. (2010). The behavioral phenotype of the Angelman syndrome. *American Journal of Medical Genetics, 154C*, 432–437.

Williams, C. A., Beaudet, A. L., Clayton-Smith, J., Knoll, J. H., Kyllerman, M., Laan, L. A., et al. (2006). Angelman syndrome 2005: Updated consensus for diagnostic criteria. *American Journal of Medical Genetics, 140*, 413–418.

Williams, C. A., Driscoll, D. J., & Dagli, A. I. (2010). Clinical and genetic aspects of Angelman syndrome. *Genetics in Medicine, 12*(7), 385–395.

Angiography, Cerebral

Nathan D. Zasler[1] and Richard Kunz[2]
[1]Concussion Care Centre of Virginia, Ltd., Richmond, VA, USA
[2]Department of Physical Medicine and Rehabilitation, Virginia Commonwealth University, Richmond, VA, USA

Synonyms

Angio

Definition

Angiography is the evaluation of the blood vessels of the central nervous system and associated cervicocerebral vasculature via radiographic imaging of intravascular contrast media injected prior to the imaging procedure. Femoral or axillary non-selective approaches can be used to catheterize the aortic arch or selective means employed to catheterize the carotid artery. Digital subtraction, computed tomography (CT) scanning, and MRI techniques can be applied as adjutant imaging techniques once contrast is injected. Obstructions, stenosis, aneurysms, and A-V malformations can be identified through this technique. Finer and more selective views are accomplished by using microcatheters. Some of the disease entities studied include ischemic cerebrovascular disease, aneurysms, vascular malformations, neoplasms, and brain injuries. Angiography is the test of choice for arterial dissections and pseudoaneurysms which may be associated with classic signs of pain, bruits, and/or cranial nerve palsies. Carotid angiography is also useful for imaging of carotid-cavernous fistulas which if not found early can cause blindness and may present with an ocular bruit, scleral injection, and ocular proptosis.

Current Knowledge

Can be part of the evaluation process of patients with cerebrovascular disease or traumatic vascular insult.

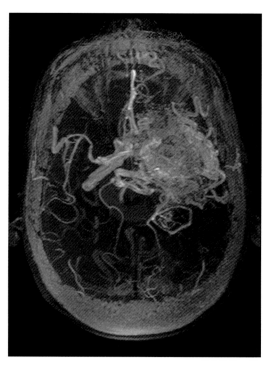

Cross-References

▶ Angioma, Cavernous Angioma
▶ Glioma
▶ Hemangioma
▶ Hemiplegia

References and Readings

Ahn, S. O., Prince, E. A., & Dubel, G. J. (2013). Basic neuroangiography: Review of technique and perioperative patient care. *Seminars in Interventional Radiology, 30*(3), 225–233.
http://www.radiologyinfo.org/en/info.cfm?pg=angiocerebral. Accessed 10/4/16.
Kaufmann, T. J., & Kallmes, D. F. (2008). Diagnostic cerebral angiography: Archaic and complication-prone or here to stay for another 80 years? *AJR: American Journal of Roentgenology, 190*(6), 1435–1437.

Angioma, Cavernous Angioma

Jennifer Tinker
Department of Neurology, Thomas Jefferson University, Philadelphia, PA, USA

Synonyms

Cavernoma; Cavernous hemangioma; Cavernous venous malformation; Cerebral cavernous malformation (CCM)

Definition

Cavernous angiomas are benign vascular malformations found within the CNS that may occur sporadically or in a familial pattern. Cavernous angiomas are also a complication of radiation therapy, especially in children. These angiomas can remain stable, enlarge over time, or bleed, and there are no factors that predict their occurrence or behavior.

Three genetic loci responsible for familial cavernous angioma (CCM1, CCM2, and CCM3) have been identified. Cavernomas are typically found supratentorially (approximately 80%), predominantly in the subcortical rolandic and temporal areas. Infratentorially, cavernous angiomas are most commonly found in the pons and cerebellar hemispheres (Sage and Blumbergs 2001). Originally thought to be relatively rare and most commonly detected during autopsy, the advent of MRI has led to an increased detection, with incidence rates now estimated between 0.02% and 0.8% of the general population. The size of the well-circumscribed, "mulberry-like" mass can range from less than 1 cm to greater than 4 cm. Prevalence rates are relatively equivalent among males and females. While it can remain asymptomatic lifelong, symptomatic presentation is most commonly seen in the third and fourth decades of life. However, newly symptomatic cases have been well reported throughout the life span. Women are more likely to present with hemorrhage and neurologic deficits (Del Curling et al. 1991).

Clinical manifestations, when present, vary significantly and generally correlate to location of the lesion. Most commonly reported symptoms include headache (6–65%), seizure (23–52%), focal neurological deficit (20–45%), and intracranial hemorrhage (13–25%) (Conway and Rigamonti 2006). Despite the regional affinity for frontal and temporal regions, no studies have specifically examined for selective neuropsychological deficits. Treatment can include observation, surgical resection, or stereotactic radiosurgery.

References and Readings

Conway, J. E., & Rigamonti, D. (2006). Cavernous malformations: A review and current controversies. *Neurosurgery Quarterly, 16*(1), 15–23.
Del Curling, O., Kelly, D. L., Elster, A. D., & Craven, T. E. (1991). An analysis of the natural history of cavernous angiomas. *Journal of Neurosurgery, 75*(5), 702.
Sage, M. R., & Blumbergs, P. C. (2001). Cavernous haemangiomas (angiomas) of the brain. *Pathological-Radiological Correlation, 45*, 247–256.

Angioplasty

Elliot J. Roth
Department of Physical Medicine and
Rehabilitation, Northwestern University,
Feinberg School of Medicine, Chicago, IL, USA

Synonyms

Coronary angioplasty; Percutaneous coronary intervention (PCI); Percutaneous transluminal angioplasty (PTA); Percutaneous transluminal coronary angioplasty (PTCA)

Definition

Angioplasty is a minimally invasive (nonsurgical) percutaneously performed clinical procedure used to dilate blood vessels narrowed or blocked by atherosclerosis. Historically, angioplasty was performed most commonly on the coronary arteries that supply blood to the heart muscle. However, recent evidence indicates its effectiveness in improving cerebral circulation in patients with acute stroke. Angioplasty may be used to treat coronary artery disease, which often presents with persistent angina (chest pain) or a myocardial infarction (heart attack), cerebrovascular disease causing stroke or transient ischemic attacks, renal artery stenosis causing kidney dysfunction, and peripheral artery disease, usually in the blood vessel of the leg. During angioplasty, a stent is placed in the vessel to keep the vessel patent.

Current Knowledge

In this procedure, a small incision is made over the skin of a peripheral artery (usually the femoral artery in the thigh), and the artery is punctured to gain access into the blood vessel. A thin catheter is then inserted into the blood vessel, and both blood vessels and catheter are visualized by radiographic fluoroscopy. The catheter is then pushed further into the vessel (guided by fluoroscopic images). When

the tip of the catheter reaches the target blood vessel, a previously folded balloon at the end of the catheter is inflated to flatten the plaque in the vessel wall, thereby reducing the blockage and expanding the diameter of the artery. Usually, a stent, a metal mesh tube of small diameter which also was on the end of the catheter, is then placed inside the vessel and expanded by manipulating the catheter tip. Many of these stents, called "drug-eluting stents," contain and secrete antiplatelet medications that assist in preventing arterial stenosis in the future. The result of the angioplasty is a dilated artery and improved blood flow through the vessel.

This procedure is done to prevent the vessel from developing narrowing or becoming blocked again. It is a relatively safe procedure, and complications are rare, but they include allergy, bleeding, clotting, stroke, kidney failure, and re-blockage of the newly opened artery. After the procedure, patients usually remain on bedrest for a short time and are instructed to use antiplatelet medications.

See Also

▶ Angiography, Cerebral
▶ Atherosclerosis
▶ Cerebrovascular Disease
▶ Coronary Disease
▶ Myocardial Infarction
▶ Peripheral Vascular Disease
▶ Stent
▶ Thrombectomy

References

Levine, G. N., Bates, E. R., Blankenship, J. C., Bailey, S. R., Bittl, J. A., Cercek, B., Chambers, C. E., Ellis, S. G., Guyton, R. A., Hollenberg, S. M., Khot, U. N., Lange, R. A., Mauri, L., Mehran, R., Moussa, I. D., Mukherjee, D., Nallamothu, B. K., & Ting, H. H. (2011). ACCF/AHA/SCAI guideline for percutaneous coronary intervention: A report of the American College of Cardiology Foundation/ American Heart Association Task Force on Practice Guidelines and the Society for Cardiovascular Angiography and Interventions. *Circulation, 124*, 2574–2609.

Anomalous Dominance

John E. Mendoza
Department of Psychiatry and Neuroscience,
Tulane Medical School and SE Louisiana
Veterans Healthcare System, New Orleans, LA,
USA

Synonyms

Mixed dominance

Definition

Anomalous dominance describes any pattern of cerebral organization of function in which the left hemisphere is *not* primarily responsible for initiating propositional speech and processing written or spoken language.

Current Knowledge

Since the left hemisphere primacy for language is typical of most right-handers (who represent the vast majority of the population), it is considered to be the "dominant" pattern of brain organization. Hence, any pattern that differs from this is considered to be *anomalous*. Most deviations occur in left-handers, approximately 30% of whom exhibit some form of anomalous dominance for language where these functions are organized either primarily in the right hemisphere ("reversed dominance") or are more bilaterally represented. Although anomalous dominance can occur in right-handers, this is rare and, when present, is often a consequence of some early developmental defect or brain trauma. Other associations that have been reported to be related to anomalous patterns of hemispheric organization of language are female gender, mixed hand preference (ambidexterity), and family history of sinistrality. In these situations, there is an increased tendency for language functions to be organized in both hemispheres. Support for this hypothesis comes in part from radiographic studies which show a tendency for males when compared with females to have greater anatomical asymmetry in the region of the frontal operculum (Broca's area) and in the temporal operculum (planum temporale), both key language areas. This apparent tendency for greater bilateral representation of language has been suggested as a possible explanation for (1) the earlier development (on average) of language in females than in males, and (2) the superior recovery of language functions following strokes seen in some left-handers.

Cross-References

▶ Dominance (Cerebral)

References and Readings

Geschwind, N., & Galaburda, A. (1985). Cerebral lateralization. *Archives of Neurology, 42,* 428–459; 521–552; 634–654.
Geschwind, N., & Galaburda, A. M. (1987). *Cerebral lateralization: Biological mechanisms, associations, and pathology.* Cambridge, MA: MIT Press.
Herron, J. (Ed.). (1980). *Neuropsychology of left-handedness.* New York: Academic.

Anomia

Anastasia Raymer
Communication Disorders and Special Education,
Old Dominion University, Norfolk, VA, USA

Synonyms

Naming impairments; Word-finding difficulties

Definition

Anomia generally refers to instances of word-finding difficulty that occur during the course of conversational discourse. It is often documented clinically in confrontation picture-naming tasks.

Current Knowledge

Anomia can occur in healthy individuals who occasionally experience difficulty retrieving an intended word during a conversation, also known as the tip-of-the-tongue state (Biedermann et al. 2008). It is a frequent occurrence in individuals with left hemisphere brain damage and aphasia (Raymer 2011). Typically associated with difficulties for nouns, anomia also can refer to difficulties in retrieving other classes of words, such as verbs and adjectives. Anomia arises from failure at any stage in the complex series of lexical processes engaged in word retrieval, including activation of semantic representations for the meaning to be conveyed and phonological representations for the form of the word to express that meaning (Tippett and Hillis 2015). These distinct processes in word retrieval engage different parts of the brain distributed throughout the left cerebral hemisphere (Race and Hillis 2015). Therefore, when brain damage occurs, anomia may take somewhat different patterns (Laine and Martin 2006). For example, in semantic anomia, failure to retrieve words is accompanied by difficulty in recognition of the same words. In contrast, phonologic anomia occurs when a word is recognized but cannot be retrieved. It is important to note that anomia and anomic aphasia are not synonymous. Anomia is the primary symptom of anomic aphasia and also can be observed in virtually all other forms of aphasia (e.g., Broca's aphasia, Wernicke's aphasia), both as initial and residual signs when other signs and symptoms of aphasia have resolved.

When anomia occurs across different forms of aphasia, a number of errors can be seen (Laine and Martin 2006). At times, the moment of anomia leads to complete inability to retrieve a word. Other times, an inappropriate word is retrieved, also known as a paraphasia. Sometimes, the error word is somehow related to the intended word in meaning (semantic paraphasia, e.g., saying "dog" for cat) or sound characteristics (phonologic paraphasia, e.g., saying "crat" for cat). Sometimes, the moment of word-finding difficulty is filled with a circumlocution or description of the intended word (e.g., "That thing that meows and has whiskers. I can't think of the name."). In severe forms

of anomia, neologisms may occur in which the uttered word may not be recognizable at all (e.g., saying "bilan" for cat).

Cross-References

▶ Circumlocution
▶ Confrontation Naming
▶ Paraphasia
▶ Semantic Paraphasia
▶ Word Finding

References and Readings

Biedermann, B., Ruh, N., Nickels, L., & Coltheart, M. (2008). Information retrieval in tip of the tongue states: New data and methodological advances. *Journal of Psycholinguistic Research, 37*, 171–198.

Laine, M., & Martin, N. (2006). *Anomia: Theoretical and clinical aspects*. New York: Psychology Press.

Race, D. C., & Hillis, A. E. (2015). The neural mechanisms underlying naming. In A. E. Hillis (Ed.), *The handbook of adult language disorders* (pp. 151–160). New York: Psychology Press.

Raymer, A. M. (2011). Naming and word retrieval problems. In L. L. LaPointe (Ed.), *Aphasia and related neurogenic language disorders* (4th ed., pp. 95–110). New York: Thieme Medical Publishers.

Tippett, D. C., & Hillis, A. E. (2015). The cognitive processes underlying naming. In A. E. Hillis (Ed.), *The handbook of adult language disorders* (pp. 141–150). New York: Psychology Press.

Anomic Aphasia

Anastasia Raymer
Communication Disorders and Special Education, Old Dominion University, Norfolk, VA, USA

Definition

Anomic aphasia is the language impairment that involves only word-finding difficulties or pure anomia in contrast to other forms of aphasia (Harnish 2015). Other language modalities typically are intact in anomic aphasia, including auditory comprehension of language, repetition of words and sentences, and spontaneous generation of sentences, yet struggle may be noted to retrieve words during sentence generation.

Current Knowledge

Anomic aphasia is a form of language disorder associated with acquired brain damage typically affecting the left cerebral hemisphere (Raymer 2011). Anomic aphasia can be manifest as a difficulty in retrieving specific intended words, often nouns, but sometimes verbs, during the course of sentence generation. The grammatical characteristics of the sentence remain intact. The moments of word retrieval difficulty lead to long pauses, insertion of filler words, or selection of wrong words (paraphasias) during conversation or other word retrieval activities, most commonly in tasks requiring individuals to name pictures. Also common in anomic aphasia is circumlocution, in which the speaker cannot think of the intended word and instead describes or provides associated information about the word.

When anomic aphasia occurs as a result of an acute neurologic event (e.g., stroke), it can be accompanied by pure alexia and difficulties with color identification (Goodglass et al. 2001). Acutely, anomic aphasia has been described following left temporal/occipital lesions (e.g., area 37) and left thalamic lesions (Race and Hillis 2015). Anomic aphasia often can be seen chronically as individuals recover from other forms of aphasia (Hoffmann and Chen 2013). In that case, the accompanying symptoms and neural correlates of anomic aphasia vary. Treatment approaches for anomic aphasia vary, including restorative approaches that attempt to facilitate recovery using typical semantic and phonologic processes engaged in word retrieval and compensatory approaches that circumvent word retrieval difficulties (Raymer 2011).

Cross-References

▶ Anomia
▶ Circumlocution

▶ Confrontation Naming
▶ Paraphasia
▶ Semantic Paraphasia
▶ Word Finding

References and Readings

Goodglass, H., Kaplan, E., & Barresi, B. (2001). *The assessment of aphasia and related disorders* (3rd ed.). Philadelphia: Lippincott, Williams, & Wilkins.

Harnish, S. M. (2015). Anomia and anomic aphasia: Implications for lexical processing. In A. M. Raymer & L. G. Rothi (Eds.), *The Oxford handbook of aphasia and language disorders*. New York: Oxford Handbooks Online.

Hoffmann, M., & Chen, R. (2013). The spectrum of aphasia subtypes and etiology in subacute stroke. *Journal of Stroke and Cerebrovascular Disease, 22,* 1385–1392.

Laine, M., & Martin, N. (2006). *Anomia: Theoretical and clinical aspects*. New York: Psychology Press.

Race, D. C., & Hillis, A. E. (2015). The neural mechanisms underlying naming. In A. E. Hillis (Ed.), *The handbook of adult language disorders* (pp. 151–160). New York: Psychology Press.

Raymer, A. M. (2011). Naming and word retrieval problems. In L. L. LaPointe (Ed.), *Aphasia and related neurogenic language disorders* (4th ed., pp. 72–86). New York: Thieme.

Anorexia Nervosa

Kristin M. Graham
Department of Physical Medicine and Rehabilitation, Virginia Commonwealth University, Richmond, VA, USA

Synonyms

Anorexia

Definition

Anorexia nervosa is defined in the *Diagnostic and Statistical Manual of Mental Disorders* (5th ed.; *DSM-5*; American Psychiatric Association 2013) as a feeding and eating disorder characterized by restrictions on eating and significantly low weight. This disorder is manifested through feelings of intense fear of gaining weight that lead to behaviors to stimulate weight loss (e.g., restricted food intake). The fear is not alleviated by weight loss. Self-perception of body weight and shape is often distorted. There are two subtypes: (1) *restricting type* in which weight loss is accomplished through dieting, caloric restriction, or excessive exercise and there is no binging/purging behavior and (2) *binge-eating/purging type* in which there are recurrent episodes of binging or purging behaviors.

Categorization

The disorder is classified with the Feeding and Eating Disorders in DSM-5.

Current Knowledge

Development and Course
The development of anorexia nervosa is common during adolescence and young adulthood and is often associated with a stressful life event. Course and outcome is highly variable (e.g., recovery after one episode, fluctuating pattern of weight gain leading to relapse). Likewise, functional consequences (e.g., social and professional functioning) vary between individuals, with some experiencing few functional consequences. Anorexia nervosa is more common in females as compared to males (female-to-male ratio, 10:1), and the prevalence rate for young females is 0.4% (APA 2013). Risk of suicidal ideation or behaviors is greater in individuals with this disorder.

Associated Features and Current Research
Individuals with anorexia nervosa often lack insight or deny it as being a problem. As such, professional intervention is often sought by family members or the individual when distressed over somatic or psychological sequelae. Significant and life-threatening medical conditions (e.g., amenorrhea, vital sign abnormalities, decreased bone mineral density), co-occurring psychological disorders (e.g., bipolar, depressive, and anxiety disorders), and obsessive-compulsive features (e.g., preoccupied thoughts of food, food hoarding) are common. There is some evidence for brain structural changes, such as increased ventricular width and cortical sulci (Uher et al. 2003). Neuropsychological functioning deficits in the areas of sustained and divided attention, working memory, inhibition, and mental flexibility have been identified in individuals with anorexia nervosa.

Assessment and Treatment
A comprehensive assessment interview for anorexia nervosa should include clinical interview, standardized self-report, interview-based measures (e.g., Eating Attitudes Test (EAT-12), Eating Disorder Inventory (EDI-3), Structured Clinical Interview for DSM-5 (SCID-5), Eating Disorder Examination (EDE)), and medical assessment (e.g., assessing for laboratory abnormalities, amenorrhea, emaciation, hypotension, and bradycardia). Additionally, information should be gathered from other sources (e.g., family members). Treatment of anorexia nervosa should include restoring healthy weight, medical treatment of physical complications, and evidence based psychotherapy (Watson & Bulik 2013). While no specific psychotherapy approach has shown superiority, treatment modalities commonly utilized and recommended include cognitive analytic therapy, cognitive behavioral therapy, and interpersonal psychotherapy. Anorexia nervosa should be differentiated from other causes of significantly low body weight or significant weight loss, such as gastrointestinal disease, substance use disorders, or other feeding and eating disorders. Additional differential diagnoses include major depressive disorder, schizophrenia, social anxiety disorder, obsessive-compulsive disorder, and body dysmorphic disorder.

See Also

▶ Avoidant/Restrictive Food Intake Disorder
▶ Body Dysmorphic Disorder

▶ Bulimia Nervosa
▶ Feeding and Eating Disorders

References and Readings

American Psychiatric Association. (2013). *Diagnostic and statistical manual of mental disorders (DSM-5 ®)*. Washington, DC: American Psychiatric Association.

Kidd, A., & Steinglass, J. (2012). What can cognitive neuroscience teach us about anorexia nervosa? *Current Psychiatry Reports, 14*(4), 415–420.

Mustelin, L., Silén, Y., Raevuori, A., Hoek, H. W., Kaprio, J., & Keski-Rahkonen, A. (2016). The DSM-5 diagnostic criteria for anorexia nervosa may change its population prevalence and prognostic value. *Journal of Psychiatric Research, 77*, 85–91.

Reville, M. C., O'Connor, L., & Frampton, I. (2016). Literature review of cognitive neuroscience and anorexia nervosa. *Current Psychiatry Reports, 18*(2), 1–8.

Surgenor, L. J., & Maguire, S. (2013). Assessment of anorexia nervosa: An overview of universal issues and contextual challenges. *Journal of Eating Disorders, 1*(1), 29.

Uher, R., Brammer, M. J., Murphy, T., Campbell, I. C., Ng, V. W., Williams, S. C. R., & Treasure, J. (2003) Recovery and chronicity in anorexia nervosa: brain activity associated with differential outcomes. *Biological Psychiatry, 54*(9), 934–942.

Watson, H. J., & Bulik, C. M. (2013). Update on the treatment of anorexia nervosa: review of clinical trials, practice guidelines and emerging interventions. *Psychological Medicine, 43*(12), 2477–2500.

Anosmia

Holly James Westervelt[1] and
Nicole C. R. McLaughlin[2]
[1]Memory and Cognitive Assessment Program, Department of Psychiatry, Rhode Island Hospital, Providence, RI, USA
[2]Butler Hospital Alpert Medical School of Brown University, Providence, RI, USA

Synonyms

Anosphrasia

Definition

Anosmia is defined as a lack of the sense of smell or an inability to detect odors of any kind. In the strictest sense, "anosmia" refers to a total lack of olfactory ability, though the term is often used more loosely to refer also to partial or diminished sense of smell. There are multiple additional terms describing olfactory abilities. *Normosmia* is the intact ability to perceive odors. *Hyposmia* is a more precise term to describe decreased ability to perceive smells, whereas *hyperosmia* is the increased ability to perceive odors. *Dysosmia* (a.k.a. *parosmia)* refers to distortions in the sense of smell, including *cacosmia* (distortion of a smell as particularly unpleasant) and *phantosmia* (an olfactory hallucination, or the sensation of a smell in the absence of a stimulus).

Epidemiology

Olfactory dysfunction is present in at least 1% of individuals under the age of 65, with some estimates suggesting total anosmia in as much as 5% of the population. Rates of impairment increase dramatically with age, with approximately 25% of older adults showing deficits in olfaction (Murphy et al. 2002). In patients presenting to chemosensory clinics, olfactory deficits are reported to be related to disability and quality of life, though most individuals with olfactory deficits are unaware of them. It is well established that throughout the lifespan, women show more acute olfactory abilities than men.

Causes

The causes of olfactory impairments are typically categorized as: (1) conductive/transport impairments, (2) sensory/sensorineural deficits, or (3) central olfactory neural impairment, though these categories are not mutually exclusive. The understanding of the potential causes of olfactory deficits will be enhanced by a brief review of the olfactory system, though it is noted that the olfactory pathways within the central nervous system (CNS) are not entirely agreed upon.

Anatomy of the Olfactory System

The sensation of smell is the brain's perception of odor in response to odorants activating olfactory receptors. Odors enter the nose, where they come in contact with the olfactory epithelium, made up of olfactory receptors. Olfactory receptor cells (first order neurons) send signals along the olfactory nerve (first cranial nerve) to the mitral cells of the olfactory bulb, where olfactory axons synapse with second-order neurons in the olfactory bulb. Each olfactory receptor type sends a signal to a particular region of the olfactory bulb. Mitral cell axons project through the olfactory tract and lateral olfactory stria to the primary olfactory cortex, which is primarily made up of the piriform cortex. Other structures receiving direct input include the anterior olfactory nucleus, olfactory tubercle, amygdala, and rostral entorhinal cortex (Gotfried and Zald 2005). Projections from these primary areas extend to secondary olfactory regions in the hippocampus, hypothalamus, thalamus, amygdala, and agranular insula, enabling encoding of odors into memory as well as emotional processing of specific odors (Gotfried and Zald 2005). There are also projections to the orbitofrontal cortex (OFC), and it is believed that the OFC mediates conscious perception of odors; lesions to this area often lead to impaired olfactory abilities (Gotfried and Zald 2005). In addition to the activation of the first cranial nerve, certain smells may also activate the trigeminal nerve (CNV), which mediates sensations associated with certain odorants, including burning, cooling, irritation, or tickling sensations. Activation of the trigeminal nerve may allow the "detection" of some odors, even in the presence of primary olfactory impairments. Cranial nerve zero (nervus terminalis) may also play some role in olfaction, though its function is poorly understood in humans.

Conductive/Transport Impairment

Olfactory impairment within this category arises from obstruction of nasal passages. Typical causes of obstruction include nasal inflammation, such as from allergies or upper respiratory infection (URI), or other structural interference, such as nasal polyps. URI is the most common cause of smell loss, and is often transient. Permanent smell loss due to URI can occur, presumably reflecting direct insult to the neuroepithelium, and becomes more likely in older age.

Sensorineural/Central Olfactory Neural Impairment

Olfactory deficits within these categories arise from damage to the neuroepithelium and/or impairment or impingement of central olfactory structures from CNS disease. There are numerous congenital, endocrine, neurological/neurodegenerative, nutritional/metabolic, and psychiatric disorders that have been shown to be associated with olfactory deficits (for a review of these causes, see Murphy et al. 2003). In addition, injury, medications (for review see Doty and Bromley 2004), environmental toxins (for review see Upadhyay and Holbrook 2004), structural lesions, and medical/surgical interventions (for review see Murphy et al. 2003) can affect neural functioning. The Table 1 provides a small sampling of disorders that can be associated with olfactory loss. Given the vast number of disorders that have shown olfactory deficits, theories have been postulated that olfactory impairment may

Anosmia, Table 1 Sampling of disorders associated with olfactory deficits

Alcoholism/Korsakoff's syndrome	Multiple sclerosis
Alzheimer's disease	Multiple system atrophy
Amyotrophic lateral sclerosis	Parkinson dementia complex of Guam
Corticobasal degeneration	Parkinson's disease
Dementia with Lewy bodies	Progressive supranuclear palsy
Diabetes mellitus	REM sleep behavior disorder
Down's syndrome	Restless leg syndrome
Frontotemporal dementia	Schizophrenia
Head injury	Sjögren's syndrome
Human immunodeficiency virus	Syphilis
Huntington's disease	Temporal lobe epilepsy
Mild cognitive impairment	Vascular dementia

be a nonspecific marker of CNS dysfunction. This is likely not the case, given that the degree of deficit can differ widely among disorders, there exists significant range of deficits among patients within disorders, and the deficits can be unrelated to disease stage or magnitude of disease symptoms in some diseases but not others. Rather, it is probable that the presence and degree of olfactory involvement is related to the relative degree of structural or biochemical damage to the specific regions of the brain involved in olfactory transduction.

Neurodegenerative Diseases Interest in olfaction in neurodegenerative disorders began most intensely in the 1980s, with a focus on Alzheimer's disease (AD) and Parkinson's disease (PD). It was initially thought that these two disorders, which were often thought of as the prototypical examples of cortical and subcortical diseases, would share an early and notable deficit. Olfactory deficits were then identified in a variety of neurodegenerative disorders, making olfactory loss a nonspecific finding, though the degree of impairment may be useful in distinguishing some disorders. The cause of olfactory deficits in neurodegenerative diseases is unknown (for a review of potential causes, see Smutzer et al. 2003). The deficits may be due at least in part to neurotransmitter system alterations, especially dopamine and acetylcholine. Damage to central processing areas is also a likely explanation, particularly involvement of the olfactory bulb and tracts, as relevant neuropathologic changes (e.g., neurofibrillary tangles, amyloid plaques, dystrophic neurites, Lewy bodies, and disproportionate neuronal loss) are often seen in these areas. Other relevant central processing areas (e.g., entorhinal cortex), however, also show neuropathologic changes, as may peripheral structures (e.g., olfactory epithelium).

Parkinson's Disease Olfactory impairment is a prominent, common, and early feature of Parkinson's disease (PD; see Doty 2003a, b, for a review). The deficits tend to be bilateral, and are more common than some of the hallmark symptoms of PD, such as tremor. Olfactory deficits may

be present before the motor symptoms become evident, and are apparent with both threshold and identification tasks. The size of the effect is astounding (ranging from 1.17 to 12.15 in a meta-analysis; Mesholam et al. 1998), though the majority of patients are not completely anosmic. Deficits do not appear to correlate with the extent of cognitive or motor involvement, do not respond to treatment, and do not appear to be progressive over time.

Other Parkinsonian Spectrum Disorders Other Parkinsonian disorders, such as corticobasal degeneration (CBD), multiple system atrophy, and progressive supranuclear palsy, are also associated with olfactory deficits, though the impairments tend to be more mild than is seen in PD (Doty 2003a, b). These findings suggest that olfactory functioning may be useful in distinguishing PD from other parkinsonian disorders, though a more recent study of olfaction in CBD raises some question of potentially more notable deficit in this disorder than was previously described (Pardini et al. 2009).

Alzheimer's Disease and Mild Cognitive Impairment There has been fairly good consistency in the literature for most of the studies examining olfaction in Alzheimer's disease (AD; see Doty 2003a, b, for a review). The size of the effect is extremely large, ranging from 0.98 to 8.55 in a meta-analysis (Mesholam et al. 1998), though, as in PD, patients are typically not completely anosmic. Odor identification deficits are always found; odor detection deficits are more inconsistently demonstrated and may be a later symptom. The odor identification deficit does not seem to be primarily due to a general cognitive deficit and deficits worsen with disease progression. Although group studies have shown consistent deficits in odor identification, it should be noted that the presence of deficits is not a universal finding among patients with AD, making odor identification tests imperfect screening instruments for the disorder.

Odor identification has also been studied recently in patients with mild cognitive impairment (MCI) and cognitively intact older adults with and without genetic risk for future cognitive decline. Several longitudinal studies have demonstrated that odor identification has a strong relationship with memory performance, even in healthy older adults performing within normal limits on cognitive measures (Devanand et al. 2000; Wilson et al. 2007). These studies also show that odor identification is a unique and significant predictor of future cognitive decline above and beyond baseline memory performance, as well as a good predictor of conversion to dementia in patients with MCI. In cross-sectional studies of MCI subtypes, patients with both amnestic and non-amnestic subtypes perform modestly worse than healthy older adults but better than patients with dementia (Devanand et al. in press; Westervelt et al. 2008). In using olfactory performance to distinguish MCI subtypes, results are mixed, though when significant differences have been found between subtypes, the magnitude of the difference is of questionable clinical significance. Together, these studies suggest that when a notable olfactory deficit is observed in patients with MCI, there is substantial risk of future decline. However, odor identification measures may not be particularly clinically useful in early detection or early differential diagnosis for the modal patient.

Dementia with Lewy Bodies Olfaction in dementia with Lewy bodies (DLB) was first described in a study that crudely measured anosmia with a brief detection task (McShane et al. 2001). Forty percent of patients with DLB were found to be anosmic, in contrast with 16% of patients with AD, and 6% of the healthy controls. The presence of smell loss was not found to be associated with concurrent AD and DLB pathology on autopsy. Subsequent studies confirmed anosmia to be more common in DLB than in AD, with anosmia present in 56–65% of patients with DLB (and some degree of smell loss in nearly 90%), but in only 11–23% of AD patients (Olichney et al. 2005; Westervelt et al. 2003). Assessment of anosmia has been shown to improve the sensitivity of diagnostic criteria for DLB, with minimal loss of specificity (Olichney et al. 2005). Combined, these few studies raise the possibility that olfactory measures may be useful in distinguishing AD from DLB.

Other Dementias Olfactory deficits have also been described in other dementias, including recent, consistent findings of smell deficits in frontotemporal dementia that are generally of the magnitude of deficits seen in AD (Luzzi et al. 2007; McLaughlin and Westervelt 2008; Pardini et al. 2009), and, in vascular dementia to a similar or lesser extent to that seen in AD (Gray et al. 2001; Knupfer and Spiegel 1986).

Head Injury Olfactory loss is fairly common following head injury (for review, see Costanza et al. 2003), with the incidence of anosmia ranging from approximately 5 to 60%. These latter estimates represent the incidence among patients with severe head injury, though total anosmia can occur even after very mild injury. Partial or unilateral loss may be less likely to be detected than total anosmia. Deficits may be caused by a variety of mechanisms, including sinus/nasal injury, shearing of the olfactory nerve, or contusion/hemorrhage in central processing regions. In regard to shear injuries, the axons of the olfactory receptor cells are particularly susceptible to injury as they pass through the body ridges of the cribiform plate. Coup and contra-coup forces are likely to result in anosmia, with occipital blows most frequently causing smell loss.

Schizophrenia Olfactory deficits have been well-studied in schizophrenia (for review, see Doty 2003a, b). Deficits have been shown to be of lesser magnitude than typically seen in AD and PD, progress with disease duration, and are most associated with negative symptoms of the disease. In patients showing olfactory deficits, the impairments appear early in the disease, perhaps in prodromal stages. There does not appear to be any notable relationship with antipsychotic medication use or cigarette smoking. Odor identification deficits correlate most strongly with measures of executive functioning in this population, rather than those of medial temporal lobe functioning. All aspects of olfaction appear to be impaired (i.e., identification, threshold, discrimination, and memory).

Evaluation

Clinical History

Obtaining a detailed clinical history is critical in assessing olfactory deficits. Symptoms should be clearly defined, and the clinician should attempt to determine the extent and duration of the perceived loss, as well as the occurrence of any event associated with the deficit (e.g., head injury, illness). Fluctuations in symptoms may be most suggestive of obstructive causes, but need to be distinguished from paroxysmal events. Medical history should be carefully assessed, as multiple medical conditions and medications may be associated with olfactory alterations. Referral for an ENT evaluation may be warranted. Olfactory hallucinations, in particular, require careful work-up as they may be indicative of seizure or tumor, and are less likely of primary psychiatric origin.

Classes of Assessment

There are three classes of olfactory assessment methods: psychophysical, electrophysiological, and psychophysiological, with psychophysical assessment being the most common and most clinically relevant.

Psychophysiological

Psychophysiological assessment of olfactory abilities relies on the measurement of changes in the autonomic nervous system after presentation of an odorous stimuli, through such methods as heart rate and blood pressure. These methods are rarely used.

Electrophysiological

Electrophysiological assessments examine electrical activity generated in response to an odorant and are primarily research tools. Electro-olfactograms (EOG) use electrodes placed on the human olfactory epithelium to directly assess olfactory abilities. Olfactory event-related potentials (ERP) are recorded from the scalp surface, measuring electroencephalographic activity after presentation of brief, precisely defined odorous stimuli. For example, chemosensory ERP's can be obtained after stimulation of olfactory nerve (olfactory ERPs) or the trigeminal nerve (somatosensory ERPs). Absence of olfactory ERPs in presence of somatosensory ERPs suggests olfactory deficits. These measures are sensitive to age and gender effects. Chemosensory evoked potentials are unable to discern where the impairment is within the olfactory pathway, but are considered among the only objective ways of establishing smell loss.

Psychophysical

Psychophysical methods are the most commonly used assessment practices in both clinical and research settings. In these techniques, stimuli are presented, and the patient or participant reports their perception (detection, discrimination, identification); this category can be further sub-divided into threshold and suprathreshold tasks.

Threshold Testing *Threshold testing* is used to determine at what concentration a patient or participant can accurately detect the presence of an odor. Two methods have been developed to determine this threshold: the method of limits procedure and the single staircase procedure. In the method of limits procedure, a low concentration of a specific odor is presented, and the concentration is increased until it can be detected. In the single staircase procedure, the concentration is increased following trials in which the participant cannot detect the odor, and decreased following correct detection. There are commercially available smell threshold tests, for example, using felt-tipped pens and squeeze bottles. Olfactometers can be used to present precise amounts of odorants through constant airflow. However, many of these techniques can be cumbersome for clinical use.

Suprathreshold Tasks *Suprathreshold tasks* include rating scales/magnitude estimation scales, odor identification tasks, and odor memory/recognition tasks. When using rating scales, the participant rates the amount of the attribute perceived (e.g., pleasantness); these may include category scales (which category describes sensation) and line scales (placement of mark on line with descriptors). When using a magnitude estimation scales, a participant will assign a number to stimuli in relation to relative intensity.

Odor Identification Tasks *Odor identification tasks* also suprathreshold tasks, require participants to identify odors, often by presenting scratch-and-sniff items, tinctures in jars, or odorant-soaked tampons. These tasks almost invariably include multiple choice options, as odor identification is otherwise extremely challenging even for individuals with intact olfactory abilities. These tasks are easy to administer and the most frequent type of task used in clinical settings, but can be somewhat costly depending on the task. The most widely used odor identification task is the University of Pennsylvania Smell Identification Task (UPSIT), which consists 40 micro-encapsulated odorants presented in a 4-option, multiple choice format. Other, briefer measures include 12-item versions (e.g., Cross-Cultural Smell Identification Test/Brief Smell Identification Test (BSIT), the BSIT-A designed especially for AD, the BSIT-B designed especially for PD) and a 3-item screen (Pocket Smell Test). The UPSIT and BSIT both have associated norms. Sniffin' Sticks includes both a threshold task and an odor identification task, and is extensively normed in European samples (Hummell et al. 2007).

Odor Memory Test *Odor memory test* involve having the individual smell an odor (or group of odors), and after a specified period of time, recognize the odor from a set of distracters. Often, novel, non-descript odors are utilized to minimize the ability to label, and interference tasks are introduced during delays to minimize rehearsal of the odor labels/qualifiers.

Other Olfactory Assessment Tools

The Sniff Magnitude Test
The sniff magnitude test is a recently developed clinical measure of olfaction based on the reflex-like reduction in sniffing that occurs in response to detection of odors (especially unpleasant odors), but does not occur when sniffing non-odorized air (Frank et al. 2003). This response is observed in people with normal sense of smell, but is absent in those with anosmia. The task involves having the patient sniff a canister that releases either a blank or an odor, while wearing a nasal cannula connected to a device to measure the negative pressure created by the sniff. The test is quick to administer (about 5 min) and has minimal, if any, reliance on cognition, linguistic ability, and familiarity of odors.

Neuroimaging Imaging, particularly MRI, is clearly important for identification of structural lesions that may be impinging on the olfactory system, or in assisting in diagnosis of other neurologic disorders that may account for smell loss. CT is frequently used in identifying sinonasal disease. MRI can also be useful in evaluating changes in olfactory bulb volume due to viral, traumatic, or idiopathic olfactory dysfunction, with good relationship demonstrated between objective olfactometry (with chemosensory evoked potentials) and bulb volume. Functional scans, in particular fMRI and PET, are also often used as research tools in studying the functional organization of olfaction. These studies have shown involvement in the amygdala, piriform cortex, OFC, insula, anterior cingulate, thalamus, caudate, subiculum, upper pons, and cerebellar vermis, with different activation patterns depending on the nature of the task (e.g., sniffing, smelling single odors, discrimination, identification, etc.).

Treatment

Treatment is most promising in patients with smell loss associated with conduction problems. For example, antibiotic treatment, steroids, and allergy management may be helpful in reducing deficits associated with inflammatory disease. Surgical removal of other obstructions, such as nasal polyps, can also be effective in restoring olfactory ability. In contrast, treatment of sensorineural/central neural problems is often less effective. Exceptions may include resection of tumors impinging on the olfactory system and, in some cases, resection of epileptogenic foci associated with olfactory seizures. Iatrogenic effects of medications are typically reversible with discontinuation of the medication and eventual improvement in smell is expected after cessation of smoking. Recent work also suggests that olfactory training may improve olfaction in some patients (Hummel et al. 2009). Zinc or vitamin therapies are at times prescribed to treat olfactory loss, but there is little evidence of benefit in the absence of associated deficiencies. Typically, the more severe and long-standing the smell loss, the less likely recovery is in sensorineural/central neural disorders. Especially for individuals who do not respond to treatment, education about the safety implications of smell loss is important, given concerns of the patient's failure to detect hazardous odors (e.g., smoke) or spoiled food. Nutritional status may also be compromised in patients with olfactory deficits, and use of flavor enhancements in foods can be helpful in improving food intake (Schiffman 2000).

Cross-References

▶ Cranial Nerves
▶ Olfaction
▶ Olfactory Bulb
▶ Olfactory Tract

References and Readings

Costanza, R. M., DiNardo, L. J., & Reiter, E. R. (2003). Head injury and olfaction. In R. L. Doty (Ed.), *Handbook of olfaction and gustation* (2nd ed.). New York: Marcel Dekker.

Devanand, D. P., Michaels-Marston, K. S., Liu, X., Pelton, G. H., Padilla, M., Marder, K., et al. (2000). Olfactory deficits in patients with mild cognitive impairment predict Alzheimer's disease at follow-up. *American Journal of Psychiatry, 157*, 1344–1405.

Devanand, D. P., Tabert, M. H., Cuasay, K., Manly, J. J., Schupf, N., Brickman, A. M., et al. (in press). Olfactory identification deficits and MCI in a multi-ethnic elderly community sample. *Neurobiology of Aging.*

Doty, R. L. (2003a). Odor perception in neurodegenerative diseases. In R. L. Doty (Ed.), *Handbook of olfaction and gustation* (2nd ed.). New York: Marcel Dekker.

Doty, R. L. (Ed.). (2003b). *Handbook of olfaction and gustation* (2nd ed.). New York: Marcel Dekker.

Doty, R. L., & Bromley, S. M. (2004). Effects of drugs on olfaction and taste. *Otolaryngologic Clinics of North America, 37*, 1229–1254.

Frank, R. A., Dulay, M. F., & Gestland, R. C. (2003). Assessment of the sniff magnitude test as a clinical test of olfactory function. *Physiology & Behavior, 78*, 195–204.

Gotfried, J. A., & Zald, D. H. (2005). On the scent of human olfactory orbitofrontal cortex: Meta-analysis and comparison to non-human primates. *Brain Research Brain Research Reviews, 50*, 287–304.

Gray, A. J., Staples, V., Murren, K., Dhariwal, A., & Bentham, P. (2001). Olfactory identification is impaired in clinic-based patients with vascular dementia and senile dementia of the Alzheimer type. *International Journal of Geriatric Psychiatry, 16*, 513–517.

Hummel, T., Rissom, K., Reden, J., Hähner, A., Weidenbecher, M., & Hüttenbrink, K. B. (2009). Effects of olfactory training in patients with olfactory loss. *Laryngoscope, 119*, 496–499.

Hummell, T., Kobal, G., Gudziol, H., & Mackay-Sim, A. (2007). Normative data for the "sniffin'sticks" including tests of odor identification, odor discrimination, and olfactory thresholds: An upgrade based on a group of more than 3000 subjects. *European Archives of Otorhinolaryngology, 264*, 237–243.

Knupfer, L., & Spiegel, R. (1986). Differences in olfactory test performance between normal aged, Alzheimer and vascular type dementia individuals. *International Journal of Geriatric Psychiatry, 1*, 3–14.

Luzzi, S., Snowden, J. S., Neary, D., Coccia, M., Provinciali, L., & Lambon Ralph, M. A. (2007). Distinct patterns of olfactory impairment in Alzheimer's disease, semantic dementia, frontotemporal dementia, and corticobasal degeneration. *Neuropsychologia, 45*, 1823–1831.

McLaughlin, N., & Westervelt, H. J. (2008). Odor identification deficits in frontotemporal dementia: A preliminary study. *Archives of Clinical Neuropsychology, 23*, 119–123.

McShane, R. H., Nagy, Z., Esiri, M. M., King, E., Joachim, C., Sullivan, N., et al. (2001). Anosmia in dementia is associated with Lewy bodies rather than Alzheimer's pathology. *Journal of Neurology, Neurosurgery, and Psychiatry, 70*, 739–743.

Mesholam, R. I., Moberg, P. H., Mahr, R. N., & Doty, R. L. (1998). Olfaction in neurodegenerative disease. A meta-analysis of olfactory functioning in Alzheimer's and Parkinson's diseases. *Archives of Neurology, 55*, 84–90.

Murphy, C., Schubert, C. R., Cruickshanks, K. J., Klein, B. E., Klein, R., & Nondahl, D. M. (2002). Prevalence of olfactory impairment in older adults. *Journal of the American Medical Association, 288*, 2307–2312.

Murphy, C., Doty, R. L., & Duncan, H. J. (2003). Clinical disorders of olfaction. In R. L. Doty (Ed.), *Handbook of olfaction and gustation* (2nd ed.). New York: Marcel Dekker.

Olichney, J. M., Murphy, C., Hofstetter, C. R., Foster, K., Hansen, L. A., Thal, L. J., et al. (2005). Anosmia is very common in the Lewy body variant of Alzheimer's disease. *Journal of Neurology, Neurosurgery, and Psychiatry, 76*, 1342–1347.

Pardini, M., Huey, E. D., Cavanagh, A. L., & Grafman, J. (2009). Olfactory function in corticobasal syndrome and frontotemporal dementia. *Archives of Neurology, 66*, 92–96.

Schiffman, S. S. (2000). Intensification of sensory properties of food for the elderly. *Journal of Nutrition, 130*, 9275–9305.

Smutzer, G. S., Doty, R. L., Arnold, S. E., & Trojanowski, J. Q. (2003). Olfactory system neuropathology in Alzheimer's disease Parkinson's disease, and schizophrenia. In R. L. Doty (Ed.), *Handbook of olfaction and gustation* (2nd ed.). New York: Marcel Dekker.

Upadhyay, U. D., & Holbrook, E. H. (2004). Olfactory loss as a result of toxic exposure. *Otolaryngologic Clinics of North America, 37*, 1185–1207.

Westervelt, H. J., Stern, R. A., & Tremont, G. (2003). Odor identification deficits in diffuse Lewy body disease. *Cognitive and Behavioral Neurology, 16*, 93–99.

Westervelt, H. J., Bruce, J. M., Coon, W. G., & Tremont, G. (2008). Odor identification in mild cognitive impairment subtypes. *Journal of Clinical and Experimental Neuropsychology, 30*, 151–156.

Wilson, R. S., Schneider, J. A., Arnold, S. E., Tang, Y., Boyle, P. A., & Bennett, D. A. (2007). Olfactory identification and incidence of mild cognitive impairment in older age. *Archives of General Psychiatry, 64*, 802–808.

Anosodiaphoria

John E. Mendoza
Department of Psychiatry and Neuroscience, Tulane Medical School and SE Louisiana Veterans Healthcare System, New Orleans, LA, USA

Definition

Anosodiaphoria is defined as the failure to fully appreciate the significance of a neurological deficit as a result of a brain lesion.

Current Knowledge

Following certain injuries to the brain, most commonly strokes in the right hemisphere, a patient may fail to recognize (deny) the resulting neurological deficit(s), such as paralysis. This latter condition is known as anosognosia. With time, patients typically show increased awareness of the deficit. For example, if asked, they might acknowledge that a stroke has occurred and that their ability to use their arm or leg has been affected. However, the patient might fail to fully appreciate the extent or functional implications of the deficit, attribute it to another more benign factor (such as being right-handed), or otherwise appear relatively unconcerned about it. This latter condition has been termed anosodiaphoria (Adair et al. 2003; Critchley 1969). Thus, while acknowledging that his arm and/or leg are/is "weak," a patient may talk about his plans to return to work in the near future, although that may be totally unrealistic, given the severity of his condition and the nature of his work. There does not appear to be any clear consensus as to the etiology of this condition, the level of denial of which might be seen to vary from one day to the next. The more common hypotheses are that the anosodiaphoria likely reflects the same type of neglect or inattention that results in the original anosognosia, only less severe, is a result of a general emotional flattening or indifference that can follow right hemispheric lesions, or a combination of the two (Heilman et al. 2003).

Cross-References

▶ Anosognosia
▶ Denial

References and Readings

Adair, J. C., Schwartz, R. L., & Barrett, A. M. (2003). Anosognosia. In K. Heilman & E. Valenstein (Eds.), *Clinical neuropsychology* (4th ed., pp. 185–214). New York: Oxford University Press.

Critchley, M. (1969). *The parietal lobes*. New York: Hafner.

Heilman, K. M., Blonder, L. X., Bowers, D., & Valenstein, E. (2003). Emotional disorders associated with neurological diseases. In K. M. Heilman & E. Valenstein (Eds.), *Clinical neuropsychology* (4th ed., pp. 447–478). New York: Oxford University Press.

Prigatano, G. P., & Schacter, D. L. (Eds.). (1991). *Awareness of deficit after brain injury*. Oxford: New York.

Anosognosia

Kenneth M. Heilman
Department of Neurology, University of Florida
College of Medicine, Center for Neurological
Studies and the Research Service of the Malcom
Randall Veterans Affairs Medical Center,
Gainesville, FL, USA

Synonyms

Self-awareness

Definition

Anosognosia is a disorder characterized by denial of illness or lack of awareness of disability.

Historical Background

In the clinic, it is very common to see patients who suffer with a neurological disease, such as stroke, but who appear to deny illness or be unaware of their disabilities. Seneca, the Stoic philosopher, noted this about 2000 years ago, but the first modern description of a patient with unawareness-denial was by von Monakow (1885). Although there were other investigators who wrote about this striking disorder, it was Babinski (1914), who coined the term *anosognosia*. This word comes from three roots: a = without, noso = disease, and gnosis = knowledge. In addition to describing patients who were unaware of their illness or disability, Babinski described other patients who appeared to be aware but remained unconcerned. He called this disorder, *anosodiaphoria*.

There are many forms of anosognosia and these forms are related to the nature of a patient's disability. When Babinski first used this term, the patients he described denied or were unaware of their hemiparesis. Anton (1898) described patients who were unable to see because they had destroyed their primary visual cortex but were unaware or denied their blindness. Patients with Korsakoff's amnesic disorder are unaware of their memory loss, and aphasic patients such as those with Wernicke's aphasia appear to be unaware of their jargon speech.

Current Knowledge

Although of great academic interest, the presence of anosognosia or anosodiaphoria has important medical implications. For example, there are now treatments for stroke that must be given within hours of the onset of symptoms. The patients who are unaware of their disabilities or undervalue their importance might not seek immediate medical attention. In addition, people who have disabilities but are not aware of these disabilities might inadvertently injure themselves and/or others. Rehabilitation works best, when patients are strongly motivated to get well. When a person is either unconcerned or unaware of their disabilities, they are not motivated, and unmotivated patients are less likely to benefit from these treatments. They might even refuse to undergo rehabilitation, and they might not take their medications that can reduce their disability or possibly prevent further possible brain damage.

Possible Mechanisms of Anosognosia for Hemiplegia

Patients with hemispheric strokes often develop an inability to use the arm-hand on the contralesional side of their body (hemiparesis). Many of these patients will be unaware of their weakness and when asked about the presence of weakness, they will deny this disability. Several, not mutually exclusive, mechanisms have been used to explain this phenomenon.

Psychological Denial Weinstein and Kahn (1955) who brought modern attention to this syndrome posited that for many people having a stroke with weakness was a psychologically traumatic event, and the means by which some people deal with this trauma is to use psychological denial. To test this hypothesis, Weinstein and Kahn studied patients who had anosognosia and found that even before their stroke, these patients frequently used this denial defense mechanism.

Some investigators have noted that anosognosia for hemiplegia is more often associated with a left than right hemiparesis. The psychological denial theory of anosognosia cannot explain this asymmetry. Many patients with left hemisphere injury, however, are aphasic and have problems with both the comprehension of questions (What is wrong with you? Are you weak?) as well as speaking-answering questions. Thus, Weinstein and Kahn thought what appeared to be a hemispheric asymmetry was induced by a sampling bias.

Using selective hemispheric anesthesia (the Wada study) and questioning the patient after they recover from anesthesia revealed that unawareness of the hemiplegia (anosognosia) was more common with the right than left hemisphere anesthesia (Gilmore et al. 1992). After the selective hemispheric anesthesia has worn off, there is no aphasia or a need for psychological denial. The right-left hemisphere asymmetries found were within subjects, and thus premorbid personality can also not account for this asymmetry. Although this study suggests that denial cannot entirely explain anosognosia for hemiplegia, denial might be used by many people to help deal with diseases and disabilities.

Failure of Feedback To know something is impaired, a person requires feedback. Many investigators have suggested that it is a failure of feedback, induced by either sensory loss (e.g., proprioception and hemianopia) or inattention neglect, spatial or personal, that accounts for anosognosia of hemiplegia. That inattention neglect that is more commonly associated with right hemisphere injury might also account for the asymmetries of anosognosia.

Studies from our laboratory have revealed when undergoing selective right hemisphere anesthesia, during the time these patients demonstrate shoulder weakness, their shoulder proprioception is intact. To learn if this disorder could be related to neglect, spatial or personal, we brought their hemiplegic left forelimb over to the right side of their body and to their right visual field. To make certain subjects see their hand, we wrote a number on their hand, and subjects were able to read these numbers. Despite

these strategies many, but not all, patients still denied weakness of that hand. Thus, a failure of feedback can only explain anosognosia in some patients. In support of this postulate, several investigators have reported dissociations between the presence of spatial neglect and anosognosia.

Asomatognosia Hypothesis While patients with personal neglect might be unaware of the parts of their body, patients with asomatognosia do not feel or claim that certain body parts belong to them. It has been posited that asomatognosia is caused by the alteration of the brain's representation of the body, a body schema. Like spatial and personal neglect, asomatognosia is more commonly associated with right than left hemisphere lesions. If patients with right hemisphere injury do not believe their left arm-hand belongs to them, they will not recognize their own weakness. During right hemispheric anesthesia, the patients with left hemiplegia were shown their left hand or someone else's left hand in a restricted view box that projected to their right visual field. The patients were asked if the hand they were viewing was their own or another person's hand. We found that there were some patients who had anosognosia who also had asomatognosia, but only a small proportion. Thus, asomatognosia can also not fully account for this disorder.

Disconnection Hypothesis When a patient with a complete callosal disconnection receives a stimulus to the left visual field or on the left side of the body and is asked to tell the examiner the nature of the stimulus, the left language-speech hemisphere often confabulates a response. Geschwind (1965) noted that large right hemisphere lesions can both injure the right hemisphere's cortex and intrahemispheric networks, as well as induce an interhemispheric disconnection. Thus, when asked about weakness, the left hemisphere which is disconnected from the right will confabulate a response – "I am not weak." The observation mentioned above, where during the right hemisphere anesthesia the patient's left hand is brought over to the right visual field and thus has access to the left language-speech-dominant hemisphere, also tests this disconnection hypothesis. As mentioned, in few patients when their arm could be visualized in the right visual field, they did recognize their weakness. In these cases, we cannot be sure if their anosognosia was induced by a failure in feedback or a disconnection. Future research will have to learn if these mechanisms can be dissociated. However, as mentioned above, this procedure only helps a small minority of patients.

Phantom Movements Limb amputation is often associated with a perception that the limb is still present, and this perception is thought to be related to the continued presence of a brain representation of that missing phantom limb. When patients with a hemiparesis are asked to move a limb, many often perceive that the paretic limb is moving, and this phantom movement in combination with impaired feedback might account for anosognosia. During selective hemispheric anesthesia (Wada test), we had blindfolded subjects with left hemiplegia attempt to raise their paretic left arm, and we then asked them to raise their right (non-paretic) arm to the same level as they perceived the left arm. Some of the patients we tested did raise their right arm, suggesting that they had phantom movements, but we found no significant relationship between phantom movements and anosognosia.

Intentional Motor Disorder Patients with right hemisphere lesions often demonstrate contralesional limb akinesia also called motor neglect. Many of these patients do not attempt to spontaneously move their akinetic arm, and while less common some do not even attempt to move this arm to command. Limb akinesia can occur both with and without a hemiplegia. Patients with limb akinesia might not discover that they are weak because they do not attempt to move this left arm. If they do not attempt to move this arm, they will not experience a dissociation between their expectations and performance, and it is this dissociation that alerts people that there is a problem. Providing external motivation such as suggestions or commands might entice patients to attempt a movement, and with these commands some patients do discover their

weakness. Electromyographic studies have also provided evidence in support of this akinesia hypothesis.

Summary Based on the above discussion, it appears that several mechanisms might contribute to the presence of anosognosia for hemiplegia.

Possible Mechanisms of Anosognosia for Amnesia and Cortical Blindness

Damage to three interconnected brain networks can produce amnesia, an impairment in the episodic memory system: (1) the medial temporal lobe – Papez circuit (e.g., hippocampus, entorhinal and perirhinal cortex, fornix, the mammillary bodies, the mammillothalamic tract, the anterior thalamus, and the retrosplenial cortex); (2) the dorsomedial thalamus; and (3) the basal forebrain (medial septal nucleus and the diagonal band of Broca), which provide acetylcholine to the hippocampus. Amnesic patients with medial temporal lesions are often aware of their disability, and patients with damage to the basal forebrain and to the medial thalamus are often unaware of their memory deficit.

The reason for this dichotomy is not fully known, but the dorsomedial thalamic nucleus is heavily connected with the frontal lobes, and damage to this dorsomedial nucleus induces frontal dysfunction. Damage to the basal forebrain is also often associated with frontal dysfunction. Frontal lobe dysfunction is often associated with impaired recall but not recognition, suggesting that the problem is not with the consolidation of memories but rather retrieval. The patients with amnesia from a thalamic or basal forebrain injury more often confabulate memories than do those with medial temporal lobe damage. Since these patients retrieve memories and have no means of testing these memories' veracity, they might be unaware that their recall is incorrect, and therefore they might be unaware of their memory disorder.

Blindness Patients with Anton's syndrome have blindness from damage to their primary visual cortex, usually from stroke. These patients often deny their blindness, confabulate responses, and are unaware they are blind, anosognosic. The reason why these patients are not aware of their blindness is not known. We examined a patient with Anton's syndrome who had intact visual imagery. Perhaps since these patients have intact visual imagery and cannot receive visual input, this imagery is mistaken for online input.

Possible Mechanisms for Unawareness of Aphasia

Patients with Wernicke's aphasia speak in jargon, cannot comprehend, name, or repeat. Many are not aware that they are aphasic and that they are speaking in jargon. For example, we saw a patient, who, when speaking jargon, became angry when he was not understood. It has been posited that Wernicke's aphasia is induced by injury to the phonological lexicon – a store of learned word sounds. To be aware that an error has been made, a person needs to have a normal representation of the targeted behavior. Since patients with Wernicke's aphasia have destroyed their representations of word sounds when they speak jargon, they have no representations with which to compare their speech and are thus unaware of their errors.

We have also reported patients who appear to have an intact input lexicon (e.g., can understand speech) but who make phonological errors and are not aware that they made these errors. If these patients' speech is recorded and played back to them, they do detect their errors, suggesting that their unawareness might have been related to not being able to closely attend to their output. These aphasic patients might have focused their attention on what they were attempting to say rather than how they said it.

Future Directions

Anosognosia, the failure to recognize a disease or a disability, might delay treatment, interfere with rehabilitation, and put people in danger. Patients might be anosognosic for a variety of neurological disorders such as weakness, sensory loss, personal and spatial neglect, memory loss, and aphasia. There appears to be a variety of mechanism that might account for anosognosia including psychological denial, impaired and false feedback, alterations of the body schema, failures to test systems,

and to initiate behaviors. Future research is needed. In addition to continuing to define and test possible mechanisms, effective treatments for these disorders are needed.

Cross-References

▶ Attention
▶ Consciousness
▶ Impaired Self-Awareness

References and Readings

Anton, G. (1898). Blindheit nach beiderseitiger Gehirnerkrankung mit Verlust der Orienterung in Raume. *Mitt. Ver. Arzte Steirmark, 33*, 41–46.
Babinski, J. (1914). Contribution à l'etude des troubles mentaux dans l'hémiplégie organique cérébrale (anosognosie). *Revue Neurologique, 27*, 845–847.
Clare, L., & Halligan, P. (Eds.). (2006). *Pathologies of awareness: Bridging the gap between theory and practice*. New York: Psychology Press.
Geschwind, N. (1965). Disconnexion syndromes in animals and man. *Brain, 88*(237–294), 585–644.
Gilmore, R. L., Heilman, K. M., Schmidt, R. P., Fennell, E. M., & Quisling, R. (1992). Anosognosia during Wada testing. *Neurology, 42*, 925–927.
Prigatano, G. P., & Schacter, D. L. (1991). *Awareness of deficit after brain injury: Clinical and theoretical issues*. New York: Oxford University Press.
von Monakow, C. (1885). Experimentelle und pathologisch-anatomische Untersuchungen über die Beziehungen der sogenannten Sehphäre zu den infrakorticalen Opticuscentren und zum N. opticus. *Archiv für Psychiatrie und Nervenkrankheiten, 16*, 151–199.
Weinstein, E. A., & Kahn, R. L. (1955). *Denial of illness: Symbolic and physiological aspects*. Springfield: Charles C. Thomas.

Anoxia

Bruce J. Diamond
Department of Psychology, William Paterson University, Wayne, NJ, USA

Synonyms

Severe hypoxia; Severe oxygen deficiency

Definition

Hypoxia refers to a decrease in oxygen supply rather than a complete loss of oxygenation (Jones 2015). Anoxia refers to an extreme hypoxia or deficiency in the oxygenation of the arterial blood of sufficient severity to result in permanent neurologic damage (Webster 2006). This vulnerability to severely reduced oxygenation is based on the fact that the brain has little to no reserve of oxygen or glucose, consequently an anoxic episode of 4–6 min can result in neuronal cell death or necrosis because of impairment in cellular metabolism (Zillmer and Spiers 2001).

Etiology

Anoxia can result from a number of conditions including cardiac arrest, carbon monoxide poisoning, stroke, brain injury, and complications due to anesthesia. It is thought that cells exposed to anoxia release glutamate. The CA1 cells of the hippocampus contain high concentrations of glutamate and are particularly vulnerable to subnormal oxygenation levels. Therefore, it appears that the action of glutamate on these cells is the putative mechanism mediating cell death in this region of the hippocampus and helps explain many of the signs and symptoms associated with anoxia (Bonner and Bonner 1991). The decreased oxygenation seen in hypoxia may be caused by airway obstruction, apnea, lung collapse, medication side effects, anemia, and heart failure (Auday et al. 2014).

Signs and Symptoms

Mild cerebral hypoxia may include the symptoms of inattentiveness, poor judgment, memory loss, and a decrease in motor coordination (NINDS 2015), while anoxia often results in impairments in memory, executive, and motor function. Signs and symptoms are likely attributable to damage to limbic and subcortical regions, in addition to the frontal lobes and the cerebellum (Golden et al. 1992).

Neuropsychological and Psychological Outcomes

Anoxia can result in impairments in anterograde memory which in its most severe form may manifest as an amnestic disorder. Presenting symptoms may also include impairments in awareness and affect as well as confabulatory behavior. Anoxia associated with cardiac arrest may include amnesia, in addition to bibrachial paresis, cortical blindness, and visual agnosia. Carbon monoxide poisoning may be associated with affective and cognitive disturbances associated with anoxia-induced dysfunction (Aminoff et al. 2005). Vulnerability to cognitive impairments in response to decreased arterial oxygenation is supported by the finding that experimental induction of hypoxia in healthy subjects showed decrements of 10–36% in neurocognitive processes that are vulnerable to oxygen deprivation including verbal and visual memory, processing speed, executive function psychomotor speed, reaction time, complex attention, and cognitive flexibility (Turner et al. 2015).

Cross-References

▶ Carbon Monoxide Poisoning
▶ Glutamate
▶ Hippocampus

References and Readings

Aminoff, M. J., Simon, R. P., & Greenberg, D. A. (2005). *Clinical neurology*. New York: McGraw-Hill.

Auday, B. C., Buratovich, M. A., Marrocco, G. F., & Moglia, P. (Eds.). (2014) *Salem health Magill's medical guide* (7th ed., p. 1188). Ipswich: Grey House Publishing

Bonner, J. S., & Bonner, J. J. (1991). *The little black book of neurology: A manual for neurologic house officers* (2nd ed.). St Louis: Mosby-Year Book.

Cavendish, M., Bernabeo, P., Esposito, M. (2008). *Diseases and disorders* (1st ed., pp. 121-122). Tarrytown: Marshall Cavendish Corporation.

Golden, C. J., Zillmer, E. A., & Spiers, M. V. (1992). *Neuropsychological assessment and intervention*. Springfield: Charles C. Thomas.

Jones, K. (Ed.) (2015). *Brain disorders sourcebook* (4th ed., pp. 3306-3307). Detroit: Omnigraphics Inc.

NINDS. (2015). NINDS cerebral hypoxia information page. National Institute of Neurologic Disorders and Stroke website. http://www.ninds.nih.gov/disorders/anoxia/anoxia.htm. Updated 14 Feb 2014; Accessed 29 May 2014.

Turner, C. E., Barker-Collo, S. L., Connell, C. J., & Gant, N. (2015). Acute hypoxic gas breathing severely impairs cognition and task learning in humans. *Physiology & Behavior, 142*, 104–110.

Webster. (2006). *Webster's new explorer medical dictionary (new edition)*. Springfield: Merriam-Webster.

Zillmer, E. A., & Spiers, M. V. (2001). *Principles of neuropsychology*. Belmont: Wadsworth/Thomson Learning.

Anterior Cerebral Artery

Bruce J. Diamond and Keith Happawana
Department of Psychology, William Paterson
University, Wayne, NJ, USA

Synonyms

ACA; Cerebral artery

Definition

The anterior cerebral artery (ACA) arises as the medial branch of an anterior bifurcation of the internal carotid artery (ICA) at later embryonic stages of development (Menshawi et al. 2015). The ACA supplies the anterior four-fifths of the medial surface of the cerebral hemisphere, frontal and parietal lobes, the anterior four-fifths of the corpus callosum, and a narrow strip of the superior, lateral surface of the cerebral hemisphere (Zhou et al. 2013), as well as the front portion of the diencephalon (Rea 2015). Three major vascular areas supply the head of the caudate nucleus, i.e., Heubner's artery, the anterior lenticulostriate arteries (from the proximal section of the anterior cerebral artery), and the lateral lenticulostriate arteries (from the middle cerebral artery) (Mizuta and Motomura 2006). Various motor areas are supplied by the ACA including the supplementary motor complex, the anterior and middle cingulate cortex, and the rostral section of the corpus callosum. The

ACA is also part of the vasculature of the Circle of Willis, arising from trifurcations implicated by an anastomosis created by the ICAs (Vrselja et al. 2014). Thus, when blood supply from the ACA is impeded (anterior cerebral artery syndrome), symptomatology varies with the degree and location of restriction within the ACA (Vrselja et al. 2014).

Categories

The ACA is structurally delineated by five distinct segments, commonly referred to as segments A1–A5. A1 branches from the ICA bifurcation and extends to also entail the anterior communicating artery (ACoA). The A2 segment extends from the ACoA to the bifurcation forming the pericallosal and callosomarginal arteries. Heubner's artery (which supplies the internal capsule) usually arises at the beginning of A2 near the ACoA. Branching from Heubner's artery are the orbitofrontal artery (medial frontal basal) and the frontopolar artery (polar frontal) (which rises after the orbitofrontal artery and is close to A2's span over the corpus callosum). A2 mimics the length and contours of the genu and rostrum in the corpus callosum. A3, known as the pericallosal artery, extends posteriorly in the pericallosal sulcus to form the internal superior and inferior parietal arteries, as well as the precuneal artery (Lawton and Mirzadeh 2012). The callosal marginal artery branches out from the pericallosal artery. A3 is also known to form anastomoses with neighboring arteries. A4 and A5 segments are also known as the supracallosal and postcallosal segments (respectively) and outline the body of the corpus callosum, the division between them being located at the plane of the coronal suture (Lawton and Mirzadeh 2012).

Medical, Neuropsychological, and Psychological Symptoms

Infarctions in the territory of this artery are associated with a variety of clinical signs and symptoms including gait, limb sensation, abulia, lack of spontaneous activity, urinary incontinence, and frontal and memory impairments, in addition to emotional dysregulation (apathy) (Brust 1995). Associated aneurysms are found relatively frequently in patients with ACA variations (Uchino et al. 2006). The effects of ACA occlusion vary in severity depending on if the recurrent artery of Heubner is present. Spastic arms, flaccid legs, and brisk reflexes may occur if the Heubner artery is present. Blockage in the proximal segment can result in upper motor neuron pathology of the face. If branches to the olfactory bulb and tract are affected, anosmia may result. Extensive anterior cerebral artery occlusion can affect micturition. If occlusion affects blood flow to the frontal lobe or corpus callosum, apathy may result. Less severe occlusions may only affect the lower limbs with signs such as reduced sensation, lack of power, up-going plantar reflexes, and brisk reflexes (Rea 2015). In ACA stroke cases, patients may present with difficulties in performing volitional hand movements, while movements in response to external stimuli are preserved. In the chronic stage (median follow-up of 83.5 days), improvements in the initiation of voluntary movements may occur, although signs of disturbed motor control may persist (Brugger et al. 2015).

Cross-References

▶ Anterior Communicating Artery

References and Readings

Arboix, A., García-Eroles, L., Sellarés, N., Raga, A., Oliveres, M., & Massons, J. (2009). Infarction in the territory of the anterior cerebral artery: Clinical study of 51 patients. *BMC Neurology, 9*(1), 30.

Brugger, F., Galovic, M., Weder, B. J., & Kägi, G. (2015). Supplementary motor complex and disturbed motor control – A retrospective clinical and lesion analysis of patients after anterior cerebral artery stroke. *Frontiers in Neurology, 6,* 209.

Brust, J. C. M. (1995). Agitation and delirium. In J. Bogousslavsky & L. Caplan (Eds.), *Stroke syndromes* (pp. 134–139). Cambridge: Cambridge University Press.

Lawton, M. T., & Mirzadeh, Z. (2012). Surgical management of anterior communicating and anterior cerebral artery aneurysms. In H. H. Schmidek & W. H. Sweet (Eds.), *Operative neurosurgical techniques, indications, methods, and results* (5th ed., pp. 882–896). Philadelphia: Saunders/Elsevier.

Menshawi, K., Mohr, J. P., & Gutierrez, J. (2015). A functional perspective on the embryology and anatomy of the cerebral blood supply. *Journal of Stroke, 17*(2), 144.

Mizuta, H., & Motomura, N. (2006). Memory dysfunction in caudate infarction caused by Heubner's recurring artery occlusion. *Brain and Cognition, 61*(2), 133–138.

Rea, P. (2015). Blood supply of the brain and clinical issues. In B. V. Elsevier (Ed.), *Essential clinical anatomy of the nervous system* (pp. 99–119). London: Academic Press.

Uchino, A., Nomiyama, K., Takase, Y., & Kudo, S. (2006). Anterior cerebral artery variations detected by MR angiography. *Neuroradiology, 48*(9), 647–652.

Vrselja, Z., Brkic, H., Mrdenovic, S., Radic, R., & Curic, G. (2014). Function of circle of Willis. *Journal of Cerebral Blood Flow and Metabolism, 34*(4), 578–584.

Vrselja, Z., Brkic, H., & Curic, G. (2016). Penetrating arteries of the cerebral white matter: The importance of vascular territories of delivering arteries and completeness of circle of Willis. *International Journal of Stroke, 11*(3), NP36–NP37.

Zhou, X. Y., Chen, L., & Zhang, S. Q. (2013). Nonfluent aphasia and cognitive impairment caused by anterior cerebral artery infarction. *CNS Neuroscience & Therapeutics, 19*(12), 987–989.

Anterior Cingulate Cortex

Ronald A. Cohen[1,2] and
Anna MacKay-Brandt[3,4]
[1]Department of Clinical and Health Psychology, College of Public Health and Health Professions, University of Florida, Gainesville, FL, USA
[2]Center for Cognitive Aging and Memory, McKnight Brain Institute, University of Florida, Gainesville, FL, USA
[3]Nathan S. Kline Institute for Psychiatric Research, Orangeburg, NY, USA
[4]Taub Institute for Research on Alzheimer's Disease and the Aging Brain, Columbia University, New York, NY, USA

Synonyms

ACC

Structure

The anterior cingulate cortex (ACC) is a meso-cortical paralimbic area located anterior to the corpus callosum and posterior to the prefrontal cortex. The ACC was once viewed as a single limbic structure, forming an important part of the "Papez" circuit, though in reality analysis of its cytoarchitecture indicates that it consists of regions with different cell types. Its cell characteristics are agranular and therefore are distinct from the cortex.

The ACC encompasses several Brodmann areas, including areas 24, 25, 32, and 33. The ACC wraps around the corpus callosum, having the appearance of a collar or belt. In fact, the term cingulum means belt in Latin. A large volume of the ventral ACC consists of Area 24, which merges with the posterior cingulate cortex (Area 23) along the posterior half of the corpus callosum. The division between the ACC and posterior cingulate is undifferentiated to a large extent, though these areas can be separated based on the cortical layer IV in the posterior cingulate. Anterior to Area 24 is the subgenual cortex (Area 25), which may be considered to be distinct from other ACC areas. Anterior to this region is the dorsal ACC, including areas 32 and 33. The mid-anterior section of the ACC is often termed mid-cingulate (mACC), while the more posterior section is termed perigenual cingulate (pACC). These areas have distinct cell characteristics, and there is strong evidence of functional differences across subareas of the ACC.

Primary afferent input to the ACC is received via axons from the midline and intralaminar thalamic nuclei, with the anterior nucleus receiving input from mamillary neurons, which in turn has projections from the subiculum. The ACC is associated with a large white-matter bundle, the cingulum, through which signals are transmitted to other limbic areas. As a paralimbic area, the ACC is a transition area between subcortical and limbic structures, such as the amygdala and cortical areas, most notably in the frontal lobes. The posterior ACC has heavy input from the amygdala, whereas the mid-ACC receives greater input from parietal areas.

Connections between the ACC and the mesial, ventral, and orbital frontal areas appear to be particularly important for emotional and behavioral regulation.

Function

Current knowledge regarding the functions of the ACC has its origins in the psychosurgical efforts of the mid-twentieth century. At that time, the role of the frontal lobes in emotion and behavioral control were recognized, and frontal lobotomy was experimented with as a means of treating a variety of psychiatric conditions, including severe depression and schizophrenia. While frontal lobotomy resulted in a reduction in agitation and other severe psychiatric symptoms, surgical removal of the frontal lobe caused severe cognitive dysfunction. Given that the orbital frontal region was considered to be particularly important for the control of impulses and emotional regulation, subsequent psychosurgical approaches typically restricted ablation to these areas, often through leukotomy. Unfortunately, patients undergoing this procedure often exhibited marked personality change, with flattening of affect, apathy, and other undesirable effects. A third generation of psychosurgical procedures ensued with efforts to target brain areas more selectively. The ACC was a point of focus because of its association with both limbic areas as well as the frontal cortex. Beginning in the late 1950s, cingulotomy was developed as an alternative to frontal ablation. Early studies suggested that it had few adverse cognitive effects and that it seemed helpful for certain patients, particularly those with intractable obsessive-compulsive symptoms, chronic pain, and opiate dependence. There was also some evidence that it was helpful for patients with severe chronic depression, though the basis for these effects may relate to reductions in emotional tension, obsessive thought processes, and other depression-associated problems.

Literature on the psychosurgical effects of cingulotomy provided compelling evidence that the ACC plays a role in human emotional experience and regulation. Furthermore, there is also evidence that the ACC influences autonomic nervous system response, including heart rate, blood pressure, and galvanic skin response, with these responses showing alterations in the rate of habituation following cingulotomy (Cohen et al. 1994). Yet, most early studies of the effects of cingulotomy suggested that the ACC had little impact on intellectual ability or most neuropsychological functions. Postsurgery patients tended not to experience significant memory, language, or visual change. Subsequent controlled studies indicated that while these functions are largely spared following cingulotomy, there are alterations in some attention-related functions, most notably attentional focus, intention, and response selection and control (Cohen et al. 2001). These changes correspond with reductions in emotional tension and distress and also a tendency for reduced self-initiation of behavior (Cohen et al. 2001).

Recent experimental evidence suggests a functional dissociation between the posterior and middle ACC. The mid-ACC plays a role in response selection and control, including intention and planning to act or to engage in cognitive operations. It has also been implicated in processing new motor programs, working memory, and mismatch detection. In contrast, the posterior ACC appears to play a more direct role in emotional processing, though these areas are likely highly interconnected, enabling the integration of emotional and attentional processes (Bush et al. 2000).

Interest in the functional significance of ACC increased dramatically with the advent of functional neuroimaging methods. Activation of the ACC is evident across a wide range of tasks. In fact, it is among the most responsive areas of the brain on fMRI. This probably reflects the fact that it plays an increased role when tasks require motivation and drive to complete and where there is demand for attentional effort and focus.

The ACC plays a significant role in response to the conflict during cognitive tasks associated with decision making and the need to resolve competing or discrepant information (Botvinick et al. 1999). Some cognitive neuroscientists argue that conflict monitoring is the primary function of the ACC, though it seems likely that this capacity is closely associated with the broader functions of regulation of drive, emotion, attention, and response intention; and selection, initiation, and persistence relative to situational demands.

Illness

Focal brain diseases affecting only the ACC are rare. However, the ACC is vulnerable to the effects of tumor, stroke, and other neurological conditions involving anterior cortical infarction or mass action. Unilateral ablation of the ACC in laboratory studies of primates, and also secondary to stroke, has been shown to produce hemineglect syndrome, providing further evidence that the ACC plays an important role in attention. There is evidence of ACC dysfunction secondary to atrophy associated with neurodegenerative conditions, such as Alzheimer's disease, which may contribute to symptoms of apathy and behavioral inertia in certain patients. However, these changes are usually part of a much more global pattern of brain abnormality.

The ACC plays a more obvious role in psychiatric illness and also the range of normal behavior. Activation of the ACC occurs in association with increased levels of distress and emotional tension and anxiety. It also tends to be associated with obsessive rumination and preoccupation with internal states and signals, such as pain and impulses to seek reward. Accordingly, the ACC has been implicated in substance abuse, including opiate addiction and nicotine dependence. Citalopram binds to the serotonin transporter at very high levels in the posterior ACC, which may account for the effects of this type of drug on reducing mood, anxiety, and pain symptoms. There is also evidence that functional response of the ACC varies as a function of risk-reward dynamics, appetitive state, and motivation. Neuroimaging studies have begun to point to its role in a variety of behavior problems, such as obesity and inactivity.

Cross-References

▶ Apathy
▶ Executive Functioning
▶ Psychotherapy

References and Readings

Ballentine Jr., H. T., Levey, B. A., Dagi, T. F., & Diriunas, I. B. (1977). Neurosurgical treatment in psychiatry, pain, and epilepsy. In W. H. Sweet, S. Obrador, & J. G. Martin-Rodriques (Eds.), *Cingulotomy for psychiatric illness: Report of 13 years experience* (pp. 333–353). Baltimore: University Park Press.

Botvinick, M., Nystrom, L. E., Fissell, K., Carter, C. S., & Cohen, J. D. (1999). Conflict monitoring versus selection-for-action in anterior cingulate cortex. *Nature, 402*(6758), 179–181.

Bush, G., Luu, P., & Posner, M. I. (2000). Cognitive and emotional influences in anterior cingulate cortex. *Trends in Cognitive Sciences, 4*(6), 215–222.

Cohen, R. A., Kaplan, R. F., Meadows, M. E., & Wilkinson, H. (1994). Habituation and sensitization of the orienting response following bilateral anterior cingulotomy. *Neuropsychologia, 32*(5), 609–617.

Cohen, R. A., Kaplan, R. F., Zuffante, P., Moser, D. J., Jenkins, M. A., Salloway, S., et al. (1999). Alteration of intention and self-initiated action associated with bilateral anterior cingulotomy. *Journal of Neuropsychiatry and Clinical Neurosciences, 11*(4), 444–453.

Cohen, R. A., Paul, R., Zawacki, T. M., Moser, D. J., Sweet, L., & Wilkinson, H. (2001). Emotional and personality changes following cingulotomy. *Emotion, 1*(1), 38–50.

Devinsky, O., Morrell, M. J., & Vogt, B. A. (1995). Contributions of anterior cingulate cortex to behaviour. *Brain, 118*(Pt. 1), 279–306.

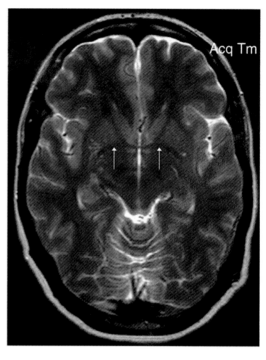

Anterior Commissure, Fig. 1

Definition

A relatively small commissure in the basal forebrain lying above the optic chiasm and anterior to the main columns of the fornix that connects homologous areas of the middle and inferior temporal gyri, including parts of the olfactory cortices (Fig. 1).

Anterior Commissure

John E. Mendoza
Department of Psychiatry and Neuroscience, Tulane Medical School and SE Louisiana Veterans Healthcare System, New Orleans, LA, USA

Synonyms

Interhemispheric commissure

Anterior Communicating Artery

Bruce J. Diamond
Department of Psychology, William Paterson University, Wayne, NJ, USA

Synonyms

ACoA; Communicating artery

Description

The anterior communicating artery (ACoA) inter-connects the two anterior cerebral arteries just rostral to the optic chiasm and resides at the anterior portion of the Circle of Willis.

Ruptured ACoA aneurysms may impact a variety of neurologic, neuropsychological, and psychological functions. This may, in part, be due to the fact that the perforating branches of the ACoA supply the anterior hypothalamus, mesial anterior commissure, lamina termininalis, and areas implicated in executive function, memory, and affect (e.g., fornix and basal forebrain, septal nuclei, nucleus accumbens, diagonal band, and the medial substantia innominata) (DeLuca and Diamond 1995; Sawada and Kazui 1995). The profound memory disorders that can be associated with ACoA aneurysm rupture do not appear to directly involve neuroanatomic areas traditionally implicated in amnesia, which makes the ACoA artery of both clinical and theoretical interest.

Etiology

ACoA aneurysms may develop as a result of trauma, infections, degenerative diseases, or a congenital defect (Parkin and Leng 1993). Aneurysms often become symptomatic as a result of subarachnoid hemorrhage (SAH) following rupture (Riina et al. 2002). SAH has an overall incidence of 10 to 16 per 100,000 and is a major cause of mortality and morbidity (Clinchot et al. 1994).

Mechanisms

Ruptured ACoA aneurysms alter the hemodynamic circulation of the anterior portion of the Circle of Willis, often resulting in cerebral infarction and impairments in cognition, personality, and activities of daily living (ADL's) (DeLuca and Diamond 1995; McCormick 1984). Damage to the basal forebrain region may account for many of the cognitive impairments that are observed in ACoA aneurysm due to the fact that the basal forebrain region contains cholinergic neurons that project to the hippocampus and amygdala, via the medial forebrain bundle to the entire cerebral cortex. Damage to this area would potentially interfere with cholinergic activation of structures and circuits implicated in memory within the medial temporal lobe (Schnider and Landis 1995). Moreover, vascular compromise of the perforating branches of the ACoA are believed to adversely impact a variety of cognitive domains (e.g., executive function, memory, and affect) that are innervated by these vascular branches. Personality changes following ACoA aneurysm are thought to result from frontal lobe dysfunction in the medio-basal zones along the distribution of the anterior cerebral artery. The subcallosal perforating artery (ScA) has been implicated in personality changes and short-term memory impairments with stroke in the vascular territory of the ScA associated with ischemia involving the anterior columns of the fornix and the genu of the corpus callosum (Meila et al. 2015). Neurocomputational models of hippocampal function may also provide insight into possible mechanisms of action mediating learning impairments in ACoA aneurysm. One such model shows that simulating the loss of acetylcholine in the hippocampal region (as in ACoA aneurysm) results in slower acquisition learning (Moustafa et al. 2012).

Epidemiological Factors

Rupture of cerebral aneurysms strikes at a mean age of 50 years and accounts for 5–10% of all strokes (Dombovy et al. 1998), and approximately 85–95% of all aneurysms develop at the anterior portion of the cerebral arterial supply, primarily at the Circle of Willis (Adams and Biller 1992; Ropper et al. 2005). The ACoA is one of the most common sites of cerebral aneurysm and is the most frequent site of cerebral infarct following aneurysm rupture (DeLuca and Diamond 1995; McCormick 1984). About 30–40% of cerebral aneurysms affect the ACoA artery and 90% of cases are asymptomatic (Beeckmans et al. 1998;

A

Manconi et al. 2001). Various reports suggest that the incidence of rupture is highest between 40 and 70 years of age (McCormick 1984; Sethi et al. 2000) and that rupture occurs more frequently in females (i.e., 60% of cases) (Adams and Biller 1992). Some work suggests that risk factors such as age, gender, and no alcohol consumption influence the site of the aneurysm. For example, men have ruptured aneurysms more often at the ACoA compared to the PCoA (Lindner et al. 2010).

Natural History, Prognostic Factors, and Outcomes

The risk of ACoA aneurysm formation appears to be determined by a number of independent risk factors, including clinical, morphological, and hemodynamic. That is, smoking, asymmetry of A1 segments >40%, low blood flow pulsatility, and the angle between A1 and A2 segments $\leq 100°$ have been identified as the strongest independent risk factors (Kaspera et al. 2014). Surgical and/or endovascular procedures should pay special attention to the subcallosal perforating artery given its putative role in disturbances in cognition and personality. With respect to impairment and chronicity, acute ACoA patients are more impaired than chronic ones with differences most notable on tests of executive and memory function.

Relationships between recovery of executive function and temporal gradients in retrograde amnesia have been reported, with improvements in executive function accompanied by parallel improvements in the severity of retrograde amnesia. Improvement in the recall of complex visual-spatial information and an enhanced ability to benefit from an executive learning strategy have also been reported in the absence of improvement on traditional measures of memory or executive function (Diamond et al. 1997a). Recovery from neuropsychological disturbances is generally poorer in patients with ventral frontal lesion compared to those with basal forebrain and striate lesions.

Surgical outcome and prognosis following aneurysms depend on multiple factors (e.g., initial clinical status, localization of aneurysm, age,

and the morphological characteristics of the aneurysm). Comparisons of clipping versus endovascular embolization procedures have shown that, in a number of studies, clipped patients have more severe cognitive impairments than embolization patients and that 33% of clipped patients had impairments in memory and executive functioning (Chan et al. 2002). There is a report of a complete third nerve palsy following a ruptured ACoA aneurysm resulting from an interpeduncular hematoma. The patient did, however, fully recover 3 months after the coiling procedure (Balossier et al. 2012).

Generally, the severity of cognitive impairment has predictive value for functional status particularly with respect to levels of required supervision at discharge (Saciri and Kos 2002). Some work suggests that recovery of executive function and not short- and long-term memory may, in fact, be the best predictor of the ability to return to work (DeLuca and Diamond 1995).

Neuropsychological and Psychological Outcomes

Neuropsychological

It is generally concluded that verbal intellectual skills, language functions, visuo-spatial skills, and attention/concentration are within normal limits or only mildly impaired, although complex concentration appears to be reduced in ACoA aneurysm. An increased sensitivity to interference may be a defining feature among ACoA amnesics and between ACoA amnesics and diencephalic-mesial and temporal amnesics. More severe impairments are seen in delayed versus immediate memory and in executive function (DeLuca and Diamond 1995). Impairments in spatio-temporal discrimination appear similar to other populations with frontal lobe dysfunction (Schacter 1987). Implicit memory involving data- and concept-driven retrieval processes and behavioral and physiological indices (Diamond et al. 1996) appear to be relatively intact, although the evidence is sparse. Procedural memory on serial reaction time and mirror-reading tasks also appears to be preserved. Spatial working memory in ACoA patients has been reported to be impaired, and the impairment profile is similar to patients with temporal lobe excisions. ACoA patients have displayed impairments in semantic memory, and difficulties in both the acquisition and recall of verbal information showing little initial learning, a passive learning style, a flat learning slope, and impaired recognition discrimination, in addition to emitting a high number of intrusions and false positives (Diamond et al. 1997b).

ACoA amnesics (i.e., with putative basal forebrain damage) have exhibited impairments in delay eyeblink classical conditioning (Myers et al. 2001), event-related potentials (ERPs), and in prospective remembering. Discrimination, in addition to emitting a high number of intrusions and false positives (Diamond et al. 1997b). While semantic memory impairment is generally associated with lesion of the anterior temporal lobe, there is a recent case of a patient with severely impaired semantic knowledge and anterograde amnesia after bilateral ischemic lesion of the fornix and of the basal forebrain following clipping of an ACoA aneurysm. This appears to have been mediated by functional disconnection of the temporal lobe and associated temporal hypometabolism as verified by PET imaging (Solcà et al. 2015). ACoA patients have shown impairments in information processing and autobiographical memory (especially for events associated with context). ACoA amnesics (i.e., with putative basal forebrain damage) have exhibited impairments in delay eyeblink classical conditioning (Myers et al. 2001), event-related potentials (ERPs), and in prospective remembering. In addition, patients with subarachnoid hemorrhage secondary to ruptured ACoA aneurysms have exhibited deficits in decision-making under ambiguity, with clipped patients, but not coiled patients, showing deficits in making decisions in comparison with controls (Escartin et al. 2012).

Psychological

Confabulation is observed in a subset of ACoA aneurysm patients and is manifested by statements or actions that involve unintentionally false or distorted memories (Moscovitch and Melo 1997). This may be due to a generalized impairment in source monitoring (Turner et al. 2010).

Two distinct types of confabulation are generally recognized in the literature, spontaneous and provoked (Kopelman 1987), and the key difference between them is that in spontaneous confabulation the confabulation guides actions. Recovery from confabulation appears to parallel improvement in temporal context confusion, and recovery can occur in the absence of significant improvement on traditional tests of memory and executive function. Interestingly, while confabulation associated with ACoA aneurysm is well known, a clinical condition known as "Phantabulation" was recently reported. It is characterized by the purposeful interaction with contextually appropriate imagined objects. It was hypothesized that that these episodes depended on a combination of phenomena, including a top-down mechanism involving florid visual-imagery, facilitated by cortical release secondary to frontal damage and enhanced by an associated malfunction of the fronto-parietal pathway resulting in real and functionally appropriate imagined objects being confused (Cocchini et al. 2014).

With respect to psychosocial outcomes, a significant percentage of SAH survivors are left with cognitive, emotional, and behavioral changes that can profoundly impact their daily lives. Compared with controls, SAH patients display an increased incidence of mood disturbance, cognitive impairment, and lower levels of independence, and participation on measures that reflect social functioning. Levels of productive employment are generally reduced and many patients show clinically significant posttraumatic stress symptomatology (see Table 1 for a list of neuropsychological and psychological impairments).

Assessment and Treatment

Given the wide range of impairments associated with ACoA aneurysm, it may be advisable for clinicians to use assessments that focus on those impairments that are most salient and have the greatest impact on activities of daily living

Anterior Communicating Artery, Table 1 Neuropsychological and psychological impairments associated with ACoA aneurysm

Awareness, self-monitoring, mood, personality	Memory/learning	Cognitive/executive, electrophysiological
Disorders of awareness	Semantic memory	Complex attention
Spontaneous confabulation	Prospective memory	Cognitive estimation
Provoked confabulation	Visuo-spatial	Decision-making under ambiguity
Phantabulation	Working memory	Dual task performance
Anosognosia	Recall	Concentration
Intrusions	Spatial working memory	Proactive interference/vulnerability to interference
Source monitoring	Delayed memory	Verbal fluency
Mood	Impaired initial learning	Executive dysfunction
Motor/sensory	Passive learning style	Autonomic and event-related potentials (ERP)
Paraparesis syndrome	Flat learning slope	Electrocardiogram (ECG)
Visuomotor skill learning	Delay eyeblink conditioning	Delayed ERP (P300): Auditory
Alien hand syndrome	Acquisition	Delayed ERP (P300): Visual
Visual-sensory function (unruptured aneurysms)	Recognition	Prolonged QTc intervals
Third cranial nerve palsy	Language	Dichotic listening

(ADLs). Impairments in memory, executive function, and attention/concentration as well as mood figure prominently following ACoA aneurysm rupture and should be part of routine assessment. For example, assessments should examine set-shifting (e.g., Wisconsin Card Sort Test (WCST) and Trails B), verbal and visual fluency (e.g., CFT/FAS and Design Fluency Test), verbal recall and recognition (e.g., California Verbal Learning Test (CVLT)), visual recall (e.g., Rey-Osterreith Complex Figure Test (ROCFT)), sustained attention (e.g., Cancellation Test), information processing speed (e.g., n-back tasks), and impaired abstraction (e.g., Cognitive Estimation Test (CET)).

In some cases, modification of existing assessment tools can be an effective way to enhance the assessment process. For example, the Rey-Osterrieth Organizational and Extended Memory (ROEM) test, which is a modification of the ROCFT, was reported to help identify mechanisms underlying the nature of the impaired memory in ACoA amnesics by using measures of recall and recognition (e.g., subunit recognition, spatial arrangement, and whole figure recognition). Moreover, encoding and recall were improved by using an executive organizational strategy, in addition to identifying patients who were more likely to benefit from such an intervention (Diamond et al. 1997a; Prigatano and DeLuca 1999).

Some work suggests that cognitive rehabilitation can help increase compensatory strategies for attention and memory dysfunction and that rehabilitation can help improve professional activities as well as ADLs with positive rehabilitation outcomes primarily associated with changes in memory and attention. In a mixed sample of SAH patients, a majority of survivors who receive inpatient rehabilitation attain physical independence but impairments in cognition and ADLs persist in upwards of 40% of the patients (Dombovy et al. 1998). Patients have generally shown impairments 1–5 years post-stroke, in visual short-term memory, reaction-time, verbal long-term memory, concentration, and language and information processing. Evaluation several years after SAH associated with ACoA aneurysm rupture has shown that cognitive problems negatively correlate with the level of community integration and that impairments in visual memory, verbal memory, and executive function are most frequently observed. Therefore, while being characterized as having a good outcome, many ACoA patients continue to exhibit persistent cognitive impairments that negatively impact psychosocial functioning (Ravnik et al. 2006).

Cross-References

▶ Activities of Daily Living (ADL)
▶ Amnesia
▶ Aneurysm
▶ Anterior Cerebral Artery
▶ Confabulation
▶ Executive Functioning
▶ Rey Complex Figure Test

References and Readings

Adams, H. P., & Biller, J. (1992). Hemorrhagic intracranial vascular disease. In A. B. Baker & R. J. Joynt (Eds.), *Clinical neurology* (Vol. 2). Philadelphia: J. B. Lippincott.

Balossier, A., Postelnicu, A., Khouri, S., Emery, E., & Derlon, J. M. (2012). Third nerve palsy induced by a ruptured anterior communicating artery aneurysm. *British Journal of Neurosurgery, 26*(5), 770–772.

Beeckmans, K., Vancoillie, P., & Michiels, K. (1998). Neuropsychological deficits in patients with an anterior communicating artery syndrome: A multiple case study. *Acta Neurologica Belgica, 98*(3), 266–278.

Chan, A., Ho, S., & Poon, W. S. (2002). Neuropsychological sequelae of patients treated with microsurgical clipping or endovascular embolization for anterior communicating artery aneurysm. *European Neurology, 47*, 37–44.

Clinchot, D. M., Kaplan, P., Murray, D. M., & Pease, W. S. (1994). Cerebral aneurysms and arteriovenous malformations: Implications for rehabilitation. *Archives of Physical Medicine and Rehabilitation, 75*(12), 1342–1351.

Cocchini, G., Lello, O., McIntosh, R. D., & Della Sala, S. (2014). Phantabulation: A case of visual imagery interference on visual perception. *Neurocase, 20*(5), 581–590.

Cummings, J. L., & Trimble, M. R. (1995). *A concise guide to neuropsychiatry and behavioral neurology.* Washington, DC: American Psychiatric Press.

DeLuca, J., & Diamond, B. J. (1995). Aneurysm of the anterior communicating artery: A review of neuroanatomical and neuropsychological sequelae. *Journal of Clinical and Experimental Neuropsychology, 17*(1), 100–121.

Diamond, B. J., Mayes, A. R., & Meudell, P. (1996). Autonomic and recognition indices of aware and unaware memory in amnesics and healthy subjects. *Cortex, 32*, 439–459.

Diamond, B. J., DeLuca, J., & Kelley, S. M. (1997a). Executive and memory impairment in patients with anterior communicating artery aneurysm. *Brain and Cognition, 35*, 340–341.

Diamond, B. J., DeLuca, J., & Kelley, S. M. (1997b). Verbal learning in anterior communicating artery aneurysm and multiple sclerosis patients: Performance on the California verbal learning test. *Applied Neuropsychology, 4*, 89–98.

Dombovy, M. L., Drew-Cates, J., & Serdans, R. (1998). Recovery and rehabilitation following subarachnoid haemorrhage: Part II. Long-term follow-up. *Brain Injury, 12*(10), 887–894.

Escartin, J., Juncadella, G., & de Miquel, R. (2012). Decision-making impairment on the Iowa gambling task after endovascular coiling or neurosurgical clipping for ruptured anterior communicating artery aneurysm. *Neuropsychology, 26*(2), 172–180.

Kaspera, W., Ładziński, P., Larysz, P., Hebda, A., Ptaszkiewicz, K., Kopera, M., & Larysz, D. (2014). Morphological, hemodynamic, and clinical independent risk factors for anterior communicating artery aneurysms. *Stroke; a Journal of Cerebral Circulation, 45*(10), 2906–2911. https://doi.org/10.1161/STROKEAHA.114.00605.

Kopelman, M. D. (1987). Two types of confabulation. *Journal of Neurology, Neurosurgery and Psychiatry, 50*(11), 1482–1487.

Lindner, S. H., Bor, A. S. E., & Rinkel, G. J. E. (2010). Differences in risk factors according to the site of intracranial aneurysms. *Journal of Neurology, Neurosurgery & Psychiatry, 81*(1), 116–118.

Manconi, M., Paolino, E., Casetta, I., & Granieri, E. (2001). Anosmia in a giant anterior communicating artery aneurysm. *Archives of Neurology, 58*(9), 1474–1475.

McCormick, W. F. (1984). Pathology and pathogenesis of intracranial saccular aneurysms. *Seminars in Neurology, 4*(3), 291–303.

Meila, D., Saliou, G., & Krings, T. (2015). Subcallosal artery stroke: Infarction of the fornix and the genu of the corpus callosum. The importance of the anterior communicating artery complex. Case series and review of the literature. *Neuroradiology, 57*(1), 41–47. https://doi.org/10.1007/s00234-014-1438-8.

Moscovitch, M., & Melo, B. (1997). Strategic retrieval and the frontal lobes: Evidence from confabulation and amnesia. *Neuropsychologia, 35*(7), 1017–1034.

Myers, C. E., DeLuca, J., Schultheis, M. T., Schnirman, G. M., Ermita, B. R., Diamond, B. J., Warren, S. G., & Gluck, M. (2001). Impaired delay eyeblink classical conditioning in individuals with anterograde amnesia resulting from anterior communicating artery aneurysm. *Behavioral Neuroscience, 115*(3), 560–570.

Parkin, A., & Leng, R. C. (1993). *Neuropsychology of the amnestic syndrome.* Hove: Lawrence Erlbaum.

Prigatano, G., & DeLuca, J. (1999). Methodological issues in research on neuropsychological and intellectual assessment. In P. C. Kendall, J. Butcher, & G. Holmbeck (Eds.), *Handbook of research methods in clinical psychology* (pp. 241–250). New York: Wiley.

Ravnik, J., Starovasnik, B., Šešok, S., Pirtošek, Z., Švigelj, V., Bunc, G., et al. (2006). Long-term cognitive deficits in patients with good outcomes after aneurysmal sub-arachnoid hemorrhage from anterior communicating artery. *Croatian Medical Journal, 47*, 253–263.

Riina, H. A., Lemole, G. M., Jr., & Spetzler, R. F. (2002). Anterior communicating artery aneurysms. *Neurosur-gery, 51*(4), 993–996.

Ropper, A. H., Brown, R. H., Adams, R. D., & Victor, M. (2005). *Adams & Victor's principles of neurology*. New York: McGraw-Hill.

Saciri, B. M., & Kos, N. (2002). Aneurysmal subarachnoid haemorrhage: Outcomes of early rehabilitation after surgical repair of ruptured intracranial aneurysms. *Journal of Neurology, Neurosurgery, and Psychiatry, 72*(3), 334–337.

Sawada, T., & Kazui, S. (1995). Anterior cerebral artery. In J. Bogousslavsky & L. Caplan (Eds.), *Stroke Syn-dromes* (pp. 235–246). Cambridge: Cambridge University Press.

Schacter, D. L. (1987). Implicit memory: History and cur-rent status. *Journal of Experimental Psychology. Learning, Memory, and Cognition, 13*, 501–518.

Schnider, A., & Landis, T. (1995). Memory loss. In J. Bogousslavsky & L. Caplan (Eds.), *Stroke syn-dromes* (pp. 145–150). Cambridge, MA: Cambridge University Press.

Sethi, H., Moore, A., Dervin, J., Clifton, A., & MacSweeney, J. E. (2000). Hydrocephalus: Compari-son of clipping and embolization in aneurysm treat-ment. *Journal of Neurosurgery, 92*(6), 991–994.

Solcà, M., Di Pietro, M., Schnider, A., & Leemann, B. (2015). Impairment of semantic memory after basal forebrain and fornix lesion. *Neurocase, 21*(2), 198–205.

Turner, M., Cipolotti, L., & Shallice, T. (2010). Spontane-ous confabulation, temporal context confusion and reality monitoring: A study of three patients with ante-rior communicating artery aneurysms. *Journal of the International Neuropsychological Society, 16*(6), 984–994.

Anterograde Amnesia

Ginette Lafleche and Mieke Verfaellie
Memory Disorders Research Center, VA Boston Healthcare System and Boston University School of Medicine, Boston, MA, USA

Short Description or Definition

The term "anterograde amnesia" refers to an inability to acquire or retain memories of the ongoing events of one's life (i.e., autobiograph-ical information) or factual (semantic) informa-tion to which one was exposed following the onset of amnesia. In contrast to this, implicit memory (such as the acquisition of simple habits or skills like riding a bicycle) is preserved in amnesia.

Brief Historical Background

Current scientific understanding of anterograde amnesia originated with the study of patient HM. In 1953, at age 27, HM underwent bilateral resection of the medial temporal lobes for alle-viation of refractory seizures, which had wors-ened following a head injury he had suffered at age 9. The resection was successful in reducing his seizures, but, unexpectedly, following the treatment, he was unable to remember his nor-mal daily activities. For example, he could not remember the content of a conversation or even having had a conversation, minutes after it ended. He was unable to remember his regular caregivers, even though he could converse and interact normally with them when they were present. These findings established that intact medial temporal lobes are critical for establishing new memories: HM's medial tem-poral lobe resection had left him with a dense anterograde amnesia. In addition to his antero-grade amnesia, HM also had difficulties remem-bering information acquired prior to his surgery (▶ Retrograde Amnesia). Initial observations suggested that his retrograde amnesia was lim-ited to approximately 2 years prior to the oper-ation. However, more recent findings indicate that he had a more lengthy retrograde amnesia that extended into the distant past (Steinvorth et al. 2005). Yet, in spite of his memory difficul-ties, HM showed preservation of intelligence, attention, language function, and social skills. Subsequent neuropsychological studies of HM and other amnesic individuals have further informed our current understanding of both impaired and preserved memory function in amnesia (Corkin 1984).

Neuropsychology of Anterograde Amnesia

Patients suffering from anterograde amnesia have great difficulty in bringing to mind new information that they were exposed to after the onset of their amnesia. Although these patients have preserved short-term memory, in that they can hold in mind a current topic of conversation and can repeat a string of digits with no delay, if there is a distraction or delay, memory for the information is lost. Episodic memory (i.e., memory for personal events) is severely impaired, and, as a result, patients no longer form an ongoing record of their lives. For example, it is common for patients to forget what they ate for lunch only minutes after they finished eating. In the same vein, in the laboratory, patients will typically forget material they learned minutes earlier in a session, such as images presented on a computer or the details of a story. The precise nature of this memory loss depends on the site and extent of damage. For example, impaired verbal recall results from damage to the left medial temporal lobe whereas impaired nonverbal recall results from right-sided damage. With bilateral damage, both verbal and nonverbal memory problems will ensue. In addition to loss of episodic memory, patients also experience difficulty learning and remembering new facts or concepts (semantic memory). The degree of impairment in new semantic learning is also a function of the extent of the medial temporal lobe lesion. Patients with injury limited to the hippocampus are able to acquire some new facts and concepts post-morbidly, even if inefficiently, but patients with more extensive medial temporal lobe damage show minimal ability to do so (Verfaellie 2000). Together, episodic and semantic memory comprise declarative (or explicit) memory and are what the plain term "memory" refers to in common usage. An important insight to arise from the study of patients with anterograde amnesia is that not all forms of long-term memory are impaired. Forms of memory that do not require deliberate reference to a prior experience, often referred to as nondeclarative (or implicit) memory, remain intact.

Failure of declarative memory in amnesia can arise from a number of different etiologies. These include anoxia, herpes simplex encephalitis (HSE), anterior communicating artery aneurysm (ACoA), Wernicke-Korsakoff syndrome (WKS), and stroke. The amnesia is a direct consequence of damage to the medial temporal lobes, (i.e., HSE, anoxia), the midline diencephalon (WKS, stroke), basal forebrain structures (ACoA), or some of the fiber tracts that link these regions. These amnesias are usually permanent. In contrast, in transient global amnesia (TGA), there is temporary dysfunction of memory-related brain structures including the hippocampal formation and thalamus. Episodes of TGA typically last no more than 24 h, after which the patient's new learning returns to normal, but a permanent amnesic gap remains for the period of the attack (see entry ▶ "Litigation").

The ability to remember newly encountered information depends on a number of stages, including the processing and representation of immediate experience (encoding), the transfer of that encoded information to long-term storage (consolidation), and its re-manifestation in consciousness upon deliberate recall (retrieval) at a later time. Disruption of any one of these stages could lead to anterograde amnesia. In patients with medial temporal or diencephalic lesions, encoding and retrieval are thought to be relatively intact. Such patients perform normally on intelligence tests and on short-term memory tests, suggesting adequate encoding (Baddeley 1995). Furthermore, impaired retrieval is unlikely to be the cause of their failed explicit memory, because memories from many years ago can still be retrieved. Therefore, it is assumed that their impairments reflect deficient consolidation. The medial temporal lobes, through interactions with neocortical regions, are thought to be critical for consolidation. They bind together into a coherent representation the different aspects of an event that are neocortically represented (Eichenbaum 2006).

Generally, the size of the causative brain lesion is directly proportional to the density of the amnesia, but the specific location of the lesion will also impact on the nature of the memory impairment.

For example, if the damage is limited to the hippocampal formation, performance on recall tasks is impaired, but performance on recognition tasks can remain intact (Mayes et al. 2002). To account for these findings, it has been suggested that two distinct processes contribute to explicit memory: recollection and familiarity. Recollection is thought to enable the conscious recovery of contextually specific information about an event (e.g., recalling the full context of how you met someone for the first time on a particular street last December in New York). Familiarity enables retrieval of context-free information through a feeling of "knowing" (e.g., having the feeling that you have met someone previously without remembering where or when you met them). Whereas performance on recall tasks depends on the ability to retrieve contextually relevant information (recollection), performance on recognition tasks can be supported by either recollection or familiarity. Thus, the preserved recognition performance observed in patients with limited hippocampal lesions is thought to reflect preserved familiarity, despite impaired recollection. The dissociation between recollection and familiarity is supported by findings from neuroimaging (Diana et al. 2007) and neuropsychological studies (Zita-Patai et al. 2015) that suggest that the hippocampus is critical for recollection whereas familiarity is supported by the perirhinal cortex. If the damage extends beyond the hippocampus to include other medial temporal lobe structures such as the perirhinal cortex, then both recollection and familiarity are affected, leading to striking impairments on tests of recognition as well as recall.

In some cases, for example, in patients with amnesia due to anoxia or rupture of an aneurysm of the anterior communicating artery, frontal lobe impairments may be superimposed on the core amnesia (▶ Amnestic Syndromes). This can lead to exacerbation of the anterograde amnesia by additional impairments in encoding and retrieval. Executive functions such as planning, organizing, monitoring, and control of attention, all depend on the integrity of the frontal lobes. Executive impairments will interfere with the ability to mentally manipulate and organize information during

deliberate encoding and will also disrupt initiation and evaluation of memory search during effortful retrieval. The latter can lead to unusually high levels of intrusions in recall or false alarms in recognition, and this is referred to as enhanced susceptibility to false memory.

Despite such pervasive impairments in declarative memory, patients with anterograde amnesia show intact performance in a variety of forms of nondeclarative (implicit) memory. These include procedural learning (the acquisition of new skills or habits), eyeblink conditioning (learning to blink the eyes in response to a tone because of the repeated association of the tone with an air puff to the eye), and repetition priming (improved accuracy or speed of performance for stimuli to which an individual was recently exposed) (Verfaellie and Keane 2002). These forms of nondeclarative memory depend on neural circuits in the basal ganglia, cerebellum, or neocortex that remain spared in amnestic syndromes (Squire 1994).

Evaluation

Anterograde amnesia refers to a severe and permanent inability to learn new information in the presence of otherwise normal intelligence, attention span, perception, reasoning, and language ability. The evaluation of anterograde amnesia must therefore, as a first step, include a comprehensive neuropsychological work-up to determine whether other areas of cognitive functioning are intact and, if not, whether any deficits found contribute to the memory disorder. With regard to assessment of memory functioning itself, there are a variety of standardized tests available. Lezak et al. (2004) provide a comprehensive review of the most commonly used ones. Assessing performance on recall and recognition tests is an essential component of the evaluation, because their comparison can reveal the nature of the memory processes that are affected. Both verbal and nonverbal memory should be examined, and memory should be tested both shortly after learning and following a longer delay, to assess the rate of forgetting. Other factors of diagnostic importance are a patient's sensitivity to interference and his or her ability to use organizational strategies at encoding and retrieval. While a comprehensive assessment of anterograde memory typically includes a variety of different tests, each developed for a specific purpose, the use of a single standardized memory battery that evaluates all major aspects of new learning can provide a good overview of memory functioning. The Wechsler Memory Scale-III and Wechsler Memory Scale-IV (Wechsler 1997, 2009) are probably the most widely used instruments for this purpose. In addition to indices of immediate and delayed memory, they provide an index of short-term memory, and, in patients with anterograde amnesia, a significant discrepancy in performance is to be expected between the short-term and long-term memory measures.

Treatment

Rehabilitation interventions in amnesia aim at increasing day-to-day functional adaptation and independence. A wide array of intervention techniques is available, and the choice among them should be informed by cognitive factors such as premorbid abilities and skills as well as postmorbid neuropsychological strengths and weaknesses, including the severity of amnesia. Relevant non-cognitive factors include premorbid lifestyle and habits and educational background. Other contributing factors include insight and motivation, which are essential for any treatment choice, because the absence of either will undermine rehabilitation efforts.

Remediation of patients with severe amnesia relies largely on those aspects of memory that are preserved, such as procedural learning and priming. Techniques that capitalize on procedural learning use repetition to drill skills and habits that range from essential activities of daily living to simple assembly tasks and cognitive skills. Such skill learning is frequently involved when teaching a patient to use an external memory aid, such as a memory notebook, calendar, diary,

appointment book, or written reminders. The memory notebook is a preferred compensatory instrument for amnesics because it is divided into sections that are personally tailored to a patient's life (i.e., daily tasks, future plans, notes section, and so on). More sophisticated technology, in the form of computerized paging systems, electronic assistants, alarms, and timers, is most useful for individuals who had some proficiency in the use of such devices premorbidly.

Other methods promote the use of strategies that make use of preserved priming abilities. These approaches typically use structured presentation of the to-be-learned material whereby patients are encouraged to guess the correct answer based on cues. One such approach uses trial and error learning, and once a correct answer is generated, cues are gradually reduced until the correct answer can be spontaneously generated. A drawback of a trial and error approach, however, is that it allows for the generation of incorrect responses during the learning phase. There is now considerable evidence that the generation of errors may interfere with subsequent learning of the correct response. Therefore, the use of errorless learning techniques is preferable, in which cues are used that prevent the occurrence of errors (Kessels and Haan 2003).

For patients with milder memory impairments, strategies aimed at strengthening the impaired form of memory are more appropriate. Such patients may benefit from rehearsal and relearning of the material. Spaced repetitions across different time intervals and different spatial locations are especially beneficial as they enhance the likelihood that information will be richly encoded, thus enhancing the chances that a freestanding memory will be integrated with preexisting memories. For patients whose memory impairment reflects impairment in effortful encoding and retrieval, techniques that promote enhanced organization (e.g., chunking, thematic organization) and elaboration (e.g., verbal mnemonics, visual imagery) at the time of learning may be useful. In a sense, elaboration provides the learner with alternative retrieval routes that may enhance recall.

Cross-References

▶ Amnesia
▶ Retrograde Amnesia

References and Readings

Baddeley, A. D. (1995). The psychology of memory. In A. D. Baddeley, B. A. Wilson, & F. N. Watts (Eds.), *Handbook of memory disorders* (pp. 3–25). New York: John Wiley & Sons.

Corkin, S. (1984). Lasting consequences of bilateral medial temporal lobectomy: Clinical course and experimental findings in H. M. *Seminars in Neurology, 4,* 249–259.

Diana, R. A., Yonelinas, A. P., & Ranganath, C. (2007). Imaging recollection and familiarity in the medial temporal lobe: A three-component model. *Trends, 11*(9), 379–386.

Eichenbaum, H. (2006). Memory binding in hippocampal relational networks. In H. D. Zimmer, A. Mecklinger, & U. Linderberger (Eds.), *Handbook of binding and memory: Perspectives from cognitive neuroscience* (pp. 25–51). New York: Oxford University Press.

Kessels, R. P. C., & Haan, E. H. F. (2003). Implicit learning in memory rehabilitation: A meta-analysis on errorless learning and vanishing cues methods. *Journal of Clinical and Experimental Neuropsychology, 25*(6), 805–814.

Lezak, M. D., Howieson, D. B., & Loring, D. W. (2004). *Neuropsychological assessment* (4th ed.). New York: Oxford University Press.

Mayes, A. R., Holdstock, J. S., Isaac, C. L., Hunkin, N. M., & Roberts, N. (2002). Relative sparing of item recognition memory in a patient with adult-onset damage limited to the hippocampus. *Hippocampus, 12,* 325–340.

Scolville, W. B., & Milner, B. (1957). Loss of recent memory after bilateral hippocampal lesions. *Journal of Neurology, Neurosurgery and Psychiatry, 20*(11), 11–21.

Squire, L. S. (1994). Declarative and nondeclarative memory: Multiple brain systems supporting learning and memory. In D. L. Schacter & E. Tulving (Eds.), *Memory systems 1994* (pp. 203–232). Cambridge, MA: MIT Press.

Steinvorth, S., Levine, B., & Corkin, S. (2005). Medial temporal lobe structures are needed to re-experience remote autobiographical memoires: Evidence from H.M. And W.R. *Neuropsychologia, 43,* 479–496.

Verfaellie, M., Koseff P., & Alexander, M. P. (2000). Acquisition of novel semantic information in amnesia: effects of lesion location. *Neuropsychologia, 38,* 484–492.

Verfaellie, M., & Keane, M. M. (2002). Impaired and preserved memory processes in amnesia. In L. R. Squire & D. L. Schacter (Eds.), *Neuropsychology of memory* (3rd ed., pp. 35–46). New York: Guilford Press.

Wechsler, D. (1997). *Wechsler memory scale – third edition. Administration and scoring manual.* San Antonio: The Psychological Corporation, Pearson, Inc.

Wechsler, D. (2009). *Wechsler memory scale – Fourth edition, Administration and scoring manual.* San Antonio: The Psychological Corporation, Pearson, Inc.

Zita-Patai, E., Gadian, D. G., Cooper, J. M., Dzieciol, A. M., Mishkin, M., & Vargha-Kadem, F. (2015). Extent of hippocampal atrophy predicts degree of deficit in recall. *Proceedings of the National Academy of Sciences, 112*(41), 12830–12833.

Anterolateral System

John E. Mendoza
Department of Psychiatry and Neuroscience, Tulane Medical School and SE Louisiana Veterans Healthcare System, New Orleans, LA, USA

Synonyms

ALS; Spinothalamic tract

Definition

One of two ascending pathways in the spinal cord that carry conscious sensory information from the upper and lower extremities, trunk, and posterior portion of the head to the brain (the other being the lemniscal system).

Current Knowledge

Of the two ascending somatosensory pathways (the other being the posterior columns or lemniscal system) the anterolateral system (ALS) is the more primitive and polysynaptic and is primarily responsible for the sensations of pain, temperature, and crude ("less well defined") or simple touch. Input into the ALS is derived from both specialized cutaneous receptors and free nerve endings in the skin. These sensory impulses then travel centrally (toward the cord) in the peripheral nerves. Just outside the cord, the peripheral nerves bifurcate into the dorsal and ventral nerve roots. The dorsal roots, which carry sensory information, then synapse in the gray matter of the cord (dorsal horns) on the same side in which they enter. Secondary fibers then cross the midline of the cord in the ventral white commissure and ascend in the ventral-lateral portion of the spinal cord as the ventral and lateral spinothalamic tracts. While these two tracts were once described as carrying different and distinct types of sensory information, the current thinking is that they have extensive functional overlap and hence should be considered as a single anterolateral system. These second-order fibers of the ALS ascend in the ventral lateral portion of the cord and then in the lateral and later in the dorsolateral portions of the brainstem. These ascending pathways continue to ventral posterior lateral nucleus of the thalamus. From the thalamus, third-order neurons project to the somatosensory cortices in the parietal lobes of the brain. Because the nerve fibers making up the ALS cross the midline within a few vertebral segments of where they enter the cord, lesions affecting the ALS will result in contralateral deficits.

Cross-References

► Medial Lemniscus

References and Readings

Mendoza, J. E., & Foundas, A. L. (2008). The somatosensory systems. In J. E. Mendoza & A. L. Foundas (Eds.), *Clinical neuroanatomy – A neurobehavioral approach* (pp. 23–47). New York: Springer.

Anticholinergic

Mary Pat Murphy
MSN, CRRN, Paoli, PA, USA

Synonyms

Anticholinergic medications

Definition

Anticholinergic agents alter the balance of neurotransmitters in the central and peripheral nervous system inhibiting parasympathetic nerve impulses. Specifically, the agents diminish acetylcholine and allow for the increase of dopamine. Anticholinergic medications are divided into three categories based on their specific receptor targets in the nervous system and in other sites in the body: antimuscarinic, ganglionic blockers, and neuromuscular blockers. The receptor subtypes affect the brain, salivary glands, smooth muscle, and ciliary muscles of the eye. Categories of medications are clinically used for the antimuscarinic effects and include medications for urinary spasmodics and overactive bladder, anticholinergic antiparkinson's agents, antivertigo medications, gastrointestinal antispasmodics, mydriatic medications, and medications for bronchospasm. Another group of medications not primarily targeting the cholinergic receptors include sedating antihistamines, tricyclic antidepressants, muscle relaxants, some antipsychotics, antiarrhythmics, and antiemetics. Neuropsychologists should be aware of the medications their patients are taking and the potential impact on neuropsychological test results. It is necessary to differentiate between medication side effects and true consequences or neurologic disorder.

Current Knowledge

Anticholinergic medications are used in treating a variety of medical conditions. Anticholinergic drugs are used in treating a variety of conditions including Parkinson's disease and other Parkinsonian-like disorders, gastrointestinal disorders such as diverticulitis, respiratory disorders such as asthma, and genitourinary disorders such as prostatitis (Tables 1 and 2).

Side Effects

Anticholinergic side effects can be caused by a wide range of medications. Anticholinergic

Anticholinergic, Table 1 Anticholinergic medications clinically used for the antimuscarinic effects

Medications for neurogenic bladder including urge incontinence, for overactive bladder	Oxybutynin (Ditropan), tolterodine (Detrol), trospium (Sanctura), solifenacin (VESIcare), darifenacin (Enablex)
Anticholinergic antiparkinson's medication	Benztropine (Cogentin), trihexyphenidyl (Artane)
Antivertigo medication	Meclizine (Antivert), scopolamine (Transderm Scop)
Gastrointestinal antispasmodics medications	Diphenoxylate/atropine (Lomotil), belladonna (Donnatal)
Medications for bronchospasm	Tiotropium (Spiriva), ipratropium (Atrovent)

Anticholinergic, Table 2 Anticholinergic medications not primarily targeting the cholinergic receptors

Sedating antihistamines	Diphenhydramine (Benadryl), hydroxyzine (Vistaril), cyproheptadine (Periactin)
Tricyclic antidepressants	Amoxapine (Asendin), amitriptyline (Elavil), desipramine (Norpramin), imipramine (Tofranil), nortriptyline (Pamelor)
Certain antipsychotics	Clozapine (Clozaril), olanzapine (Zyprexa), risperidone (Risperdal)
Muscle relaxants	Dantrolene (Dantrium), cyclobenzaprine (Flexeril)

medications have peripheral and central side effects including dry mouth, blurred vision, urinary retention or difficulty initiating voiding, constipation or bowel obstruction, decreased sweating, increased heart rate, ataxia, increased body temperature, agitation, confusion, delirium, memory impairment, decreased attention, dizziness, and drowsiness.

Certain populations are at greater risk for adverse events related to anticholinergic medications. They include older adults who already experience a decrease in acetylcholine production, men with benign prostatic hypertrophy, patients with glaucoma, and individuals with dementia who are already taking cholinesterase inhibitors.

The elderly and patients with brain injury are often prescribed medications with anticholinergic

properties to address medical issues for bladder management, increased muscle tone, and behavior (atypical antipsychotics). There may be a cumulative effect of taking multiple medications which act on the cholinergic system. Anticholinergic side effects in older adults include an increase in delirium, diminished ADLs, and decrease in cognition (Fick et al. 2003; Han et al. 2001).

Cross-References

▶ Acetylcholine
▶ Dopamine
▶ Neurotransmitters

References and Readings

Fick, D. M., Cooper, J. W., Wade, W. E., Waller, J. L., Maclean, J. R., & Beers, M. H. (2003). Updating the beers criteria for potentially inappropriate medication use in older adults: Results of a US consensus panel of experts. *Archives of Internal Medicine, 163*(22), 2716–2724.

Han, L., McCusker, J., Cole, M., Abrahamowicz, M., Primeau, F., & Élie, M. (2001). Use of medications with anticholinergic effect predicts clinical severity of delirium symptoms in older medical inpatients. *Archives of Internal Medicine, 161*(8), 1099–1105.

Lieberman, J. A. (2004). Managing anticholinergic side effects. *Journal of Clinical Psychiatry, 6*(Suppl. 2), 20–23.

Anticholinesterase Inhibitors

JoAnn Tschanz[1,2] and Elizabeth K. Vernon[1]
[1]Department of Psychology, Utah State University, Logan, UT, USA
[2]Center for Epidemiologic Studies, Utah State University, Logan, UT, USA

Synonyms

Acetylcholinesterase inhibitors; ACHE inhibitors; AchEIs; CHEIs; Cholinesterase inhibitors

Definition

A class of substances that target the cholinergic neurotransmitter system and are often used in the treatment of memory disorders such as Alzheimer's disease (AD). Nonclinical uses include agricultural applications such as pesticides and military applications such as the development of neurotoxins. Acetylcholine is normally released by the presynaptic neuron and activates receptors on the postsynaptic cell. Acetylcholinesterase is the primary enzyme that breaks down acetylcholine in the synaptic cleft. Agents such as cholinesterase inhibitors block the activity of this enzyme, allowing the neurotransmitter substance to remain in the synaptic cleft longer to stimulate postsynaptic receptors (see Cholinesterase Inhibitors).

Current Knowledge

Clinical Indications

Cholinesterase inhibitors (CHEI) are often used in the treatment of memory and other cognitive disorders. In AD, degeneration of brain cholinergic neurons has been associated with progressive cognitive deterioration. Since cholinesterase inhibitors do not reverse or stop the progressive degeneration of cholinergic neurons, their effectiveness is greatest early in the course of AD while existing neurons are able to continue to produce and release acetylcholine (Orgogozo 2003). The newest addition to the CHEI class, Namzaric is a combination of donepezil and memantine. CHEIs are moderately effective on improvement of cognitive processes, functional abilities, and possibly neuropsychiatric symptoms. Other compounds such as memantine (which acts on the glutamatergic system) have been approved for use in moderate to severe dementia. These drugs do not stop the progression of AD or stop the degeneration of cholinergic neurons, but can temporarily reduce the degree of cognitive impairment.

Formulation and Side Effects

Several cholinesterase inhibitors are available. The primary mode of intake is oral, although a cutaneous route through a dermal patch has been developed. Common side effects of cholinesterase inhibitors include nausea, vomiting, diarrhea, and anorexia. Less common are insomnia and cardiovascular symptoms such as bradycardia. Drug tolerability may be enhanced by varying dosing and titration rates to achieve therapeutic levels (Orgogozo 2003).

Other Applications

In addition to its distribution in the brain, acetylcholine is also the neurotransmitter substance at the neuromuscular junction and sympathetic and parasympathetic nervous systems. Thus, acetylcholine plays an important role in the body's motor and autonomic functions. Anticholinesterase inhibitors developed for agricultural or military applications affect these systems by causing an accumulation of acetylcholine at synapses, leading to excessive excitation of muscles, cessation of muscle contraction (due to overexcitation), and autonomic symptoms such as sweating and bronchial constriction and congestion. Therefore, anticholinesterase inhibitors may also be potent neurotoxins for use as insecticides or in warfare (Feldman et al. 1997; Iversen et al. 2008).

See Also

▶ Acetylcholine
▶ Alzheimer's Disease
▶ Cholinesterase Inhibitors

References and Readings

Feldman, R. S., Meyer, J. S., & Quenzer, L. F. (1997). Acetylcholine. In *Principles of Neuropsychopharmacology* (pp. 246–249). Sunderland: Sinauer Associates, Inc.

Iversen, L. L., Iversen, S. D., Bloom, F. E., & Roth, R. H. (2008). Acetylcholine. In *Introduction to Neuropsychopharmacology* (pp. 128–149). New York: Oxford University Press.

Orgogozo, J.-M. (2003). Treatment of Alzheimer's disease with cholinesterase inhibitors. An update on currently used drugs. In K. Iqbal & B. Winblad (Eds.), *Alzheimer's disease and related disorders: Research advances* (pp. 663–675). Bucharest: Ana Asian Intl. Acad. of Aging.

Anticoagulation

Elliot J. Roth
Department of Physical Medicine and Rehabilitation, Northwestern University, Feinberg School of Medicine, Chicago, IL, USA

Synonyms

Antithrombotic therapy

Definition

Anticoagulation refers to the prevention of blood from clotting. An anticoagulant is a chemical that prevents coagulation. The body contains a number of naturally occurring physiological anticoagulants, but other anticoagulants are used as pharmacological agents to prevent and treat thrombotic disorders such as coronary artery disease causing ischemic heart disease, cerebrovascular disease causing stroke, peripheral arterial disease causing limb ischemia, and venous thromboembolic disease.

Commonly used anticoagulation medications include warfarin (Coumadin®), heparin and low molecular weight heparin compounds such as enoxaparin (Lovenox®), tinzaparin (Innohep®), and dalteparin (Fragmin®). New oral anticoagulants, which use a different mechanism of action, have recently gained widespread use. These medications include apixaban (Eliquis®), dabigatran (Pradaxa®), edoxaban (Savaysa®), and rivaroxaban (Xarelto®).

Current Knowledge

Dosages of warfarin can be adjusted using blood tests that measure the levels of certain clotting functions which can be used to monitor the effectiveness of the medication regimen. Optimum ranges for the results of these tests are available for specific conditions and clinical situations. The newer anticoagulants offer the advantages of fixed dosing, minimal food and drug interactions, and lack of requirement for blood test monitoring.

Predictably, adverse effects of all anticoagulants are largely hemorrhagic in nature. Prolonged bleeding from simple superficial lacerations, and more serious internal hemorrhage into gastrointestinal system, brain, or muscles in the pelvis or leg, occurs with greater frequency depending on the type and level of anticoagulation. Rarely, a paradoxical thrombotic disorder might occur as a *result* of using one of these medications. On balance, the benefits of using certain anticoagulants in selected situations outweigh the risks of the medications but primarily in controlled circumstances when clinical monitoring is feasible and when the patient does not have risk of falls, injuries, or other contraindications.

See Also

► Atherosclerosis
► Central Venous Thrombosis
► Cerebral Embolism
► Novel Oral Anticoagulants
► Thrombosis
► Venous Thrombosis
► Warfarin (Coumadin)

References

Dentali, F., Douketis, J. D., Gianni, M., Lim, W., & Crowther, M. A. (2007). Meta-analysis: Anticoagulant prophylaxis to prevent symptomatic venous thromboembolism in hospitalized medical patients. *Annals of Internal Medicine, 146,* 278–288.

Kearon, C., Akl, E. A., Ornelas, J., Blaivas, A., Jimenez, D., et al. (2016). Antithrombotic therapy for VTE disease: CHEST guideline and expert panel report. *Chest, 149,* 315–352.

van der Hulle, T., Kooiman, J., den Exter, P. L., Dekkers, O. M., Klok, F. A., & Huisman, M. V. (2014).

Effectiveness and safety of novel oral anticoagulants as compared with vitamin K antagonists in the treatment of acute symptomatic venous thromboembolism: A systematic review and meta-analysis. *Journal of Thrombosis and Haemostasis, 12,* 320–328.

Anticonvulsants

Mary Pat Murphy
MSN, CRRN, Paoli, PA, USA

Synonyms

Antiepileptic drugs (AED)

Definition

A group of medications used in the management of epilepsy.

Current Knowledge

The selection of an AED depends on the type of seizure, age of patient, and gender. According to the literature, monotherapy is the goal for the treatment of epilepsy, choosing medications targeting seizure control with fewest side effects. Monotherapy also makes it easier to monitor side effects. Usually, if one drug fails, another medication is trialed. If the initial AED fails, the physician typically will wean this medication and try another first-line drug. If monotherapy fails, polytherapy may be tried. The physician will maximize the first-line dose and then add a second-line medication. General monitoring for AEDs includes the frequency and severity of seizures, adverse events and side effects, and monitoring of plasma. The chart below identifies FDA indications for commonly used AEDs (Table 1).

Mechanism of Action for AEDs

Phenytoin, carbamazepine, lamotrigine, gabapentin, topiramate, and valproate block sodium channel and impede generation of high-frequency action potentials. Some of the drugs may also reduce high-threshold calcium currents, resulting in a decrease in excitatory transmitter release. In therapeutic ranges, barbiturates and diazepam derivatives enhance GABA responses. Topiramate may enhance GABAergic inhibition. Gabapentin may promote nonsynaptic GABA release. Phenobarbital is a long-acting barbiturate with sedative, hypnotic, and anticonvulsant properties. It acts on the GABA receptors, increasing synaptic inhibition. This has the effect of elevating the seizure threshold and reducing the spread of seizure activity in the brain. Phenobarbital may also inhibit calcium channels.

Anticonvulsants, Table 1 Commonly used AED

	Partial seizures	Tonic-clonic	Absence
First-line drugs	Carbamazepine	Valproate	Ethosuximide
	Phenytoin	Phenytoin	Valproate
	Valproate	Carbamazepine	
	Topiramate	Topiramate	
Second-line drugs (alternative therapy)	Primidone	Lamotrigine	
	Gabapentin	Gabapentin	
	Phenobarbital	Primidone	Clonazepam
	Primidone	Phenobarbital	Primidone
	Valproate	Topiramate	
	Felbamate (use when other alternative medications have failed)	Felbamate (use when other alternative medications have failed)	

First-Line Medications

Valproate (Depakote)

Indication
Labeled indications include control of epilepsy (seizure disorders). As an AED, it can be used as monotherapy and adjunctive treatment of tonic-clonic, partial complex seizures, and simple and complex absence seizures. It can be used as an adjunctive treatment in patients who have multiple types of seizures.

Contraindications
The medication should be prescribed cautiously for individuals with liver disease and urea cycle disorders and for pregnant women.

Adverse Events/Side Effects
Weight gain, thrombocytopenia, and elevated liver enzymes may be dose related. When initially starting the medication, patients may complain of nausea and diarrhea. Hyperammonemia has been reported and may be present despite normal liver function testing. In the elderly, there is a possible increase in somnolence.

Drug Interactions
Medications that **may increase valproate levels** include felbamate, rifampin, and chlorpromazine; medications that valproate may affect include carbamazepine, amitriptyline, nortriptyline, clonazepam, ethosuximide, lamotrigine, phenobarbital, phenytoin, tolbutamide, and lorazepam.

Phenytoin (Dilantin)

Indication
Phenytoin is the oldest and one of the most effective medications in the treatment of a wide range of seizure types. The labeled use is for tonic-clonic and partial complex seizures. It is often used as a first-line drug choice for monotherapy. The usual dose is 300 to 400 mg/day. An extended-release capsule allows for one-time-a-day dosing. The therapeutic range is 10–20.

Adverse Events/Side Effects
Phenytoin can be administered intravenously. As a result, **specific adverse events/side effects** can include hypotension, bradycardia, dysrhythmias, and cardiac changes, as well as venous irritation and thrombophlebitis.

Other **adverse events/side effects** include gingival hyperplasia, hirsutism, rash, hepatitis, megaloblastic anemia, thrombocytopenia, Stevens-Johnson syndrome, systemic lupus erythematosus, and folic acid deficiency.

Drug Interactions
Drug interactions are many and include (but are not limited to) chloramphenicol, dexamethasone, doxycycline, furosemide, haloperidol, meperidine, methadone, oral contraceptives, theophylline, and warfarin. Non-AEDs that affect phenytoin levels include alcohol, antacids, folic acid, rifampin, tube feedings, alcohol, cimetidine, fluoxetine, imipramine, INH, omeprazole, propoxyphene, sulfonamides, and trazadone.

Carbamazepine (Tegretol)

Indication
Carbamazepine is indicated as a first-line drug for use as an anticonvulsant for partial seizures, generalized tonic-clonic, and mixed seizures, but not absence seizures. It is generally nonsedating within therapeutic range. It is also indicated in the treatment of trigeminal neuralgia.

Adverse Events/Side Effects
Adverse events associated with carbamazepine include aplastic anemia and agranulocytosis. Pretreatment hematology testing should be completed to obtain a baseline. The patient should be monitored and treatment should be discontinued with hematology changes. Stevens-Johnson syndrome (an exfoliating dermatitis) has been reported. Carbamazepine has mild anticholinergic properties, so patients with intraocular eye pressure should be monitored. Carbamazepine should not be used in pregnant women. Patients should be cautioned against drinking alcohol.

In the beginning of treatment, patients report side effects including dizziness, drowsiness, nausea, and vomiting.

Medications that Affect Carbamazepine Plasma Levels

Drugs that increase plasma levels include cimetidine, danazol, macrolides, erythromycin, troleandomycin, fluoxetine, nefazodone, loratadine, terfenadine, INH, propoxyphene, verapamil, grapefruit juice, protease inhibitors, and valproate. Medications that **decrease** carbamazepine plasma levels include cisplatin, felbamate, rifampin, phenobarbital, phenytoin, primidone, methsuximide, and theophylline.

Topamax (Topiramate)

Topiramate is considered effective as a monotherapy for individuals with partial complex or generalized tonic-clonic seizures. It is also effective as an adjunctive treatment for partial complex and generalized tonic-clonic seizures.

Adverse Events/Side Effects

Metabolic acidosis is an **adverse event** associated with topiramate. Conditions that predispose individuals include renal disease, severe respiratory disorders, status epilepticus, and diarrhea. Measurement of baseline and periodic sodium bicarbonate is recommended. Other side effects/adverse events include kidney stones, paresthesia of the extremities, acute myopia and glaucoma, decreased sweating and hyperthermia, cognitive-related dysfunction, psychiatric/behavioral disturbances, and somnolence or fatigue.

Drug Interactions

Concomitant administration of topiramate and valproate has been associated with hyperammonemia. Topiramate concentrations affect phenytoin and valproate. Topiramate concentrations are affected by phenytoin, carbamazepine, valproate, and lamotrigine.

Ethosuximide (Zarontin) has been approved for absence (petit mal) seizures. Adverse events/side effects include blood dyscrasias; decreased cognition including drowsiness, dizziness, irritability, hyperactivity, and fatigue; and ataxia. There have been reports of increased tonic-clonic seizures.

Second-Line Medications

Gabapentin (Neurontin)

Gabapentin is effective as an adjunctive therapy in the treatment of partial seizures with and without generalization.

Adverse Events/Side Effects

Adverse events/side effects include dizziness, ataxia, weight gain, GI upset, somnolence, and other symptoms of CNS depression.

Drug Interactions

Antacids decrease their bioavailability.

Lamotrigine (Lamictal)

Lamotrigine is effective as monotherapy for individuals with partial complex seizures; it is also considered effective as an adjunctive therapy for partial complex seizures and generalized tonic-clonic seizures. It is thought to inhibit voltage-sensitive sodium channel mechanisms. It is well tolerated and does not seem to have cognitive altering side effects. A therapeutic plasma concentration has not been established for lamotrigine.

Side Effects/Adverse Events

Side effects/adverse events include rash, fatigue, dizziness, diplopia, and ataxia. Angioedema, nystagmus, and hematuria also may occur.

Drug Interactions

Medications that **decrease** lamotrigine's effectiveness include carbamazepine, valproate, phenobarbital, primidone, and acetaminophen.

Felbamate (Felbatol) has been approved for adjunctive therapy or monotherapy for individuals with partial complex or tonic-clonic seizures. This medication is recommended when other therapies have been tried and have failed.

Adverse Events/Side Effects

This medication potentially causes aplastic anemia or hepatotoxicity and should be used with extreme care by a knowledgeable physician when other therapies have been tried. Other side effects/adverse events include anorexia, vomiting, and insomnia.

Drug Interactions

Felbatol affects phenytoin, valproate, and carbamazepine concentrations.

Barbiturates (Second Line)

Phenobarbital

Indication

Labeled indications include control of epilepsy (seizures disorders) and as a sedative/hypnotic medication for short-term treatment of insomnia. As an AED, it can be used as monotherapy in the treatment of generalized (tonic-clonic), simple, or partial complex seizures, for myoclonic epilepsy, and for neonatal and febrile seizures in children. It has also been prescribed for eclamptic seizures during pregnancy.

Contraindications

The medication should be prescribed cautiously for individuals with liver disease, CHF, and hypovolemic shock and for pregnant women. The medication does cause both physical and psychological drug dependence; for this reason, it is not a first-line medication of choice for individuals with drug dependence. If prescribed for sleep, it should not be used longer than 2 weeks and prescribed for the elderly because of its long half-life. Patients should avoid alcohol and other CNS depressants while taking phenobarbital. Other contraindications include preexisting CNS depression, severe uncontrolled pain (may mask symptoms), porphyria, and severe respiratory disease with obstruction or dyspnea. Abrupt discontinuation may cause seizures.

Adverse Events/Side Effects

Adverse effects include sedation, ataxia, and cognitive impairment and may cause a paradoxical effect including hyperactivity and problems with sleep, megaloblastic anemia (responds to folic acid) and rash, exfoliative dermatitis, and Stevens-Johnson syndrome.

Non-AEDs Affected by Phenobarbital

Phenobarbital may interfere with the effectiveness of *acetaminophen* and increase liver damage. The effectiveness of beta-blockers except atenolol, levobunolol, metipranolol, and nadolol, oral contraceptives, chloramphenicol, chlorpromazine, cimetidine, corticosteroids, cyclosporine, desipramine, doxycycline, folic acid, griseofulvin, haloperidol, meperidine, methadone, nortriptyline, quinidine, theophylline, and warfarin may be compromised when taking phenobarbital.

Non-AEDs Affecting Phenobarbital Levels

Chloramphenicol, propoxyphene, and quinine may increase phenobarbital levels. Chlorpromazine, folic acid, and prochlorperazine may decrease phenobarbital levels. There may be increased toxicity with benzodiazepines, CNS depressants, and methylphenidate.

Primidone (Mysoline) is related in structure to barbiturates. It is used in the management of tonic-clonic, partial complex, and focal seizures. The adverse events/side effects and drug interactions are similar to phenobarbital.

Benzodiazepines

This class of medication is not typically used as first-line medications. As a class, they can produce CNS depression and behavioral changes. Other adverse reactions include tachycardia, chest pain, headache, constipation, nausea, and ataxia.

Medications include the following:

Clonazepam (Klonopin) is effective as an adjunctive medication for individuals with absence, tonic-clonic, and myoclonic seizures. Diazepam (Valium) and Lorazepam (Ativan) can be used to treat status epilepticus.

Cross-References

▶ Epilepsy
▶ GABA
▶ Seizure

References and Readings

Lanctôt, K., Herrmann, N., Mazzotta, P., Khan, L., & Ingber, N. (2004). GABAergic function in Alzheimer's disease: Evidence for dysfunction and potential as a therapeutic target for the treatment of behavioural and psychological symptoms of Dementia. *Canadian Journal of Psychiatry, 49*(7), 439–453.

MacQueen, G., & Young, T. (2003). Cognitive effects of atypical antipsychotics: focus on bipolar spectrum disorders. *Bipolar Disorders, 5*, 53–61.

Yasseen, B., Colantonio, A., & Ratcliff, G. (2008). Prescription medication use in persons many years following traumatic brain injury. *Brain Injury, 22*(10), 752–757.

Antidepressant Discontinuation Syndrome

Cynthia Rolston
Department of PM&R, Virginia Commonwealth University-Medical College of Virginia, Richmond, VA, USA

Synonyms

Antidepressant discontinuation symptoms; Antidepressant withdrawal syndrome (not preferred)

Definition

Antidepressant discontinuation syndrome (ADS) is cluster of physical and psychological symptoms that may arise after sudden discontinuation (either end of use or change in formulation) of antidepressant medication of any class, including tricyclic antidepressants (TCAs), monoamine oxidase inhibitors (MAOIs), serotonin-specific reuptake inhibitors (SSRIs), SNRIs (serotonin norepinephrine reuptake inhibitors), and others (including noradrenergic and specific serotonergic antidepressant).

Categorization

ADS is classified under medication-induced movement disorders in the *Diagnostic and Statistical Manual of Mental Disorders* (5th ed.; DSM-5; American Psychiatric Association 2013).

Current Knowledge

Clinical Presentation and Diagnosis

Consensus does not yet exist on diagnostic criteria for ADS. Symptoms begin abruptly (within days), continue only briefly even if untreated (24 h–3 days), and rapidly resolve (within 48 h) when antidepressant medication is reintroduced. Common symptoms include dizziness, headache, nausea, gastrointestinal upset, lethargy, anxiety, agitation, dysphoria, irritability, poor concentration, and sleep problems. Ataxia, electrical shock-like sensations, extrapyramidal symptoms, and overt manic or hypomanic symptoms have also been reported. ADS is differentiated from depression resurgence by certain unique symptoms (e.g., "electric shock" sensations, nausea, nightmares) and by occurrence when treatment is ongoing, but when the composition of treating agent is changed (i.e., generic or different brand). Risk of ADS is minimal if treatment has lasted less than 6 weeks (Harvey and Slabbert 2014) and there is no evidence to suggest that a longer course of antidepressant treatment is associated with increased risk of ADS (Baldwin et al. 2007).

Little is known how ASD events impact the long-term management of depression. Understanding ADS is essential, given widespread antidepressant use paired with high rates of nonadherence. Implications of misdiagnosis may include physical discomfort, psychosocial problems, inappropriate interventions, and reluctance to use psychotropic medications.

Incidence

The likelihood of ADS is impacted by an agent's half-life: the shorter half-life, the greater the risk of ADS (Warner et al. 2006). The highest incidence of ASD is reported for TCA clomipramine (21.5–100%; Leujoyeux and Ades 1997), and the lowest for fluoxetine (almost 0%; Wilson and Lader 2015). Further research is needed on how patient factors such as age and sex impact the course of ASD.

Underlying Mechanism

The mechanisms of ASD are unclear, but symptoms clusters covary with specific antidepressant classes. TCAs, impacting serotonergic and cholinergic pathways, may result in gait or balance problems, or tremors (Shelton 2006). MAOIs affect the alpha2-adrenergic and dopaminergic receptors, causing risk for agitation and psychosis (Warner et al. 2006). A novel agent called agomelatine does not seem to cause ADS; its unique profile may allow for further clarification of the mechanism underlying ADS (Harvey and Slabbert 2014).

Treatment Recommendations

Expert guidelines advise psychoeducation regarding ADS prior to prescribing and discontinuing antidepressant medication, with close monitoring during a gradual taper (Cleare et al. 2015; Schatzberg et al. 1997). At a minimum, a 4-week taper is suggested, with more rapid tapering for lower doses and longer half-life agents like fluoxetine. Sparse research exists on the role psychotherapy may play, but a small study suggests that cognitive-behavioral therapy may provide patients with useful support and skills through the discontinuation process (Cromarty et al. 2011).

See Also

▶ Antidepressants
▶ Depressive Disorder
▶ Major Depression
▶ Minor Depressive Disorder

References and Readings

American Psychiatric Association. (2013). *Diagnostic and statistical manual of mental disorders* (5th ed.). Arlington: American Psychiatric Association Publishing.

Baldwin, D. S., Montgomery, S. A., Nil, R., & Lader, M. (2007). Discontinuation symptoms in depression and anxiety disorders. *International Journal of Neuropharmacology, 10*(1), 73–84.

Cleare, A., Pariante, C. M., Young, A. H., Anderson, I. M., Christmas, D., Cowen, P. J., et al. (2015). Evidence-based guidelines for treating depressive disorders with antidepressants: A revision of the 2008 British Association for Psychopharmacology guidelines. *Journal of Psychopharmcaology, 29*(5), 459–525.

Cromarty, P., Jonsson, J., Moorhead, S., & Freeston, M. H. (2011). Cognitive behaviour therapy for withdrawal from antidepressant medication: A single case series. *Behavioral and Cognitive Psychotherapy, 39*(1), 77–97.

Harvey, B. H., & Slabbert, F. N. (2014). New insights on the antidepressant discontinuation syndrome. *Human Psychopharmacology, 29*(6), 503–516.

Lejoyeux, M., & Ades, J. (1997). Antidepressant discontinuation: A review of the literature. *Journal of Clinical Psychiatry, 58*(Suppl. 7), 11–15.

Schatzberg, A. F., Haddad, P., Kaplan, E. M., Lejoyeux, M., Rosenbaum, J. F., Young, A. H., & Zajecka, J. (1997). Serotonin reuptake inhibitor discontinuation syndrome: A hypothetical definition. Discontinuation consensus panel. *Journal of Clinical Psychiatry, 58*(Suppl. 7), 5–10.

Shelton, R. C. (2006). The nature of the discontinuation syndrome associated with antidepressant drugs. *The Journal of Clinical Psychiatry, 67*(Suppl. 4), 3–7.

Warner, C. H., Bobo, W., Warner, C., Reid, S., & Rachal, J. (2006). Antidepressant discontinuation syndrome. *American Family Physician, 74*(3), 449–456.

Wilson, E., & Lader, M. (2015). A review of the management of antidepressant discontinuation symptoms. *Therapeutic Advances in Psychopharmacology, 5*(6), 357–368.

Antidepressants

Joshua M. Matyi[1] and JoAnn Tschanz[1,2]
[1]Department of Psychology, Utah State University, Logan, UT, USA
[2]Center for Epidemiologic Studies, Utah State University, Logan, UT, USA

Definition

Antidepressants are a class of medications that are used primarily in the treatment of clinically severe mood and anxiety disorders. The majority of effective antidepressants currently in use enhance neurotransmission of serotonin and/or norepinephrine. Generally, this is achieved by blocking the reuptake of the neurotransmitter substance(s), inhibiting the enzymes responsible for its metabolism, or directly stimulating the postsynaptic receptors (Iversen et al. 2009). Several antidepressants are also used in treating generalized anxiety disorder, panic disorder, and obsessive-compulsive disorder (Bourin and Lambert 2002). Other conditions for which antidepressants have demonstrated efficacy include eating disorders (Powers and Bruty 2009), neuropathic pain (O'Connor and Dworkin 2009), stress incontinence, nocturnal enuresis, ejaculatory disorders (Michel et al. 2006), migraine headaches, fibromyalgia (Stone et al. 2003), attention deficit hyperactivity disorder (Chung et al. 2002), smoking cessation, insomnia, and possibly pathological gambling (Grant and Grosz 2004).

There are several classes of antidepressant medications. Tricyclic antidepressants (TCAs) block the reuptake of monoaminergic neurotransmitters in the synaptic cleft, and monoamine oxidase inhibitors (MAOIs) inhibit their metabolism in the presynaptic cell. Other compounds are more selective in blocking the reuptake of specific neurotransmitters [selective serotonin reuptake inhibitors (SSRIs) and noradrenergic reuptake inhibitors (NRIs)]. Compounds with dual serotonergic and noradrenergic actions that have better tolerability have also been developed (Iversen et al. 2009).

Regardless of the type of antidepressant, the compounds are similar in their effectiveness and the time course of their effects. Generally, the lag between the initiation of antidepressant treatment and alleviation of symptoms generally takes two to six weeks for the maximal response. The delay in treatment response suggests that the therapeutic effects may result from "downstream" events that reflect the brain's adaptation to treatment (Iversen et al. 2009). Alternative treatments with a shorter treatment lag are under active investigation (see "Future Directions").

Antidepressant medications differ in their profile of side effects. First-generation MAOIs, which inhibit the activity of both MAO-A and MAO-B, were known for potentially serious side effects if patients also consumed foods containing tyramine (fermented products such as wine or cheese). Potential effects included headache, hypertension, cerebral hemorrhage, and death. Newer generation MAOIs that act more selectively on MAO-A do not require the dietary restriction from tyramine-containing foods. Side effects associated with TCAs include dry mouth, urinary retention, sedation, orthostatic hypotension, constipation, blurred vision, and weight gain. Additionally, a concern regarding TCAs is the narrow therapeutic index, thus raising the risk of death with overdose due to Q-T prolongation. By contrast, SSRIs do not carry the same health concerns as those of the TCAs or MAOIs. Common side effects of SSRIs include nausea, headache, anxiety, sexual dysfunction, and, the topic of much controversy, a possible increase in suicidal ideation and behavior (see "Current Knowledge"). Side effects reported with the mixed SSRI-NRI compound venlafaxine include headache, dry mouth, sedation, hypertension, and constipation (Iversen et al. 2009).

Current Knowledge

Approximately 60–70% of persons treated with antidepressants show a positive response. The lack of response in 30–40% of depressed individuals (at least to SSRIs) may, in part, reflect the effects of genes. Variations in the serotonin transporter gene (often referred to as 5-HTTLPR) modify the response of depressed persons to SSRIs. Compared to those with a long (L) allele of this gene, persons with a short allele exhibit poorer response to SSRI treatment. Variations in 5-HTTLPR may also influence the experience of side effects (Horstmann and Binder 2009).

The response rate to placebo in clinical trials of antidepressants is relatively high, ranging from 30% to 50%. The placebo response is greater among individuals with mild depressive symptoms, and recent meta-analyses of clinical trials of second-generation antidepressants indicate significant treatment effects only among those with severe symptoms (Kirsch et al. 2008; Fournier et al. 2010).

Significant concerns of an increased risk of suicidal ideation and behavior (suicidality) have arisen over the use of new-generation antidepressants. In 2006, the US Food and Drug Administration (FDA) issued a standing "black box" advisory on SSRIs and other antidepressants regarding an increased risk for suicidality in the first few months of treatment among pediatric through young adult patients (FDA 2007). However, the research surrounding the FDA advisory has received substantial criticism (Isacsson and Rich 2014). The observed increase in suicidal behavior is in contrast to epidemiological data that indicate reduced rates of *completed* suicides. Additionally, subsequent studies have shown no association between SSRI treatment and suicide risk in youths (Gibbons et al. 2012; Strawn et al. 2015). Some have hypothesized that the higher risk of suicidality with antidepressant treatment likely occurs in a subset of high-risk patients with agitated major depression or unrecognized bipolar disorder (Rihmer and Akiskal 2006).

Future Directions

More research is needed to examine the safety of antidepressant treatment in pediatric and young adult populations. Thorough characterization of patients may help clarify whether certain subgroups are more vulnerable to develop suicidal behaviors while receiving antidepressants. Additionally, antidepressants are not effective for 30–40% of depressed patients. Current work is exploring alternative treatments, for example, testing antagonists of NMDA glutamate receptors for an antidepressant effect (Dale et al. 2015). Initial studies with ketamine, an NMDA antagonist, show a significant antidepressant effect within two hours (Skolnick et al. 2009). In addition to a more rapid treatment effect, it is hoped that glutamate-based therapies will alleviate depressive symptoms among those unresponsive to current treatments. Other neurobiological systems have also been implicated in antidepressant studies, such as GABAergic, cholinergic, opioid,

and the hypothalamic-pituitary axis (HPA) (Dale et al. 2015). Furthermore, there is increasing evidence regarding the relationship between depression and processes such as neuronal plasticity and neuroinflammation; future research is directed toward expanding potential therapeutic targets.

References and Readings

Bourin, M., & Lambert, O. (2002). Pharmacotherapy of anxious disorders. *Human Psychopharmacol clin Exp, 17*, 383–400.

Chung, B., Suzuki, A. R., & McGough, J. J. (2002). New drugs for treatment of attention-deficit/hyperactivity disorder. *Expert Opinion Emerging Drugs, 7*, 269–276.

Dale, E., Bang-Andersen, B., & Sánchez, C. (2015). Emerging mechanisms and treatments for depression beyond SSRIs and SNRIs. *Biochemical pharmacology, 95*(2), 81–97.

Fournier, J. C., DeRubeis, R. J., Hollon, S. D., Dimidjian, S., Amsterdam, J. D., Shelton, R. C., & Fawcett, J. (2010). Antidepressant drug effects and depression severity: A patient-level meta-analysis. *JAMA, 303*, 47–53.

Gibbons, R. D., Brown, C. H., Hur, K., Davis, J. M., & Mann, J. J. (2012). Suicidal thoughts and behavior with antidepressant treatment: Reanalysis of the randomized placebo-controlled studies of fluoxetine and venlafaxine. *Archives of General Psychiatry, 69*(6), 580–587.

Grant, J. E., & Grosz, R. (2004). Pharmacotherapy outcome in older pathological gamblers: A preliminary investigation. *Journal of Geriatric Psychiatry and Neurology, 17*, 9–12.

Horstmann, S., & Binder, E. B. (2009). Pharmacogenomics of antidepressant drugs. *Pharmacology and Therapeutics, 124*, 57–73.

Isacsson, G., & Rich, C. L. (2014). Antidepressant drugs and the risk of suicide in children and adolescents. *Pediatric Drugs, 16*(2), 115–122.

Iversen, L. L., Iversen, S. D., Bloom, F. E., & Roth, R. H. (2009). *Antidepressants and anxiolytics. Introduction to neuropsychopharmacology* (pp. 306–335). New York: Oxford University Press.

Kirsch, I., Deacon, B. J., Huedo-Medina, T. B., Scoboria, A., Moore, T. J., & Johnson, B. T. (2008). Initial severity and antidepressant benefits: A meta-analysis of data submitted to the food and drug administration. *PlOS Medicine, 5*, e45.

Michel, M. C., Ruhe, H. G., de Groot, A. A., Castro, R., & Oelke, M. (2006). Tolerability of amine uptake inhibitors in urologic diseases. *Current Drug Safety, 1*, 73–85.

O'Connor, A. B., & Dworkin, R. H. (2009). Treatment of neuropathic pain: An overview of recent guidelines. *Am Journal of Medicine, 122*, S22–S32.

Powers, P. S., & Bruty, H. (2009). Pharmacotherapy for eating disorders and obesity. *Child Adolescent Psychiatric Clinics of North America, 18*, 175–187.

Rihmer, Z., & Akiskal, H. (2006). Do antidepressants t(h)reat(en) depressives? Toward a clinical judicious formulation of the antidepressant-suicidality FDA advisory in light of declining national suicide statistics from many countries. *Journal of Affective Disorders, 94*, 3–13.

Skolnick, P., Popik, P., & Trullas, R. (2009). Glutamate-based antidepressants: 20 years on. *Trends in Pharmacological Sciences, 30*, 563–569.

Stone, K. J., Viera, A. J., & Parman, C. L. (2003). Off-label applications for SSRIs. *American Family Physician, 68*, 498–504.

Strawn, J. R., Welge, J. A., Wehry, A. M., Keeshin, B., & Rynn, M. A. (2015). Efficacy and tolerability of antidepressants in pediatric anxiety disorders: A systematic review and meta-analysis. *Depression and Anxiety, 32*(3), 149–157.

U.S. Food and Drug Administration. (2007). FDA proposes new warnings about suicidal thinking, behaviour in young adults who take antidepressant medications. Retrieved from http://www.fda.gov/NewsEvents/Newsroom/PressAnnouncements/2007/ucm108905.htm

Antihistamines

Maya Balamane[1] and
Stephanie A. Kolakowsky-Hayner[2]
[1]Mount Sinai Brain Injury Research Center, San Francisco, CA, USA
[2]Department of Rehabilitation Medicine, Icahn School of Medicine at Mount Sinai, New York, NY, USA

Synonyms

Histamine antagonist; Inverse histamine agonists

Definition

Antihistamines have multiple clinical indications including allergic conditions (rhinitis, dermatoses, atopic dermatitis, contact dermatitis, allergic conjunctivitis, hypersensitivity reactions to drugs, mild transfusion reactions, and urticaria), chronic idiopathic urticaria, motion sickness, vertigo, and insomnia. Antihistamines are most commonly used to treat allergies; H_1 receptor inverse agonists typically reduce swelling and vasodilation within the nasal area. H_1 receptor antagonists include cetirizine, diphenhydramine also known as Benadryl, desloratadine, doxylamine, ebastine, fexofenadine, loratadine, pheniramine, and promethazine. H_2 inverse agonists reduce gastric acid and are used to treat ulcers and reflux. H_2 receptor antagonists include cimetidine, famotidine, lafutidine, nizatidine, ranitidine, and roxatidine. H_3 and H_4 receptor antagonists are experimental in nature and are being investigated for their cognitive enhancing and immunomodulation abilities. H3 receptors reside mostly on neurons, so antagonists to these receptors could treat cognitive impairment, schizophrenia, sleep disorders, epilepsy, and neuropathic pain. H4 receptors reside mostly on hemopoietic cells, so their antagonists might treat inflammatory diseases, pruritus, dermatitis, asthma, and arthritis. Additionally, antihistamines may be used to treat off-label issues such as motion sickness, anxiety, and insomnia. Neuropsychologists must be aware of the potential effects of antihistamines on the physical, emotional, and cognitive functioning of their patients. Side effects of antihistamine use may include dry nose and mouth, drowsiness, dizziness, headache, upset stomach, loss of appetite, irritability, motor slowness, diminished processing speed, and impaired visual skills. Antihistamine effects are exacerbated by the use of alcohol and other substances, which in turn will be of further detriment to neuropsychological testing.

Cross-References

▶ Pharmacodynamics
▶ Pharmacokinetics
▶ Psychopharmacology

References and Readings

Hindmarch, I., & Shamsi, Z. (1999). Antihistamines: Models to assess sedative properties, assessment of sedation, safety and other side-effects. *Clinical & Experimental Allergy, 29*, 133–142.

Matsushita, A., Seike, M., Okawa, H., Kadawaki, Y., & Ohtsu, H. (2012). Advantages of histamine H4 receptor antagonist usage with H1 receptor antagonist for the treatment of murine allergic contact dermatitis. *Experimental Dermatology, 21*(9), 714–7155.

Parsons, M., & Ganellin, C. (2006). Histamine and its receptors. *British Journal of Pharmacology, 147*, S127–S135.

Theunissen, E., Vermeeren, A., van Oers, A., van Maris, I., & Ramaekers, J. (2004). A dose-ranging study of the effects of mequitazine on actual driving, memory and psychomotor performance as compared to dexchlorpheniramine, cetirizine and placebo. *Clinical & Experimental Allergy, 34*(2), 250–258.

Thurmond, R. L. (2015). The histamine H_4 receptor: From orphan to the clinic. *Frontiers in Pharmacology, 6*, 65.

van Ruitenbeek, P., Vermeeren, A., Smulders, F., Sambeth, A., & Riedel, W. (2009). Histamine H_1 receptor blockade predominantly impairs sensory processes in human sensorimotor performance. *British Journal of Pharmacology, 157*(1), 76–85.

Vuurman, E., Rikken, G., Muntjewerff, N., de Halleux, F., & Ramaekers, J. (2004). Effects of desloratadine, diphenhydramine, and placebo on driving performance and psychomotor performance measurements. *European Journal of Clinical Pharmacology, 60*(5), 307–313.

Zlomuzica, A., Ruocco, L., Sadile, A., Huston, J., & Dere, E. (2009). Histamine H_1 receptor knockout mice exhibit impaired spatial memory in the eight-arm radial maze. *British Journal of Pharmacology, 157*(1), 86–91.

Antihypertensives

Mary Pat Murphy
MSN, CRRN, Paoli, PA, USA

Definition

Antihypertensives are pharmacologic agents used to lower blood pressure to normal levels or near normal levels. The initiation and intensity of drug treatment depends on blood pressure level, the individual's risk factors (smoking, dyslipidemia, diabetes mellitus, older than 60, male, postmenopausal women, and family history of cardiovascular disease for women under 65 and men under 55 years of age), and target organ damage (e.g., strokeor TIA, nephropathy, peripheral artery disease, retinopathy) or cardiovascular disease. Cardiovascular risks decrease when the blood pressure is below 139/89. Typical agents for treating hypertension include diuretics, beta-blockers, ACE (angiotensin-converting enzyme) inhibitors, calcium channel blockers, peripheral alpha selective blockers, central alpha2 agonists, direct vasodilators, and adrenergic antagonists.

Current Knowledge

Hypertension is a risk factor for stroke, myocardial infarction, renal failure, congestive heart failure, progressive atherosclerosis, and dementia. Treatment reduces the risks of heart disease as well as cardiovascular morbidity. For stage I hypertension, the blood pressure ranges from 140/90 to 159/99; for stage II and stage III blood pressure, the systolic number is greater than 160 and diastolic is greater than 100.

Monotherapy is preferred initially. The first line of treatment is beta-blockers and diuretics for uncomplicated hypertension individuals who do not have preexisting coronary disease, diabetes, or proteinuria. In patients with diabetes mellitus, renal disease, or CHF, ACE inhibitors and angiotensin receptor antagonists are the appropriate initial therapy. Typically, the patient is started on a low dose of long-acting, once-daily drug, and the dose is titrated until the blood pressure is lowered. If blood pressure is not controlled with the dose of a single drug, a second agent from a different class is recommended. Combination therapy provides more rapid control of hypertension and is recommended for patients with stages II and III hypertension. Triple-drug therapy may be required if the blood pressure control is not achieved. Some patients have resistant hypertension. A fourth line of medications may be required.

Classes of Antihypertensives

Diuretics
Diuretics decrease blood pressure by causing diuresis, which results in decreased blood volume,

cardiac output, and stroke volume. They fall into three categories: thiazides, loop diuretics, and potassium-sparing diuretics. **Thiazide's** onset of action occurs within 2–3 h. Their half-life is 8–12 h allowing for once-daily dosing. Trade names include Hygroton, Hydrodiuril, Lozol, and Zaroxolyn.

Loop diuretics act in the loop of Henle in the kidney and are less effective in the long term. Their duration is 6 h. These agents are indicated with CHF or nephrotic syndrome. Bumex, Edecrin, Lasix, and Demadex are trade names.

Potassium-sparing agents cause minimal diuresis and are relatively ineffective in lowering the blood pressure. The medications correct thiazide-induced potassium and magnesium losses. Medication trade names include Midamor, Aldactone, and Dyrenium.

Adverse Events

Most complications occur related to dose and duration of use. Hypokalemia is a side effect, but can be managed with potassium chloride or use of potassium-sparing agents.

Acute gouty arthritis, muscle cramps, development of diabetes, nocturia or incontinence, and sun sensitivity have been noted as clinical side effects.

Beta-Blocking Agents

Beta1-receptors are located in the heart and kidneys and regulate heart rate and cardiac contractility. Beta2-receptors regulate bronchodilation and vasodilation. Beta-blockers decrease blood pressure by blocking the beta-receptors. Some beta-blockers are cardioselective, that is, they do not block the beta2-receptors and, therefore, do not cause bronchoconstriction. These medications include Lopressor, Kerlone, Tenormin, Sectral and Zebeta, Corgard, Inderal, and Cartrol.

Side Effects

The most common side effects of beta-blockers are fatigue, dizziness, bronchospasm, nausea, and vomiting. Beta-blockers should not be discontinued abruptly but should be tapered over 14 days to prevent withdrawal which includes unstable angina, myocardial infarction, and death.

ACE Inhibitors

This class of antihypertensives inhibits ACE which converts angiotensin I to II – a potent vasoconstrictor. This is a first-line therapy for patients with diabetes and proteinuria. Medications include Lotensin, Capoten, Vasotec, Monopril, Zestril, Univasc, Accupril, Altace, and Mavik.

Side effects include cough, hypotension, hyperkalemia, rash, loss of taste, leukopenia, and neutropenia. They are contraindicated in pregnancy and for patients with bilateral real artery stenosis.

Calcium Channel Blockers

Calcium channel blockers relax the cardiac and smooth muscle by blocking calcium channels that allow calcium into the cells. The result is vasodilation. They also decrease the heart rate and slow cardiac conduction. Medications include Calan, Cardizem, Norvasc, Plendil, Procardia Cardene, Sular, and DynaCirc.

Side Effects

Side effects include GI upset, edema, and hypotension. Rare side effects include bradycardia, CHF, and AV block. Other adverse effects include dizziness, headache, shortness of breath, gingival hyperplasia, and edema.

Contraindications

Calcium channel blockers should not be prescribed for individuals with second- and third-degree heart block or left ventricular dysfunction.

Other Classes of Antihypertensives

Peripheral alpha1-receptors (Cardura, Minipress, and Hytrin), central alpha2 (Clonidine, Aldomet, Tenex, and Wytension), direct vasodilators (Apresoline and Loniten), and adrenergic antagonists (Serpasil, Ismelin and Hylorel) are the remaining categories of antihypertensives. They are mainly used as second- and third-line medications.

Cross-References

▶ Psychopharmacology
▶ Stroke
▶ Transient Ischemic Attack

References and Readings

August, P. (2003). Initial treatment of hypertension. *New England Journal of Medicine, 348*, 610–617.
Cranwell-Bruce, L. (2008). Antihypertensives. *Medsurg Nursing, 17*(5), 337–341.
Ernst, M., & Moser, M. (2009). Use of diuretics in patients with hypertension. *New England Journal of Medicine, 361*, 2153–2164.
Houston, M. C., Pulliam Meador, B., & Moore Schipani, L. (2000). *Handbook of antihypertensive therapy* (10th ed.). Philadelphia: Hanley & Belfus.
Staessen, J., & Birkenhager, W. (2005). Evidence that new antihypertensives are superior to older drugs. *Lancet, 366*(9489), 869–871.

Antiplatelet Therapy

Elliot J. Roth
Department of Physical Medicine and Rehabilitation, Northwestern University, Feinberg School of Medicine, Chicago, IL, USA

Synonyms

Platelet anti-aggregant drugs

Definition

Antiplatelet therapy uses specific pharmacological agents (antiplatelet drugs) to inhibit the ability of platelets to clump together to form blood clots or thromboses, primarily in arteries. Antiplatelet therapy is commonly used in people with atherosclerosis (narrowing of the arteries). Platelets are naturally occurring cells (actually, portions of cells) that circulate in the blood. They clump, or aggregate, under certain conditions to initiate the formation of blood clots. These platelet clumps are then further bound together by the protein, fibrin. Together, the fibrin and the platelet clump comprise the thrombus or blood clot. Thrombi are useful in that they stop bleeding in normal circumstances. When there is a break in an artery, allowing blood to leave the vessel, platelets become activated by attaching to the wall of the blood vessel at the site of the bleeding and by attracting fibrin and other coagulation factors to the area to stop the bleeding. However, if the blood clot forms *inside* the artery, it can block the flow of blood to the tissue that is supplied by the artery, which can result in tissue damage. A clot forming in the coronary artery causes ischemic heart disease (which may present as angina or myocardial infarction), and when the blood clot forms in the carotid or cerebral arteries, it may cause a stroke.

Current Knowledge

Many studies have demonstrated the effectiveness of aspirin and other antiplatelet agents in preventing heart attack and stroke. This favorable effect is based on the ability of these agents to inhibit the chemicals that cause platelets to clump together initiating blood clot formation.

Aspirin is the prototypical antiplatelet agent. Other currently available antiplatelet agents include ticlopidine (Ticlid ®), clopidogrel (Plavix®), and dipyridamole (Persantine ®). Recently, a newer antiplatelet drug, ticagrelor (BRILINTA®), became available. Occasionally, the drugs are used in combination with each other or with anticoagulants. The most common side effect of all of these medications is bleeding.

See Also

▶ Anticoagulation
▶ Atherosclerosis
▶ Cerebrovascular Disease
▶ Coronary Disease
▶ Ischemic Stroke
▶ Myocardial Infarction
▶ Novel Oral Anticoagulants
▶ Peripheral Vascular Disease
▶ Stent

References

Jhansi, K., & Vanita, P. (2014). A review on antiplatelet drugs and anticoagulants. *Advance Pharmacoepidemiology Drug Safety, 3,* R003.

Tran, H., & Anand, S. S. (2004). Oral antiplatelet therapy in cerebrovascular disease, coronary artery disease, and peripheral arterial disease. *Journal of the American Medical Association, 292,* 1867–1874.

White, H. D. (2011). Oral anti-platelet therapy for atherothrombotic disease: Current evidence and new directions. *American Heart Journal, 161,* 450–461.

Antipsychotics

Helen M. Carmine
ReMed, Paoli, PA, USA

Synonyms

Antipsychotic medications; Atypicals (antipsychotics); Conventional antipsychotics; High-potency/low-potency groups of antipsychotics; Neuroleptics; Standard antipsychotics

Definition

Antipsychotic agents are used for the treatment of psychotic disorders, severe mental illnesses, and mood/behavior disorders not responsive to other medication/behavioral interventions. Broader application/often "off-label" are used to address thought/behavior disorders in various populations including adults with dementia, traumatic brain injury, developmental disorders with behavioral symptoms unresponsive to other treatments, and individuals with depression who are not responsive to antidepressant therapy alone. Specifically in TBI populations, according to B.C. McDonald et al. (2002), neuroleptics agents may have a role in individuals whose cognition and behaviors are disorganized and who are agitated. Another study by Ahmed and Fuiji (1998) identified that individuals who have a brain injury experience a two- to fivefold greater risk of developing psychosis than the general population and may require treatment with atypical antipsychotics to help restore behavioral and cognitive stability.

Historical Background

Antipsychotic medications according to Preston et al. (2006) have "truly revolutionized" the treatment of psychotic disorders. Conventional/typical antipsychotics act primarily through blockade of dopamine D2 receptors. Chlorpromazine(Thorazine), a phenothiazine, was first used in 1952 as a postoperative agent, but quickly became a standard treatment for sedation, reducing psychotic symptoms of psychiatric patients, and soon many other "phenothiazines" were developed (Preston et al. 2006). The role of dopamine 2 postsynaptic receptor blockade led to the development of future dopamine blockers that are chemically targeted to reduce and selectively block/weakly block dopamine to minimize side effects. Since that time, off-label use of these agents has benefited other populations. These agents were called "neuroleptics" because as a result of their dopamine blockade, they also lead to other neurological side effects/undesired effects. The newer antipsychotics, known as "atypicals," are strong serotonin blockers (5-HT2A and 5-HT2C) and produce varying degrees of dopamine blockade, weakly blocking D2 receptors and D1 receptors, and also act on the serotonin, dopamine, and GABA neurotransmitter systems. This multiple pathway approach may help with the individualization and selection of the best agent based on the individual's response.

Current Knowledge

Standard antipsychotics have been used since the 1950s for their sedating effects on individuals with psychosis/psychotic symptoms. As phenothiazines were known to produce these effects as postoperative sedation agents, the sedating effect led to the development of additional standard antipsychotic agents produced and utilized through the 1980s, including, but not limited to, agents such as Thorazine, Mellaril, Stelazine, Prolixin, Navane, and Trilafon. These standard antipsychotic agents were divided into high- and low-potency groups based on their profiles indicating desirable/undesirable effects including sedation, anticholinergic/parasympathetic side effects including urinary and bowel retention, dry mouth and cardiovascular effects, and extrapyramidal symptoms as a result of their dopamine blockade, their effects on sympathetic blockade/alpha adrenergic blockade leading to hypotension and dizziness, and the effects of neurotransmission leading to involuntary movements (tardive dyskinesias) and extrapyramidal symptoms. Other adverse effects noted with typical antipsychotics include lowering seizure threshold, thermal dysregulation, hormonal dysregulation including hyperprolactinemia, and a fatal but rare side effect known as neuroleptic malignant syndrome characterized by fever, rigidity, and confusion. Obviously, all medication agents require close monitoring and may also require other agents to address undesired effects, or lowering of the antipsychotic agent or change in administration time to minimize untoward effects.

Newer "atypical" or "novel" agents with Clozaril (Clozapine) as the first agent in this category have been noted to be effective in significantly reducing the symptoms of psychosis, particularly when other agents are unsuccessful, by targeting specific dopamine receptors or blocking/inhibiting reuptake of serotonin. The most significant difference is in the reduction of the negative symptoms and the lower risk of developing tardive dyskinesias. However, Clozaril's effects on the bone marrow may lead to a severe blood disorder, agranulocytosis. Clozaril requires adherence to an FDA protocol for complete blood count/ANC monitoring based on threshold values. Newer atypical agents were developed to improve the reduction of negative symptoms, improve cognition, and decrease risk of tardive dyskinesias and other neurological changes resulting from these agents.

Newer "atypical/novel" antipsychotic agents have included Risperidone, Zyprexa, Seroquel, Geodon, Abilify, and, most recently, Saphris.

However, with these newer "atypical antipsychotics," other concerning side effects have been exposed including metabolic changes leading to alterations in carbohydrate and lipid metabolism, possible diabetes, and excessive weight gain. All of these newer agents require routine monitoring of weight, blood sugar, and lipid profile studies to control the potential adverse effects while achieving improvement in both positive and negative symptoms of psychosis. Treatment duration with these agents is individually maximized based on response to reduction in positive symptoms of chronic thought disorders/psychosis. Shorter treatment durations may be possible in acute onset of delirium, acute psychoses, or brief reactive psychosis.

Future Directions

The use of the newer atypical agents has been shown to produce a reduction in hostility and aggression in schizophrenic patients, elderly patients with dementia, and empirically with individuals experiencing aggression and agitation in TBI. The next generation of agents will be directed at further reducing overall side effects while maximizing treatment response and symptom reduction while returning to optimal daily functioning and cognitive, mood, and behavioral stability.

Cross-References

▶ Neuroleptics
▶ Psychopharmacology
▶ Psychotic Disorder

References and Readings

Ahmed, I. I., & Fuiji, D. (1998). Posttraumatic Psychosis. *Seminars in. Clinical Neuropsychology, 3*(1), 23–33.

McDonald, B. C., Flashman, L. A., & Saykin, A. J. (2002). Executive dysfunction following traumatic brain injury: neural substrates and treatment strategies. *NeuroRehabilitation, 17*(4), 333–344.

Meredith, C., Jaffe, C., Ang-Lee, K., & Saxon, A. (2005). Implications of chronic methamphetamine use:

A literature review. *Harvard Review of Psychiatry, 13*(3), 141–154.

Preston, J., O'Neal, J. H., & Talaga, M. C. (2006). *Child and adolescent clinical psychopharmacology made simple*. Oakland: New Harbinger Publications.

Savitz, J., van der Merwe, L., Stein, D., Solms, M., & Ramesar, R. (2008). Neuropsychological task performance in bipolar spectrum illness: genetics, alcohol abuse, medication and childhood trauma. *Bipolar Disorders, 10*(4), 479–494.

Voruganti, L., & Awad, A. (2004). Neuroleptic dysphoria: Towards a new synthesis neuroleptic dysphoria. *Psychopharmacology, 171*(2), 121–132.

Wozniak, J., Block, E., White, T., Jensen, J., & Schulz, S. (2008). Clinical and neurocognitive course in early-onset psychosis: a longitudinal study of adolescents with schizophrenia-spectrum disorders. *Early Intervention in Psychiatry, 2*(3), 169–177.

Antisocial Personality Disorder

Cynthia Rolston
Department of PM&R, Virginia Commonwealth University-Medical College of Virginia, Richmond, VA, USA

Synonyms

Dyssocial personality disorder; Psychopathy; Sociopathy

Definition

Antisocial personality disorder (ASPD) is characterized by gross and guiltless disregard for and violation of others' rights, present since age 15 and persisting in adulthood. *Diagnostic and Statistical Manual of Mental Disorders* (5th ed.; DSM-5; American Psychiatric Association 2013) criteria include:

- Nonconformity to social norms, unlawful behavior.
- Deceitful, impulsive, irresponsible, and reckless behavior.
- Irritability and aggressiveness, with no remorse.

The symptoms must not present exclusively in the course of schizophrenic or bipolar disorders. Individuals with ASPD often display superficial charm initially but then treat others with disdain and contempt.

Categorization

ASPD is classified with the Cluster B Personality Disorders in DSM-5.

Current Knowledge

Prevalence

Prevalence estimates range from 0.2% to 3.3%, with men outnumbering women 3:1 (APA 2013). Higher rates of ASPD occur in males with alcohol abuse, individuals in substance abuse clinics and prisons, and people in adverse socioeconomic conditions.

Clinical Correlates

Adolescent conduct disorder (CD) often predates ASPD, with earlier onset predictive of poor prognosis (Black 2015). ASPD symptoms may be less evident with age. Substance Abuse (SA) is common in ASPD. Men with SA and ASPD may report more antisocial behaviors if they have a history of childhood trauma (Sher et al. 2015). Women with SA and ASPD may be at risk for committing violent acts in intimate relationships (Dykstra et al. 2015). Women have higher rates of aggressiveness and irritability (versus violence), greater overall impairment, lower social support, more emotional neglect in childhood, sexual abuse, and other victimization (Alegria et al. 2013). Cognitive performance and criminal behavior patterns differed in inmates with ASPD and psychopathy compared to those with only ASPD, suggesting ASPD and psychopathy are distinct, although frequently co-occurring (Riser and Kosson 2013).

Physiology and Neuropsychology

A "highly heritable common factor" may account for ASPD criteria interrelations (Rosenström et al. 2017). In one study, genetics accounted for 71% of the stability of ASPD, whereas environmental factors impacted phenotypic expression of the condition (Reichborn-Kjennerud et al. 2015). Monoamine oxidase A (MAO-A) has been linked to deregulation of prefrontal regions and serotonergic systems in this population (Kolla et al. 2016). ASPD has also been associated with reduced grey matter volume in the frontal cortex (Rautiainen et al. 2016), reduced cortical thickness, increased surface area, and diminished frontotemporal network activity (Jiang et al. 2016; Liu et al. 2014).

Assessment and Treatment

ASPD may be assessed through clinical interview, records review, self-report measures, and objective personality measures such as the Minnesota Multiphasic Personality Inventory (MMPI) or the Millon Clinical Multiaxial Inventory (MCMI). Most individuals with ASPD do not seek help for characterological concerns, but they may seek treatment for depression, anxiety, or SA. ASPD treatment typically focuses on reducing negative and destructive behaviors. Empirical supported psychotherapeutic interventions include impulsive lifestyle counseling (Thylstrup and Hesse 2016), affect management and problem solving (Black et al. 2016), mentalization-based treatment emphasizing appreciation of others' mental states (Bateman et al. 2016), and mindfulness-based treatment to reduce aggression (Velotti et al. 2016). Pharmacological treatments may include clozapine, ACE inhibitors, and opioid antagonists for treatment of endogenous opioid system dysfunction.

See Also

▶ Conduct Disorder
▶ Hare Psychopathy Checklist
▶ Personality Disorders
▶ Substance Abuse

References and Readings

Alegria, A. A., Blanco, C., Petry, N. M., Skodol, A. E., Liu, S. M., Grant, B., & Hasin, D. (2013). Sex differences in antisocial personality disorder: Results from the national epidemiological survey on alcohol and related conditions. *Personality Disorders, 4*(3), 214–222. https://doi.org/10.1037/a0031681.

American Psychiatric Association. (2013). *Diagnostic and statistical manual of mental disorders* (5th ed.). Arlington: American Psychiatric Association Publishing.

Bateman, A., O'Connell, J., Lorenzini, N., Gardner, T., & Fonagy, P. (2016). A randomised controlled trial of mentalization-based treatment versus structured clinical management for patients with comorbid borderline personality disorder and antisocial personality disorder. *BMC Psychiatry, 16*, 304-016-1000-9. https://doi.org/10.1186/s12888-016-1000-9.

Black, D. W. (2015). The natural history of antisocial personality disorder. *Canadian Journal of Psychiatry Revue Canadienne De Psychiatrie, 60*(7), 309–314.

Black, D. W., Simsek-Duran, F., Blum, N., McCormick, B., & Allen, J. (2016). Do people with borderline personality disorder complicated by antisocial personality disorder benefit from the STEPPS treatment program? *Personality and Mental Health, 10*(3), 205–215. https://doi.org/10.1002/pmh.1326.

Dykstra, R. E., Schumacher, J. A., Mota, N., & Coffey, S. F. (2015). Examining the role of antisocial personality disorder in intimate partner violence among substance use disorder treatment seekers with clinically significant trauma histories. *Violence Against Women, 21*(8), 958–974. https://doi.org/10.1177/1077801215589377.

Jiang, W., Li, G., Liu, H., Shi, F., Wang, T., Shen, C., ... Shen, D. (2016). Reduced cortical thickness and increased surface area in antisocial personality disorder. *Neuroscience, 337*, 143–152. https://doi.org/10.1016/S0306-4522(16)30434-1.

Kolla, N. J., Dunlop, K., Downar, J., Links, P., Bagby, R. M., Wilson, A. A., et al. (2016). Association of ventral striatum monoamine oxidase-A binding and functional connectivity in antisocial personality disorder with high impulsivity: A positron emission tomography and functional magnetic resonance imaging study. *European Neuropsychopharmacology: The Journal of the European College of Neuropsychopharmacology, 26*(4), 777–786. https://doi.org/10.1016/j.euroneuro.2015.12.030.

Liu, H., Liao, J., Jiang, W., & Wang, W. (2014). Changes in low-frequency fluctuations in patients with antisocial personality disorder revealed by resting-state functional MRI. *PloS One, 9*(3), e89790. https://doi.org/10.1371/journal.pone.0089790.

Rautiainen, M. R., Paunio, T., Repo-Tiihonen, E., Virkkunen, M., Ollila, H. M., Sulkava, S., et al. (2016). Genome-wide association study of antisocial personality disorder. *Translational Psychiatry, 6*(9), e883. https://doi.org/10.1038/tp.2016.155.

Reichborn-Kjennerud, T., Czajkowski, N., Ystrom, E., Orstavik, R., Aggen, S. H., Tambs, K., et al. (2015). A longitudinal twin study of borderline and antisocial personality disorder traits in early to middle adulthood. *Psychological Medicine, 45*(14), 3121–3131. https://doi.org/10.1017/S0033291715001117.

Riser, R. E., & Kosson, D. S. (2013). Criminal behavior and cognitive processing in male offenders with antisocial personality disorder with and without comorbid psychopathy. *Personality Disorders, 4*(4), 332–340. https://doi.org/10.1037/a0033303.

Rosenström, T., Ystrom, E., Torvik, F. A., Czajkowski, N. O., Gillespie, N. A., Aggen, S. H., . . . Reichborn-Kjennerud, T. (2017). Genetic and environmental structure of DSM-IV criteria for antisocial personality disorder: A twin study. *Behavior Genetics.* https://doi.org/10.1007/s10519-016-9833-z.

Sher, L., Siever, L. J., Goodman, M., McNamara, M., Hazlett, E. A., Koenigsberg, H. W., & New, A. S. (2015). Gender differences in the clinical characteristics and psychiatric comorbidity in patients with antisocial personality disorder. *Psychiatry Research, 229*(3), 685–689. https://doi.org/10.1016/j.psychres.2015.08.022.

Thylstrup, B., & Hesse, M. (2016). Impulsive lifestyle counseling to prevent dropout from treatment for substance use disorders in people with antisocial personality disorder: A randomized study. *Addictive Behaviors, 57,* 48–54. https://doi.org/10.1016/j.addbeh.2016.02.001.

Velotti, P., Garofalo, C., D'Aguanno, M., Petrocchi, C., Popolo, R., Salvatore, G., & Dimaggio, G. (2016). Mindfulness moderates the relationship between aggression and antisocial personality disorder traits: Preliminary investigation with an offender sample. *Comprehensive Psychiatry, 64,* 38–45. https://doi.org/10.1016/j.comppsych.2015.08.004.

Anxiety

Joel W. Hughes
Department of Psychology, Kent State University, Kent, OH, USA

Synonyms

Fear

Definition

Anxiety is an unpleasant state characterized by affective, cognitive, and physiological elements such as fear, worry, apprehension, and tension.

Anxiety is similar to the emotion of fear, although the function of chronic anxiety is often to avoid or mask true fear through mechanisms of anxiety such as worry and anticipation of negative future outcomes. The physiological manifestations of anxiety include increased blood pressure; increased breathing rate (often shallow); increased heart rate; other cardiac symptoms (e.g., pain, "skipped" beats); gastrointestinal distress including nausea, stomach aches, increased motility of the gut, and diarrhea; and generalized bodily distress such as fatigue and pain. Cognitively, anxiety is frequently characterized by an overestimation of the probability of a negative future outcome and an exaggeration of the consequences of the negative outcome. For example, an anxious person may believe that it is likely that they will fail a test with catastrophic consequences.

Anxiety often occurs in response to external stressors. It can be a normal reaction to stress, in which case anxiety can help coping behavior by focusing attention, mobilizing energy, and increasing goal-directed behavior. However, anxiety can also be a reaction to internal (physiological) cues or a generalized and pervasive mood without identifiable precipitants. When anxiety is an excessive reaction, or present in the absence of any true challenges or dangers, it is considered pathological. Individuals with pathological levels of anxiety are typically high in "trait" anxiety, which is a stable and enduring tendency to respond with anxiety to a wide variety of situations. Individuals high in trait anxiety are often also high in neuroticism.

Historical Background

Anxiety is basic to human experience and has been documented and treated since the beginning of recorded history. The relation between anxiety and health complaints has been recognized since the seventeenth century, although psychiatric nosology did not become well developed until the last century. A number of anxiety disorders have been delineated in contemporary psychiatric writings and are described in the most recent edition of the *Diagnostic and Statistical Manual of Mental Disorders* published by the American Psychiatric Association.

Current Knowledge

Although anxiety can be learned, it is thought to have a biological basis in the amygdala and hippocampus. When individuals are exposed to potentially dangerous or harmful stimuli, brain imaging often shows increased activity in the amygdala accompanied by participant reports of increased anxiety. Excessive anxiety can also compromise performance on neuropsychological tests, especially by interfering with attention and cognitive efficiency.

When suspected, the level of anxiety should be assessed. Anxiety is often measured using the Beck Anxiety Inventory or Hamilton Anxiety Scale. They do not diagnose anxiety disorders but give a dimensional measure of anxiety.

There are a number of recognized anxiety disorders in the contemporary psychiatric nosology (i.e., DSM 5). They are (alphabetically):

Agoraphobia
Generalized anxiety disorder
Panic disorder
Selective mutism
Separation anxiety disorder
Social anxiety disorder
Specific phobia

Additional anxiety-related disorders in the current diagnostic system such as obsessive compulsive disorder and posttraumatic stress disorder have been reclassified into new sections of the diagnostic and statistical manual of mental disorders (DSM-5[®]).

Effective treatment of anxiety almost always involves exposure to the feared stimulus. Treatments are based on the principles of classical conditioning, and the goal is to extinguish the fear response through exposure and habituation. Exposure can be in vivo or imaginal, and therapy frequently uses cognitive techniques to modify anxiety-generating cognitions. Anxiolytic medication is also often prescribed.

Cross-References

▶ Anxiolytics
▶ Beck Anxiety Inventory

References and Readings

Allen, L. B., McHugh, R. K., & Barlow, D. H. (2008). Emotional disorders: A unified protocol. In D. H. Barlow (Ed.), *Clinical handbook of psychological disorders: A step-by-step treatment manual* (4th ed., pp. 216–249). New York: Guilford Press.

American Psychiatric Association. (2000). *Diagnostic and statistical manual of mental disorders* (4th ed.), Text Revision. Washington, DC: American Psychiatric Association.

American Psychiatric Association. (2013). *Diagnostic and statistical manual of mental disorders (DSM-5[®])*. Arlington: American Psychiatric Publishing.

Beck, A. T., & Steer, R. A. (1990). Manual for the Beck anxiety inventory. San Antonio, TX: Psychological Corporation.

Maier, W., Buller, R., Philipp, M., & Heuser, I. (1988). The Hamilton anxiety scale: Reliability, validity and sensitivity to change in anxiety and depressive disorders. *Journal of Affective Disorders, 14*(1), 61–68.

Anxiolytics

Chava Creque[1] and
Stephanie A. Kolakowsky-Hayner[2]
[1]Department of Psychology and Neuroscience, University of Colorado Boulder, Boulder, CO, USA
[2]Department of Rehabilitation Medicine, Icahn School of Medicine at Mount Sinai, New York, NY, USA

Synonyms

Anti-anxiety drugs; Anti-anxiety medications

Definition

Anxiolytics are prescription drugs used to reduce the severity and extent of symptoms due to anxiety-related disorders. The most commonly prescribed anxiolytic drugs are benzodiazepines, drugs used to treat generalized anxiety disorder, panic attacks, phobias, and other ongoing issues of excessive fear and dread. Medical illness often associated with high levels of anxiety also includes brain injury, heart disease, and COPD. There are six approved benzodiazepines in the USA today including the popular diazepam (Valium), lorazepam (Ativan), and alprazolam (Xanax). Anxiolytics are designed to impact neurotransmitters in the amygdala by increasing gamma-aminobutyric acid (GABA), an inhibitory neurotransmitter that diminishes the fear response. Other drugs with anxiolytic effects include selective serotonin reuptake inhibitors (SSRIs).

Neuropsychologists must be aware of the potential effects of anxiolytics on the physical, emotional, and cognitive functioning of their patients. Anxiolytics are highly addictive and are often abused when used as a recreational drug. Patients may also become dependent on their medication if on increased doses for long periods of time. Side effects of anxiolytics may include excessive drowsiness to the point of sedation; suicidal thoughts; unexplained excitement, rage, anger, or hostility; confusion and cognitive slowing; balance and dizziness issues; diminished motor and visual skills; breathing issues; and memory impairment. Negative side effects may impact neuropsychological testing and treatment, and these effects should be considered in treatment planning and recommendations. Clinicians should also take into account patient age, medication dose, and concurrent medications, all of which can have an impact on neuropsychological performance of someone under the influence of anxiolytic medication.

Cross-References

▶ Benzodiazepines
▶ Diazepam
▶ GABA
▶ Psychopharmacology

References and Readings

Cosci, F., Schruers, K., Faravelli, C., & Griez, E. (2004). The influence of alcohol oral intake on the effects of 35% CO_2 challenge: A study in healthy volunteers. *Acta Neuropsychiatrica, 16*(2), 107–109.

Deacon, R., Bannerman, D., & Rawlins, J. (2002). Anxiolytic effects of cytotoxic hippocampal lesions in rats. *Behavioral Neuroscience, 116*(3), 494–497.

Harmer, C. J. (2012). Have no fear: The neural basis of anxiolytic drug action in generalized social phobia. *Biological Psychiatry Journal, 73*(4), 300–301.

Karl, T., Duffy, L., Scimone, A., Harvey, R., & Schofield, P. (2007). Altered motor activity, exploration and anxiety in heterozygous neuregulin 1 mutant mice: Implications for understanding schizophrenia. *Genes, Brain, and Behavior, 6*(7), 677–687.

Lanctôt, K., Herrmann, N., Mazzotta, P., Khan, L., & Ingber, N. (2004). GABAergic function in Alzheimer's disease: Evidence for dysfunction and potential as a therapeutic target for the treatment of behavioural and psychological symptoms of dementia. *Canadian Journal of Psychiatry, 49*(7), 439–453.

McHugh, S., Deacon, R., Rawlins, J., & Bannerman, D. (2004). Amygdala and ventral hippocampus contribute differentially to mechanisms of fear and anxiety. *Behavioral Neuroscience, 118*(1), 63–78.

Stein, R. A., & Strickland, T. L. (1998). A review of the neuropsychological effects of commonly used prescription medications. *Archives of Clinical Neuropsychology, 13*(3), 259–284.

Treit, D., & Menard, J. (1997). Dissociations among the anxiolytic effects of septal, hippocampal, and amygdaloid lesions. *Behavioral Neuroscience, 111*(3), 653–658.

Apathy

Laura L. Frakey
Memorial Hospital of Rhode Island and Alpert Medical School of Brown University, Pawtucket, RI, USA

Synonyms

Abulia; Amotivational; Anhedonia; Negative symptom

Short Description or Definition

In the vernacular, the word apathy generally refers to indifference or a lack of feeling or concern. In clinical settings, "apathy" is often conceptualized as a lack of drive or motivation, a lack of responsiveness (behavioral or emotional) to stimuli or a lack of initiation, or a reduction in self-generated, purposeful behavior.

Epidemiology

Apathy has been described in a variety of psychiatric, neurological, and medical conditions including depression, schizophrenia, Alzheimer's disease, frontotemporal dementia, mild cognitive impairment (MCI), Parkinson's disease, progressive supranuclear palsy, Huntington's disease, cortical basal degeneration, dementia with Lewy bodies, stroke, vascular dementia, cerebral autosomal dominant arteriopathy with subcortical infarcts and leukoencephalopathy (CADASIL), traumatic brain injury (TBI), anoxic encephalopathy, Wernicke-Korsakoff syndrome, hydrocephalus, human immunodeficiency virus (HIV), multiple sclerosis, apathetic hyperthyroidism, chronic fatigue syndrome, vitamin B12 deficiency, Lyme disease, and drug intoxication and withdrawal.

Following an extensive review of the literature, van Reekum et al. (2005) summarized the prevalence rates of apathy in many of the above-named conditions derived from studies which employed a variety of assessment measures (see below). Combining data from multiple studies, these authors report point prevalence rates of 60.3% in Alzheimer's disease, 46.7% in TBI, 60.3% in persons with focal frontal lesions, 33.8% in vascular dementia, 34.7% post-stroke, 22.2% in dementia with Lewy bodies, 29.8% in HIV, 20.5% in multiple sclerosis, and 53.3% in patients with major depression. Studies examining apathy in other neurological conditions have found prevalence rates of 41% in CADASIL (Reyes et al. 2009), 90% in frontotemporal dementia, 91% in progressive supranuclear palsy, 59% in Huntington's disease (Levy et al. 1998), and 54% in Parkinson's disease (Aarsland et al. 2007). Apathy is also one of the most commonly observed neuropsychiatric symptoms in MCI (Apostolova and Cummings 2008).

While the above-described findings relate to clinic-based samples, apathy has also been reported in a community-based sample of older adults with prevalence rates of 1.4% in cognitively normal elderly, 3.1% in mild cognitive syndrome, and 17.3% in dementia (Onyike et al. 2007). Apathy also appears to be quite common in nursing home settings, with one study reporting a prevalence rate of 84.1% (Wood et al. 2000). Apathy may also appear as an adverse effect of some prescription drugs, including selective serotonin reuptake inhibitors (SSRIs) (Hoehn-Saric et al. 1990).

Natural History, Prognostic Factors, and Outcomes

The word apathy comes from the Greek word "apatheia" meaning an "absence of feeling." The Stoic philosophers used this term to connote the total freedom from emotions and passions which were thought to compromise rationality and the desired state of mental tranquility. However, over the centuries, the term apathy came to refer to a lack of reactivity and became viewed as pathological rather than desirable.

While apathy can be observed as a symptom associated with a variety of psychiatric, neurological, and medical conditions, some authors have argued that apathy, in some circumstances, may represent a neuropsychiatric syndrome as well. Marin (1990) defined an apathy syndrome as a loss of motivation which could not be attributed to emotional distress, intellectual impairment, or a diminished level of consciousness. In contrast, apathy as a symptom was defined as a loss of motivation due to a disturbance of intellect, emotion, or level of consciousness (Marin 1990). Apathy is not considered an independent syndrome in the current DSM-V, though it does appear as a nonspecific symptom for several other disorders.

Prognostically, there is evidence to suggest that apathy may be associated with more severe impairment and negative outcomes. For example, a longitudinal study examining apathy in persons with Alzheimer's disease found apathy at baseline was associated with faster cognitive and functional decline at follow-up (Starkstein et al.

2006) There is also some evidence that apathy may precede the development of Alzheimer's disease. One longitudinal study of patients with MCI found that those patients who converted to Alzheimer's disease had higher rates of apathetic symptomatology (91.7%) than those patients who did not convert (26.9%) (Robert et al. 2006). Apathy has also been found to be significantly associated with lower cognitive functioning and more severe motor symptoms in persons with Parkinson's disease (Pedersen et al. 2009). Apathetic symptomatology has also been found to be negatively associated with functional improvement in rehabilitation settings after strokes (Hama et al. 2007) and increased risk for mortality in nursing home residents with dementia (van Dijk et al. 1994).

Studies have also found that apathy is associated with decreased performance of activities of daily living (ADLs) in persons with stroke (Mayo et al. 2009; Starkstein et al. 1993), vascular dementia (Zawacki et al. 2002), frontotemporal dementia (Kipps et al. 2009), dementia with Lewy bodies (Ricci et al. 2009), and major depression (Steffens et al. 1999). Alzheimer's disease patients with apathy are more likely to be impaired on basic activities of daily living (dressing, bathing, toileting, transferring, walking, and eating) than nonapathetic Alzheimer's disease patients, even when matched on degree of cognitive impairment (Albert et al. 1996; Stout et al. 2003). In addition, apathy has been found to account for 27% of the variance in instrumental activities of daily living scores (medication management, shopping, finances) in patients with Alzheimer's disease (Boyle et al. 2003).

Finally, apathy does not only impact the patient. Due to impairments in motivation, individuals with apathy can require more support and management, which can in turn result in increased caregiver burden and stress. The caregivers of patients with Alzheimer's disease-related apathy have been shown to report significantly elevated levels of distress and perceived burden compared to those who are caring for less apathetic patients with a similar level of cognitive impairment (Kaufer et al. 1998). Caregiver distress secondary

to neuropsychiatric symptoms, including apathy, has been implicated in the eventual institutionalization of many patients with Alzheimer's disease (Scott et al. 1997; Steele et al. 1990).

Neuropsychology and Psychology of Apathy

In clinical practice and research, apathy is often mistaken for depression, though it is a distinct syndrome that can be distinguished from depression (Levy et al. 1998; Marin 1991; Starkstein et al. 2001). The syndromes of depression and apathy share some symptoms (Table 1) and may co-occur in that same individual making diagnosis challenging (Damsio and Van Hosen 1983). For example, an apathetic demented patient who presents with fatigue, sleep disturbance, poor appetite and weight loss, poor concentration, and anhedonia may be diagnosed with major depressive disorder even in the absence of dysphoria (Ishii et al. 2009). A number of studies have found apathy to be correlated with high scores on various depression measures (Rabkin et al. 2000; Ready et al. 2003; Starkstein et al. 2006). However, this correlation may be due to the fact that many clinical measures of depression include questions assessing symptoms of both apathy and depression, which may lead to misdiagnosis.

Apathy, Table 1 Apathy vs. Depression

Symptoms of apathy	Overlapping symptoms	Symptoms of depression
Loss of motivation and initiation	Lack of interest in events or activities	Dysphoria
Lack of persistence	Lack of energy	Hopelessness
Diminished emotional reactivity	Psychomotor slowing	Guilt
Reduced social engagement	Fatigue	Pessimism
	Poor insight	Suicidal ideation
		Loss of appetite
		Sleep problems

Apathy may be distinguished from depression by the absence of dysphoric mood symptoms such as sadness, guilt, hopelessness, and helplessness. The difference in mood states, dysphoric vs. emotionally indifferent, is the most useful characteristic in making a differential diagnosis between apathy and depression. Apathy can be thought of as a syndrome of primary motivational loss and diminished emotional reactivity, while depression reflects a syndrome of mood disturbance.

The mechanisms of apathy are not fully understood, though most theories suggest it involves disruption of the frontal-subcortical neural circuit. This circuit begins with the anterior cingulate cortex, and continues to the ventral striatum, the globus pallidus, and the thalamus, before loping back to the anterior cingulate cortex. It has been hypothesized that neuropathological changes and alterations in regional chemistry, especially acetylcholine, dopamine, and serotonin, in this circuit are responsible for the clinical manifestation of apathy (David et al. 2008; Franceschi et al. 2005; Landes et al. 2001; Mega and Cummings 1994). Apathy with impaired motivation and indifference has most strongly been associated with damage to anterior cingulate cortex (ACC) (Damsio and Van Hosen 1983). In the most extreme cases, damage to the ACC results in akinetic mutism and a complete loss of initiation and motivation. Single photon emission computed tomography (SPECT) studies of patients with Alzheimer's disease found that apathy was strongly and inversely correlated with right anterior cingulate activity (Benoit et al. 1999) or with a bilateral reduction in cingulate activity (Migneco et al. 2001).

Frontal regions have also been implicated in the manifestation of apathy. Neuroimaging studies have found apathy in AD patients to be correlated with hypoperfusion in frontotemporal regions (Benoit et al. 1999; Craig et al. 1996). In one study, apathetic stroke patients showed reduced regional cerebral blood flow in right dorsolateral prefrontal cortex and left frontotemporal regions (Okada et al. 1997). Subcortical regions may also be implicated in the presence of apathy. In one study, apathy was seen in 80 stroke patients with lesions to the posterior limb of the internal capsule (Starkstein et al. 1993). Apathy has also

been observed with lesions to right hemisphere subcortical structures following TBI (Finset and Andersson 2000).

Evidence from neuropsychological studies suggests apathy may be associated with cognitive impairment, in particular executive dysfunction. Apathetic patients with Alzheimer's disease have been shown to have greater executive functioning deficits, abilities thought to be mediated by the frontal lobes, than depressed patients with Alzheimer's disease (Kuzis et al. 1999). Another study found apathetic patients with Alzheimer's disease showed significantly greater deficits on measures of executive functioning but performed similarly on other neuropsychological measures not dependent on executive function (McPherson et al. 2002). Apathy has also been associated with executive dysfunction in other clinical populations, including TBI (Andersson and Bergedalen 2002), Parkinson's disease (Starkstein et al. 1992), progressive supranuclear palsy (Litvan et al. 1998), and HIV (Castellon et al. 2000).

Evaluation

Formal assessment measures for apathy focus on those symptoms of apathy that are distinct from depression. The most commonly employed assessment instruments for apathy in clinical and research settings include the Apathy Evaluation Scale (AES), the Neuropsychiatric Inventory (NPI), and the Frontal Systems Behavior Scale (FrSBe). Less commonly used but validated measures include the Dementia Apathy Interview and Rating, the Lille Apathy Rating Scale, the Apathy Inventory, the Behavior Rating Scale for Dementia, and the Scale for the Assessment of Negative Symptoms in Alzheimer's Disease. Of note, while several of these measures include self-report versions, these may fail to identify apathy in patients with reduced insight, and therefore informant measures may be more helpful in assessing for apathy.

The AES comes in a clinician-administered version, an informant version, and a self-report version, all of which have been shown to have satisfactory reliability (Marin et al. 1991). The clinician-administered version of this measure (AES-C) is a semi-structured interview which includes 18 items and is focused on behavior that has been present during the past month. Each item falls into one of four categories (cognitive, behavior, emotional, or others) and is rated on a four-point Likert scale with higher scores representing a greater degree of apathy. A recent study examined the clinician-administered version (AES-C) and found it to be valid and reliable for identifying and quantifying apathy and found that using a cutoff score of 40.5 resulted in good sensitivity and moderate specificity (Clarke et al. 2007a, b).

The FrSBe (Grace and Malloy 2001) was specifically designed to assess for behavioral changes associated with frontal lobe dysfunction and comes in a self-report and informant version. These questionnaires consist of 46 items and ask the respondent to rate the patient's behavior on each item using a five-point Likert scale. Respondents are asked to rate the patient's behavior both before and after the onset of illness or injury. Subscales assess apathy, disinhibition, and executive dysfunction. This allows for an estimation of the extent to which current problem behaviors represent a change from premorbid functioning. T-scores greater than 65 are clinically significant. The FrSBe has been shown to be reliable, valid, and sensitive to behavior change due to frontal lobe damage (Grace et al. 1999), Alzheimer's disease (Stout et al. 2003), TBI (Lane-Brown and Tate 2009), and a variety of other neurological conditions.

The NPI is a structured interview conducted with an informant designed to assess for the presence of 12 neuropsychiatric symptoms, including apathy (Cummings 1997). A positive response to a screening question indicates the presence of the symptom and leads to further questions about the behavior and eventual ratings of the symptom severity (mild, moderate, or severe) and the amount of caregiver distress it causes. The Neuropsychiatric Inventory Questionnaire (NPI-Q) (Kaufer et al. 2000) is a self-administered questionnaire completed by a caregiver or informant that assesses for the presence of the same 12 symptoms and asks for ratings of severity and

caregiver distress using the same rating scale as the NPI interview. Importantly, both of these versions of the NPI include separate questions for depression and apathy. The NPI asks caregivers to consider whether the behavior has been present for the past month. The NPI has been shown to have good reliability and validity; however, unlike the other measures discussed, there is no recommended cutoff score for clinical significance. Of note, while the AES and FrSBe provide more nuanced assessments of apathy, the NPI is the most widely reported measure of apathy reported in the literature. This is likely due to the fact that the NPI assesses for a wide array of neuropsychiatric symptomatology, and is often used in intervention studies for a variety of conditions of which apathy may be one symptom, but not a cardinal feature, of a disorder.

Treatment

Nonpharmacologic interventions for apathy tend to focus on introducing new sources of interest and stimulation. Pet therapy, art therapy, and physical therapies may be useful in decreasing apathy, though the efficacies of these interventions have not been examined in a systematic fashion with apathetic patients. Increasing opportunities for socialization and encouraging participation in social activities may also be helpful. Patients should be encouraged to be as functionally autonomous as possible. Sensory deficits and pain should be managed so these do not interfere with activities. Implementing exercise programs and scheduled activities may also be beneficial in enhancing initiation and motivation. While there have been few studies on behavioral interventions specifically for apathy, there is some evidence that behavioral therapy may be helpful in reducing apathetic symptomatology. One randomized controlled study comparing "reminiscence therapy" (a treatment modality designed to facilitate recall of experiences from the past to promote intrapersonal and interpersonal functioning) to a time and attention control group (one-on-one time with an activity therapist) found that apathy was reduced for both groups of patients with dementia (Politis et al. 2004). Another study showed that individualized functional and occupational training reduced apathy in patients with mild-to-moderate stage dementia (Lam et al. 2009). Behavioral activation (BA) therapy is an intervention which focuses on alleviating depression by increasing the individual's exposure to rewarding and reinforcing stimuli by increasing activation and decreasing barriers and avoidance of activation (Dimidjian and Davis 2009). This behavioral approach includes goal-setting, activity scheduling, problem solving, and self-monitoring to get patients to become more active and thus increase exposure to reward and positive reinforcement to combat depressive symptomatology. It has been shown to be comparable to cognitive behavior therapy and pharmacotherapy (paroxetine) in reducing depressive symptomatology in placebo-controlled studies (Dimidjian et al. 2006; Sturmey 2009). While this intervention has not been examined in the treatment of apathy, its focus on increased activity and exposure to pleasant, rewarding experiences would appear to be particularly well-suited to address the lack of interest, motivation, and anhedonia that characterize apathy. Future research may show this to be a promising intervention for both depression and apathy.

Psychoeducation for families and caregivers can also be beneficial. Oftentimes, apathy is mischaracterized as a "willful behavior" (e.g., stubbornness or laziness) by caregivers who do not recognize that these behaviors are related to neurological, psychiatric, and medical comorbidities. Educating families on the underlying causes for a patient's low initiation and motivation may help lessen perceived caregiver burden and stress.

Currently, there is no FDA-approved pharmacological intervention for apathy; however, many different medications, including acetylcholinesterase inhibitors, psychostimulants, dopaminergic drugs, and atypical antipsychotics, have been used "off-label" to treat apathetic symptomatology.

Methylphenidate and dextroamphetamine are psychostimulant medications that are commonly used to treat attention deficit/hyperactivity disorder (AD/HD) and narcolepsy. These medications have also been used to treat apathy in Alzheimer's disease, normal pressure hydrocephalus, Parkinson's disease, cerebrovascular accidents, and depression (Chatterjee and Fahn 2002; Jansen et al. 2001; Keenan et al. 2005; Padala et al. 2007b; Spiegel et al. 2009). However, most of the evidence for the efficacy of these medications in apathy comes from case report or case series. These medications can also have negative side effects, including insomnia, loss of appetite, anxiety, and higher blood pressure, which may deter their use with vulnerable populations (Ishii et al. 2009). Other "stimulating" medications such as modafinil (Padala et al. 2007a) and selegiline (Newburn and Newburn 2005) have been reported to reduce apathy in case studies. A small double-blind placebo-controlled study assessing for the effects of modafinil used in conjunction with a cholinesterase inhibitor medication on apathy in a sample of individuals with mild-to-moderate stage Alzheimer's disease failed to find significant group differences. Indeed, both groups (treatment and control) showed small reductions in caregiver-reported symptoms of apathy following this 8-week trial suggesting that a "placebo effect" was observed (Frakey et al. 2012).

Reductions in apathy with the use of dopaminergic agents such as bromocriptine (Powell et al. 1996) and amantadine (Swanberg 2007; Van Reekum et al. 1995) have been reported in a few case studies, but no randomized clinical trials have been conducted to date. Apathetic-type symptoms and behavior may be seen in schizophrenic patients with negative symptoms. Atypical antipsychotic medications such as risperidone, olanzapine, and clozapine have been shown to be helpful in reducing negative symptoms in schizophrenia (van Reekum et al. 2005); however, none of the studies to date have specifically examined apathy, and these medications can be associated with serious negative side effects such as tardive dyskinesia, akathisia, extrapyramidal symptoms, and orthostatic hypotension.

As previously noted, apathy is the most common neuropsychiatric symptom associated with Alzheimer's disease, and modest improvements in apathy have been seen in patients with Alzheimer's disease who are treated with acetylcholinesterase inhibitor medications (Cummings 2000; Mega et al. 1999). Currently, there are three acetylcholine inhibitor medications approved for use in the United States: donepezil, galantamine, and rivastigmine. A meta-analysis identified 14 randomized, placebo-controlled trials of monotherapy with these medications in patients with Alzheimer's disease that reported a behavioral outcome (Rodda et al. 2009). Of these, only four were specifically designed to assess behavioral outcomes, and the rest used behavioral outcomes as secondary measures. Overall, 3 of the 14 studies reviewed reported a statistically significant improvement in overall score on the Neuropsychiatric Inventory, and only one found a significant reduction in apathy, specifically (Gauthier et al. 2002).

A recent study investigated whether a sustained cholinergic challenge, such as treatment with a cholinergic precursor choline alphoscerate and the cholinesterase inhibitor medication donepezil, could improve apathy symptoms in patients with Alzheimer's disease (Rea et al. 2015). The researchers examined changes in apathy ratings on the NPI in participants in the randomized double-blind ASCOMALVA study (Association Between the Cholinesterase Inhibitor Donepezil and the Cholinergic Precursor Choline Alphoscerate in Alzheimer's Disease). Results indicated that subjects treated with the combination of drugs had lower apathy scores after 12 and 24 months as compared to the control group. A similar trend was observed for caregiver ratings of distress with reductions noted in the stress level of the caregivers of participants receiving the combination of medications as compared to their control counterparts. Interestingly, the effects on apathy symptoms were unrelated to the level of cognitive impairment, as measured by the Mini-Mental Status Exam (MMSE) and Alzheimer's Disease Assessment Scale Cognitive Subscale (ADAS-cog), but may have been related to pretreatment level of executive dysfunction. Specifically, those participants with normal range baseline performance on the frontal assessment battery (FAB) were the ones who showed lower apathy after 12, 18, and 24 months of treatment.

There does appear to be increasing recognition of the prevalence of apathy, its impact on patients and their families, and its importance in neuropsychiatric research. This recognition appears to be fueling an interest in developing a more rigorous approach to clinical research on apathy. Recognizing the need for reliable identification of apathy and seeking ways to improve communication in both research and treatment of apathy, the Centre Memoire de Ressources et de Recherche organized a task force to develop a formal diagnostic criteria for apathy which they hoped would be used to facilitate research in apathy (Robert et al. 2009). Along those lines, Radakovic et al. (2015) recently conducted a systematic review of the literature to provide an overview of apathy scales which had been validated in generic and specific neurodegenerative disorders and to compare that methodological quality and psychometric properties of these scales to provide recommendations for the use of several instruments with some specific neurodegenerative disorders. Finally, Cummings et al. (2015), citing increased interest in new therapeutic options for apathy, recently published a position paper offering recommendations for the design and development of clinical studies investigating treatment of apathy in Alzheimer's disease and Parkinson's disease as well as a wider range of disorders.

See Also

▶ Abulia
▶ Akinetic Mutism
▶ Anterior Cingulate Cortex
▶ Avolition
▶ Major Depression
▶ Motivation

Further Reading

Aarsland, D., Bronnick, K., Ehrt, U., De Deyn, P. P., Tekin, S., Emre, M., & Cummings, J. L. (2007). Neuropsychiatric symptoms in patients with Parkinson's disease and dementia: Frequency, profile and associated care giver stress. *Journal of Neurology, Neurosurgery, and Psychiatry, 78*, 36–42.

Albert, S. M., Del Castillo-Castaneda, C., Sano, M., Jacobs, D. M., Marder, K., Bell, K., et al. (1996). Quality of life in patients with Alzheimer's disease as reported by patient proxies. *Journal of the American Geriatrics Society, 44*(11), 1342–1347.

Andersson, S., & Bergedalen, A. M. (2002). Cognitive correlates of apathy in traumatic brain injury. *Neuropsychiatry, Neuropsychology, and Behavioral Neurology, 15*(3), 184–191.

Apostolova, L. G., & Cummings, J. L. (2008). Neuropsychiatric manifestations in mild cognitive impairment: A systematic review of the literature. *Dementia and Geriatric Cognitive Disorders, 25*(2), 115–126.

Benoit, M., Dygai, I., Migneco, O., Robert, P. H., Bertogliati, C., Darcourt, J., et al. (1999). Behavioral and psychological symptoms in Alzheimer's disease. Relation between apathy and regional cerebral perfusion. *Dementia and Geriatric Cognitive Disorders, 10*(6), 511–517.

Boyle, P. A., Malloy, P. F., Salloway, S., Cahn-Weiner, D. A., Cohen, R., & Cummings, J. L. (2003). Executive dysfunction and apathy predict functional impairment in Alzheimer disease. *The American Journal of Geriatric Psychiatry, 11*(2), 214–221.

Castellon, S. A., Hinkin, C. H., & Myers, H. F. (2000). Neuropsychiatric disturbance is associated with executive dysfunction in hiv-1 infection. *Journal of the International Neuropsychological Society, 6*(3), 336–347.

Chatterjee, A., & Fahn, S. (2002). Methylphenidate treats apathy in Parkinson's disease. *The Journal of Neuropsychiatry and Clinical Neurosciences, 14*(4), 461–462.

Clarke, D. E., Reekum, R., Simard, M., Streiner, D. L., Freedman, M., & Conn, D. (2007a). Apathy in dementia: An examination of the psychometric properties of the apathy evaluation scale. *The Journal of Neuropsychiatry and Clinical Neurosciences, 19*(1), 57–64.

Clarke, D. E., Van Reekum, R., Patel, J., Simard, M., Gomez, E., & Streiner, D. L. (2007b). An appraisal of the psychometric properties of the clinician version of the apathy evaluation scale (aes-c). *International Journal of Methods in Psychiatric Research, 16*(2), 97–110.

Craig, A. H., Cummings, J. L., Fairbanks, L., Itti, L., Miller, B. L., Li, J., et al. (1996). Cerebral blood flow correlates of apathy in Alzheimer disease. *Archives of Neurology, 53*(11), 1116–1120.

Cummings, J. L. (1997). The neuropsychiatric inventory: Assessing psychopathology in dementia patients. *Neurology, 48*(5 Suppl 6), S10–S16.

Cummings, J. L. (2000). The role of cholinergic agents in the management of behavioural disturbances in Alzheimer's disease. *The International Journal of Neuropsychopharmacology, 3*(7), 21–29.

Cummings, J., Friedman, J. H., Garibaldi, G., Jones, M., Macfadden, W., Marsh, L., & Robert, P. H. (2015). Apathy in neurodegenerative diseases: Recommendations on the design of clinical trials. *Journal of Geriatric Psychiatry and Neurology, 28*(3), 159–173.

Damsio, A. R., & Van Hosen, G. W. (1983). Emotional disturbances associated with focal lesions of the frontal lobe. In K. M. Heilman & P. Satz (Eds.), *Neuropsychology of human emotion*. New York: Guilford Press.

David, R., Koulibaly, M., Benoit, M., Garcia, R., Caci, H., Darcourt, J., et al. (2008). Striatal dopamine transporter levels correlate with apathy in neurodegenerative diseases a spect study with partial volume effect correction. *Clinical Neurology and Neurosurgery, 110*(1), 19–24.

Dimidjian, S., & Davis, K. J. (2009). Newer variations of cognitive-behavioral therapy: Behavioral activation and mindfulness-based cognitive therapy. *Current Psychiatry Reports, 11*(6), 453–458.

Dimidjian, S., Hollon, S. D., Dobson, K. S., Schmaling, K. B., Kohlenberg, R. J., Addis, M. E., et al. (2006). Randomized trial of behavioral activation, cognitive therapy, and antidepressant medication in the acute treatment of adults with major depression. *Journal of Consulting and Clinical Psychology, 74*(4), 658–670.

Finset, A., & Andersson, S. (2000). Coping strategies in patients with acquired brain injury: Relationships between coping, apathy, depression and lesion location. *Brain Injury, 14*(10), 887–905.

Frakey, L. L., Salloway, S., Buelow, M., & Malloy, P. F. (2012). A randomized, double-blind, placebo-controlled trial of modafinil for the treatment of apathy in individuals with mild-to-moderate stage Alzheimer's disease. *The Journal of Clinical Psychiatry, 73*(6), 796–801.

Franceschi, M., Anchisi, D., Pelati, O., Zuffi, M., Matarrese, M., Moresco, R. M., et al. (2005). Glucose metabolism and serotonin receptors in the frontotemporal lobe degeneration. *Annals of Neurology, 57*(2), 216–225.

Gauthier, S., Feldman, H., Hecker, J., Vellas, B., Ames, D., Subbiah, P., et al. (2002). Efficacy of donepezil on behavioral symptoms in patients with moderate to severe Alzheimer's disease. *International Psychogeriatrics, 14*(4), 389–404.

Grace, J., & Malloy, P. F. (2001). *Frontal systems behavior scale. Professional manual*. Lutz: Psychological Assessment Resources.

Grace, J., Stout, J. C., & Malloy, P. F. (1999). Assessing frontal lobe behavioral syndromes with the frontal lobe personality scale. *Assessment, 6*(3), 269–284.

Hama, S., Yamashita, H., Shigenobu, M., Watanabe, A., Hiramoto, K., Kurisu, K., et al. (2007). Depression or apathy and functional recovery after stroke. *International Journal of Geriatric Psychiatry, 22*(10), 1046–1051.

Hoehn-Saric, R., Lipsey, J. R., & McLeod, D. R. (1990). Apathy and indifference in patients on fluvoxamine and fluoxetine. *Journal of Clinical Psychopharmacology, 10*(5), 343–345.

Ishii, S., Weintraub, N., & Mervis, J. R. (2009). Apathy: A common psychiatric syndrome in the elderly. *Journal* of the American Medical Directors Association, 10(6), 381–393.

Jansen, I. H., Olde Rikkert, M. G., Hulsbos, H. A., & Hoefnagels, W. H. (2001). Toward individualized evidence-based medicine: Five "n of 1" trials of methylphenidate in geriatric patients. *Journal of the American Geriatrics Society, 49*(4), 474–476.

Kaufer, D. I., Cummings, J. L., Christine, D., Bray, T., Castellon, S., Masterman, D., et al. (1998). Assessing the impact of neuropsychiatric symptoms in Alzheimer's disease: The neuropsychiatric inventory caregiver distress scale. *Journal of the American Geriatrics Society, 46*(2), 210–215.

Kaufer, D. I., Cummings, J. L., Ketchel, P., Smith, V., MacMillan, A., Shelley, T., et al. (2000). Validation of the npi-q, a brief clinical form of the neuropsychiatric inventory. *The Journal of Neuropsychiatry and Clinical Neurosciences, 12*(2), 233–239.

Keenan, S., Mavaddat, N., Iddon, J., Pickard, J. D., & Sahakian, B. J. (2005). Effects of methylphenidate on cognition and apathy in normal pressure hydrocephalus: A case study and review. *British Journal of Neurosurgery, 19*(1), 46–50.

Kipps, C. M., Mioshi, E., & Hodges, J. R. (2009). Emotion, social functioning and activities of daily living in frontotemporal dementia. *Neurocase*, 1–8.

Kuzis, G., Sabe, L., Tiberti, C., Dorrego, F., & Starkstein, S. E. (1999). Neuropsychological correlates of apathy and depression in patients with dementia. *Neurology, 52*(7), 1403–1407.

Lam, L. C., Lui, V. W., Luk, D. N., Chau, R., So, C., Poon, V., et al. (2009). Effectiveness of an individualized functional training program on affective disturbances and functional skills in mild and moderate dementia-a randomized control trial. *International Journal of Geriatric Psychiatry, 25*(2), 133–141.

Landes, A. M., Sperry, S. D., Strauss, M. E., & Geldmacher, D. S. (2001). Apathy in Alzheimer's disease. *Journal of the American Geriatrics Society, 49* (12), 1700–1707.

Lane-Brown, A. T., & Tate, R. L. (2009). Measuring apathy after traumatic brain injury: Psychometric properties of the apathy evaluation scale and the frontal systems behavior scale. *Brain Injury, 23*(13–14), 999–1007.

Levy, M. L., Cummings, J. L., Fairbanks, L. A., Masterman, D., Miller, B. L., Craig, A. H., et al. (1998). Apathy is not depression. *The Journal of Neuropsychiatry and Clinical Neurosciences, 10*(3), 314–319.

Litvan, I., Cummings, J. L., & Mega, M. (1998). Neuropsychiatric features of corticobasal degeneration. *Journal of Neurology, Neurosurgery, and Psychiatry, 65*(5), 717–721.

Marin, R. S. (1990). Apathy: A neuropsychiatric syndrome. *The Journal of Neuropsychiatry and Clinical Neurosciences, 3*(3), 243–254.

Marin, R. S., Biedrzycki, R. C., & Firinciogullari, S. (1991). Reliability and validity of the apathy evaluation scale. *Psychiatry Research, 38*(2), 143–162.

Mayo, N. E., Fellows, L. K., Scott, S. C., Cameron, J., & Wood-Dauphinee, S. (2009). A longitudinal view of apathy and its impact after stroke. *Stroke, 40*(10), 3299–3307.

McPherson, S., Fairbanks, L., Tiken, S., Cummings, J. L., & Back-Madruga, C. (2002). Apathy and executive function in Alzheimer's disease. *Journal of the International Neuropsychological Society, 8*(3), 373–381.

Mega, M. S., & Cummings, J. L. (1994). Frontal-subcortical circuits and neuropsychiatric disorders. *The Journal of Neuropsychiatry and Clinical Neurosciences, 6*(4), 358–370.

Mega, M. S., Masterman, D. M., O'Connor, S. M., Barclay, T. R., & Cummings, J. L. (1999). The spectrum of behavioral responses to cholinesterase inhibitor therapy in Alzheimer disease. *Archives of Neurology, 56*(11), 1388–1393.

Migneco, O., Benoit, M., Koulibaly, P. M., Dygai, I., Bertogliati, C., Desvignes, P., et al. (2001). Perfusion brain spect and statistical parametric mapping analysis indicate that apathy is a cingulate syndrome: A study in Alzheimer's disease and nondemented patients. *NeuroImage, 13*(5), 896–902.

Newburn, G., & Newburn, D. (2005). Selegiline in the management of apathy following traumatic brain injury. *Brain Injury, 19*(2), 149–154.

Okada, K., Kobayashi, S., Yamagata, S., Takahashi, K., & Yamaguchi, S. (1997). Poststroke apathy and regional cerebral blood flow. *Stroke, 28*(12), 2437–2441.

Onyike, C. U., Sheppard, J. M., Tschanz, J. T., Norton, M. C., Green, R. C., Steinberg, M., et al. (2007). Epidemiology of apathy in older adults: The cache county study. *The American Journal of Geriatric Psychiatry, 15*(5), 365–375.

Padala, P. R., Burke, W. J., & Bhatia, S. C. (2007a). Modafinil therapy for apathy in an elderly patient. *The Annals of Pharmacotherapy, 41*(2), 346–349.

Padala, P. R., Burke, W. J., Bhatia, S. C., & Petty, F. (2007b). Treatment of apathy with methylphenidate. *The Journal of Neuropsychiatry and Clinical Neurosciences, 19*(1), 81–83.

Pedersen, K. F., Larsen, J. P., Alves, G., & Aarsland, D. (2009). Prevalence and clinical correlates of apathy in Parkinson's disease: A community-based study. *Parkinsonism & Related Disorders, 15*(4), 295–299.

Politis, A. M., Vozzella, S., Mayer, L. S., Onyike, C. U., Baker, A. S., & Lyketsos, C. G. (2004). A randomized, controlled, clinical trial of activity therapy for apathy in patients with dementia residing in long-term care. *International Journal of Geriatric Psychiatry, 19*(11), 1087–1094.

Powell, J. H., al-Adawi, S., Morgan, J., & Greenwood, R. J. (1996). Motivational deficits after brain injury: Effects of bromocriptine in 11 patients. *Journal of*

Neurology, Neurosurgery, and Psychiatry, 60(4), 416–421.

Rabkin, J. G., Ferrando, S. J., van Gorp, W., Rieppi, R., McElhiney, M., & Sewell, M. (2000). Relationships among apathy, depression, and cognitive impairment in hiv/aids. *The Journal of Neuropsychiatry and Clinical Neurosciences, 12*(4), 451–457.

Radakovic, R., Harley, C., Abrahams, S., & Starr (2015). A systematic review of the validity and reliability of apathy scales in neurodegenerative conditions. International Psychogeriatrics, 27(6), 903–923.

Rea, R., Carotenuto, A., Traini, E., Fasananro, M., & Amenta, F. (2015). Apathy treatment in Alzheimer's disease: Interim results of the ascomalva trial. *Journal of Alzheimer's Disease, 48*, 377–383.

Ready, R. E., Ott, B. R., Grace, J., & Cahn-Weiner, D. A. (2003). Apathy and executive dysfunction in mild cognitive impairment and Alzheimer disease. *The American Journal of Geriatric Psychiatry, 11*(2), 222–228.

van Reekum, R., Stuss, D. T., & Ostrander, L. (2005). Apathy: Why care? *The Journal of Neuropsychiatry and Clinical Neurosciences, 17*(1), 7–19.

Reyes, S., Viswanathan, A., Godin, O., Dufouil, C., Benisty, S., Hernandez, K., et al. (2009). Apathy: A major symptom in cadasil. *Neurology, 72*(10), 905–910.

Ricci, M., Guidoni, S. V., Sepe-Monti, M., Bomboi, G., Antonini, G., Blundo, C., et al. (2009). Clinical findings, functional abilities and caregiver distress in the early stage of dementia with lewy bodies (dlb) and Alzheimer's disease (ad). *Archives of Gerontology and Geriatrics, 49*(2), e101–e104.

Robert, P. H., Berr, C., Volteau, M., Bertogliati, C., Benoit, M., Sarazin, M., et al. (2006). Apathy in patients with mild cognitive impairment and the risk of developing dementia of Alzheimer's disease: A one-year follow-up study. *Clinical Neurology and Neurosurgery, 108*(8), 733–736.

Robert, P., Onyike, C. U., Leentjens, A. F. G., Dujardin, K., Aalten, P., Starkstein, S., Verhey, F. R. J., Yessavage, J., Clement, J. P., Drapier, D., Bayle, F., Benoit, M., Boyer, P., Lorca, P. M., Thibaut, F., Gauthier, S., Grossberg, G., Vellas, B., & Byrne, J. (2009). Proposed diagnostic criteria for apathy in Alzheimer's disease and other neuropsychiatric disorders. *European Psychiatry, 24*, 98–104.

Rodda, J., Morgan, S., & Walker, Z. (2009). Are cholinesterase inhibitors effective in the management of the behavioral and psychological symptoms of dementia in Alzheimer's disease? A systematic review of randomized, placebo-controlled trials of donepezil, rivastigmine and galantamine. *International Psychogeriatrics, 21*(5), 813–824.

Scott, W. K., Edwards, K. B., Davis, D. R., Cornman, C. B., & Macera, C. A. (1997). Risk of institutionalization among community long-term care clients with dementia. *Gerontologist, 37*(1), 46–51.

Spiegel, D. R., Kim, J., Greene, K., Conner, C., & Zamfir, D. (2009). Apathy due to cerebrovascular accidents successfully treated with methylphenidate: A case series. *The Journal of Neuropsychiatry and Clinical Neurosciences, 21*(2), 216–219.

Starkstein, S. E., Mayberg, H. S., Preziosi, T. J., Andrezejewski, P., Leiguarda, R., & Robinson, R. G. (1992). Reliability, validity, and clinical correlates of apathy in Parkinson's disease. *The Journal of Neuropsychiatry and Clinical Neurosciences, 4*(2), 134–139.

Starkstein, S. E., Fedoroff, J. P., Price, T. R., Leiguarda, R., & Robinson, R. G. (1993). Apathy following cerebrovascular lesions. *Stroke, 24*(11), 1625–1630.

Starkstein, S. E., Petracca, G., Chemerinski, E., & Kremer, J. (2001). Syndromic validity of apathy in Alzheimer's disease. *The American Journal of Psychiatry, 158*(6), 872–877.

Starkstein, S. E., Jorge, R., Mizrahi, R., & Robinson, R. G. (2006). A prospective longitudinal study of apathy in Alzheimer's disease. *Journal of Neurology, Neurosurgery, and Psychiatry, 77*(1), 8–11.

Steele, C., Rovner, B., Chase, G. A., & Folstein, M. (1990). Psychiatric symptoms and nursing home placement of patients with Alzheimer's disease. *The American Journal of Psychiatry, 147*(8), 1049–1051.

Steffens, D. C., Hays, J. C., & Krishnan, K. R. (1999). Disability in geriatric depression. *The American Journal of Geriatric Psychiatry, 7*(1), 34–40.

Stout, J. C., Wyman, M. F., Johnson, S. A., Peavy, G. M., & Salmon, D. P. (2003). Frontal behavioral syndromes and functional status in probable Alzheimer disease. *The American Journal of Geriatric Psychiatry, 11*(6), 683–686.

Sturmey, P. (2009). Behavioral activation is an evidence-based treatment for depression. *Behavior Modification, 33*(6), 818–829.

Swanberg, M. M. (2007). Memantine for behavioral disturbances in frontotemporal dementia: A case series. *Alzheimer Disease and Associated Disorders, 21*(2), 164–166.

van Dijk, P. T., Dippel, D. W., & Habbema, J. D. (1994). A behavioral rating scale as a predictor for survival of demented nursing home patients. *Archives of Gerontology and Geriatrics, 18*(2), 101–113.

Van Reekum, R., Bayley, M., Garner, S., Burke, I. M., Fawcett, S., Hart, A., et al. (1995). N of 1 study: Amantadine for the amotivational syndrome in a patient with traumatic brain injury. *Brain Injury, 9*(1), 49–53.

Wood, S., Cummings, J. L., Hsu, M. A., Barclay, T., Wheatley, M. V., Yarema, K. T., et al. (2000). The use of the neuropsychiatric inventory in nursing home residents. Characterization and measurement. *The American Journal of Geriatric Psychiatry, 8*(1), 75–83.

Zawacki, T. M., Grace, J., Paul, R., Moser, D. J., Ott, B. R., Gordon, N., et al. (2002). Behavioral problems as predictors of functional abilities of vascular dementia patients. *The Journal of Neuropsychiatry and Clinical Neurosciences, 14*(3), 296–302.

Aphasia

Janet P. Patterson
Audiology and Speech-Language Pathology
Service, VA Northern California Health Care
System, Martinez, CA, USA

Short Description or Definition

"Aphasia is an acquired communication disorder caused by brain damage, characterized by impairments of language modalities; speaking, listening, reading and writing; it is not the result of a sensory or motor deficit, a general intellectual deficit, confusion or a psychiatric disorder" (Hallowell and Chapey 2008, p. 3). Aphasia is typically acquired suddenly as a result of a stroke or traumatic brain injury but can appear more slowly accompanying other neurological events such as tumor or disease. When aphasia develops slowly over time and is the only behavioral symptom present, the diagnosis is primary progressive aphasia (PPA). Aphasia is often classified according to the appearance of a constellation of behavioral symptoms including impairment in auditory comprehension, reading comprehension, naming, production of grammatically correct sentences, repetition, writing, and presence of paraphasic (substitution) sound or word errors (e.g., saying *table* for *chair* or *pork* for *fork*). Aphasia disrupts communication ability, sometimes so severely that a person with aphasia withdraws from social interaction and other times only minimally so that the person with aphasia continues his or her life activities.

Aphasia Classification

Many systems have been proposed to classify aphasia types (Kertesz 1979). Each system represents a theoretical perspective of aphasia and identifies aphasia types according to a constellation of behavioral characteristics. Classification systems can be dichotomous (e.g., fluent vs. nonfluent or comprehension deficit vs. production deficit), anatomically based (e.g., Boston classification system of aphasia types, such as Broca's aphasia), and behaviorally based (e.g., Schuell's system of multimodality, unidimensional impairment, such as aphasia with visual involvement), can be based on severity (e.g., mild, moderate, or severe), or can follow a processing model (e.g., cognitive neuropsychological model of naming; Kay et al. 1996). Classification systems are useful for a general understanding of an individual's communication ability; however, controversy exists regarding their clinical utility. Some individuals with aphasia show symptoms that match more than one type of aphasia, and others show symptoms that do not fit into any of the classification categories. Studies examining classification report 35–70% success in classifying participants as one aphasia type (Caramazza 1984; Crary et al. 1992). Table 1 shows three classification systems, with general characteristics of each aphasia type.

Epidemiology

Aphasia resulting from stroke occurs in approximately 30% of the 15 million people worldwide who experience a stroke each year. In the United States alone, 80,000 new occurrences of aphasia appear each year, and at any point in time, approximately one million people are living with aphasia following stroke. Aphasia resulting from traumatic brain injury and other causes is difficult to estimate.

Natural History, Prognostic Factors, and Outcomes

Reports of language disorder following brain injury have existed for hundreds of years, initially as case reports. Paul Broca and Carl Wernicke in the late 1800s presented clinical data relating behavioral and anatomical information, localizing language ability to the left hemisphere, and

Aphasia, Table 1 Three examples of aphasia classification systems showing aphasia types and general characteristics of each type

Dichotomous classification	
Type	**Characteristics**
Nonfluent aphasia	Limited speech output
	Effortful speech output
	Content words retained; function words omitted
	May or may not have articulation difficulties
	Melodic contour altered
Fluent aphasia	Approximates normal rate and sentence length
	Content words omitted in severe fluent aphasia
	Circumlocution present in mild fluent aphasia
	Melodic contour preserved

Anatomical and behavioral classification	
Type	**Characteristics**
Broca's aphasia	Nonfluent aphasia; expressive aphasia
	Effortful output
	Reduced phrase length and syntactic complexity; content words usually preserved
	Auditory comprehension may or may not be impaired
	Impairments in reading, writing, naming, and repetition
	Right hemiplegia often present
Wernicke's aphasia	Fluent aphasia; receptive aphasia
	Auditory comprehension often impaired
	Impairments also may appear in reading, writing, naming, and repetition
	Paraphasic errors
	Melodic contour retained
Conduction aphasia	Fluent aphasia
	Auditory comprehension preserved
	Impairment in repetition
	Naming may be impaired
	Error recognition typically preserved
Global aphasia	Nonfluent aphasia
	Impairments in auditory comprehension, reading, writing, naming, and repetition
	Limited functional communication often preserved
Anomic aphasia	Fluent aphasia
	Auditory and reading comprehension and repetition typically preserved
	Word retrieval deficit
Transcortical motor aphasia	Nonfluent aphasia
	Auditory comprehension and naming may be impaired
	Repetition preserved
	Paraphasic errors and perseveration present
Transcortical sensory aphasia	Fluent aphasia
	Auditory comprehension impaired
	Paraphasic errors
	Repetition preserved
	Naming may be impaired

(*continued*)

Aphasia, Table 1 (continued)

Behavioral classification	
Type	**Characteristics**
Simple aphasia	Mild impairment
	Multimodality impairment (spoken language; speech; reading; writing)
	No specific perceptual, sensorimotor, or dysarthric components
Aphasia with visual involvement	Mild aphasia
	Central impairment of visual modality
Aphasia with persisting dysfluency	Mild aphasia
	Verbal dysfluency
Aphasia with scattered findings	Moderate aphasia
	Impairments in one or more modalities
	Functional communication preserved
Aphasia with sensorimotor involvement	Severe aphasia
	Impaired output
Aphasia with intermittent auditory imperception	Severe aphasia
	Impaired auditory comprehension
Irreversible aphasia syndrome	Severe aphasia
	Impairments in all modalities (comprehension of spoken language; speech; reading; writing)

ultimately having their names adopted to identify anatomical areas in the brain related to patterns of language deficit. Current studies of persons with aphasia use neuroimaging techniques to further elucidate the behavioral and anatomical relationship.

Aphasia in the first few months after a stroke is the acute stage and is often characterized by spontaneous recovery of language and communication deficits. In the chronic stage, an individual learns to live with aphasia and returns to life activities. Prognosis for recovery is variable and dependent upon both internal patient factors (e.g., severity of aphasia, type and extent of lesion, or concomitant medical problems), external factors (e.g., family support or communication interaction opportunities), and other ambient experiences (McClung et al. 2010). Personal variables such as age, education, and gender do not systematically influence prognosis (Basso 1992; Pedersen et al. 2004; Plowman et al. 2012).

Aphasia recovery occurs most rapidly immediately following the brain injury as the brain begins to heal itself. Studies have shown that recovery also continues for years post-stroke and following treatment (Moss and Nicholas 2006). Outcome measures documenting change are impairment based (e.g., change in naming ability) or activity/participation based (e.g., increased participation in social activities), following the World Health Organization's International Classification of Functioning, Disability and Health (ICF; WHO 2001). In addition to measuring functional communication outcomes, patient-reported outcomes (PRO) are gaining importance as a component of patient-oriented treatment (Hula et al. 2015). Some persons with aphasia recover to near-normal premorbid language and communication performance, while others remain severely aphasic. Almost every person has the potential for some level of functional communication, from being an independent communicator in a variety of communication interactions to being dependent upon an alternative or augmentative communication system or a conversational partner (Hachioui et al. 2013).

Models of Language, Communication, and Aphasia

Numerous models serve to guide assessment and treatment of persons with aphasia and foster understanding of how aphasia affects persons with aphasia and their family members. Theoretical influences underpinning these models range from impairment-based models, such as cognitive neuropsychological models of language processing, to models based on psychosocial theory, such as the A-FROM (Kagan et al. 2008). Cognitive neuropsychology brought to aphasia evaluation and treatment a set of models of human cognitive mechanisms and processes thought to underlie language performance. An individual's performance on several linguistic tasks is examined for patterns of impaired and spared cognitive processes in order to infer the cognitive architecture that underlies the performance. For example, in a model of lexical processing, the linguistic tasks might be lexical recognition (word/nonword identification), auditory comprehension (pointing to a named word), and naming a picture (confrontation naming). An individual who scores high on auditory comprehension and reading words tasks but low on confrontation naming may be inferred to show a deficit in phonological output lexicon but have an intact semantic system and ability to use phonic skills to read a word. That is, the individual may have intact semantic knowledge and be aware of the phonological form of a word and be able to read it but lack the phonological skills to generate the verbal label. The pattern of performance is important to note and serves to direct treatment to the impaired processes, using the spared processes as strengths. Cognitive neuropsychological models of language processing frequently used in aphasia assessment and treatment, however, are not without criticism as being descriptive and not prescriptive and requiring time-consuming assessment.

In contrast to the deficit-specific models of cognitive neuropsychology, other models recognize the importance of an individual's psychosocial state, quality of life, functional communication abilities, and communication network. Tanner (2003) proposed an eclectic approach to examine the psychology of aphasia from three perspectives: effects of brain injury, psychological defenses and coping styles, and responses to loss. This view speaks to the importance of an individual's premorbid personal characteristics, their ability to adjust to change, and their external support network as they and their family learn to live with aphasia. Several models and tools exist to guide assessment and treatment in these areas. For example, quality-of-life scales ask questions about topics such as family support and general outlook on life (e.g., communication-related quality-of-life scale; Cruice et al. 2003). An important model, the A-FROM (Living with Aphasia: Framework for Outcome Measurement; Kagan et al. 2008) espouses an integrated approach to aphasia assessment. The A-FROM clarifies outcomes in five domains: participation, aphasia severity, language and communication environment, personal factors/identity, and life with aphasia. Social network diagrams illustrate the breadth and depth of an individual's support and communication networks (e.g., Blackstone and Berg 2003).

While aphasia tests are founded on specific models of language, communication, or cognition, assessment and treatment activities often reflect a combination of impairment-based and activity/participation-based models.

Evaluation

Approaches to evaluation of aphasia vary with the conceptualization of aphasia.

Some approaches take an impairment-based approach, viewing aphasia as a disorder of selected abilities, while others, such as the Life Participation Approach to Aphasia (LPAA 2000) take an activity/participation approach, viewing aphasia as a disruption to communication and placing the person with aphasia and his or her family at the center of clinical decision-making activities. Schuell et al. (1964) proposed assessment based on the definition of aphasia as language deficit that crosses all modalities, all of which are examined in the *Minnesota Test for the Differential Diagnosis of Aphasia* (Schuell 1965). Chapey (2008) suggested that evaluation stem from a cognitive stimulation model, which views communication as a problem-solving and decision-making task. Following the World

Health Organization ICF (2001), models of assessment and treatment typically incorporate information at levels of impairment and activity/participation.

In contrast to language-based evaluation tools, some approaches to evaluation consider the circumstances in which treatment will be conducted. Group treatment has gained popularity in recent years, recognizing the value of social connectedness, and some assessment tools examine the social desires and needs of a person with aphasia (Avent 1997; Kearns and Elman 2008). Lubinski (2008) discussed an environmental model, suggesting that clinicians consider physical and social environments of a person with aphasia to enhance treatment effects. Finally, psychosocial models of intervention focus on integrating an individual into a communicating society and promoting their participation in personally relevant activities (Simmons-Mackie 2008). Regardless of the approach, in order to understand the linguistic and communicative abilities and needs of an individual, it is important to conduct evaluation within a culturally sensitive framework.

Three types of aphasia tests are commonly used to assess language and communication abilities in persons who have aphasia: screening tests (short assessments that may be administered at bedside), comprehensive aphasia tests (batteries containing several subtests to examine language behavior such as naming, reading, and writing), and tests of specific linguistic or communicative function (e.g., syntactic function or naming) (Patterson 2008). In addition, assessment of aphasia and its impact on a person's life include testing cognitive abilities (e.g., memory), testing executive functioning (e.g., divided attention), observing a person in activities of daily communication, and interviewing the person with aphasia and family members about the impact of aphasia on life participation and functional communication.

In aphasia assessment, it is as important to determine the presence or absence of aphasia and the presence of concomitant disorders, as it is to classify aphasia type, describe aphasia symptoms, and understand how the aphasia affects the individual and family. Sometimes only some of these goals can be achieved. Examples of disorders that may accompany aphasia but that are not aphasia are apraxia of speech, dysarthria, dementia, memory impairment, or psychiatric problems. These concomitant disorders will affect treatment planning and task selection. Medical conditions, such as diabetes, cardiovascular disease, and any medications the patient takes, may affect performance and should also be noted in the assessment report.

Sometimes people with aphasia experience depression, and several scales have been developed to screen for depression. Some have a linguistic bias or rely on caregiver report, while others have been adapted to be "aphasia friendly" and not depend exclusively on complex written sentences. Three examples of instruments to examine depression are the Stroke Aphasia Depression Questionnaire (SADQ) (Lincoln et al. 2000), the Aphasia Depression Questionnaire (Benaim et al. 2004), and the Visual Analog Mood Scale (Stern et al. 1997). The SADQ while designed for persons with aphasia has a linguistic bias and is intended to rely on caregiver report. The ADQ is a nine-item tool used to assess poststroke depression in persons who are hospitalized after a stroke. The VAMS is an example of a nonlinguistic mood scale used for self-report of depressive symptoms.

The goals of evaluation will vary depending upon factors such as severity of aphasia, age, and time post-onset. For example, an individual with mild aphasia who anticipates returning to work should have an assessment that includes detailed information on linguistic processing and a job task analysis to determine the linguistic requirements of the position. This information may be used to determine the individual's ability to return to a job, to identify communication requirements of the job, and to guide employment-related treatment. In contrast, evaluation for an individual with severe aphasia and concomitant severe apraxia of speech may require an evaluation focused on functional communication strategies to use with familiar communication partners within a contained environment.

Treatment

The acute stage of aphasia is the first few months after a stroke as the brain recovers from injury and is often characterized by spontaneous recovery of language and communication deficits, while in the chronic stage of aphasia, an individual learns to live with aphasia and returns to life activities. There are many well-validated, effective techniques for aphasia rehabilitation, particularly for chronic aphasia. These range from general stimulation approaches to treatments aimed at specific signs of aphasia and are chosen according to the patient's individual needs, goals, aphasia characteristics, and etiology. For aphasia due to acute-onset causes (e.g., vascular etiologies or trauma), therapy has been demonstrated to be effective both early after onset (Carpenter and Cherney 2016) and in the chronic stage. For aphasia due to progressive etiologies, therapy has been shown to be effective in maintaining functional communication and maximizing quality of communication life to the extent possible given the medical diagnosis (Beeson et al. 2011).

Pharmacological intervention for aphasia may be undertaken for direct treatment of the language deficit or administered to address a concomitant disorder, such as depression. Although research in this area is encouraging, to date, no pharmacologic treatment has emerged as consistently improving linguistic function without adverse side effects (Greener et al. 2001; Murray and Clark 2006; Troisi et al. 2002).

Treatment for aphasia historically focused primarily on restitution of function using impairment-based treatment techniques, with treatment targets such as word or sentence production or writing. Examples of these treatment techniques are Melodic Intonation Therapy, a semantic or phonologic cueing hierarchy, and confrontation naming. More recently, treatment goals have expanded to include activity/participation-based treatments such as functional communication and group therapy. Examples of activity/participation treatment methods are book groups for persons with aphasia (with the linguistic level of the book modified to be aphasia friendly), reciprocal scaffolding (e.g., Avent et al. 2009), and supported conversation (e.g., Kagan et al. 2001).

Recently intensive treatment has become a focus for aphasia rehabilitation. Intensive treatment can be measured by the amount and frequency of delivery of a treatment protocol. Warren et al. (2007) suggest using cumulative intervention intensity (a produce of dose of treatment, frequency, and total duration) to equate intensity across various treatments. Evidence supports intensive treatment for aphasia under careful considerations of treatment protocol and patient characteristics. Intensive treatment can be effective at all stages of recovery from aphasia. Another form of intensive treatment is the Intensive Comprehensive Aphasia Program (ICAP; Babbitt et al. 2015) where individuals with aphasia spend several hours each day for a few weeks completing multiple treatment activities.

The four principles of evidence-based practice, current best practices, clinical expertise, client/patient values, and context of treatment, guide treatment planning. Clinical practice research and clinical trials support the efficacy and effectiveness of aphasia therapy. Systematic reviews, such as the one for constraint-induced language therapy (Cherney et al. 2008), and meta-analyses (e.g., Robey 1998) report the evidence from group studies and single-subject research studies for a specific treatment or aphasia therapy in general. Cherney and Robey (2008) and the Academy of Neurological Communication Disorders and Sciences (ANCDS 2016) present analyses of treatment effect sizes of aphasia treatment for specific treatment areas such as syntax and language comprehension.

Cross-References

- ▶ Agnosia
- ▶ Agrammatism
- ▶ Agraphia
- ▶ American Speech-Language-Hearing Association (ASHA)
- ▶ Anarthria

- Anomic Aphasia
- Aphasia Tests
- Apraxia of Speech
- Augmentative and Alternative Communication (AAC)
- Boston Diagnostic Aphasia Examination
- Boston Naming Test
- Broca, Pierre Paul (1824–1880)
- Broca's Aphasia
- Conduction Aphasia
- Crossed Aphasia
- Cue
- Dysarthria
- Evidence-Based Practice
- Fluent Aphasia
- Global Aphasia
- Goodglass, Harold (1920–2002)
- Kaplan, Edith (1924–2009)
- Melodic Intonation Therapy
- Multilingual Aphasia Examination
- Neurosensory Center Comprehensive Examination for Aphasia
- Paragrammatism
- Paraphasia
- Pragmatic Communication
- Progressive Aphasia
- Semantic Paraphasia
- Speech-Language Therapy
- Subcortical Aphasia
- Telegraphic Speech
- Transcortical Motor Aphasia
- Transcortical Sensory Aphasia
- Wernicke, Karl (1848–1905)
- Wernicke–Lichtheim Model of Aphasia
- Wernicke's Aphasia
- Western Aphasia Battery

References and Readings

Academy of Neurological Communication Disorders and Sciences. (2016). Practice guidelines of the ANCDS: Evidence based practice guidelines for the management of communication disorders in neurologically impaired individuals. http://www.ancds.org/index.php?option=com_content&view=article&id=9&Itemid=9. Accessed 25 Feb 2016.

Avent, J. R. (1997). *Manual of cooperative group treatment for aphasia*. New York: Elsevier.

Avent, J., Patterson, J., Lu, A., & Small, K. (2009). Reciprocal scaffolding treatment: A person with aphasia as clinical teacher. *Aphasiology, 23*, 110–119.

Babbitt, E. M., Worrall, L., & Cherney, L. R. (2015). Structure, processes, and retrospective outcomes form and intensive comprehensive aphasia program. *American Journal of Speech-Language Pathology, 24*, S854–S863.

Basso, A. (1992). Prognostic factors in aphasia. *Aphasiology, 6*(4), 337–348.

Beeson, P. M., King, R. M., Bonakdarpour, B., Henry, M. L., Chou, H., & Rapcsak, S. Z. (2011). Positive effects of language treatment for the logopenic variant of primary progressive aphasia. *Journal of Molecular Neuroscience, 45*, 724–736.

Benaim, C., Cailly, B., Perennou, D., & Pellissier, J. (2004). Validation of the aphasic depression rating scale. *Stroke, 35*, 1692–1969.

Blackstone, S., & Hunt Berg, S. (2003). *Social networks: A communication inventory for individuals with complex communication needs and their communication partners*. Monterey, CA: Augmentative Communication Inc.

Caramazza, A. (1984). The logic of neuropsychological research and the problem of patient classification in aphasia. *Brain and Language, 21*(1), 9–20.

Carpenter, J., & Cherney, L. R. (2016). Increasing aphasia treatment in an acute inpatient rehabilitation setting programme: A feasibility study. *Aphasiology, 30*(5), 542–565.

Chapey, R. (2008). Cognitive stimulation: Stimulation of recognition/comprehension. Memory, and convergent, divergent, and evaluative thinking. In R. Chapey (Ed.), *Language intervention strategies in aphasia and related neurogenic communication disorders* (5th ed., pp. 469–506). Philadelphia: Wolters Kluwer.

Chapey, R., Duchan, J. F., Elman, R. J., Garcia, L. J., Kagan, A., Lyon, J., et al. (2008). Life participation approach to aphasia: A statement of values for the future. In R. Chapey (Ed.), *Language intervention strategies in aphasia and related neurogenic communication disorders* (5th ed., pp. 279–289). Philadelphia: Wolters Kluwer.

Cherney, L. R., & Robey, R. R. (2008). Aphasia treatment: Recovery, prognosis and clinical effectiveness. In R. Chapey (Ed.), *Language intervention strategies in aphasia and related neurogenic communication disorders* (5th ed., pp. 186–202). Philadelphia: Wolters Kluwer.

Cherney, L. R., Patterson, J. P., Raymer, S. M., Frymark, T., & Schooling, T. (2008). Evidence-based systematic review: Effects of intensity of treatment and constraint-induced language therapy for individuals with stroke-induced aphasia. *Journal of Speech-Language-Hearing Research, 51*, 1282–1299.

Crary, M. A., Werta, R. T., & Deal, J. L. (1992). Classifying aphasias: Cluster analysis of western aphasia battery and Boston diagnostic aphasia examination results. *Aphasiology, 6*(1), 29–36.

Cruice, M., Worral, L., Hickson, L., & Murison, R. (2003). Finding focus for quality of life with aphasia: Social and emotional health, and psychological well-being. *Aphasiology, 17*, 333–353.

Davis, G. A. (2006). *Aphasiology: Disorders and clinical practice*. Englewood Cliffs, NJ: Prentice Hall.

Greener, J., Enderby, P., & Whurr, R. (2001). Pharmacological treatment for aphasia following stroke. *Cochrane Database of Systematic Reviews*, (4), Article No.: CD000424. https://doi.org/10.1002/14651858. CD000424.

Hachioui, H. E. L., Lingsma, H. F., van de Sandt-Koenderman, M., Dippel, D. W. J., Kousdstaal, P. J., & Visch-Brink, E. G. (2013). Recovery of aphasia after stroke: A 1-year follow-up study. *Journal of Neurology, 260*, 166–171.

Hallowell, B., & Chapey, R. (2008). Introduction to language intervention strategies in aphasia. In R. Chapey (Ed.), *Language intervention strategies in aphasia and related neurogenic communication disorders* (5th ed., pp. 3–19). Philadelphia: Wolters Kluwer.

Kagan, A., Black, S. E., Duchan, J. F., Simmons-Mackie, N., & Square, P. (2001). Training volunteers as conversational partners using "Supported Conversation for Adults with aphasia" (SCA): A controlled trial. *Journal of Speech-Language-Hearing Research, 44*, 624–638.

Kagan, A., Simmons Mackie, N., Rowland, A., Huijbregts, M., Shumway, E., McEwen, S., et al. (2008). Counting what counts: A framework for capturing real-life outcomes of aphasia intervention. *Aphasiology, 22*(3), 258–280.

Kay, J., Lesser, R., & Coltheart, M. (1996). Psycholinguistic assessments of language processing in aphasia (PALPA): An introduction. *Aphasiology, 10*, 159–215.

Kearns, K., & Elman, R. (2008). Group therapy for aphasia: Theoretical and practical considerations. In R. Chapey (Ed.), *Language intervention strategies in aphasia and related neurogenic communication disorders* (5th ed., pp. 376–398). Philadelphia: Wolters Kluwer.

Kertesz, A. (1979). *Aphasia and associated disorders: Taxonomy localization and recovery*. New York: Grune & Stratton.

Lincoln, N. B., Sutcliffe, L. M., & Unsworth, G. (2000). Validation of the Stroke Aphasic Depression Questionnaire (SADQ) for use with patients in hospital. *Clinical Neuropsychological Assessment, 1*, 88–96.

LPAA Project Group. (2000). Life participation approach to aphasia: A statement of values for the future. *The ASHA Leader, 5*, 4–6.

Lubinski, R. (2008). Environmental approach to adult aphasia. In R. Chapey (Ed.), *Language intervention strategies in aphasia and related neurogenic communication disorders* (5th ed., pp. 319–349). Philadelphia: Wolters Kluwer.

McClung, J. S., Gonzalez Rothi, L. J., & Nadeau, S. E. (2010). Ambient experience in restitutive treatment of aphasia. *Frontiers in Human Neuroscience, 4*, Article 183, 1–19.

Moss, A., & Nicholas, M. (2006). Language rehabilitation in chronic aphasia and time postonset: A review of single-subject data. *Stroke, 37*, 3043–3051.

Murray, L. L., & Clark, H. M. (2006). *Neurogenic disorders of language: Theory driven clinical practice (chap. 10)*. Clifton Park, NY: Thompson Delmar Learning.

Patterson, J. P. (2008). Assessment of language disorders in adults. In R. Chapey (Ed.), *Language intervention strategies in aphasia and related neurogenic communication disorders* (pp. 64–160). Baltimore: Wolters Kluwer.

Pedersen, P. M., Jorgensen, H. S., Nakayama, H., Raaschou, H. O., & Olsen, T. S. (2004). Aphasia in acute stroke: Incidence, determinants, and recovery. *Annals of Neurology, 38*, 659–666.

Plowman, E., Hentz, B., & Ellis Jr., C. (2012). Post-stroke aphasia prognosis: A review of patient-related and stroke-related factors. *Journal of Evaluation in Clinical Practice, 18*, 689–694.

Robey, R. R. (1998). A meta-analysis of outcomes in the treatment of aphasia. *Journal of Speech-Language-Hearing Research, 41*, 172–187.

Schuell, H. H. (1965). *Minnesota test for differential diagnosis of aphasia*. Minneapolis: University of Minnesota Press.

Schuell, H., Jenkins, J., & Jimenez-Pabon, E. (1964). *Aphasia in adults*. New York: Harper medical Division.

Simmons-Mackie, N. (2008). Social approaches to aphasia intervention. In R. Chapey (Ed.), *Language intervention strategies in aphasia and related neurogenic communication disorders* (5th ed., pp. 290–318). Philadelphia: Wolters Kluwer.

Stern, R. A., Arruda, J. E., Hooper, C. R., Wolfner, G. D., & Morey, C. E. (1997). Visual analog mood scales to measure internal mood state in neurologically impaired patients: Description and initial validity evidence. *Aphasiology, 11*, 59–71.

Tanner, D. C. (2003). Eclectic perspectives on the psychology of aphasia. *Journal of Allied Health, 32*, 256–260.

Troisi, E., Paolucci, E., Silvestrini, M., Matteis, M., Vernieri, F., Grasso, M. G., et al. (2002). Prognostic factors in stroke rehabilitation: The possible role of pharmacological treatment. *Acta Neurologica Scandinavica, 105*, 100–106.

Warren, S. F., Fey, M. E., & Yoder, P. J. (2007). Differential treatment intensity research: A missing link to creating optimally effective communication interventions. *Mental Retardation and Developmental Disabilities Research Reviews, 13*, 70–77.

World Health Organization. (2001). *International classification of functioning, disability and health*. Geneva: Author. http://www.who.int/classifications/icfbrowser/. Accessed 30 Mar 2010.

Aphasia Diagnostic Profiles

Janet P. Patterson
Audiology and Speech-Language Pathology
Service, VA Northern California Health Care
System, Martinez, CA, USA

Description

The Aphasia Diagnostic Profiles (ADP; Helm-Estabrooks 1992) is an impairment-based measure (World Health Organization 2001) designed to assess language and communication skills in persons with aphasia, primarily following stroke. The ADP consists of nine subtests, each of which yields a standard score and percentiles. The subtests assess speech, language, and communication in all modalities (verbal and written), and the test emphasizes conversational interaction; verbal instructions to the patient are written in an informal style in the manner of conversation (e.g., "Well now that's out of the way, I'm going to turn on the tape recorder").

Responses are typically scored on a five-point scale: immediately correct, mostly correct, some correct, fully incorrect, and no response. Scores from the subtests are combined to produce five profiles describing the level of impairment of aphasia. The profiles are the Aphasia Classification Profile, the Aphasia Severity Profile, the Alternative Communication Profile, the Error Profiles, and the Behavioral Profile. Other scores of interest are the ADP Phrase length (average length of longest three phrases), Information Units (new pieces of information), and Index of Wordiness (Correct Information Units relative to total number of words). Table 1 shows the titles and a brief description of the nine subtests and five profiles.

The ADP is used to classify an individual's aphasia type as nonfluent, borderline fluent, or fluent. Using the lexical retrieval score, ADP phrase length, auditory comprehension score, and repetition score, the ADP further classifies the aphasia type as global, mixed nonfluent, Broca's, transcortical motor, Wernicke's,

Aphasia Diagnostic Profiles, Table 1 Aphasia diagnostic profiles: nine subtests and five profiles

ADP subtests	
Subtest	Description
Personal information	Verbal response to questions
Writing	Complete patient information sheet
Reading	Read items on patient information sheet
Fluency	Produce connected speech in three contexts
Naming	Name familiar pictured items
Auditory language comprehension	Answer questions – word, sentence, and story levels
Repetition	Repeat words and phrases
Elicited gestures	Pretend to complete action
Singing	Sing three familiar songs
ADP profiles	
Profile	Description
Aphasia classification profile	Identifies aphasia type (based on the Boston classification system)
Aphasia severity profile	Indicates specific strengths and weaknesses
Alternative communication profile	Identifies patient's strongest response modalities and guides therapy
Error profiles	Identifies the communicative value of a patient's responses
Behavioral profile	Indexes the patient's overall emotional state during testing

transcortical sensory, conduction, or anomic aphasia, following the conventions of the Boston aphasia classification system.

The ADP was created in part to address the need for a comprehensive aphasia battery that could be administered in a relatively brief time (40–50 min) in a medical setting. The manual is clearly written with explicit administration and scoring instructions. The record form is easy to use and facilitates the completion of the profile scores.

Historical Background

The ADP was first published in 1992 and since then has been frequently used in clinical and research activities. Numerous studies of aphasia treatment use the ADP as a measure of behavior change following intervention.

Psychometric Data

The ADP manual reported that it was standardized on 290 adults with neurological impairments (222 potentially aphasic adults) and 40 nonaphasic adults. The median age of these individuals was 70 years. The manual further reported reliability coefficients (inter-item consistency) for subtest raw scores that ranged from 0.73 (behavioral score) to 0.96 (repetition), with most of the coefficients in the 0.90 s. Test-retest coefficients ranged from 0.64 (elicited gestures) to 0.91 (information units). The ADP has a strong theoretical and psychometric foundation but has not been subjected to additional psychometric evaluation.

Clinical Uses

Three characteristics make the ADP a valuable clinical assessment tool: the theoretical foundation and close relationship to the Boston aphasia classification system, the structure of the test and clarity of the administration manual, and the amount of administration and scoring time required. It is also notable that both verbal and nonverbal modalities of communication are included in the assessment. One limitation of the ADP is that it does not examine any linguistic, psycholinguistic, or neuropsychological behavior in detail; additional tests in specific areas would be required to obtain in-depth information as part of an extensive diagnostic evaluation.

Cross-References

▶ Anomia
▶ Anomic Aphasia
▶ Aphasia

▶ Aphasia Tests
▶ Boston Diagnostic Aphasia Examination
▶ Broca's Aphasia
▶ Conduction Aphasia
▶ Global Aphasia
▶ Goodglass, Harold (1920–2002)
▶ Kaplan, Edith (1924–2009)
▶ Repetition
▶ Speech/Communication Disabilities
▶ Speech-Language Therapy
▶ Transcortical Motor Aphasia
▶ Transcortical Sensory Aphasia
▶ Wernicke, Karl (1848–1905)
▶ Wernicke's Aphasia

References and Readings

Helm-Estabrooks, N. (1992). *Aphasia diagnostic profiles.* Austin: Pro Ed.
World Health Organization. (2001). *International classification of functioning, disability and health..* http://www.who.int/classifications/icfbrowser/.

Aphasia Tests

Janet P. Patterson
Audiology and Speech-Language Pathology Service, VA Northern California Health Care System, Martinez, CA, USA

Synonyms

Aphasia assessment; Aphasia diagnosis; Aphasia evaluation

Description

Tests of aphasia are used to diagnose the type and severity of aphasia and related disorders and to plan intervention for the speech, language, and communication deficits demonstrated by persons who have aphasia following brain injury (PWA). Three types of aphasia tests are commonly used to assess language and communication abilities in PWA: screening tests, comprehensive aphasia batteries, and tests of specific linguistic or communicative function (Patterson 2008, 2015). In addition, assessment of aphasia and its impact on a person's life includes testing cognitive abilities and related disorders (e.g., memory), testing executive functioning (e.g., attention and planning), observing a person in activities of daily communication (e.g., social functional communication or work-related communication), interviewing the person with aphasia and family members, assessing quality of communication life and communication participation, and determining an individual's candidacy for use of alternative and augmentative communicative systems (e.g., an alphabet board to spell words, drawing, or a commercially available device).

Historical Background

Aphasia has been assessed more or less systematically for many years. Clinical observation was the earliest method of assessment, and the first standardized test was published in 1926 by Henry Head. In the ensuing years, several comprehensive aphasia tests and specific linguistic tests appeared. Each comprehensive test is based upon a theoretical model of aphasia, and although the tests contain common subtests (e.g., sentence repetition), the test results and aphasia diagnoses vary. For example, the *Minnesota Test for Differential Diagnosis of Aphasia* (Schuell 1965) assesses language performance across several modalities and rests upon Schuell's theory of aphasia as a unitary reduction in language across modalities with or without accompanying perceptual or motor deficits. In contrast, the *Boston Diagnostic Aphasia Examination* (Goodglass et al. 2001) relates speech and language behavioral deficits to neurological lesions. With yet a different perspective, Luria (1966) proposed a comprehensive examination for aphasia through nonstandardized observation of language performance in several modalities, but without specific subtests.

In recent years, several tests have emerged to assess specific language or communication functions in PWA, or to complete testing in a shorter period of time. For example, the *ASHA-FACS* (Frattali et al. 1995) assesses functional communication skills such as participating in conversation, while the *Reading Comprehension Battery for Aphasia – 2* (LaPointe and Horner 1998) evaluates reading performance in several contexts, such as single words and paragraphs. *The Aphasia Rapid Test* (Azur et al. 2013) is a bedside scale developed for administration in acute stroke settings.

Psychometric Data

The availability of psychometric data for aphasia tests ranges from prolific and well documented for some tests to minimal or nonexistent for others, and the data appear in scholarly journals as well as in the test manuals. Spreen and Risser (2003) and Strauss et al. (2006) provide overviews of psychometric data for many general aphasia tests and supplemental language tests. Few studies, and none recently, compare psychometric data across tests. In evaluating a general or supplemental test for aphasia, several factors should be considered, including size and definition of the standardization sample; reports of item, concurrent and predictive validity; test-retest, interrater and intrarater reliability; report of raw score means, standard deviations, ranges, and standard error of measurement; information about test development, examiner qualifications, administration instructions, scoring, and interpretation; and normative data.

Although it is difficult to judge which of the many aphasia tests best meets all the factors mentioned above, five tests are frequently used in clinical settings and have the most psychometric data published about them: *Boston Diagnostic Aphasia Examination, Boston Naming Test, Token Test* (and *Revised Token Test*), *the Comprehensive Aphasia Test,* and *Western Aphasia Battery.*

Clinical Uses

Screening Tests for Aphasia

Screening tests for aphasia are brief and may be administered at bedside. Their purpose is to rapidly determine the presence of aphasia or the need for further assessment. A screening test may be independent (e.g., *Quick Assessment for Aphasia*; Tanner and Culbertson 1999) or a shortened form of a comprehensive aphasia battery, such as the *Western Aphasia Battery* (WAB; Kertesz 2006).

Comprehensive Aphasia Batteries

A comprehensive aphasia battery is based on a theoretical model of aphasia and contains several subtests. For example, the *Boston Diagnostic Aphasia Examination* (Goodglass et al. 2001a, b) has 34 subtests, and the performance pattern is used to classify an individual with an aphasia type (e.g., Broca's aphasia). Although some subtests of comprehensive aphasia batteries may appear similar, the data obtained from each of the subtests and the resulting aphasia diagnosis will vary according to the theoretical model of aphasia which underlies the test. Other comprehensive aphasia batteries are the *Comprehensive Aphasia Test* (Swinburn et al. 2004; *the Western Aphasia Battery* (Kertesz 2006), *the Multilingual Aphasia Examination* (Benton et al. 1994), and *the Neurosensory Center Comprehensive Examination for Aphasia* (Spreen and Benton 1977).

Tests of Specific Linguistic or Communication Function

Tests of specific functions provide detailed information about a person's abilities in one area of linguistic or communication ability and are particularly useful for persons who have severe or minimal aphasia and for whom comprehensive aphasia batteries would understate communication strengths and weaknesses. Three examples are the *Revised Token Test* (McNeil and Prescott 1978) for auditory comprehension, the *Boston Naming Test* (Goodglass et al. 2001b) for oral naming, and the *Psycholinguistic Assessments of Language Processing in Aphasia* (Kay et al. 1992) The PALPA uses a cognitive neuropsychological model of language to understand the deficit at the various stages of language processing.

Tests of Cognitive-Communication Abilities and Related Functions

Tests of cognitive-communicative abilities related to language functions have been included as part of comprehensive aphasia batteries (e.g., the *Raven's Progressive Matrices* (Raven et al. 1995) as part of the Cortical Quotient in the WAB) or administered independently (e.g., *Wechsler Memory Scale*; Wechsler 2009).

Tests of Functional Communication

Functional communication abilities in PWA are assessed through observation or the use of specific tests. Functional communication includes verbal and nonverbal methods of conveying information in activities of daily living, such as reading signs, greeting individuals, and participating in conversation. Functional communication assessed through observation can be contextually bound, such as assessing conversation with familiar or unfamiliar partners. Tests of functional communication are intended to simulate activities of daily living but typically are acontextual. Two examples of tests of functional communication are the *Communicative Activities of Daily Living – 2* (Holland et al. 1999) and the *Assessment of Language-Related Functional Activities* (Baines et al. 1999).

Functional communication can also be assessed in a contextually sensitive manner through checklists or scales, as observed by clinicians or reported by persons with aphasia or their family members. Prutting and Kirchner (1987) published the pragmatic protocol which is a list of communicative acts that are rated as appropriate, inappropriate, or no opportunity to observe. The third rating type is important in assessing functional communication because not all communicative acts can be observed within an interaction. Other examples of checklists or scales are the *Functional Assessment of Communication Skills for Adults* (ASHA FACS; Frattali et al. 1995), the *Functional Communication Profile* (FCP; Sarno 1969), the *Communicative Confidence Rating Scale for Aphasia* (CCRSA; Babbitt and Cherney 2010), and the *Communicative Effectiveness Index* (CETI; Lomas et al. 1989).

Related to but non-synonymous with functional communication is quality of life, or more specific to aphasia, quality of communication life (QCL). QCL examines the impact of a communication disorder on life aspects of a person with aphasia, for example, participation in social, vocational, or educational activities, communication with friends and family, and development of satisfying relationships. Examples of tools to measure QCL are the *Quality of Communication Life Scale* (ASHA QCL; Paul et al. 2004), the *Stroke and Aphasia Quality of Life Scale-39* (SAQOL-39; Hilari et al. 2003), and the *Assessment for Living with Aphasia* (ALA; Simmons-Mackie et al. 2014).

Patient-Reported Outcomes

Patient-reported outcomes (PRO) as a status report on a health condition have gained importance in understanding assessment and treatment. In addition to measuring patient reports of communication, a PRO in aphasia testing also measures the physical, cognitive, and psychological burdens of stroke on the person with aphasia and family members. Two examples of aphasia assessment PRO tools are the *Aphasia Communication Outcome Measure* (ACOM; Hula et al. 2015) and the *Burden of Stroke Scale* (BOSS; Doyle et al. 2004).

Cross-References

▶ Activities of Daily Living (ADL)
▶ Aphasia
▶ Augmentative and Alternative Communication (AAC)
▶ Boston Diagnostic Aphasia Examination
▶ Boston Naming Test

▶ Luria, Alexander Romanovich (1902–1977)
▶ Multilingual Aphasia Examination
▶ Neurosensory Center Comprehensive Examination for Aphasia
▶ Wechsler Memory Scale All Versions
▶ Western Aphasia Battery

References and Readings

Azur, C., Leger, A., Arbizu, C., Henry-Amar, F., Chomel-Guillame, S., & Samson, Y. (2013). The aphasia rapid test: An NIHSS-like aphasia test. *Journal of Neurology, 260*(8), 2110–2117.

Babbitt, E. M., & Cherney, L. R. (2010). Communication confidence in persons with aphasia. *Topics in Stroke Rehabilitation, 17*(3), 197–206.

Baines, K. A., Martin, K. W., & Heeringa, H. M. (1999). *ALFA: Assessment of Language Related Functional Activities*. Austin: Pro-Ed.

Benton, A. L., Hamsher, K., Rey, G. J., & Sivan, A. B. (1994). *Multilingual Aphasia Examination (MAE-3)*. Lutz: Psychological Assessment Resources Inc (PAR).

Davis, G. A. (2007). *Aphasiology: Disorders and clinical practice* (2nd ed.). Boston: Pearson Allyn & Bacon.

Doyle, P. J., McNeil, M. R., Mikolic, J. M., Prieto, L., Hula, W. D., Lustig, A. P., Ross, K. B., Wambaugh, J. L., Gonzalez-Rothi, L. J., & Elman, R. J. (2004). The Burden of Stroke Scale (BOSS) provides valid and reliable score estimates of functioning and well-being in stroke survivors with and without communication disorders. *Journal of Clinical Epidemiology, 57*, 997–1007.

Frattali, C. M., Thompson, C. K., Holland, A. L., Wohl, C. B., & Ferketic, M. M. (1995). *The American Speech-Language-Hearing Association Functional Assessment of Communication Skills in Adults*. Rockville: The American Speech-Language-Hearing Association.

Goodglass, H., Kaplan, E., & Weintraub, S. (2001a). *Boston Naming Test* (2nd ed.). Austin: Pro-Ed.

Goodglass, H., Kaplan, E., & Baressi, B. (2001b). *Boston Diagnostic Aphasia Examination* (3rd ed.). San Antonio: Psychological Corporation.

Head, H. (1926). *Aphasia and kindred disorders of speech*. New York: MacMillan.

Hilari, K., Byng, S., Lamping, D. L., & Smith, S. C. (2003). Stroke and Aphasia Quality of Life Scale-39 (SAQOL-39): Evaluation of acceptability, reliability, and validity. *Stroke, 34*(8), 1944–1950.

Holland, A. L., Frattali, C. M., & Fromm, D. (1999). *Communicative Activities of Daily Living* (2nd ed.). San Antonino: Psychological Corporation.

Hula, W. D., Doyle, P. J., Stone, C. A., Hula, S. N. A., Kellough, S., Wambaugh, J. L., Ross, K. B.,

Schumacher, J. G., & St. Jacque, A. (2015). The Aphasia Communication Outcome Measure (ACOM): Dimensionality, item bank calibration, and initial validation. *Journal of Speech, Language, and Hearing Research, 58,* 906–919.

Kay, J., Lesser, R., & Coltheart, M. (1992). *Psycholinguistic Assessments of Language Processing in Aphasia.* London: Taylor & Francis Group.

Kertesz, A. (2006). *Western Aphasia Battery.* New York: Grune & Stratton.

LaPointe, L. L., & Horner, J. (1998). *Reading Comprehension Battery for Aphasia (RCBA-2).* San Antonio: Pearson.

Lomas, J., Pickard, L., Bester, S., Elbard, H., Finlayson, A., & Zoghaib, C. (1989). The Communicative Effectiveness Index: Development and psychometric evaluation of a functional communication measure for adult aphasia. *Journal of Speech and Hearing Disorders, 54,* 113–124.

Luria, A. R. (1966). *Higher cortical functions in man.* New York: Basic Books.

McNeil, M. R., & Prescott, T. E. (1978). *Revised Token Test.* Austin: Pro-Ed.

Patterson, J. P. (2008). Assessment of language disorders in adults. In R. Chapey (Ed.), *Language intervention strategies in aphasia and related neurogenic communication disorders* (5th ed., pp. 64–160). Baltimore: Wolters Kluwer.

Patterson, J. P. (2015). Aphasia assessment. In A.M. Raymer & L. Gonzalez-Rothi (Eds.). *The Oxford handbook of aphasia and language disorders.* New York: Oxford University Press.

Paul, D., Fratalli, C. M., Holland, A. L., Thompson, C. K., Caperton, C. J., & Slater, S. C. (2004). *Quality of Communication Life Scale.* Rockville: American Speech-Language-Hearing Association (ASHA).

Prutting, C., & Kirchner, D. (1987). A clinical appraisal of the pragmatic aspects of language. *Journal of Speech and Hearing Disorders, 52,* 105–119.

Raven, J., Court, J., & Raven, J. C. (1995). *Raven's Progressive Matrices.* San Antonio: The Psychological Corporation.

Sarno, M. T. (1969). *The Functional Communication Profile.* New York: Institute of Rehabilitation Medicine, New York University Medical Center.

Schuell, H. (1965). *Minnesota Test for Differential Diagnosis of Aphasia.* Minneapolis: University of Minnesota Press.

Spreen, O., & Benton, A. L. (1977). *Neurosensory Center Comprehensive Examination for Aphasia.* Victoria: University of Victoria Neuropsychology Laboratory.

Spreen, O., & Risser, A. H. (2003). *Assessment of aphasia.* Oxford: Oxford University Press.

Strauss, E., Sherman, E. M. S., & Spreen, O. (2006). *A compendium of neuropsychological tests: Administration, norms and commentary* (3rd ed.). Oxford: Oxford University Press.

Swinburn, K., Porter, G., & Howard, D. (2004). *Comprehensive Aphasia Test.* Hove: Psychology Press, Inc.

Tanner, D.C. & Culbertson, W. (1999). *Quick Assessment for Aphasia.* Oceanside CA: Academic Communication Associates, Inc.

Wechsler, D. M. (2009). *Wechsler Memory Scale* (4th ed.). San Antonio: Psychological Corporation.

AphasiaBank/TalkBank

Roberta DePompei
School of Speech-Language Pathology and Audiology, University of Akron, Akron, OH, USA

Definition

The AphasiaBank/TalkBank is a federally funded project that supplies interested professionals with information about aphasia from both a practical and research (data based) perspective.

It is a shared database of multimedia interactions for the study of communication in aphasia. Access to AphasiaBank is through www.AphasiaBank.com. While some information can be seen immediately, access to the data in AphasiaBank is password protected and restricted to members of the AphasiaBank consortium group.

Researchers and clinicians working with aphasia who are interested in joining the consortium should read the Ground Rules and then send email to macw@cmu.edu with contact information and affiliation.

Aphonia

Lyn S. Turkstra
School of Rehabilitation Science, McMaster University, Hamilton, ON, Canada

Synonyms

Mutism

Definition

Aphonia is the complete absence of voice, i.e., adduction and vibration of the vocal folds are insufficient for vocal production. Aphonia may be associated with vocal fold paralysis; trauma; severe cases of inflammation, edema, or scarring of the vocal folds; benign or malignant diseases of the vocal folds that interfere with vocal fold closure; neurologically based movement disorders (e.g., spasmodic dysphonia); overuse of the voice; or somatoform disorders (e.g., in forms of elective mutism). Aphonia may be intermittent or episodic. For example, individuals with spasmodic dysphonia may have periodic, abnormal abduction or adduction of the vocal folds that may be perceived as voice breaks. Individuals who stutter also may have periodic voice breaks, in this case associated with tight adduction of the vocal folds.

When voice loss is incomplete, or when vocal quality is affected without complete loss of voice (e.g., if the voice is hoarse), it is referred to as dysphonia. Aphonia and dysphonia refer specifically to abnormal sound output from the phonatory sound source (i.e., the larynx) and should be distinguished from anarthria or dysarthria, which are disorders of articulation, i.e., related to the movements of the tongue, lips, jaw, and soft palate. Accordingly, dysphonia or aphonia can occur independently from anarthria or dysarthria.

Cross-References

▶ Dysphonia

References and Readings

Merati, A., & Bielamowicz, S. (Eds.). (2007). *Textbook of voice disorders*. San Diego: Plural Publishing.
Stemple, J. C., Glaze, L. E., & Klaben, B. G. (2000). *Clinical voice pathology, theory & management* (3rd ed.). Thompson Learning (now Florence: Cengage Learning).

Apolipoprotein E

John DeLuca
Research Department, Kessler Foundation, West Orange, NJ, USA

Definition

Apolipoprotein E (ApoE) is a polymorphic plasma glycoprotein that transports cholesterol and other lipids and has been shown to be involved in the growth and repair of neurons. There is also some evidence to suggest that ApoE is involved in lipid redistribution after demyelination. The ApoE protein is mapped to chromosome 19 and is polymorphic with three major isoforms, each of which translates into three alleles of the gene: ApoE-2, ApoE-3, and ApoE-4. ApoE-2 is associated with the genetic disorder type III hyperlipoproteinemia. There is also some evidence that this allele may serve as a protective role in the development of Alzheimer's disease (AD). ApoE-3 is found in approximately 64% of the population and is considered as the "neutral" ApoE genotype. ApoE-4 has been implicated in atherosclerosis and AD and impaired cognitive functioning. More specifically, ApoE-4 has been shown to be a major risk factor for development of AD and has been associated with subtle neuropsychological deficits in preclinical AD. Brain changes associated with ApoE-4 in AD include increased counts of amyloid plaques and neurofibrillary tangles, smaller medial temporal lobe structures, reduced glucose metabolism, and depletion of cholinergic markers in the hippocampus, frontal, and temporal cortices. ApoE-4 has also been associated with adverse recovery after traumatic brain injury (TBI). Persons with TBI with the ApoE-4 allele are ten times more likely to develop AD than those without the ApoE-4 allele. In multiple sclerosis, ApoE-4 has been found to be associated with rapid disease progression and increased cognitive impairment, although the findings for cognitive impairment have been inconsistent.

Cross-References

▶ Alzheimer's Disease

References and Readings

Plomin, R., Defries, J. C., Craig, I. W., & McGuffin, P. (2003). *Behavioral genetics in the postgenomic era.* Washington, DC: American Psychological Association.

Apoptosis

Kathleen L. Fuchs
Department of Neurology, University of Virginia
Health System, Charlottesville, VA, USA

Synonyms

Programmed cell death

Definition

Apoptosis is both a normal developmental process to rid the body of overproduced cells as well as a sign of pathology in mature neural systems. Apoptosis involves activation of caspases - proteins that cleave other proteins in order to inactivate or modulate them to trigger "pro-death" molecular pathways. The resulting cellular debris is then removed by microglia in the central nervous system. Abnormal protein cleavage and cell death has been implicated in neurodegenerative disorders such as Alzheimer's disease as well as autoimmune disorders such as multiple sclerosis.

Cross-References

▶ Alzheimer's Disease
▶ Multiple Sclerosis

References and Readings

Hengartner, M. O. (2000). The biochemistry of apoptosis. *Nature, 407,* 770–776.
Yuan, J., & Yankner, B. A. (2000). Apoptosis in the nervous system. *Nature, 407,* 802–809.

Appalic Syndrome

Dona Locke
Psychiatry and Psychology, Mayo Clinic, Scottsdale, AZ, USA

Synonyms

Persistent vegetative state; Unresponsiveness wakefulness syndrome

Definition

Apallic syndrome is an older term that was first replaced by **persistent vegetative state**. More recently, **unresponsive wakefulness syndrome (UWS)** is the proposed nomenclature. The syndrome is a clinical condition describing patients who fail to show voluntary motor responsiveness in the presence of eyes-open wakefulness. Patients show reflexive behavior such as spontaneous breathing, but no signs of awareness of the self or the environment. A thorough clinical evaluation may be required to distinguish between UWS and other conditions, including coma, brain death, and locked-in syndrome.

Cross-References

▶ Brain Death
▶ Coma
▶ Locked-in Syndrome
▶ Minimally Conscious State
▶ Minimally Responsive State

References and Readings

(1994). Medical aspects of the persistent vegetative state-first of two parts. *NEJM, 330,* 1499–1508.

Multi-society task force on PVS (1994). Medical aspects of the persistent vegetative state-second of two parts. *NEJM, 330,* 1572–1579.

Laureys, S., Celesia, G. G., Cohadon, F., Lavrijsen, J., et al. (2010). Unresponsive wakefulness syndrome: A new name for the vegetative state or apallic syndrome. *BMC Medicine, 8,* 68.

van Erp, W., Lavrijsen, J. C. M., van de Laar, F. A, Vos, P . E., Laureys S., Koopmans, R. T. C. M. (2014). The vegetative state/unresponsiveness wakefulness syndrome: A systematic review of prevalence studies. *European Journal of Neurology, 21,* 1361–1368.

Apperceptive Visual Agnosia

John E. Mendoza
Department of Psychiatry and Neuroscience, Tulane Medical School and SE Louisiana Veterans Healthcare System, New Orleans, LA, USA

Definition

Inability or marked difficulty in visually identifying an object or picture of an object as a result of impaired perceptual abilities. In apperceptive agnosia, in addition to problems in the visual identification of an object, patients show impairment in reproducing (e.g., by drawing) the object or image and even matching the item to a similar one within a visual array. This contrasts with associative visual agnosia in which identification may also be impaired but the patient can usually render a reasonable representation (e.g., a drawing or graphomotor copy) of the object that cannot be visually identified and can visually match it to a sample. Apperceptive visual agnosia likely results from a defect in the secondary association areas of the visual cortex and is usually found in patients who complain of general loss or reduction in visual acuity.

Cross-References

▶ Associative Visual Agnosia

References and Readings

Bauer, R. M., & Demery, J. A. (2003). Agnosia. In K. Heilman & E. Valenstein (Eds.), *Clinical neuropsychology* (4th ed., pp. 236–295). New York: Oxford University Press.

DeRenzi, E., & Spinnler, H. (1966). Visual recognition in patients with unilateral cerebral disease. *Journal of Nervous and Mental Disease, 142,* 513–525.

DeRenzi, E., Scotti, G., & Spinnler, H. (1969). Perceptual and associative disorders of visual recognition. Relationship to the side of the cerebral lesion. *Neurology, 19,* 634–642.

Appercetive Agnosia

Talia R. Seider[1,2], Ronald A. Cohen[1,2] and Adam J. Woods[1,2,3]
[1]Department of Clinical and Health Psychology, College of Public Health and Health Professions, University of Florida, Gainesville, FL, USA
[2]Center for Cognitive Aging and Memory, McKnight Brain Institute, University of Florida, Gainesville, FL, USA
[3]Department of Neuroscience, University of Florida, Gainesville, FL, USA

A failure to recognize a stimulus due to impaired perceptual abilities, although elementary sensory functions (acuity, color vision, etc.) are intact. Though most cases of apperceptive agnosia are visual, auditory and tactile cases have also been reported. Patients with visual apperceptive agnosia are a heterogeneous group who typically have damage in visual association cortices and appear to have a profound visual deficit. While both apperceptive and associative agnosics have difficulty with object naming, they can be differentiated in that the associative agnosic will be able to copy a drawing of the object, while the apperceptive agnosic will have difficulty drawing it or matching it to a visually similar stimulus.

References and Readings

Bauer, R. M. (2012). Agnosia. In K. M. Heilman & E. Valenstein (Eds.), *Clinical neuropsychology* (5th ed., pp. 238–295). New York: Oxford University Press.

DeRenzi, E., Scotti, G., & Spinnler, H. (1969). Perceptual and associative disorders of visual recognition. Relationship to the side of the cerebral lesion. *Neurology, 19*, 634–642.

Shelton, P. A., Bowers, D., Duara, R., & Heilman, K. M. (1994). Apperceptive visual agnosia: a case study. *Brain and Cognition, 25*(1), 1–23.

Applied Behavior Analysis

Michael J. Hartman and Tiffany Kodak
Department of Psychology, University of
Wisconsin-Milwaukee, Milwaukee, WI, USA

Introduction to Applied Behavior Analysis

Applied behavior analysis (ABA) is a science in which principles of behavior are applied to problems of social importance (Cooper et al. 2007). Behavior analysts seek to predict and control behavior, and they are interested in analyzing and identifying environmental events surrounding behavior. Several categories of environmental events are important in the prediction and control of a given behavior. These include: (a) the broader environmental context in which behavior occurs (e.g., employees behave differently while in the workplace than at a holiday party), (b) motivational variables (e.g., asking for a glass of water is more likely to occur following a strenuous workout), (c) events that correlate with the availability of consequences for a response (e.g., turning the handle on a doorknob and pulling the door open will be successful if the deadbolt is unlocked), and (d) the consequence(s) of a response (e.g., touching a hot stove may result in an aversive state and will be less likely to occur in the future; Fisher et al. 2011). With insight into the environmental variables surrounding the behavior of interest, behavior analysts can predict behavior and alter responding based on manipulations of one or more of these variables.

Whereas some scientists in other fields of psychology assume that human behavior is indicative of underlying cognitive mechanisms, behavior analysts do not. That is, behavior is studied as a subject matter in its own right. Nevertheless, a common misconception in other fields is that behavior analysts deny the existence of covert (unobservable) behavior such as thinking. However, behavior analysts affirm the existence of covert behavior under the premise that these events are governed by the same laws that govern overt (observable) behavior (Moore 2009).

Several dimensions define the field of ABA and were described in a seminal article by Baer et al. (1968). These dimensions stipulate that applied behavior analytic research is (a) applied, defined as addressing socially significant problems; (b) behavioral, defined as using the behavior of the organism as the subject matter; (c), analytic, defined as using objective and controlled designs that engender clear demonstrations of a functional relation between an independent variable (e.g., a behavioral intervention) and target behavior; (d) technological, defined as providing precise descriptions of experimental methods in sufficient detail so that the procedure can be replicated by other behavior analysts; (e) conceptually systematic, defined as linking the results of the study to behavioral principles in order to produce a body of science; (f) effective, defined as showing changes in behavior that are observable via visual inspection of graphical displays and are clinically significant, and contrasts other areas in psychology in which statistical significance is used to determine intervention efficacy; and (g) generalizable, defined as behavior that occurs across settings and people, is durable over time, and when the effects of intervention spread across behavior. Studies which meet these criteria are described as consistent with an applied behavior analysis.

Operant and Classical Conditioning

The science of ABA is based on the fact that behaviors are learned (Fisher et al. 2011). There exist two mechanisms through which organisms learn: operant conditioning and classical conditioning. Both learning processes describe changes in the probability of a response given specific environmental events and learning histories.

Classical conditioning is the process by which responses occur because of learned associations between neutral stimuli and stimuli that automatically elicit a response (Chance 2014). For example, a puff of air in the eye (i.e., an unconditioned stimulus) elicits the reflex of blinking (i.e., an unconditioned response). A neutral stimulus (e.g., a clicking sound) can become a conditioned stimulus and elicit an eyeblink if the sound consistently precedes a puff of air into the eye. Though this chapter focuses on operant conditioning, classical conditioning has been used successfully to address socially significant issues (e.g., Whitehead et al. 1976).

Operant conditioning involves changes in the probability of a behavior as a function of consequences that follow the behavior (Miltenberger 2012). Thus, operant behavior is selected, altered, and maintained by consequences. The effects that consequences have on behavior are either reinforcing or punishing. That is, a specific behavior is *more* likely to occur in the future if a reinforcer tends to follow the behavior, and a specific behavior is *less* likely to occur in the future if an aversive consequence tends to follow the behavior, respectively. Importantly, consequences are defined as reinforcers or punishers based on their effects on behavior.

Components of Applied Behavior Analysis

An early step in the analysis of behavior is to develop definitions of the behavior of interest, which are referred to as operational definitions. Subjective terms (e.g., anxiety) to define behavior are avoided; rather, behavior is objectively described so that it can be reliably measured by multiple observers. Further, behavior analysts utilize direct measurement systems (e.g., observing an individual during specified intervals) rather than indirect measurement systems (e.g., self-reports, personality inventories) to collect data on the behavior of interest. A common direct measurement method is to record the frequency of a target behavior during which observers record each occurrence of a response. For example, head-hitting is often recorded using a frequency method, as it is readily discernable when this target behavior is and is not occurring. Behavior analysts also measure the duration of behavior to record the amount of time an individual engages in a target response. This method is best for recording behavior that may occur less often but is problematic due to the duration of time spent engaging in the behavior (e.g., crying). To ensure that measurement systems are reliable, behavior analysts assess interobserver agreement which provides an estimate of agreement on the occurrence of behavior across multiple observers. This type of reliability provides verification of the level of accuracy in the data collected on the target behavior.

Once behavior is precisely defined and can be reliably measured, the goal of most behavioral assessments is to identify the variables responsible for operant behavior (discussed above). To guide these investigations, researcher use a model of operant behavior referred to as the three-term contingency. This model asserts that behavior is controlled by both (a) antecedent events, which set the occasion for behavior to occur (e.g., the removal of a preferred activity or the introduction of a demand) and (b) consequence events, which follow behavior.

Michael (1982) further refined the field's understanding of the three-term contingency with the addition of a second antecedent variable, referred to as motivating operations (MOs). Motivating operations are events that alter the probability of a response (i.e., behavior-altering effect) and the value of a consequence that typically follows the behavior (i.e., the value-altering effect). For example, MOs that increase the probability of a response and value of a consequence are referred to as establishing operations (EOs), and MOs that decrease the probability of a response and value of a consequence are referred to as abolishing operations (AOs). Consistent with the conceptual framework of behavior analysis, MOs fluctuate based on changes in an organism's environment. For example, lengthy periods of sleep deprivation increase the probability of behavior that typically produces sleep (e.g., lying in bed) and the value of sleep.

Functional relationships between environmental variables and behavior are analyzed using single-subject experimental designs, which are carefully designed to aid in the identification of such relationships (Fisher et al. 2011). Further, single-subject designs help to ensure that ABA research continually abides to the tenets discussed in Baer et al. (1968). That is, single-subject designs permit an evaluation of the extent to which observed differences in behavior following the introduction of intervention reflect clinically significant differences for all individuals in an experimental group. The single-subject design is preferable to the group design because an emphasis is placed on the importance of a beneficial intervention outcome for each individual, not a statistically significant outcome for group means. Participants who do not demonstrate a clinically significant treatment effect may receive additional interventions that are tailored to the individual. Furthermore, individuals serve as their own control from which repeated measures of behavior are compared. The purpose of a single-subject design is to permit a valid demonstration of the prediction and control over behavior.

A common experimental design that behavior analysts use to demonstrate a functional relationship is a reversal design (Bailey and Burch 2002). In this design, the independent variable is introduced and removed systematically to demonstrate its effect on the dependent variable. The strength of the relationship between variables can be determined by the magnitude of change in behavior. Experimental control is shown within the reversal design when behavior "turns on" with the introduction of independent variable and "turns off" when the independent variable is removed.

Strategies for Behavior Change

As discussed previously, the main goal of applied behavior analysis is to solve problems of social significance using behavioral principles. Researchers and clinicians alike have identified three categories for tactics to modify behavior. Broadly, and with some overlap, these tactics serve the purpose to (a) increase the prevalence of a desired behavior, (b) decrease the prevalence of problem behavior, and/or (c) bring a target behavior under contextual control so that it occurs in some contexts but not others (referred to as stimulus control).

Increasing Behavior. Behavioral treatment packages often identify responses that are desirable or appropriate. For example, a child with an intellectual disability may have limited communication. In such a scenario, it is beneficial to teach functional communication skills that the individual can emit to interact effectively in his or her environment (e.g., ask for a snack, have a conversation). Common strategies that are used to increase behavior include prompts and differential reinforcement. A prompt is any stimulus that produces the target response (Miltenberger 2012). A prompt is provided by an instructor to help the learner perform the appropriate behavior so that the behavior can produce a reinforcing consequence, which will increase the probability of the occurrence of the appropriate behavior in the future. For example, an adult uses a model prompt with a child by showing (modeling) how to zip up her coat, and the child has the opportunity to imitate the adult's model thereafter.

Differential reinforcement occurs when one behavior produces the reinforcing consequence and another behavior does not produce the reinforcing consequence (Vladescu and Kodak 2010). For example, during early instruction for a novel skill, an instructor may provide a reinforcer following a prompted correct response (e.g., asking for help with a task after the adult provides a prompt to demonstrate how to ask for help). However, as the learner begins to acquire the skill, the instructor uses differential reinforcement and only independent correct responses (e.g., asking for help without the instructor's prompt) produce the reinforcer.

Decreasing Behavior. Behavior analysts frequently provide intervention to individuals who are referred for services due to problem behavior that is of concern to the people in the person's life (e.g., parents, school staff). For example, individuals may engage in self-injurious behavior that produces bodily harm (Toussaint and Tiger 2012). Other, frequently treated topographies of problem behavior include aggression, disruption, pica (eating of inedible substances), tantrums, among others. To effectively treat problem behavior, it is critical to identify the function of the problem behavior (i.e., the cause of the behavior). The function of problem behavior is commonly identified by an assessment called a functional analysis (Iwata et al. 1982/1994). The functional analysis includes test conditions that manipulate one antecedent and consequence for behavior, such as the availability of attention or brief breaks from completing difficult tasks. The rate of behavior in these test conditions is compared to a control condition in which no consequences are provided for problem behavior and antecedents are arranged to decrease the likelihood of problem behavior (e.g., the individual has preferred items, attention, and no demands are given). The test condition(s) that produces high rates of behavior is identified as the function (i.e., cause) of problem behavior.

Once the function of problem behavior is identified, behavior analysts provide function-based treatment (Iwata et al. 1994). That is, treatment is arranged to ensure that problem behavior no longer produces reinforcement. Extinction is the process by which a previously reinforced response no longer contacts reinforcement (i.e., the contingency between response and reinforcement is removed). Other interventions, such as differential reinforcement, are combined with extinction to teach an individual to engage in an alternative, appropriate behavior to produce reinforcement rather than engaging in problem behavior (Cooper et al. 2007).

Stimulus Control. Some behaviors may only present as inappropriate because of the context in which they occur. For example, reading out loud may be acceptable while in the privacy of one's own home, whereas reading out loud during a standardized achievement test at school may be considered problematic. Stimulus control refers to the extent to which behavior is controlled by antecedent stimuli (Balsam 1993). Stimulus control exists along a continuum from strong (i.e., behavior is *only* emitted in the presence of a specific antecedent stimulus) to weak (i.e., behavior is emitted in the presence of many antecedent stimuli). Stimulus control is typically established through differential reinforcement of behavior; that is, behavior in the presence of a stimulus is reinforced, and behavior in the absence of the stimulus is not reinforced. For example, we learn to pick up the telephone and say hello when it rings (i.e., when answering the telephone is likely to be reinforced by talking to the person calling) and not when it is silent (which is unlikely to result in a conversation with another person).

Maintenance and Generalization

A critical component of behavioral intervention is strategies to promote the maintenance and generalization of behavior change. Applied behavior analysts have developed several techniques to enhance the maintenance of target responses and have further refined an understanding of generalization from one of passive measurement to one of active programing (Stokes and Baer 1997).

Maintenance. When skills are first taught, responses are typically acquired under a dense schedule of reinforcement. A schedule of reinforcement refers to when reinforcement is available for a target response. This schedule can fluctuate from continuous (reinforcement is provided following *every* response) to intermittent (reinforcement is provided following *some* responses). Following the acquisition of a target response, maintenance involves thinning of the reinforcement schedule (i.e., responding does not produce reinforcement as often) and removing some or all components of the intervention. This transition in schedule density and intervention components is important as it helps to promote lasting behavior change.

Generalization. Generalization occurs when behavior is emitted in contexts similar in some ways to the context(s) present during training (Miltenberger 2012). Behavior analysts are interested in stimulus generalization and response generalization. Stimulus generalization occurs when a newly acquired behavior occurs in a novel setting, with people who did not participate in intervention, and in the presence of other novel stimuli. For example, if a child learns to ask her teacher to go to the bathroom, the skill has generalized if the child asks her parents if she can go to the bathroom at a restaurant and successfully uses the toilet despite differences in aspects of the toilet and toilet-paper dispenser. Response generalization occurs when novel responses occur under conditions that are similar to the training context. For example, an individual may be taught the response, "hello" when encountering a peer and, following the acquisition of the response, may then emit the response, "hi" without any direct training. There are numerous strategies that behavior analysts use to increase the likelihood that skills generalize following training, as described by Stokes and Baer (1977).

Applications of Applied Behavior Analysis

Applied behavior analysis has proliferated as an effective field in addressing socially significant problems in a variety of contexts. Behavior analytic practices have been successfully applied to address problems of social importance for individuals with developmental and intellectual disabilities, mental illness, traumatic brain injury, drug and alcohol addictions, gambling, feeding disorders, severe problem behavior, among others. ABA-based practices have also been incorporated into many other fields including education, medicine, occupational, physical, and speech therapy, counseling, business, government, rehabilitation, and gerontology, to name a few. ABA-based treatment has also gleaned considerable support from federal agencies (e.g., Centers for Disease Control, National Institutes

of Mental Health), state committees (e.g., New York State Department of Health), and professional organizations (e.g., American Academy of Child and Adolescent Psychiatry, American Association on Intellectual and Developmental Disabilities, and the Association for Science in Autism Treatment).

Resources on Applied Behavior Analysis

To learn more about the evidence for ABA, readers should refer to several websites and reports, including the National Autism Center's website (http://www.nationalautismcenter.org/reports/), the National Professional Development Center (NCPD) on Autism Spectrum Disorder (http://autismpdc.fpg.unc.edu/), the What Works Clearinghouse (http://ies.ed.gov/ncee/wwc/), and Overview and Summary of Scientific Support for Applied Behavior Analysis (Hagopian et al. 2015; https://www.kennedykrieger.org/patient-care/patient-care-programs/inpatient-programs/neurobehavioral-unit-nbu/applied-behavior-analysis/positions).

References

Baer, D. M., Wolf, M. M., & Risley, T. R. (1968). Some current dimensions of applied behavior analysis. *Journal of Applied Behavior Analysis, 1*, 91–97. https://doi.org/10.1901/jaba.1968.1-91.

Bailey, J. S., & Burch, M. R. (2002). *Research methods in applied behavior analysis.* Thousand Oaks: Sage.

Balsam, P. B. (1988). Selection, representation, and equivalence of controlling stimuli. In R. C. Atkinson, R. J. Herrnstein, G. Lindzey, & R. D. Luce (Eds.), *Stevens' handbook of experimental psychology* (2. ed., pp. 111–166). New York: Wiley.

Chance, P. (2014). *Learning and behavior* (7th ed.). Belmont: Wadsworth Cengage Learning.

Cooper, J. O., Heron, T. E., & Heward, W. L. (2007). *Applied behavior analysis* (2nd ed.). Upper Saddle River: Pearson.

Fisher, W. W., Piazza, C. C., & Roane, H. S. (2011). *Handbook of applied behavior analysis.* New York: Guilford Press.

Hagopian, L. P., Hardesty, S. L., & Gregory, M. K. (2015). Overview and summary of scientific support for applied behavior analysis. Retrieved from https://www.kennedykrieger.org/sites/default/files/patient-care-files/aba-scientific-support-9-2015.pdf

Iwata, B. A., Pace, G. M., Cowdery, G. E., & Miltenberger, R. G. (1994). What makes extinction work: An analysis of procedural form and function. *Journal of Applied Behavior Analysis, 27*, 131–144. https://doi.org/10.1901/jaba.1994.27-131.

Iwata, B. A., Dorsey, M. F., Sliffer, K. J., Bauman, K. E., & Richman, G. S. (1994/1982). Toward a functional analysis of self-injury. Journal of Applied Behavior Analysis, *27*, 19–209. https://doi.org/10.1901/jaba.1994.27-197.

Michael, J. (1982). Distinguishing between discriminative and motivational functions of stimuli. *Journal of the Experimental Analysis of Behavior, 37*, 149–155. https://doi.org/10.1901/jeab.1982.37-149.

Miltenberger, R. G. (2012). *Behavior modification: Principles and procedures* (5th ed.). Belmont, CA: Thomson Wadsworth.

Moore, J. (2009). Why the radical behaviorist conception of private events is interesting, relevant, and important. *Behavior and Philosophy, 37*, 21–37.

Stokes, T. F., & Baer, D. M. (1997). An implicit technology of generalization. *Journal of Applied Behavior Analysis, 10*, 349–367. https://doi.org/10.1901/jaba.1977.10-349.

Toussaint, K. A., & Tiger, J. II. (2012). Reducing covert self-injurious behavior maintained by automatic reinforcement through a variable momentary DRO procedure. *Journal of Applied Behavior Analysis, 45*, 179–184. https://doi.org/10.1901/jaba.2012.45-179.

Vladescu, J. C., & Kodak, T. (2010). A review of recent studies on differential reinforcement during skill acquisition in early intervention. *Journal of Applied Behavior Analysis, 43*, 351–355. https://doi.org/10.1901/jaba.2010.43-351.

Whitehead, W. E., Lurie, E., & Blackwell, B. (1976). Classical conditioning of decreases in human systolic blood pressure. *Journal of Applied Behavior Analysis, 9*, 153–157. https://doi.org/10.1901/jaba.1976.9-153.

Apraxia

Douglas I. Katz
Department of Neurology, Boston University School of Medicine, Braintree, MA, USA

Definition

The inability to correctly carry out a learned, skilled motor act despite the preserved capability of the sensorimotor system to produce the intended movement.

Current Knowledge

Apraxia is thought to involve a loss of representations or the inability to adequately access representations of learned movements and motor skills in the damaged brain. This may lead to a loss of recall of the concept or configuration of the movement or the inability to transform or implement the representational knowledge of the movement into a well-coordinated, properly configured, and sequenced gesture. The diagnosis of apraxia requires the exclusion of cognitive and sensorimotor impairments that may affect the ability to carry out the motor skill, such as arousal, attention, intention, language deficits or weakness, discoordination, movement disorders, and sensory loss.

Assessment: Assessment for apraxia involves asking a patient to carry out pantomimes of movements (e.g., "show me how you would salute . . . brush your teeth with a toothbrush. . . blow out a candle"). If the response in not correct, the examiner may evaluate the patient's response to imitation of the movement or ability to produce the movement using actual objects or tools. The patient may also be tested for recognition of skilled movements produced by the examiner.

Classification of apraxia: Apraxias may be differentiated by the body elements involved in the impaired movement, using the terms *limb apraxia, oral or buccofacial apraxia, trunk* or *axial apraxia.* These disorders have different neuroanatomical underpinnings and may occur separately in different individuals. For instance, patients with oral apraxia may demonstrate normal function on tests of limb praxis.

Apraxia has been subclassifed into *ideational apraxia, ideomotor apraxia,* and *limb-kinetic apraxia* (Liepmann 1900). *Ideational apraxia* is a loss of the conception of a gesture or skilled movement. In this form, the patient does not seem to know what to do, and the motor activity is not facilitated by the use of actual objects. *Ideomotor apraxia* affects the implementation of the movement, producing spatial and timing errors. The patient seems to know what to do but cannot carry the movement out properly.

Limb-kinetic apraxia is the inability to make finely graded, precise limb movements. It has been difficult to separate this form of apraxia from motor dysfunction related to elemental motor disturbance, and it remains controversial that this is actually an apraxic disorder of learned skilled movement.

Neuropathological localization: Apraxias are almost always associated with lesions in the dominant hemisphere. The left parietal lobe is most often implicated in limb apraxia in right-handers. Portions of the frontal lobes, including the supplementary motor area, have been implicated in some forms of apraxia. Lesions in and around Broca's area are most often implicated in cases of oral apraxia. Lesions affecting transmission of information between the cerebral hemispheres, including lesions of the corpus callosum, may lead to apraxia of just the left limbs because of disconnection of movement engrams in the left hemisphere from motor control areas in the right hemisphere (*callosal apraxia*).

Other disorders: A number of disorders have labels that include the term "apraxia" but have no relationship with apraxia according to the usual definition. These include *dressing apraxia*, difficulty orienting clothes to the body, often associated with left neglect, and usually occurring with superior parietal right hemisphere lesions; *constructional apraxia*, difficulty drawing or copying pictures or designs; *gait apraxia*, difficulty initiating or maintaining a normal gait pattern as can be seen in normal pressure hydrocephalus; and *apraxia of gaze*, difficulty directing eye movements as seen in Balint's syndrome. *Apraxia of speech* is a disorder that affects the sequencing of sounds in words and syllables. It can be developmental or acquired, and people with this disorder have difficulty coordinating articulatory motor activities necessary for speech. It is controversial whether this represents an apraxia consistent with the definitions described above or a subtype of language or elemental motor disorders affecting articulatory sequencing.

Cross-References

▶ Balint's Syndrome
▶ Broca's Aphasia
▶ Frontal Lobe
▶ Movement Disorders
▶ Supplementary Motor Area (SMA)

References and Readings

De Renzi, E. (1990). Apraxia. In F. Boller & J. Grafman (Eds.), *Handbook of neuropsychology* (Vol. 2, pp. 245–263). New York: Elsevier.

Heilman, K. M. (1997). Disorders of skilled movements: Limb apraxia. In T. E. Feinberg & M. J. Farah (Eds.), *Behavioral neurology and neuropsychology* (pp. 227–235). New York: McGraw Hill.

Liepmann, H. (1900). Das Krankheitsbild der Apraxie (motorische Asymbolie) auf Grund eines Falles von einseitiger Apraxie. *Monatschrift Psychiatrie und Neurologic, 8*, 15–44, 102–132, 182–197.

Rothi, L. J. G., & Heilman, K. M. (1997). *Apraxia: The neuropsychology of action.* East Sussex: Psychology Press.

Apraxia of Speech

Julie L. Wambaugh
Veterans Affairs Salt Lake City Healthcare System, University of Utah, Salt Lake City, UT, USA

Synonyms

Historically, acquired apraxia of speech (AOS) has been known under a variety of terminological designations (e.g., aphemia, phonemic disintegration, cortical dysarthria, dyspraxia of speech). Currently, there are no acceptable synonyms in use. The descriptor, "stroke induced" (SI), has occasionally been used to specify AOS resulting from stroke (e.g., SI-AOS). Primary progressive apraxia of speech (PPAOS) is used to designate AOS associated with neurodegenerative disease.

Definition

AOS is a neurologic, motoric disorder of speech production that is characterized by slowed rate of speech, difficulties in sound production, and disrupted prosody. AOS is not a disorder of language, although it rarely occurs without aphasia. Consequently, there is no impairment of comprehension or production of language in pure AOS.

Categorization

AOS currently does not have subcategories but is differentiated relative to onset and progression: PPAOS (primary progressive) or AOS/SI-AOS (sudden onset with improving or stable course). Childhood apraxia of speech (CAS) is a related disorder, but not a category of AOS.

Epidemiology

Duffy (2013) reported that AOS was the primary communication disorder in 6.9% of 8101 cases of neurologic motor speech disorders. As a secondary diagnosis (e.g., accompanying aphasia), AOS can be expected to occur more frequently.

Natural History, Prognostic Factors, and Outcomes

The establishment of AOS as a distinct clinical entity is typically credited to Dr. Fredrick Darley, who in the late 1960s stimulated much of the early discussion and research concerning the nature and characteristics of this disorder. Since that time, the definition and descriptors of AOS have continued to evolve, with continuing research efforts being likely to result in further refinement of our knowledge concerning this disorder.

The most frequent cause of AOS is cerebral vascular accident involving the language-dominant hemisphere of the brain. Other causes of focal brain damage (e.g., penetrating head injury, neoplasm resection) may also result in AOS. Areas of injury that have been most often associated with AOS include regions in the premotor cortex (notably, the left posterior, inferior frontal gyrus), supplementary motor area, parietal lobe, and insula (see Wambaugh and Shuster (2008) for a review). PPAOS has been associated with tauopathies such as corticobasal degeneration, progressive supranuclear palsy, and amyotrophic lateral sclerosis (Duffy 2013).

Little objective evidence exists concerning the natural course of AOS, including the factors affecting prognosis. Duffy (2013) indicates that mutism associated with AOS rarely lasts beyond a few days or weeks unless other speech, language, or cognitive deficits are also present.

Treatment can be expected to result in the improvement in symptoms of AOS, even when AOS is chronic. Treatment guidelines for AOS have been developed, which provide effectiveness ratings for different types of treatment based on the existing published evidence (see below; Wambaugh et al. 2006a, b).

Neuropsychology and Psychology of AOS

AOS is a neurogenic, motoric speech disorder that is characterized by reduced rate of speech, disrupted production of speech sounds, and disordered prosody. These symptoms may be accompanied by behaviors such as articulatory groping (silent and/or audible), speech initiation difficulties, increasing number of sound errors with increasing word length or phonetic complexity, awareness of speech errors, and motoric perseverations. Its severity ranges from a total inability to speak to negligible speech disruptions (McNeil et al. 2009; Wambaugh et al. 2006a).

AOS is thought to be caused by difficulties in the process of translating correctly selected and ordered sounds into previously learned movement information necessary for the implementation of intended speech movements. That is, it is assumed that phonology is intact at the linguistic level of processing.

However, there is difficulty in accessing stored movement plans/programs needed to articulate correctly chosen sounds. These difficulties cause disruptions in the selection, positioning, and movement timing of the articulators (e.g., tongue, lips, etc.). Consequently, sound productions may be inaccurate, transitions between sounds may be disrupted, and prosody may be abnormal. Sound durations as well as the intervals between sounds, syllables, and words tend to be prolonged.

Controversy continues to exist concerning error variability in AOS. Early diagnostic criteria included highly variable error patterns. Over the period of several decades, relative consistency in the location and type of errors replaced high variability as a diagnostic characteristic (following findings by McNeil et al. 1995). However, more recent investigations have called into question the use of relative error consistency as diagnostic criteria (e.g., Staiger et al. 2012). Currently, observations of error variability (or consistency) in AOS appear to be influenced by numerous factors such type of stimuli, method of stimulus presentation, method of variability measurement, AOS severity, and the presence or absence of aphasia.

AOS typically occurs with aphasia and rarely occurs without it. The symptoms of AOS, however, are not attributable to disruptions in language. AOS may also occur with another motor speech disorder, dysarthria. Unlike the dysarthrias, AOS is not associated with problems with muscle tone, weakness, reflexes, or sensory processing.

Evaluation

Diagnosis of AOS requires that the primary symptoms of reduced rate of speech, distorted sound production, and disrupted prosody be present. Behaviors such as difficulties with speech initiation or articulatory groping (see above) may also be observed but should not be used alone for purposes of differential diagnosis (Wambaugh et al. 2006a). Screening for AOS typically involves eliciting a variety of speech samples and determining the presence or absence of AOS

symptoms. For example, Duffy (2013) provides a tool that may be used to evaluate speech production across tasks such as sound, monosyllabic word, multisyllabic word, and sentence repetition, repeated word productions, alternate and sequential motion rates, reading aloud, and connected speech production. The Apraxia Battery for Adults-second edition (Dabul 2000) also provides tasks that may be used for examining speech production in adults with suspected AOS. However, the criteria for diagnosis of AOS provided by this test will not differentiate AOS from aphasia with phonemic paraphasia.

Treatment

Behavioral treatment has been demonstrated to have positive outcomes for persons with AOS. The AOS practice guidelines report revealed four general approaches to AOS treatment: (1) articulatory-kinematic treatments (techniques focused on improving articulation of sounds), (2) rate/rhythm control treatments (therapies involving manipulating rate of speech production or imposing an external rhythm on speech), (3) alternative/augmentative communication approaches (therapies involving training the use of methods/devices for supplementing or replacing speech), and (4) intersystemic facilitation/reorganization treatments (therapies utilizing a relatively intact system/modality such as singing or gesturing to facilitate speech production) (Wambaugh et al. 2006b). On the basis of objective evaluation of the existing evidence, the AOS guideline developers determined that articulatory-kinematic approaches were "probably effective" rate/rhythm control approaches and intersystemic approaches were "possibly effective"; and AAC approaches had insufficient support to warrant a rating. A systematic review of AOS treatment reports published from 2004 through 2012 serves as an update to the guidelines (Ballard et al. 2015). The systematic review revealed that the majority of treatment investigations covering the 9-year period reviewed provided evidence concerning articulatory-kinematic treatments.

Findings from a few reports of transcranial direct current stimulation (tDCS) paired with behavioral therapy suggest that neuromodulary treatments may have promise in the treatment of AOS.

Cross-References

▶ Aphasia
▶ Dysarthria
▶ Paraphasia

References and Readings

Ballard, K., Wambaugh, J., Duffy, J., Layfield, C., Maas, E., Mauszycki, S., & McNeil, M. (2015). Updated treatment guidelines for acquired apraxia of speech: A systematic review of intervention research between 2004 and 2012. *American Journal of Speech-Language Pathology, 24*, 316–337. https://doi.org/10.1044/2015_AJSLP-14-0118.

Dabul, B. (2000). *Apraxia battery for adults* (2nd ed.). Austin: Pro-ed.

Duffy, J. R. (2013). *Motor speech disorders: Substrates, differential diagnosis, and management* (3rd ed.). St. Louis: Elsevier Mosby.

Marangolo, P., Marinelli, C. V., Bonifazi, S., Fiori, V., Ceravolo, M. G., Proviniali, L., & Tomaiuolo, F. (2011). Electrical stimulation over the left inferior frontal gyrus (IFG) determines long-term effects in the recovery of speech apraxia in three chronic aphasics. *Behavioural Brain Research, 225*(2), 498–504.

Marangolo, P., Fiori, V., Cipollari, S., Campana, S., Razzano, C., DiPaola, M., Koch, G., & Caltagirone, C. (2013). Bihemispheric stimulation over left and right inferior frontal region enhances recovery from apraxia of speech in chronic aphasia. *European Journal of Neuroscience, 38*(9), 3370–3377.

McNeil, M. (2002). Apraxia of speech: From concept to clinic. *Seminars in Speech and Language, 23*(4), 221–222.

McNeil, M. R., Odell, K. H., Miller, S. B., & Hunter, L. (1995). Consistency, variability, and target approximation for successive speech repetitions among apraxic, conduction aphasic, apraxic dysarthric speakers. *Clinical Aphasiology, 23*, 39–55.

McNeil, M. R., Robin, D. A., & Schmidt, R. A. (2009). Apraxia of speech: Definition and differential diagnosis. In M. R. McNeil (Ed.), *Clinical management of sensorimotor speech disorders* (2nd ed., pp. 249–268). New York: Thieme.

Staiger, A., Finger-Berg, W., Aichert, I., & Ziegler, W. (2012). Error variability in apraxia of speech:

A matter of controversy. *Journal of Speech, Language, and Hearing Research, 55*, S1544–S1561.

Wambaugh, J. L., & Shuster, L. I. (2008). The nature and management of neuromotor speech disorders accompanying aphasia. In R. Chapey (Ed.), *Language intervention strategies in aphasia and related neurogenic communication disorders* (5th ed., pp. 1009–1042). Philadelphia: Lippincott Williams & Wilkins.

Wambaugh, J. L., Duffy, J. R., McNeil, M. R., Robin, D. A., & Rogers, M. (2006a). Treatment guidelines for acquired apraxia of speech: A synthesis and evaluation of the evidence. *Journal of Medical Speech Language Pathology, 14*(2), xv–xxxiii.

Wambaugh, J. L., Duffy, J. R., McNeil, M. R., Robin, D. A., & Rogers, M. (2006b). Treatment guidelines for acquired apraxia of speech: Treatment descriptions and recommendations. *Journal of Medical Speech Language Pathology, 14*(2), xxxv–ixvii.

Aprosodia

Kate Krival
Speech Pathology, School of Health Sciences, Edinboro University of Pennsylvania, Edinboro, PA, USA

Definition

Aprosodia is a deficit in comprehending or expressing prosody, i.e., variations in pitch, loudness, or rhythm of speech used in addition to words to convey specific meaning and emotional information (Monrad-Krohn 1948; Leon and Rodriguez 2008; Wymer et al. 2002). Aprosodia is traditionally characterized as *linguistic* or *affective* (Wymer et al. 2002). Linguistic prosody aids meaning, e.g., con*vict* vs. con*vict* or *the dog and the cat in the cage are mine* vs. *the dog, and the cat in the cage, are mine* allow unambiguous discrimination of the semantic target. Affective prosody conveys attitude, e.g., incredulity, sadness, or anger, e.g., depending on the prosodic intonation, *oh, yeah, I'm just great* may be a sincere expression of a good feeling or an equally sincere communication that the speaker is angry or frustrated. Linguistic aprosodia is associated with both left and right hemisphere lesions; affective aprosodia is more consistently associated with lesions of the right hemisphere (Baum and Pell 1999; Pell 2006; Ross and Monnot 2008). Additionally, the basal ganglia appear to play a key role in processing and further distributing the meaning associated with the prosodic characteristics (Cancelliere and Kertesz 1990; Pell and Leonard 2003).

Clinically, aprosodia is most often considered in terms of whether receptive, expressive, or both aspects of prosodic ability are diminished in an individual. However, Ross and various colleagues have proposed a categorization system for the aprosodias, which is similar to that used to categorize aphasia types. The system is based on a combination of deficit profile and site-of-lesion information: *motor* (in the area of the frontal operculum), *sensory* (posterior temporal operculum), *conduction* (arcuate fasciculus), *transcortical* (anterior or posterior watershed), or *global* deficits (Ross 1981, 2000; Ross and Monnot 2008). For example, an individual with motor aprosodia might not express affective or emotional prosody when speaking; one with sensory aprosodia might not recognize the affective meaning of prosodic signals in another's speech. These nondominant hemisphere anatomic correlates of prosodic deficits do have modest empirical support (see Ross and Monnot 2008 for a summary of related investigations). Ross' *motor aprosodia* should not be confused with prosodic production impairments that arise from deficits in speech production due to dysarthria (Duffy 2005).

Assessment of aprosodia is generally accomplished through careful observation; however, the Florida Affect Battery (Bowers et al. 1998) and the Aprosodia Battery (Ross et al. 1997) may be useful additions to standard testing regimes.

Until recently, management of aprosodic impairments has received little attention in the literature. However, emerging evidence suggests that behavioral therapies may have some effect (Ballard et al. 2010; Bellon-Harn et al. 2007; Bellon-Harn 2011; Bornhofen and McDonald 2008; Jones et al. 2009; Leon et al. 2005; Rosenbek et al. 2004; Rosenbek et al. 2006; Russell et al. 2010). For recent analysis of this literature, descriptions of selected approaches, and suggested future directions in research, see Hargrove (2013).

Cross-References

▶ Apraxia of Speech
▶ Dysarthria
▶ Prosody

References

Baum, S. R., & Pell, M. D. (1999). The neural bases of prosody: Insights from lesion studies and neuroimaging. *Aphasiology, 13*, 581–608.
Ballard, K. J., Robin, D. A., McCabe, P., & McDonald, J. (2010). A treatment for dysprosody in childhood apraxia of speech. *Journal of Speech, Language, and Hearing Research, 53*, 1227–1245.
Bellon-Harn, M. (2011). Targeting prosody: A case study of an adolescent. *Communication Disorders Quarterly, 2*, 109–117.
Bellon-Harn, M., Harn, W. E., & Watson, G. D. (2007). Targeting prosody in an eight-year-old child with high-functioning autism during an interactive approach to therapy. *Child Language Teaching and Therapy, 23*, 157–179.
Bornhofen, C., & McDonald, S. (2008). Comparing strategies for treating emotion perception deficits in traumatic brain injury. *Journal of Head Trauma Rehabilitation, 23*(2), 103–115.
Bowers, D., Blonder, L., & Heilman, K. M. (1998). *The Florida Affect Battery*. Gainesville: University of Florida Brain Institute.
Cancelliere, A. E. B., & Kertesz, A. (1990). Lesion localization in acquired deficits of emotional expression and comprehension. *Brain and Cognition, 13*(2), 133–147.
Duffy, J. R. (2005). *Motor speech disorders: Substrates, differential diagnosis, and management*. St. Louis: Mosby.
Hargrove, P. M. (2013). Pursuing prosody interventions. *Clinical Linguistics & Phonetics, 27*(8), 647–660.
Jones, H. N., Plowman-Prine, E. K., Rosenbek, J. C., Shrivastay, R., & Wu, S. S. (2009). Fundamental frequency and intensity mean and variability before and after two behavioral treatments for aprosdia. *Journal of Medical Speech-Language Pathology, 17*, 45–52.
Leon, S. A., & Rodriguez, A. D. (2008). Aprosodia and its treatment. *Perspectives on Neurophysiology and Neurogenic Speech and Language Disorders, 18*, 66–72.
Leon, S. A., Rosenbek, J. C., Crucian, G. P., Heiber, B., Holiway, B., Rodriguez, A. D., et al. (2005). Active treatments for aprosodia secondary to right hemisphere stroke. *Journal of Rehabilitation Research and Development, 42*(1), 93–102.

Monrad-Krohn, G. H. (1948). Dysprosody or altered 'melody of language'. *Brain, 70*, 405–415.

Pell, M. D. (2006). Cerebral mechanisms for understanding emotional prosody in speech. *Brain and Language, 96*(2), 221.

Pell, M. D., & Leonard, C. L. (2003). Processing emotional tone from speech in Parkinson's disease: a role for the basal ganglia. *Cognitive, Affective, & Behavioral Neuroscience, 3*(4), 275–288.

Rosenbek, J. C., Crucian, G. P., Leon, S. A., Hieber, B., Rodriguez, A. D., Holiway, B., et al. (2004). Novel treatments for expressive aprosodia: A phase I investigation of cognitive linguistic and imitative interventions. *Journal of the International Neuropsychological Society: JINS, 10*(5), 786–793.

Rosenbek, J. C., Rodriguez, A. D., Hieber, B., Leon, S. A., Crucian, G. P., Ketterson, T. U., Ciampitti, M., Singletary, F., Heilman, K. M., & Gonzalez-Rothi, L. J. (2006). Effect of two treatments for aprosodia secondary to acquired brain injury. *Journal of Rehabilitation Research and Development, 43*, 379–390.

Ross, E. D. (1981). The aprosodias: Functional-anatomical organization of the affective components of language in the right hemisphere. *Archives of Neurology, 38*, 561–569.

Ross, E. D. (2000). Affective prosody and the aprosodias. In M. M. Mesulam (Ed.), *Principles of behavioral and cognitive neurology.* New York: Oxford University Press.

Ross, E. D., & Monnot, M. (2008). Neurology of affective prosody and its functional-anatomic organization in right hemisphere. *Brain and Language, 104*(1), 51–74.

Ross, E. D., Thompson, R. D., & Yenkosky, J. P. (1997). Lateralization of affective prosody in brain and the callosal integration of hemispheric language functions. *Brain and Language, 56*, 27–54.

Russell, S., Laures-Gore, J., & Patel, R. (2010). Treating expressive aprosodia: A case study. *Journal of Medical Speech-Language Pathology, 18*, 115–120.

Wymer, J. H., Lindman, L. S., & Booksh, R. L. (2002). A neuropsychological perspective of aprosody: Features, function, assessment and treatment. *Applied Neuropsychology, 9*(1), 37–47.

Arachnoid Cyst

Barbara Spacca[1] and Andrew Brodbelt[2]
[1]Anna Meyer Children's Hospital, Florence, Italy
[2]The Walton Centre NHS Foundation Trust, Liverpool, UK

Synonyms

Temporal lobe agenesis

Short Description or Definition

Arachnoid cysts are benign intracranial space occupying lesions. An arachnoid membrane surrounds a collection of clear fluid, identical to cerebrospinal fluid (CSF). Arachnoid cysts present due to mass effect, sudden hemorrhage, or incidentally.

Categorization

Arachnoid cysts are classified according to their location as intracranial or spinal. Intracranial arachnoid cysts can be further subclassified (Table 1). Middle fossa cysts (MFAC) can also be classified according to their size and distortion of surrounding structures based on Galassi classification (Galassi et al. 1982). Type I cysts are small, biconvex, and have no mass effect (Fig. 1a); type II cysts have a rectangular shape and involve proximal and intermediate segments of the Sylvian fissure (Fig. 1b); type III cysts entirely involve the Sylvian fissure and can produce midline shift (Fig. 1c). Arachnoid cysts may also be classified as primary congenital or acquired (Di Rocco 1990; Oberbauer 1999). Midline posterior fossa arachnoid cysts must not be confused with the Dandy-Walker complex. The Dandy-Walker complex describes hypoplasia or agenesis of the cerebellar vermis, associated hydrocephalus, structural anomalies such as agenesis of the corpus callosum (occurring in 68% of patients), and a post fossa arachnoid cyst-like structure that is not a true arachnoid cyst (Wilkinson and Winston 2008).

Epidemiology

Arachnoid cysts are estimated to account for 1% of all nontraumatic intracranial lesions and are incidentally found in 1 per 1,000 autopsies (Boop and Teo 2000; Di Rocco 1990; Oberbauer 1999; Wilkinson and Winston 2008). They present in the first two decades of life, with a mean age at diagnosis of 6 years. There is a male predominance (2–3:1). Arachnoid cysts are mainly

Arachnoid Cyst, Table 1 Frequency and distribution of intracranial arachnoid cysts (Rengachary et al. 1978)

Position	Incidence (%)	Position	Incidence (%)
Supratentorial	76.8	Infratentorial	23.2
Middle cranial fossa	38.6	Cerebellopontine angle	15.7
Sellar, intrasellar, suprasellar	13.3	Vermal	6.3
Convexity	11.5	Clival	1.2
Interhemispheric fissure	8.3		
Quadrigeminal plate	5.1		

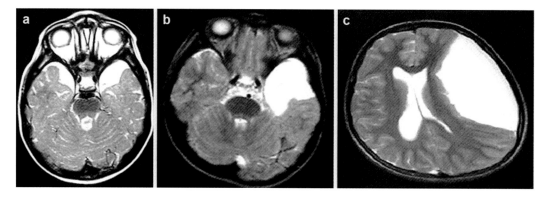

Arachnoid Cyst, Fig. 1 Classification of middle fossa arachnoid cysts. (**a**) Bilateral type I middle fossa arachnoid cyst demonstrating small size, biconvex appearance, and absence of mass effect; (**b**) type II middle fossa arachnoid cysts are rectangular; (**c**) type III middle fossa arachnoid cyst are large and often have significant mass effect

localized to one side, but case reports of bilateral cysts have been described (Ziaka et al. 2008). Familial presentations occur (glutaric aciduria type I) (Jamjoom et al. 1995).

Etiology/Pathology

Microscopic examination demonstrates splitting of the arachnoid membrane at the margin of the cyst, a thick layer of collagen, hyperplastic arachnoid cells, and numerous blood vessels in the cyst wall, and an absence of traversing trabeculae although fine blood vessels may be present (Miyajima et al. 2000; Rengachary and Watanabe 1981). Arachnoid cysts can communicate or be separated from the subarachnoid space (SAS) but appear to contain fluid similar in composition to CSF (Miyajima et al. 2000; Rengachary and Watanabe 1981; Yildiz et al. 2005).

Originally thought to be due to congenital hypoplasia of the brain (e.g., temporal lobe agenesis), this concept has been questioned, as postoperative imaging confirms that the brain expands after cyst decompression (Fig. 2). Most arachnoid cysts are now considered to be the result of a defect in early fetal development. Between the sixth and the eight week of gestation, the meninx primitiva differentiates into the pia and arachnoid mater. Congenital duplication or splitting of the arachnoid layer at this time is thought to lead to the formation of primary congenital arachnoid cysts (Bright 1831; Gosalakkal 2002; Miyajima et al. 2000; Rengachary and Watanabe 1981; Schachenmayr and Friede 1978, 1979) (Fig. 3).

Imaging and endoscopic evidence exists demonstrating that at least in some arachnoid cysts, enlargement is due to a unidirectional valve-type mechanism (Gosalakkal 2002; Miyajima et al. 2000; Santamarta et al. 1995; Schroeder and Gaab 1997). A secretory mechanism from the cyst wall has been suggested, although others have disputed this because of a lack of microscopic evidence of secretion including pinocytosis (Go et al. 1984; Gosalakkal 2002; Schachenmayr and Friede

Arachnoid Cyst,
Fig. 2 Middle fossa
arachnoid cyst both before
(**a**) and after (**b**) surgery.
Note the significant brain
re-expansion, an
observation used to refute
the suggestion of a
congenital hypoplastic
origin

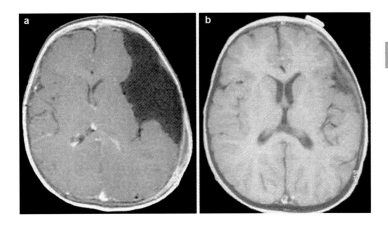

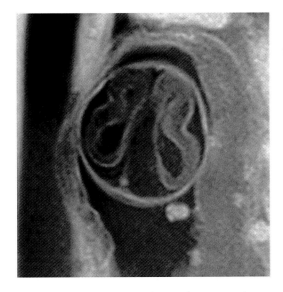

Arachnoid Cyst, Fig. 3 Fetal magnetic resonance image
demonstrating an interhemispheric arachnoid cyst

1979). Water movement along an osmotic pressure gradient due to repeated small intracystal
hemorrhage has also been suggested (Di Rocco
1990). Arachnoid cysts can also be acquired
following hemorrhage, head injury, or surgery
(Kutlay et al. 1998).

Natural History, Prognostic Factors, Outcomes, Symptoms, and Signs

The natural history of arachnoid cysts is
unpredictable. Cysts can grow in size, remain
stable, rarely reduce, or disappear completely.
Spontaneous hemorrhage or hemorrhage occurring after minor head injury have been
described. In patients with middle fossa arachnoid cysts, the annual risk of symptomatic hemorrhage is less than 0.1% (Parsch et al. 1997).
Hemorrhage can be asymptomatic, or, at worst,
present as a life-threatening acute subdural
hematoma. Subdural hygromas can also develop
due to the rupture of the cyst wall. Symptomatic
patients may complain of symptoms related to
raised ICP or specific to the cyst location.
Described symptoms and signs include irritability, lethargy, headache, nausea, vomiting, diplopia, papilledema, cranial nerve dysfunction, and,
in infants, macrocrania, a tense fontanelle,
displayed sutures, failure to thrive, or to reach
developmental milestones.

In MFAC, bone deformities are common with
large cysts and usually consist of macrocrania,
temporal bone thinning, and bossing. Less commonly, downward displacement of the temporal
floor and upward and forward displacement of the
lesser wing of the sphenoid may lead to proptosis
and in extreme cases visual loss, facial numbness,
and ocular palsies. Long tract compression can
lead to sensory and motor limb signs. Seizures
are common, occurring in up to 40% of patients.
Developmental delays, behavioral disorders,
memory, and attention dysfunction have also
been described (Boop and Teo 2000; Di Rocco
1990; Oberbauer 1999; Wilkinson and Winston
2008).

Patients with sellar and suprasellar cysts typically present with endocrine dysfunction, manifesting as failure to thrive or precocious puberty. Optic pathway compression can result in the loss of visual fields or acuity, while hypothalamic pressure can produce eating and behavioral disorders. Thinning and displacement of the floor of the sella turcica and an empty sella can be observed with intrasellar cysts. Rarely, Suprasellar cysts compressing the third ventricle present with "bobblehead doll" syndrome, whose pathogenesis is unknown, consisting in involuntary movement of the head forward and backward at a rate of two to three times/s (Hagebeuk et al. 2005). Cerebral convexity cysts often present with cranial deformity and asymmetry alone. Quadrigeminal plate cysts (Fig. 4) can present with obstructive hydrocephalus or upward gaze palsies. Spinal arachnoid cysts usually present with myelopathy or nerve root compression (Di Rocco 1990).

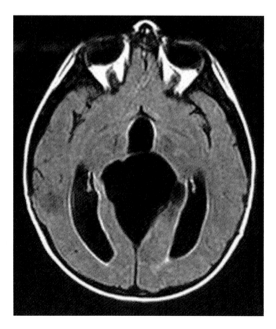

Arachnoid Cyst, Fig. 4 Quadrigeminal plate arachnoid cyst

Neuropsychology and Psychology of Arachnoid Cysts

Large arachnoid cysts may present with failure to reach developmental milestones and psychomotor delay. Cases of dementia in adults have been reported (Harsh et al. 1986). Cerebellar signs may be misdiagnosed as motor delay. MFAC and convexity cysts can be associated with cognitive problems, developmental delay, behavioral disorders, and memory and attention deficits in up to 7.8% of patients (Arai et al. 1996). Symptoms can be potentiated with antiepileptic drugs and sedatives. The relationship between arachnoid cysts and developmental and behavior problems is poorly understood. Functional magnetic resonance imaging demonstrates no alterations in blood-oxygen-level-dependent responses (BOLD) yet single-photon emission computed tomography (SPECT) images can demonstrate reduced cerebral blood flow and glucose metabolism even in the contralateral hemisphere (Wilkinson and Winston 2008). Pre- and postoperative cognitive testing, in small series, demonstrate improved performance in specific tasks after treatment, suggesting that arachnoid cysts may suppress cognitive and cortical function (Baroey Raeder et al. 2005; Wester and Hugdahl 2003). However, larger series do not support significant clinical improvement after surgery in patients with severe developmental and behavior problems (Arai et al. 1996; Levy et al. 2003). In patients with developmental delay, behavioral disorders, and an arachnoid cyst, or in very young patients with large cysts, preoperative neuropsychological testing, EEG, and/or SPECT may have a role in supporting surgical intervention (Wilkinson and Winston 2008).

Evaluation

Diagnosis and follow-up are based on clinical evaluation and imaging. Arachnoid cysts appear as cavities filled with fluid with the same characteristics as CSF, surrounded by a thin wall that is not calcified and does not enhance after contrast. Magnetic resonance imaging (MRI) is the diagnostic tool of choice because of image resolution for the cyst and surrounding anatomy (Wilkinson and Winston 2008).

Treatment

Indications

Arachnoid cysts causing a focal neurological deficit, raised ICP, or enlarging should be treated. The management of asymptomatic patients or patients with functional symptoms, such as seizures and developmental delay, is controversial.

Asymptomatic cysts without mass effect may have a lower risk of bleeding if treated (Wilkinson and Winston 2008; Parsch et al. 1997). Seizure control may be improved, but a causal link is not always apparent. Currently, treatment in patients with severe developmental delay does not appear to confer a significant functional improvement (Arai et al. 1996; Levy et al. 2003).

Surgical Options

Three surgical options exist. These include shunt insertion, open exploration, or endoscopic fenestration (Lena et al. 1996; Kaufman and Park 2000). Commonly, a cystoperitoneal shunt is placed, although revision rates due to infection or system failure remain at 20–40% at 8 years (Arai et al. 1996; Oberbauer et al. 1992). Cyst fenestration consists of opening a window in both the superficial and deep walls of the cyst to allow communication between the cyst and the subarachnoid space (Figs. 5 and 6). Both microsurgical and endoscopic approaches demonstrate improvement in up to 90% of patients (Karabatsou et al. 2007; Levy et al. 2003; Spacca et al. 2009). Endoscopic fenestration is less invasive, and series suggest reduced morbidity (Karabatsou et al. 2003; Spacca et al. 2009). Treatment of an associated subdural hemorrhage or hygroma may lead to the resolution of the arachnoid cyst (Parsch et al. 1997).

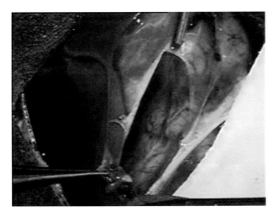

Arachnoid Cyst, Fig. 5 Intraoperative photograph demonstrating microsurgical fenestration of an arachnoid cyst

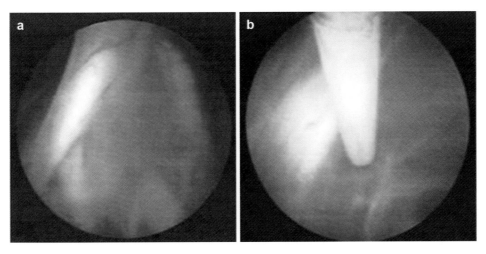

Arachnoid Cyst, Fig. 6 Appearance before (**a**) and during (**b**) endoscopic fenestration of a middle fossa arachnoid cyst

References and Readings

Arai, H., Sato, K., Wachi, A., Okuda, O., & Takeda, N. (1996). Arachnoid cysts of the middle cranial fossa: Experience with 77 patients who were treated with cystoperitoneal shunting. *Neurosurgery, 39*(6), 1108–1113.

Baroey Raeder, M., Helland, C. A., Hugdahl, K., & Wester, K. (2005). Arachnoid cysts cause cognitive deficits that improve after surgery. *Neurology, 64,* 160–162.

Boop, F. A., & Teo, C. (2000). Congenital intracranial cysts. In D. G. McLane (Ed.), *Pediatric neurosurgery* (pp. 489–498). Philadelphia: W.B. Saunders.

Bright, R. (1831). Reports of medical cases selected with a view of illustrating the symptoms and cure of diseases by a reference to morbid anatomy. In R. Longman, B. Orme, P.-R. Green, et al. (Eds.), *Diseases of the brain and nervous system* (pp. 437–439). London: W.B. Saunders.

Di Rocco, C. (1990). *Arachnoid cysts*. In *Youmans: Neurological surgery (1299–1323)*. Philadelphia: WB Saunders Company.

Galassi, E., Tognetti, F., Gaist, G., Fagioli, L., Frank, F., & Frank, G. (1982). CT scan and metrizamide CT cisternography in arachnoid cysts of the middle cranial fossa: Classification and pathophysiological aspects. *Surgical Neurology, 17*(5), 363–369.

Go, K. G., Houthoff, H. J., Blaauw, E. H., Havinga, P., & Hartsuiker, J. (1984). Arachnoid cysts of the sylvian fissure. Evidence of fluid secretion. *Journal of Neurosurgery, 60*(4), 803–813.

Gosalakkal, J. A. (2002). Intracranial arachnoid cysts in children: A review of pathogenesis, clinical features, and management. *Pediatric Neurology, 26*(2), 93–98.

Hagebeuk, E. E., Kloet, A., Grotenhuis, J. A., & Peeters, E. A. (2005). Bobble-head doll syndrome successfully treated with an endoscopic ventriculo-cystocisternostomy. Case report and review of the literature. *Journal of Neurosurgery, 103*(3 Suppl), 253–259.

Harsh, G. R., Edwards, M. S. B., & Wilson, C. B. (1986). Intracranial arachnoid cysts in children. *Journal of Neurosurgery, 64,* 835–842.

Jamjoom, Z. A., Okamoto, E., Jamjoom, A. H., Al-Hajery, O., & Abu-Melha, A. (1995). Bilateral arachnoid cysts in the Sylvian region in female siblings with glutaric aciduria type I. *Journal of Neurosurgery, 82,* 1078–1081.

Karabatsou, K., Hayhurst, C., Buxton, N., O'Brien, D. F., & Mallucci, C. L. (2007). Endoscopic management of arachnoid cysts: An advancing technique. *Journal of Neurosurgery, 106*(6 Suppl pediatrics), 455–462.

Kaufman, B. A., & Park, T. S. (2000). Treatment of arachnoid cysts. In D. G. McLane (Ed.), *Pediatric neurosurgery* (pp. 499–504). Philadelphia: WB Saunders.

Kutlay, M., Colak, A., Demircan, N., & Akin, O. N. (1998). Iatrogenic arachnoid cyst with distinct clinical picture as a result of bone defect in the floor of the middle cranial fossa: Case report. *Neurosurgery, 43*(5), 1215–1218.

Lena, G., Erdincler, P., Van Calenberg, F., Genitori, L., & Choux, M. (1996). Arachnoid cysts of the middle cranial fossa in children. A review of 75 cases, 47 of which have been operated in a comparative study between membranectomy with opening of cisterns and cystoperitoneal shunt. *Neurochirurgie, 42*(1), 29–34.

Levy, M. L., Wang, M., Aryan, H. E., Yoo, K., & Meltzer, H. (2003). Microsurgical keyhole approach for middle fossa arachnoid cyst fenestration. *Neurosurgery, 53*(5), 1138–1145.

Miyajima, M., Arai, H., Okuda, O., Hishii, M., Nakanishi, H., & Sato, K. (2000). Possible origin of suprasellar arachnoid cysts: Neuroimaging and neurosurgical observations in nine cases. *Journal of Neurosurgery, 93*(1), 62–67.

Oberbauer, R. W. (1999). Intracranial and intraspinal cysts. In M. Choux, C. Di Rocco, A. D. Hockley, & M. L. Walker (Eds.), *Pediatric neurosurgery* (pp. 137–149). London: Churchill Livingstone.

Oberbauer, R. W., Haasa, J., & Pucher, R. (1992). Arachnoid cysts in children: A European co-operative study. *Child's Nervous System, 8,* 281–286.

Parsch, C. S., Krauss, J., Hofmann, E., Meixensberger, J., & Roosen, K. (1997). Arachnoid cysts associated with subdural hematomas and hygromas: Analysis of 16 cases, long-term follow-up and review of the literature. *Neurosurgery, 40*(3), 483–490.

Rengachary, S. S., & Watanabe, I. (1981). Ultrastructure and pathogenesis of intracranial arachnoid cysts. *Journal of Neuropathology and Experimental Neurology, 40*(1), 61–83.

Rengachary, S., Watanabe, I., & Brackett, C. (1978). Pathogenesis of intracranial arachnoid cysts. *Surgical Neurology, 9,* 139–144.

Santamarta, D., Aguas, J., & Ferrer, E. (1995). The natural history of arachnoid cysts: Endoscopic and cine-mode MRI evidence of a slit-valve mechanism. *Minimally Invasive Neurosurgery, 38*(4), 133–137.

Schachenmayr, W., & Friede, R. L. (1978). Fine structure of arachnoid cysts. *Journal of Neuropathology and Experimental Neurology, 38,* 434–446.

Schachenmayr, W., & Friede, R. L. (1979). Fine structure of arachnoid cysts. *Journal of Neuropathology and Experimental Neurology, 38*(4), 434–446.

Schroeder, H. W., & Gaab, M. R. (1997). Endoscopic observation of a slit-valve mechanism in a suprasellar prepontine arachnoid cyst: Case report. *Neurosurgery, 40*(1), 198–200.

Spacca, B., Kandasamy, J., Mallucci, C. L., & Genitori, L. (2010). Endoscopic treatment of middle fossa arachnoid cysts: A series of forty patients treated in two centres. *Childs Nerv Syst, 26*(2), 163–72.

Wester, K., & Hugdahl, K. (2003). Verbal laterality and handedness in patients with intracranial arachnoid cysts. *Journal of Neurology, 250,* 36–41.

Wilkinson, C. C., & Winston, K. R. (2008). Congenital arachnoid cysts and the Dandy-Walker complex. In A. L. Albright, I. F. Pollack, & P. D. Adelson (Eds.), *Principles and practice of pediatric neurosurgery* (pp. 162–186). New York: Thieme.

Yildiz, H., Erdogan, C., Yalcin, R., Yazici, Z., Hakyemez, B., Parlak, M., et al. (2005). Evaluation of communication between intracranial arachnoid cysts and cisterns with phase-contrast cine MR imaging. *AJNR – American Journal of Neuroradiology, 26*(1), 145–151.

Ziaka, D. S., Kouyalis, A. T., Boviatsis, E. J., & Sakas, D. E. (2008). Asymptomatic massive subdural hematoma in a patient with bitemporal agenesis and bilateral temporal arachnoid cysts. *The Southern Medical Journal, 101*(3), 324–326.

Arbitration

Robert L. Heilbronner
Chicago Neuropsychology Group, Chicago, IL, USA

Definition

Arbitration is an alternative means of settling a dispute by impartial person(s) without proceeding to a court trial. It is sometimes preferred as a means of settling a matter in order to avoid the expense, delay, and acrimony of litigation. There is no discovery, and there are simplified rules of evidence in arbitration. The arbitrator(s) are selected directly by the parties or are chosen in accordance with the terms of the contract in which the parties have agreed to use a court-ordered arbitrator(s) or an arbitrator(s) from the American Arbitration Association. If there is no contract, usually each party chooses an arbitrator, and the two arbitrators select a third to comprise the panel. When parties submit to arbitration, they agree to be bound by and comply with the arbitrators' decision. The arbitrators' decision is given after an informal proceeding where each party presents evidence and witnesses. Arbitration has long been used in labor, construction, and securities regulation but is gaining popularity in other disputes.

Cross-References

▶ Mediation

References and Readings

The Federal Arbitration Act 9 U.S.C. Section 1 et seq., (1925).

Arcuate Fasciculus

Martin R. Graf
Department of Neurosurgery, Virginia Commonwealth University Medical Center, Richmond, VA, USA

Definition

The arcuate fasciculus is a large bundle of nerve fibers that curves around the lateral sulcus to connect Broca's area in the frontal cortex to Wernicke's area located in the posterior portion of the temporal lobe. This white matter pathway is essential for language processing in which the arcuate fasciculus connects the region associated with the ability to produce spoken language, Broca's area, to that of the ability to process spoken words that are heard which is associated with Wernicke's area. This language loop is located in the left hemisphere in approximately 90% of the population. Lesions disrupting the arcuate fasciculus result in conduction aphasia, which is characterized by paraphasic errors in which incorrect words or sounds are substituted and word repetition is impaired, although these individuals generally show reasonably normal speech and comprehension.

Cross-References

▶ Superior Longitudinal Fasciculus

References and Readings

LaPointe, L. L. (2005). *Aphasia and related neurogenic language disorders*. New York: Thieme.

Aripiprazole

Cristy Akins[1] and Efrain Antonio Gonzalez[2,3]
[1]Mercy Family Center, Metarie, LA, USA
[2]College of Psychology, Nova Southeastern
University, Fort Lauderdale, FL, USA
[3]Utah State University, Logan, UT, USA

Generic Name

Aripiprazole, Aripiprazole lauroxil

Brand Name

Abilify, Abilify Maintena, Aristada (extended release, injectable)

Class

Atypical neuroleptic

Proposed Mechanism(s) of Action

Partial agonism at dopamine 2 receptors. Also inhibits 5HT2a receptors, thus increasing presynaptic release of related catecholamines.

Indication

Schizophrenia, bipolar (mixed/manic), adjunctive for major depressive disorder, and autistic irritability in children and teens.

Off-Label Use

Other psychotic disorders, acute mania, bipolar maintenance, bipolar depression, behavioral disturbances associated with dementias, behavioral disturbances in children and adolescents, and impulse control disorders.

Side Effects

Serious
Neuroleptic malignant syndrome and seizures.

Common
Insomnia, dizziness, activation, akathisia, nausea, and vomiting.

References and Readings

Centerwatch: https://www.centerwatch.com/drug-information/fda-approved-drugs/therapeutic-area/17/psychiatry-psychology.
Physicians' Desk Reference (71st ed.). (2017). Montvale: Thomson PDR.
Stahl, S. M. (2007). *Essential psychopharmacology: The prescriber's guide* (2nd ed.). New York: Cambridge University Press.

Additional Information
Drug Interaction Effects: http://www.drugs.com/drug_interactions.html.
Drug Molecule Images: http://www.worldofmolecules.com/drugs/.
Free Drug Online and PDA Software: www.epocrates.com.
Free Drug Online and PDA Software: www.medscape.com.
Gene-Based Estimate of Drug interactions: http://mhc.daytondcs.com:8080/cgibin/ddiD4?ver=4&task=getDrugList.
Pill Identification: http://www.drugs.com/pill_identification.html.

Arithmetic Reasoning

J. Zhou[1] and R. Sands[2]
[1]School Psychology, The Chicago School of Professional Psychology, Chicago, IL, USA
[2]Legal Psychology (Psychology and Law), Neuropsychology, Clinical Psychology,
The Chicago School of Professional Psychology, Chicago, IL, USA

Synonyms

Numerical reasoning; Quantitative reasoning

Definition

Mathematical reasoning is the mathematical methodology of axiomatic reasoning, logical deduction, and formal inference.

Current Knowledge

Research in evolutionary genetics and neuroscience suggests important neurological differences between mathematical capacities that are evolutionary primitive (e.g., counting) and those (e.g., arithmetic) that are more culturally taught (Geary 1995). Empirical data demonstrate that mathematical reasoning and language are functionally and neuroanatomically independent, suggesting (a) there is a common and domain-general syntactic mechanism that underpins both language and mathematics, but that mathematical expressions can gain direct access to this system without translation into a language format, and (b) autonomous, domain-specific syntactic mechanisms exist for language and mathematics (Varley et al. 2005). Studies on sex differences provide evidence that mathematical reasoning develops from a set of biologically based cognitive capacities that males and females share (Spelke 2005). Male infants show no advantage over females in the processing of objects, space, or numbers. Highly selected male and female students show equal ability to learn mathematics. However, other studies found male advantage in arithmetical reasoning mediated by male advantages in both computational fluency and spatial cognition.

Cross-References

▶ Abstract Reasoning
▶ Academic Competency
▶ Academic Skills
▶ Problem Solving

References and Readings

Geary, D. C. (1995). Reflections on evolution and culture in children's cognition: Implications for mathematical development and instruction. *American Psychologist, 50*(1), 24–37.

Spelke, E. (2005). Sex differences in intrinsic aptitude for mathematics and science? *American Psychologist, 60*(9), 950–958.

Varley, R. A., Klessinger, N. J. C., Romanowski, C. A. J., & Siegal, M. (2005). Agrammatic but numerate. *Proceedings of the National Academy of Science of the United States of America, 102*, 3519–3524.

Zhou, Z. (2011). Mathematical reasoning. In J. S. Kreutzer, J. Deluca, & B. Caplan (Eds.), *Encyclopedia of clinical neuropsychology*. New York: Springer.

Arousal

Ronald A. Cohen
Department of Clinical and Health Psychology, College of Public Health and Health Professions, University of Florida, Gainesville, FL, USA
Center for Cognitive Aging and Memory, McKnight Brain Institute, University of Florida, Gainesville, FL, USA

Synonyms

Cortical activation; Cortical arousal; Delirium; Wakefulness

Definition

The psychological and physiological state of wakefulness, excitement, and/or activation enables readiness for action, increased sexual desire, and readiness. From a neuropsychological perspective, arousal refers to the tonic state of cortical activity elicited by the subcortical reticular formation that results in increased wakefulness, alertness, muscle tone, and autonomic response (e.g., heart rate and respiration). Mobilization of arousal including autonomic resources is necessary for the performance of both volitional and non-volitional tasks. Further, arousal varies across sleep stages, emotional states, and cognitive tasks. It is a broad construct encompassing many physiological processes and meaning requires context.

Historical Background

The concept of arousal played a key role in many of the earliest psychological theories. Physiologists of the nineteenth century, such as Brücke, focused on the basis of bioenergetics as they attempted to understand the basis of cell function. This influenced Freud who posited that bioenergetics were the driving forces underlying psychological experience and behavior and accounted for his construct of "Id." William James proposed that emotional experience involved the labeling of arousal and behavioral response associated with affective stimuli. Later, Walter Cannon coined the term fight or flight response, describing mobilization of arousal systems to threat. Classical conditioning theory was also routed in Pavlov's observations of autonomic and behavioral unconditioned response to stimuli, such as foods that have appetitive value (i.e., unconditioned stimuli). His concept of the orienting response was one of the first constructs that directly linked arousal and learning to an attentional response. Subsequently, arousal became a key construct in the development of the field of psychophysiology in its efforts to characterize the relationship between psychological experience and physiological response. The demonstration by Moruzzi and Magoun (1949) shows that the brain-stem reticular formation plays a key role in generating brain activation as evident by electroencephalography. This spurred subsequent neurophysiological inquiry into the factors underlying arousal and their mediation of higher-order cognitive functions. Early efforts to understand the actions of neurotransmitters in the brain were closely linked to the concept of arousal, based on the effects of norepinephrine on the sympathetic nervous system response and wakefulness. Pribram and McGuinness (1975) posited dissociations between arousal, activation, and effort in the

control of attention, an important theoretical neuropsychological work that tied these processes to underlying brain mechanisms. Heilman and Valenstein's (1979) attention-arousal hypothesis proposed that the arousal associated with reticular activation interacted with a number of distinct cortical and subcortical systems involved in the control of attention and that unilateral brain lesions across these brain systems occur in patients with hemineglect syndrome.

Current Knowledge

The concept of arousal has evolved substantially from its original conception. Some neuroscientists argue that the concept has outlived its usefulness because the term arousal is used to refer to a broad range of different behavioral and physiological phenomena with very different underlying mechanisms. This has led to overgeneralization of the construct. Yet, arousal continues to have an important role in neuropsychological theories. There is compelling evidence that brain stem and subcortical activity influences cortical activity and also autonomic response and that visceral activity influences these brain systems. At a behavioral and phenomenological level, arousal provides a construct that links the more primitive bioenergetic responses of the brain with higher cortical functions. This is most obvious when considering levels of consciousness that can range from deep sleep or coma to normal wakefulness to states of extreme excitement, hyperactivity, or agitation. Altered arousal is a key feature of delirium that can occur due to transient disruptions in brain function due to metabolic or drug influences.

Stimulation of the sympathetic nervous system and an increase in the secretion of epinephrine and norepinephrine increase the brain activity as evidenced by EEG recordings, along with behavioral response toward greater wakefulness, where drugs like barbiturates and alcohol have the opposite effect. Tasks that require intense focused attention to perform, that are stressful, or that require rapid response for adequate performance tend to result in increased fast wave EEG activity as well as autonomic nervous system responses such as increased heart rate and respiration, metabolic activity, and a diversion of blood from the gastrointestinal system to skeletal muscle. These responses are associated with a readiness to respond, a key element of attention; the specific nature of this attention response depends on whether the task demands involve passive vigilance or more effortful directed attention.

There is now strong evidence that multiple neural systems are involved in the maintenance, control, and allocation of arousal throughout the cortex. At least four neurotransmitter systems (acetylcholine, norepinephrine, dopamine, and serotonin) mediate the energetic state of the brain, though a variety of peptides influence the neural response across specific brain systems. While, hierarchically, the arousal originates in the brainstem, the nuclei of the hypothalamus play a critical role in the specificity of arousal relative to specific appetitive behaviors. For example, while damage to the reticular system of the brain stem often results in coma, hypothalamic nuclei such as the suprachiasmatic nucleus exert control over wakefulness, by maintaining circadian rhythm. Furthermore, the arousal associated with drives such as eating and sexual response are directly governed by hypothalamic functions, with higher level limbic (e.g., amygdala) and cortical control. And, further, vagal inputs, both efferent and afferent fibers, are important conduits for the communication of visceral system activity as well as motor activation associated with brainstem, hypothalamic, and higher cortical systems. These complex interactions have been implicated in a number of cognitive and emotional processes. Peripheral and central interactions in the process of social engagement have been described by the Polyvagal Theory (Porges 1995). The central autonomic network interacts with these systems to manage and interpret arousal components to support behavioral requirements (Benarroch 1993).

The most obvious clinical manifestations of disordered arousal occur in conjunction with delirium. However, factors that influence the level of arousal have direct effects on performance, as described at the turn of the last century in the Yerkes-Dodson law. There are data from a wide range of cognitive, behavioral, and neuropsychological studies supporting the principle that task performance varies as a function of arousal, with optimal performance occurring at some intermediate level. Pathological states that cause lethargy usually reduce attentional performance. Similarly, drugs, anxiety, or other factors that lead to excessive arousal also have detrimental consequences on performance. Disturbances of arousal are commonly associated with both intoxication and withdrawal from drugs like alcohol and barbiturates, electrolyte imbalances, trauma to brain from closed head injury, and various neurological disorders including encephalitis, tumors, advanced Alzheimer's disease, and stroke. Conditions that affect the brain stem, hypothalamus, thalamus, limbic areas (e.g., amygdala), and frontal and temporal lobes are most likely to alter arousal and thereby affect attention too.

From a neuropsychological perspective, arousal is an important factor influencing the intensity of attentional focus and also the ability of people to sustain attention. Kahneman (1973) proposed that arousal is a governing factor underlying attentional capacity. Cohen's (2014) four-factor attention framework and other neuropsychological theories of attention posit that capacity limitations associated with the overall level of behavioral and physiological arousal constrain attention by influencing the intensity of focus that is possible, which in turn affects other aspects of attention, most notably sustained performance.

Future Directions

Arousal appears to be a necessary and durable construct within neuropsychology. Yet, some of the concerns of neuroscientists regarding the overuse and overgeneralization of the term have merit. As knowledge increases regarding the functional neuroanatomy of specific white-matter pathways projecting from subcortical to cortical regions, there will be a need for further refinement of the arousal construct. Efforts to more clearly demonstrate the linkage between behavioral and physiological arousal in the clinical context are needed, given that they are not always obviously coupled. The example of decreased frontal lobe activation associated with hyperactivity and impulsivity in attention deficit disorder illustrates that this is complex system and construct. At this point in time, arousal is typically not directly assessed as part of neuropsychological evaluations, except through behavioral observation. However, with advances in the functional neuroimaging, it is possible to demonstrate both activation and deactivation of particular brain regions and to observe how these responses change in association with not only momentary task demands but also tonic state of arousal. Accordingly, in the future physiological measurement of arousal and activation across brain systems, it is likely to be a more common element of standard neuropsychological assessment.

Cross-References

▶ Attention
▶ Consciousness
▶ Orienting Response
▶ Reticular Activating System
▶ Yerkes-Dodson Law

References and Readings

Benarroch, E. E. (1993). The central autonomic network: Functional organization, dysfunction, and perspective. *Mayo Clinic Proceedings, 68*(10), 988–1001.
Cohen, R. A. (2014). *Neuropsychology of attention* (2nd ed.). New York: Springer.
Heilman, K. M., & Valenstein, E. (1979). Mechanisms underlying hemispatial neglect. *Annals of Neurology, 5*(2), 166–170.
Kahneman, D. (1973). *Attention and effort*. Englewood Cliffs: Prentice-Hall.
Moruzzi, G., & Magoun, H. W. (1949). Brain stem reticular formation and activation of the EEG. *Electroencephalography and Clinical Neurophysiology, 1*(4), 455–473.
Porges, S. W. (1995). Orienting in a defensive world: Mammalian modifications of our evolutionary heritage. A polyvagal theory. *Psychophysiology, 32*, 301–318.
Pribram, K., & McGuinness, D. (1975). Arousal, activation, and effort in the control of attention. *Psychological Review, 82*(2), 116–149.

Arterial Gas Embolism

Ben Dodsworth
PM&R, University of South Florida, Tampa, FL, USA

Synonyms

Arterial air embolism

Definition

Arterial gas embolism refers to the obstruction of an arterial (oxygen-rich) blood vessel caused by gas bubbles forming within or entering into the blood vessel. The effect can be devastating in cases where the gas bubbles are sufficient to cause ischemia (lack of blood flow) to a vital organ such as the heart or brain. Common causes include lung trauma and severe decompression sickness as a result of ascending rapidly from a dive or to a high altitude. Symptoms may consist of loss of consciousness, altered mental status, seizures, and extremity weakness, with the risk of complications such as kidney failure, cardiac arrest, brain injury secondary to oxygen deprivation, and death. Treatment begins with immediate administration of 100% oxygen, followed by the use of a recompression chamber (Bove 2015).

See Also

▶ Decompression Sickness

References and Readings

Bove, A. A., MD, PhD. (2015, Oct). Arterial gas embolism. Retrieved January 24, 2017. From http://www.merckmanuals.com/professional/injuries-poisoning/injury-during-diving-or-work-in-compressed-air/arterial-gas-embolism

Arteriovenous Malformation (AVM)

Bruce J. Diamond and Joseph E. Mosley
Department of Psychology, William Paterson
University, Wayne, NJ, USA

Synonyms

Brain arteriovenous malformation; Cerebral malformation; Vascular malformation

Short Description or Definition

Arteriovenous malformations (AVMs) are irregular, anomalous, abnormal, or faulty formations or structures connecting the arteries and veins (Webster 2006). Intracranial hemorrhage is a potential complication in patients with arteriovenous malformations of the brain (AMB) (Stapf et al. 2006).

Etiology

AVMs arise about 3 weeks after conception, at the time when blood vessels are dividing into veins and arteries (Stein and Wolpertson 1980). It has been suggested that AVMs are dynamic and have the ability to grow, regress, and regenerate following obliteration by surgery or radiosurgery (Moftakhar et al. 2009). It is hypothesized that the altered expression of more than 900 genes is involved in the pathogenesis of AVMs (Moftakhar et al. 2009).

Epidemiology

AVMs are the most common type of clinically significant vascular malformation, occurring almost exclusively in the brain and can involve extension of vessels from the subarachnoid space into brain parenchyma (Frosch et al. 2005). AVM sizes may vary from a few millimeters to several centimeters (Warlow 2001), with males being affected twice as frequently as females. Epidemiological and imaging research report that about 50% of patients with AMB present with hemorrhage and the other 50% either present with nonfocal symptoms or display no symptoms (Choi and Mohr 2005). A multicenter study examining the incidence of newly diagnosed brain AVM's reported 1.12–1.42 cases per 100,000 person-years (Abecassis et al. 2014).

Mechanisms

Due to chronic hypoperfusion associated with cerebral AVM, translocation of eloquent neurological functions to other brain areas (i.e., cortical plasticity) can occur. Cortical plasticity appears to be influenced by both AVM pathogenesis and the nature of the intervention (Ding et al. 2015). Cognitive improvements have been attributed to improved cerebral blood flow and reduction of hypoperfusion (Lantz and Meyers 2008).

Neuropsychological and Psychological Outcomes

The occurrence of cognitive impairments in AVM is difficult to determine (Lantz and Meyers 2008) because much of the data have been pooled from patients with ruptured and unruptured AVMs. Patients with AVM may exhibit below normal performance on tests of intelligence, attention, and memory (Lantz and Meyers 2008). Patients with AVMs are more likely to report developmental learning disorders than patients with tumors or aneurysms, with AVM patients reporting four times the rate of learning disability compared to the normal population (Lantz and Meyers 2008; Lazar et al. 1999). This finding may suggest that disorders of learning and intellectual function may serve as a marker for early cerebral dysfunction in patients with AVMs (Lazar et al. 1999). With respect to outcomes, some research has demonstrated postsurgical improvement in patients' neuropsychological functioning, including better performance on tasks requiring executive function (Lantz and Meyers 2008). Researchers have also demonstrated brain reorganization of language function in patients with AVMs by using Wada testing (intracarotid amobarbital sodium and xylocaine procedure), magnetic resonance imaging, and functional magnetic resonance imaging (Lantz and Meyers 2008). Other research has demonstrated structural reorganization involving the motor cortex (Lantz and Meyers 2008) (Fig. 1).

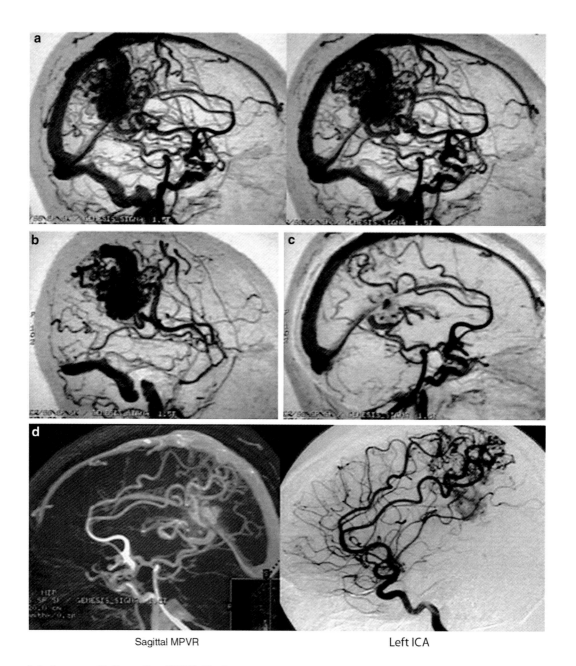

Sagittal MPVR   Left ICA

Arteriovenous Malformation (AVM), Fig. 1

Assessment and Treatment

The AVM is often recognized clinically between the ages of 10 and 30, presenting as a seizure disorder, an intracerebral hemorrhage, a subarachnoid hemorrhage, a nonspecific or migraine headache, and less frequently, as pulsatile tinnitus (Al-Shahi and Warlow 2001; Frosch et al. 2005; Warlow 2001). The most commonly affected site is the middle cerebral artery, particularly its posterior branches; however, AVMs may occur anywhere along the midbrain, cerebellum, or spinal cord (Frosch et al. 2005). Because AVMs expose patients to the risk of permanent neurological deficits or death, surgical intervention may be necessary (Zhao et al. 2005). Clinicians must consider a variety of factors, including lesion size, location, and angioarchitecture in determining the appropriate approach to treatment (Abecassis et al. 2014). The decision to treat involves evaluating the risks of subsequent intracranial hemorrhage versus the immediate risks resulting from intervention (Abecassis et al. 2014). A randomized trial of unruptured brain AVMs (ARUBA 2014) concluded that pharmacological therapy for neurological symptoms alone may be superior to surgical intervention for prevention of stroke, neurological disability, or death (Mohr et al. 2014). Surgery may result in severe neuropsychological complications for some patients, including executive dysfunction and aphasia (Lantz and Meyers 2008; Zhao et al. 2005). However, advances in interventional neuroradiology and stereotactic radiosurgery (SRS) have provided alternatives to traditional microsurgery, such as gamma knife SRS and proton beam radiosurgery (Ropper et al. 2005; Zhao et al. 2005). It should be noted that the treatment of giant cerebral AVMs (>6 cm in diameter) may require endovascular embolization as an adjunct to surgical intervention (Zhao et al. 2005).

Cross-References

▶ Anterior Communicating Artery
▶ Gamma Knife
▶ Intracarotid Sodium Amobarbital Test
▶ Radiosurgery, Stereotactic Radiosurgery
▶ Shunts
▶ Wada Test

References and Readings

Abecassis, I., Xu, D., Batjer, H., & Bendok, B. (2014). Natural history of brain arteriovenous malformations: A systematic review. *Neurosurgical Focus, 37*(3), 1–11.

Al-Shahi, R., & Warlow, C. (2001). A systematic review of the frequency and prognosis of arteriovenous malformations of the brain in adults. *Brain, 124*, 1900–1926.

Aminoff, M. J., Greenberg, D. A., & Simon, R. P. (2005). *Clinical neurology.* New York: McGraw-Hill.

Ding, D., Starke, R. M., Liu, K. C., & Crowley, R. W. (2015). Cortical plasticity in patients with cerebral arteriovenous malformations. *Journal of Clinical Neuroscience, 22*(12), 1857–1861.

Frosch, M. P., Anthony, D. C., & De Girolami, U. (2005). The central nervous system. In V. Kumar, A. K. Abbas, & N. Fausto (Eds.), *Pathologic basis of disease* (pp. 1347–1420). Philadelphia: Elsevier.

Lantz, E. R., & Meyers, P. M. (2008). Neuropsychological effects of brain arteriovenous malformations. *Neuropsychology Review, 18*, 167–177.

Lazar, R. M., Connaire, K., Marshall, R. S., Pile-Spellman, J., Hacein-Bey, L., Solomon, R. A., et al. (1999). Developmental deficits in adult patients with arteriovenous malformations. *Archives of Neurology, 56*, 103–106.

Moftakhar, P., Hauptman, J. S., Malkasian, D., & Martin, N. A. (2009). Cerebral arteriovenous malformations. Part 1: Cellular and molecular biology. *Neurosurgical Focus, 26*(5), 1–15.

Mohr, J., Parides, M., Stapf, C., Moquete, E., Moy, C., Overbey, J., Al-Shahi Salman, R., Vicaut, E., Young, W., Houdart, E., Cordonnier, C., Stefani, M., Hartmann, A., von Kummer, R., Biondi, A., Berkefeld, J., Klijn, C., Harkness, K., Libman, R., Barreau, X., & Moskowitz, A. (2014). Medical management with or without interventional therapy for unruptured arteriovenous malformations (ARUBA): A multicenter, non-blinded, randomized trial. *Lancet, 15*(383), 614–621.

Ropper, A. H., Brown, R. H., Adams, R. D., & Victor, M. (2005). *Adams & Victor's principles of neurology.* New York: McGraw-Hill.

Stapf, C., Mast, H., Sciacca, R. R., Choi, J. H., Khaw, A. V., Connolly, E. S., Pile-Spellman, J., & Mohr, J. P. (2006). Predictors of hemorrhage in patients with untreated brain arteriovenous malformation. *Neurology, 66*(9), 1350–1355.

Stein, B. M., & Wolpertson, S. M. (1980). Arteriovenous malformations of the brain. I: Current concepts and treatments. *Archives of Neurology, 37*, 69–75.

Warlow, C. (2001). Stroke, transient ischemic attacks, and intracranial venous thrombosis. In M. Donaghy (Ed.), *Brain's diseases of the nervous system* (pp. 775–896). New York: Oxford University Press.

Webster. (2006). *Webster's new explorer medical dictionary (new edition)*. Springfield: Merriam-Webster.

Zhao, J., Wang, S., Li, J., Qi, W., Sui, D., & Zhao, Y. (2005). Clinical characteristics and surgical results of patients with cerebral arteriovenous malformations. *Surgical Neurology, 63*, 156–161.

Articulation

Janet P. Patterson
Audiology and Speech-Language Pathology Service, VA Northern California Health Care System, Martinez, CA, USA

Definition

Articulation is (1) the juncture between bones or cartilages in the skeleton of a vertebrate and (2) the movement pattern and relationship of oral structures such as the tongue and lips, to produce the sounds of speech. Speech sound articulation develops gradually and consistently across children of all cultures, and the earliest sounds made by infants are undifferentiated. As a child matures and motor control becomes increasingly well-coordinated, the child's speech becomes intelligible within the linguistic community.

Speech sound articulation is evaluated through tests of single sounds and words, and in contexts such as oral reading and conversation. Speech sound articulation disorders can disrupt speech intelligibility temporarily or for extended periods of time.

Cross-References

▶ Apraxia of Speech
▶ Articulation Disorders
▶ Ataxia
▶ Dysarthria
▶ Dystonia

▶ Phoneme
▶ Phonics
▶ Phonology
▶ Speech-Language Pathology

References and Readings

http://www.asha.org/public/speech/disorders/SpeechSound Disorders/

Hulit, L. M., & Howard, M. R. (2005). *Born to talk: An introduction to speech and language development* (4th ed.). Boston: Pearson A & B.

Plante, E., & Beeson, P. M. (2013). *Communication and communication disorders: A clinical introduction* (4th ed.). Boston: Pearson A&B.

Articulation Disorders

Pamela Garn-Nunn[1] and Carney Sotto[2]
[1]Department of Pharmacology, Virginia Commonwealth University, Richmond, VA, USA
[2]College of Allied Health Sciences, University of Cincinnati, Cincinnati, OH, USA

Short Description or Definition

An articulation disorder is a failure to acquire or difficulty producing a speech sound or sounds of a particular language by the expected normative age due to some type of motoric production problem. Speech sound errors in articulation disorders include:

Substitutions: replacing a standard speech sound with a different standard speech sound, e.g., *w abbit* for *r abbit*, *thpoon* for spoon, or *bery* for *very*.

Omissions/Deletions: a standard speech sound is not produced and is deleted or omitted, e.g., *ba* for bat, *gin* for *green*. (Widespread omissions often indicate a phonological disorder.)

Distortions: the replacement of a standard speech sound by a nonstandard sound. The sound may be slightly changed, e.g., *s* in *soup* sounds "slushy" or "lateralized." A, lisp is a distortion.

Additions: insertion of a sound or syllable into a word, e.g., *cart* for *car* or *bə lack for black*. Additions are the least commonly occurring type of articulation error.

While some of these sound changes are common for toddlers and early preschoolers, children should master the speech sounds of English by the age of 8.

NOTE: Individuals whose sound substitutions or omissions reflect a dialectic variation or acquisition of English as a second language are not considered to have an articulation disorder.

Categorization

An articulation disorder is a type of speech sound disorder. It is associated with a motoric inability to produce a speech sound or sounds (rather than a failure to acquire the speech sound rules of a particular language) by the expected normative age (see ▶ "Phonological Disorder"). Articulation and phonological disorders can co-occur.

Epidemiology

Incidence figures are available for speech sound disorders, of which articulation disorders are one type. Figures cited for preschoolers are 8–9% with approximately 5% still demonstrating a speech sound disorder by first grade. Incidence of speech sound disorders in children is higher than in adults. Some children will outgrow their errors, while others will require treatment from a speech-language pathologist to develop understandable speech (see "Evaluation").

During the process of speech development, articulation disorders occur more often in children with

- Genetic syndromes such as Down syndrome or other syndromes associated with cognitive delays
- Childhood apraxia of speech
- Neurological disorders such as cerebral palsy

- Orofacial anomalies such as cleft palate
- Myofunctional disorders (sometimes referred to as tongue thrust disorders)

In some cases, no definitive etiological factor will be found.

For school-aged children, articulation disorders can be a continuation of an earlier phonological or articulation problem or the result of some type of neurological injury. Similarly, in adults, a speech sound disorder can consist of residual errors of an earlier disorder or a new disorder due to a variety of neurological causes. Please refer ▶ "Dysarthria" and ▶ "Apraxia" for further information on these adult causes of speech sound disorders.

Natural History, Prognostic Factors, and Outcomes

A child's acquisition of the speech sounds is a gradual process. Correct articulation can depend not only on motor skills and perceptual development but also the sound makeup and length of a word. Nevertheless, research indicates that the following sounds should be mastered by the ages indicated (Table 1):

- Vowels: should all be acquired by age 3 with the exception of the *er* sound in words like *b ir d* and *hamm er*.
- Consonants: these represent ages of *mastery*; prior to these ages, correct production will vary.

Articulation Disorders, Table 1 Ages by which children have mastered sounds

By age 3:	p m h w b (emerging between ages 1½ and 3)
By age 3½:	k g d t f y (girls only) (emerging between ages 2 and 3½)
By age 4:	y (boys)
By age 5:	s-blends (emerging between ages 3½ and 5)
By age 5½:	v
By age 6:	sh ch j (girls)
By age 7:	sh ch j (boys) th (as in *th*at)
By age 8:	r s ng l z th (as *in* thumb) zh (as in me*a*sure)

For children who do not meet these milestones, testing and possible treatment by a certified speech–language pathologist is highly recommended. A person who continues to exhibit articulation errors past age 8 should also be evaluated unless their sound usage is characteristic of a dialect or first language.

Neuropsychology and Psychology of Disorder

In some cases, an articulation disorder may be associated with damage to the central or peripheral nervous system. Specific neurological correlates usually are not found except in cases of dysarthria or apraxia. When misunderstood, some children may react by refusing to speak or withdrawing from others. Children who are unable to communicate due to an articulation disorder can become frustrated and act out because they cannot make basic needs and wants known. The child's family can also become frustrated at their inability to communicate with their child. However, this type of behavior is much more likely to occur in conjunction with phonological disorders rather than articulation disorders. For adults with speech sound disorders due to apraxia or dysarthria, the effect on communication will depend on the number of sounds affected, the degree of speech understandability, and the patient's reaction to the communication problem.

Evaluation

Evaluation of articulation disorders is designed to determine:

1. Existence of a problem
2. Nature of the problem (sounds in error, patterns intelligibility)

3. Possible etiology(ies) of the problem, e.g., structural problem or neurological disorder
4. Probable course of treatment
5. Prognosis

To meet these goals, the following components should be included in an evaluation for speech sound disorders:

1. Case history
2. Hearing screening
3. Oral mechanism evaluation
4. Phonemic sound-by-position articulation tests
5. Conversational speech sample
6. Statement of intelligibility
7. Language testing
8. Other tests as appropriate

Treatment

For patients with simple articulation disorders, a traditional, phonetic approach can be successful. Please refer ► "Phonological Disorder" and ► "Articulation Disorders" for more information on treatment.

Cross-References

► Apraxia
► Dysarthria
► Phonological Disorder
► Phonology
► Speech Sound Disorder

References and Readings

American Speech-Language-Hearing Association. (2007). Speech sound disorders: Articulation and phonological disorders. www.asha.org/public/speech/disorders/SpeechSoundDisorders.
American Speech-Language-Hearing Association. (2008). Incidence and prevalence of communication disorders and hearing loss in children (2008 edition). www.asha.org/members/research/reports/children.

Asenapine

Efrain Antonio Gonzalez
College of Psychology, Nova Southeastern
University, Fort Lauderdale, FL, USA
Utah State University, Logan, UT, USA

Generic Name

Asenapine

Brand Name
Saphris

Class
Antipsychotics, second generation, and mood stabilizer

Proposed Mechanism(s) of Action

Combination of central dopamine D2 and serotonin 5-HT2A receptor antagonism (sublingual)

Indication

For the treatment of schizophrenia and manic or mixed bipolar 1 episodes.

Off-Label Use

Agitation associated with a myriad of psychiatric conditions and dementia. Borderline personality disorder. Disruptive behavioral disorders associated with childhood.

Side Effects

Serious
Increased risk of mortality in elderly patients with dementia-related psychosis, mania. Extrapyramidal symptoms, prolongation of QT interval, and agranulocytosis.

Common
- Headache, dizziness, somnolence, dry mouth, nausea, tachycardia, diarrhea, orthostatic hypotension, and weight gain

References and Readings

Cutler, A. J., Kalali, A. H., Weiden, P. J., Hamilton, J., & Wolfgang, C. D. (2008). Four-week, double-blind, placebo- and ziprasidone-controlled trial of iloperidone in patients with acute exacerbations of schizophrenia. *Journal of Clinical Psychopharmacology, 28*(2 Suppl 1), S20–S28.

Kane, J. M., Lauriello, J., Laska, E., Di Marino, M., & Wolfgang, C. D. (2008). Long-term efficacy and safety of iloperidone: Results from 3 clinical trials for the treatment of schizophrenia. *Journal of Clinical Psychopharmacology, 28*(2 Suppl 1), S29–S35.

Kongsamut, S., Roehr, J. E., Cai, J., Hartman, H. B., Weissensee, P., Kerman, L. L., Tang, L., & Sandrasagra, A. (1996). Iloperidone binding to human and rat dopamine and 5-HT receptors. *European Journal of Pharmacology, 317*(2–3), 417–423.

Physicians' desk reference (71st ed.) (2017). Montvale: Thomson PDR.

Potkin, S. G., Litman, R. E., Torres, R., & Wolfgang, C. D. (2008). Efficacy of iloperidone in the treatment of schizophrenia: Initial phase 3 studies. *Journal of Clinical Psychopharmacology, 28*(2 Suppl 1), S4–11.

Sainati, S. M., Hubbard, J. W., Chi, E., Grasing, K., & Brecher, M. B. (1995). Safety, tolerability, and effect of food on the pharmacokinetics of iloperidone (HP 873), a potential atypical antipsychotic. *Journal of Clinical Pharmacology, 35*(7), 713–720.

Stahl, S. M. (2007). *Essential psychopharmacology: The prescriber's guide* (2nd ed.). New York: Cambridge University Press.

Szczepanik, A. M., Brougham, L. R., Roehr, J. E., Conway, P. G., Ellis, D. B., & Wilmot, C. A. (1996). Ex vivo studies with iloperidone (HP 873), a potential atypical antipsychotic with dopamine D2/5-hydroxytryptamine2 receptor antagonist activity. *The Journal of Pharmacology and Experimental Therapeutics, 278*(2), 913–920.

Weiden, P. J., Cutler, A. J., Polymeropoulos, M. H., & Wolfgang, C. D. (2008). Safety profile of iloperidone: A pooled analysis of 6-week acute-phase pivotal trials. *Journal of Clinical Psychopharmacology, 28*(2 Suppl 1), S12–S19.

Additional Information

Drug Interaction Effects. http://www.drugs.com/drug_interactions.html.

Drug Molecule Images. http://www.worldofmolecules.com/drugs/.

Free Drug Online. www.medscape.com.

Free Drug Online and PDA Software. www.epocrates.com.

Free Drug Online Centerwatch. https://www.centerwatch.com/drug-information/fda-approved-drugs/therapeutic-area/17/psychiatry-psychology.

Gene-Based Estimate of Drug interactions. http://mhc.daytondcs.com:8080/cgibin/ddiD4?ver=4&task=getDrugList.

Pill Identification. http://www.drugs.com/pill_identification.html.

ASHA Quality of Communication Life Scale

Diane Paul
Clinical Issues in Speech-Language Pathology,
American Speech-Language-Hearing
Association, Rockville, MD, USA

Synonyms

ASHA QCL; QCL

Description

The American Speech–Language–Hearing Association (ASHA) *Quality of Communication Life Scale* (QCL) was designed to assess the impact of a communication disorder on an adult's relationships and interactions with communication partners and on participation in social, leisure, work, and educational activities. The World Health Organization (WHO) defines quality of life as individuals' "perception of their position in life in the context of the culture and value systems in which they live and in relation to their goals, expectations, standards and concerns" (WHOQCL Group 1995). ASHA defines Quality of Communication Life as "…the extent to which a person's communication acts, as constrained within the boundaries drawn by personal and environmental factors, and as filtered through this person's perspective, allow meaningful participation in life situations" (Paul et al. 2004). The QCL is intended to be used as part of a comprehensive communication assessment in conjunction with measures of impairment and functional communication skills, such as the ASHA *Functional Assessment of Communication Skills for Adults* (ASHA FACS; Frattali et al. 1995; Frattali et al. 2017).

Rationale

The QCL emerged from the widespread need by speech–language pathologists for a reliable and valid instrument to determine the quality of life and participation in daily life activities as a result of a communication disorder. Other measures of quality of life were available (see Frattali 1998; Hirsch and Holland 2000 for a summary) and a few measures assessed a single aspect of communication, such as voice (*Voice Handicap Index*; Jacobson et al. 1997) or hearing (*Hearing Handicap Inventory for the Elderly*; Ventry and Weinstein 1982). However, no other measures were designed specifically for evaluating communication-related quality of life for adults with communication disorders. The development of the QCL was supported, in part, from a grant awarded to ASHA from the US Department of Education, National Institute on Disability and Rehabilitation Research (No. H133G970055).

Development and Testing

Pilot Test

A pilot test was conducted to determine the appropriateness of the QCL items for adults with neurogenic communication disorders. The pilot test included healthcare settings from different areas of the country and with a diverse caseload mix, including patients with aphasia, cognitive–communication disorder, and dysarthria. The subjects, 31 male and 26 female, had a mean age of 58.1 years and showed a range in severity of communication disorder, education, and employment. The 35 pilot test items were grouped into the following domains: (1) relationships/social life, (2) interests and leisure, (3) vocational and school life, and (4) autonomy and well-being. There also was an item related to overall quality of life. Subjects marked their responses on a vertical 10-cm scale. The scale was a vertical line because of a concern that patients with neurogenic communication disorders might experience visual field neglect. A factor analysis showed that the domains did not reflect how the items were related. Results also showed that using a ruler to measure the placement of the client rating added 25 min per subject. Modifications based on the pilot tests results included developing a new scoring system that did not necessitate the use of a ruler, omitting items that could not be scored reliably, and changing the domains. A question was added to ask about the subject's affect or mood at the time of administration.

Field Test

The field test was designed to determine test validity, intra-rater reliability, consistency of responses, and usability. The field test had 19 items in three domains: (1) socialization/activities, (2) confidence/self-concept, and (3) roles and responsibilities. The item to assess general well-being remained on the field test version of the QCL. Two items were repeated to provide a measure of response consistency. Field test sites included a range of healthcare settings from different geographic areas in the United States. Eighty-six subjects (61% male and 39% female) with a mean age of 57.2 years participated in the field test. Most of the subjects had a primary diagnosis of left hemisphere stroke (70.9%) or traumatic brain injury (16.3%) with a primary communication disorder of aphasia (70.9%), cognitive–communication disorder (16.3%), or dysarthria (12.8%) across severity levels. Each subject completed the QCL, with assistance if needed, and also completed a measure of well-being, the *Affect Balance Scale* (ABS; Bradburn 1969). Examiners also had the option to complete a posttest interview asking subjects to rate the importance of selected test items. Data analyses consisted of correlation coefficients for each test item, each domain mean score, and total score

with the item score for general well-being. The correlation between the total score and the item score for general well-being score was significant at 0.59. The correlation between domain mean scores and the item score for general well-being was significant for socialization/activities (0.49) and confidence/self-concept (0.54). Intra-rater reliability was moderate to high and consistency of response was considered to be acceptable. The correlation between the total score for the ABS and the QCL was low (0.09) and was not statistically significant, suggesting that the ABS and QCL measure different constructs. A factor analysis showed a strong relationship among most of the test items; 16 of the 19 items loaded under one factor. The data did not support categorization into three distinct domains. The field test results indicated that the QCL is a valid measure of quality of communication life for adults with neurogenic communication disorders. All items were included in the final version of the QCL, except the two duplicate items.

Clinical Use

The target population for the QCL is adults with neurologically based communication disorders, including aphasia, cognitive–communication disorder, and dysarthria.

The following materials are included with the QCL:

- Manual detailing the rationale, development, and testing of the QCL and administration and scoring instructions
- Case example with completed demographics form and score sheet
- Demographics form
- Test items with rating scale
- Score sheet
- Administration form

The QCL consists of a sample item, practice item, and the following 18 test items:

1. I like to talk with people.
2. It's easy for me to communicate.

3. My role in the family is the same.

4. I like myself.

5. I meet the communication needs of my job or school.

6. I stay in touch with family and friends.

7. People include me in conversations.

8. I follow news, sports, and stories on TV/movies.

9. I use the telephone.

10. I see the funny things in life.

11. People understand me when I talk.

12. I keep trying when people don't understand me.

13. I make my own decisions.

14. I am confident that I can communicate.

15. I get out of the house and do things.

16. I have household responsibilities.

17. I speak for myself.

18. In general, my quality of life is good.

The QCL takes approximately 15 min to administer. It was designed to be completed in a short time, recognizing the time constraints on clinicians. Patients with more severe communication impairments may take longer to complete the QCL and may need more assistance. The clinician may assist by reading the test items and making the mark on the rating scale to help the patient. The information derived from the QCL about the psychosocial, vocational, and educational effects of a communication impairment can assist with treatment planning, goal setting, counseling, progress monitoring, and documentation of treatment outcomes.

References

Bradburn, N. M. (1969). *The structure of psychological well-being*. Chicago: Aldine.

Frattali, C. M. (1998). Measuring modality-specific behaviors, functional abilities, and quality of life. In C. M. Frattali (Ed.), *Measuring outcomes in speech-language pathology* (pp. 55–88). New York: Thieme.

Frattali, C. M., Thompson, C. K., Holland, A. L., Wohl, C. B., & Ferketic, M. M. (1995). *American speech-language-hearing association functional assessment of communication skills for adults*. Rockville, MD: American Speech-Language-Hearing Association.

Frattali, C. M., Thompson, C. K., Holland, A. L., Wohl, C. B., Wenck, C. J., Slater, S. C., & Paul, D. (2017). *Americn speech-language-hearing association func-tional assessment of communication skills for adults*. Rockville, MD: American Speech-Language-Hearing Association.

Hirsch, F. M., & Holland, A. L. (2000). Beyond activity: Measuring participation in society and quality of life. In L. E. Worrall & C. M. Frattali (Eds.), *Neurogenic communication disorders: A functional approach* (pp. 35–54). New York: Thieme.

Jacobson, B. H., Johnson, A., Grywalski, C., Silbergliet, A., Jacobson, G., & Benninger, M. S. (1997). Voice handicap index (VHI): Development and validation. *American Journal of Speech-Language Pathology, 6*, 66–70.

Paul, D. R., Frattali, C. M., Holland, A. L., Thompson, C. K., Caperton, C. J., & Slater, S. C. (2004). *Quality of communication life scale*. Rockville, MD: American Speech-Language-Hearing Association.

The WHOQOL Group. (1995). The World Health Organization quality of life assessment (WHOQOL): Position paper from the World Health Organization. *Social Science and Medicine, 41*(10), 1403–1409.

Ventry, I. M., & Weinstein, B. E. (1982). The Hearing Handicap Inventory for the Elderly: A new tool. *Ear and Hearing, 3*, 128–134.

Readings

American Speech-Language-Hearing Association. (n.d.). *National outcomes measurement system* (NOMS). Available from www.asha.org/NOMS.

Aphasia Institute. (2013). *Assessment for living with aphasia toolkit (ALA)—second edition*. Toronto, Ontario, Canada: Author. Retrieved from http://www.aphasia.ca/shop/assessment-for-living-with-aphasia-toolkit/

Bose, A., McHugh, T., Schollenberger, H., & Buchanan, L. (2009). Measuring quality of life in aphasia: Results from two scales. *Aphasiology, 23*(7–8), 797–808.

Dalemans, R., de Witte, L. P., Lemmens, J., van den Heuvel, W. J. A., & Wade, D. T. (2008). Measures for rating social participation in people with aphasia: A systematic review. *Clinical Rehabilitation, 22*(6), 542–555.

Golper, L. C., & Frattali, C. M. (2012). *Outcomes in speech-language pathology: Contemporary theories, models, and practices* (2nd ed.). New York: Thieme.

Hilari, K., Byng, S., Lamping, D. L., & Smith, S. C. (2003). Stroke and Aphasia Quality of Life Scale-39 (SAQOL-39): Evaluation and acceptability, reliability, and validity. *Stroke, 34*(8), 1944–1950.

Kagan, A., Simmons-Mackie, N., Rowland, A., Huijbregts, M., Shumway, E., McEwen, S., . . . Sharp, S. (2008). Counting what counts: A framework for capturing real-life outcomes of aphasia intervention. *Aphasiology, 22*, 258–280.

Post, M. W. M., Boosman, H., van Zandvoort, M. M., Passier, P. E. C. A., Rinkel, G. J. E., & Visser-Meily, J. M. A. (2011). Development and validation of a short version of the Stroke Specific Quality of Life Scale. *Journal of Neurology, Neurosurgery & Psychiatry, 82*(3), 283–286.

Ashworth Spasticity Scale (and Modified Version)

Kari Dunning
Department of Rehabilitation Sciences,
University of Cincinnati, Cincinnati, OH, USA

Synonyms

AS; MAS

Description

The Ashworth Scale (AS) and Modified Ashworth Scale (MAS) measure spasticity. During the administration of both AS (Ashworth 1964) and MAS (Bohannon and Smith 1987), the examiner passively moves the joint being tested and rates the perceived level of resistance in the muscle groups opposing the movement. Both scales are single-item measures ranging from 0 to 4, where 0 indicates no increase in muscle tone and 4 indicates that the affected part is rigid in flexion or extension. The AS is considered an ordinal scale, whereas the MAS is considered a nominal scale due to ambiguity created by the addition of the 1+ grade between 1 and 2 (Pandyan et al. 1999).

Historical Background

The AS was first described by Ashworth in 1964 (Ashworth 1964) and was subsequently modified with the addition of a 1+ grade by Bohannon in 1987 with the intent to increase sensitivity (Bohannon and Smith 1987). However, this addition may have decreased the reliability of the MAS for heavier limbs (see below) (Ansari et al. 2008; Pandyan et al. 1999; Platz et al. 2005).

Psychometric Data

Inter- and intra-rater reliability of the AS and MAS show wide variation (Pandyan et al. 1999;
Platz et al. 2005), which cannot be attributed to any one factor (Platz et al. 2005), although some evidence suggests that the inter-rater reliability of the MAS is lower for heavier limbs (Ansari et al. 2008; Pandyan et al. 1999; Platz et al. 2005). Both scales have demonstrated responsiveness to treatment (Platz et al. 2005).

Spasticity is characterized by an involuntary muscle activity (Pandyan et al. 2005) and has been traditionally defined as a velocity-dependent increase in muscle tone due to a hyperactive stretch reflex (Lance 1980). The construct validity of the AS and MAS as spasticity assessments is inadequate because they do not address velocity dependence. Rather, these scales measure passive resistance to movement (hypertonia), which is influenced by spasticity but also altered by biomechanical factors unrelated to involuntary muscle activation (Fleuren et al. 2009; Pandyan et al. 1999; Platz et al. 2005). Thus, AS and MAS scores are only moderately associated with reflexes (Platz et al. 2005) and electromyographic assessments (Fleuren et al. 2009; Pandyan et al. 1999; Platz et al. 2005) and more strongly associated with objective measures of resistance (Fleuren et al. 2009; Pandyan et al. 1999; Platz et al. 2005).

Clinical Uses

Despite the fact that the AS and MAS are actually only valid assessments of hypertonia (Fleuren et al. 2009; Pandyan et al. 1999; Platz et al. 2005), these scales are the most commonly used clinical tools to assess spasticity (Pandyan et al. 1999; Platz et al. 2005). Both scales have been used to describe treatment response for persons with a wide range of upper motor neuron disorders, including traumatic brain injury, stroke, multiple sclerosis, cerebral palsy, and spinal cord injury (Platz et al. 2005).

Cross-References

▶ Severe Brain Injury
▶ Spinal Cord Injury

References and Readings

Ansari, N. N., Naghdi, S., Arab, T. K., & Jalaie, S. (2008). The interrater and intrarater reliability of the modified Ashworth scale in the assessment of muscle spasticity: Limb and muscle group effect. *NeuroRehabilitation, 23*(3), 231–237.

Ashworth, B. (1964). Preliminary trial of carisoprodol in multiple sclerosis. *Practitioner, 192*, 540–542.

Bohannon, R. W., & Smith, M. B. (1987). Interrater reliability of a modified Ashworth scale of muscle spasticity. *Physical Therapy, 67*(2), 206–207.

Fleuren, J. F., Voerman, G. E., Erren-Wolters, C. V., et al. (2009). Stop using the Ashworth scale for the assessment of spasticity. *Journal of Neurology, Neurosurgery, and Psychiatry, 81*(2), 46–52.

Lance, J. W. (1980). Symposium synopsis. In R. G. Feldman, R. R. Young, & W. P. Koella (Eds.), *Spasticity: Disordered motor control* (pp. 485–494). Chicago: Year Book Medical Publishers.

Pandyan, A., Johnson, G., Price, C., Curless, R., Barnes, M., & Rodgers, H. (1999). A review of the properties and limitations of the Ashworth and modified Ashworth scales as measures of spasticity. *Clinical Rehabilitation, 13*(5), 373–383.

Pandyan, A. D., Gregoric, M., Barnes, M. P., et al. (2005). Spasticity: Clinical perceptions, neurological realities and meaningful measurement. *Disability and Rehabilitation, 27*(1–2), 2–6.

Platz, T., Eickhof, C., Nuyens, G., & Vuadens, P. (2005). Clinical scales for the assessment of spasticity, associated phenomena, and function: A systematic review of the literature. *Disability and Rehabilitation, 27*(1–2), 7–18.

ASIA Impairment Scale

Amitabh Jha
TBIMS National Data and Statistical Center, Craig Hospital, Englewood, CO, USA

Synonyms

ASIA (American Spinal Injury Association) exam; Frankel scale; International Standards for Neurological Classification of Spinal Cord Injury

Description

The *International Standards for Neurological Classification of SCI (ISNCSCI)* is a widely accepted and readily administered guide to document neurological function after spinal cord injury (SCI) and is intended to be a standard for measuring neurological outcomes in both clinical and research settings. Briefly, these standards utilize a two-step process consisting of a specific neurological examination followed by a classification procedure based on the results of the exam. The systematic neurological examination assesses sensory and motor function of each spinal segmental level. Sensation of light touch and pinprick (PP) stimuli is scored as 0 for absent, 1 for impaired, and 2 for normal. Motor function is scored on a scale of 0 for total paralysis to 5 for normal strength. All 28 dermatomes are tested bilaterally for sensory function, and ten key muscles are tested bilaterally for motor function, yielding sensory/light touch (LT) and sensory/pinprick (PP) summed scores ranging from 0 to 112 and motor summed scores ranging from 0 to 100. The neurological level is assigned as the lowest level with normal neurological function. In addition, the ASIA Impairment Scale (AIS) grade classification, an indicator of injury "completeness" similar to the Frankel scale, is assigned based on this information. AIS A denotes a complete injury with no sensory or motor function below the level of injury. Incomplete injuries are graded as AIS B if there is sensory but no motor function below the injury level, AIS C if there is some motor sparing, AIS D for substantial motor sparing, and AIS E for normal neurological examination (Fig. 1).

Historical Background

ISNCSCI has been used extensively in clinical practice and research since 1982. The standards and accompanying reference manual have undergone sequential revisions, most recently in 2000 and 2003, respectively.

Psychometric Data

Published studies have found total motor score ICCs from 0.98 to 0.99 for intra-rater reliability

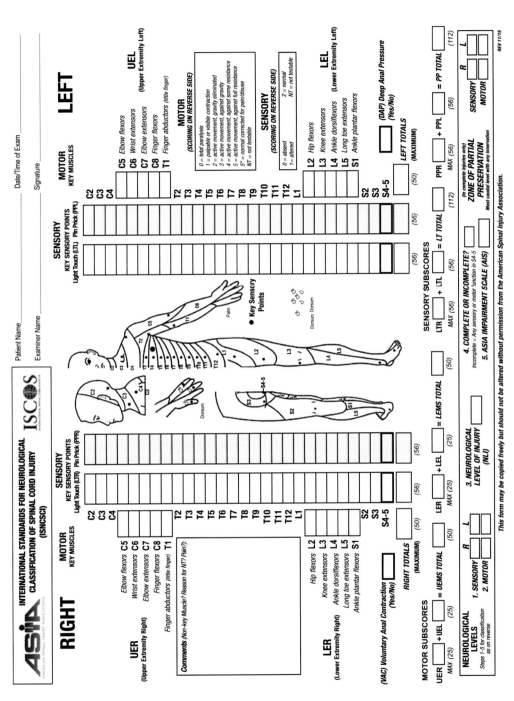

ASIA Impairment Scale, Fig. 1 International Standards for Neurological Classification of Spinal Cord Injury (ISNCSCI)

and 0.97 for inter-rater reliability. Total sensory intra-rater reliability score has ranged from 0.76 to 0.98 and 0.88 to 0.96 for inter-rater. One study reported agreement on individual muscles with Kappas ranging from 0.46 to 0.89 for each myotome (elbow extensors had the worst agreement), 0.06 to 0.83 for dermatome assessment using pinprick (wrist extensors with worst agreement), and 0.23 to 1 when assessed using light touch (wrist extensors with worst agreement).

Clinical Uses

The exam is used to document sensory and motor function after SCI. It has been used to diagnose SCI, as an outcome measure in studies to treat spinal cord pathology, as well as a tool to predict outcomes such as independence with activities of daily living, employment, life satisfaction, and life expectancy.

Cross-References

▶ Sensorimotor Assessment
▶ Spinal Cord Injury

References and Readings

American Spinal Injury Association. (2002). *International standards for neurological classification of spinal cord injury (revised 2002)*. Chicago: American Spinal Injury Association.

American Spinal Injury Association. (2003). *Reference manual for the international standards for neurological classification of spinal cord injury (revised 2003)*. Chicago: American spinal injury association.

Furlan, J. C., Fehlings, M. G., Tator, C. H., & Davis, A. M. (2008). Motor and sensory assessment of patients in clinical trials for pharmacological therapy of acute spinal cord injury: Psychometric properties of the ASIA standards. *Journal of Neurotrauma, 25*(11), 1273–1301.

Jonsson, M., Tollback, A., Gonzales, H., & Borg, J. (2000). Inter-rater reliability of the 1992 international standards for neurological and functional classification of incomplete spinal cord injury. *Spinal cord, 38*, 675–679.

Kirshblum, S. C., Memmo, P., Kim, N., Campagnolo, D., & Millis, S. (2002). Comparison of the revised 2000 American spinal injury association classification

standards with the 1996 guidelines. *American journal of Physical Medicine & Rehabilitation, 81*(7), 502–505.

Mulcahey, M. J., Gaughan, J., Betz, R. R., & Johansen, K. J. (2007). The international standards for neurological classification of spinal cord injury: Reliability of data when applied to children and youths. *Spinal Cord, 45*(6), 452–459.

Asomatognosia

John E. Mendoza
Department of Psychiatry and Neuroscience, Tulane Medical School and SE Louisiana Veterans Healthcare System, New Orleans, LA, USA

Synonyms

Disturbance of body schema

Definition

Disturbance in the normal awareness of one's own body, typically characterized by one or more of the following symptoms: (1) a tendency to ignore or neglect one side of the body, (2) a failure to recognize or difficulty in identifying a specific part of the body (usually a limb or part of a limb), (3) difficulty in differentiating the right from the left side of the body, or (4) recognizing an impairment in a part of the body (*anosognosia*).

Current Knowledge

Asomatognosia most commonly results from acute or subacute brain lesions and may affect one or both sides of the body. Unilateral neglect generally involves an entire side of the body, more commonly the left. This might be reflected in a failure to shave the affected side of the face, putting a glove only on one hand, or reduced use of the involved limb for certain activities, even though it is physically capable of doing so. If a limb is paralyzed, the patient may either deny or minimize the impairment (*anosognosia*), or may even deny ownership of the affected limb. If the affected side or a part of the body is stimulated, the individual may report that the homologous area on the intact side was touched (*allesthesia*). Patients may also have difficulty localizing or identifying parts of their own body (*autotopagnosia*). This is most commonly expressed as difficulty naming or identifying individual fingers (especially the three middle digits) either of their own hands or those of others (*finger agnosia*). This deficit is usually expressed bilaterally. *Right-left disorientation* is generally also considered a form of asomatognosia. Here, the individual has difficulty reliably identifying the right and left sides of his or her own body or those of the examiner.

Although asomatognosia strictly refers to impaired awareness or attention to parts of one's own body, personal neglect often extends into extrapersonal space. Thus, a patient may fail to attend to visual or auditory stimuli on the affected side, despite intact visual fields or the fact that auditory stimuli enter both ears. This can be very disconcerting for family members if they are not made aware of these phenomena, perhaps believing the patient is purposely ignoring their presence.

Unilateral neglect or anosognosia-type disorders are most commonly found, following acute lesions (such as strokes) of the right hemisphere. Although improvement is typically seen over time, subtle degrees of deficit may persist indefinitely. By contrast, those deficits that present bilaterally (such as finger agnosia and right-left disorientation) are usually the result of posterior left-hemispheric lesions.

Cross-References

▶ Allesthesia
▶ Anosognosia
▶ Autotopagnosia
▶ Finger Agnosia
▶ Right Left Disorientation

References and Readings

Feinberg, T., Venneri, A., Simone, A., Fan, Y., & Northoff, G. (2010). The neuroanatomy of asomatognosia and somatoparaphrenia. *Journal of Neurology, Neurosurgery, and Psychiatry, 81*(3), 276–281.

Hecaen, H., & Albert, M. L. (1978). *Human neuropsychology* (pp. 303–330). New York: Wiley.

Heilman, K. M., Watson, R. T., & Valenstein, E. (2003). Neglect and related disorders. In K. Heilman & E. Valenstein (Eds.), *Clinical neuropsychology* (pp. 296–346). New York: Oxford University Press.

Kortte, K. B., & Wegener, S. T. (2004). Denial of illness in medical rehabilitation populations: Theory, research and definitions. *Rehabilitation Psychology, 49*, 187–199.

Prigatano, G. P., & Schacter, D. L. (1991). *Awareness of deficit after brain injury: Clinical and theoretical issues*. New York: Oxford University Press.

Asperger's Disorder

Micah O. Mazurek[1] and Stephen M. Kanne[2]
[1]Curry School of Education, University of Virginia, Charlottesville, VA, USA
[2]Thompson Center for Autism and Neurodevelopmental Disorders, University of Missouri, Columbia, MO, USA

Synonyms

Asperger syndrome

Definition

Asperger's disorder refers to a neurodevelopmental disorder, defined in the DSM-IV and more recently removed in the DSM-5, associated with impairment in social relatedness and repetitive or restricted behaviors and interests. Social difficulties characteristic of Asperger's disorder include nonverbal aspects of social interaction (e.g., eye contact, gestures, and facial expressions) as well as social and emotional reciprocity (e.g., sharing interests, taking turns, and demonstrating empathy). Behaviorally, individuals with

Asperger's disorder often exhibit intense and narrow circumscribed interests, insistence on sameness or routine, and behavioral rigidity (American Psychiatric Association 1994). While overall level of intellectual functioning (i.e., IQ) is not impaired in individuals with Asperger's disorder, their cognition is often compromised in other areas such as executive functioning (see Neuropsychology and Psychology of Asperger's Disorder).

Categorization

Asperger's disorder first appeared in DSM-IV (1994) as a separate diagnostic category but has since been removed in the most recent version (DSM-5; American Psychiatric Association 2013). Asperger's disorder was previously classified in the DSM-IV as one of five separate pervasive developmental disorders (which also included autistic disorder, Rett's disorder, childhood disintegrative disorder, and pervasive developmental disorder not otherwise specified, PDD NOS). To meet DSM-IV criteria for Asperger's disorder, an individual needed to demonstrate impairment in social interaction (exhibiting at least two out of four possible symptoms) and restricted and repetitive patterns of behaviors or interests (exhibiting at least one out of four possible symptoms). In addition, an individual must *not* have had a history of developmental delays in language, cognition, or adaptive functioning. Of note, the criteria for Asperger's disorder were identical to those for autistic disorder (i.e., autism) in the areas of social impairment and restricted and repetitive behavior. However, autistic disorder required an additional criterion of impairment in communication (i.e., delays in language development, impairment in conversation, stereotyped language, or lack of pretend play). Additionally, there was not a requirement in the criteria for autistic disorder that cognitive, language, and adaptive development fall within the normal range in childhood as was the case in Asperger's disorder (American Psychiatric Association 1994).

The DSM-IV criteria for Asperger's disorder gave rise to a number of difficulties that reduced its clinical utility and made it difficult to demonstrate its etiological independence. For example, individuals meeting criteria for Asperger's disorder almost always demonstrated difficulties with reciprocal conversation, meaning that they would have also met criteria for autistic disorder. As a result, the diagnosis demonstrated poor specificity and poor reliability across clinicians. Additionally, individuals with Asperger's disorder were not distinguishable from individuals with high functioning autism across a number of studies. For these reasons, Asperger's disorder was removed as a distinct diagnostic category in DSM-5 (see Ozonoff 2012 for review).

This decision to remove Asperger's disorder was met with controversy among some researchers, clinicians, and community members. A primary concern was that individuals previously diagnosed with Asperger's disorder may no longer meet criteria for autism spectrum disorder (ASD) under the new DSM-5. However, studies have found that most individuals meeting DSM-IV criteria for Asperger's disorder also meet DSM-5 criteria for ASD (Huerta et al. 2014). To further allay these concerns, DSM-5 criteria specify that "individuals with a well-established DSM-IV diagnosis of autistic disorder, Asperger's disorder, or pervasive developmental disorder not otherwise specified should be given the diagnosis of autism spectrum disorder" (American Psychiatric Association 2013, p. 51). Although no longer recognized as a distinct category, the term "Asperger's disorder" will be used for simplicity in the sections that follow to describe individuals who met previous criteria for the disorder.

Epidemiology

Prevalence estimates have varied widely from 0.3/1000 to 6/1000 (see Mattila et al. 2007 for review). Based on a review of the literature, Fombonne (Fombonne and Tidmash 2003, 2005) estimated the prevalence rate for Asperger's disorder to be approximately 2/10,000. Such wide variations in prevalence rates are likely due to differences in diagnostic procedures and operational definitions used in each study. In fact, rates from the same study varied from 1.6/1000 to 2.9/1000 depending on the specific criteria used for diagnosis (Mattila et al. 2007). In terms of sex differences, males are overrepresented in Asperger's disorder, with an estimated sex ratio of 4:1 (see Schopler et al. 1998 for review).

Natural History, Prognostic Factors, and Outcomes

Asperger's disorder took its name from the Austrian physician, Hans Asperger, whose 1944 paper on "autistic psychopathy" described a group of children who showed deficits in social behaviors, insistence on sameness, a lack of nonverbal communication, repetitive movements, and average intelligence. Asperger (in 1944) and Leo Kanner (in 1943), although unaware of one another's work, were the first to describe this cluster of symptoms. While Leo Kanner's seminal work describing autistic behaviors was the subject of much discussion and resulted in the eventual inclusion of autism in the DSM (in 1980), Asperger's paper did not receive wide attention after publication and was not translated into English until 1991 (see Frith 1991). After the appearance of autism in the DSM-III, it became apparent that there was a group of individuals who did not meet the criteria for the narrowly defined definition of infantile autism, but who demonstrated deficits in social interaction and repetitive behaviors. As a result, Wing (1981) published an influential paper reintroducing Asperger's original ideas and arguing for broadening the definition of autism to include Asperger's disorder on the autism continuum. Eventually, a separate diagnosis of Asperger's disorder was added to the fourth edition of the DSM (1994). Since that time, debate continued as to whether or not Asperger's disorder should remain a separate diagnosis from autism. The prevailing current view is that Asperger's disorder and autism are not distinctly different and that Asperger's disorder may simply represent a specific phenotype or subgroup of the autism

spectrum. As a result, Asperger's disorder is often used synonymously with the term "high-functioning autism" (which typically refers to individuals meeting criteria for Autistic Disorder whose IQ levels are above 70). Ultimately, these issues resulted in the decision by the DSM-5 Neurodevelopmental Disorders Workgroup to remove Asperger's disorder as a separate diagnosis, and to consolidate previous PDD subgroups into a single category. The intention of this change was to retain a single diagnostic category (i.e., ASD), while allowing for characterization of variability in severity and symptom presentation within both social-communication and restricted and repetitive behavior domains.

With regard to developmental course, Asperger's disorder was generally diagnosed much later than autistic disorder, with an average age of diagnosis being 11 years (possibly due to the lack of early developmental delays). Individuals diagnosed with Asperger's disorder exhibited a continuous course of symptoms throughout the life span, although for some individuals symptoms improved substantially as a result of early intervention (see Frith 2004 for review). Research into prognostic factors and outcome in Asperger's disorder is sparse, particularly since it was only recognized as an official diagnosis for a brief period of time; however, IQ and language ability have been found to be strong predictors of outcomes in autism spectrum disorders in general (see Magiati et al. 2014 for review).

Neuropsychology and Psychology of Asperger's Disorder

By definition, social interactions are impaired in individuals with Asperger's disorder. However, the underlying processes by which social interactions are disrupted have been the source of recent attention. First, there is clear evidence that individuals with Asperger's disorder have impairments in their ability to understand complex emotions and a resulting inability to recognize and empathize with others' feelings. Individuals with Asperger's disorder also have impairments in what is known as "theory of mind." As such, they have difficulty automatically attributing mental states to others. Although there were no formal criteria concerning communication skills for Asperger's disorder according to DSM-IV, clinical and research accounts highlight the presence of social communication difficulties. Specifically, difficulties with pragmatic language and difficulties with turn-taking in conversation are common (see Klin et al. 2000 for review).

Asperger's disorder is also associated with cognitive features that affect functioning outside the social domain. Studies have shown that individuals with Asperger's disorder have very uneven cognitive profiles. One explanation for this common finding is that these individuals have "weak central coherence." That is, they are more likely to process information as discrete units rather than processing them as a unified whole. There is some evidence that bottom-up processing occurs without accompanying top-down control. As a result, high levels of details are perceived, while global information may be missed (see Frith 2004). Studies have also shown consistent deficits in overall executive function among individuals with Asperger's disorder. Specifically, poor performance has been shown on both the Wisconsin Card Sorting Test and the Tower of Hanoi. Particular deficits have been noted in the ability to shift response set and in overall planning. Consistent with this, individuals with Asperger's disorder are often described as having difficulty adjusting to changes in routine or task demands and as having a strong need for sameness (see Klin et al. 2000).

Some studies, including Wing's (1981) original description, have found significantly higher verbal IQ scores than performance IQ scores among individuals with Asperger's disorder (the reverse of which was often found in individuals who met DSM-IV criteria for autistic disorder). Motor clumsiness has also been observed among children with Asperger's disorder since Hans Asperger's original paper, although it has never been a part of the formal diagnostic criteria (see Frith 1991). As a result, researchers have been interested in potential similarities between Asperger's disorder and nonverbal learning disorders (NVLD) or right hemispheric dysfunction.

These profiles are marked by relative strengths at rote verbal skills, with deficits in social understanding and motor coordination. While there is a great deal of overlap among these conditions, empirical findings have been equivocal. Some studies have found visual-spatial impairments (with strengths in Verbal IQ) in Asperger's disorder, while others have not demonstrated this pattern (see Klin et al. 2000). Given recent diagnostic changes, further work with more specific subtyping criteria is needed to continue to understand potential phenotypic and neuropsychological differences within the ASD population.

Coexisting Conditions

In addition to the core symptoms, Asperger's disorder may also be accompanied by co-occurring disorders. Studies have shown that a large percentage of children with Asperger's disorder also exhibit problems with attention and impulse control (similar to those found in ADHD). In adolescence and adulthood, case studies indicate relatively high rates of depression, anxiety, and bipolar disorder among individuals with Asperger's disorder (see Ghaziuddin 2002 for review). Individuals with Asperger's disorder also have significant adaptive impairments (see Saulnier and Klin 2007).

Evaluation

Diagnostic assessment of high functioning ASD (previously Asperger's disorder) is best conducted using multiple methods and observers. Due to the complexity of the disorder, and its effects on broad areas of functioning, interdisciplinary assessment is recommended. First, because ASD is a neurodevelopmental disorder, parent report of early history and development, as well as structured observations of current behavior, are essential. Currently, the two "gold-standard" tools for diagnosis of ASD are the Autism Diagnostic Interview-Revised (ADI-R) and the Autism Directed Observation Schedule – 2nd Edition (ADOS-2). These are the most widely studied measures in the field, and reliability and validity have been well established. The ADI-R is a comprehensive interview that assesses past and current functioning in the areas of communication, social interaction, and restricted or repetitive behavior. The ADOS-2 is another diagnostic tool that allows for clinic-based observations across various structured activity- and conversation-based interactions. A number of other scales were previously developed to specifically assess Asperger's disorder, but systematic research is lacking (see Matson & Boisjoli 2008; Mesibov et al. 2001 for review). The removal of Asperger's disorder as a distinct diagnostic category in DSM-5 may further limit their utility.

In addition to assessing the core symptoms of ASD, assessment should focus on cognitive, adaptive, and communication skills. General measures of intelligence, such as the *Wechsler Scales* and the *Stanford Binet Intelligence Scales* are useful in assessing overall functioning as well as particular strengths and weaknesses. Additionally, it is helpful to include measures of visual-spatial and visual-motor processing, particularly since skills in these areas were typically weaker in prior studies of individuals with Asperger's disorder. Given common deficits in executive function and attention, neuropsychological assessment of these functions is recommended. Measures of social communication and pragmatic language, and adaptive skills, also add information to the clinical picture and help inform intervention recommendations (see Klin et al. 2000 for review).

Treatment

There is, as of yet, no available treatment that provides a "cure" for the core impairments of ASD. However, there are a number of interventions that target specific symptoms. For addressing social deficits, there have been several promising studies of social competence interventions among children and adolescents with Asperger's disorder and high functioning ASD. Such interventions can be delivered in educational or outpatient clinic-based settings, and typically include cognitive and behavioral components (including direct instruction, modeling skills, and skills practice) (see Klin et al. 2000).

Educationally, students with Asperger's disorder often benefit from modifications and supports provided through special education. Although services vary widely based on the region, they may range from specialized schools designed to serve students with Asperger's disorder to modifications within general education classrooms. Some students may get benefit and support from paraprofessional aides in the classroom, while others may require only slight academic modifications. Most students with Asperger's disorder benefit greatly from communication interventions aimed at improving pragmatic and social skills (see Klin et al. 2000; Mesibov et al. 2001 for review).

Family support, parent training, and instruction on behavior management strategies can also be helpful when disruptive behaviors accompany the clinical picture. Recent research has also shown that both individual and group-based cognitive behavioral therapy is effective in the treatment of co-occurring symptoms of anxiety in individuals with Asperger's disorder and high functioning ASD (Danial and Wood 2013; Sukhodolsky et al. 2013). Individual work with counselors or mental health professionals could also focus on social and communication skills training as well as bolstering adaptive functioning. In addition, medications may be prescribed to treat associated symptoms (particularly inattention, depression, and anxiety).

Cross-References

▶ Nonverbal Learning Disabilities

References and Readings

American Psychiatric Association. (1994). *Diagnostic and statistical manual of mental disorders* (4th ed.). Washington, DC: American Psychiatric Publishing.
American Psychiatric Association. (2013). *Diagnostic and statistical manual of mental disorders* (5th ed.). Washington, DC: American Psychiatric Publishing.

Danial, J. T., & Wood, J. J. (2013). Cognitive behavioral therapy for children with autism: Review and considerations for future research. *Journal of Developmental & Behavioral Pediatrics, 34*(9), 702–715.

Fombonne, E. (2005). The changing epidemiology of autism. *Journal of Applied Research in Intellectual Disabilities, 18,* 281–294.

Fombonne, E., & Tidmarsh, L. (2003). Epidemiologic data on Asperger disorder. *Child and Adolescent Psychiatric Clinics of North America, 12,* 15–21.

Frith, U. (Ed.). (1991). *Autism and Asperger syndrome.* Cambridge: Cambridge University Press.

Frith, U. (2004). Emanuel miller lecture: Confusions and controversies about Asperger syndrome. *Journal of Child Psychology and Psychiatry, 45,* 672–686.

Ghaziuddin, M. (2002). Asperger syndrome: Associated psychiatric and medical conditions. *Focus on Autism and Other Developmental Disabilities, 17,* 138–144.

Huerta, M., Bishop, S. L., Duncan, A., et al. (2014). Application of DSM-5 criteria for autism spectrum disorder to three samples of children with DSM-IV diagnoses of pervasive developmental disorders. *American Journal of Psychiatry.* https://doi.org/10.1176/appi.ajp.2012.12020276.

Klin, A., Volkmar, F. R., & Sparrow, S. (Eds.). (2000). *Asperger syndrome.* New York: The Guilford Press.

Magiati, I., Tay, X. W., & Howlin, P. (2014). Cognitive, language, social and behavioural outcomes in adults with autism spectrum disorders: A systematic review of longitudinal follow-up studies in adulthood. *Clinical psychology review, 34*(1), 73–86.

Matson, J. L., & Boisjoli, J. A. (2008). Strategies for assessing Asperger's syndrome: A critical review of data based methods. *Research in Autism Spectrum Disorders, 2,* 237–248.

Mattila, M., Kielinen, M., Jussila, K., Linna, S., Bloigu, R., Ebeling, H., et al. (2007). An epidemiological and diagnostic study of Asperger syndrome according to four sets of diagnostic criteria. *Journal of the American Academy of Child & Adolescent Psychiatry, 46,* 636–646.

McLaughlin-Cheng, E. (1998). Asperger syndrome and autism: A literature review and meta-analysis. *Focus on Autism and Other Developmental Disabilities, 13,* 234–245.

Mesibov, G. B., Shea, V., & Adams, L. W. (2001). *Understanding Asperger syndrome and high-functioning autism.* New York: Kluwer Academic/Plenum Publishers.

Ozonoff, S. (2012). Editorial perspective: Autism Spectrum disorders in DSM-5 – An historical perspective and the need for change. *Journal of Child Psychology and Psychiatry, 53*(10), 1092–1094.

Saulnier, C. A., & Klin, A. (2007). Brief report: Social and communication abilities and disabilities in higher functioning individuals with autism and Asperger syndrome. *Journal of Autism and Developmental Disorders, 37*(4), 788–793.

Schopler, E., Mesibov, G. B., & Kunce, L. J. (Eds.). (1998). *Asperger syndrome or high-functioning autism?* New York: Plenum Press.

Sukhodolsky, D. G., Bloch, M. H., Panza, K. E., et al. (2013). Cognitive-behavioral therapy for anxiety in children with high-functioning autism: A meta-analysis. *Pediatrics, 132*(5), e1341–e1350.

Wing, L. (1981). Asperger's syndrome: A clinical account. *Psychological Medicine, 11,* 115–130.

Assessment of Life Habits (LIFE-H)

Jessica Fish
Medical Research Council Cognition and Brain Sciences Unit, Cambridge, UK

Synonyms

The abbreviation LIFE-H is consistent, but version numbers are often appended (e.g., LIFE-H 1.0, 2.0, 3.0, 3.1)

Description

The Assessment of Life Habits (LIFE-H) is a self-report measure of social participation of people with disabilities. The original version of the scale consisted of 298 items; later versions have reduced the number of items to 240 (version 3.0). Various short forms are also available (55–77 items), with the most recent being the 77-item version 3.1. The long form is said to take between 20 and 120 min to complete and the short form, 20–60 min. In the short form (version 3.1), items are organized into 12 categories: nutrition, fitness, personal care, communication, housing, mobility (classified as activities of regular living) and responsibilities, interpersonal relationships, community life, education, employment, and recreation (classified as social roles). The long form includes 31 subsections, essentially covering the listed domains with a greater degree of specificity. Each item is rated on a 4-point "level of accomplishment" scale (with an additional option to state "not applicable,") a 5-point "level of satisfaction" scale, as well as a rating regarding the type and level of assistance required (i.e., no assistance, assistive device, adaptation, human assistance). A score for each item is obtained with reference to a scoring template included in the manual, grading according to the level of difficulty and level of assistance. Item scores range from 0 (not accomplished) to 9 (performed with no difficulty and no assistance), with mid-scale examples being 3 (performed with difficulty and human assistance) and 6 (performed with difficulty and technical aid or adaptation). Scores can then be weighted by the number of applicable activities to obtain domain-level scores, or a simple formula can be used to obtain an overall score.

Historical Background

Noreau, Fougeyrollas, and Tremblay (2005) stated that the LIFE-H was developed to assess social participation in people with disabilities, regardless of the nature of those disabilities, and based upon the Disability Creation Process model, which views handicap as "the situational result of the interaction of two causal dimensions: the characteristics of the individual and those of the environment." Version 2.0 of the scale was developed following a content validity study that involved 12 experts in rehabilitation medicine evaluating the scale (in terms of clarity and pertinence of content, classifications used in the measurement scales, etc.); modifications included reversing the scoring of the accomplishment section such that higher scores reflected the competence in the activity. Version 3.0 incorporated a greater number of items within particular domains and added additional filter questions to some sections (e.g., if you are not currently employed, skip to section x). Version 3.1 is a short form based upon version 3.0.

Psychometric Data

Fougeyrollas et al. (1998) reported that the LIFE-H v1.0 demonstrated acceptable internal consistency in adults and children (intra-class correlation (ICCs) > 0.5 for each life habit) and good test-retest reliability in children and adults with spinal cord injury (ICC children $r = 0.73$ and adults $r = 0.74$). Inter-rater reliability was examined in a group of 20 stroke patients (Beaulieu et al. 1996; Cited in Noreau et al. 2002), with ICCs for 6/12 "accomplishment" ratings of life habits above 0.6 and 10/12 "satisfaction" ratings for life habits above 0.6. Similar findings have been reported for inter-rater reliability of LIFE-H scores for people with physical disabilities, with ICCs of $r > 0.75$ for 7/10 categories and $r = 0.89$ for the whole scale (Noreau et al. 2004).

Several studies have examined the predictive validity of the LIFE-H. Desrosiers et al. (2003) presented evidence of the convergent validity of the LIFE-H in the form of high correlations with the Functional Autonomy Measurement System (SMAF) and moderate correlations with the Functional Independence Measure (FIM). Further, LIFE-H scores were lower in stroke patients than neurologically healthy controls. A comprehensive review of the psychometric properties of the LIFE-H was performed by Figueiredo et al. (2010).

Clinical Uses

The LIFE-H is available in Dutch, English, and French versions. Adapted forms suitable for use with children aged 0–4 and 5–13 are available (for which a proxy respondent is required). The LIFE-H has been used to evaluate social participation in many patient groups, including children with cerebral palsy, adults with spinal cord injury, traumatic brain injury, and stroke.

Cross-References

▶ Functional Autonomy Measurement System
▶ Functional Independence Measure

References and Readings

Desrosiers, J., Rochette, A., Noreau, L., Bravo, G., Hébert, R., & Boutin, C. (2003). Comparison of two functional independence scales with a participation measure in post-stroke rehabilitation. *Archives of Gerontology and Geriatrics, 37*(2), 157–172.

Desrosiers, J., Noreau, L., Rochette, A., Bravo, G., & Boutin, C. (2002). Predictors of handicap situations following post-stroke rehabilitation. *Disability and Rehabilitation, 24*(15), 774–785.

Figueiiredo, S., Korner-Bitensky, N., Rochette, A., & Desrosiers, J. (2010). Use of the LIFE-H in stroke rehabilitation: A structured review of its psychometric properties. *Disability and Rehabilitation, 32,* 705–712.

Fougeyrollas, P., Noreau, L., Bergeron, H., Cloutier, R., Dion, S. A., & St-Michel, G. (1998). Social consequences of long term impairments and disabilities: Conceptual approach and assessment of handicap. *International Journal of Rehabilitation Research, 21*(2), 127–141.

More information is available on http://ripph.qc.ca/en/assessment-tools/introduction/life-h. Accessed 25 Feb 2017.

Noreau, L., Fougeyrollas, P., & Vincent, C. (2002). The LIFE-H: Assessment of the quality of social participation. *Technology and Disability, 14*(3), 113–118.

Noreau, L., Desrosiers, J., Robichaud, L., Fougeyrollas, P., Rochette, A., & Viscogliosi, C. (2004). Measuring social participation: Reliability of the LIFE-H in older adults with disabilities. *Disability and Rehabilitation, 26*(6), 346–352.

Rochette, A., Desrosiers, J., & Noreau, L. (2001). Association between personal and environmental factors and the occurrence of handicap situations following a stroke. *Disability and Rehabilitation, 23*(13), 559–569.

Assessment of Motor Process Skills

Kelli Williams Gary
Department of Occupational Therapy,
Virginia Commonwealth University, Richmond, VA, USA

Synonyms

AMPS

Description

The Assessment of Motor Process Skills (AMPS) is a standardized observational assessment widely used by occupational therapists to measure the quality of performance in activities of daily living (ADL) of persons across the age spectrum beginning at 2 years. Specifically, the AMPS tests functions that relate to purposeful, goal-oriented daily life tasks that a person wants, needs, and is expected to perform; it does not evaluate neuromuscular, biomechanical, cognitive, and psychosocial impairments (Fisher and Jones 2011). The current version of the assessment contains 110 calibrated ADL tasks that permit evaluation of 36 skills (16 motor, 20 process); AMPS-trained raters must observe two or more specific tasks in 10–20 min increments.

A multi-perspective approach is used to rate each task by observing various motor and process skills in terms of physical effort, efficiency, safety, and independence. The 16 motor skills reflect ability to use body positions, obtain and hold objects, move self and objects, and sustain performance during ADL task performance. The 20 process skills are used to assess ability to sustain performance, apply knowledge, temporal organization, organize space and objects, and adapt performance. Scores are based on observation of the client from certified raters (Fisher and Jones 2011). Motor and process skills are rated simultaneously utilizing a 4-point ordinal criterion referenced rating scale with the highest score denoting competent performance, followed by questionable, inefficient, and markedly inefficient performance. AMPS computer scoring software converts ordinal raw scores of easy skill items for persons of low ability and hard skill items for persons of high ability along a single common equal-interval linear scale (Fisher 2006).

Historical Background

The genesis of the AMPS is found in the psychiatric assessment of clients with schizophrenia and depression in Halifax, Canada (Fisher and

Bernspång 2007). In 1994, Anne G. Fisher, ScD, OTR, and colleagues from the Division of Occupational Therapy, Umeå University in Umeå, Sweden, further developed the idea of this assessment into a specific more standardized tool. At least 20 countries use the AMPS, and the use in these countries have increased applicability across populations, diagnoses, disabilities, cultural background, nationality, and age groups by adding additional tasks (Fisher 2006). The seventh version was published in 2011 along with updated software to facilitate occupation-based documentation and intervention planning (Fisher and Jones 2011).

Psychometric Data

The AMPS has robust psychometric properties. Interrater and intrarater reliability are high with 95% of calibrator raters demonstrating goodness of fit to the many faceted Rasch model. Test-retest reliability is high on a diagnostically heterogeneous sample of older adults with $r = 0.90 - 0.91$ for AMPS process scale and motor scale, respectively (Doble et al. 1999). Internal studies have found good validity of the AMPS when applied to groups of different racial, ethnic, and cultural backgrounds, across gender, and with multiple diagnoses (Stauffer et al. 2000; Fisher 2006; Wæhrens and Fisher 2007).

Clinical Uses

(Fisher 2006) states, "the AMPS provides occupational therapy practitioners with a powerful and sensitive tool that can assist with planning effective ADL interventions and documenting change." Because of the AMPS' unique and innovative design, occupational performance is evaluated based on the familiarity and relevance of the tasks to the client's daily life needs. Therefore, the environment should be naturalistic and approximate the conditions in which the client can comfortably perform tasks. Settings for AMPS observation can vary based on the space available and can include fully equipped clinic kitchens, laundry rooms, outdoor, and the client's own room in the hospital or nursing home.

The primary advantage of the AMPS is that it can be used with persons of virtually any age, diagnosis, or disability. However, the scope and breadth of evidence for AMPS use is limited in psychiatric, neurologic, and pediatric settings. Geriatric settings have offered the most research evidence for those with cognitive impairments and dementias, followed by a sizable proportion of research for people with learning disabilities (Hitch 2007).

Cross-References

▶ Activities of Daily Living (ADL)
▶ Instrumental Activities of Daily Living
▶ Occupational Therapy

References and Readings

Doble, S. E., Fisk, J. D., Lewis, N., & Rockwood, K. (1999). Test-retest reliability of the assessment of motor and process skills. *Occupational Therapy Journal of Research, 19*, 203–215.

Fisher, A. G. (2006). *Assessment of motor and process skills. Vol. 1: Development, standardization, and administration manual* (6th ed.). Fort Collins: Three Star Press.

Fisher, A. G., & Bernspång, B. (2007). Response to: A critique of the Assessment of Motor and Process Skills (AMPS) in mental health practice. *Mental Health Occupational Therapy, 12*, 10–11.

Fisher, A. G., & Jones, B. J. (2011). *The assessment of motor and process skills (AMPS)* (7th ed., rev., Vols. 1 & 2). Fort Collins: Three Star Press.

Hitch, D. (2007). A reply from Danielle Hitch to the Fisher and Bernspång response to: A critique of the assessment of motor and process skills (AMPS) in mental health practice. *Mental Health Occupational Therapy, 12*, 14.

Stauffer, L. M., Fisher, A. G., & Duran, L. (2000). ADL performance of black Americans and white Americans on the assessment of motor and process skills. *American Journal of Occupational Therapy, 54*, 607–613.

Wæhrens, E. E., & Fisher, A. G. (2007). Improving quality of ADL performance after rehabilitation among persons with acquired brain injury. *Scandinavian Journal of Occupational Therapy, 14*, 250–257.

Assisted Living

Jay Behel
Department of Behavioral Sciences, Rush
University Medical Center, Chicago, IL, USA

Synonyms

Domiciliary care; Residential care

Definition

Assisted living is a care arrangement that provides intermittent supervision and instrumental support to individuals unable to live independently but not requiring the level of care provided in conventional nursing facilities.

Current Knowledge

Assisted living arrangements may take place in structured assisted living facilities, small group homes, or an individual's own home or the home of a family member. These arrangements have as their goal the preservation of a degree of autonomy and privacy at home or in a home-like setting. When sited in one's home, assistance may be provided by a combination of paid caregivers, family members, and other paid or unpaid assistants to help with housekeeping, laundry, cooking, and transportation. Assistance provided may include supervision for safety, medication management, meal preparation, and accompaniment and assistance during community-based activities. Assisted living facilities may also offer social activities and specialized services for individuals with cognitive impairment. There is a growing interest in using technology to cost-effectively provide "ambient" assistance to older adults and people with disabilities both in formal assisted living settings and in homes. Basic Activities of Daily Living (BADL) such as hands-on bathing, dressing, and feeding usually are not considered a part of an assisted living arrangement as the consistent need for such basic care is often seen as an indication that a traditional nursing facility or a home-based parallel thereof is the more appropriate level of care. Assisted living typically is not covered by private health insurance or Medicare, and access to such care may be limited by an individual's finances.

Although there has been increased scholarly attention to assisted living in recent years, this work includes topics as disparate as end-of-life care and social networking in assisted living settings speaks to the continued need for well-articulated, shared definitions for discussing these care arrangements.

See Also

▶ Life Care Planning

References and Readings

Stone, R. I., & Reinhard, S. C. (2007). The place of assisted living in long-term care and related service systems. *Gerontologist, 47*(Spec No. 3), 23–32.

Assistive Technology

Diane Cordry Golden[1] and Amy S. Goldman[2]
[1]Association of Assistive Technology Act Programs, Delmar, NY, USA
[2]Association of Assistive Technology Act Programs (ATAP), Springfield, IL, USA

Definition

Assistive technology (AT) is a term used to refer to both AT devices and AT services. A formal, legal definition of AT devices and services was first published in the Technology-Related Assistance for Individuals with Disabilities Act of 1988 as follows:

assistive technology device means any item, piece of equipment, or product system, whether acquired commercially, modified, or customized, that is used to increase, maintain, or improve functional capabilities of individuals with disabilities

assistive technology service means any service that directly assists an individual with a disability in the selection, acquisition, or use of an assistive technology device

AT devices include a vast array of items such as wheelchairs, eyeglasses, hearing aids, Braille printers, electronic note-takers and organizers, augmentative communication systems, text-to-speech software, speech synthesizers, adaptive keyboards, alternative pointing devices, voice recognition software, aids for daily living, etc. AT services include evaluation/assessment services, selecting, fitting, customizing, and repairing devices, delivering training and technical assistance supports, and coordinating funding and other necessary interventions to support device acquisition and use.

The definition of AT devices and services has remained unchanged through numerous reauthorizations of the Assistive Technology Act and has been adopted in other statutes, such as the Individuals with Disabilities Education Act. The same definition has also been used in promulgating federal rules, such as the Electronic and Information Technology Accessibility Standards developed pursuant to Section 508 of the Rehabilitation Act (https://www.access-board.gov/guidelines-and-standards/communications-and-it/about-the-section-508-standards/section-508-standards).

Historical Background

A precise history of AT is difficult to depict because of the diversity of devices and services included in the definition of AT. The history of hearing aids can be traced back to Alexander Graham Bell's pioneering work on development of the telephone. Modern wheelchairs are patterned after the first folding, tubular steel wheelchair developed in the 1930s; while the first dedicated wheelchair (called an invalids chair) is thought to have been invented four centuries ago for Phillip II of Spain. Some devices were developed as AT and evolved into mainstream technology. For example, in 1948 the National Bureau of Standards developed specifications for a low-cost reliable talking-book machine for the blind that became the tape recorder. Conversely, some items developed as mainstream technology became AT such as voice recognition software originally developed for dictation that is used by individuals with motor disabilities who are unable to use a keyboard for computer access.

In recent years, technology use has become more commonplace for everyone. Similarly, AT use is now more frequent across the disability spectrum, addressing deficits in hearing, vision, motor, social, organizational, cognitive, speech, language, information processing, etc. Especially critical today is the use of information technology (IT), including telecommunications. IT use is now critical to success in education, employment, independent living, and community integration and AT is the interface that makes IT accessible.

Rationale or Underlying Theory

Today, AT intervention is rooted in the disability rights movement and self-determination efforts of individuals with disabilities and their advocates. These initiatives helped to delineate the difference between the medical/rehabilitation and independent living models of intervention for individuals with disabilities. The medical model identifies a physical or mental impairment or lack of certain skills and treatment is delivered to remediate the deficit(s). With the medical model, the locus of the problem lies with the individual and the goal is to "fix" the individual in some way through professional treatment. Under the independent living model, the problem is defined as a lack of supports and accommodations, inaccessibility, and/or autonomy – the problem lies with the environment or the interaction with the environment, rather than within the person. In this model, AT plays a major role in addressing/ameliorating interaction difficulties, typically without overtly attempting to "fix" the disability itself (DeJong 1979; Pelka 1997).

Goals and Objectives

AT goals and objectives begin with a primary focus on ameliorating and/or compensating for a specific functional deficit. For example, electronic organizers can be used to address memory or information processing problems; text-to-speech software can be used to address reading deficits; augmentative communication systems can be used to address communication limitations, etc. In most cases, secondary goals are also targeted for outcomes including increasing academic success, fostering gainful employment, supporting independent community living, decreasing inappropriate behaviors, etc. With expanding legal mandates for integration of individuals with disabilities into all societal settings (Individuals with Disabilities Education Act, Section 504 of the Rehabilitation Act, and the Americans with Disabilities Act), AT goals and objectives continue to expand into new outcome areas.

Treatment Participants

AT is an appropriate intervention option to consider when functional limitations are encountered. Candidacy for AT is not limited by age, disability diagnosis, or severity/combination of deficits. There are no prerequisites for AT consideration and AT should not be relegated to a "last resort" intervention after all other interventions have been tried and abandoned.

AT can address a variety of human functions and is frequently grouped into areas such as vision, hearing, communication, daily living, computer access, learning/cognition, environmental adaptations, mobility/seating/positioning, vehicle modifications, and recreation/leisure. For almost all functional limitations, there is a range

of AT intervention that can be considered as a treatment option (Cook and Hussey 2001).

Treatment Procedures

Consideration for AT begins with assessment by a qualified team of individuals who are knowledgeable about the individual, their strengths and limitations and the range of potential AT options available to address the individual's functional needs. Best practice includes conducting structured device trials with various AT devices in the environment(s) in which the individual will be using the technology (e.g., home, school, work, community, etc.). This allows for comparative analysis of different device features and functions to determine which best addresses the individual's needs.

Once AT has been acquired for an individual, training and support must be provided for the user, their family, and other critical individuals such as teachers, therapists, etc. More complex AT (computer-based software applications, assistive listening systems, augmentative communication devices, etc.) frequently requires significant investment of time and resources in initial programming, fitting, and set-up, in addition to training on device use (Galvin and Scherer 1996).

Efficacy Information

Efficacy research on AT includes basic documentation of changes in functional skill areas (those the AT is intended to address) and potential secondary improvements in academic, social, behavioral, and other areas. Much of this efficacy is self-evident and is reported by the AT users themselves (Scherer 1993).

No discussion of AT efficacy would be complete without addressing the issues of device abandonment and cost/benefit. For many types of AT, consumer discontinuing use of the device after acquisition has been a historic problem (Wessels et al. 2003). Factors shown to mitigate abandonment include active consumer and family involvement in the selection and implementation of AT and the relative advantage of AT within the array of intervention options available (Alper and Raharinirina 2006; Riemer-Reiss and Wacker 2000).

As technology continues to improve, the problem of device abandonment steadily abates. Today, the greater challenge is in justifying the cost/benefit of AT to secure funding from private insurance, local, state, federal, and other funding sources. Some types of AT, such as durable medical equipment, have a longer history of cost/benefit data including prevention of secondary disabilities making funding more readily available. Other types of AT, such as electronic organizers used to remediate/compensate for cognitive limitations, are relatively new with little cost/benefit data making funding difficult to secure (Gillette and DePompei 2004; Hart et al. 2004).

Outcome Measurement

The field of AT outcomes is quite young with most published work emerging in the 1990s. Two of the first focused articles on evaluating AT outcomes posed the questions "Are we ready to answer the tough questions?" and "Do we understand the commitment?" (DeRuyter 1995; Trachtmann 1994). In these articles, the authors postulated that stakeholders and AT providers must be prepared to show how their devices/services make a difference in the lives of individuals who receive an AT intervention.

Today, outcome measurement is occurring in all AT service areas (medicine, education, employment/vocational rehabilitation, and independent living) through a variety of interdisciplinary activities. Some are driven by policy needs, in particular, accountability for public dollars spent on AT (e.g., Medicare, Medicaid, special education, vocational rehabilitation, etc.) and justification for private insurance expenditures on AT. Others are driven by an overarching goal of quality service delivery and continuous program improvement.

The most direct outcome measure for AT intervention is demonstration of functional skills, independence, well-being, and quality of life. Administration of standardized assessments in the aided condition (using AT) can be useful in measuring outcomes in discreet skill areas (e.g., auditory discrimination, memory, expressive communication, etc.). In addition, some global assessment of AT outcomes can be helpful such as the Psychosocial Impact of Assistive Devices Scales (PIADS) (Jutai and Day 2002), the Quebec User Evaluation of Satisfaction with Assistive Technology (QUEST) (Demers et al. 1996), and similar instruments. A number of online resources are also available with extensive data on AT outcome tools and research such as the Adaptive Technology Resource Center (http://www.adaptech.org/en), the Assistive Technology Outcomes Measurement System (ATOMS) Project (www.uwm.edu/CHS/atoms), the Consortium for Assistive Technology Outcomes Research, and the Quality Indicators for Assistive Technology Services (www.qiat.org).

Qualifications of Treatment Providers

AT intervention can be provided by an extensive list of professionals, usually specialists in the type of the AT provided. For example, hearing aids are typically provided by audiologists or hearing instrument dispensers, eyeglasses by optometrists and ophthalmologists, etc. However, as the AT becomes less "prescriptive" in nature, the range of providers expands. Electronic note-takers and organizers can be provided by a whole host of providers, special educators, rehabilitation counselors, behavior therapists, occupational therapists, AT practitioners, etc. The Rehabilitation Engineering and Assistive Technology Association of North America (RESNA) administers a certification program for Assistive Technology Professionals (ATPs) with associated standards of practice (www.resna.org/certification).

Cross-References

▶ Americans with Disabilities Act of 1990
▶ Augmentative and Alternative Communication (AAC)

▶ Independent Living Centers
▶ Individuals with Disabilities Education Act
▶ Section 504 of the Rehabilitation Act of 1973

References and Readings

Alper, S., & Raharinirina, S. (2006). Assistive technology for individuals with disabilities: A review and synthesis of literature. *Journal of Special Education Technology, 21*(2), 47–64.

Cook, A., & Hussey, S. (2001). *Assistive technologies: Principles and practice* (2nd ed.). California: Mosby Year-Book, Inc.

DeJong, G. (1979). Independent living: From social movement to analytic paradigm. *Archives of Physical Medicine and Rehabilitation, 60*, 435–446.

Demers, L., Weiss-Lambrou, R., & Ska, B. (1996). Development of the Quebec user evaluation of satisfaction with assistive technology (QUEST). *Assistive Technology, 8*, 3–13.

DeRuyter, F. (1995). Evaluating outcomes in assistive technology: Do we understand the commitment? *Assistive Technology, 7*(1), 3–16.

Galvin, J. C., & Scherer, M. J. (1996). *Evaluating, selecting and using appropriate assistive technology.* Gaithersburg: Aspen Publishers, Inc.

Gillette, Y., & DePompei, R. (2004). The potential of electronic organizers as a tool in the cognitive rehabilitation of young people. *NeuroRehabilitation, 19*(3), 233–243.

Hart, T., Buchhofer, R., & Vaccaro, M. (2004). Portable electronic devices as memory and organizational aids after traumatic brain injury: A consumer survey study. *Journal of Head Trauma Rehabilitation, 19*(5), 351–365.

Jutai, J., & Day, H. (2002). Psychosocial impact of assistive devices scale (PIADS). *Technology and Disability, 14*(3), 107–111.

Pelka, F. (1997). *ABC-CLIO companion to the disability rights movement.* Santa Barbara: ABC-CLIO, Inc.

Riemer-Reiss, M. L., & Wacker, R. R. (2000). Factors associated with assistive technology discontinuance among individuals with disabilities. *Journal of Rehabilitation, 66*(3), 44–50.

Scherer, M. J. (1993). *Living in the state of stuck: How technology impacts the lives of people with disabilities.* Cambridge, MA: Brookline Books.

Trachtmann, L. (1994). Outcome measures: Are we ready to answer the tough questions? *Assistive Technology, 6*, 91–92.

Wessels, R., Dijcks, B., Soede, M., Gelderblom, G. J., & De Witte, L. (2003). Non-use of provided assistive technology devices, a literature overview. *Technology and Disability, 15*(4), 231–238.

Association Areas

Maryellen Romero
Department of Psychiatry and Behavioral Sciences, Tulane University School of Medicine, New Orleans, LA, USA

Synonyms

Association cortex

Definition

It is recognized that the brain is neither holistic nor rigidly localized with respect to cognitive functions. However, higher-order cognitive capabilities depend on specialized regions within the brain that *process*, *link* or *integrate* elementary or new, as well as stored, information into increasingly complex wholes. Such regions are termed *association areas* and are thought to be the neuroanatomical substrate for such higher functions as memory, emotion, perception, language, spatial and problem-solving skills, as well as the planning and execution of behavioral responses.

Three major association areas are recognized:

1. *Frontal association cortices*, as the name implies, are located in the more anterior aspects of the frontal lobes and include dorsolateral, orbitofrontal, and premotor areas. While various feedback loops are likely involved including those from the posterior and limbic association areas, conceptually, the initial decisions and planning regarding executive or motor responses to a given situation are generally thought to flow from the prefrontal (most anterior) cortices to the premotor cortex that organizes, coordinates, and sequences the actions essential to the successful completion of the response. From there, commands are believed to be forwarded to the primary motor area (precentral gyrus) that then actually

executes the motor response. The orbitofrontal cortex is shared with *limbic association cortex* (see below) that underscores the importance of the integration of emotion, memory, and behavior. Lesions to prefrontal association cortices often affect self-monitoring, planning, and executive functions, including behavioral inhibition.

2. The *limbic association cortex* includes ventromedial frontal lobe, medial parietal lobe, temporal pole, and cingulate and parahippocampal areas. Integration of information from the hypothalamus, other limbic or paralimbic structures, and secondary sensory association areas is received and projected to other areas of the cortex, including the prefrontal cortex discussed above, again permitting the integration of emotions, cognition and perceptions, and memory. Dysfunction is often expressed as emotional/behavioral dysregulation and memory impairment.

3. The locations of the *parieto-temporal-occipital association cortices* are described by their names and are typically divided into secondary and tertiary areas. The former are *unimodal* in nature (respond more or less exclusively to a single sensory modality) and lie adjacent to their respective primary cortical sensory projection areas. They are thought to be responsible for further integrating and processing sensory input into potentially meaningful percepts. Hence, lesions of these secondary association areas will commonly result in modality-specific perceptual disturbances or agnosias. By contrast, the tertiary or heteromodal association areas receive input from all sensory modalities. Because of this and their central location, they are sometimes referred to as the PTO (parietal-temporal-occipital) cortex. Because of their crossed or multimodal inputs, these latter areas, which are very highly developed in man, are thought to represent the foundations for higher-order conceptual and intellectual abilities, including abstraction, language, and visual-spatial and mathematical problem solving, any or all of which can be adversely affected by lesions to these areas.

Cross-References

▶ Association Pathways
▶ Heteromodal Cortex
▶ Secondary Cortex
▶ Unimodal Cortex

References and Readings

Kupermann, I. (1991). Localization of higher cognitive and affective functions: The association cortices. In E. R. Kandel, J. H. Schwartz, & T. M. Jessel (Eds.), *Principles of neural science* (3rd ed., pp. 823–838). East Norwalk: Appleton & Lange.

Mendoza, J. E., & Foundas, A. F. (2008). *Clinical neuroanatomy: A behavioral approach*. New York: Springer.

Mesulam, M.-M. (2000). *Principles of behavioral and cognitive neurology*. New York: Oxford University Press.

Pandya, D. N., & Seltzer, B. (1982). Association areas of the cerebral cortex. *Trends in Neurosciences, 5*, 385–390.

Pandya, D. N., & Yeterian, E. H. (2003). Cerebral cortex: Architecture and connections. In *Encyclopedia of the neurological sciences* (pp. 594–604). Amsterdam: Elsevier Science.

Association for Postdoctoral Programs in Clinical Neuropsychology (APPCN)

Jacobus Donders
Mary Free Bed Rehabilitation Hospital, Grand Rapids, MI, USA

Membership

The Association of Postdoctoral Programs in Clinical Neuropsychology (APPCN) is an organization of over 75 member programs that offer comprehensive, integrated postdoctoral residencies.

Major Areas or Mission Statement

The mission of APPCN is to foster the provision of advanced specialty education and training to promote the competencies that are necessary for practice in the specialty of clinical neuropsychology (Boake et al. 2002). APPCN programs prepare residents for certification by the American Board of Clinical Neuropsychology (ABCN). Successful completion of an APPCN residency is sufficient to demonstrate that one has met the ABCN didactic requirements for board certification.

Landmark Contributions

Formally incorporated in 1992, APPCN contributed to the Houston Conference, which established that completion of 2 years of formal postdoctoral residency training is a uniform requirement for entry into the professional practice of clinical neuropsychology (Hannay et al. 1998). In more recent years, APPCN has been a key representative to interorganizational groups like the Clinical Neuropsychology Synarchy and the Inter-organizational Summit on Education and Training.

Major Activities

APPCN is not an accrediting organization, a role which is left to the Commission on Accreditation of the American Psychological Association (APA). However, a growing number of the APPCN members are currently accredited by APA as a postdoctoral specialty program in clinical neuropsychology. Details about individual APPCN member programs, including focus on adult *v.* pediatric neuropsychology, accreditation status, primary diagnostic groups served, and other characteristics, are available on the APPCN website.

The major standards for program membership in APPCN include the following: (1) the duration of training is for a minimum of 2 years, or for an equivalent time on no less than a half-time basis, at a fixed site with regular, on-site supervision; (2) the program includes an organized and integrated combination of at least 50% clinical service, at least 10% didactic/educational activities, and at least 10% research or other scholarly activities; and (3) the program director is board-certified in clinical neuropsychology through the American Board of Professional Psychology (ABBP-CN). One of the major accomplishments of APPCN is the development and implementation, in collaboration with National Matching Services, of a computerized system for matching of applicants for postdoctoral residency training in clinical neuropsychology to programs that offer such training. This electronic system, instituted in 2001, is the most fair to applicants, and the most efficient for programs, with all APPCN programs that have open positions in any given year taking part in this electronic match. Postdoctoral programs that are not members of APPCN are also allowed to participate as long as they meet APPCN standards #1 and #2 above, and if they agree to respect all other conditions of the match, including prohibition of preemptive offers, and adherence to the binding nature of the match outcomes. Further details are available at http://www.natmatch.com/appcnmat/.

APPCN is dedicated to education of aspiring neuropsychologists about what it takes to become a competitive candidate for postdoctoral residency training. For this purpose, several educational seminars are offered on a regular basis, some in collaboration with other organizations, such as Division 40 (▶ "Clinical Neuropsychology") of the APA and the Association of Neuropsychology Students in Training (ANST). Over the past several years, APPCN program directors have also consistently provided a "special topic presentation" about postdoctoral residency training at the annual meeting of the National Academy of Neuropsychology (NAN).

APPCN has also strived to make the process of education and evaluation as part of postdoctoral residency training in clinical neuropsychology more standardized. For this purpose, a 50-item written examination has been developed by APPCN to be used with residents who are near completion of their first postdoctoral training year, to evaluate their knowledge of major content areas like functional neuroanatomy, adult and pediatric syndromes, psychometrics, etc. This exam is not intended to give residents a "grade"; rather, it is to be used as an educational tool, to identify relative strengths and weaknesses in the residents' working knowledge base, so that the relative lacunae can be addressed during the subsequent training year. During that second year, APPCN member programs also have the opportunity to start preparing residents for board certification, by means of ethics vignettes and mock oral "fact finding" case materials that are very similar in format and level of difficulty to those used by ABPP-CN.

Finally, the most recent initiative of APPCN has involved advocacy with the United States Department of Veterans Affairs for the development of more postdoctoral training programs in clinical neuropsychology, primarily because of the high number of traumatic brain injuries among US service personnel involved in the combat in Iraq. When more than a dozen of these training programs became available in the Fall of 2007, APPCN contacted the programs, provided mentoring as needed, and waived their first-time participation fee in the electronic match. APPCN has also continued to offer assistance to new programs as they seek specialty accreditation through the APA. APPCN will continue to embrace additional organized and integrated postdoctoral training programs in clinical neuropsychology.

Cross-References

▶ American Board of Clinical Neuropsychology (ABCN)

▶ American Board of Professional Psychology (ABPP)
▶ American Psychological Association (APA)

References and Readings

Boake, C., Yeates, K. O., & Donders, J. (2002). Association of Postdoctoral Programs in clinical neuropsychology: Update and new directions. *The Clinical Neuropsychologist, 16*, 1–6.

Hannay, H. J., Bieliauskas, L., Crosson, B. A., Hammeke, T. A., Hamsher, K., & Koffler, S. P. (1998). The Houston conference on specialty education and training in clinical neuropsychology. *Archives of Clinical Neuropsychology, 13*, 157–250.

Association Pathways

John E. Mendoza
Department of Psychiatry and Neuroscience, Tulane Medical School and SE Louisiana Veterans Healthcare System, New Orleans, LA, USA

Definition

Fiber pathways that lie within the cerebrum that connect one part of the cerebral cortex with another *within the same hemisphere*. Association pathways are thus contrasted with *commissures* that generally interconnect homologous areas of the two halves of the brain, and *projection pathways* that are fiber tracts interconnecting cortical and subcortical structures. They may be very long (typically termed *fasciculi*) or very short. The latter may consist of "U"-shaped fibers connecting one gyrus with an adjacent one or horizontal connections within a gyrus itself (e.g., *bands of Baillarger*). These various pathways allow different areas of the brain to communicate with one another. Some of the major association pathways are shown in Fig. 1.

Association Pathways,
Fig. 1

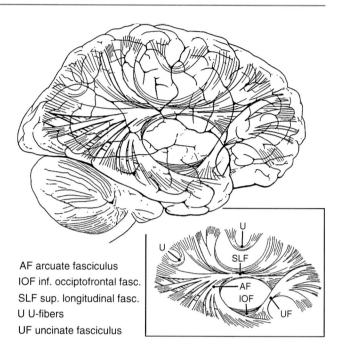

AF arcuate fasciculus
IOF inf. occiptofrontal fasc.
SLF sup. longitudinal fasc.
U U-fibers
UF uncinate fasciculus

Cross-References

▶ Commissures, Cerebral
▶ Projection Pathways

Associational Fibers

Melissa J. McGinn
Anatomy and Neurobiology, Virginia
Commonwealth University School of Medicine,
Richmond, VA, USA

Synonyms

Arcuate fibers

Definition

Associational fibers are bundles of white matter
that connect various cortical regions within the

same cerebral hemisphere. The most prevalent
type of white matter tract found in the cortex,
associational fibers permit bidirectional communication between different cortical areas, thus
allowing the cortex to function as a coordinated
whole. Associational fibers predominantly arise
from cortical layer III pyramidal neurons and
can be classified as either short associational
fibers, which connect adjacent gyri within the
same lobe, or long associational fibers,
interconnecting more distant regions located in
different lobes. The major long associational
fibers tracts in the brain include the superior
longitudinal fasciculus, arcuate fasciculus, uncinate fasciculus, and cingulum.

Cross-References

▶ Arcuate Fasciculus
▶ Association Pathways
▶ Cerebral Cortex
▶ Cingulum
▶ Superior Longitudinal Fasciculus
▶ White Matter

Associative Visual Agnosia

John E. Mendoza
Department of Psychiatry and Neuroscience,
Tulane Medical School and SE Louisiana
Veterans Healthcare System, New Orleans, LA,
USA

Definition

Regardless of modality, an associative agnosia
implies that although perception is intact, the particular stimulus has no meaning ("associative" value)
to the individual. The stimulus can neither be named
nor linked to other personal or sensory experiences.
Hence, *associative visual agnosia* refers to the
inability to identify or categorize a visually presented stimulus despite adequate visual perception.

Current Knowledge

Individuals with this disorder should be able to
match the visual stimulus to a sample and copy or
draw what is seen, thus distinguishing *associative*
from *apperceptive* visual agnosia. In the latter condition, visual object recognition is also impaired,
but primarily as a result of a disturbance of perception. In addition to having difficulty naming visually presented objects, a patient suffering from
associative visual agnosia would likely be unable
to describe their use or purpose, or indicate to
which category of objects they may belong. However, in pure visual associative agnosia, identification should be possible if the patient were allowed
to hold the object(s) (tactile recognition).

An associative visual agnosia may differentially affect recognition of objects, words, colors,
or faces. In visual agnosia for words (also known
as *pure alexia* or *pure word blindness*), visual
word recognition is impaired. But the individual
may be able to "read" if allowed to trace the letters
with a finger, thus permitting tactile or kinesthetic
recognition of individual letters. In associative
color agnosia, the individual may be able to

match colors, but neither name them nor identify
objects with which they might be associated (such
as cherries or apples for the color red). Facial
agnosia (*prosopagnosia*) is a bit complex in that
one may differentiate the inability to make discriminations among unfamiliar faces (thought to be
more of a perceptual problem) from an inability to
recognize familiar faces (generally considered an
associative problem). Thus, in the latter instance,
while the patient might be able to match the face or
picture of a familiar person to one within an array of
pictures, he would not be able to identify the face or
the picture as that of his wife, his daughter, or other
famous person with whom he might be familiar.

While the specific lesions causing specific
associative visual agnosias are not well defined,
they are generally thought to represent a disconnection type syndrome involving the temporal,
occipital, and/or parietal regions of the left hemisphere with some disruption of fiber pathways or
connections between the unimodal (visual) and
heteromodal cortices.

Cross-References

▶ Alexia
▶ Apperceptive Visual Agnosia
▶ Color Agnosia
▶ Color Anomia
▶ Disconnection Syndrome
▶ Heteromodal Cortex
▶ Prosopagnosia
▶ Unimodal Cortex

References and Readings

Bauer, R. M., & Demery, J. A. (2003). Agnosia. In
   K. Heilman & E. Valenstein (Eds.), *Clinical neuropsychology* (4th ed., pp. 236–295). New York: Oxford
   University Press.
DeRenzi, E., & Spinnler, H. (1966). Visual recognition in
   patients with unilateral cerebral disease. *Journal of
   Nervous and Mental Disease, 142*, 513–525.
DeRenzi, E., Scotti, G., & Spinnler, H. (1969). Perceptual
   and associative disorders of visual recognition. Relationship to the side of the cerebral lesion. *Neurology,
   19*, 634–642.

Astasia-Abasia

Douglas I. Katz
Department of Neurology, Boston University
School of Medicine, Braintree, MA, USA

Synonyms

Blocq's disease

Definition

An inability to stand and walk in a normal and coordinated manner. Astasia means inability to maintain standing, and abasia refers to impaired coordination of gait. The term is usually applied to unusual, often bizarre patterns of gait and stance that appear to have no neuropathophysiologic basis. Conversion disorder is frequently the underlying cause. Patients may sway in a staggering, unstable manner, often catching themselves before falling. This syndrome is also referred to as Blocq's disease.

Cross-References

▶ Abasia
▶ Gait Disorders
▶ Psychogenic Disorder

References and Readings

Morris, J. G., Mark de Moore, G., & Herberstein, M. (2006). Psychogenic gait: An example of deceptive signaling. In C. R. Cloninger & M. Hallett (Eds.), *Psychogenic movement disorders: Neurology and neuropsychiatry.* Philadelphia: Lippincott Williams & Wilkins.
Okun, M. S., & Koehler, P. J. (2007). Paul Blocq and (psychogenic) astasia abasia. *Movement Disorders, 22,* 1373–1378.

Astereognosis

Melissa Amick
Department of Psychiatry and Human Behavior,
Brown University, Providence, RI, USA

Synonyms

Object agnosia; Tactile agnosia

Short Description or Definition

Astereognosis is defined as the inability to identify objects through touch without visual input.

Categorization

Astereognosis has been subdivided into primary and secondary recognition deficits. Primary recognition deficits, also called morphognosia, reflect impairments in recognizing the physical features of the object (e.g., weight or texture). Secondary recognition deficits reflect a specific impairment in object recognition with spared primary recognition (for review, see De Renzi 1982).

Epidemiology

Astereognosis can be common after stroke with one report indicating that up to 90% of patients demonstrate astereognosis (Connell et al. 2008). Damage to the cortical regions important for haptic input integration can cause astereognosis. This disorder, therefore, is common and can occur in the presence of many neurological disorders including brain (e.g., Knecht et al. 1996) or spinal cord tumors (Lesoin et al. 1986) and traumatic brain injury (Hom and Reitan 1982).

Natural History, Prognostic Factors, and Outcomes

Connell et al. (2008) followed 58 stroke survivors over a period of 6 months (baseline, 2, 4, and 6 months), and at each time period, participants completed the Nottingham Sensory Assessment (see below). Stereognosis significantly improved during the observation period, with the greatest changes occurring within the first 4 months (baseline relative to 4-month performance). Regression analyses indicated that stroke severity and motor performance of the upper limb were predictive of the presence of impaired stereognosis at the baseline assessment.

Neuropsychology and Psychology of Astereognosis

Astereognosis can occur after injury to either the left or right hemisphere. A specialized role for the right hemisphere in stereognosis has been proposed; however this finding has not been consistently observed (for review, see Zaidel 1998 and De Renzi 1982). Initially astereognosis was thought to be due to damage to the primary somatosensory cortex; however, posterior parietal lesions have also been associated with this impairment (Knecht et al. 1996).

Evaluation

Astereognosis is often examined with non-standardized methods. In the typical neurological examination, astereognosis is assessed by asking the patient to identify an object through touch without visual input. Common objects used for identification can include coins, keys, paper clips, or screws. For patients with hemiparesis, the examiner may manipulate the patient's hand to assist in object identification. Standardized assessments of astereognosis do exist. The Tactile Form Recognition Test from the Halstead-Reitan Neuropsychological Test Battery (Reitan and Wolfson 1993) requires participants to manipulate a flat plastic shape with one hand obscured from vision, while the other hand points to the same shape mounted on a board with three other potential distractors. In the Benton Stereognosis Test (Benton 1969), ten cards with fine-grain, sandpaper figures pasted on top are felt by the participant out of view. The participant has 30 s to explore the card and 45 s to respond. Responses are made by pointing to the corresponding line drawing mounted in full view of the respondent. The Nottingham Sensory Assessment includes an assessment of astereognosis (Gaubert and Mockett 2000). In this task, the participant is blindfolded and asked to name the object placed in his/her hand. Presentation of the objects is time limited. Objects to be identified include coins, comb, sponge, pencil, scissors, a cup, and a glass. Responses are scored on a scale of 0–2 depending upon the quality of the verbal response.

Treatment

Astereognosis has been observed to spontaneously improve over time (Connell et al. 2008). One study has found that stereognosis improves following systematic hand retraining in stroke survivors who were at least 2 years post stroke. Yekutiel and Guttman (1993) had 25 participants receive three 45-min hand-retraining sessions weekly for a period of 6 weeks. The therapy was customized for each participant, but everyone received education to improve insight about their impairment, and exercises were intended to be appropriately challenging and designed to promote self-efficacy, used vision and the less affected hand to aid sensory function, and provided frequent breaks and novel stimuli. Unlike the control group, the patient group showed a statistically significant improvement on the stereognosis assessment. These findings suggest that functional gains through therapy can occur in the years following stroke.

Cross-References

References and Readings

Benton, A. L. (1969). *Stereognosis test; Manual of instructions*. Victoria: Neuropsychology Laboratory, Department of Psychology, University of Victoria.

Connell, L. A., Lincoln, N. B., & Radford, K. A. (2008). Somatosensory impairment after stroke: Frequency of different deficits and their recovery. *Clinical Rehabilitation, 22*, 758–767.

De Renzi, E. (1982). *Disorders of space exploration and cognition*. New York: Wiley.

Gaubert, C. S., & Mockett, S. P. (2000). Inter-rater reliability of the Nottingham method of stereognosis assessment. *Clinical Rehabilitation, 14*(2), 153–159.

Hom, J., & Reitan, R. M. (1982). Effect of lateralized cerebral damage upon contralateral and ipsilateral sensorimotor performances. *Journal of Clinical Neuropsychology, 4*(3), 249–268.

Knecht, S., Kunesch, E., & Schnitzler, A. (1996). Parallel and serial processing of haptic information in man: Effects of parietal lesions on sensorimotor hand function. *Neuropsychologia, 34*, 669–687.

Lesoin, F., Rousseaux, M., Martin, H. J., Petit, H., & Jomin, M. J. (1986). Astereognosis and amyotrophy of the hand with neurinoma of the second cervical nerve root. *Neurology, 233*, 57–58.

Lincoln, N. B., Crow, J. L., Jackson, J. M., Waters, G. R., Adams, S. A., & Hodgson, P. (1991). The unreliability of sensory assessment. *Clinical Rehabilitation, 5*, 273–282.

Reitan, R. M., & Wolfson, D. (1993). *The Halstead-Reitan neuropsychological test battery: Theory and clinical interpretation*. Tucson: Neuropsychology Press.

Yekutiel, M., & Guttman, E. J. (1993). A controlled trial of the retraining of the sensory function of the hand in stroke patients. *Journal of Neurology, Neurosurgery, and Psychiatry, 56*, 241–244.

Zaidel, E. (1998). Stereognosis in the chronic split brain: Hemispheric differences, ipsilateral control and sensory integration across the midline. *Neuropsychologia, 36*, 1033–1047.

Astrocytoma

Robert Rider[1] and Carol L. Armstrong[2]
[1]Department of Psychology, Drexel University, Philadelphia, PA, USA
[2]Child and Adolescent Psychiatry and Behavioral Sciences, The Children's Hospital of Philadelphia, Philadelphia, PA, USA

Definition

Astrocytomas are the most frequently diagnosed tumors, are usually slow growing, and may develop a cystic component. Arising in astrocytic cells anywhere throughout the central nervous system, they may occur in any age group but are most frequently diagnosed in middle-aged males. The highest incidence of brain stem astrocytomas is found in children. Grading systems focus on the degree of resemblance to normal astrocytes, with higher grades associated with more rapid growth and greater likelihood of metastasis. Three common types of astrocytomas are low-grade astrocytomas, which are often benign and tend to occur in the cerebellum (especially in children) but may also occur in the cerebrum in adults; anaplastic astrocytomas, which are malignant; and glioblastoma multiforme, which are thought to arise from astrocytomas and are the most malignant.

The specific symptoms associated with astrocytomas depend on the region of the CNS that is affected. A low-grade astrocytoma may remain quiescent throughout the lifespan of the person, especially when diagnosed at a young age, but the effects of surgery and radiation on the region of the tumor may cause progressive injury; surgical effects on brain and behavior tend to occur within a year after surgery, but radiation effects may cause progression of the deficits caused by the original tumor location for decades after. In cases of progressive cognitive injury in patients with high-grade supratentorial astrocytomas, deterioration in information processing speed, attention, working memory, long-term memory, and executive functioning has been reported. The extent of injury is in part dependent on the size of the tumor and how much normal tissue it has invaded. In cases of cerebellar gliomas (astrocytomas and medulloblastomas), the location of the tumor in the cerebellum again predicts the type of deficit, for example, visuospatial memory and attention, anxiety with left cerebellar tumors, and verbal memory and fluency in right cerebellar tumors.

Cross-References

- ► Fibrillary Astrocytoma
- ► Oligoastrocytoma
- ► Pilocytic Astrocytoma and Juvenile Pilocytic Astrocytoma

References and Readings

Bosma, I., Vos, M. J., Heimans, J. J., Taphoorn, J. B., Aaronson, N. K., Postma, T. J., et al. (2007). The course of neurocognitive functioning in high-grade glioma patients. *Neuro-Oncology, 9*(1), 53–62.

Iuvone, L., Peruzzi, L., Colosimo, C., Tamburrini, G., Caldarelli, M., DiRocco, C., et al. (2011). Pretreatment neuropsychological deficits in children with brain tumors. *Neuro-Oncology, 13*(5), 517–524.

Louis, D., Ohgaki, H., Cavenee, W., & Wiestler, O. (2007). *WHO classification of tumours of the central nervous system* (4th ed.). Louis: World Health Organization.

Moitra, E., & Armstrong, C. L. (2013). Neural substrates for heightened anxiety in children with brain tumors. *Developmental Neuropsychology, 38*(5), 337–351.

Asymmetry

Maryellen Romero
Department of Psychiatry and Behavioral Sciences, Tulane University School of Medicine, New Orleans, LA, USA

Synonyms

Hemispheric specialization

Definition

Asymmetry is the discordance between the right and left sides of the brain in respect to structure and/or function.

Current Knowledge

Although not initially linked to brain asymmetry, the first behavioral asymmetry that was likely noted was the superiority of motor skills exhibited by one hand, most commonly the right, over the other. The next real breakthrough with regard to asymmetry is generally thought to have occurred in the nineteenth century with the discovery that acquired language deficits (aphasia) were typically associated with lesions of the left hemisphere. Since then, other asymmetries, both functional and structural, have been identified with regard to the two cerebral hemispheres.

Structural Asymmetries

Structural asymmetries of the brain were first noted around the beginning of the twentieth century, but it was not until the late 1960s that these were first strongly correlated with functional differences between the hemispheres. In a study of 100 postmortem brains, Geschwind and Levitsky (1968) noticed that the planum temporale, located in the temporal operculum, was larger in 65% of the brains studied as compared with only 11% in which the right was larger. They concluded that this difference was likely related to the left hemisphere's association with the production of language in most individuals. Subsequent studies have demonstrated that this asymmetry can be shown to present even prior to birth, reinforcing the genetic predisposition to left-hemispheric dominance for language.

Since the advent of more sophisticated imaging techniques that allow for large-scale in vivo studies of the brain, other structural differences have been documented. The inferior frontal gyrus in the left hemisphere, corresponding to Broca's area, has been shown to be more highly developed on the left side for most individuals. The gyri and sulci associated with the motor strip (Brodmann's area 4) are more prominent in the left hemisphere of right-handers. Fairly consistent differences in the lateral fissure have been found, with the posterior ascending ramus of this sulcus making a more abrupt upward turn in the right hemisphere as compared with the left. This would suggest likely differences in the distribution of the supramarginal and angular gyri in the inferior parietal lobules of the two hemispheres. Even on a more microlevel, differences in the size and organization of individual cells or cell columns have been identified in the two hemispheres.

It is reasonable to speculate that some structural differences likely relate to functional differences between the two hemispheres, particularly behaviors such as language and handedness. However, functional asymmetries have either been demonstrated or are suspected well beyond those which can currently be explained by structural differences. The following represent a sampling of some of the functional differences that have been observed.

Functional Asymmetries

It has been well established that language expression and comprehension are normally mediated primarily, if not exclusively, by the left hemisphere, even among left-handers. However, the right hemisphere has also been shown to play an important role in communication. Verbal communication is not just about using words in sentences or paragraphs; emotional tone or nuances of the speaker often convey important meaning. In some communications, such as those with a sarcastic intent, the real message is carried by the tone rather than by the words, which, if interpreted literally, might actually convey a very different message. The ability to use as well as interpret these emotional components of speech, known as prosody, is primarily mediated by the right hemisphere; damage to this side of the brain may produce various forms of *aprosodia*. With regard to using or interpreting the language of others, the right hemisphere is also believed to play an important role in identifying the central theme or point of the discourse of others and being able to stay on

point when speaking or writing. It appears to be important in appreciating verbal (as well as nonverbal) humor and in detecting meaning from the differential inflections given to individual words in speech.

In addition to words, numbers also have their own symbolic meaning. Hence, as might be expected, the ability to use numbers is thought to be a function normally carried out by the left hemisphere, the disturbance of which following a lesion to the left hemisphere may be defined as *acalculia* (*dyscalculia*). However, most complex arithmetic operations also have a spatial component. For example, precise alignment of rows and columns of numbers is critical in mathematical operations, whether completed mentally or on paper. These spatial relations can be disturbed following right-hemispheric lesions, resulting in what has been termed *spatial dyscalculia*.

It is known that the hemisphere contralateral to the hand being used to carry out some motor tasks is immediately responsible for the execution of these movements. However, the motor programs or engrams for overlearned motor skills are believed to reside in the left hemisphere, certainly for the vast majority of right-handers, as well as many left-handers. Thus, any lesion that either directly interferes with those engrams or the ability of that information to reach the premotor cortex of either hemisphere can result in an impaired performance, especially if the individual is asked to demonstrate the action in the absence of the actual object. This latter condition is referred to as an *ideomotor apraxia*.

Perceptual abilities appear to be differentially distributed between the two hemispheres. It has already been noted that the left hemisphere is normally the leading hemisphere in interpreting verbal (semantic) information, while the right appears to be better adapted to processing certain types of emotional cues. It seems that the right hemisphere is also the more proficient in processing many types of visual-spatial or visual-gestalt information. Thus, the right hemisphere has been found to be generally superior in carrying out certain constructional tasks, making judgments regarding the orientation of lines in space, in making discriminations regarding *unfamiliar* faces, and in recognizing familiar tunes or environmental sounds. On the other hand, the left hemisphere appears to be the leading hemisphere when it comes to perception of certain aspects of one's own body. Problems of right-left orientation and difficulty recognizing individual fingers of one's hands (*finger agnosia*) are typically associated with lesions of the left inferior parietal lobule. Functional MRI studies have demonstrated consistent activation of right hemisphere structures during tests of *vigilance* and *directed* attention. However, *divided* attention tasks have been shown to selectively activate left prefrontal cortex. PET imaging studies have demonstrated increased blood flow in the right prefrontal and superior parietal cortex during tasks requiring *sustained* attention, regardless of the type of stimulus (verbal, visual, etc.) or where it is introduced (left vs. right).

Differences between the two hemispheres have also been demonstrated in learning and memory tasks and other cognitive domains. Of the two, the left hemisphere has been more strongly associated with learning verbal information. While many studies have shown that the right hemisphere is perhaps better at learning certain "nonverbal" or "visual-spatial" type information, the findings are generally less robust compared to the left hemisphere and verbal memory. One frequent explanation for this is that when faced with any memory task, humans have a natural tendency to try to verbally encode the stimulus, thus bringing the left hemisphere into play.

It has also been suggested that the two hemispheres play different roles in attention. The much more frequent association of disorders such as *unilateral neglect* and *anosognosia* with right hemispheric lesions has led to the hypothesis that while, as might be expected, the left hemisphere attends to the right side of space (both personal and extrapersonal), the right hemisphere focuses on both right and left space.

Finally, the association of the right hemisphere and emotional expression would appear to go beyond the affective intonations of speech as described above. It is commonly observed, both by health-care professionals as well as the spouses and other family members of persons with brain injury that individuals with right hemisphere lesions often behave differently than those with left-sided lesions. While the latter seem to remain emotionally attached, even if that emotion is often one of anger, frustration, or sadness, right hemispherically damaged patients are more likely to be described as apathetic, indifferent, emotionally flat, both in terms of their verbal and facial expressions and their interpersonal relationships.

Cross-References

▶ Anosognosia
▶ Directed Attention
▶ Dominance (Cerebral)
▶ Language
▶ Wada Test

References and Readings

Corballis, P. M. (2003). Visuospatial processing and the right-hemisphere interpreter. *Brain and Cognition, 53*, 171–176.

Davidson, R. J. (1992). Emotion and affective style: Hemispheric substrates. *Psychological Science, 3*, 39–43.

Davidson, R. J., & Hugdahl, K. (Eds.). (1996). *Brain asymmetry*. Cambridge, MA: Bradford Books.

Gazzaniga, M. S. (2000). *The new cognitive neurosciences*. Boston: MIT Press.

Gazzaniga, M. S., Ivry, R. B., & Mangun, G. R. (2002). *Cognitive neuroscience: The biology of the mind*. New York: W. W. Norton & Company.

Geschwind, N., & Levitsky, W. (1968). Left-right asymmetry in temporal speech region. *Science, 161*, 186–187.

Good, C. D., Johnsrude, I., Ashburner, J., Henson, R. N. A., Friston, K. J., & Frackowiak, R. S. J. (2001). Cerebral asymmetry and the effects of sex and handedness on brain structure: A voxel-based morphometric analysis of 465 normal adult human brains. *NeuroImage, 14*, 685–700.

Kinsbourne, M. (Ed.). (1978). *Asymmetrical function of the brain*. New York: Cambridge University Press.

Mendoza, J. E., & Foundas, A. L. (2008). *Clinical neuroanatomy: A neurobehavioral approach*. New York: Springer.

Ross, E. (2000). Affective prosody and the aprosodias. In M. Mesulam (Ed.), *Principles of behavioral and cognitive neurology*. New York: Oxford University Press.

Walsh, K. (1994). *Neuropsychology: A clinical approach*. New York: Churchill Livingstone.

Ataxia

Anna DePold Hohler[1] and
Marcus Ponce de Leon[2]
[1]Boston University Medical Center, Boston,
MA, USA
[2]Madigan Army Medical Center, Tacoma,
WA, USA

Synonyms

Clumsiness

Definition

Ataxia describes a lack of coordination while performing voluntary movements. It is associated with damage to the cerebellum or its afferent or efferent pathways. It may appear as clumsiness, inaccuracy, or instability. It may affect any part of the body. When ataxia affects the arms and hands, it may cause tremor due to overcorrection of inaccurate movements. It may produce dysmetria or an inability to gauge distance correctly. It may cause past-pointing when an attempted reach overshoots the target. It may also cause dysdiadochokinesia or poor performance of regular, repeated movements. Cerebellar injury may contribute to nystagmus, hyper- and hypometric saccades, scanning speech, titubation, and difficulties with gait and balance.

Current Knowledge

There are a number of different types of damage to the cerebellum. These range from fixed damage (e.g., stroke, trauma, hypoxic injury) to chemical, metabolic, and degenerative. Cerebellar injury related to vitamin deficiency (e.g., E, B12, and thiamine) may be reversible and should be identified and treated. Metabolic diseases such as Hartnup's, Refsum's, and the mitochondrial disorders are less treatable. A deficiency of Coenzyme Q10 has been described in patients with cerebellar ataxia, usually with childhood onset and often associated with seizures. The symptoms may respond to Coenzyme Q10 treatment. There are a number of hereditary cerebellar ataxias. Most of the autosomal recessive and autosomal dominant ataxias have no treatments. An exception is vitamin E deficiency, which is an autosomal recessive disorder. It is due to a mutation in the gene coding for the alpha tocopherol transfer protein located on the long arm of chromosome 8. It is characterized by childhood onset of ataxia, dysarthria, areflexia, proprioceptive deficits, extensor plantar responses, and skeletal deformities.

The episodic ataxias, which are inherited in an autosomal dominant fashion, may also have some symptomatic treatment regimens. Episodic ataxia type 1 is related to a chromosome 12 mutation in the potassium channel gene. Clinically, the disease manifests with episodes of ataxia lasting seconds to minutes. Patients may also suffer from myokymia during and between attacks of ataxia. The ataxia may be induced by startle or exercise. Episodic ataxia type 2 is related to a defect located on chromosome 19. It is due to a mutation in a voltage-dependent calcium channel. Clinically, patients present with nystagmus. Attacks last minutes to hours and may be induced by a change in posture. Patients may also complain of vertigo. As the disease progresses, ataxia becomes permanent.

Epidemiology

Ataxia is a common sign associated with inherited, acquired, toxic, and traumatic events.

Natural History

The genetic syndromes that are associated with ataxia tend to be progressive. Individuals with static insults such as strokes or trauma may show improvement in function over time.

Neuropsychology

Cerebellar syndromes may be associated with cognitive slowing.

Evaluation includes a detailed neurological examination, magnetic resonance imaging, and laboratory investigation for reversible or genetic causes.

Treatment depends on the underlying insult.

Cross-References

► Cerebellum
► Dysdiadochokinesia

References and Readings

Gilman, S. (2004). Clinical features and treatment of cerebellar disorders. In R. L. Watts & W. C. Koller (Eds.), *Movement disorders* (2nd ed., pp. 723–736). New York: McGraw-Hill.

Atherosclerosis

Elliot J. Roth
Department of Physical Medicine and
Rehabilitation, Northwestern University,
Feinberg School of Medicine, Chicago, IL, USA

Synonyms

Arteriosclerotic vascular disease or ASVD; Atheromatous plaque; Hardening of the arteries

Definition

Atherosclerosis is the progressive pathological process of buildup of plaque inside the blood vessels, resulting in blockage of blood flow through the vessels.

Current Knowledge

The plaque that causes atherosclerosis is comprised of fatty substances, cholesterol, cells, calcium, and fibrin, a stringy material found normally in the blood to help clot the blood. The plaque formation process stimulates the cells of the artery wall to produce substances that then accumulate in the vessel wall. Fat builds up within these cells and around them, and they form connective tissue and calcium. The artery wall thickens, the artery's diameter is reduced, and blood flow and oxygen delivery are decreased. Plaques can rupture or crack open, causing the sudden formation of a blood clot (thrombosis). Atherosclerosis can cause angina or myocardial infarction if it blocks the blood flow in the coronary arteries that supply the heart muscle, stroke if it blocks the carotid arteries that supply the brain, kidney disease if it blocks the renal arteries or gangrene possibly leading to amputation if it blocks the peripheral arteries that supply the limbs.

Atherosclerosis may be asymptomatic for many years. Risk factors for this disease have been well studied. It is thought that atherosclerosis is caused by a response to damage to the endothelium from high cholesterol, high blood pressure, and cigarette smoking. A person who has all three of these risk factors is eight times more likely to develop atherosclerosis than is a person who has none. Physical inactivity, diabetes, and obesity are also risk factors for atherosclerosis. Heredity, advancing age, and racial background are less-significant risk factors.

Treatment options include lifestyle changes, use of lipid-lowering and other drugs, angioplasty, and various surgical procedures, depending on the location of the plaque. Many lifestyle changes that prevent disease progression also prevent the onset of the disease; these include a low-fat, low-cholesterol diet, weight loss, exercise, blood pressure control, diabetes management, and smoking cessation.

Cross-References

► Angioplasty
► Anticoagulation
► Antiplatelet Therapy
► Cerebrovascular Disease

- ▶ Cholesterol
- ▶ Coronary Disease
- ▶ Ischemic Stroke
- ▶ Myocardial Infarction
- ▶ Peripheral Vascular Disease
- ▶ Stent
- ▶ Thrombolysis
- ▶ Thrombosis

References and Readings

Stary, H. C., Chandler, A. B., Dinsmore, R. E., Fuster, V., Glagov, S., Insull, W., et al. (1995). A definition of advanced types of atherosclerotic lesions and a histological classification of atherosclerosis: A report from the Committee on Vascular Lesions of the Council on Arteriosclerosis, American Heart Association. *Circulation, 92*, 1355–1374.

Atkins v. Virginia

Robert L. Heilbronner
Chicago Neuropsychology Group, Chicago, IL, USA

Synonyms

Mental retardation defense

Historical Background

Daryl Atkins and William Jones abducted Eric Nesbitt from a convenience store, and after finding only $60 in his wallet, Atkins and Jones used Nesbitt's vehicle to drive to an ATM and forced him to withdraw $200. Thereafter, Atkins and Jones drove Nesbitt to an isolated location where he was shot eight times and subsequently died. Atkins and Jones were quickly tracked down by police, and in custody, it was determined that Jones' story claiming that Atkins pulled the trigger was more coherent than Atkins' story implicating Jones as the shooter.

Thus, Atkins was charged and convicted of abduction, armed robbery, and capital murder. This took place despite the results of an IQ test completed by a clinical psychologist, in which Atkins' score of 59 placed him in the mildly mentally retarded range. Nonetheless, he was sentenced to death.

The Supreme Court of Virginia was in agreement with the judgment of the trial court, and the appeal was taken to the US Supreme Court. In July of 2002, the US Supreme Court reversed the judgment of the trial court and the Supreme Court of Virginia and referred the case back to the sentencing court to render a sentence other than the death penalty. The US Supreme Court ruled that the punishment was excessive and thus prohibited by the eighth Amendment as cruel and unusual if it is not "graduated and proportioned to the offense." An excessive judgment is judged by current societal standards. Thus, society's standards of decency, albeit subject to change, must prove that they are influenced by "objective factors to the maximum possible extent." Furthermore, it was ruled that mental retardation does not preclude a person's capability to discriminate right from wrong, though mental retardation does lead to a diminished capacities to process and comprehend information, reduces communication abilities, and decreases one's ability to learn from mistakes and experiences, reason logically, inhibit impulses, and understand the emotions and behaviors of others. The US Supreme Court concluded that mentally retarded individuals are not exempt from criminal sanctions, though a decrease in personal culpability is warranted. Thus, due to the conclusions that the purposes of retribution and deterrence are not accomplished in the execution of mentally retarded individuals, coupled with the increased risk that the death penalty will be imposed erroneously, the US Supreme Court ruled that the eighth Amendment precludes execution of mentally retarded persons.

Despite the court's ruling, in July of 2005, a Virginia jury determined that Atkins was intelligent enough to be executed due to the fact that another IQ score had been recorded at above 70.

Moreover, the prosecution claimed that his poor performance in school was related to use of alcohol and drugs and that earlier assessments of his IQ were "tainted." Thus, Atkins was set to be executed on 2 December 2005. However, the decision was recently reversed again by the Virginia Supreme Court, as a result of state procedural grounds.

Current Knowledge

Forensic psychological and neuropsychological assessments of mentally retarded individuals being considered for the death penalty are highly important. Specifically, the US Supreme Court did not specify the degree of mental retardation required to circumvent the death penalty and instead left such determinations up to the discretion of the states. It is important to note that subaverage intelligence alone does not warrant a label of mental retardation. Impairments in adaptive functioning and evidence of mental retardation prior to the age of 18 years are needed for a diagnostic determination of mental retardation.

Cross-References

► Intellectual Disability
► Intelligence

References and Readings

Atkins v. Virginia, 153 L. Ed 2d 335 (2002).
Cunnningham, M. D., & Goldstein, A. M. (2003). Sentencing determinations in death penalty cases. In A. Goldstein (Ed.), *Forensic psychology (vol 11). Handbook of psychology*. Hoboken: Wiley.
Denney, R. L. (2005). Criminal responsibility and other criminal forensic issues. In G. Larrabee (Ed.), *Forensic neuropsychology: A scientific approach*. New York: Oxford University Press.
Melton, G. B., Petrila, J., Poythress, N. G., & Slobogin, C. (2007). *Psychological evaluations for the courts: A handbook for mental health professionals and lawyers* (3rd ed.). New York: Guilford Press.

Atomoxetine

Efrain Antonio Gonzalez
College of Psychology, Nova Southeastern University, Fort Lauderdale, FL, USA
Utah State University, Logan, UT, USA

Generic Name

Atomoxetine

Brand Name

Strattera

Class

ADHD agents

Proposed Mechanism(s) of Action

Inhibits the presynaptic reuptake of norepinephrine and theoretically increases dopamine in the prefrontal cortex via the same mechanism.

Indication

Attention deficit/hyperactivity disorder.

Off-Label Use

Treatment-resistant depression and anxiety.

Side Effects

Serious
Increased cardiac rate, potential hypertension, orthostatic hypotension, rare liver damage, potential for induction of mania, and suicidal ideation.

Common

Sedation in children, decreased appetite, dry mouth, constipation, nausea, vomiting, dysmenorrhea, erectile dysfunction, and impaired libido.

References and Readings

Physicians' Desk Reference (71st ed.). (2017). Montvale: Thomson PDR.

Stahl, S. M. (2007). *Essential psychopharmacology: The prescriber's guide* (2nd ed.). New York: Cambridge University Press.

Additional Information

Drug Interaction Effects: http://www.drugs.com/drug_interactions.html.

Drug Molecule Images: http://www.worldofmolecules.com/drugs/.

Free Drug Online and PDA Software: www.epocrates.com.

Free Drug Online and PDA Software: www.medscape.com.

Gene-Based Estimate of Drug interactions: http://mhc.daytondcs.com:8080/cgibin/ddiD4?ver=4&task=getDrugList.

Pill Identification: http://www.drugs.com/pill_identification.html.

Atrophy

JoAnn Tschanz[1,2] and Stephanie Behrens[1]
[1]Department of Psychology, Utah State University, Logan, UT, USA
[2]Center for Epidemiologic Studies, Utah State University, Logan, UT, USA

Synonyms

Degenerative; Wasting

Definition

Atrophy is a loss of cells of any tissue. In the brain, atrophy refers to a loss of neurons that may be generalized (e.g., diffuse atrophy) or focal, reflecting

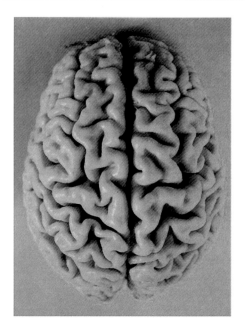

Atrophy, Fig. 1 Displays diffuse atrophy of the cerebral hemispheres. Note the shrunken gyri and prominent, widened sulci (Photo courtesy of Steven S. Chin, M.D., Ph.D., University of Utah Health Sciences Center)

circumscribed regional loss. Focal atrophy may occur as a result of trauma or cerebrovascular lesions, for example. Generalized atrophy may occur with neurodegenerative conditions such as Alzheimer's disease. With atrophy, there is also corresponding loss of neural connections (synapses). Visual features of atrophy include sulcal widening, shrunken gyri, and enlarged ventricles. Atrophy may be viewed on gross inspection of the brain post-mortem or antemortem with structural imaging techniques such as MRI or CT scan. Figure 1 displays diffuse brain atrophy of the cerebral hemispheres viewed from the top.

References and Readings

Smits, L. L., Tijms, B. M., Benedictus, M. R., Koedam, E. L. G. E., Koene, T., Reuling, I. E. W., Barkhof, F., Scheltens, P., Pijnenburg, Y. A. L., Wattjes, M. P., & van der Flier, W. M. (2014). Regional atrophy is associated with impairment in distinct cognitive domains in Alzheimer's disease. *Alzheimer's & Dementia, 10*, S299–S305.

Attendant Care

Amy J. Armstrong
Department of Rehabilitation Counseling,
Virginia Commonwealth University, Richmond,
VA, USA

Definition

Attendant care involves the provision of services to assist individuals with mental and/or physical disabilities in the performance and/or conduct of activities of daily living in order to maximize community inclusion and independent living. The intent of attendant care is to promote independence, participation, sustainability, and quality of life of the individual while also preventing or reducing the impact of medical problems. Typically, the individual receiving attendant services is unable to perform such tasks independently or may perform them with great difficulty. Attendant services include but are not limited to activities such as bathing, dressing, feeding, toileting, transferring, mobility, cooking, cleaning, and laundering. Services may also relate to sustaining health such as dispensing medications. However medical services typically are not provided by personel care attendants.

Attendant care may be provided by a family member such as a spouse, partner, sibling, or parent or by a hired employee. Typically, attendant care is provided by persons who have been trained to provide the service/s within the home and/or community. The independent living model of attendant care contends that individuals with disabilities should be empowered, to the highest degree possible, to recruit, screen, and hire, train, and terminate their respective personal attendants, thereby ensuring self-determination and choice. Additional considerations related to the provision of attendant care include where and how to locate and access quality service providers, adequate training of an attendant, and financial issues including paying a competitive wage to personal attendants (Rodriguez-Banister 2006). Funding sources of attendant care may include private resources, such as health insurance, auto insurance, and worker's compensation, or public resources such as Medicaid, Department of Vocational Rehabilitation, Department of Veterans Affairs, crime victims compensation, and/or other state-funded programs.

Federal legislation provides regulations that are relevant to attendant care services. For example, The Home and Community-Based Services, as mandated by 1915 (i) and 1915 (c), provides for long-term community-based services and state-wide waivers under the Medicaid program, focused upon an individual's right to live an independent life, within a community of choice. Subpart K, Part 441 of the Community First Choice Option, CMS-2337 F implements Section 2401 of the Affordable Care Act. Subpart K provides for the development of state plans to provide home and community attendant services and supports. Developing familiarity with relevant legislation on the federal and state levels as well as the policies and procedures of specific funders of attendant care is necessary for those providing professional and family-based supports for eligible individuals.

Cross-References

▶ Assisted Living

References and Readings

Federal Register. Medicaid Program; Community First Choice Program, Subpart K. https://www.federalregister.gov/articles/2012/05/07/2012-10294/medicaid-program-community-first-choice-option#h-57

Rodriguez-Banister, K. (2006). *The personal care attendant guide: The art of finding, keeping, or being one.* New York: Demos Medical Publishing.

Attention

Ronald A. Cohen
Department of Clinical and Health Psychology,
College of Public Health and Health Professions,
University of Florida, Gainesville, FL, USA
Center for Cognitive Aging and Memory,
McKnight Brain Institute, University of Florida,
Gainesville, FL, USA

Synonyms

Concentration; Focus; Vigilance

Definition

Cognitive processes that enable the selection of, focus on, and sustained processing of information. The object of attention can either be environmental stimuli actively being processed by sensory systems, or associative information and response alternatives generated by ongoing cognitive activity.

Historical Background

Attention is subjectively self-evident to all people, and terms that referred to attention-type experiences have been described by philosophers through the ages. The concept of attention is strongly linked in the philosophy to the nature of consciousness, self-awareness, and most theories of the "mind." Accordingly, attention has been the subject of psychological inquiry from the beginning of this scientific discipline. The writings of William James captured this fact, as evident from this well-known excerpt from his *Principles of Psychology* (1898).

Everyone knows what attention is. It is the taking possession by the mind, in clear and vivid form, of one out of what seem several simultaneously possible objects or trains of thought. Focalization, concentration, of consciousness are of its essence. It implies withdrawal from some things in order to deal effectively with others.

While written over 100 years ago, this description very succinctly captures essential aspects of the phenomena of attention, and remains apropos even today. The understanding of cognitive, behavioral, and neuropsychological bases, influences, and effects of attention have dramatically evolved since the time of William James. Yet, the underlying subjective and behavioral experiences characterized by James and the other psychologists of his time remain largely consistent with current phenomenology of attention. Different types of attention were described, such as directed, divided, focused, sustained, selective, and volitional attention, many of which continue to be used to describe the varieties of attentional experience. The primary limitation of these early efforts was the lack of experimentation that would have enabled operationalizing of these constructs and understanding of the processes underlying them.

Following the initial efforts of early psychologists to study attention from perspectives of structuralism and functionalism, a rather long period ensued dominated by behaviorism during which cognitive processes, like attention, were largely viewed as outside of the realm of empirical psychological inquiry. Attention was considered to be a construct that could be explained by more basic behavioral principles, such as discrimination learning, cue dominance, anticipation, and expectation. Classical conditioning theory provided an essential framework for behavioral analysis of attention, as the orienting response to novel stimuli, and its subsequent habituation, provided the behavioral and neural building blocks for simple forms of attention, in the absence of long-term memory formation (i.e., conditioning). The concepts of motivation and drive which played a major role in neobehaviorism, also helped to bridge attention theory and learning principles.

Information theory (Shannon and Weaver 1949), which evolved out of technological advances in radio communication and also radar detection during World War II, was a major impetus for the subsequent re-emergence of cognitive science. In particular, the application of information processing models and signal detection methods to the study of communication led to a resurgence of research interest in attention. This is not surprising considering the fact that signal detection and selection, the basic elements of almost all theories of selective attention, are also central to information and communication theory. This approach emphasized the probabilistic nature of information detection and selectivity, a conceptual departure from earlier psychophysical methods used to study perception. The application of information processing approaches to the study of attention was a logical step, as one of the primary problems for any communication or information processing system is reducing the total amount of incoming signal to manageable levels to enable subsequent processing of this information.

Broadbent (1958) proposed the first formal model of selective attention based on the information processing theory. He maintained that attention occurs because there is an information "bottleneck" as the large quantity of environmental information that is available during parallel processing is subject to channel capacity limitations later in the stream of processing due to serial processing constraints. Broadbent posited that the primary requirement for attention to occur was a filtering process (as shown in Fig. 1) that occurred soon after sensory registration and served to separate relevant from irrelevant signals in order to enable meaningful information to be available for subsequent serial processing through limited capacity information channels. This model presumed a somewhat passive system by which this filtering occurred, with selection driven by the salience of the stimuli themselves. However, the nature of this filtering process was not fully operationalized in this initial model. In the years

that followed, a number of variations on this model of attention were proposed by other investigators working in the newly emerging field of cognitive psychology.

Most notably, Treisman proposed an attenuation theory of attention, which was similar to Broadbent's model in which he postulated a single process that occurred early in the information processing stream, soon after sensory registration (Treisman and Gelade 1980). According to attenuation theory, selective attention requires distinguishing between messages on the basis of their physical characteristics, such as location, intensity, and pitch, as well as content. In this model of attention, stimuli naturally differ in their threshold for activating awareness of a stimulus, and the process of attention effectively decreases (i.e., attenuates) the strength (e.g., loudness) of irrelevant stimuli. This attenuation process was considered to occur in conjunction with a feature integration process that enabled perceptual experience. This line of research was noteworthy for the use of dichotic listening paradigms in which attention is divided between the two ears, and information must be selected from one of the two channels of input.

The bottleneck models proposed by Broadbent and Treisman proposed that selection occurs at a very early stage of processing soon after sensory registration, thereby linking attention squarely with sensory selection. Essentially, selective attention filters inhibits focus on information occurring in the unattended ear in dichotic listening experiments before semantic analysis and other cognitive processes have time to occur. Other investigators (e.g., Deutsch and Deutsch (1963) argued that attention is strongly influenced by the response demands of a situation and that it likely occurred at a later stage of processing, and

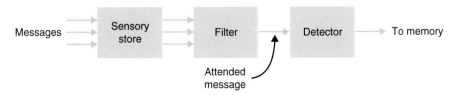

Attention, Fig. 1 Model depicting filtering process as proposed by Broadbent (1958)

that in reality both ears analyze incoming information semantically, though response demands creates a bias toward one ear over the other. This led to heated debates in the 1960s and 1970s over the location of the bottleneck. While considerable experimental evidence indicated that early sensory selection occurs prior to a point in time when semantic information has been processed, there is also other paradigms that demonstrate that in most situations selection is greatly influenced by semantics and the response requirements that exist.

Subsequent researchers took this a step further by demonstrating that capacity limitations constrain attention and the intensity of attentional focus that is possible at any given point in time. Kahenman's (1983) capacity theory of attention proposed that people's capacity for attentional focus is not static, but instead varies as a function of factors such as the reward characteristics of the task, arousal level, and other biological determinants. This theory of attention was extremely important in that it brought to the forefront the fact that attention should not be conceptualized in purely mechanical terms as was the case in early attention models based solely on information processing theory. Rather attention needed to be viewed in the context of the biological factors that drive it. This helped to catalyze an emphasis on the study of focused attention, a shift that coincided with information coming from psychophysiological studies that showed linkages between arousal, activation, and effort in the control of attention (Pribram and McGuinness 1979).

A large body of cognitive studies of attention followed this pioneering work. Several of these are particularly important in a historical context. Posner (1979) made an important distinction between overt and covert shifts of attention that occur in the context of visual selective attention. Overt attention is characterized by the act of intentionally directing attention (i.e., looking) toward a stimulus, whereas covert attention occurs without intention when focus is drawn to a particular stimulus or location, typically as a result of cues or other types of information of which the person may have little conscious awareness. Posner also refined the use of chronometric methods to demonstrate the costs associated with these attention shifts. His research also made a distinction between two primary processes, selection and focus, that were necessary to account attention's intensity and spatial distribution.

Shiffrin and Schneider (1979) conducted seminal studies that distinguished automatic from controlled attention. They varied the number of targets to be detected and the consistency of target location based on either fixed or variable memory demands. By creating greater variability in task characteristics, subjects could not rely on memory to facilitate performance, which slowed their response time. Under these conditions, automaticity was no longer feasible. Besides demonstrating the distinction between automatic and controlled attention, these findings also illustrated the relationship between attention and memory, and set the stage for a long line of research examining working memory in relationship to attention.

Neuropsychological Models and Frameworks

Over the past two decades, research efforts have been directed at organizing these varieties of attention into coherent frameworks. Furthermore, researchers have proposed neuropsychological models of attention that seek to characterize the functional neuroanatomic systems involved in attention, the processes for which these systems are responsible, and also how these functional brain areas interact. The models described below are not meant to be an exhaustive review of the literature in this regard, but rather highlights some of the key elements of current theoretical frameworks and the extent to which there is consistency across models.

Alan Mirsky provided one of the first neuropsychological frameworks to account for what he described as the "elements" of attention. This framework proposed five elements of attention: (1) selection, (2) focus, (3) execute, (4) switch, and (5) sustain. This theoretical framework was derived from factor analyses of neuropsychological test results obtained from a large sample from his clinical practice.

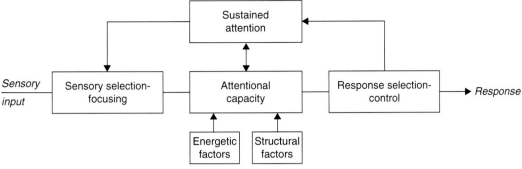

Attention, Fig. 2 Simplified neuropsychological model of the components of attention

Cohen (1993) proposed a similar component process framework of attention that hypothesized four primary components of attention (Fig. 2): (1) sensory selective attention; (2) response intention, selection, and control; (3) capacity-focus; and (4) sustained attention. A primary goal of Cohen's model was to include components reflecting similar levels of analysis. The components of this framework were also derived from factor analysis of clinical neuropsychological data with efforts made to retain only the minimum number of factors necessary to account for maximum variance in the data, with an effort to make conservative interpretation of the component processes associated with each factor. Each component was hypothesized to be a function of other more basic subcomponent processes. This model posits that these four components of attention are not completely orthogonal or functionally independent, but instead rather share common component subprocesses, processes depending on the task at hand. A simplified version of the model is shown.

In everyday situations, attention depends on the interaction of all four of these component processes. However, for some tasks, the primary demand may be for sustained attention or vigilance, whereas for another task it may be efficient use of available attention capacity and the intensity of focus. Similarly, some tasks that are weighted more demand for sensory selective attention, while others place greater demand on response intention and selection. In other words, while these four components need to be accounted for in explaining attention across all situations,

particular tasks may require minimal demands for sustained attention, but intense demands on capacity and focus. Validation efforts directed at this framework have shown the principal factors to be highly reliable, internally consistent, and valid with respect to their weighting relative to specific brain disorders and conditions. For example, patients with attention-deficit disorder have greatest impairment on tasks requiring sustained attention, whereas patients with diminished speed of processing have greatest problems on tasks requiring capacity and focus. It is noteworthy that the analyses conducted by both Mirsky and Cohen yielded very similar factor structures and validity data, providing strong evidence that four to five primary components processes exist that account for most varieties of attention. These attentional component processes are described in greater detail below.

Selective Attention

A fundamental aspect of all attentional processes is that it is selective. Attention enables the selective deployment of cognitive resources for the processing of information from either the external environment or internal cognitive processes or associative representations. Attention also requires a shift from less salient information. Processes that enable or facilitate the selection of salient information for further cognitive processing are collectively referred to as *selective attention* (Treisman 1969; Triesman and Geffen 1967). Individuals are constantly flooded with an infinite number of signals from both outside and within. By reducing the amount of information that will receive additional processing, attention constrains incoming information to the individual's available capacity at a given point in time, thereby keeping the level of information to be processed at a manageable level. While selective attention is necessary and beneficial for cognitive function, there are costs associated with selectively attending. By attending to a particular stimulus, the likelihood of detecting other potentially relevant stimuli or choosing an alternative response strategy is reduced. Optimal selective attention depends on the system being flexible and adaptive, with the capacity to select and focus on certain stimuli, but then to shift to other stimuli or cognitive processing when task conditions change. Selective attention thereby serves as a gating mechanism for the flow of information processing and the control of behavior.

Response Selection and Control

Attention has traditionally been viewed as a process closely related to perceptual processing. It prepares the individual for sensory intake, perceptual analysis, and integration with other cognitive processes. Yet, there are many situations in which attention is not directed at incoming sensory information, but rather selection response alternatives, and the control of responding once a selection has been made. Even when a task primarily requires selective attention, there are usually coexisting response demands. While sensory selection may be automatically elicited by the occurrence of salient external stimuli, more often than not the act of attending is linked to a planned, goal-directed course of action. In this regard, attention and responding are directed to obtain information that will optimize behavior.

The processes associated with response selection and control range from simple behavioral orienting, such as turning one's head in response to a sound source to more complex cognitive processes involving intention, planning, and decision making. Response selection and control form the basis for what humans typically experience as volitional action. Before responding, individuals generate a large number of response alternatives. These response alternatives are evaluated prior to

making an actual motor response, leading to response bias, that is, the probability of selecting specific responses.

The attentional processes involved in response selection and control are related to a broader class of cognitive processes, commonly referred to as *executive functions* (Fuster 1989; Luria 1966). Several processes associated with response generation underlie executive control: intention, selection, initiation, inhibition, facilitation, and switching. Not only do these processes account for the control of simple motor responses, they also provide the foundation for more complex cognitive processes, such as planning, problem solving, and decision making, as well as conceptual processes such as categorization, organization, and abstraction. Executive control is strongly dependent on the actions of prefrontal-subcortical systems. Executive control is dependent on the ability of the system to act with intention, to initiate responding, to inhibit responding based on new information, and to efficiently shift from one response alternative to another in accordance with changing environmental demands.

Focused Attention and Capacity Limitations

Attention is also characterized by having intensity and by the extent to which it is allocated in either a focal or diffuse manner. The intensity of attentional focus is a function of both situational and task demands and organismic factors, such as motivation and drive. Focused attention is constrained by capacity limitations (Kahneman 1973) that limit the intensity of focus that is possible on a moment-by-moment basis. Attentional capacity is influenced by both structural and energetic factors (Cohen 1993). Energetic capacity limitations tend to be state dependent and reflect the changing energetic conditions of the brain, including motivation, and the incentives to attend that are present in the situation. Structural factors tend to be more stable and dependent on each person's intrinsic information processing capacity. Factors that influence structural capacity include the processing speed capacity that is a function of the integrity of neural transmission, memory encoding, storage and retrieval limitations, and temporal-spatial processing dynamics that vary across people. Given these factors that limit attentional capacity, focused attention varies relative to the cognitive demands and type of information to be processed, and situational incentive. Focused attention can occur relative to either sensory selective attention, or intention and response selection, and in fact often involves the coordination of sensory and response selection. Such coordination is quite effortful (Pribram and McGuinness 1975). Arousal and activation vary as a function of the existing demands for focused attention, with greater activation occurring when there is more utilization of available capacity because of the need to focus.

Automatic Versus Controlled Attention

An important distinction exists between automatic and controlled attentional processing (Schneider and Shiffrin 1977; Hasher and Zacks 1979). Automaticity occurs most commonly in the context of sensory selective attention, particularly for tasks requiring simple detection of a target from a set of stimuli, and also on tests of attention span. With automaticity, there is usually relatively little demand placed on attentional capacity, and often attention can occur without much awareness or subjective effort (e.g., attending to other cars while driving on an empty highway). Automaticity can be interfered with increase in size and complexity of the environment to be attended to. Spatial selective attention is particularly well suited for automatic attentional processing since visual information typically occurs in parallel with a vast array of information reaching the brain almost instantaneously. Automaticity is more difficult to achieve for tasks that require sequential cognitive operations, though some degree of automaticity may be attainable through practice. Controlled attention is typically required for tasks in which there are working memory demands, or other requirement of other cognitive processes, such as memory encoding and retrieval, rapid processing speed, or executive control. The demand for focused intensity varies as a function of requirements for controlled attention that exist for a particular task. Generally,

response intention, selection, and control are not very amenable to automatic attentional processing, as behavioral responding typically requires complex motor sequencing with executive control demands. However, the fact people are able to perform certain tasks such as typing or playing a musical instrument with considerable automaticity illustrates that automaticity is attainable for well-learned motor programs.

Sustained Attention

Attention varies as a function of the temporal dynamics of the task to be performed and the situation, and all humans experience some degree of performance variability, particularly when long periods of sustained performance are required. Sustained attention refers to processes that enable the maintenance of performance over time. Compared to other cognitive processes, such as language and visual perception, attention is inherently variable by necessity, as it must be responsive to changing stimulus conditions, task demands, and motivational and energetic states. Problems with sustained attention commonly occur on tasks requiring attentional persistence for long durations when there are high levels of demand for effortful processing. All people have limits in their capacity for sustained attention. Sitting in a 1-h lecture is not a problem for most bright college students, but even the brightest students would encounter tremendous difficulties sustaining their focus for a lecture that lasted 12 consecutive hours.

Vigilance refers to sustained attention directed toward specific targets, in which a state of readiness is required to detect and respond to stimuli occurring at variable and often infrequent intervals (e.g., Colquhoun and Baddeley 1967; Corcoran et al. 1977). Detecting rare targets with lengthy intervals between responses can be difficult. This type of sustained attention is quite common in everyday life. For example, a watchman may spend the entire night attending to the possibility of an intruder without this event ever occurring. Attention to low-frequency events has different processing requirements than responding to high-frequency events and, for many people, is more difficult. Vigilance and sustained attention are under the influence of sustained motivational level, boredom, and fatigue, which are sensitive to the dynamics of temporal tasks.

Current Clinical and Experimental Evidence

Neuropsychological Studies

Twenty years ago the clinical and experimental neuropsychological literature on impairments of attention associated with neurological and psychiatric disorders affecting the brain was quite limited. Much of the neuropsychological focus on attention was on the assessment of attention span in the context of psychometric analysis of performance on tests such as digit span. This probably reflected the fact that adequate attention was once viewed more as a necessary condition for other cognitive functions to occur optimally, but not particularly important in its own right in considerations of brain-behavior relationships. This attitude has changed dramatically, and attention is now widely regarded as a critical cognitive process that reflects not only the interface between both the external environment and internal cognitive functions, but also moment-by-moment information processing. A literature review conducted about two decades ago revealed less than 500 studies focused on the neuropsychology of attention. Recent literature reviews suggest that this number is now over 40, 000. This increase in interest in attention reflects the fact that: (1) attention disturbances are one of the most common by-products of brain, (2) attention is closely tied to the human experiences of consciousness, awareness, and cognitive control, (3) major advances have occurred in the methodology for studying and assessing attention, and (4) for a number of reasons, there has been an increased societal interest in attention disturbances, perhaps in part because of the intense information processing demands and pace of life that people now experience.

Impairments of attention may be either specific or nonspecific. Specific impairments occur when only aspect of attention is affected. Often this occurs when impaired attention is directly associated with a particular type of cognitive operation, such as spatial processing. These impairments are often associated with focal brain disturbances affecting specific cortical or subcortical systems necessary for the cognitive operation. Nonspecific disturbances of attention are much more common, often occurring due to disorders that affect arousal, motivation, or other factors that reduce attentional capacity, and as a result of more diffused nonlocalized brain disorders. Both types of attentional disturbance provide insights into the cognitive processes of attention and the brain mechanisms that underlie these processes. Though localized lesions provide the best vehicle for analysis of the role of specific brain structures in attentional control, nonspecific attentional impairments illustrate the influence of metabolic and neurotransmitter abnormalities on information processing rate, arousal, and other energetic and structural factors that may affect attentional capacity and focus. Attentional capacity is a direct function of level of consciousness, making this an essential part of the clinical assessment of attention. Levels of consciousness range from normal states of alertness and awareness to coma.

A brief summary of the attentional disturbances associated with several common neurological and psychiatric conditions is provided below. For more detailed consideration see Cohen (1993).

Stroke and Neglect Syndrome

Unilateral stroke affecting the nondominant cortex often causes hemi-neglect syndrome, perhaps the most well known and dramatic form of attention disturbance. The defining feature of neglect syndrome is the failure to attend to, respond to, or be aware of stimuli on one side of space. Many variants of neglect syndrome may be observed clinically. Most patients with neglect exhibit impairments of sensory selective attention, although some may have primary problems with hemi-spatial response selection and control. Experimental investigations have confirmed the role of attention in hemi-neglect syndrome. Manipulation of attentional parameters demonstrates that symptoms of hemi-neglect change as attentional demands are modified (Kaplan et al. 1990). Regardless of which attentional process is most affected, all patients with neglect syndrome have a fundamental disorder involving the spatial distribution and allocation of attention.

Alzheimer's and Neurodegenerative Dementias

Attention disturbance is usually not described as a primary feature of Alzheimer's disease (AD) and historically tended to be viewed as one cognitive function that was largely spared. This conclusion is misleading. While patients with early-stage AD typically do not show overt symptoms of severe inattention, they frequently have marked difficulty with focused attention and executive control, particularly when tasks required controlled attentional processing. This reflects a distinction between performance on tests of simple and complex attention, as conclusions about spared attention in AD have often been based on the observation of preserved attention span on tests such as digit span. Patients with early AD are often usually alert, energetic, and able to maintain their general focus on the assessment process. Yet, most will have considerable difficulty on tasks requiring focused and divided attention, suppression of interference (e.g., Stroop), information processing speed and efficiency (e.g., Symbol Coding), and working memory. As the disease progresses, performance becomes impaired on most tasks requiring effortful attentional processing. Pervasive disturbance eventually develops affecting all aspects of attention, including self-awareness.

Multiple Sclerosis

Multiple sclerosis (MS), one of the most common neurologic in young adults, often affects learning, memory, and executive control. Given the fact that the disease affects the myelin of the white matter, deficits in these areas are often strongly associated with attentional impairments and slowed inefficient information processing. Attentional capacity is typically reduced with performance decrements usually evident under conditions of increased informational load. Fatigue is the most common of all symptoms in MS and is associated not only with motor effort but also with attending to and performing cognitive tasks. Patients with MS experience difficulty maintaining consistent effort on tasks.

HIV

Similar to MS, HIV-infected patients who have not developed severe AIDS dementia typically show primary impairments in the areas of psychomotor and information processing speed, focused and sustained attention, and executive functioning. This reflects the fact that when not adequately treated, HIV tended to initially have greatest effects on subcortical systems, including the basal ganglia.

Closed Head Injury

The most common effects of closed head trauma are diffuse axonal damage due to shearing forces and frontal lobe disturbances. Consequently, attention and executive dysfunction are among the most common associated cognitive problems. Persistent distractibility, poor concentration, apathy, and fatigability are prominent sequelae. Deficits of arousal and poor performance on measures of selective, focused, divided and sustained attention, processing speed, and executive functioning tend to occur, which may contribute to associated learning and memory retrieval problems as well.

Epilepsy

Transient changes in the level and quality of consciousness, common in seizure disorder, typically cause marked alterations in attention around the time of the seizure. During the time between seizures, patients with epilepsy may have greater problems than healthy individuals on tests of focused and divided attention. These deficits appear to be related in part to slowed speed of processing and its effects on attentional capacity. Pharmacological effects associated with anticonvulsant therapy likely contribute in part to these attentional effects.

Metabolic Disturbances

Factors that affect the metabolic function often cause delirium, or more subtle alterations in attention and arousal. Accordingly, metabolic disturbance is one of the most common reasons for transient alterations in attention among people without other neurological or psychiatric illness. Metabolic disturbances that affect the brain can be the result of a wide variety of factors, including drug effects and systemic illnesses, such as liver and kidney disease, and diabetes.

Psychiatric Disorders

Difficulties with focused and sustained attention are extremely common among patients with psychiatric disorders, including affective disorders (major depression and bipolar disturbance) and schizophrenia. Severe anxiety states can also interfere with attention. A strong relationship exists between expenditure of effort and performance on tests of attention and other demanding cognitive functions for patients with major affective disorders. Impairments tend to be somewhat proportional to severity of depression, with performance improving when the depression resolves. Diminished attentional capacity is particularly evident on tasks that require psychomotor speed, attentional focus, and effortful demands for mental control. Abnormal attention is also a central feature of schizophrenia, as filtering of irrelevant stimuli and thoughts has long been considered to be a major element of the disorder, which has been linked to the dopamine system. Schizophrenics often encounter difficulties on tests of sensory selective attention because of their susceptibility to distraction. Slowed reaction time and processing speed also contribute to problems with attentional capacity, and both focused and sustained attention (Nuechterlein 1977).

Attention-Deficit Disorder (ADD)

A developmental disorder of attention, ADD is the most widely recognized of all attention disturbance. Problems with sustained attention and distractibility are key features of the disorder, along with hyperactivity among a subset of children. While there is general agreement regarding the existence of ADD, there continues to be considerable debate about its manifestations and pathophysiology, particularly in light of the fact that ADD tends to occur along with other comorbid conditions.

Primate Studies

Understanding of the neural substrates of attention was greatly enhanced by the use of neurophysiological methods in primates. The value of these studies is that they provided directed recording of electrical activity from brain areas implicated in attention both by past clinical studies of patients with neurological disorders and also ablation studies involving laboratory animals. In the 1970s, Robert Wurtz, Michael Goldberg and their colleagues (Wurtz et al. 1982) began electrophysiological studies from the brain of monkeys trained on specific attention paradigms. The earliest of these studies showed that the superior colliculus exhibits increased firing rates during visual attention, providing the first direct evidence of the involvement of a neural area in this process. Subsequently, a large number of studies were conducted that showed the contribution of other brain regions, particularly in posterior visual areas to specific aspects of visual selective attention. This work both confirmed the role of areas like the inferior parietal cortex that had been suspected of being involved in visual selective attention based on studies of hemi-neglect syndrome. Over time, there has been increasing emphasis on the role of frontal brain systems in relationship to these posterior brain areas. There is now a large body of research on this topic, supporting to general conclusions about selective attention: (1) Visual selective attention is controlled by multiple interacting brain areas that comprise a functional system. (2) Selective attention involves not only posterior visual brain areas, but also frontal-striatal systems that provide executive response control. Active investigation continues using primate models with particular emphasis on source analysis of how particular types of neurons are tuned to optimize attention to particular types of signals. This research has been instrumental in characterizing the functional brain systems governing attention in humans.

Functional Neuroimaging

Attention was one of the first cognitive functions to be demonstrated through the use of functional imaging methods, such as functional MRI and PET. The fact that attentional parameters can be easily manipulated in the context of the scanner and that attention reflects the moment-by-moment information processing of the brain makes it very conducive to study through functional brain imaging. These efforts have largely confirmed the involvement of inferior parietal and frontal brain systems in attention, with studies showing the relative contribution of specific areas in selective, focused, and sustained attention. This is a rapidly growing area of neuropsychological inquiry. To date, results of functional neuroimaging experiments have largely supported evidence from earlier cognitive, neuropsychological, psychophysiological, and primate studies with respect to the neural substrates of attention.

Clinical Assessment Considerations

Although an essential cognitive process, attention is more difficult to directly observe or measure than other cognitive functions like language, visual perception, or memory. Attention fluctuates in accordance with changes in task demands and the processing capacity of the patient over time. Unlike other cognitive functions, performance may be quite different across different points in time, and it is this variability that in fact defines attention. Attention is often situation specific. This accounts for why some children with ADD perform well in a controlled laboratory setting, despite reports of gross problems with inattention in school or the home.

Unlike most other cognitive processes, attention primarily serves a facilitative function. Attention enhances or inhibits perception, memory, motor output, and executive functions, including problem solving. Yet, attention is always measured as a function of performance on tasks that also loads on one or more of these other cognitive domains. Therefore, pure tests of attention do not exist, and attention usually must be assessed within the context of performance on tasks that load on one or more these other domains. Attentional performance is often assessed as derived measure obtained by comparing performance across tasks that control for key attentional parameters (e.g., target-distractor ratio). Absolute performance often provides less informative measures of performance inconsistencies in the assessment of attention. For example, how performance varies as a function of time, spatial characteristics, or memory load provides more information about attentional dynamics than simply considering total errors on a visual detection task. Since attention is not the by-product of a unitary process, or a single sensory modality, it cannot be adequately assessed on the basis of findings from one specific test. For example, conclusions based on digit span performance are misguided. Attentional assessment requires a multifactorial approach. The specific attention measures used in an evaluation depends on the overall level of functioning of the particular patient. For patients with global cognitive dysfunction, it may be difficult to use certain tasks that require overly complex responses. For patients with relatively high overall cognitive abilities, tasks should be chosen that require multiple component processes. If the patient is able to perform well on these tasks, then severe attention disturbance involving specific attentional component processes can be ruled out. The Stroop and Trail-Making tests are examples of tasks that require multiple attentional processes. If impairments are found on such tasks, then more extensive testing of specific component processes can be conducted. When possible, efforts should be made to use tasks that incorporate signal detection methods, even when not evaluating sensory selective attention per se. This methodology provides the best means of accurately summarizing performance relative to all types of possible errors, and easily integrates with response time measures.

Attentional Parameters that Should be Considered A thorough assessment of attention should be based on analysis of data from a comprehensive battery of attentional tests that sample underlying component processes (Cohen 1993). Accordingly, tasks should be used that are differentially sensitive to the following attentional parameters: (1) spatial characteristics, (2) temporal dynamics, (3) memory demands, (4) processing speed requirements, (5) perceptual complexity, (6) demands for response sequencing and control, (7) cognitive complexity of the task, (8) effort required to complete task, and (9) task salience, relevance, and reward value.

While multifactor neuropsychological assessment provides the best means of evaluating attentional impairments, a comprehensive attentional evaluation may not be feasible in everyday clinical practice, because of time constraints, the patient's overall severity of cognitive impairment, or the fact that other cognitive functions must be assessed in greater detail because of the referral questions. Consequently, clinicians should be aware of the information that can be obtained from different levels of attentional assessment. A few primary tests of attention should be included in all neuropsychological evaluations. The continuous performance test (CPT) paradigm provides an excellent measure for assessing sustained attention and other related indices. Tests of focused and selective attention are also now widely available. Several attention batteries have also been developed that may facilitate the comprehensive assessment of the elements of attention.

Future Directions

Real-time functional brain-imaging methods will enhance the ability of neuropsychologists in the future to assess moment-by-moment variations in attention associated with task performance. There continues to be the need to attentional batteries that are theoretically coherent and provide assessment of the component processes that govern attention.

Cross-References

▶ Attention Deficit Hyperactivity Disorder
▶ Automaticity
▶ Consciousness
▶ Directed Attention
▶ Divided Attention
▶ Effort
▶ Focused Attention
▶ Habituation
▶ Hemi-attention Syndrome
▶ Intention Tremors
▶ Orienting Response
▶ Selective Attention Models
▶ Sustained Attention

References and Readings

Cohen, R. A. (1993). *Neuropsychology of Attention.* New York: Plenum.
Cohen, R. A., Meadows, M. E., Kaplan, R. F., & Wilkinson, H. (1994). Habituation and sensitization of the OR following bilateral cingulate damage. *Neuropsychologia, 32*(5), 609–617.
Colquhoun, W. P., & Baddeley, A. D. (1967). Influence of signal probability during pretraining on vigilance decrement. *Journal of Experimental Psychology, 73*, 153–155.
Desimone, R., & Gross, C. G. (1979). Visual areas in the temporal cortex of the macaque. *Brain Research, 178,* 363–380.
Deutsch, J. A., & Deutsch, D. (1963). Attention: Some theoretical considerations. *Psychological Review, 70*, 80–90.
Fuster, J. M. (1989). *The prefrontal cortex: Anatomy, physiology, and neuropsychology of the frontal lobe.* New York: Raven.
Goldberg, M. E., & Bushnell, M. D. (1981). Behavioral enhancement of visual response in monkey cerebral cortex. II. Modulation in frontal eye fields specifically related to saccades. *Journal of Neurophysiology, 46*, 783–787.
Hasher, L., & Zacks, R. T. (1979). Automatic and effortful processes in memory. *Journal of Experimental Psychology: General, 108*, 356–388.
Heilman, K. M., Bowers, D., Coslett, H. B., & Watson, R. T. (1983). Directional hypokinesia in neglect. *Neurology, 2*(33), 104.
Heilman, K. M., Watson, R. T., & Valenstein, E. (1993). Neglect and related disorders. In K. M. Heilman & E. Valenstein (Eds.), *Clinical neuropsychology* (3rd ed., pp. 279–336). New York: Oxford University Press.
Heilman, K. M., Watson, R. T., Valenstein, E., & Goldberg, M. E. (1988). Attention: Behavior and neural mechanisms. *Attention, 11*, 461–481.

James, W. (1890). *The principles of psychology* (Vol. 1, pp. 403–404). New York: Henry Holt.

Kahneman, D. (1973). *Attention and effort.* Englewood Cliffs: Prentice-Hall.

Kahneman, D., & Treisman, A. (1984). Changing views of attention and automaticity. In R. Parasuraman & D. R. Davies (Eds.), *Varieties of attention.* New York: Academic.

Kaplan, R. F., Verfaellie, M., DeWitt, L. D., & Caplan, L. R. (1990). Effects of changes in stimulus contingency on visual extinction. *Neurology, 40*(8), 1299–1301.

Mattingley, J. B., Bradshaw, J. L., Bradshaw, J. A., & Nettleton, N. C. (1994). Residual rightward attentional bias after apparent recovery from right hemisphere damage: Implications for a multi-component model of neglect. *Journal of Neurology, Neurosurgery & Psychiatry, 57*(5), 597–604.

Mesulam, M. A. (1981). A cortical network for directed attention and unilateral neglect. *Archives of Neurology, 10,* 304–325.

Parasuraman, R. (1984). Sustained attention in detection and discrimination. In R. Parasuraman & D. R. Davies (Eds.), *Varieties of attention* (pp. 243–289). New York: Academic.

Pardo, J. V., Fox, P. T., & Raichle, M. E. (1991). Localization of a human system for sustained attention by positron emission tomography. *Nature, 349*(6304), 61–64.

Posner, M. I., & Cohen, Y. (1984). Facilitation and inhibition in shifts of visual attention. In H. Bouma & D. Bowhuis (Eds.), *Attention and performance X.* Hillsdale: Erlbaum.

Posner, M. I., Walker, J. A., Friedrich, F. A., & Rafal, R. D. (1987). How do the parietal lobes direct covert attention? *Neuropsychologia, 25*(1A), 135–145.

Pribram, K. H., & McGuinness, D. (1975). Arousal, activation, and effort in the control of attention. *Psychological Review, 82,* 116–149.

Schneider, W., & Shiffrin, R. M. (1977). Controlled and automatic human information processing: I. Detection, search, and attention. *Psychological Review, 84,* 1–66.

Shannon, C. E., & Weaver, W. (1949). *The mathematical theory of communication.* Urbana: The University of Illinois Press.

Treisman, A., & Gelade, G. (1980). A feature-integration theory of attention. *Cognitive Psychology, 12,* 97–136.

Verfaellie, M., Bowers, D., & Heilman, K. M. (1988). Attentional factors in the occurrence of stimulus-response compatibility effects. *Neuropsychologia, 26,* 435–444.

Watson, R. T., Heilman, K. M., Cauthen, J. C., & King, F. A. (1973). Neglect after cingulotomy. *Neurology, 23,* 1003–1007.

Wurtz, R. H., Goldberg, M. E., & Robinson, D. L. (1982). Brain mechanisms of visual attention. *Scientific American, 246*(6), 124–135.

Attention Deficit Hyperactivity Disorder

Kevin M. Antshel[1] and Russell A. Barkley[2]
[1]Department of Psychology, Syracuse University, Syracuse, NY, USA
[2]Virginia Treatment Center for Children and Virginia Commonwealth University Medical Center, Richmond, VA, USA

Synonyms

ADD; ADHD; ADHD, combined; ADHD, predominantly hyperactive-impulsive type; ADHD, predominantly inattentive type; Attention deficit disorder; Hyperkinetic disorder

Short Description or Definition

Attention deficit/hyperactivity disorder (ADHD) is characterized by developmentally inappropriate levels of inattention and/or hyperactivity-impulsivity, which most often arise in early to middle childhood, result in functional impairment across multiple domains of daily life activities, and remain relatively persistent over time.

Categorization

DSM-5 defines three ADHD presentations: predominantly inattentive (ADHD-I), predominantly hyperactive/impulsive (ADHD-H/I), and combined (ADHD-C). ADHD-C is the most prevalent subtype in clinically referred samples yet the true population prevalence of ADHD-C and ADHD-I is likely comparable, each accounting for roughly half of the ADHD cases (Wilcutt 2012). ADHD-H/I is less common, is most often observed in preschool and early elementary school-age children, and is probably just the earlier developmental stage to the C-presentation in many instances. In general, hyperactive-impulsive symptoms decline more steeply as children age (although feelings of restlessness may persist), but inattentive symptoms remain relatively constant.

Children with ADHD-H/I and ADHD-C are at higher risk for disruptive behavior. Youth with ADHD-I is at higher risk for learning disorders, anxiety, and possibly depression. While some argue that ADHD-I is a distinct disorder from ADHD-C and ADHD-H/I, others have not found consistent differences between the subtypes on neuropsychological or laboratory measures. Though diagnosed as a categorical disorder, ADHD may actually represent an extreme end along a normal continuum for the traits of attention, inhibition, and the regulation of motor activity.

Epidemiology

The population prevalence of ADHD is estimated to be 5% of school-age children and 2–4% of adults (Polanczyk et al. 2007). ADHD is a worldwide disorder found in most countries with rates similar to those found in North America. ADHD is more prevalent in males in childhood yet this sex discrepancy wanes in adulthood. Differences across ethnic groups within the North America are sometimes found but seem to be more a function of social class than ethnicity. ADHD is heritable; parents and siblings of individuals with ADHD have between and five- and tenfold increased risk of developing ADHD. Environmental risk factors associated with ADHD include prenatal maternal smoking or alcohol use, low birth weight, and exposure to environmental toxins.

Natural History, Prognostic Factors, and Outcomes

The syndrome of attention difficulties, impulsive behavior, and overactivity has been known since the late 1700s and certainly since the early 1900s. Numerous attempts have been made at definition and nomenclature, including Strauss syndrome, minimal brain dysfunction or damage, hyperkinetic child syndrome (or hyperkinesis), and attention deficit disorder with and without hyperactivity.

ADHD can exist without other psychiatric disorders in 20–30% of ADHD cases (Barkley 2014) but is more often associated with comorbidity. Oppositional defiant disorder (45–65%) is the most common psychiatric comorbidity in ADHD. As many as half of these oppositional children will progress to conduct disorder such as lying, stealing, fighting, and otherwise violating the rights of others. Major depressive disorder (20–30%) and anxiety disorders (20–30%) are also relatively common comorbid conditions in pediatric ADHD.

Longitudinal research following children with ADHD into adulthood suggests that approximately two-thirds of children with ADHD continue to show impairing symptoms as they age (Faraone et al. 2006). The fact that some children *do not* continue to have an ADHD diagnosis may be due in part to the finding that ADHD symptoms decline as a function of age in typically developing populations. However, it may also simply reflect that DSM symptoms and symptom thresholds may be developmentally inappropriate and too restrictive, respectively, to be applied outside of childhood. For example, DSM-5 inattentive symptoms are more common in adolescents than DSM-5 hyperactive/impulsive symptoms. While this may infer that inattention persists more than hyperactivity/impulsivity, it may also simply reflect the developmental insensitivity of the DSM-5 symptoms.

Genetics also appear to be a large factor in those who continue to demonstrate clinically significant ADHD post-childhood versus those whose symptoms are in remission. For example, prevalence rates of ADHD among the relatives of children with persistent ADHD are significantly higher than rates in relatives of children with remitted ADHD. In addition, a history of major depressive disorder in childhood is a predictor of the syndromic persistence of ADHD into adolescence, as is having a below average IQ.

By definition, individuals with ADHD need to be functionally impaired in two or more domains of major life activities. In children, academic, social, and family functioning domains are the most frequently impaired (MTA Collaborative Group 1999). Educational impairments including academic underachievement and learning disabilities are well documented in the pediatric ADHD literature.

In adolescents and young adults, academic impairments continue to persist; young adults with ADHD completed fewer years of education, with nearly one-fourth failing to complete high school (Kuriyan et al. 2013). Compared to children with ADHD who are followed into adulthood, clinically diagnosed adults with ADHD appear to have higher intellectual levels and have done better academically (Barkley 2014). In addition to educational impairments, impairments in domains such as occupational, dating/marital relations, financial management, driving, child-rearing, managing a household, and maintaining health are also consistently reported in adults with ADHD. For example, employer ratings are lower for adults with ADHD, and adults with ADHD have more part-time employment and change jobs more often (Barkley et al. 2007).

There are some data to suggest that ADHD is *more* functionally impairing than most other outpatient psychiatric disorders in these domains. While the relationship between ADHD symptoms and impairment in children with ADHD is modest ($r = 0.3$), these relationships may be more robust in adults ($r = 0.7$) (Barkley et al. 2007).

Neuropsychology and Psychology of ADHD

A meta-analysis suggested that children with ADHD have an IQ about nine points lower than typically developing peers (Frazier et al. 2004). Similar data have been reported in adults with ADHD. Lower performance on the Wechsler Processing Speed and Working Memory indices may account for a substantial portion of the IQ differences noted between children/adults with ADHD and community controls.

Controlled processing deficits are commonly observed in both pediatric and adult ADHD. Children and adults with ADHD perform less well on laboratory tasks that assess vigilance, motoric inhibition, organization, planning, complex problem solving, and verbal learning and memory. Both children and adults with ADHD perform less well on tasks that require vigilance, or the ability to sustain attention.

Response inhibition has been hypothesized to play a central role in ADHD. Continuous performance test (CPT) commission errors are a common laboratory measure of this construct. Unlike attention deficits which seem to emerge more reliably in rare target CPTs like the Gordon Diagnostic System (Gordon 1983), response inhibition deficits emerge more reliably in higher signal probabilities such as the Conners CPT-3rd edition (Conners 2014). Several studies have reported that adults with ADHD make more errors of commission on high signal CPTs relative to both clinical and community control participants.

Executive functioning deficits are present in both pediatric and adult ADHD. Thus, it is surprising that performance on one of the most well-established tests of executive functioning, the Wisconsin Card Sorting Test (WCST; Heaton et al. 1993), is not impaired in adults with ADHD. Multiple studies have failed to report a significant difference between adults with ADHD and community controls on WCST categories completed and number of errors, both perseverative and non-perseverative (see Hervey et al. 2004 for a meta-analysis).

Verbal fluency is impaired in adult ADHD. The most widely used verbal fluency task in adult ADHD populations has been the Controlled Oral Word Association Test (Benton et al. 1983). Multiple studies have reported significant differences between community controls and adults with ADHD.

Given the importance of attention and working memory to memory encoding and storage, it is not surprising that adults with ADHD have been demonstrated to have memory deficits. They also appear to have more difficulty managing auditory/verbal information relative to visual information. Although differences emerge between adults with ADHD and community controls on the WAIS-IV Digit Span, the effect size of the differences is much larger on the California Verbal

Learning Test-2nd edition (Delis et al. 2000). For example, adults with ADHD perform less well on overall rates of learning, recall, recognition, and semantic clustering. The weaker performance on the semantic clustering index may indicate failure to adopt a strategy.

Finally, both children and adults with ADHD demonstrate reward dysregulation. Individuals with ADHD have decision-making impairments related to a preference for immediate rather than delayed rewards that are thought to be independent of the deficits in cognitive control.

Evaluation

The American Academy of Child and Adolescent Psychiatry (Pliszka 2007) has established guidelines for the assessment and treatment of ADHD. No neurological, genetic, neuropsychological, or behavioral tests have sufficient positive and negative predictive power to accurately classify ADHD cases with sufficient success to recommend them for clinical diagnosis. Clinical diagnosis is based largely on careful history taking, use of structured interviews containing DSM-5 criteria for ADHD and related disorders, and the expert knowledge of the clinician in the differential diagnosis among other mental disorders. Paramount in the evaluative process for children and adolescents is the time to listen to parental and patient concerns; probe for details concerning nature, onset, and course; elaborate the specific impairments resulting from these concerns; and place them in the larger framework of the clinical taxonomy of mental disorders. The clinical interview is then supplemented with the use of parent and teacher behavior rating scales to assess developmental deviance of symptoms, screening of intelligence and academic achievement skills by standardized testing, brief observation of the child during unstructured and structured activities, contact with school personnel concerning classroom functioning, and compilation of prior school and mental health records available on the child.

Other sources of information essential for the diagnostic process are behavioral rating scales or checklists on which normative data are available. These include "broadband" questionnaires, such as the Behavioral Assessment System for Children-3rd edition (Reynolds and Kamphaus 2015) or Child Behavior Checklist (Achenbach and Rescorla 2001) for screening the major dimensions of childhood psychopathology (e.g., anxiety, depression, attention, hyperactivity, aggression, etc.). "Narrowband" questionnaires specifically evaluate the symptoms of ADHD as set forth in DSM-5. Rating scales can reliably, validly, and efficiently measure *DSM-5*-based ADHD symptoms. Some examples of instruments demonstrating appropriate psychometric properties with a strong normative base include the ADHD Rating Scale-5th edition (DuPaul et al. 2016) and the Conners Rating Scales-3rd edition (Conners 2008).

The diagnostic process for adults is very similar to the process for children and adolescents. Structured diagnostic interviews such as the Diagnostic Interview for Adult ADHD-2nd edition (DIVA-2; Kooij and Francken 2010) along with ADHD rating scales such as the World Health Organization Adult ADHD Self-Report Scale (ASRS; Kessler et al. 2005) for patients and collateral reporters (e.g., spouse) are commonly utilized.

A number of specific tests have been devised to provide objective measures of a subject's vigilance and impulse control, such as the Gordon Diagnostic System, Conners Continuous Performance Test, or the Test of Variables of Attention (Greenberg 2015), among others. Research suggests that these tests are not especially accurate at classifying individuals as having ADHD; while the presence of abnormal scores on such tests indicates the presence of a disorder in as many as 90% of individuals who perform poorly, such scores cannot indicate the specific disorder present (Barkley and Grodzinsky 1994). Moreover, the ecological validity of these tests is low thus precluding the ability to predict from the test scores how the individual will function in more natural settings, such as home, school, and work. These tests are therefore not recommended for routine diagnostic evaluations for individuals with ADHD, although they may be used in clinics specializing in ADHD as part of research or drug trials. More useful information is likely to be obtained from the clinical interview and the rating scales discussed above.

Treatment

Treatment for ADHD in children typically involves three components: parent and child education and support, classroom accommodations, and medication. Substantial evidence exists to show that training parents in child behavior management skills can be of significant benefit in the reduction of parent-child conflict and improvement in child success within the home (MTA Collaborative Group 1999). The school setting frequently requires adjustment to meet the special needs of the child with ADHD. School interventions often include alterations to the curriculum and workload to better mesh with the limited attention, persistence, and disorganization of the child with ADHD, increases in sources of positive reinforcement for work productivity, occasional use of immediate and systematic negative consequences for disruptive or inappropriate behavior, and implementation of a daily school behavior report card (the ratings on which are linked to a home token economy).

The mainstay of treatment for many children with ADHD is medication, frequently psychostimulants. Three classes of medication appear to be useful for management of ADHD, these being psychostimulants (methylphenidate, amphetamines), noradrenergic reuptake inhibitors (atomoxetine), and antihypertensive medications (clonidine, guanfacine).

Stimulant medications, especially extended release formulations, are a frontline management strategy in pediatric ADHD; approximately 70% of children with ADHD will show an efficacious response to stimulant medications (Spencer et al. 1996). The side effects of stimulants are fairly benign, short-lived, dose related, and often managed through dose or timing adjustments or by switching to a different delivery system or stimulant.

Atomoxetine is a nonstimulant approved for management of ADHD. Atomoxetine is an exclusive noradrenergic reuptake inhibitor and is a Schedule II controlled substance with low potential for abuse, making it more convenient than the stimulants for prescribing. Clonidine and guanfacine are $alpha_2$-noradrenergic agonists that are FDA approved for treating ADHD and are more effective for the management of hyperactive-impulsive ADHD symptomatology.

In adults, stimulant medications are effective in approximately 70% of individuals with ADHD (Spencer et al. 1996). Atomoxetine is FDA approved and prescribed most often for adults with ADHD and comorbid depression or for those with a comorbid substance use disorder.

Managing psychiatric comorbidity is a significant component of pediatric ADHD. The same dictum appears central to managing ADHD in adults. While "uncomplicated" ADHD exists in about 25% of the adults with ADHD, most adults with ADHD have significant psychiatric comorbidity that requires clinical attention and management. One aspect in which the psychiatric comorbidity is evident in treatment strategies is pharmacotherapy. Although the evidence for the efficacy of polypharmacy is limited at this time, multiple researchers have asserted that polypharmacy may be more likely in adult ADHD than pediatric ADHD.

Similar to pediatric ADHD, a psychosocial treatment component is typically recommended in adult ADHD. What constitutes the psychosocial component, however, appears to be somewhat different in adult ADHD relative to pediatric ADHD. For example, neither cognitive behavioral therapy (CBT) nor cognitive therapy has much research support in pediatric ADHD. Nonetheless, there are some data to suggest that CBT may be more efficacious in adolescents and adults with ADHD (Antshel et al. 2014; Boyer et al. 2015; Safren et al. 2010; Solanto et al. 2010). For example, in the adult ADHD literature, there is some evidence that CBT is efficacious for reducing functional impairments in adults concurrently treated with stimulants.

Cross-References

References and Readings

Achenbach, T. M., & Rescorla, L. A. (2001). *The manual for the ASEBA school-age forms & profiles*. Burlington: University of Vermont, Research Center for Children, Youth, and Families.

Antshel, K. M., Faraone, S. V., & Gordon, M. (2014). Cognitive behavioral treatment outcomes in adolescent ADHD. *Journal of Attention Disorders, 18*, 483.

Barkley, R. A. (2013). *Taking charge of ADHD: The complete authoritative guide for parents* (3rd ed.). New York: Guilford.

Barkley, R. A. (2014). *Attention deficit hyperactivity disorder: A handbook for diagnosis and treatment* (4th ed.). New York: Guilford Press.

Barkley, R. A., & Grodzinsky, G. M. (1994). Are tests of frontal lobe functions useful in the diagnosis of attention deficit disorders? *Clinical Neuropsychology, 8*, 121–139.

Barkley, R., Murphy, K., & Fischer, M. (2007). *ADHD in adults: What the science says*. New York: Guilford Press.

Benton, A. L., Hamsher, S. K., & Sivan, A. B. (1983). *Multilingual aplasia examination* (2nd ed.). Iowa City: AJA Associates.

Boyer, B. E., Geurts, H. M., Prins, P. J., & Van der Oord, S. (2015). Two novel CBTs for adolescents with ADHD: The value of planning skills. *European Child and Adolescent Psychiatry, 24*, 1075–1090.

Conners, C. K. (2008). *Conners' rating scales* (3rd ed.). North Tonawanda: Multi-Health Systems.

Conners, C. K. (2014). *Conners continuous performance test* (3rd ed.). North Tonawanda: Multi-Health Systems.

Delis, D. C., Kramer, J. H., Kaplan, E., & Ober, B. A. (2000). *California verbal learning test – second edition. Adult version*. San Antonio: Psychological Corporation.

DuPaul, G. J., Power, T. J., Anastopoulos, A. D., & Reid, R. (2016). *ADHD rating scale—5 For children and adolescents: Checklists, norms, and clinical interpretation*. New York: Guilford Press.

Faraone, S. V., Biederman, J., & Mick, E. (2006). The age dependent decline of attention deficit/hyperactivity disorder: A meta-analysis of follow-up studies. *Psychological Medicine, 36*, 159–165.

Frazier, T., Demaree, H., & Youngstrom, E. (2004). Meta-analysis of intellectual and neuropsychological test performance in attention-deficit/hyperactivity disorder. *Neuropsychology, 18*, 543–555.

Gordon, M. (1983). *The Gordon diagnostic system*. DeWitt: Gordon Systems.

Greenberg, L. (2015). *Test of variables of attention – version 8*. Odessa: Psychological Assessment Resources.

Heaton, R. K., Chelune, G. J., Talley, J. L., Kay, G. G., & Curtiss, G. (1993). *Wisconsin card sorting test manual: Revised and expanded*. Odessa: Psychological Assessment Resources.

Hervey, A. S., Epstein, J. N., & Curry, J. F. (2004). Neuropsychology of adults with attention-deficit/hyperactivity disorder: A meta-analytic review. *Neuropsychology, 18*, 485–503.

Kessler, R. C., Adler, L., Ames, M., Demler, O., Faraone, S., Hiripi, E., Howes, M. J., Jin, R., Secnik, K., Spencer, T., Ustun, T. B., & Walters, E. E. (2005). The World Health Organization Adult ADHD Self-Report Scale (ASRS): A short screening scale for use in the general population. *Psychological Medicine, 35*, 245–256.

Kooij, J.J.S., & Francken, M.H. (2010). *DIVA 2.0. Diagnostic interview Voor ADHD in adults bij volwassenen [DIVA 2 0 diagnostic interview ADHD in adults]*. The Hague, Netherlands: DIVA Foundation.

Kuriyan, A. B., Pelham, W. E., Molina, B. G., Waschbusch, D. A., Gnagy, E. M., Sibley, M. H., Babinski, D. E., Walther, C., Cheong, J. W., Yu, J., & Kent, K. M. (2013). Young adult educational and vocational outcomes of children diagnosed with ADHD. *Journal of Abnormal Child Psychology, 41*, 27–41.

MTA Collaborative Group. (1999). A 14-month randomized clinical trial of treatment strategies for attention-deficit/hyperactivity disorder. The MTA Cooperative Group. Multimodal treatment study of children with ADHD. *Archives of General Psychiatry, 56*(12), 1073–1086.

Nigg, J. (2006). *What causes ADHD: Understanding what goes wrong and why*. New York: Guilford.

Pliszka, S. (2007). Practice parameter for the assessment and treatment of children and adolescents with attention-deficit/hyperactivity disorder. *Journal of the American Academy of Child and Adolescent Psychiatry, 46*(7), 894–921.

Polanczyk, G., de Lima, M. S., Horta, B. L., Biederman, J., & Rohde, L. A. (2007). The worldwide prevalence of ADHD: A systematic review and metaregression analysis. *American Journal of Psychiatry, 164*, 942–948.

Reynolds, C., & Kamphaus, R. (2015). *Behavior assessment system for children, third edition (BASC-3)*. San Antonio: Pearson.

Safren, S. A., Sprich, S., Mimiaga, M. J., Surman, C., Knouse, L., Groves, M., & Otto, M. W. (2010). Cognitive behavioral therapy vs relaxation with educational support for medication-treated adults with ADHD and persistent symptoms: A randomized controlled trial. *Journal of the American Medical Association, 304*, 875–880.

Solanto, M. V., Marks, D. J., Wasserstein, J., Mitchell, K., Abikoff, H., Alvir, J. M., & Kofman, M. D. (2010). Efficacy of meta-cognitive therapy for adult ADHD. *American Journal of Psychiatry, 167*, 958–968.

Spencer, T., Biederman, J., Wilens, T., Harding, M., O'Donnell, D., & Griffin, S. (1996). Pharmacotherapy of attention-deficit hyperactivity disorder across the life cycle. *Journal of the American Academy of Child and Adolescent Psychiatry, 35*, 409–432.

Wilcutt, E. (2012). The prevalence of DSM-IV attention-deficit/hyperactivity disorder: A meta-analytic review. *Neurotherapeutics, 9*, 490–499.

Attention Network Test (ANT)

Michael S. Worden
Department of Neuroscience, Brown University, Providence, RI, USA

Attention is often subdivided by researchers into a number of separate systems. Although there is certainly some interaction between them, these systems play different roles in terms of their effect on information processing and the control of behavior. Further, there is evidence that different attentional systems are associated with different, largely nonoverlapping brain regions and rely to a large extent on different neurotransmitter systems. One such framework advanced by Michael Posner and colleagues defines three separate attention systems or networks: alerting, orienting, and executive control.

The *alerting system* is responsible for helping the organism reach and maintain an alert state. This state, which is separate from arousal, is characterized by a readiness to perceive and process incoming stimuli. The alerting system has been associated with superior parietal, right frontal, and thalamic brain regions and the norepinephrine neurotransmitter system.

The *orienting system* is responsible for selecting and giving preference to specific sensory information, often in terms of spatial location. Attentional orienting in space may be done overtly by, for example, moving the head or covertly, that is, without moving the eyes or head. For example, a football player might look down the field with his eyes while attending covertly to the location and movements of other players in his peripheral vision. Attended items are generally processed faster and more accurately than nonattended items. Brain areas that have been linked to the orienting system include areas of the parietal cortex and the frontal eye fields, and the cholinergic neurotransmitter system appears to play an important role.

The *executive attention system* is involved in monitoring one's performance in the context of current task demands and providing control signals that help other systems adapt to changing contexts and conflicting information. Executive attention is especially important for detecting and responding to situations in which there is stimulus-response conflict. Such conflict arises when two or more stimuli or two or more aspects of the same stimulus are associated with different behavioral responses. A common example is the Stroop task in which subjects are presented with printed words, and they must name the color of the ink in which the word is printed (e.g., red ink) when the word itself spells out a different color (e.g., BLUE). Brain areas implicated in the executive attention system include frontal midline regions such as the anterior cingulate cortex and the lateral prefrontal cortex. The neurotransmitter dopamine is important in the functioning of this network.

The *attention network task (ANT)* was developed by Jin Fan, Michael Posner, and colleagues at the Sackler Institute for Developmental Psychobiology. Using subtractive methodology, the ANT is designed to assess each of these three attentional networks using a single reaction-time paradigm. The fundamental task of the participant is simple. On each trial, the participant looks at a small *fixation cross* in the center of a computer screen and a small arrow, called the *target*, is briefly displayed either above or below the fixation. The participant is required to respond by pressing one of two buttons as quickly and accurately as possible indicating whether the arrow is pointing to the left or right. On some presentations, the target is preceded by a briefly presented cue stimulus while on other trials it is presented with no advanced warning. These cues are either predictive or non-predictive. *Orienting cues* are presented either above or below the central fixation and indicate the location at which the upcoming arrow will be shown. *Non-orienting cues* are presented either at the center of the screen or else both above and below fixation simultaneously. Both types of cues indicate that the target is about to appear but only orienting cues provide information regarding the location of the impending target. Finally, in some cases, the target arrow is flanked on either side by other stimuli. These *flanking stimuli* may be arrows pointing in the same direction as the target (called congruent trials) or they may be arrows pointing in the opposite direction as the target (called incongruent trials).

The efficiency of the three attention networks may be assessed independently for each participant by use of the subtractive method. Both reaction time and accuracy may be examined. To assess the alerting network, scores from trials in which no cue was presented are compared to scores from trials in which there was a cue presented. The difference in mean reaction times between these two trial types constitutes an *efficiency score* for the alerting network and is indicative of the extent to which the alerting network was able to use the information provided by the cue to improve behavioral performance. In a similar manner, an efficiency score for the orienting network may be derived by subtracting mean scores from trials with orienting cues from the scores for trials with non-orienting cues. Both of these trial types include a cue so there should be no difference in terms of a contribution from the alerting network. The difference in scores measures the degree to

which the orienting system could take advantage of the predictive cues to orient to a specific spatial location. In the case of the non-orienting cues, the participant could not predict whether the target would appear above or below the fixation point and therefore could not improve performance by orienting to one or the other spatial location. An efficiency score is derived for the executive attention system by comparing scores on trials with congruent flankers to trials with incongruent flankers. Subjects will tend to be slower and less accurate for incongruent trials than for congruent trials, and the size of these differences indicates the extent to which the individual is able to suppress conflicting response tendencies.

A number of intriguing findings have come from studies that have utilized the ANT. Supporting the notion that the three attention networks assessed by the ANT constitute independent systems, a large-scale study of over 200 individuals found that there was very little correlation in efficiency scores among the three networks. In other words, the particular score of an individual on any one of the three attention networks does not tend to predict the individual's scores on the other two networks. A high efficiency score for the alerting network, for example, does not suggest what one's scores are likely to be for either the orienting or executive attention networks. Using electroencephalographic (EEG) recordings from the surface of the scalp, it was found that each of these three attention systems is associated with distinct patterns of neural oscillations. A number of variations on the original ANT have been developed to address specific questions and for the study of special populations. For example, child-friendly versions of the ANT that use cartoon pictures of fish instead of arrows have been used to study the development of attention systems.

Attentional deficits are a hallmark of many psychiatric and neurological disorders. The ANT has been used to assess the relative impact of many disorders on the different attention systems and to help distinguish between or establish subtypes of particular disorders. Among others, variations on the ANT have proven useful in the study of attention deficit hyperactivity disorder, Alzheimer's disease, autism, borderline personality disorder, traumatic brain injury, substance abuse, and schizophrenia.

References and Readings

Fan, J., McCandliss, B. D., Sommer, T., Raz, A., & Posner, M. I. (2002). Testing the efficiency and independence of attentional networks. *Journal of Cognitive Neuroscience, 14*(3), 340–347.

Fan, J., McCandliss, B. D., Fossella, J., Flombaum, J. I., & Posner, M. I. (2005). The activation of attentional networks. *NeuroImage, 26*(2), 471–479.

http://www.sacklerinstitute.org/users/jin.fan/

Posner, M. I., & Rothbart, M. K. (2007). Research on attention networks as a model for the integration of psychological science. *Annual Review of Psychology, 58*, 1–23.

Attention Training

McKay Moore Sohlberg
Communication Disorders and Sciences,
University of Oregon, Eugene, OR, USA

Synonyms

Attention process training; Direct attention training; Process training

Definition

Attention training is based on the premise that attentional abilities can be improved by activating particular aspects of attention through a stimulus drill approach. The repeated stimulation of attentional systems via graded attention exercises is hypothesized to facilitate changes in attentional functioning. Most attention training programs assume that aspects of cognition can be isolated and discretely targeted with training exercises.

Current Knowledge

The aspects of attention that are trained vary widely among interventions and frequently depend upon a theoretical model of attention. Attention models, regardless of their operational framework, appear to include functions related to sustaining attention over time (vigilance), capacity for information, shifting attention, speed of processing, and screening out distractions. Some attention efficacy studies evaluate attention interventions that focus on particular attention components such as reaction time and sustained attention for visual information (e.g., Ponsford and Kinsella 1988). Other efficacy studies use attention training programs that include hierarchical tasks to address a continuum of attention components from basic sustained attention to more complex mental control (e.g., Park et al. 1999; Sohlberg et al. 2001).

Evidence supports the effectiveness of attention training beyond the effects of nonspecific cognitive stimulation for patients with traumatic brain injury or stroke during the postacute phase of recovery and rehabilitation (Butler et al. 2008; Cicerone et al. 2000), and preliminary evidence suggests attention training helps alleviate symptoms in psychiatric disorders such as schizophrenia (e.g., Knowles et al. 2016). Recent studies have sought to investigate underlying changes in neural processes following attention training (e.g., Hopfinger 2017). Evidence-based practice guidelines for attention training were generated from examination of the intervention research literature (Sohlberg et al. 2003). Analysis of nine Class I and Class II studies suggested that certain aspects of attention training are helpful in improving attention performance in some adults with traumatic brain injury. Treatment parameters found to influence positive outcomes included high frequency of attention training, combining attention training with metacognitive training (e.g., self-monitoring and strategy training), and individualizing training to match the client's attention profile. The effects of attention training may be relatively small or task-specific, and the research encourages clinicians to actively facilitate and monitor the impact of attention training on functional, everyday activities.

Cross-References

▶ Attention
▶ Neuropsychological Rehabilitation
▶ Plasticity
▶ Process Training

References and Readings

Butler, R. W., Copeland, D. R., Fairclough, D. L., Mulhern, R. K., Katz, E. R., Kazak, A. E., et al. (2008). A multicenter, randomized clinical trial of a cognitive remediation program for childhood survivors of a pediatric malignancy. *Journal of Consulting and Clinical Psychology, 76*(3), 367–378.

Cicerone, K. D., Dahlberg, C., Kamar, K., Langenbahn, D. M., Malec, J. F., Bergquist, T. F., et al. (2000). Evidence-based cognitive rehabilitation: Recommendations for clinical practice. *Archives of Physical Medicine & Rehabilitation, 81*, 316–321.

Galbiati, S., Recla, M., & Pastore, V. (2009). Attention remediation following traumatic brain injury in childhood and adolescence. *Neuropsychology, 23*(1), 40–49.

Hopfinger, J. (2017). Introduction to special issue: Attention and plasticity. *Cognitive Neuroscience, 8*, 69–71.

Knowles, M., Foden, P., El-Deredy, W., & Wells, A. (2016). A systematic review of efficacy of the attention training technique in clinical and nonclinical samples. *Journal of Clinical Psychology, 72*, 999–1025.

Park, N. W., & Ingles, J. L. (2001). Effectiveness of attention rehabilitation after acquired brain injury: A meta-analysis. *Neuropsychology, 15*, 199–210.

Park, N. W., Proulx, G., & Towers, W. M. (1999). Evaluation of the attention process training programme. *Neuropsychological Rehabilitation, 9*, 135–154.

Sohlberg, M. M., McLaughlin, K. A., Pavese, A., Heidrich, A., & Posner, M. (2001). Evaluation of attention process training and brain injury education in persons with acquired brain injury. *Journal of Clinical and Experimental Neuropsychology, 22*, 656–676.

Sohlberg, M. M., Avery, J., Kennedy, M., Ylvisaker, M., Coelho, C., Turkstra, L., & Yorkston, K. (2003). Practice guidelines for direct attention training. *Journal of Medical Speech Language Pathology, 11*(3), 19–39.

Attentional Blink

Eric S. Porges
Department of Clinical and Health Psychology, University of Florida, Gainesville, FL, USA
Center for Cognitive Aging and Memory, McKnight Brain Institute, University of Florida, Gainesville, FL, USA
Department of Neurology, University of Florida, Gainesville, FL, USA

Definition

Attentional blink (AB) is a phenomenon primarily reported in the visual domain (Horváth and Burgyán 2011), in which attention to a primary target results in a reduced likelihood of identifying a secondary target presented a short duration after. The effect is most pronounced in a 200–600 ms window after the initial target is presented (Nieuwenstein et al. 2009). The classic paradigm involves the rapid serial visual presentation (RSVP) of letters, with a primary target letter and secondary target letter embedded within the RSVP. When the secondary target in the RSVP appears during the AB window, the likelihood of successful identification is dramatically reduced. If the secondary target is presented outside the 200–600 ms window, a deficit in identification does not occur. The initial reports of the AB reported that the effect depended on the inclusion of distractor letters in the RSVP (Raymond et al. 1992), though more recent reports have suggested that this may not be the case (Visser 2007). Mechanistically, the AB is thought to reflect a constraint in the ability of the nervous system to deploy selective attention (Dux and Marois 2009) and not to be constrained by sensory limitations.

References and Readings

Dux, P. E., & Marois, R. (2009). The attentional blink: A review of data and theory. *Attention, Perception & Psychophysics, 71*(8), 1683–1700. https://doi.org/10.3758/APP.71.8.1683.

Horváth, J., & Burgyán, A. (2011). Distraction and the auditory attentional blink. *Attention, Perception, & Psychophysics, 73*(3), 695–701. https://doi.org/10.3758/s13414-010-0077-3.

Nieuwenstein, M. R., Potter, M. C., & Theeuwes, J. (2009). Unmasking the attentional blink. *Journal of Experimental Psychology. Human Perception and Performance, 35*(1), 159–169. https://doi.org/10.1037/0096-1523.35.1.159.

Raymond, J. E., Shapiro, K. L., & Arnell, K. M. (1992). Temporary suppression of visual processing in an RSVP task: an attentional blink? *Journal of Experimental Psychology. Human Perception and Performance, 18*(3), 849–860. Retrieved from http://www.ncbi.nlm.nih.gov/pubmed/1500880.

Visser, T. A. W. (2007). Masking T1 difficulty: Processing time and the attentional blink. *Journal of Experimental Psychology: Human Perception and Performance, 33*(2), 285–297. https://doi.org/10.1037/0096-1523.33.2.285.

Attentional Response Bias

Ronald A. Cohen
Department of Clinical and Health Psychology,
College of Public Health and Health Professions,
University of Florida, Gainesville, FL, USA
Center for Cognitive Aging and Memory,
McKnight Brain Institute, University of Florida,
Gainesville, FL, USA

Synonyms

Behavioral predisposition; Beta (β); Response tendency

Definition

Attentional response bias refers to the tendency or increased likelihood of selecting one response over others.

Summary

The concept of response bias is essential when considering or assessing attention, as it accounts for the fact that attentional selection is not only affected by sensitivity of the perceptual system to certain stimuli in the environment but also to an inclination to respond in one manner versus another to these stimuli. Response bias is a primary element of signal detection theory, which maintains that signal detection, and more broadly the accuracy of attention to target stimuli, is not only a function of discriminability (d') associated with perceptual sensitivity but also the tendency to either respond or not respond in the situation (Beta). Response bias may be determined by various factors related to a given person's behavioral disposition, including their tendency to be accepting of errors of one type or another. A person who is inclined to never make an incorrect response will tend to miss targets while attending, but will have few false-positive errors of responding when a response was not called for. Conversely, a person with a response bias of never missing a target will tend to miss fewer targets, but will make many more false positive responses. While overall stimulus detection accuracy (d') is largely a function of perceptual and attentional selection processes that occur quite early after initial sensory registration, attentional response bias can be influenced by factors occurring at various stages of cognitive processing, including the response demands inherent in the situation. Response bias can be altered by changing physiological (e.g., wakefulness) and psychological-emotional state, incentives, and a variety of other factors. The fact that response bias plays an important role in signal detection and sensory selection more broadly provides evidence for the involvement of attentional processes in addition to sensory registration and perception. This is reinforced by the fact that response biases play a major role when sustained attention and vigilance are required over time, with this bias subject to change under conditions of fatigue. The concept of response bias has its roots in statistical theory, specifically the distinction between type I and II errors. When assessing attention in a clinical context, it is essential that both discriminability and response bias be determined in order to fully assess the performance characteristics. Tasks designed to assess sustained attention, such as continuous performance tests, usually provide measures of response bias as a way of fully measuring and characterizing error types associated with attention disturbances. Brain disorders that impair frontal lobe function often affect response bias with greater propensity to false-positive errors reflecting impulsivity. However, disturbances of intention associated damage to the frontal cortex and other brain regions can cause reductions in spontaneous behavior and behavioral inertia, which would tend to increase the likelihood of missing targets during attention tasks. This response tendency is also common with psychiatric disorders, most notably major depression. There has been a recent surge in therapeutic approaches aimed at modifying attentional response bias. Malingering is often assessed by determining if there are extreme response biases that fall outside the range of disturbances observed in patients with neurological or psychiatric disorders.

Cross-References

▶ Attention
▶ Continuous Performance Tests
▶ Malingering
▶ Signal Detection Theory

References and Readings

Cohen, R. A. (2014). *Neuropsychology of attention* (2nd ed.). New York: Plenum Publishing.
Green, D. M., & Swets, J. A. (1989). *Signal detection theory and psychophysics*. Los Altos: Peninsula Publishing.
Heeren, A., De Raedt, R., & Koster, E. H. W. (2013). The (neuro) cognitive mechanisms behind attention bias modification in anxiety: Proposals based on theoretical accounts of attentional bias. *Frontiers in Human Neuroscience*. Lausanne. journal.frontiersin.org
Heilbronner, R. L., Sweet, J. J., & Morgan, J. E. (2009). *American Academy of Clinical Neuropsychology consensus conference statement on the neuropsychological assessment of effort, response bias, and malingering*. *The clinical neuropsychologist*. New York: Taylor and Francis.
Newman, D. P., O'Connell, R. G., & Bellgrove, M. A. (2013). *Linking time-on-task, spatial bias and hemispheric activation asymmetry: A neural correlate of rightward attention drift*. Neuropsychologia: Elsevier: Amsterdam.

Attorney

Moira C. Dux
US Department of Veteran Affairs, Baltimore, MD, USA

Definition

An attorney is defined as one who is legally appointed on another's behalf. An attorney-at-law is an individual who has achieved the necessary educational requirements (J.D.) and is licensed to practice law by the highest court of a state or some other forms of jurisdiction. In civil cases (e.g., personal injury, medical malpractice), there are plaintiff and defense attorneys. The plaintiff attorney represents the injured party (e.g., plaintiff) in an action against the party they allege to be responsible for the damages; the defense attorney represents the defendant (e.g., insurance company, hospital, and doctor). In criminal matters, there are prosecution and defense attorneys. The prosecuting attorney represents the party (e.g., federal, state, or local government) who has accused and wants to convict the offender of some type of criminal action (e.g., murder, assault). The defense attorney represents the party (e.g., defendant) who has been accused of committing the crime.

Cross-References

▶ Litigation

References and Readings

Larrabee, G. (2005). *Forensic neuropsychology: A scientific approach*. New York: Oxford University Press.
Stern, B. H., & Brown, J. (2007). *Litigating brain injuries*. New York: Thomson Reuters.

Atypical Teratoid/Rhabdoid Tumor (AT/RT)

Jennifer Tinker
Department of Neurology, Thomas Jefferson University, Philadelphia, PA, USA

Definition

Atypical teratoid/rhabdoid tumor (AT/RT) is a rare, highly malignant tumor of early childhood, most commonly diagnosed in infants who are less than 3 years. First described by Rorke and colleagues in 1987, the AT/RT received its designation because of its complex histological components. Prognosis is extremely poor with a median survival of 6–11 months. Factors associated with improved prognosis include supratentorial location, localized disease at the time of presentation, and complete resection (Torchia et al. 2015). Over half of AT/RTs identified are located within the posterior fossa (brainstem, cerebellum, and predominantly the cerebellopontine angle) (Rorke et al. 1996). Roughly one-fourth are supratentorial and 8% may be multifocal. Clinical presentation varies largely by tumor location and size. Infants, in particular, may present with nonspecific symptoms, including lethargy, vomiting, and failure to thrive. Older children (>3 years of age) may demonstrate more specific problems, including head tilt, diplopia, cranial nerve palsy, headache, and hemiplegia (Rorke and Biegel 2000). Often histologically confused with PNET/medulloblastoma.

Cross-References

▶ Medulloblastoma
▶ Primitive Neuroectodermal Tumor

References and Readings

Lefkowitz, I. B., Rorke, L. B., & Packer, R. J. (1987). Atypical teratoid tumor of infancy: Definition of an entity. *Annals of Neurology, 22*, 56–65.

Rorke, L. B., & Biegel, J. A. (2000). Atypical teratoid/rhabdoid tumour. In P. Kleihues & W. K. Cavenee (Eds.), *World health organization classification of tumours. Pathology & genetics. Tumours of the nervous system* (pp. 145–148). Lyons: IARC Press.

Rorke, L. B., Packer, R. J., & Biegel, J. A. (1996). Central nervous system atypical teratoid/rhabdoid tumors of infancy and childhood: Definition of an entity. *Journal of Neurosurgery, 85*, 56–65.

Torchia, J., et al. (2015). Molecular subgroups of atypical teratoid rhabdoid tumours in children: An integrated genomic and clinicopathological analysis. *Lancet Oncology, 16*(5), 569–582.

Auditory Agnosia

John E. Mendoza
Department of Psychiatry and Neuroscience, Tulane Medical School and SE Louisiana Veterans Healthcare System, New Orleans, LA, USA

Synonyms

Auditory-sound agnosia; Auditory-verbal agnosia; Pure word deafness

Definition

Rare condition in which sounds, although heard, are not properly interpreted and thus have little or no meaning for the patient.

Current Knowledge

When present, auditory agnosia is usually primarily limited to impaired recognition of either language sounds or nonlanguage (environmental) sounds. The former is known as *auditory-verbal agnosia* or *pure word deafness*. No commonly used term is applied to the latter. In either condition, appreciation of certain aspects of musical sounds might also be compromised (*amusia*). For this syndrome to be diagnosed, other higher-order deficits that might more readily explain the deficit (such as aphasic disorder) should be ruled out. In auditory-verbal agnosia, there is impairment of one's ability to process, interpret, or comprehend speech sounds or spoken language. Patients may report that it is like hearing someone speaking in a foreign language. Reading, writing, and speaking are intact, although speaking may be slightly problematic due to the distortions in auditory feedback heard as speech is attempted. In auditory-verbal agnosia (pure word deafness), the ability to match nonspeech or "environmental" sounds (e.g., a barking dog, the ringing of a bell, or a train whistle) to corresponding pictures may remain intact. Conversely, one may have difficulties identifying or matching nonspeech sounds, while retaining the ability to process and interpret spoken language. Some degree of impairment in one's ability to recognize musical sounds is commonly, but not invariably, present in these disorders. Select patients may have difficulty recognizing familiar tunes or melodies, while retaining their ability to produce them spontaneously. Others may be impaired at matching tones, rhythms, or timbre, for example, identifying the sound of a particular musical instrument.

Auditory agnosia is thought to result from either (1) unilateral or bilateral lesions of the unimodal (secondary) auditory association cortex in the middle portions of the superior temporal gyrus and/or (2) a disconnection syndrome involving the primary auditory cortex (Heschl's gyrus) of one hemisphere and the subcortical projections from the opposite hemisphere to the unimodal auditory association cortex on that same side. Such lesions would allow elementary sounds to be heard (as one or both of Heschl's gyri are intact), but would produce impaired higher-level processing due to damage or inaccessibility to the unimodal cortex. With critically placed bilateral lesions of the superior temporal gyri, an agnosia for all types of complex auditory input may be present. Auditory-verbal agnosia is more likely to result from left-sided lesions as described above, while auditory agnosia for nonspeech sounds is more likely to be associated with right hemispheric lesions. Agnosia for musical sounds may also be differentially affected, but in an even less consistent manner.

Cross-References

▶ Agnosia
▶ Amusia
▶ Disconnection Syndrome

References and Readings

Bauer, R. M., & Demery, J. A. (2003). Agnosia. In K. Heilman & E. Valenstein (Eds.), *Clinical neuropsychology* (4th ed., pp. 236–295). New York: Oxford University Press.

Slevc, L., & Shell, A. (2015). Auditory agnosia. In M. Aminoff, F. Boller, & D. Swaab (Eds.), *Handbook of clinical neurology* (Vol. 129, pp. 573–587).

Auditory Comprehension

Kelly Knollman-Porter
Department of Speech Pathology and Audiology, Miami University, Oxford, OH, USA

Definition

The ability to decode and understand spoken language at the word (e.g., Stop!), sentence (e.g., Turn left at the next intersection), and discourse (e.g., conversation) levels. Linguistic factors influencing auditory comprehension can include a word's frequency of occurrence (e.g., cat vs. omnivore), semantic or acoustic similarities to competing words (e.g., car vs. bus), sentence length, and syntactic complexity. Attention, auditory memory, and a listener's ability to apply the spoken word to previous experiences or knowledge base can influence effective and efficient auditory comprehension. Auditory comprehension can be impaired to varying degrees following acquired neurogenic disorders such as stroke, traumatic brain injury, and dementia.

Cross-References

▶ Aphasia
▶ Attention
▶ Language

References and Readings

Brookshire, R. H. (Ed.). (2007). *Introduction to neurogenic communication disorders* (7th ed.). St. Louis: Mosby.

Helm-Estabrooks, N., Albert, M. L., & Nicholas, M. (Eds.). (2014). *Manual of aphasia and aphasia therapy* (3rd ed.). Austin: Pro-Ed.

Auditory Cortex

John E. Mendoza
Department of Psychiatry and Neuroscience, Tulane Medical School and SE Louisiana Veterans Healthcare System, New Orleans, LA, USA

Definition

That portion of the cerebral cortex devoted exclusively to the processing of input from the medial geniculate nuclei (auditory information).

Current Knowledge

Located in the superior portion of the temporal lobe of each hemisphere, the auditory cortex consists of both primary (*idiotypic*) and secondary (*unimodal homotypic*) cortices. The former is located in the temporal operculum (Brodmann's area 41 and part of 42) and is referred to as Heschl's gyrus. The primary auditory cortex receives direct input from the medial geniculate nuclei of the thalamus, which it is thought to process auditory input at a very basic level with little, if any, distinction between the right and left hemispheres. The secondary auditory cortex (primarily Brodmann's area 22) surrounds the primary cortex and, for the most part, is located in the lateral portion of the superior temporal gyrus. The posterior portion of this secondary cortex in the left hemisphere constitutes *Wernicke's area*. These secondary cortices are thought to be responsible for the further refinement of auditory input, organizing it into meaningful or potentially meaningful percepts.

Lesions of Wernicke's area (left hemisphere) are associated with severe comprehension and other language-related deficits, whereas comparable lesions in the right hemisphere may be associated with difficulty recognizing or interpreting nonlanguage sounds. Such lesions in the right hemisphere might help account for the inability of some patients to comprehend or interpret the emotional tones or inflections in spoken language, which may convey more meaning than the actual words themselves (i.e., receptive aprosodia).

Cross-References

▶ Aprosodia
▶ Auditory Agnosia
▶ Homotypic Cortex
▶ Idiotypic Cortex

Auditory Discrimination

Kelly Broxterman[1], Beth Kuczynski[2], Stephanie A. Kolakowsky-Hayner[3] and Alyssa Beukema[1]
[1]School Psychology, The Chicago School of Professional Psychology, Chicago, IL, USA
[2]Imaging of Dementia and Aging (IDeA) Laboratory, Department of Neurology and Center for Neuroscience, University of California, Davis, CA, USA
[3]Department of Rehabilitation Medicine, Icahn School of Medicine at Mount Sinai, New York, NY, USA

Synonyms

Auditory processing

Definition

Auditory discrimination is part of phonology, which is one of the five components of language.

It is the ability to recognize differences in phonemes (the smallest unit of sound in a language), including the ability to identify words and sounds that are similar and those that are different. Auditory discrimination tests are performed to measure a person's phonological awareness, such as the ability to compare and contrast speech sounds, separate and blend phonemes, identify phonemes within spoken words, and combine phonemes into spoken words. Impaired auditory discrimination should be addressed early in child development, as it is pertinent to learning. Auditory discrimination ability or phonological awareness skills are correlated with reading performance.

Cross-References

▶ Central Auditory Processing Disorder
▶ Language
▶ Phonemic Awareness
▶ Phonological Disorder
▶ Phonology

References and Readings

Fromkin, V., & Rodman, R. (1974). *An introduction to language*. New York: Holt, Rinehart and Winston.
Gordon-Brannan, M. E., & Weiss, C. E. (2008). *Clinical management of articulatory and phonologic disorders* (3rd ed.). Philadelphia: Lippincott Williams & Wilkins.
Moller, A. R. (2000). *Hearing: Its physiology and pathophysiology*. San Diego: Academic Press.
Ouimet, T., & Balaban, E. (2009). Auditory stream biasing in children with reading impairments. *Dyslexia, 16*, 45–65.
Sharma, M., Purdy, S. C., & Kelly, A. S. (2009). Comorbidity of auditory processing, lauguage, and reading disorders. *Journal of Speech Language and Hearing Research, 52*, 706–722.
Warren, R. M. (1999). *Auditory perception: A new synthesis* (2nd ed.). New York: Cambridge University Press.
Warren, R. M. (2008). *Auditory perception: An analysis and synthesis* (3rd ed.). New York: Cambridge University Press.

Auditory Pathway

Woon N. Chow
Department of Pathology, Microbiology, and Immunology, Vanderbilt University Medical Center, Nashville, TN, USA

Definition

The auditory neural pathway in the central nervous system transmits and processes sound signals from the ear to the cortex. The configuration of the pathway is multisynaptic and bilaterally projecting.

Current Knowledge

From the Outer Ear to the Cochlear Nuclei
Sound is transmitted as longitudinal waves through the air, enters the outer ear, and vibrates the tympanic membrane. The three "tiny bones" of the middle ear, the ossicles (malleus, incus, and stapes), amplify and transmit these vibrations to the oval window, producing waves in the scala vestibuli, a fluid-filled compartment within the coil-shaped cochlea of the inner ear. These fluid waves distort the stiff basilar membrane. Residing on this membrane, hair cells within the organ of Corti transduce the minute movements of the membrane into the graded release of glutamate onto the peripheral processes of bipolar afferent fibers, whose cell bodies are located in the spiral ganglion. The central processes exit the base of the cochlea, form the auditory trunk of the vestibulocochlear nerve (eighth cranial nerve, CN VIII), and project ipsilaterally to the ventral and dorsal cochlear nuclei in the brainstem.

From the Cochlear Nuclei to the Superior Olivary Nuclei
Fibers from the dorsal cochlear nucleus decussate to the contralateral inferior colliculus via the lateral lemniscus. Fibers from the ventral cochlear nuclei project ipsilaterally to the superior olivary nucleus and also decussate via the trapezoid body to the contralateral superior olivary nucleus. This circuit

provides temporal and intensity differences in the horizontal plane between right and left ear to aid in sound source localization. Because of the bilateral nature of these afferent projections, central lesions rarely result in total unilateral hearing loss.

From the Superior Olivary Nuclei to the Medial Geniculate Nuclei

Afferent fibers from the superior olivary nuclei merge with other audition-associated ascending fibers and project via the lateral lemniscus to the inferior colliculus. The inferior colliculus receives bilateral inputs from almost all audition-related nuclei and acts as an almost obligatory relay in the ascending auditory pathway. It is here that horizontally oriented and vertically oriented sound source localization data is fully and finally integrated. Ascending fibers from the inferior colliculus project ipsilaterally to the last subcortical relay station, the medial geniculate nucleus.

Located in the posteroinferior portion of the thalamus, the medial geniculate nucleus is a relay between the inferior colliculus in the brainstem and the auditory cortex. The medial geniculate nucleus plays a role in directing and maintaining attention.

From the Medial Geniculate Nuclei to Heschl's Gyri

Outputs from the medial geniculate nucleus project via the internal capsule to the ipsilateral primary auditory cortex located in the posterior portion of the superior temporal gyrus of Heschl. At the cortical level, detected sound is finally perceived. Bilateral lesions of the auditory cortex remove the conscious perception of sounds, but because of extensive subcortical processing, an individual may still react reflexively to a sound without actually "hearing" it.

Tonotopic Mapping

One idea of note is tonotopy, which is the spatial arrangement of where particular frequencies of sound are relayed and processed within the auditory system. In the cochlea, high-frequency sounds are detected by hair cells at the base and low-frequency sounds at the apex. This tonotopic organization is preserved systematically all the way up to the primary auditory cortex, where higher-frequency sounds are mapped to a more medial location on the superior temporal gyrus, whereas lower-frequency sounds are mapped to a more anterolateral location.

Cross-References

► Auditory Cortex
► Auditory System
► Cochlea
► Cochlear Nuclei (Dorsal and Ventral)
► Heschl's Gyrus
► Inferior Colliculi
► Internal Capsule
► Lateral Lemniscus
► Medial Geniculate Nuclei
► Trapezoid Body
► Vestibulocochlear Nerve

Auditory Processing

Scott L. Decker and Rachel M. Bridges
Department of Psychology, University of South Carolina, Columbia, SC, USA

Definition

Auditory processing is used to describe the manner in which sound waves are transformed into neurological impulses and subsequently decoded by the primary auditory cortex in the temporal lobe of the brain. Simply put, object vibration causes surrounding molecules of air to condense and pull apart, producing waves that travel away from the object. Receptor cells within our ears will be stimulated if the vibration ranges between approximately 30 and 20,000 times per second (Carlson 2007). These waves will then be perceived as sound.

There are three dimensions of sound: pitch, loudness, and timbre. The pitch of an auditory stimulus is determined by the frequency of repetitive (cyclic) vibrations per second (Hertz); a "high-pitch" sound has a high frequency of vibrations per second, whereas a "low-pitch" sound has a low frequency of vibrations per second. The loudness, or intensity, of a sound determines if it is perceived as "loud" or "soft" – vigorous vibrations of an object produce more intense sound waves, resulting in louder sounds. Finally, timbre is the quality of sound, which further differentiates two sounds (e.g., voice vs. piano) when they have identical pitch and loudness.

Our ears are able to detect stimuli, determine the spatial location of those stimuli (by differentiating interaural time and interaural sound intensity; Gazzaniga et al. 2014), and recognize the identity of such stimuli.

References and Readings

Carlson, N. R. (2007). *Physiology of behavior* (8th ed.). Boston: Pearson.
Gazzaniga, M. S., Ivry, R. B., & Mangun, G. R. (2014). *Cognitive neuroscience: The biology of the mind* (4th ed.). New York: W.W. Norton & Company.

Auditory Selective Attention Test

Elena Polejaeva[1] and Adam J. Woods[2,3,4]
[1]Department of Clinical and Health Psychology, University of Florida, Gainesville, FL, USA
[2]Department of Clinical and Health Psychology, College of Public Health and Health Professions, University of Florida, Gainesville, FL, USA
[3]Center for Cognitive Aging and Memory, McKnight Brain Institute, University of Florida, Gainesville, FL, USA
[4]Department of Neuroscience, University of Florida, Gainesville, FL, USA

The Auditory Selective Attention Test (ASAT) was developed by Gopher and Kahneman in Israel and translated into English in 1976 by Mihal and Barrett. The primary focus of the ASAT within these studies, as well as much of the research that has followed, was to examine individual differences in selective attention as related to the operator's driving and flight operation performance (Gopher and Kahneman 1971; Mihal and Barrett 1976). Selective auditory attention is often tested by a dichotic listening task such as the ASAT. Dichotic listening tasks require the examinee to focus in on relevant auditory information while ignoring irrelevant auditory information that is being presented. The most updated version of the ASAT was compiled by Arthur and Doverspike in 1993.

The ASAT is administered through an audio player where the examinee listens to the instructions as well as the entire test through headphones. The examinee is instructed to repeat the message they hear back to the examiner immediately after each trial. A tone cue is presented at the beginning of each trial to identify whether the individual should focus on the left or right ear input. A 250 Hz cue indicates that the examinee should attend to the left ear sound, while a 2500 Hz cue tone indicates that the participant should attend to the right ear sound. There is a practice portion to the ASAT comprised of four messages. Overall, the examinee hears 24 dichotic messages that consist of various combinations of number and letter pairs. Once the cue is presented, 16 pairs (a single-digit number and a letter) are presented at the rate of two per second. Auditory stimuli are presented on both sides but not simultaneously. Thus, the examinee must attend to the input direction denoted by the cue prior to the trial while ignoring the stimuli presented from the other direction (left/right). The examinee is instructed to immediately repeat the numbers they heard aloud to the examiner at the completion of each trial. The examinee has five seconds to do so before the next trial begins. The next portion of the ASAT presents another cue followed by three pairs of numbers that the examinee must attend to. These pairs are preceded by an additional pair of letters, two additional pairs, or no pairs. Once again the examinee must repeat the numbers they heard at the end of each trial (Doverspike et al. 1986).

Scores for the ASAT can be subdivided into a variety of categories: sum of correct items, errors, directionality of cue performance accuracy, and part one or two of the test. The error scores are further subdivided into omission, intrusion, and switching errors. An omission error occurs when the examinee does not report a number that was presented in the cue designated ear. An intrusion error indicates that the number reported was not part of the message or not reported in the correct sequence. Switching errors occur when the examinee omits the cue's direction to switch attention from one ear to another (Doverspike et al. 1986).

A reliability study of the ASAT was conducted with a sample of 20 undergraduate students where the ASAT was administered at an initial time point and then again two weeks later. The results were r = 0.71 for total errors, r = 0.81 for omissions, and r = 0.39 for intrusions. However, a practice effect seemed to be present since performance increased from the initial test (Doverspike et al. 1986). Studies that examined correlations between the various outcome scores for the ASAT showed mixed results ranging from 0.2 to 0.8 (Avolio et al. 1981).

As noted earlier, the ASAT was initially used as a predictive factor on how individuals performed in flight school. Two of the ASAT scores were significantly correlated with flight school performance at r = 0.26 and r = 0.36 (Gopher and Kahneman 1971). The ASAT has additionally been used to predict traffic accidents. A study of bus drivers' attention and driving accidents found that ASAT scores significantly correlated with accidents at r = 0.29–0.37 (Kahneman et al. 1973). Mihal and Barrett utilized the ASAT as a predictive factor for vehicle accidents and found a moderate correlation (Mihal and Barrett 1976). Another study supported these results via their own findings of poorer performance on the ASAT as a predictor of vehicular accident involvement with r = 0.24, p < 0.01 and at r = 0.20, p < 0.01 in cases where the accident was that individual's fault (Arthur and Doverspike 1992). A more extensive review and critique of studies examining predicting factors in traffic accidents was conducted by Wahlberg and includes a summary of studies utilizing the ASAT as a predictor variable (Wahlberg 2003).

References

Arthur, W. J., & Doverspike, D. (1992). Locus of control and auditory selective attention as predictors of driving accident involvement: A comparative longitudinal investigation. *Journal of Safety Research, 23*, 73–80.

Arthur, W. J., & Doverspike, D. (1993). *ASAT: The Auditory Selective Attention Test manual*. Psychology Department: Texas A&M University.

Aviolio, B. J., Alexander, R. A., Barrett, G. V., & Sterns, H. L. (1981). Designing a measure of visual selective attention to assess individual differences in information processing. *Applied Psychological Measurement, 5*, 29–41.

Doverspike, D., Cellar, D., & Barrett, G. V. (1986). The auditory selective attention test: A review of field and laboratory studies. *Educational and Psychological Measurement, 46*, 1095–1104.

Gopher, D., & Kahneman, D. (1971). Individual differences in attention and the prediction of flight criteria. *Perceptual and Motor Skills, 33*, 1335–1342.

Kahneman, D., Ben-Ishai, R., & Lotan, M. (1973). Relation of a test of attention to road accidents. *Journal of Applied Psychology, 58*, 113–115.

Mihal, W., & Barrett, G. V. (1976). Individual differences in perceptual information processing and their –relation to automobile accident involvement. *Journal of Applied Psychology, 61*, 229–233.

Wahlberg, A. E. (2003). Some methodological deficiencies in studies of traffic accident predictors. *Accident Analysis and Prevention, 35*, 473–486.

Auditory System

Maryellen Romero
Department of Psychiatry and Behavioral Sciences, Tulane University School of Medicine, New Orleans, LA, USA

Structure

The structure and function of the human auditory system was first postulated by the physicist George Ohm more than 100 years ago. Dr. Ohm theorized that the auditory system's main function was to translate complex sound material into highly specialized vibratory signals that could then be processed in the brain and recoded as recognizable entities. At a very basic level, the auditory system might be considered as being composed of three primary structures and their interconnections. The first of these is the ear, which itself is typically divided into three components. The outer or external ear is that which is visible, the *pinna* and the *auditory meatus* or ear canal which terminates at the *tympanic membrane* or ear drum. Next is the middle ear which primarily consists of a linked series of three small bones, the *malleus, incus*, and *stapes*, which act together as a system of levers. The former is attached to the tympanic membrane and the latter to the oval window of the inner ear. The middle ear is connected to the oral cavity by the eustachian tube which allows for equalization of pressure on either side of the tympanic membrane. The semicircular canals, the vestibule, and the cochlea comprise the inner ear. The first two constitute the end organs for the vestibular system, whereas the *cochlea* and *organ of Corti* contained within it represent the origin of the nerve impulses that eventually are translated into sounds.

The second set of structures in the auditory system is the brainstem nuclei associated with hearing. The *dorsal* and *ventral cochlear nuclei* located in the region of the pontine-medullary junction represent the origin of the second-order auditory fibers. Next in line are the *superior olivary nuclei*, which lie in the pons and are the first nuclear group to receive auditory input from both ears. The next and final *major* nucleus concerned with hearing in the brain stem is the *inferior colliculus*, a paired structure in the dorsal portion of the midbrain.

The brain itself might be considered the third portion of the auditory system. The two most critical structures here are the medial geniculates of the thalamus, and Heschl's gyri (Brodmann's area 41) which lie in the temporal operculum (within the lateral fissure) of each hemisphere. It is this last structure, in conjunction with its adjacent secondary auditory cortices, which is responsible for processing the auditory input into meaningful information.

Finally, there are the major pathways that interconnect these various structures. The auditory portion of the vestibulo-cochlear nerve (CN VIII) is the first-order neuronal pathway in the auditory system. It has its origins in the organ of Corti and terminates in the dorsal and ventral cochlear nuclei. The *acoustic stria* (dorsal, ventral, and intermediate) form the second-order neurons of the auditory system. What is important to note is that while most fibers cross the midline, some remain ipsilateral, thus at a very early stage there is bilateral input from each ear. The *trapezoid body* of the pons represents one such major crossing of these auditory fibers (primarily those from the ventral acoustic stria). Most of these second-order fibers synapse in the superior olivary nuclei, although some proceed directly to the inferior colliculi. The *lateral lemniscus*, again consisting of both crossed and uncrossed fibers, interconnects the superior olivary nuclei with the inferior colliculi. From there, the *brachium of the inferior colliculi* carries auditory signals to the medial geniculates which, in turn, project ipsilaterally to the primary auditory cortices. It should be noted that, due to the arrangement of the auditory pathways, by the time these signals reach the cortex they are derived from both ears, with approximately 60% coming from the contralateral ear and 40% from the ipsilateral one.

Function

Joseph Fourier, a French mathematician, identified the physical and mathematical properties of sound waves and described the transformation of such stimuli into frequency, amplitude, and phase, which govern discrete elements of sound such as loudness and pitch. In its raw, unprocessed state, sound exists in the form of vibration that results in alterations in the pressure of the air in the immediate environment. These alterations in pressure take the form of waves that have a specific *frequency* or combination of frequencies as well as intensity. The *frequency* of the sound wave, as measured by hertz (Hz) is the major determinant of the *pitch* of the resulting sound, experienced by the listener as high or low. The *amplitude* of the wave, or its height, is the major determinant of the *loudness* of the resulting sound, measured in *decibels (dB)*. The human ear is capable of capturing sound over a considerable frequency range, approximately 20–20,000 Hz.

The transduction of sound waves into the perception of sound is complex. Vibrations entering the *external auditory meatus* strike the *tympanic membrane*, causing it to vibrate. This vibration is transferred directly to the *ossicles*; first the *malleus*, which is attached to the *tympanic membrane*, followed by the *incus* and then the *stapes* which sets the oval window of the inner ear in motion. The vibration is then picked up by the fluids (perilymph and endolymph) of the cochlea, first setting the perilymph of the scala vestibuli and then the endolymph of the organ of Corti and basilar membrane upon which its rests, and finally the perilymph of the scala tympani from where it is dissipated via the round window of the inner ear. In the course of this activity, the basilar membrane is differentially affected depending on the frequency of the waves causing the hair cells along its length to be stimulated, initiating patterns of nerve impulses that correspond to the particular pitch. This very discrete information is picked up by the *auditory nerve* (CN VIII) in the form of bioelectrical nerve impulses, which then are propagated through the various pathways described above until eventually reaching the cerebral cortex where they are eventually interpreted as speech or other sounds.

Illness

Damage to any part of the auditory system, from cerumen (wax) in the auditory canal to bilateral cortical lesions (exceedingly rare) can result in hearing deficits. Because of the multiple crossings and ipsilateral connections within the system, hearing loss which is confined to one ear normally implies damage no higher than the cochlear nuclei. Pure word deafness (intact hearing with the inability to understand spoken language without other major aphasic deficits) can result from a relatively rare occurrence of damage to Heschl's gyrus on the left and a dissociation of input to the secondary association areas from the non-dominant hemisphere. Damage at intermediate levels may result in poor localization of sounds. Aside from ponto-medullary strokes, unilateral (or bilateral) hearing loss is most commonly the result of damage to the middle or inner ear or the nerves that emanate from the latter. Any of many causes could be the problem, from prolonged exposure to loud noises, trauma, infections, medications, and, of course, simply aging. While formal assessments of hearing loss are best left to audiologists, a gross assessment of hearing acuity is important to better understand why a particular patient may be having difficulty either on examination of mental status or coping at home or on the job. Given a hearing loss, neurologists will often try to differentiate its particular nature. Two types of peripheral hearing loss (i.e., not due to a lesion of the brain stem or above) are typically identified, conductive and sensorineural. The former, which is generally more amenable to treatment, is a result of a problem with the external or middle ear, while the latter implies damage to the inner ear. These can often be distinguished by a couple of procedures using a tuning fork (preferably 512 Hz). In the first, the ability of the patient to hear the vibration is tested by comparing air to bone conduction (*Rinne test*). Here the base of the vibrating tuning fork is applied to the mastoid process just behind the ear. When the sound is said to have dissipated, the ends of the fork are immediately moved near the auditory canal (air conduction). If the problem is in the middle ear, the sound will not be heard. Conversely, if the sound is heard better via air than bone conduction, a sensorineural (inner ear) deficit is suspected. It should be noted that for normals, air conduction will be superior to bone conduction, but one should be looking for relative differences in acuity, not absolute auditory thresholds as the latter will likely lowered in the affected ear. A second procedure is to press the base of the tuning fork on the middle of the forehead. If there is a sensorineural loss, the sound will be localized to the unaffected ear, while it will be localized (sound louder) in the affected ear in a conductive hearing loss. This latter procedure is referred to as the *Weber test*.

Another common problem associated with hearing is *tinnitus*, a buzzing, ringing, or other repetitive noxious sound in one or both ears. It can be relatively brief or chronic. If the latter, it can be very disturbing to the patient. The causes can be multiple, including certain drugs (e.g., aspirin), after effects of exposure to loud noises, infections, or occasionally may represent the initial symptoms of a more serious condition such as a brainstem tumor. Unfortunately, treatment options for this condition are quite limited. Having background noise, such as music, is often helpful.

A

Cross-References

▶ Aphonia
▶ Auditory Cortex
▶ Auditory Pathway
▶ Cochlea
▶ Pure Word Deafness
▶ Tinnitus
▶ Weber Test

References and Readings

Bradley, W. G., Daroff, R. B., Fenichel, G. M., & Jankovic, J. (2004). *Neurology in clinical practice: Principles of diagnosis and management* (4th ed.). Philadelphia: Butterworth-Heinemann.
Wilson-Pauwek, L., Akesson, E. J., Stewart, P. A., & Spacey, S. D. (2002). *Cranial nerves in health and disease*. Hamilton: B.C. Decker.

Auditory Verbal Learning

Nancy S. Foldi[1,2], Clara Vila-Castelar[1], Emnet Gammada[1], Joan C. Borod[3,4] and Heidi A. Bender[4]
[1]Department of Psychology, Queens College and The Graduate Center, The City University of New York, New York, NY, USA
[2]Department of Medicine, Winthrop University Hospital, Stony Brook School of Medicine, Mineola, NY, USA
[3]Department of Psychology, Queens College and The Graduate Center of the City University of New York (CUNY), New York, NY, USA
[4]Department of Neurology, Icahn School of Medicine at Mount Sinai, New York, NY, USA

Description

An auditory verbal learning task typically requires individuals to hear a list of items, learn those items, and recall and/or recognize them at a later time. These tasks assess acquisition and retrieval components of memory, including encoding, learning characteristics, storage, consolidation over short- or long-time intervals, and subsequent access to the information either by free retrieval or recognition. The nature of the test composition, the instructions to the individual, and the scoring dictate what conclusions are drawn from the specific task administered.

Auditory verbal learning tasks (AVLTs) are widely used in both clinical and research settings and constitute a hallmark of memory assessment. Different tests include the California Verbal Learning Test-II (CVLT-II; Delis et al. 2000), Hopkins Verbal Learning Test-R (HVLT-R; Brandt and Benedict 2001), World Health Organization/UCLA Auditory Verbal Learning Test (WHO/UCLA AVLT; Maj et al. 1993), Rey Auditory Verbal Learning Test (RAVLT; Schmidt 1996), Neuropsychological Assessment Battery (NAB; Stern and White 2003), list learning in the Center to Establish Registry for Alzheimer's Disease (CERAD; Morris et al. 1989; Welsh et al. 1991), Repeatable Battery for the Assessment of Neuropsychological Status (Randolph et al. 1998), and *Wide Range Assessment of Memory and Learning – Second Edition* (WRAML-2; Sheslow and Adams 2003). Other commonly used list-learning tasks, e.g., the Alzheimer's Disease Assessment Scale – Cognition (ADAS-COG; Rosen et al. 1984) and the Free and Cued Selective Reminder Task (FCSRT; Buschke et al. 2006; Grober et al. 1997), are not solely auditory, as they include visual presentation of words or pictures of items.

List-learning tasks can share many common features. To capture the characteristics of learning and memory – and not just attentional skill – the number of words included in the list should exceed the typical working memory span (7 ± 2 items; Miller 1956). The learning phase is the presentation of the list either once or across multiple trials. Following each trial, the examinee is asked to recall as many items as possible. Once the learning is complete, a short-time interval elapses, usually including interference tasks designed to prevent rehearsal of the list items. The examinee is then asked to recall items from the list, constituting a short-term recall. After another longer distractor-filled interval, a second recall is requested. These short- and long-term retrieval assessments capture the examinee's ability to store, consolidate, and maintain information, as well as to retrieve it on command. Tests can also include a multiple- or forced-choice task to facilitate access, capturing the items that were encoded but could not be accessed on free retrieval.

Despite these commonalities, instruments vary in content and administration. List construction on some tests (e.g., CVLT-II, HVLT-R, WHO/CVLT AVLT, and NAB) incorporates semantic categories, whereas others do not (e.g., RAVLT, CERAD, RBANS, WRAML-2, and ADAS-COG). Examinees are not initially informed of semantic categories, in order to determine whether they can exploit categorical information to their advantage and facilitate their ability to organize, encode, or learn more items. To ensure and document that any particular item is fully encoded with semantic knowledge, the FCSRT, for example, adopts an alternate use of semantic organization by cueing examinees with the overarching semantic category while the word is being learned and by prompting the category immediately afterward. Another variation among tests is the use of interference lists. For instance, after the initial learning phase of the target list in the CVLT-II and NAB, an alternate list is administered, designed to share some but not all of the semantic categories. This helps to address susceptibility to proactive and retroactive interference and source learning. Other tests (e.g., HVLT-R) do not have prescribed interference tasks, although other word lists or naming tasks should be avoided. Delayed recall is commonly tested after a 20–30 min interval. There are various methods to assess the knowledge of target list items. Examinees can report items on free recall, identify target words among a list of distracters (CVLT-II, HVLT-R, NAB, RBANS, and WRAML-2), or identify targets in forced- (CVLT-II) or multiple-choice (FCSRT) recognition trials. While most tasks use recognition after short- (NAB) or long-term (CVLT-II and HVLT-R) free recall, one test (ADAS-COG) relies exclusively on the immediate recognition to assess learning.

AVLTs reveal significant information about learning and retrieval processes. The multiple trial exposure generates an individual's learning curve, indicating whether information learned on an earlier trial is consistently maintained and later appended with new information. Learning characteristics, such as serial position effects (i.e., recall from primacy and recency list positions), provide insight into an individual's learning. For instance, the dual-storage model (Glanzer and Cunitz 1966; Raaijmakers 1981) suggests that items from primacy list positions are thought to reflect long-term storage relying on successful semantic encoding, whereas recent items remain in immediate working memory. The position of an item in the list, known as a distinctiveness feature (Neath 1993), can also aid in later recall, the first or last items – which have only one adjacent item – are learned and retained more easily. Susceptibility to proactive and/or retroactive interference of the alternate list or shared semantic categories of target items can be analyzed. Long-term retention of verbal information can be parsed into storage and retrieval components via examination of free recall versus recognition scores.

Historical Background

Word lists have been used to assess learning and memory for well over a century. Ebbinghaus (1885) observed and described the serial position phenomenon. Eduoard Claparède (Boake 2000) assessed learning and memory in his work on child pedagogy in 1916 using a 15-item word list, which was adapted by André Rey to develop the RAVLT in 1941. The RAVLT, first published in France, has been adapted since its development and modified for use in multiple languages. A RAVLT manual (Schmidt 1996) was published to provide standard instructions on administration, scoring, and interpretation. The original CVLT (Delis et al. 1987) incorporated semantic categories, scorings of learning characteristics, the use of semantic strategy, and contrast measures of learned and retrieved items. The CVLT-II revision (Delis et al. 2000) adopted new norms.

Lists have been developed to address the needs of populations of different ages, cultures, and diseases. The CVLT-Children's Version (Delis et al. 1994) is appropriate for children in the age group of 5–16 years. The HVLT-R (Brandt and Benedict 2001) contains six alternate forms designed for longitudinal, repeated testing and incorporates delayed recall and recognition trials. Some AVLTs are targeted for certain populations using age-appropriate words (e.g., CVLT-C). Shorter forms have also been adopted for more impaired individuals (e.g., CVLT-II, Short Form; Delis et al. 2000). The WHO/UCLA AVLT was designed to better evaluate examinees worldwide (Maj et al. 1993). In this instrument, the authors were careful to select words that were familiar across multiple cultures. Similar to the CVLT-II, the words comprising the WHO/UCLA AVLT can be classified into universally familiar categories (i.e., body parts, animals, tools, household objects, and transportation vehicles). Of note, the WHO/UCLA AVLT is a component of the Neuropsychological Screening Battery for Hispanics (Ponton et al. 1996). A similar approach was adopted when developing the International Shopping List (Lim 2009), a list-learning task to assess individuals from diverse cultural and language groups (i.e., English, French, Malay, and Chinese-speaking cultures).

Psychometric Data

Norms

Normative data for different AVLTs span an age range of 5–97 years. For example, the NAB has been normed on individuals up to 97 years of age; similarly, the WRAML-2 is used in children and adults and has been normed for individuals between 5 and 90 years of age. Standardization samples include healthy adults of different language or culture groups, stratified by age, sex, ethnicity, educational level, and/or geographic region of a country (e.g., northeast of the United States). Many tests (e.g., CVLT-II and CERAD) have been normed for European, Asian, and Southeast Asian groups. Direct translation of a word list into other languages should be avoided, as words may have been selected to accommodate word frequency within a language or appropriateness within a culture. There are also norms for many neurological and psychiatric populations.

Reliability

Verbal learning tests are used to evaluate memory performance over time. Test-retest reliability using the same version of the test has been evaluated for 1-month as well as 1-year intervals. Many tests have adopted alternate or multiple forms (e.g., CVLT-II or RBANS). Whereas alternate versions can reduce practice effects, there is evidence that these effects are not completely eliminated (Houx et al. 2002) due to procedural learning. Therefore, examiners must be very aware of practice effects. Even after 2 years, healthy older adults showed practice effects on the CVLT-II (Blasi et al. 2009). For within-subject test-retest measures, reliable change indices (RCI; Iverson 2001) have been applied to changes of AVLT scores in some populations, e.g., pre- and posttemporal lobe epilepsy surgery (Shah et al. 2015), progression in multiple sclerosis (Andersson-Roswall 2012), and dementia (Gonçalves et al. 2015).

Validity

Construct validity of AVLTs has also been examined. For example, a factor analysis in a sample of children with traumatic brain injury using the CVLT-C yielded four factors: attention span, learning efficiency, delayed recall, and inaccurate recall (Mottram and Donders 2005). Also, while AVLTs are not interchangeable because administrations vary significantly, correlations among word lists have been documented (e.g., RAVLT and CVLT-II, Crossen and Wiens 1994; HVLT-R and CVLT-II, see Lacritz and Cullum 1998) demonstrating that these tests measure common constructs.

Clinical Uses

AVLTs are ubiquitous in assessments of memory-impaired populations. Amnesic disorders, degenerative dementias (including Alzheimer's, Parkinson's, and Huntington's disease), mild cognitive impairment, temporal lobe epilepsy, traumatic brain injury, depression, and focal stroke are diseases that have not only benefitted from these tests but also have promoted refinements and further development to extend our knowledge of the neuropsychological and neural underpinnings of memory function. Such tests have been instrumental in assessing change in memory over time, as well as being very sensitive in discriminating between healthy and memory-impaired groups. A vast literature demonstrates the sensitivity of these tests to the detection of prodromal Alzheimer's disease.

These instruments evaluate both qualitative and quantitative, procedural aspects of verbal learning and provide detailed information about an individual's capacity to acquire, consolidate, store, and retrieve information, thus revealing significant aspects of the learning and retrieval processes. Learning characteristics, particularly primary and recency serial position effects (Foldi et al. 2003), are highly informative in differentiating clinical populations and provide insight about cognitive learning, as well as neurostructural substrates of behavioral changes in preclinical disease (Bruno et al. 2013; Egli et al. 2014). A detailed step-by-step exploration of each individual's learning process enables the clinician or researcher to identify specific areas of vulnerability and can guide intervention strategies.

Cross-References

► California Verbal Learning Test (California Verbal Learning Test-II)
► Consortium to Establish a Registry on Alzheimer's Disease
► Hopkins Verbal Learning Test
► Memory
► Neuropsychological Assessment Battery
► Rey Auditory Verbal Learning Test, Rey AVLT

References and Readings

Andersson-Roswall, L., Malmgren, K., Engman, E., & Samuelsson, H. (2012). Verbal memory decline is less frequent at 10 years than at 2 years after temporal lobe surgery for epilepsy. *Epilepsy & Behavior, 24*(4), 462–467. https://doi.org/10.1016/j.yebeh.2012.05.015.

Blasi, S., Zehnder, A. E., Berres, M., Taylor, K. I., Spiegel, R., & Monsch, A. U. (2009). Norms for change in episodic memory as a prerequisite for the diagnosis of mild cognitive impairment (MCI). *Neuropsychology, 23,* 189–200. https://doi.org/10.1037/a0014079.

Boake, C. (2000). Edouard Claparède and the auditory verbal learning test. *Journal of Clinical and Experimental Neuropsychology, 22,* 286–292. PMID: 10779842.

Brandt, J., & Benedict, R. (2001). *Hopkins verbal learning test-revised.* Lutz: Psychological Assessment Resources.

Bruno, D., Reiss, P. T., Petkova, E., Sidtis, J. J., & Pomara, N. (2013). Decreased recall of primacy words predicts cognitive decline. *Archives of Clinical Neuropsychology, 28*(2), 95–103. https://doi.org/10.1093/arclin/acs116.

Buschke, H., Sliwinski, M. J., Kuslansky, G., Katz, M., Verghese, J., & Lipton, R. B. (2006). Retention weighted recall improves discrimination of Alzheimer's disease. *Journal of the International Neuropsychological Society, 12,* 436–440. PMID: 16903137.

Crossen, J. R., & Wiens, A. N. (1994). Comparison of the auditory-verbal learning test (AVLT) and California verbal learning test (CVLT) in a sample of normal subjects. *Journal of Clinical and Experimental Neuropsychology, 16*(2), 190–194. PMID: 8021306.

Delis, D. C., Kramer, J. H., Kaplan, E., & Ober, B. A. (1987). *California verbal learning test: Adult version.* New York: The Psychological Corporation.

Delis, D. C., Kramer, J., Kaplan, E., & Ober, B. A. (1994). *California verbal learning test – Children's version.* San Antonio: Pearson.

Delis, D. C., Kaplan, E., Kramer, J. H., & Ober, B. A. (2000). *California verbal learning test – II* (2nd ed.). San Antonio: The Psychological Corporation.

Ebbinghaus, H. (1885). *Memory: A contribution to experimental psychology* (H. A. Ruger & C. E. Bussenenues, Trans., 1913). New York: Teachers College, Columbia University.

Egli, S. C., Beck, I. R., Berres, M., Foldi, N. S., Monsch, A. U., & Sollberger, M. (2014). Serial position effects are sensitive predictors of conversion from MCI to Alzheimer's disease dementia. *Alzheimer's & Dementia, 10*(5 Suppl), S420–S424. https://doi.org/10.1016/j.jalz.2013.09.012.

Foldi, N. S., Brickman, A. M., Schaefer, L. A., & Knutelska, M. E. (2003). Distinct serial position profiles and neuropsychological measures differentiate late life depression from normal aging and Alzheimer's disease. *Psychiatry Research, 120,* 71–84. PMID: 14500116.

Glanzer, M., & Cunitz, A. R. (1966). Two storage mechanism in free recall. *Journal of Verbal Learning and Verbal Behavior, 5,* 351–360.

Gonçalves, C., Pinho, M. S., Cruz, V., Pais, J., Gens, H., Oliveira, F., Santana, I., Rente, J., & Santos, J. M. (2015). The Portuguese version of Addenbrooke's cognitive examination-revised (ACE-R) in the diagnosis of subcortical vascular dementia and Alzheimer's disease. *Neuropsychology, Development and Cognition Section B: Aging, Neuropsychology & Cognition, 22*(4), 473–485. https://doi.org/10.1080/13825585.2014.984652.

Grober, E., Merling, A., Heimlich, T., & Lipton, R. B. (1997). Free and cued selective reminding and selective reminding in the elderly. *Journal of Clinical and Experimental Neuropsychology, 19*, 643–654. PMID: 9408795.

Houx, P. J., Shepherd, J., Blauw, G. J., Murphy, M. B., Ford, I., Bollen, E. L., et al. (2002). Testing cognitive function in elderly populations: The PROSPER study. *Journal of Neurology, Neurosurgery, and Psychiatry, 73*, 385–389. PMCID 1738070.

Iverson, G. L. (2001). Interpreting change on the WAIS III/WMS III in clinical samples. *Clinical Neuropsychology, 16*, 183–191. PMID 1459018.

Lacritz, L. H., & Cullum, C. M. (1998). The hopkins verbal learning test and CVLT: A preliminary comparison. *Archives of Clinical Neuropsychology, 13*(7), 623–628. PMID 14590623.

Lim, Y.Y., Prang, K.H., Cysique, L. A., Pietrzak, R.H., Snyder, P.J., & Maruff, P. (2009). A method for cross-cultural adaptation of a verbal memory assessment. *Behavior Research Methods, 41*(4), 1190–1200.

Maj, M., D'Elia, L., Satz, P., Janssen, R., Zaudig, M., Uchiyama, C., et al. (1993). Evaluation of two new neuropsychological tests designed to minimize cultural bias in the assessment of HIV-1 seropositive persons: A WHO study. *Archives of Clinical Neuropsychology, 8*, 123–135. PMID 14589670.

Miller, G. A. (1956). The magical number seven plus or minus two: some limits on our capacity for processing information. *Psychol Rev, 63*(2), 81–97.

Morris, J. C., Heyman, A., Mohs, R. C., Hughes, J. P., van Belle, G., Fillenbaum, G., et al. (1989). The consortium to establish a registry for Alzheimer's disease (CERAD). Part I. Clinical and neuropsychological assessment of Alzheimer's disease. *Neurology, 39*, 1159–1165.

Mottram, L., & Donders, J. (2005). Construct validity of the California verbal learning test-children's version (CVLT-C) after pediatric traumatic brain injury. *Psychological Assessment, 17*, 212–217. PMID 16029108.

Neath, I. (1993). Distinctiveness and serial position effects in recognition. *Memory & Cognition, 21*(5), 689–698.

Ponton, M. O., Satz, P., Herrera, L., Ortiz, F., Urrutia, C. P., Young, R., et al. (1996). Normative data stratified by age and education for the neuropsychological screening battery for hispanics (NeSBHIS): Initial report. *Journal of the International Neuropsychological Society, 2*, 96–104. PMID 9375194.

Raaijmakers, J. G. W., & Shiffrin, R. M. (1981). Search of associative memory. *Psychological Review, 88*(2), 93–134.

Randolph, C., Tierney, M. C., Mohr, E., & Chase, T. N. (1998). The repeatable battery for the assessment of neuropsychological status (RBANS): Preliminary clinical validity. *Journal of Clinical and Experimental Neuropsychology, 20*(3), 310–319. https://doi.org/10.1093/arclin/acu070.

Rosen, W. G., Mohs, R. C., & Davis, K. L. (1984). A new rating scale for Alzheimer's disease. *American Journal of Psychiatry, 141*, 1356–1364. PMID 6496779.

Schmidt, M. (1996). *Rey auditory verbal learning test: A handbook*. Los Angeles: Western Psychological Services.

Shah, U., Desai, A., Ravat, S., Muzumdar, D., Godge, Y., Sawant, N., … Jain, N. (2015). Memory outcomes in mesial temporal lobe epilepsy surgery. *International Journal of Surgery*. 10.1016/j.ijsu.2015.11.037.

Sheslow, D., & Adams, W. (2003). *Wide range assessment of memory and learning–revised (WRAML-2). Administration and technical manual*. Wilmington: Wide Range.

Stern, R. A., & White, T. (2003). *Neuropsychological assessment battery*. Lutz: Psychological Assessment Resources.

Welsh, K., Butters, N., Hughes, J., Mohs, R., & Heyman, A. (1991). Detection of abnormal memory decline in mild cases of Alzheimer's disease using CERAD neuropsychological measures. *Archives of Neurology, 48*, 278–281. PMID 200185.

Zygouris, S., & Tsolaki, M. (2015). Computerized cognitive testing for older adults: A review. *American Journal of Alzheimer's Disease and Other Dementias, 30*(1), 13–28. https://doi.org/10.1177/1533317514522852.

Augmentative and Alternative Communication (AAC)

Amy S. Goldman
Association of Assistive Technology Act Programs (ATAP), Springfield, IL, USA

Definition

Augmentative and alternative communication (AAC) is a set of procedures and processes by which an individual's communication skills can be maximized for functional and effective communication. AAC approaches supplement or replace natural speech with aided options that incorporate the use of some type of device ranging from simple picture communication systems to complex speech generating devices and/or unaided options that involve only the individual's body, such as sign language. AAC may be used to augment understanding as well as written or oral expression. A "multimodal" approach that includes both devices and unaided strategies may be most effective in meeting the individual's communication needs.

Historical Background

Prior to about 1970, AAC was not a widely accepted intervention technique and could even be described as contraindicated in the professional literature. At that time, it was thought that the act of vocal production was a critical building block of human language development. As a result, interventionists believed that providing an alternative to speech production would deter speech (and thus language) development because the child would choose to use the "easier" alternative mechanism (Bates 1976; Fourcin 1975).

In the late 1960s and in the 1970s, research evidence indicated speech was actually a secondary component to language function and that robust receptive and expressive language could be developed without vocal production. In many cases, the use of alternatives to speech production was found to actually support (and in no way deter) vocal production (Schlosser and Wendt 2008; Silverman 1980; Zangari et al. 1994). In 1980, the American Speech-Language-Hearing Association (ASHA) established an Ad Hoc Committee on Communication Processes and Nonspeaking Persons that developed a position statement outlining the concept of AAC as a set of intervention techniques using a variety of symbol sets and communication interaction behaviors. This became the framework for the field of AAC today.

At about the same time, new computer technologies were exploding onto the scene creating previously unimaginable opportunities for AAC device development. The Trace Research and Development Center, part of the College of Engineering at the University of Wisconsin-Madison, was formed in 1971 to address the communication needs of people with severe disabilities who were nonspeaking. The Center was an early leader and innovator in the augmentative communication field and pioneered development of electronic communication aids in the 1970s and 1980s that became prototypes for the speech generating devices (SGDs) of today (Vanderheiden 1978; Vanderheiden and Grilley 1976).

Most recently, the emergence of affordable mobile technologies and "apps" that can be configured to serve as an AAC device have increased the awareness and availability of technological solutions to significant communication impairment. Advances in access technologies such as eyegaze and eye tracking and emerging work in the area of brain–computer interface continue to offer solutions to those whose communication disability is accompanied by significant physical disability.

Rationale or Underlying Theory

Today, the widespread acceptance of AAC is a valid intervention option to develop viable means of effective communication for any individual with limited "natural" speech, as well as to enhance comprehension for those who are not hearing impaired, but who have difficulty understanding spoken language. In 1992, the National Joint Committee for the Communication Needs of Persons with Severe Disabilities issued a Communication Bill of Rights that unequivocally states, "All persons, regardless of the extent or severity of their disabilities, have a basic right to affect, through communication, the conditions of their own existence." Revised in 2016, a set of 15 specific rights are described in the Bill of Rights including, "the right to have access to functioning AAC (augmentative and alternative communication) and other AT (assistive technology) services and devices at all times."

Goals and Objectives

Most of the early history of AAC focused on individuals with neuromotor impairments that limited oral-motor skills such as cerebral palsy and amyotrophic lateral sclerosis (ALS). However, with the passage of landmark legislation such as the Education of Handicapped Children's Act (P.L. 94–142), Section 504 of the Rehabilitation Act, and later the Americans with Disabilities Act, individuals with all types of disabilities have become more integrated into education, employment, community living, and society in general. This change created a widespread need for individuals with all types of disabilities to have an effective, functional communication system. More complex and efficient AAC systems have been developed to meet this need with some specifically focused on individuals with neuropsychological disabilities such as autism (Glennen and DeCoste 1997). While the core goal of AAC is to provide effective communication, related objectives can include decreasing problem behaviors and increasing successful education (e.g., literacy), employment, and community living outcomes.

Treatment Participants

Early in the history of AAC, two misconceptions thrived regarding candidacy for AAC – that a set of prerequisite skills (usually cognitive and motor) was required before AAC could be considered and AAC should only be implemented after all traditional forms of speech therapy had failed. Both have been proven unsubstantiated as many successful AAC users have severe motor and/or cognitive impairments, and research has shown no justification for waiting to implement AAC as it can support speech development (Shane and Bashir 1980). As a result, candidacy for AAC is not limited by age, disability diagnosis or prerequisite cognitive or motor skills. Individuals who can benefit from AAC may be of all ages, including infants and toddlers with disabilities and may have diagnoses including apraxia, dysarthria, aphasia, autism, ALS, cerebral palsy, multiple sclerosis, Parkinsons, intellectual disabilities, etc.

Treatment Procedures

The challenges for those providing intervention are maintaining current knowledge of the vast array of available AAC device options, appropriately matching the skill sets of individuals with disabilities to available AAC systems (hardware, software/apps [language system]), securing funding to acquire the system, improving communication opportunities and environments, and providing supports sufficient to ensure effective use of the system.

Consideration for aided AAC intervention begins with assessment by a qualified team of individuals who are knowledgeable about the individual and his other strengths and limitations especially in the areas of speech, language, and motor skills. One or more team members should be knowledgeable about the range of potential AAC alternatives available and those that are viable options to meet the individual's communication needs. Appropriate practice in assessment includes conducting structured device trials with various AAC devices in the environment(s) in which the individual will be using the technology (e.g., home, school, community, etc.). This allows for comparative analysis of different device features and functions to determine which best address the individual's functional communication needs, answer any clinical questions about the device-person "match" that remain after the formal assessment, and establish user preferences, as appropriate.

The result of an AAC assessment is identification of the system features appropriate for an individual including specification of device input features (selection techniques), language system, representational format (picture/symbol/orthography), and output features. Once an appropriate AAC system has been acquired, training and support for the user, their family, and others (e.g., teachers, therapists, etc.) must be implemented. More complex AAC systems frequently require customization as part of user support services. Short- and long-term communication goals should be developed using the AAC system and therapy services implemented to support goal achievement (Beukleman et al. 2007; Beukelman and Mirenda 2013; www.aac-rerc.com).

Efficacy Information

Efficacy research on AAC ranges from observation of changes in functional communication skills to potential secondary improvements in academic, social, behavioral, and other areas. For individuals with limited or no functional communication, an AAC system that delivers basic communication ability can be deemed effective by self-verification of communication occurring (Fried-Oken and Bersani 2000). Beyond this basic gauge of AAC efficacy, research has been done on a variety of specific outcomes such as decreasing problem behaviors through the use of AAC (Vaughn and Horner 1995), enhancing the rate of AAC communication, (Venkatagiri 1993), and even nuances such as speech synthesizer intelligibility (Mirenda and Beukelman 1990) all in an effort to support AAC efficacy.

Seminal work on AAC efficacy done by Ralf Schlosser (2003) addressed a wide range of AAC efficacy issues including the role of AAC in facilitating or hindering natural speech development, literacy development in AAC users, and the effects of speech output (use of speech generating devices). In 2001, Medicare began coverage of speech generating devices (SGDs) based on acceptance of AAC efficacy research. Since then, a number of private insurance carriers have followed suit and now cover SGDs as do most state Medicaid programs. In 2015, Medicare affirmed that communication augmentation may include text, stating "We believe that a written message or phone message from an individual lacking the ability to speak serves the same purpose in communicating with individuals not in close proximity to the patient as generation of speech does in communicating with individuals who are in close proximity to the patient."

Outcome Measurement

Current technologies may include built in (or the option to add-on) language activity monitoring systems that can provide ongoing data as to device usage and message construction as well as quantitative data on selection rates. The most direct outcome measure for AAC intervention is demonstration of effective and efficient communication, for a variety of communicative purposes and with a variety of communication partners AAC.

Qualifications of Treatment Providers

AAC intervention is typically provided by speech-language pathologists (SLPs) who are licensed by states as health care providers, educated at the graduate level in the study of human communication, its development and its disorders. Medicare requires an SLP who provides AAC assessments or treatment to hold the Certificate of Clinical Competence (CCC) in speech-language pathology from the American Speech-Language-Hearing Association. In addition to SLPs, some other types of professional providers may be members of the intervention team providing AAC services, especially in the educational environment, e.g., special educators, occupational therapists, assistive technology practitioners, etc. (ASHA 2004).

Cross-References

▶ Articulation
▶ Articulation Disorders
▶ Assistive Technology
▶ Speech
▶ Speech Sound Disorder
▶ Speech/Communication Disabilities
▶ Speech-Language Pathology
▶ Speech-Language Therapy

References and Readings

AAC-RERC. (2011). Mobile devices and communication apps: An RERC white paper. Downloaded from http://aac-rerc.psu.edu/index.php/pages/show/id/46
American Speech-Language-Hearing Association. (2004). *Preferred practice patterns for the profession of speech-language pathology* [Preferred Practice Patterns]. Available from www.asha.org/policy.
American Speech-Language-Hearing Association. Augmentative and alternative communication decisions. Downloaded 2. 23. 2018.
Bates, E. (1976). *Language and context: The acquisition of pragmatics*. New York: Academic.
Beukelman, D., & Mirenda, P. (2013). *Augmentative & alternative communication: Supporting children& adults with complex communication needs* (4th ed.). Baltimore: Paul H. Brookes Publishing Company.

Beukleman, D., Garrett, K., & Yorkston, K. (2007). *Augmentative and alternative communication strategies for adults with acute or chronic medical conditions.* Baltimore: Paul H. Brookes Publishing Company.

Brady, N. C., Bruce, S., Goldman, A., Erickson, K., Mineo, B., Ogletree, B. T., Paul, D., Romski, M., Sevcik, R., Siegel, E., Schoonover, J., Snell, M., Sylvester, L., & Wilkinson, K. (2016). Communication services and supports for individuals with severe disabilities: Guidance for assessment and intervention. *American Journal on Intellectual and Developmental Disabilities, 121*(2), 121–138.

Brumberg, J. S., Pitt, K. M., Mantie-Kozlowski, A., & Burnison, J. D. (2018). Brain–computer interfaces for augmentative and alternative communication: A tutorial. *American Journal of Speech-Language Pathology, 27*(1), 1–12. https://doi.org/10.1044/2017_AJSLP-16-0244.

Centers for Medicare and Medicaid Services. (2015). National coverage determination of speech generating devices. Available from https://www.cms.gov/medicare-coverage-database/details/medicare-coverage-document-details.aspx?MCDId=26&mcdtypename=National+Benefit+Category+Analyses&MCDIndexType=3&bc=AgAEAAAAAAAAAA%3d%3d&#final

Fourcin, A. J. (1975). Language development in the absence of expressive speech. In E. H. Lenneberg & E. Lenneberg (Eds.), *Foundations of language development* (Vol. II). New York: Academic.

Fried-Oken, M., & Bersani, H. (2000). *Speaking up and spelling it out: Personal essays on augmentative and alternative communication.* Baltimore: Paul H. Brookes Publishing Company.

Glennen, S. L., & DeCoste, D. C. (1997). *Handbook of augmentative and alternative communication.* San Diego: Singular Publishing Group.

Hill, K., Kovacs, T., & Shin, S. (2015). Critical issues using brain-computer interfaces for augmentative and alternative communication. *Archives of Physical Medicine and Rehabilitation, 96*(3), S8–S15.

Mirenda, P., & Beukelman, D. (1990). A comparison of intelligibility among the natural speech and seven speech synthesizers with listeners from three age groups. *Augmentative and Alternative Communication, 6*, 61–68.

National Joint Committee for the Communication Needs of Persons With Severe Disabilities. (1992). *Guidelines for meeting the communication needs of persons with severe disabilities* [Guidelines]. Available from www.asha.org/policy or www.asha.org/njc.

Schlosser, R. W. (2003). *The efficacy of augmentative and alternative communication: Toward evidence-based practice.* San Diego: Academic.

Schlosser, R. W., & Wendt, O. (2008). Effects of augmentative and alternative communication intervention on speech production in children with autism: A systematic review. *American Journal of Speech-Language Pathology, 17*, 212–230.

Shane, H., & Bashir, A. S. (1980). Election criteria for the adoption of an augmentative communication system: Preliminary considerations. *Journal of Speech and Hearing Disorders, 45*, 408–414.

Silverman, F. (1980). *Communication for the speechless.* Englewood Cliffs: Prentice-Hall.

Vanderheiden, G. C. (1978). *Non-vocal communication resource book.* Baltimore: University Park Press.

Vanderheiden, G. C., & Grilley, K. (1976). *Non-vocal communication techniques and aids for the severely physically handicapped.* Austin: Pro-Ed.

Vaughn, B., & Horner, R. (1995). Effects of concrete versus verbal choice systems on problem behavior. *Augmentative and Alternative Communication, 11*, 89–92.

Venkatagiri, H. S. (1993). Efficiency of lexical prediction as a communication acceleration technique. *Augmentative and Alternative Communication, 9*, 161–167.

Zangari, C., Lloyd, L. L., & Vicker, B. (1994). Augmentative and alternative communication: A historic perspective. *Augmentative and Alternative Communication, 10*, 27–59.

Aura

Kenneth R. Perrine
Neurological Surgery, Weill Cornell Medicine, New York, NY, USA

Definition

An *aura* is a *paroxysmal* episode that occurs before several types of neurologic events. It is a type of warning heralding the onset of the *ictal* event such as a migraine or an epileptic seizure. Auras usually last longer in migraines (up to minutes) than in seizures (typically several seconds). Episodes longer in duration or more remote from the *ictus* in both migraine and seizures are called *prodromes*. In epilepsy, this *simple partial seizure* (focal seizure with retained awareness/responsiveness)[1] can lead to a *complex partial seizure* (focal seizure with altered/dyscognitive awareness/responsiveness), or a *generalized tonic-clonic seizure* (bilateral convulsive seizure).

---

[1] The International League Against Epilepsy suggested new terminology for seizure types (Berg et al. 2010). These new terms have not yet been fully adopted but are given in parentheses.

In both disorders, auras can represent any disruption of networks limited to one hemisphere, the specific phenomena of which arise from the localization of their onset in the brain. The term aura is attributed to the Roman physician Galen (130–200AD) who reportedly overheard a boy say just before a seizure that he felt a cool breeze, "aura" in Latin (Haynes and Bennett 1992).

Current Knowledge

Auras can consist of disruptions or activations of primary sensory modalities (touch, hearing, smell, taste, vision), including paresthesias (somatosensory hallucinations that feel like tingling or "pins and needles") or numbness, unformed (noises, distortions) or formed (voices, songs, commercial jingles) auditory hallucinations or transient deafness, and olfactory or gustatory hallucinations (usually noxious, such as burned rubber). Visual hallucinations are especially common in migraine and can include loss of vision such as blind spots or hemianopsia (loss of vision on one side), positive phenomena such as "scintillating scotoma" (flickering spots of light that may begin centrally and extend to arcs of flickering white or colored lights), or zigzag or other geometric lines or patterns. Formed visual hallucinations can occur (especially in epilepsy), which are usually described as animals or cartoon characters. Visual distortions can also occur, such as macropsia/micropsia (seeing objects larger/smaller) and telescopia/micropsia (seeing objects farther away/closer). In epilepsy, more complex somatosensory auras can occur, such as a rising epigastric sensation (feeling the stomach rising up to the mouth) or ineffable "feelings" that the patient cannot elucidate. Complex experiential psychic auras can also occur (especially in epilepsy), such as déjà vu, out-of-body experiences, depersonalization, derealization, bizarre perceptual phenomena, etc. Psychological symptoms such as anxiety, panic, and fear are also common. In migraines, auras are thought to be caused by the vascular phenomena causing the headache. Of note, migraine auras can occur without any subsequent headache. In epilepsy, auras are actually *simple partial seizures* (focal partial seizures with retained awareness/responsiveness) produced by epileptiform electrical discharges that affect just one brain region alone; they do not disrupt consciousness and can be recalled by the patient after the ictus.

Cross-References

► Epilepsy
► Simple Partial Seizure

References and Readings

Berg, A. T., Berkovic, S. F., Brodie, M. J., Buchhalter, J., Cross, J. H., van Emde, B. W., Engel, J., French, J., Glauser, T. A., Mathern, G. W., Moshe, S. L., Nordli, D., Plouin, P., & Scheffer, I. E. (2010). Revised terminology and concepts for organization of seizures and epilepsies: Report of the ILAE Commission on Classification and Terminology, 2005–2009. *Epilepsia, 51*(4), 676–685.

Haynes, S. D., & Bennett, T. L. (1992). Historical perspective and overview (p. 7). In T. L. Bennett (Ed.), *The Neuropsychology of Epilepsy*. New York: Plenum Press.

www.epilepsyfoundation.org

www.ilae.org

Wyllie, E. (Ed.). (2015). *Wyllie's treatment of epilepsy: Principles and practice* (6th ed.). New York: Lippincott Williams & Wilkins.

Autism Diagnostic Interview, Revised

So Hyun Kim[1] and Catherine Lord[2]
[1]Yale Child Study Center, Yale School of Medicine, New Haven, CT, USA
[2]Center for Autism and the Developing Brain, New York-Presbyterian Hospital/Westchester Division, White Plains, NY, USA

Synonyms

ADI-R

Description

The current edition of the *Autism Diagnostic Interview-Revised* (ADI-R; Rutter et al. 2003) is a standardized, semistructured, and investigator-based interview for parents or caregivers of individuals with autism. It provides a diagnostic algorithm for the ICD-10 definition of autism (World Health Organization [WHO] 1992) and DSM-IV (American Psychiatric Association [APA] 1993). The interview is appropriate for the diagnostic assessment of any person within the age range extending from early childhood to adult life, provided that they have a nonverbal mental age above 2 years. The ADI-R includes 93 items in three domains of functioning – language/communication, reciprocal social interactions, and restricted, repetitive, and stereotyped behaviors and interests, as well as other aspects of behaviors. Up to 42 of the interview items are systematically combined to produce a formal, diagnostic algorithm for autism as specified by the authors, or a general diagnosis of autism spectrum disorders (ASD) as used in several collaborative studies (Risi et al. 2006). All items in the ADI-R are coded in terms of whether the behavior is "currently" occurring, and whether it "ever" occurred, or occurred during a specifically defined period in preschool years. The diagnostic algorithm is based on the "ever/most abnormal" codes in preschool years, but current scores can be used to facilitate a clinical diagnosis.

Most of the ADI-R pertains to behaviors that are rare in individuals who do not have ASD and/or who do not have profound intellectual disabilities. Thus, numerical estimates of the typical scores of general population have not been obtained. Researchers have used scores in the domains or overall as estimates of severity of autistic symptoms. However, the validity of this approach has not been directly tested. Scores have been published for many research populations but not yet systematically dimensionalized.

Historical Background

The WPS Edition of the ADI-R (2003) is a modified version of the 1994 version (Lord et al. 1994), which was based on the original Autism Diagnostic Interview (ADI; Le Couteur et al. 1989). The 1994 version was somewhat shorter than the original in order to make the interview more appropriate for clinical, as well as research, usage. The diagnostic algorithm developed for the 1994 version remains unaltered (apart from minor changes in age cutoff). However, a recent study has suggested that alternative algorithms developed based on machine learning techniques show slightly improved validity compared to the original algorithms (Bone et al. 2016). In addition, new algorithms have been developed specifically for toddlers and preschoolers with ASD (Kim and Lord 2012; Kim et al. 2013). The new algorithms have shown improved sensitivity and specificity compared to the original algorithms for these young children from 12 to 47 months of age.

Psychometric Data

Psychometric properties for the original ADI were provided for a carefully selected, blindly interviewed and coded, sample of 16 autistic and 16 mentally handicapped children and adults covering a range of IQs and chronological ages. Inter-rater reliability was assessed for a sample of ten children with autism and ten without, with multi-rater kappas ranging from 0.55 to 0.94 for each item and intraclass correlations above 0.94 for all subdomain and domain scores. The majority of individual items showed good discriminative validity showing diagnostic differences across autistic and mentally handicapped groups (Le Courteur et al. 1989).

Psychometric properties for the current ADI-R were provided for a carefully selected, blindly interviewed and coded, sample of 25 autistic and 25 mentally handicapped children ranged in chronological age from 36 to 59 months, with mental ages ranging from 21 to 74 months. Inter-rater reliability was assessed, with multirater kappas ranging from 0.63 to 0.89 for each item and intraclass correlations above 0.92 for all subdomain and domain scores. Following the initial standardization study of the ADI-R, a further study was undertaken of a separate sample of

53 children with autism and 41 nonautistic children with mental handicap or language impairments (Lord et al. 1993). Inter-rater reliability was as high as the initial study, with multirater kappas ranging from 0.62 to 0.96 for individual items. Test-retest reliability was very high, with all coefficients being in the 0.93–0.97 range. Majority of individual items showed good discriminative validity showing diagnostic differences across autistic and mentally handicapped groups (see Lord et al. 1994). The algorithm cutoffs were determined by identifying the point within each area that yielded the best combination of sensitivity and specificity both exceeding 0.90.

Clinical Uses

The ADI-R offers a profile of a child in different areas including language/communication, reciprocal social interactions, and restricted, repetitive, and stereotyped behaviors and interests based on the parents' detailed descriptions of the history and behaviors of the child. It can provide a comprehensive description of a child both currently and in earlier ages but must be used in conjunction with observations and/or direct testing in making a diagnosis of ASD. The ADI-R can provide a useful structure to obtain history and understand a parent's perspective on their children's symptoms associated with ASD but requires approximately 2 h to administer and substantial practice to do so reliably.

The *Diagnostic Algorithms* are sets of rules that allow classification of patterns of behavior according to whether or not they meet the current DSM-IV or ICD-10 diagnostic criteria of autism and nonautistic ASD. One caveat for clinical users is that they should be aware that diagnostic algorithm result and a true clinical diagnosis are not the same. Clinical diagnosis is based on multiple sources of information, including direct observation. Thus, even though the ADI-R provides broader contexts including the information about history or functioning of a child than observations, ADI-R alone cannot be used to make a complete standard diagnosis.

Current Behavior Algorithms can be used to assess the participant's current behavior. This can be used in clinical settings to assess changes brought about by intervention or changes reflecting increasing developmental maturity or changing life circumstances.

The ADI-R should only be used by appropriately experienced clinicians. Interviewers must be familiar with the concepts of ASD and relevant behaviors. Training workshops and videotapes are available to help clinicians understand the scoring and administration of the ADI-R.

Cross-References

▶ Autism Diagnostic Observation Schedule
▶ Autistic Disorder
▶ Childhood Autism Rating Scales
▶ Modified Checklist for Autism in Toddlers, Revised, with Follow-Up (M-CHAT-R/F), also M-CHAT

References and Readings

American Psychiatric Association. (1993). *Options book for DSM-IV.* Washington, DC: Author.

Bone, D., Biship, S., Black, M. P., Goodwin, M. S., Lord, C., & Narayanan, S. S. (2016). Use of machine learning to improve autism screening and diagnostic instruments: Effectiveness, efficacy, and multi-instrument fusion. *Journal of Child Psychology and Psychiatry, 57*(8), 927–937.

DiLavore, P., Lord, C., & Rutter, M. (1995). The prelinguistic autism diagnostic observation schedule (PL-ADOS). *Journal of Autism and Developmental Disorders, 25,* 355–379.

Kim, S. H., & Lord, C. (2012). New autism diagnostic interview-revised algorithms for toddlers and young preschoolers from 12 to 47 months of age. *Journal of Autism and Developmental Disorders, 42*(1), 82–93.

Kim, S. H., Thurm, A., Shumway, S., & Lord, C. (2013). Multisite study of new autism diagnostic interview-revised (ADI-R) algorithms for toddlers and young preschoolers. *Journal of Autism and Developmental Disorders, 43*(7), 1527–1538.

Le Couteur, A., Rutter, M., Lord, C., Rios, P., Robertson, S., Holdgrafer, M., et al. (1989). Autism diagnostic interview: A semistructured interview for parents and caregivers of autistic persons. *Journal of Autism and Developmental Disorders, 19,* 363–387.

Lord, C., Rutter, M., & Le Couteur, A. (1994). Autism diagnostic interview-revised: A revised version of a diagnostic interview for caregivers of individuals with possible pervasive developmental disorders. *Journal of Autism and Developmental Disorders, 24*(5), 659–685.

Risi, S., Lord, C., Gotham, K., Corsello, C., Chrysler, C., Szatmari, P., et al. (2006). Combining information from multiple sources in the diagnosis of autism spectrum disorders. *Journal of the American Academy of Child and Adolescent Psychiatry, 45*, 1094–1103.

Rutter, M., Le Couteur, A., & Lord, C. (2003). *Autism diagnostic interview-revised.* Los Angeles: Western Psychological Services.

World Health Organization. (1992). *The ICD-IO classification of mental and behavioral disorders: Clinical descriptions and diagnostic guidelines.* Geneva: Author.

Autism Diagnostic Observation Schedule

So Hyun Kim[1] and Catherine Lord[2]
[1]Yale Child Study Center, Yale School of Medicine, New Haven, CT, USA
[2]Center for Autism and the Developing Brain, New York-Presbyterian Hospital/Westchester Division, White Plains, NY, USA

Synonyms

ADOS

Description

The *Autism Diagnostic Observation Schedule* (ADOS; Lord et al. 2001) is a semistructured, standardized assessment of communication, social interaction, and play or imaginative use of materials for individuals who have been referred because of possible autism spectrum disorders (ASD). As part of the schedule, planned social occasions, referred to as "presses" (Lord et al. 1989), are created in which a range of social initiations and responses is likely to appear. In the same way, communication opportunities are designed to elicit a range of interchanges. Play situations are included to allow observation of a range of imaginative activities

and social role-play. A variety of structured activities and materials, and less structured interactions, provide standard contexts within the ADOS in which the social, communicative, and other behaviors relevant to the understanding of ASD are observed.

The previous version of the ADOS-Generic consisted of four Modules (Module 1–4). The newly revised ADOS-2 now includes five Modules (Toddler Module, Module 1–4; Lord et al. 2012). Each Module is appropriate for children and adults at different developmental and language levels, ranging from no expressive or receptive use of words, to fluent, complex language in an adult. Only one Module, lasting about 30 min, is administered to any individual at a given point of time. In the ADOS, the examiner uses the Module that best matches the expressive language skills of the individual child or adult in order to make judgments about social and communicative abilities as independent as possible from the effects of absolute level of language delay. Each Module has its own protocol, which contains a schedule of activities designed for use with children or adults at particular developmental and language levels. Recently, the Toddler Module of the ADOS was developed for use in children between 12 and 30 months of age in addition to the original four Modules (Lord et al. 2012).

Module 1 is intended for children who do not use spontaneous phrase speech consistently. It consists of 10 activities with 29 accompanying ratings. Module 2 is intended for children with some flexible phrase speech who are not verbally fluent. It consists of 14 activities with 28 accompanying ratings. Module 3 provides 13 activities and 28 ratings. It is intended for verbally fluent children for whom playing with toys is age-appropriate. The operational definition of verbal fluency is the spontaneous, flexible use of sentences with multiple clauses that describe logical connections within a sentence. It requires the ability to talk about objects or events not immediately present. Module 4 contains the socioemotional questions, along with interview items about daily living and additional tasks. It is intended for verbally fluent adults and for adolescents who are not interested in playing with toys such as action figures (usually over 12–16 years).

This Module consists of 10–15 activities with 31 accompanying ratings. The difference between Modules 3 and 4 lies primarily in whether information about social communication is acquired during play or through a conversational interview. It is important to note that adolescents or adults may feel uncomfortable when presented with the toys for young children that are available in Modules 1 and 2; suggestions for modifying the earlier Modules to be appropriate for older children or adults who are less verbal are available from the authors. In addition to the four Modules, the Toddler Module is intended for children between 12 and 30 months of age who should have a nonverbal age equivalent of at least 12 months and be walking independently. It consists of 11 activities with 41 accompanying ratings (Lord et al. 2012).

The ADOS provides the diagnostic algorithms that are sets of rules that allow classification of autism or ASD. Separate diagnostic algorithms for each Module can be generated using subsets of items in each Module. Items and the thresholds for the classification of autism and of ASD in the algorithms differ for each Module. However, the general principles and procedures for computation are the same across Modules and similar to the DSM-IV (American Psychiatric Association 1993) and ICD-10 (World Health Organization 1992). The algorithms for Module 1, 2, and 3 were recently revised from the previous algorithms (Gotham et al. 2007). Reflecting recent research, the revised algorithms now consist of two new domains, Social Affect and Restricted, Repetitive Behaviors, combined to one score to which thresholds are applied, resulting in generally improved predictive validity compared to the previous algorithms. The Module 1 consists of no words and some words algorithms by language level. The Module 2 includes "Younger than 5" and "Greater or Equal to 5" algorithms by chronological age. Module 3 includes a single algorithm. All items appearing on the new algorithms contribute to a single score with two classification thresholds, one for autism and another for ASD. There are the Toddler Module algorithms for children between 12 and 30 months, who do not have phrase speech; once children have developed phrase speech, they should be administered Module 2. Since differential diagnosis can be challenging especially in toddlers, the toddler Module algorithms generate range of concern (little-or-no concern; mild-to-moderate concern; moderate-to-severe concern) rather than strict classifications.

Most of the ADOS pertains to behaviors that are rare in individuals who do not have ASD and/or who do not have profound intellectual disabilities. Thus, numerical estimates of the typical scores of general population have not been obtained. Both algorithm total and domain scores for Toddler Module, Module 1–3 have now been calibrated for children with ASD to yield a standard severity score based on a large sample (see below; Esler et al. 2015; Gotham et al. 2009; Hus et al. 2014).

Historical Background

In its present form, the current WPS Edition of the ADOS-2 (Lord et al. 2012) is a second edition of the original ADOS, which was a combination of two similar diagnostic instruments: the 1989 version of the ADOS (Lord et al. 1989) and the *Pre-Linguistic* ADOS (PL-ADOS; DiLavore et al. 1995). The ADOS was first introduced in the 1980s as a method of standardizing direct observations of social behavior, communication, and play in children suspected of having autism. It was intended to be administered to children between the ages of 5 and 12, who had expressive language skills at least at the 3-year-old level. It was proposed as a complementary instrument to the Autism Diagnostic Interview (ADI; Le Couteur et al. 1989), an investigator-based parent or caregiver interview that yielded a description of history, as well as current functioning, in areas of development related to autism. Because children under age 5 constitute the bulk of referrals for a first diagnosis of autism, there was a need to extend the age and verbal limits of the ADOS to be appropriate for younger and nonverbal children. The PL-ADOS was then created based on the growing interest in using the instruments in clinical settings, which addressed the concerns of parents and fit the abilities of children functioning at infant and toddler levels. As a result, it included more flexible, briefer activities and greater use of play materials for nonverbal young children that served as a downward extension for the ADOS, rather than a replacement. The PL-ADOS was effective in discriminating 2–5-year-old-children with autism from children with non-autism spectrum developmental delays (DiLavore et al. 1995). However, it tended to be underinclusive for children with autism who had some expressive language. Thus, a tool was required to address the needs of children who fell between the PL-ADOS and ADOS in language skills. Furthermore, the ADOS consisted primarily of activities intended for school-age children. Additional or alternative tasks were needed for adolescents and adults. The current edition of the ADOS was designed in response to these factors. The current ADOS differs from the preceding instruments in a way that it is aimed at providing standard contexts for the observation of behavior for a broader developmental and age range of individuals suspected of having autism. Thus, the current ADOS includes additional items developed for verbally fluent, high-functioning adolescents and adults as well as younger and nonverbal children.

However, even though this updated version of the ADOS did indeed extend the usefulness of the original ADOS below a language level of 3 years, research has indicated that it remained of limited value for children with nonverbal mental age below 16 months. Thus, a standardized diagnostic measure applicable for infant and young toddlers was also needed for early identification (Gotham et al. 2007). The recent development of the Toddler Module, now included in the ADOS-2, reflects this need for the measure to be applicable to very young children from 12 to 30 months.

The original algorithms included two domains, social interaction and communication. Recently, Gotham et al. (2007) revised algorithms for Module 1, 2, and 3, the existing social and communication domains were merged, and the domain of Restricted Repetitive Behaviors (RRB) was newly included. The revised algorithms resulted in increased specificity and sensitivity proving increased diagnostic validity compared to the previous algorithms. Furthermore, even though the inclusion of the RRB domain did not improve predictive value of the ADOS in differentiating individuals with autism from those with pervasive developmental disorder – not otherwise specified (PDD-NOS; also referred as ASD), it aided in distinguishing PDD-NOS from non-spectrum cases.

Psychometric Data

Psychometric properties for the original ADOS were provided for a carefully selected, blindly interviewed and coded, sample of 223 children and adults with autistic disorder (autism), pervasive developmental disorder – not otherwise specified (PDD-NOS) or non-spectrum (NS) diagnoses. Inter-rater reliability was assessed, with mean multirater kappas of all items for each Module ranging from .65 to .78 and intraclass correlations above .82 for all subdomain and domain scores. Test-retest reliability varied by subdomain ranging from .59 to .82. In the original sample, the ADOS algorithms generally achieved 94% correct classification. The exceptions were the ASD versus non-spectrum (NS) Module 2 specificity of 87% and Module 3 sensitivity of 90%, and the PDD-NOS versus NS Module 2 specificity of 88% and sensitivity of 89% and Module 3 sensitivity of 80% (Lord et al. 2001).

Psychometric properties for the newly revised algorithms were provided for a sample of 1,139 different participants. The revised algorithms resulted in increased specificity in classifying non-autism ASD in lower functioning populations, evidenced by the 12–31% increase in specificity for children without any words (depending on nonverbal mental age) and the modest gain in specificity for older children who have not progressed beyond phrase speech. During Module 1, no words improved in each diagnostic comparison (e.g., from the sensitivity of 19–50% for children with nonverbal mental age of 15); the specificity of both Module 2 groups improved for non-autism ASD versus NS (e.g., from 77% to 83% for children greater or equal to 5). For autism versus non-spectrum and for ASD versus NS, the new and old algorithms performed approximately equally well in terms of sensitivity. For non-autism ASD versus non-spectrum, sensitivity of the new algorithm was somewhat lower in Module 1, no words (as was necessary to raise specificity; e.g., 100% in old algorithm versus 97% in new algorithm for children under nonverbal mental age under 15), but it showed improvement from the old algorithm in the higher-functioning Module 1 (AUT versus NS; from 88% to 97%) and Module 2 (ASD versus NS; from 76% to 84%) cells. Inter-rater reliability on the ADOS was monitored through joint administration and scoring by two different examiners for at least 1 in 10 cases and, in some cases, through scoring of videotapes. Agreement remained at greater than 85% (Gotham et al. 2007).

Psychometric properties for the Toddler Module were provided for a sample of 182 different participants. The sensitivity of each algorithm ranged from 83% to 91% and specificity from 86% to 94%. Inter-rater item and domain reliability was greater than .71, and inter-rater algorithm reliability ranged from .60 to .90. Intraclass correlations ranged from .74 to .99 for all algorithm domains and total scores (Lord et al. 2012).

Clinical Uses

Use of the ADOS is related to the examiner's clinical skills and experience with the instrument. Examiners need to be sufficiently familiar with the ratings and the activities so that they can focus their attention on observation of the individual being assessed, rather than on administration of tasks. The examiner should have sufficient practice in observation of ASD symptoms and scoring of the ADOS items, as well as in administering the activities. Examiners are encouraged to attend workshops, use videotapes, or work with colleagues to obtain inter-rater reliability before administering the ADOS for clinical or research purposes (Lord et al. 2001). Examiners should note that the Toddler Module and Module 1 are always administered with parents or caregivers in

the room, which provides an opportunity to show a parent, examples of behaviors that define ASD, and get information from a parent about the validity of the child's behaviors during the testing session. Because the ADOS consists of codings made from a single observation, it does not include information about history or functioning in other contexts. This means that the ADOS alone cannot be used to make a complete standard diagnosis, but used in conjunction with other testing.

Lord and her colleagues suggested several strategies that clinicians or researchers may take to measure how behaviors of an individual may have changed over time by using the ADOS item and domain scores (Lord et al. 2000). If an individual has been administered the same Module more than once, raw scores on individual items and on algorithm domains can be compared. If an individual has changed Modules, raw scores on items that remain constant across Modules (about two thirds of each contiguous Module) can be compared, yet comparison of raw domain scores is not meaningful. However, the ADOS calibrated scores developed by Gotham et al. (2009) can be used in this case to compare assessments across Modules and time. The calibrated scores have more uniform distributions across age- and language-groups compared to raw totals, which make it possible to compare children's scores longitudinally across distinct algorithms. Thus, calibrated scores can be useful in clinical settings to test treatment responsiveness and other clinical outcomes in individuals with ASD. However, as calibrated scores may not be sensitive enough to capture the changes that occur over the course of treatment, development of a new measure adapted from the ADOS, which has been designed to capture treatment responsiveness, brief observation of social communication change (BOSCC), is currently underway. Besides the calibrated scores for the algorithm totals, domain calibrated scores separate for social communication and restricted and repetitive behaviors have been also developed (Esler et al. 2015; Hus et al. 2014).

In addition, it was suggested that more detailed coding of communication samples or particular behaviors (e.g., pragmatics, sentence structure, gestures) may also be carried out from videotapes of the ADOS. Other observational coding schemes that address specific aspects of behavior in more detail may also be applied using the ADOS as a way of obtaining a discrete sample of behavior in standard contexts. Often, clinicians carrying out diagnostic assessments may wish to make programming suggestions for parents/caregivers, therapists, or teachers. Many of the activities and codes of the earlier Modules have fairly straightforward implications both for how to teach an individual child and for the content of appropriate goals. For example, Module 1 provides opportunities for children to make requests in a number of circumstances, including requests for action (i.e., the examiner to blow a balloon), requests for food, requests to continue a social game, and requests for an object or activation of that object (i.e., operating a bubble gun). Noting how children make requests and in what circumstances they are most easily able to communicate their interest or needs, allows the clinician to create goals to teach new request behaviors and to help the children generalize existing behaviors across contexts. Generating programming goals from Modules 3 and 4 may be somewhat more complex, because fewer codes describe specific behaviors that may be usefully taught in a direct fashion. Realizing the degree to which adults with autism have limited insight into the nature of social relationships, or having the opportunity to observe adolescents describing the emotions of the main characters in a story, can be helpful in representing the strengths they may have and difficulties they experience in social interaction.

Cross-References

▶ Autism Diagnostic Interview, Revised
▶ Autistic Disorder
▶ Childhood Autism Rating Scales
▶ Modified Checklist for Autism in Toddlers, Revised, with Follow-Up (M-CHAT-R/F), also M-CHAT

References and Readings

American Psychiatric Association. (1993). *Options book for DSM-IV*. Washington, DC: Author.

DiLavore, P., Lord, C., & Rutter, M. (1995). Pre-linguistic autism diagnostic observation schedule (PL-ADOS). *Journal of Austism and Developmental Disorders, 25*, 355–379.

Esler, A. N., Bal, V. H., Guthrie, W., Wetherby, A., Weismer, S. E., & Lord, C. (2015). The autism diagnostic observation schedule, toddler module: Standardized severity scores. *Journal of Autism and Developmental Disorders*, 1–17.

Gotham, K., Risi, S., Pickles, A., & Lord, C. (2007). The autism diagnostic observation schedule: Revised algorithms for improved diagnostic validity. *Journal of Autism and Developmental Disorders, 37*, 613–627.

Gotham, K., Pickles, A., & Lord, C. (2009). Standardizing ADOS scores for a measure of severity in autism spectrum disorders. *Journal of Autism and Developmental Disorders, 39*(5), 693–705.

Hus, V., Gotham, K., & Lord, C. (2014). Standardizing ADOS domain scores: Separating severity of social affect and restricted and repetitive behaviors. *Journal of Autism and Developmental Disorders, 44*(10), 2400–2412.

Le Couteur, A., Rutter, M., Lord, C., Rios, P., Robertson, S., Holdgrafer, M., et al. (1989). Autism diagnostic interview: A semistructured interview for parents and caregivers of autistic persons. *Journal of Autism and Developmental Disorders, 19*, 363–387.

Lord, C., Rutter, M., Goode, S., & Heemsbergen, J. (1989). Autism diagnostic observation schedule: A standardized observation of communicative and social behavior. *Journal of Autism and Developmental Disorders, 19*(2), 185–212.

Lord, C., Rutter, M., & Le Couteur, A. L. (1994). Autism diagnostic interview-revised: A revised version of a diagnostic interview for caregivers of individuals with possible pervasive developmental disorders. *Journal of Autism and Developmental Disorders, 24*(5), 659–685.

Lord, C., Risi, S., Lambrecht, L., Cook, E. H., Leventhal, B. L., DiLavore, P., et al. (2000). The autism diagnostic observation schedule-generic: A standard measure of social and communication deficits associated with the spectrum of autism. *Journal of Autism and Developmental Disorders, 30*(3), 205–223.

Lord, C., Rutter, M., DiLavore, P. C., & Risi, S. (2001). *Autism diagnostic observation schedule*. Los Angeles: Western Psychological Services.

Lord, C., Rutter, M., DiLavore, P., Risi, S., Gotham, K., & Bishop, S. (2012). *Autism diagnostic observation schedule–2nd edition (ADOS-2)*. Los Angeles: Western Psychological Corporation.

World Health Organization. (1992). *The ICD-IO classification of mental and behavioral disorders: Clinical descriptions and diagnostic guidelines*. Geneva: World Health Organization.

Autistic Disorder

Fred R. Volkmar
Child Study Center, Child Psychiatry, Pediatrics
and Psychology, Yale University School of
Medicine, New Haven, CT, USA

Synonyms

Autism spectrum disorder; Childhood autism;
Infantile autism; Kanner's syndrome.

Short Description/Definition

Autistic disorder is a neurodevelopmental condition characterized by marked problems in social
interaction, communication/play, and a set of
unusual behaviors related to difficulties in tolerating change in the environment. The condition is of
early onset. In most cases, it appears to be congenital, but perhaps in 20% of cases, a period of
normal development is observed. The condition
almost always appears before 3 years of age –
usually before 2 years.

Categorization

Autism was first described by Leo Kanner in 1943
(Kanner 1943). Early controversy centered around
the idea that autism might be a form of schizophrenia, but several lines of evidence suggest this is not
the case. Changes in approaches to the definition of
autism have occurred over time. The American
Psychiatric Association (DSM-IV-TR) (APA
2000) and International (ICD-10) (World Health
Organization 1994) categorization systems define
autistic disorder in essentially the same way. The
new DSM-5 (APA 2013) adopts a new approach
with a single disorder – autism spectrum disorder
with several numeric modifiers, e.g., with Rett's.
This approach has been controversial for several
reasons in that it results (somewhat paradoxically)
in a more restricted diagnostic approach. Subtypes
previously identified, such as Asperger's disorder,

are no longer recognized but cases are
"grandfathered" in if they had a well-established
diagnosis, i.e., essentially retaining the DSM-IV
system for cases with a diagnosis. The atypical/
subthreshold category is eliminated. A new category, social communication disorder, is included
but with limited empirical justification.

Epidemiology

A number of epidemiological studies have been
undertaken around the world. Their interpretation
is complicated by methodological differences
including case finding and definitions used. The
earliest studies reported rates on the order of 1 in
2000 children, but more recent work suggests that
a figure of 1 in 800–1000 children is probably
more accurate; the broader PDD spectrum is
much more ambiguously defined and probably
affects as many as 1 in 150 children if not more
(Presmannes et al. 2014). Much debate has centered on whether autism is increasing in frequency, but this issue remains unclear despite
better methods of case detection and greater public awareness.

Rates of autistic disorder are typically three to
four times higher in boys than in girls. The nature
of this gender difference remains unclear, but
speculation has centered on lower thresholds for
expression of the condition in boys. An early
impression of increased rates in better educated
families appears to have been due to referral bias
and has not been supported by later work.

Natural History, Prognostic Factors, and Outcomes

Issues of diagnosis can be complex in infants as not
all required features may be exhibited until around
age three (Lord and Venter 1992). After that time,
diagnostic agreement increases substantially. By
school age, autistic children become more sociable
and may make significant academic gains although
behavioral difficulties are prominent. During adolescence, some children make substantial gains and
others lose skills. There is increased risk for

development of epilepsy throughout the developmental period, with peak frequencies of new onset of epilepsy in early childhood and adolescence (Volkmar and Nelson 1990).

The first studies of long-term outcome in children with autism were relatively pessimistic with only 2–3% of cases being able to achieve adult independence and self-sufficiency. Several factors appear to significantly improve prognosis: cases are now detected at early ages when intervention may be more effective (National Research Council 2001), and in many countries, educational services are now mandated. It appears that at least 20% or more of children with autism are capable of self-sufficiency in adulthood with at least another 15–20% able to be largely independent (Howlin 2005). Major predictors of long-term outcome include nonverbal cognitive ability and the capacity to use language to communicate by age five. Adaptive abilities (the ability to cope with real-world situations) are also important particularly as the person becomes older.

Neuropsychology and Psychology of Autistic Disorder

The first attempts to develop psychological models of autism centered around the notion that experiential factors might be involved. As evidence of brain involvement accumulated, theories shifted to focus on neurocognitive and brain-based mechanisms.

Several neurocognitive models/theories have been proposed. One approach posits difficulties in executive functioning skills; this model would account for some of the problems with shifting set and perseveration typical of individuals with autism (Ozonoff et al. 2005). However, deficits in these areas are not specific to autism and are not strongly related to the extent of social vulnerability. Another approach has focused on difficulties in what is termed "central coherence" or the capacity to integrate information into coherent or meaningful wholes (Happe 2005). This model centers on problems resulting from difficulties in selective attention and appreciation of social meaning. Another approach posits difficulties in

understanding and empathizing with others (Baron-Cohen 1989). This Theory of Mind hypothesis has been very productive for research. It presumes that difficulties arise as a result of an inability to understanding feelings, intention, and social meaning. Weaknesses of this approach include the fact that more able individuals with autism can solve usual theory of mind type problems; a second problem arises because many of the first features of autism appear before usual theory of mind skills are established in typically developing infants. A relatively newer approach, Enactive Mind, has attempted a synthesis of insights from studies of social cognitive information processing in autism with normal developmental perspectives (Klin et al. 2003) (Fig. 1). While Asperger's disorder was removed from DSM-5, it remains in ICD-10, and studies have now shown differences between it and higher functioning autism, e.g., Chiang et al. (2014) in a meta-analysis of IQ profiles.

A research focus on specific brain mechanisms was suggested by high rates of epilepsy and various neurological signs and symptoms (e.g., persistence of "primitive" reflexes, delayed development of hand dominance, etc.). A range of abnormalities have been found in postmortem studies. Lesion

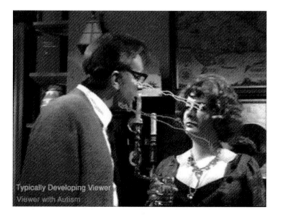

Autistic Disorder, Fig. 1 Visual focus of an autistic man and a normal comparison subject showing a film clip of a conversation. Typically developing person (*top line*) goes back and forth between the eyes in viewing a social scene, a high functioning person with autism goes back and forth between the mouths of the speakers (Reprinted with permission from Klin et al. (2002))

studies, e.g., of the amygdala or hippocampus, have produced some behaviors in monkeys similar to some of those seen in autism (Bachevalier 1996). Other studies have focused on abnormalities in the cerebellum and overall brain size, which appears to be increased in autism (Courchesne et al. 2004).

Other approaches have focused on specific neuropsychological processes. For example, Schultz and colleagues (Schultz et al. 2000) used fMRI techniques to demonstrate that more cognitively able individuals with autism process faces differently than typical controls; essentially they fail to activate the fusiform "face area." This observation is of interest given a large body of experimental work on differences in face processing in autism. Another work, e.g., using eye-tracking technology, has revealed marked differences in scanning of the environment during social situations with more able individuals with autism tending to focus on the lower half of the face or objects, thus losing a considerable amount of social-affective information (Klin et al. 2002).

Beginning with the first twin studies of autism in the late 1970s, a considerable body of work has strongly implicated genetic factors in the pathogenesis of autism. There are significantly increased rates of autism in identical twins and a higher risk in siblings both of autism and a range of other developmental problems. It appears that multiple genes are involved and several candidate genes are now being studied (Rutter 2005).

Evaluation

Evaluation of the child with autism typically involves the efforts of members of several different disciplines – psychology, speech-language pathology, medicine, occupational and physical therapy, and special education. Goals for evaluation include clarification of the diagnosis and establishment of patterns of strengths/weakness that have implications for programming. Medical evaluations are indicated to look for conditions like Fragile X syndrome and seizures sometimes associated with autism (Volkmar et al. 1999).

Treatment

Over the past decade a considerable body of work on intervention has become available. In its influential 2001 review, a panel from the US National Research Council systematically evaluated ten treatment programs for younger children with autism. Although differing in some respects, these programs shared many similarities including intensive individualized programs and structured teaching. Many, although not all, of these programs make extensive use of applied behavior analytic principles to teach basic skills, which can then be expanded. Increasing social and communication abilities are important goals. Psychotherapy is not a mainstay of treatment but is sometimes used in older and more able individuals, often problem-focused in nature.

Drug treatments can be helpful relative to certain symptoms (e.g., agitation, stereotyped mannerisms) but do not address the core social deficit (Scahill and Martin 2005).

Cross-References

▶ Applied Behavior Analysis
▶ Asperger's Disorder
▶ Behavior Modification
▶ Epilepsy
▶ Executive Functioning
▶ Intellectual Disability
▶ Social (Pragmatic) Communication Disorder
▶ TEACCH

References and Readings

American Psychiatric Association. (2000). *Diagnostic and statistical manual* (4th ed., Text Rev.). Washington, DC: APA Press.
American Psychiatric Association. (2013). *Diagnostic and statistical manual* (5th ed.). Washington, DC: APA Press.
Bachevalier, J. (1996). Brief report: Medial temporal lobe and autism: A putative animal model in primates. *Journal of Autism and Developmental Disorders, 26*(2), 217–220.
Baron-Cohen, S. (1989). The theory of mind hypothesis of autism: A reply to Boucher [comment]. *The British*

Journal of Disorders of Communication, 24(2), 199–200.

Chiang, H.-M., Tsai, L. Y., Cheung, Y. K., Brown, A., & Li, H. (2014). A meta-analysis of differences in IQ profiles between individuals with Asperger's disorder and high-functioning autism. *Journal of Autism and Developmental Disorders, 44*(7), 1577–1596.

Courchesne, E., Redcay, E., & Kennedy, D. P. (2004). The autistic brain: Birth through adulthood. *Current Opinion in Neurology, 17*(4), 489–496.

Happe, F. (2005). The weak central coherence account of autism. In F. R. Volkmar, A. Klin, R. Paul, & D. J. Cohen (Eds.), *Handbook of autism and pervasive developmental disorders* (Vol. 1, pp. 640–649). Hoboken: Wiley.

Howlin, P. (2005). Outcomes in autism spectrum disorders. In F. R. Volkmar, A. Klin, R. Paul, & D. J. Cohen (Eds.), *Handbook of autism and pervasive developmental disorders* (Vol. 2, pp. 201–222). Hoboken: Wiley.

Kanner, L. (1943). Autistic disturbances of affective contact. *Nervous Child, 2*, 217–250.

Klin, A., Jones, W., Schultz, R., Volkmar, R., & Cohen, D. (2002a). Visual fixation patterns during viewing of naturalistic social situations as predictors of social competence in individuals with autism. *Archives of General Psychiatry, 59*(9), 809–816.

Klin, A., Jones, W., Schultz, R., Volkmar, F., & Cohen, D. (2002b). Defining and quantifying the social phenotype in autism. *American Journal of Psychiatry, 159*, 895–908.

Klin, A., Jones, W., Schultz, R., & Volkmar, F. (2003). The enactive mind, or from actions to cognition: Lessons from autism. *Philosophical Transactions of the Royal Society of London, Series B: Biological Sciences, 358*(1430), 345–360.

Lord, C., & Venter, A. (1992). Outcome and follow-up studies of high-functioning autistic individuals. In E. Schopler & G. B. Mesibov (Eds.), *High-functioning individuals with autism current issues in autism* (Vol. xviii, pp. 187–199, 316). New York: Plenum.

National Research Council. (2001). *Educating young children with autism*. Washington, DC: National Academy Press.

Ozonoff, S., South, M., & Provencal, S. (2005). Executive functions. In F. R. Volkmar, A. Klin, R. Paul, & D. J. Cohen (Eds.), *Handbook of autism and pervasive developmental disorders* (3rd ed., pp. 606–627). New York: Wiley.

Presmanes Hill, A., Zuckerman, K., & Fombonne, E. (2014). Epidemiology of Autism Spectrum Disorders. In F. R. Volkmar, R. Paul, S. J. Rogers, & K. A. Pelphrey (Eds.), *Handbook of Autism and Pervasive Developmental Disorders* (p. 2). Hoboken: Wiley.

Rutter, M. (2005). Genetic influences and autism. In F. R. Volkmar, A. Klin, R. Paul, & D. J. Cohen (Eds.), *Handbook of autism and pervasive developmental disorders* (Vol. 1, pp. 425–452). Hoboken: Wiley.

Scahill, L., & Martin, A. (2005). Psychopharmacology. In F. R. Volkmar, A. Klin, R. Paul, & D. J. Cohen (Eds.), *Handbook of autism and pervasive developmental disorders* (Vol. 2, pp. 1102–1122). Hoboken: Wiley.

Schultz, R. T., Gauthier, I., Klin, A., Fulbright, R. K., Anderson, A. W., & Volkmar, F. (2000). Abnormal ventral temporal cortical activity during face discrimination among individuals with autism and Asperger syndrome. *Archives of General Psychiatry, 57*(4), 331–340.

Smith, I. C., Reichow, B., & Volkmar, F. R. (2015). The effects of DSM-5 criteria on number of individuals diagnosed with autism spectrum disorder: A systematic review. *Journal of Autism and Developmental Disorders, 45*(8), 2541–2552.

Volkmar, F. R., & Nelson, D. S. (1990). Seizure disorders in autism. *Journal of the American Academy of Child and Adolescent Psychiatry, 29*(1), 127–129.

Volkmar, F., Cook, E., Jr., Pomeroy, J., Realmuto, G., & Tanguay, P. (1999). Summary of the practice parameters for the assessment and treatment of children, adolescents, and adults with autism and other pervasive developmental disorders. *Journal of the American Academy of Child and Adolescent Psychiatry, 38*(12), 1611–1616.

World Health Organization. (1994). *Diagnostic criteria for research*. Geneva: World Health Organization.

Autobiographical Memory

Katherine Tyson
Department of Psychology, University of Connecticut, Storrs, CT, USA

Synonyms

Memory; Personal memory; Recollective memory

Definition

Autobiographical memory (AM) is the memory of events or information involving the self. Researchers generally conceptualize AM as episodic, as opposed to semantic. AMs are temporally defined (e.g., by the date of the remembered event) and involve a sense of "recollection or reliving" of the original event (Greenberg and Rubin 2003).

Historical Background

Levin et al. (1982) are sometimes credited with originating the term AM. However, AM research dates back to Francis Galton's 1879 study of his own recall of events in his personal past. Galton sampled his own episodic memories by finding associations between words and events from his past and dating those events. In 1974, Crovitz and Schiffman modified Galton's technique to create what became a widely used method for studying AM (see Rubin 1999). Their revised technique involved asking participants to think of memories associated with words presented to them. In 1983, Nigro and Neisser pioneered studies examining the effect of point of view on AM in their studies of field memories (viewed from the same viewpoint as originally experienced) and observer memories (viewed from an observer's perspective). They found that older memories were more often viewed from the observer point of view than recent memories (see Rubin 1999). Current research has spanned a variety of areas, including examining AM's functional mechanisms, studying psychopathology's potential effects on AM, and investigating AM's neuropsychological underpinnings through imaging studies.

Current Knowledge

Phenomenology

Much of the recent research on AM has concentrated on AM's function. Pillemer (1992) posited that AM has three basic functions: self-related, communicative (social), and directive (planning for present and future events) (Bluck 2003). In serving the self, AM helps people to develop a sense of coherence and continuity in defining who they are through memories. In its communicative role, AM provides the content of conversations and facilitates building intimacy in social relationships. Sharing of AMs can also inform and teach others about the sharer's world. As a directive tool, AM can help people solve problems as they examine lessons from past events and think about how future events and behavior might turn out.

As a cultural mechanism, in particular, AM helps not only to shape the individual self, but also to provide the individual with a sense of identity in relation to a wider community (Bluck 2003). In Euro-American societies, AM appears to emerge around three-and-a-half years of age, as adults begin to share memories with their children. Some cultural differences have emerged in the nature of AM. Asian societies, for example, may report fewer AMs and have fewer and later memories from earlier childhood compared to Euro-Americans. Whereas collective identity may be the focus in these societies, Americans tend to focus on creating a unique identity; AM is essential to this development of a self.

In its role of aiding self-development, AM may also drive positive perceptions of self and emotion regulation. Research by Wilson and Ross (Bluck 2003) has shown that remembering positive events often brings about a positive mood. Furthermore, the third person, observer's perspective from which people often remember negative life events gives them distance from those events, which may also promote well-being. Sharing of AMs with others may aid emotion regulation.

As a facilitator of social interaction AM helps people to reflect on and share recollections of the past with one another. Fivush et al. (Bluck 2003) have suggested that in mother-child relationships, sharing of AMs may help children to learn how to deal with and express emotions, particularly negative ones.

In its directive function, AM guides current behavior and functioning. Both everyday and traumatic memories guide people's present decisions and actions.

Methods in AM Research

Several methods have been developed for studying AM. Given its complexity and the lack of consensus about how AM works, no single method has emerged as a gold standard; rather, these methods are often used in combination.

Open-ended methods include the *word-cue method*, similar to Galton's original method. Participants are presented with cue words or other stimuli and asked to think of memories. Typically, after the cued portion of such a study, the researcher will ask the participants to date the memories. This method has tended to provide consistent results, lending support to expected findings: childhood amnesia of early life memories, retention of the memories of the most recent two decades, and for people over age 40, an increase in memories about adolescence and early adulthood (Wenzel and Rubin 2005). This cueing method is most commonly applied using the *autobiographical memory test*, first described in 1986 by Williams and Broadbent (Wenzel and Rubin 2005). A second open-ended method involves simply asking a participant about his or her life. A more structured approach, the *involuntary-memory-diary method*, asks participants to keep a diary record of involuntary AMs as they occur.

Some other methods for delving into AM are more closed-ended. The *autobiographical memory interview*, developed by Kopelman, Wilson, and Baddeley, was designed to be used with neuropsychological patients (Wenzel and Rubin 2005). The interview asks for specific kinds of memories from specific time periods. The participant is not provided a choice as to the types of memories he or she will share. In the *diary recall method*, participants record events and subsequently receive a memory test for these events. Unlike the other methods, the diary recall method can provide some measure of the accuracy of memories. A final method, the *questionnaire method,* asks participants to report on a series of properties of AMs; this method is often used in conjunction with other approaches. Recently, Sutin and Robins (2007) have developed *the memory experiences questionnaire*, a measure designed to assess a comprehensive range of dimensions of AM.

In developing methods to study such a multifaceted phenomenon as AM, researchers focus on several variables of interest. These variables include whether the memory is general or specific, latency to retrieve a memory, number of omissions (i.e., when a person does not present a specific personal memory for certain stimuli presented), age of memories, and affective tone. Studies have shown that the last of these variables, affective tone, can potentially differentiate AMs of people with psychopathology from AMs of people without psychopathology (Dalgleish and Brewin 2007).

AM and Psychopathology

In studying the relationship between psychopathology and AM, researchers have found that certain aspects of AM in clinical populations do differ from those of healthy populations. Evidence suggests that AM in patients with suicidal ideation, current or past depression, and trauma history may be overgeneral compared to the specific memories that healthy individuals recall (Hermans et al. 2006). For example, a depressed patient might report a memory of going to lunch with her mother on Tuesdays, as opposed to remembering a specific one of those Tuesday lunches.

Research also indicates that trauma and nontrauma memories differ substantially in clinical but not in healthy populations (Dalgleish and Brewin 2007). While involuntary memory may be enhanced in some clinical populations, voluntary memory is often fragmented, incomplete, and disorganized, particularly in people with a trauma history. PET and fMRI studies have suggested that the retrieval of trauma memories in PTSD patients is characterized by increased activity of limbic and paralimbic areas, including the amygdala. Additionally, researchers have found deactivation of the medial prefrontal areas and Broca's area and decreased hippocampal activity in PTSD patients when they processed emotional, rather than neutral material.

In looking at depressed individuals, studies have suggested that cues reflecting personal characteristics are more likely to promote a shift to processing of information within the long-term view of the self, increasing the likelihood that self-related semantic information will be provided in response to cues on the autobiographical memory test. In a different, but related line of research, euthymic individuals with a history of depression and patients with a borderline personality disorder retrieved less specific AMs in response to cue words that matched highly endorsed attitudes or schema. This finding suggests that an impaired retrieval of specific memories may be the result of certain cues activating generic, higher-order mental representations in people with both psychopathology histories and present diagnoses (Dalgleish and Brewin 2007; Hermans et al. 2006). Generally dysfunctional attitudes, whether in an individual exhibiting psychopathology or in a healthy individual, could play a part in an individual's inability to retrieve specific memories.

Neuropsychology

Although researchers have studied the neuropsychology of AM specifically, knowledge about the neuropsychology of memory in general is much more substantial. By looking at the broad memory literature, researchers have been able to make some claims about the neuropsychology of AM and to suggest areas for future study.

AM appears to be distributed throughout the brain. Retrieval of personally experienced events has been linked to medial temporal lobe, visual cortex, posterior parietal midline, and prefrontal cortex activity (Daselaar et al. 2008; Greenberg and Rubin 2003). AM's emotional and sensory components may involve still other brain areas.

Daselaar et al. (2008) have worked to map the time course of AM, including emotional and reliving aspects of AM. Through functional magnetic resonance imaging (fMRI), Daselaar et al. examined both initial accessing of memories and subsequent elaboration of the memories. As a person first began to recall a personal memory, hippocampal, retrosplenial, and medial and right prefrontal cortex activation occurred (Daselaar et al. 2008). As participants rated memories, brain areas associated with emotion and sensory function were activated, including the amygdala and hippocampus for initial emotion ratings, and visual cortex and ventromedial and inferior prefrontal cortex for reliving ratings. This line of research underlines AM's dynamic involvement of multiple brain areas.

The visual, auditory, and olfactory systems all appear to be potential parts of the broad AM system. Research has demonstrated that visual imagery is central to AM, especially when considering long-term visual memories (Greenberg and Rubin 2003). The medial-temporal lobes and the frontal lobes have been implicated in case study research examining visual imagery's role in AM. Auditory imagery may also be involved in AM, but so far studies have not shown autobiographical amnesias to be related specifically to damage of the auditory cortices. As with visual imagery, further research may provide more information on this aspect of AM.

In addition to its sensory dimensions, AM also seems to be closely related to language. However, with only one exception, semantic dementia, AM impairment does not seem to be related to language-related neuropsychological impairments (Greenberg and Rubin 2003). In semantic dementia, patients display better recall for recent memories than for older ones. A patient with semantic dementia experiences loss of AM, as well as a loss of the ability to maintain semantic memories in storage. While AM deficits have been documented in both Alzheimer's disease and frontotemporal dementia, the underlying cortical changes responsible for these deficits may be disease specific (Irish et al. 2017).

Future Directions

Future research on AM should concentrate on defining and specifying AM both behaviorally and through neuropsychological techniques, including functional and structural imaging. Continuing to consider and revise a conceptual model of AM, such as Pillemer's, is important to providing researchers a better, more definite way to conceptualize AM. Looking at AM cross-culturally may help to determine whether this type of memory plays distinct roles in different cultures and societies. Individual differences in AM are also an important area for study, given researchers' focus on AM as important to the formation of self. In research on psychopathology, looking at schema activation and overgeneral AMs may be important to understanding why clinical populations remember AMs differently from nonclinical populations.

Taking a closer look at the neuropsychology of AM will be necessary as we find better ways to define AM behaviorally. Correlating behavioral changes with the brain changes, we can see through imaging will be a significant area for future study so that we develop a clearer idea of what structures make up the AM circuitry in the brain.

Cross-References

▶ Declarative Memory
▶ Episodic Memory
▶ False Memory
▶ Forgetting
▶ Memory Impairment
▶ Remote Memory
▶ Working Memory

References and Readings

Bluck, S. (Ed.). (2003). Autobiographical memory: Exploring its functions in everyday life. [Special issue]. *Memory, 11*(2), 113–229.

Dalgleish, T., & Brewin, C. R. (Eds.). (2007). Autobiographical memory and emotional disorder. [Special issue]. *Memory, 15*(3).

Daselaar, S. M., Rice, H. J., Greenberg, D. L., Cabeza, R., LaBar, K. S., & Rubin, D. C. (2008). The spatiotemporal dynamics of autobiographical memory: Neural correlates of recall, emotional intensity, and reliving. *Cerebral Cortex, 18*, 217–229.

Greenberg, D. L., & Rubin, D. C. (2003). The neuropsychology of autobiographical memory. [Special issue]. *Cortex, 39*, 687–728.

Hermans, D., Raes, F., Philippot, P., & Kremers, I. (Eds.). (2006). *Autobiographical memory specificity and psychopathology*. New York: Psychology Press.

Irish, M., Landin-Romero, R., Mothakunnel, A., Ramanan, S., Hsieh, S., Hodges, J., & Piquet, O. (2017). Evolution of autobiographical memory impairments in Alzheimer's disease and frontotemporal dementia-A longitudinal neuroimaging study. *Neuropsychologia*.

Levin, H. S., Benton, A. L., & Grossman, R. G. (1982). *Neurobehavioral consequences of closed head injury*. New York: Oxford University Press.

Rubin, D. C. (Ed.). (1999). *Remembering our past: Studies in autobiographical memory*. New York: Cambridge University Press.

Sutin, A. R., & Robins, R. W. (2007). Phenomenology of autobiographical memories: The memory experiences questionnaire. *Memory, 15*(4), 390–411.

Wenzel, A., & Rubin, D. C. (Eds.). (2005). *Cognitive methods and their application to clinical research*. Washington, DC: American Psychological Association.

Automated Neuropsychological Assessment Metrics

Summer Ibarra
Rehabilitation Hospital of Indiana, Indianapolis, IN, USA

Synonyms

ANAM

Definition

The Automated Neuropsychological Assessment Metrics (ANAM) is a computer-based battery of tests designed to measure an individual's neurocognitive skills including areas such as sustained attention, processing speed, working memory, and visuospatial ability. The fourth and current version, ANAM4, consists of 22 test modules as well as forms for recording demographic information (see Fig. 1; VistaLifeSciences 2015). The entire battery of tests can be administered, or the administrator can elect to customize a subset of the ANAM tests in order to assess more specific areas of functioning (Vincent et al. 2008). The ANAM General Neuropsychological Screening Battery (ANAM-GNS), for example, consists of a subset of tests from the ANAM battery and is designed for general clinical assessment of cognition (Woodhouse et al. 2013). Additional versions specific to particular disorders (ANAM-MS [multiple sclerosis] and ANAM-TBI-MIL [TBI in a military population]) have also been developed (Settle et al. 2015; Vincent et al. 2012). The ANAM4 is available through VistaLifeSciences (2015).

Administration time can range from a few minutes for a single subtest to 90+ minutes for the entire battery (U.S. Army Medical Department 2009). In 95% of test takers in the US Department of Defense for cognitive measurement, typical administration time was

Demographics Module**	Symptoms Scale**	Sleepiness Scale**	Mood Scale II-Revised**
2-Choice reaction time*	Code substitution*	Matching grids*	Matching to sample*
Mathematical processing*	Memory search*	Running memory CPT*	Simple reaction time*
Tap left / tap right*	Procedural reaction time*	Spatial processing – sequential and simultaneous*	Switching*
Tower puzzle*	Pursuit tracking*	Stroop*	Go / No-Go*
Logical relations – Symbolic manikin*	Effort measure*		

*Performance-based measurement
**Questionnaire-type measurement

Automated Neuropsychological Assessment Metrics, Fig. 1 Automated neuropsychological assessment metrics

20–25 min (VistaLifeSciences 2015). Scoring for the ANAM is computer generated. Scores for ANAM subtests can be calculated in a variety of ways, including the percentage of correct responses (accuracy score), mean response time for accurate responses (MS), and the ratio of accuracy and speed or number of correct responses per minute (throughput score) (Jones et al. 2008). An ANAM4 Performance Report (APR), which provides full reports on current neurocognitive status as well as comparisons to previous administrations for the same individual and comparisons to various reference/normative groups, is also available (VistaLifeSciences 2015).

Historical Background

The ANAM was originally developed by the US Department of Defense as a means of monitoring changes in human performance when encountering environmental challenges but has now become a common assessment instrument for use in several clinical populations (Kane et al. 2007) and research applications (Vincent et al., 2008). The current ANAM is the result of 30+ years of research and is directly linked to older standardized test batteries, including the Unified Tri-Service Cognitive Performance Assessment Battery (Reeves et al. 2007).

Current Knowledge

Various combinations of ANAM subtests have been employed to investigate neurocognitive changes and impairment in medical and neurological conditions including acquired brain injury, multiple sclerosis, Parkinson's disease, systemic lupus erythematosus (Kane et al. 2007), migraine headache (Roebuck-Spencer et al. 2007), and Alzheimer's dementia (Levinson et al. 2005). Currently, in an effort to better identify the occurrence of traumatic brain injury (TBI), the ANAM is also being used by the US military to establish a baseline of neurocognitive functioning prior to deployment for all service members (U.S. Army Medical Department 2009).

Data from over nine studies suggest that varying combinations of ANAM subtest batteries are sensitive and specific in detecting neurocognitive change among individuals with neurological disorders (Kane et al. 2007). Common uses include screening and triage, monitoring of disease progression, and detection of treatment and medication effects (Kane et al. 2007).

Other uses of the ANAM include evaluation of cognitive functioning in determining fitness for duty, neurotoxicology, human factors engineering, and various fields of medicine such as aerospace, undersea, military operations, and sports (Reeves et al. 2007). The ANAM4-TBI, especially reaction time-based tests, has also been found to have some clinical utility in return to duty decisions in the military following concussion (Norris et al. 2013).

Advantages

The ANAM has been noted as an ideal instrument for assessing change in neurocognition (Roebuck-Spencer et al. 2007). Through randomization of stimuli, practice effects are minimized across numerous testing sessions (Roebuck-Spencer et al. 2007). Further, subtle changes in response time can be more precisely detected as compared to manual calculation of response time (Roebuck-Spencer et al. 2007). Other advantages include time efficiency and cost-effectiveness, both of which are helpful when attempting to triage large numbers of patients (Kane et al. 2007).

Limitations

Some researchers (e.g., Woodhouse et al. 2013) have suggested that use of computerized assessment measures such as the ANAM may not be appropriate for some people who exhibit clinical signs of a neurological disorder that may interfere with their ability to complete the assessment in a standardized format (i.e., wide fluctuations in attention, disinhibition, disorganized thinking, language disturbances, etc.).

Administration

Administration time can range from a few minutes for a single subtest to 90+ minutes for the entire battery (U.S. Army Medical Department 2009). Scoring for the ANAM is computer generated. Scores for ANAM subtests can be calculated in a variety of ways, including the percentage of correct responses (accuracy score), mean response time for accurate responses (MS), and the ratio of accuracy and speed or number of correct responses per minute (throughput score) (Jones et al. 2008).

Psychometrics

The subtests of the ANAM were selected from previously established assessment instruments (e.g., Walter Reed Performance Assessment Battery, the Air Force Criterion Task Set, Navy Performance Evaluation Tests for Environmental Research) with research supporting their respective sensitivity, reliability, and validity (Reeves et al. 2007). As researchers have attempted to gather psychometric data for the current ANAM, many have included only subsets of the subtests in their studies rather than the entire ANAM battery. For example, a large normative data set has been established for the ANAM-TBI-MIL (Vincent et al. 2012).

Various combinations of ANAM subtests have been shown to be both sensitive and specific in detecting cognitive changes in a number of neurological conditions (Kane et al. 2007).

Through the process of multiple baseline administrations, test-retest reliabilities across several ANAM subtest throughput scores ranged from 0.50 to 0.91 with 9 of the 10 estimates <0.77 (Short et al. manuscript in preparation).

Construct validity has been established between several of the commonly used ANAM subtests (e.g., Math, Running Memory, Code Substitution Delayed Memory, and Logical Reasoning) and more traditional measure of neurocognitive function such as Trail Making Test A&B, Animal Naming, Controlled Oral Word Association Test, and the Digits Backward and Digit Symbol subtests of the WAIS-III (Short et al. 2007). Similarly, the ANAM-GNS has demonstrated a strong relationship with the Repeatable Battery for the Assessment of Neuropsychological Status (RBANS; Woodhouse et al. 2013). Furthermore, in a mixed clinical sample, the ANAM-GNS correctly classified 87.9% of patients as impaired or not, while sensitivity and specificity was found to be 81% and 89.1%, respectively (Woodhouse et al. 2013).

Future Directions

The use of the ANAM in various fields of medicine and science continues to develop as evidenced by recent studies attempting to validate specified subsets of the ANAM battery. Examples include validation of the ANAM-sports medicine battery (ASMB) designed for surveillance and management of sports-related concussions (Cernich et al. 2007); use of ANAM tests to assess the effects of extreme environmental stressors such as high altitude, toxins, and radiation exposure (Lowe et al. 2007); and assessment of medication efficacy and potential medication side effects, specifically for CNS-active drugs (Wilken et al. 2007).

Cross-References

▶ Cognitive Functioning
▶ Concussion
▶ Mild Traumatic Brain Injury
▶ Traumatic Brain Injury (TBI)

References and Readings

Cernich, A., Reeves, D., Sun, W., & Bleiberg, J. (2007). Automated neuropsychological assessment metrics sports medicine battery. *Archives of Clinical Neuropsychology, 22S*, S101–S114.

Jones, W. P., Loe, S. A., Krach, K., Rager, R. Y., & Jones, H. M. (2008). Automated neuropsychological assessment metrics (ANAM) and Woodcock-Johnson III tests of cognitive ability: A concurrent validity study. *The Clinical Neuropsychologist, 22*, 305–320.

Kane, R. L., Roebuck-Spencer, T., Short, P., Kabat, M., & Wilken, J. (2007). Identifying and monitoring cognitive deficits in clinical populations using automated neuropsychological assessment metrics (ANAM) tests. *Archives of Clinical Neuropsychology, 22S*, S115–S126.

Levinson, D., Reeves, D., Watson, J., & Harrison, M. (2005). Automated neuropsychological assessment metrics (ANAM) measures of cognitive effects of Alzheimer's disease. *Archives of Clinical Neuropsychology, 20*, 403–408.

Lowe, M., Harris, W., Kane, R. L., Banderet, L., Levinson, D., & Reeves, D. (2007). Neuropsychological assessment in extreme environments. *Archives of Clinical Neuropsychology, 22S*, S89–S99.

Norris, J. N., Carr, W., Herzig, T., Labrie, D. W., & Sams, R. (2013). ANAM4 TBI reaction time-based tests have prognostic utility for acute concussion. *Military Medicine, 178*, 767–774.

Reeves, D. L., Winter, K. P., Bleiberg, J., & Kane, R. L. (2007). ANAM genogram: Historical perspectives, description, and current endeavours. *Archives of Clinical Neuropsychology, 22S*, S15–S37.

Roebuck-Spencer, T., Sun, W., Cernich, A. N., Farmer, K., & Bleiberg, J. (2007). Assessing change with the automated neuropsychological assessment metrics (ANAM): Issues and challenges. *Archives of Clinical Neuropsychology, 22*, S79–S87. References – ANAM.

Settle, J. R., Robinson, S. A., Kane, R., Maloni, H. W., & Wallin, M. T. (2015). Remote cognitive assessments for patients with multiple sclerosis: A feasibility study. *Multiple Sclerosis Journal, 21*, 1072–1079.

Short, P., Cernich, A., Wilken, J. A., & Kane, R. L. (2007). Initial construct validation of frequently employed ANAM measures through structural equation modeling. *Archives of Clinical Neuropsychology, 22S*, S63–S77.

Short, P., Ivins, B. J., & Kane, R. L. (n.d.). (manuscript in preparation). Reliability characteristics of select Automated Neuropsychological Assessment Metrics (ANAM) measures.

U.S. Army Medical Department. (2009). *Automated neuropsychological assessment metrics (ANAM)*. www.medicine.army.mil/prr/anam.html. Retrieved 10 Mar 2009.

Vincent, A. S., Bleiberg, J., Yan, S., Ivins, B., Reeves, D. L., Schwab, K., et al. (2008). Reference data from the automated neuropsychological assessment metrics for use in traumatic brain injury in an active duty military sample. *Military Medicine, 173*, 836–849.

Vincent, A. S., Roebuck-Spencer, T., Gilliland, K., & Schlegel, R. (2012). Automated neuropsychological assessment metrics (v4) traumatic brain injury battery: Military normative data. *Military Medicine, 177*, 256–269.

VistaLifeSciences. (2015). *ANAM FAQ.* http://www.vistalifesciences.com/anam-faq.html. Retrieved 3 Oct 2015.

Wilken, J. A., Sullivan, C. L., Lewandowski, A., & Kane, R. L. (2007). The use of ANAM to assess the side-effect profiles and efficacy of medication. *Archives of Clinical Neuropsychology, 22S*, S127–S133.

Woodhouse, J., Heyanka, D. J., Scott, J., Vincent, A., Roebuck-Spencer, T., Domboski-Davidson, K., O'Mahar, K., & Adams, R. (2013). Efficacy of the ANAM General Neuropsychological Screening battery (ANAM GNS) for detecting neurocognitive impairment in a mixed clinical sample. *The Clinical Neuropsychologist, 27*, 376–385.

Automated Neuropsychological Assessment Metrics (ANAM)

Tamara McKenzie-Hartman
Defense and Veterans Brain Injury Center, James A. Haley, VA Hospital, Tampa, FL, USA

Synonyms

ANAM4

Description

The Automated Neuropsychological Assessment Metrics (ANAM) is a computerized assessment of cognitive functioning originally developed by the Department of Defense (DoD). The ANAM was initially developed in 1984 and has undergone multiple revisions. The original version contained over 30 test modules and has four standardized batteries for the assessment of astronauts in space (ANAUT), mild traumatic brain injuries (MILD), moderate to severe traumatic brain injuries (MODERATE), or neurologically normal individuals (STANDARD) (Levinson and Reeves 1997). The ANAM's modules can be grouped into flexible or standardized fixed batteries for the assessment of cognitive changes secondary to injury, exposure, or environmental factors.

The DoD currently uses the ANAM Version 4.0 (ANAM4), which is the traumatic brain injury military battery. The ANAM4 can be administered in approximately 15–20 min and contains a specialized subset of tests and questionnaires from the full ANAM library (see Table 1). The traumatic brain injury (TBI) military battery collects demographic information and mood and sleep responses and tests cognitive domains including processing speed, working memory, visuospatial ability, and memory (Rice et al. 2011). Modules contain parameters that are modifiable (i.e., number and rate of stimuli, appearance of some stimuli, etc.), and ANAM software creates

Automated Neuropsychological Assessment Metrics (ANAM), Table 1 ANAM4 TBI battery test descriptions

Test (abbreviation)	Description
Demographics/history module (SUB)	An array of information including name, age, gender, ethnicity, education, and relevant historical and medical information are collected here. *See* Fig. 1a
TBI questionnaire (TBQ)	Questions to assess injury history and symptomatology
Sleepiness scale (SLP)	The scale provides a state and/or trait evaluation of energy-fatigue level. *See* Fig. 1b
Mood scale II-revised (MOO)	The scale assesses mood state or trait among seven categories including vigor (high energy), happiness (positive disposition), depression (dysphoria), anger (negative disposition), fatigue (low energy), anxiety (worry), and restlessness (motor agitation). *See* Fig. 1c
Simple reaction time (SRT)	The test serves as a measure of visuomotor reaction time. Simple reaction time is assessed by presenting the examinee with a series of symbols and instructing him/her to respond as quickly as possible once the target symbol appears. *See* Fig. 1d
Code substitution-learning (CDS)	Measures visual search, sustained attention, and working memory. The examinee is asked to compare a displayed symbol-digit pair against a symbol-digit key and decide whether the stimulus in question represents a correct or incorrect match. *See* Fig. 1e
Procedural reaction time (PRO)	This test measures information processing speed, visuomotor speed, and attention. The examinee is presented with a stimulus on the screen (either a 2, 3, 4, or a 5) and asked to press the left mouse key for a "low" number (either 2 or 3) or the right mouse key for a "high" number (either 4 or 5). *See* Fig. 1f
Math processing (MTH)	This task assesses basic computational skills, concentration, and working memory. The examinee is asked to solve mathematical operations requiring an addition and subtraction sequence in the form of "$x + y - z=$". The examinee must indicate if the solution to the problem is greater than or less than five. *See* Fig. 1g
Matching to sample (M2S)	The measure assesses spatial processing and visuospatial working memory. The examinee is instructed to view a pattern that is produced in eight shaded blocks in a 4×4 grid and then compare two differing patterns presented side by side. The examinee is asked to choose the pattern that matched the initial stimulus. *See* Fig. 1h
Code substitution- delayed recognition (CDD)	The test measures delayed memory. The examinee is asked to compare a displayed symbol-digit pair with previously learned symbol-digit pairs (the key). The examinee indicates whether the symbol or the digit pair is a correct or incorrect combination. *See* Fig. 1i.
Simple reaction time repeat (SR2)	The test is a repeat of the simple reaction test earlier in the battery and is used as another measure of visuomotor response speed

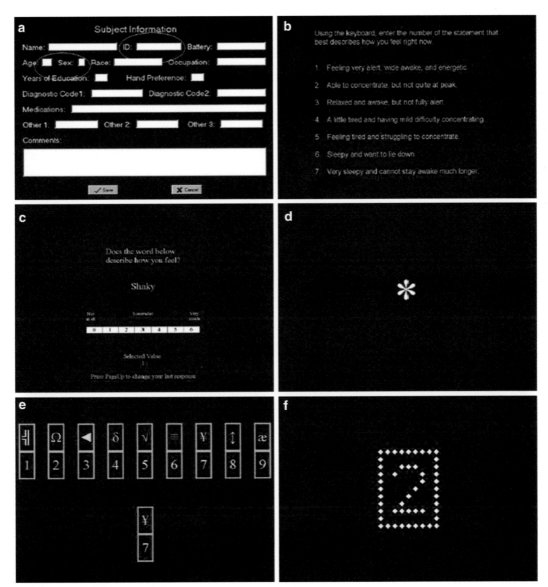

Automated Neuropsychological Assessment Metrics (ANAM), Fig. 1 (continued)

"randomized stimuli across tests sessions, thereby producing multiple alternate forms" (Reeves et al. 2007). The ANAM4 manual also reports that the test is automated and largely self-administered, requires minimally demanding motor responses (mouse click), and has millisecond timing accuracy and large capacity data collection.

ANAM operates on a variety of platforms including desktop computers, laptops, wireless networks, handheld devices, and the web. The computer keyboard and mouse are used for responding to the test. Administration procedures follow the general guidelines of the American Psychological Association (APA) and encourage a quiet, comfortable environment without distractions.

ANAM software produces a report that includes a comparison to an individual's baseline data (if available) or military normative scores. The ANAM Access Database (AADB) automates

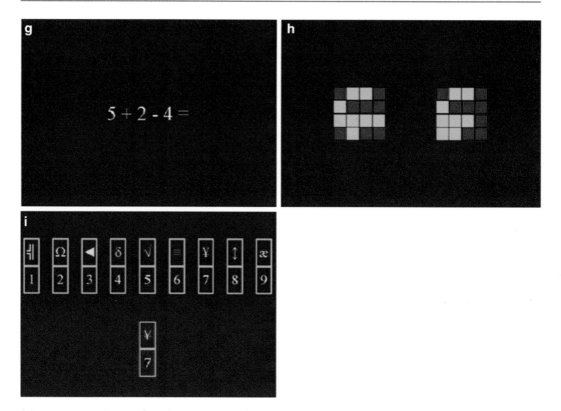

Automated Neuropsychological Assessment Metrics (ANAM), Fig. 1 ANAM4-TBI battery module visual descriptions. (a) Demographics module. (b) Sleepiness scale. (c) Mood scale. (d) Simple reaction time (SRT). (e) Code substitution-learning (CDS). (f) Procedural reaction time (PRO). (g) Math processing (MTH). (h) Matching to sample (M2S). (i) Code substitution-delayed recognition (CDD)

the import of raw and summary data and generates user interface screens that assist the examiner in viewing tables (including file and error log tables for viewing questionable raw or summary data), as well as subtest level data. Scores produced within the report include (1) mean response time for all responses, (2) percent of correct responses, (3) mean response time for correct responses, (4) standard deviation of the mean response time for all responses, (5) standard deviation of the mean response time for correct responses, (6) median response time for all responses, (7) median response time for correct responses, (8) the calculated number of correct responses per minute (also referred to as "throughput," which measures cognitive efficiency), (9) response omissions, and (10) premature responses (i.e., responses of less than 130 ms). ANAM ClinicView is a software that can also be utilized in creating tables and graphs for evaluating an individual's serial ANAM performance.

Historical Background

Development of the ANAM test battery began in 1984 and was derived from computerized tests developed by the joint military services. Prior to its development, the DoD explored initiatives dating back to the 1970s to evaluate cognition to determine the impact of chemical warfare and characterize war fighter capabilities (Reeves et al. 2007). The need for a neurocognitive assessment tool (NCAT) was underscored in the 1990s with the return of service members with persistent cognitive complaints following the Gulf War. In 1995, the Office of Military Assessment developed the first iteration of the ANAM. A research emphasis on ANAM computerized assessment following TBI beginning in 2001.

Signed into public law on January 28, 2008, Section 1673 of the National Defense Authorization Act (NDAA HR 4986) instructed the secretary of defense to establish a protocol for assessing and documenting pre-deployment cognitive functioning for service members deploying outside the USA to be later used as a reference point following a TBI (DoD 2008). In accordance with the statute, and in advance of evidence supporting any single neurocognitive assessment tool (NCAT), the ANAM was selected by a DoD consensus panel as the interim measure to be utilized pending further research. As it stands, the ANAM must be administered within 12 months prior to deployment; however, it is not routinely administered upon return from deployment unless the service member endorses having a potentially concussive event on the Post-Deployment Health Reassessment (PDHRA). The ANAM must be readministered prior to a subsequent deployment if it has been more than 12 months since the previously established baseline.

Currently, the DoD uses both the ANAM and the Immediate Post-Concussion Assessment and Cognitive Testing (ImPACT) tool to evaluate baseline and post-injury cognitive functioning. ImPACT is utilized specifically for service members who are part of the US Military Special Operations units. Studies thus far have not shown either tool to have a distinct advantage in assisting with the assessment or management of mild traumatic brain injury (mTBI) (Defense Health Board 2016). As of September 2015, the DoD has reportedly collected over 1.8 million ANAM4 test results (2016).

Psychometric Data

The ANAM4 is extensively used for the assessment of mTBI within the DoD. Research has posited that many challenges remain in improving the test's sensitivity and specificity (Coldren et al. 2012; Cole et al. 2017; Kelly et al. 2012). In a report from the Defense Health Board (2016), a number of critical findings, including

inconclusive evidence to support conducting routine pre-deployment baseline testing with the ANAM4, inconclusive evidence illustrating advantages of using the ANAM for the assessment of mTBI versus a normative dataset, limitations of the ANAM4 dataset variables, and a lack of data supporting the ANAM4's utility in consistently or significantly contributing to the long-term prognosis after a mTBI, were highlighted.

Two approaches have been used to evaluate the sensitivity of neurocognitive assessment tools to assess mild TBI with inconclusive results. One approach includes comparing performance to population normative data, and the second includes intraindividual performance that compares post-injury results to baseline performance. Arguments for both approaches have ensued (Hinton-Bayre 2015; Louey et al. 2014; Roebuck-Spencer et al. 2013; Broglio et al. 2007; Kelly et al. 2012; Iverson and Schatz 2015). Thus, the continued utility of pre-deployment baseline cognitive assessments remains uncertain.

Furthermore, the ANAM4 dataset has been criticized for the limited stratification of test data. In 2008, a reference set of baseline tests with 107,000 test scores were stratified by age and sex. Expansion efforts that include additional factors such as education, race, handedness, ethnicity, socioeconomic status, and rank with approximately 1.1 million ANAM4 test scores are reportedly being planned (Defense Health Board 2016). Due to the limitations in stratifying the data, the ANAM4 has further been criticized for an inability to accurately estimate baseline cognitive functioning for individuals who score at either the high or low ends of the cognitive spectrum.

Published studies evaluating ANAM normative data show strong age-related effects on reaction time scores (i.e., slower processing/efficiency with increased age) (Vincent et al. 2012). The effect of gender has been reported to be minimal on most subtests; however, some evidence supports faster responding among males as compared to females (Vincent et al. 2012). Some evidence also suggests that the effect of education is minimal when controlling for age; however, higher education levels have been associated with better mathematical processing (Roebuck-Spencer et al. 2008).

Early research has highlighted the lack of data supporting the ANAM's reliability and sensitivity in detecting individual impairment after a head injury. Test-retest reliability for the ANAM4 has been reported to range from 0.68 to 0.74 depending on the timeframe between assessment sessions (e.g., several months to 1 year), though a recent study reported the reliability across neurocognitive assessment tools to be "less than suggested for clinical use" (Cole et al. 2013). Other factors such as fatigue, pain, mood, effort, medication, and reported symptom severity have also been fond to negatively impact the reliability of ANAM4 test results (Bruce and Echemendia 2009; Cooper et al. 2014; Ivins et al. 2009; Suhr and Gunstad 2005). Additionally, the current policy of administering the ANAM4 in a group setting is also believed to negatively impact baseline test scores (Moser et al. 2011).

Research suggests that the ANAM4 does successfully identify cognitive deficits among concussed individuals, with specificity for individual subtests, as well as the combined battery, reported at greater than 0.80 (Register-Mihalik et al. 2013). In contrast, sensitivity was found to be low for both individual subtests and the test battery as a whole (Broglio et al. 2007; Register-Mihalik et al. 2013). Register-Mahilik and colleagues (2013) found that while sensitivity increased by 50% when the individual's symptoms were taken into account, it was not significant enough to warrant the utilization of the ANAM4 as an independent measure of mTBI. Several research studies support the simple reaction time subtest as the most sensitive and effective subtest within the ANAM, in differentiating concussed versus non-concussed service members (Bryan and Hernandez 2012; Eckner et al. 2014; Norris et al. 2013), particularly when administered within 72 h of injury (Coldren et al. 2012; Kelly et al. 2012). No studies to date assessing the usefulness of the ANAM4 in predicting long-term prognosis have been published (Defense Health Board 2016).

Some evidence supports construct validity with traditional neuropsychological measures of information processing speed, attention, and working memory (Vincent et al. 2012). However,

a recent study comparing four neurocognitive assessment tools did not support significant convergent or discriminant validity between any of the computerized measures and traditional neuropsychological tests (Cole et al. 2017). Overall, the reliability and validity for the ANAM4 are similar to other neurocognitive assessment tools (Cole et al. 2013).

Clinical Uses

The ANAM reportedly has a wide range of military and clinical applications. The predominant use of the ANAM is within the military setting to obtain pre-deployment baseline scores for comparison in the event of subsequent injury during deployment. Baseline scores on the measure are stored on a master database and are reported to be available with a quick turnaround time to any clinician who needs them. Scores obtained in theater can be compared to an individual's own baseline data so that better treatment and return-to-duty (RTD) decisions can be made (DCoE 2011).

However, while having a cognitive baseline post-injury theoretically makes sense, evidence demonstrating the advantage of this method for evaluating mTBI has been reported to be inconsistent (Defense Health Board 2015). Additionally, while the majority of ANAM tests administered are for establishment of a baseline of cognitive performance, recent findings suggest that baseline evaluation are not assessed for the majority of the population that has undergone testing post-injury. The primary explanation is that most injuries have occurred stateside (e.g., secondary to training accidents) where baseline cognitive assessments are not required (Helmick et al. 2015).

Variation across military settings exists. The US Naval Academy (USNA) also requires that their midshipmen undergo baseline cognitive testing with a slightly different version of the ANAM4 that utilizes additional subtests assessing executive functioning, visuospatial processing, working memory, and effort (Defense Health Board 2016). When midshipmen experiences a TBI, they are removed from normal activity until complete resolution of their symptoms (as assessed by repeated ANAM4 assessments); if scores remain below their baseline, they are then sent for additional testing, treatment, and recovery.

To date, the ANAM has been used to study the impact on cognition secondary to injury (i.e., TBI, blast, training exercise, anoxia/hypoxia), exposure (chemical, thermal, radiological), environmental factors (i.e., combat stress, fatigue/ sleep deprivation, heat/cold), and medication and/or rehabilitation. The ANAM has also been used to document cognitive changes secondary to multiple sclerosis, Parkinson's disease, Alzheimer's disease, TBI, and migraine headaches (Kane et al. 2007; Vincent et al. 2012).

Per DoD instruction, trained providers such as psychologists or neuropsychologists with ANAM training can interpret ANAM test results (Echemendia et al. 2013). ANAM can be administered serially (every 3–4 days) post-injury to track and document cognitive recovery and symptom resolution compared to pre-deployment levels, though research suggests questionable utility the farther out from injury (Coldren et al. 2012; Kelly et al. 2012).

The Defense and Veterans Brain Injury Center's (DVBIC) clinical recommendation suggests that those individuals with a mild concussion, no loss of consciousness (LOC), and rapidly resolving (within 1–2 h) symptoms do not typically benefit from ANAM use as part of return-to-duty decisions (DCoE 2011).

While the ANAM4 may be valuable as an indicator of cognitive functioning, it is one component of a comprehensive clinical assessment and does not provide a medical diagnosis of TBI. To this end, ANAM is not an effective tool for measuring undetected pre- or post-deployment concussions and has limited data on the impact of such factor test performance.

See Also

▶ Battlefield Assessment
▶ Defense and Veterans Brain Injury Center
▶ Military Acute Concussion Evaluation
▶ Pre-deployment Cognitive Testing

References

Broglio, S. P., Macciocchi, S. N., & Ferrara, M. S. (2007). Sensitivity of the concussion assessment battery. *Neurosurgery, 60*(6), 1050–1057. https://doi.org/10.1227/01.NEU.0000255479.90999.C0.

Bruce, J. M., & Echemendia, R. J. (2009). History of multiple self-reported concussions is not associated with reduced cognitive abilities. *Neurosurgery, 64*(1), 100–106. https://doi.org/10.1227/01.NEU.0000336310.47513.C8.

Bryan, C., & Hernandez, A. M. (2012). Magnitudes of decline on automated neuropsychological assessment metrics subtest scores relative to predeployment baseline performance among service members evaluated for traumatic brain injury in Iraq. *The Journal of Head Trauma Rehabilitation, 27*(1), 45–54. https://doi.org/10.1097/HTR.0b013e318238f146.

Coldren, R. L., Russell, M. L., Parish, R. V., Dretsch, M., & Kelly, M. P. (2012). The ANAM lacks utility as a diagnostic or screening tool for concussion more than 10 days following injury. *Military Medicine, 177*(2), 179–183. Retrieved from http://militarymedicine.amsus.org/doi/pdf/10.7205/MILMED-D-11-00278

Cole, W. R., Arrieux, J. P., Schwab, K., Ivins, B. J., Qashu, F. M., & Lewis, S. C. (2013). Test-retest reliability of four computerized neurocognitive assessment tools in an active duty militarypopulation. *Archives of Clinical Neuropsychology, 28*(7), 732–742. https://doi.org/10.1093/arclin/act040.

Cole, W. R., Arrieux, J. P., Ivins, B. J., Schwab, K. A., & Qashu, F. M. (2017). A comparison of four computerized neurocognitive assessment tools to a traditional neuropsychological test battery in service members with and without mild traumatic brain injury. *Archives of Clinical Neuropsychology*, 1–18. https://doi.org/10.1093/arclin/acx036.

Cooper, D. B., Vanderploeg, R. D., Armistead-Jehle, P., Lewis, J. D., & Bowles, A. O. (2014). Factors associated with neurocognitive performance in OIF/OEF service members with postconcussive complaints in postdeployment clinical settings. *Journal of Rehabilitation Research and Development, 51*(7), 1023–1034. https://doi.org/10.1682/JRRD.2013.05.0104.

Defense Centers of Excellence (DCoE) for Psychological Health and Traumatic Brain Injury. (2011, May). *Indications and conditions for in-theater post-injury neurocognitive assessment tool (NCAT) testing* (DCoE Clinical Recommendation). Retrieved from http://dvbic.dcoe.mil/files/resources/DCoE_Clinical_Recommendations_Post_Injury_NCAT_05-31-2011_f.pdf

Defense Health Board. (2016, February). *Review of the scientific evidence of using population normative values for post-concussive computerized neurocognitive assessments*. Retrieved from http://health.mil/Reference-Center/Reports/2016/02/10/Post-Concussive-Computerized-Neurocognitive-Assessments

Defense Health Board, Neurological/Behavioral Health Subcommittee. (2015, November). Report of the Subcommittee on the *Scientific evidence of using population normative values for post-concussive computerized neurocognitive assessments* (Decision Brief). Retrieved from http://www.health.mil/Reference-Center/Presentations/2015/11/09/Decision-Brief-NBH-Subcommittee-Automated-Neuropsychological-Assessment-Metrics-4-Tasking

Department of Defense. (2008). *National defense authorization act for fiscal year 2008 (HR 4986, section 1673)*. Retrieved from https://www.congress.gov/bill/110th-congress/house-bill/4986

Echemendia, R. J., Iverson, G. L., McCrea, M., Macciocchi, S. N., Gioia, G. A., Putukian, M., & Comper, P. (2013). Advances in neuropsychological assessment of sport-related concussion. *British Journal of Sports Medicine, 47*(5), 294–298. https://doi.org/10.1136/bjsports-2013-092186.

Eckner, J. T., Kutcher, J. S., Broglio, S. P., & Richardson, J. K. (2014). Effect of sport-related concussion on clinically measured simple reaction time. *British Journal of Sports Medicine, 48*(2), 112–118. https://doi.org/10.1136/bjsports-2012-091579.

Helmick, K. M., Spells, C. A., Malik, S. Z., Davies, C. A., Marion, D. W., & Hinds, S. R. (2015). Traumatic brain injury in the US military: Epidemiology and key clinical and research programs. *Brain Imaging and Behavior, 9*, 358–366. https://doi.org/10.1007/s11682-015-9399-z.

Hinton-Bayre, A. (2015). Normative versus baseline paradigms for detecting neuropsychological impairment following sports-related concussion. *Brain Impairment, 16*(2), 9. https://doi.org/10.1017/BrImp.2015.14.

Iverson, G. L., & Schatz, P. (2015). Advanced topics in neuropsychological assessment following sport-related concussion. *Brain Injury, 29*(2), 263–275. https://doi.org/10.3109/02699052.2014.965214.

Ivins, B. J., Kane, R., & Schwab, K. A. (2009). Performance on the automated neuropsychological assessment metrics in a nonclinical sample of soldiers screened for mild TBI after returning from Iraq and Afghanistan: A descriptive analysis. *The Journal of Head Trauma Rehabilitation, 24*(1), 24–31. https://doi.org/10.1097/HTR.0b013e3181957042.

Kane, R. L., Roebuck-Spencer, T., Short, P., Kabat, M., & Wilken, J. (2007). Identifying and monitoring cognitive deficits in clinical populations using automated neuropsychological assessment metrics (ANAM) tests. *Archives of Clinical Neuropsychology, 22*(S), 115–126. https://doi.org/10.1016/j.acn.2006.10.006.

Kelly, M. P., Coldren, R. L., Parish, R. V., Dretsch, M. N., & Russell, M. L. (2012). Assessment of acute concussion in the combat environment. *Archives of Clinical Neuropsychology, 27*(4), 375–388. https://doi.org/10.1093/arclin/acs036.

Levinson, D. M., & Reeves, D. L. (1997). Monitoring recovery from traumatic brain injury using the automated neuropsychological assessment metrics (ANAM V1. 0). *Archives of Clinical Neuropsychology, 11*(5), 419–420. https://doi.org/10.1093/arclin/12.2.155.

Louey, A. G., Cromer, J. A., Schembri, A. J., Darby, D. G., Maruff, P., Makdissi, M., & Mccrory, P. (2014). Detecting cognitive impairment after concussion: Sensitivity of change from baseline and normative data methods using the CogSport/axon cognitive test battery. *Archives of Clinical Neuropsychology, 29*(5), 432–441. https://doi.org/10.1093/arclin/acu020.

Moser, R. S., Schatz, P., Neidzwski, K., & Ott, S. D. (2011). Group versus individual administration affects baseline neurocognitive test performance. *The American Journal of Sports Medicine, 39*(11), 2325–2330. https://doi.org/10.1177/0363546511417114.

Norris, J. N., Carr, W., Herzig, T., Labrie, D. W., & Sams, R. (2013). ANAM4 TBI reaction time-based tests have prognostic utility for acute concussion. *Military Medicine, 178*(7), 767–774. https://doi.org/10.7205/MILMED-D-12-00493.

Reeves, D. L., Winter, K. P., Bleiberg, J., & Kane, R. L. (2007). ANAM® genogram: Historical perspectives, description, and current endeavors. *Archives of Clinical Neuropsychology, 22*(S1), 15–37. https://doi.org/10.1016/j.acn.2006.10.013.

Register-Mihalik, J. K., Guskiewicz, K. M., Mihalik, J. P., Schmidt, J. D., Kerr, Z. Y., & McCrea, M. A. (2013). Reliable change, sensitivity, and specificity of a multidimensional concussion assessment battery: Implications for caution in clinical practice. *The Journal of Head Trauma Rehabilitation, 28*(4), 274–283. https://doi.org/10.1097/HTR.0b013e3182585d37.

Rice, V. J., Lindsay, G., Overby, C., Jeter, A., Alfred, P. E., Boykin, G. L., . . . Bateman R. (2011, July). *Automated neuropsychological assessment metrics (ANAM) traumatic brain injury (TBI): Human factors assessment* (Army Research Lab Report ARL-TN-0440). Retrieved from http://www.dtic.mil/cgi-bin/GetTRDoc?AD=ADA549141

Roebuck-Spencer, T. M., Reeves, D. L., Bleiberg, J., Cernich, A. N., Schwab, K., Ivins, B., . . . Warden, D. (2008). Influence of demographics on computerized cognitive testing in a military sample. *Military Psychology, 20*(3), 187–203. https://doi.org/10.1080/08995600802118825.

Roebuck-Spencer, T. M., Vincent, A. S., Schlegel, R. E., & Gilliland, K. (2013). Evidence for added value of baseline testing in computer-based cognitive assessment. *Journal of Athletic Training, 48*(4), 499–505. https://doi.org/10.4085/1062-6050-48.3.11.

Suhr, J. A., & Gunstad, J. (2005). Further exploration of the effect of "diagnosis threat" on cognitive performance in individuals with mild head injury. *Journal of the International Neuropsychological Society, 11*(1), 23–29. https://doi.org/10.1017/S1355617705050010.

Vincent, A. S., Roebuck-Spencer, T., Gilliland, K., & Schlegel, R. (2012). Automated neuropsychological assessment metrics (v4) traumatic brain injury battery: Military normative data. *Military Medicine, 177*(3), 256. https://doi.org/10.7205/MILMED-D-11-00289.

Automatic Language

Roberta DePompei
School of Speech-Language, Pathology and
Audiology, University of Akron, Akron, OH,
USA

Synonyms

Nonpropositional language

Definition

Automatic language is the use of nonpropositional
language forms. Even if the patient is unable to
converse at all, he or she may produce automatic
responses. These responses may be (a) automatized
sequences, counting, reciting the alphabet, and
saying the days of the week; (b) memorized
sequences, prayers pledge of allegiance; (c) recurrent social speech, "Have a nice day" and "How are
you?"; and (d) emotional speech: cursing or a
typically stated sentence when emotionally upset.
It is important to note that these types of responses
are not clearly thought out and are not under the
cognitive control of the patient. These responses do
not represent propositional language skill and
should not be considered as a conscious attempt
to participate in conversational situations. Automatic language can be found in severe aphasias
and in many dementias. It may also occur in mental
health problems such as schizophrenia.

Cross-References

▶ Stereotypy

References and Readings

Alajouanine, T. (1956). Verbal realization in aphasia.
 Brain, 79, 1–28.
Blanken, G., & Marini, V. (1997). Where do lexical speech
 automatisms come from? *Journal of Neurolinguistics,
 10*(1), 19–31.
Chapey, R. (Ed.). (2001). *Language intervention strategies in
 aphasia and related neurogenic communication disorders*
 (4th ed.). Philadelphia: Lippincott, Williams & Wilkins.
Davis, G. A. (2014). *Aphasia and related cognitive-
 communicative disorders*. Boston: Pearson.
Papathanasiou, I., Coppens, P., & Potagas, C. (2013).
 *Aphasia and related neurogenic communication disor-
 ders*. Burlington: Jones and Bartlett Learning.

A

Automaticity

Anna MacKay-Brandt
Nathan S. Kline Institute for Psychiatric Research,
Orangeburg, NY, USA
Taub Institute for Research on Alzheimer's
Disease and the Aging Brain, Columbia
University, New York, NY, USA

Definition

A mental operation that proceeds without voluntary control and without requiring capacity or
processing resources.

Current Knowledge

Automatic processes are usually found in the context
of stimulus information that is well integrated into
the individual's memory through either a classical
conditioning, an overlearned behavior (e.g., reading),
or an evolutionarily adaptive response (e.g., orienting
response). The Stroop effect (Stroop 1935; MacLeod
1992) is a good example of the influence of automaticity on behavior. Reading becomes automatic at a
level of proficiency acquired by most school-aged
children, such that it is out of an individual's control
not to read a presented word. This involuntary
response is captured in the interference it produces
when one attempts to ignore a color word and instead
name the color of the stimulus. Color naming is
slower when the color word and the color of the
stimulus are incongruent when compared to the
stimulus which is neutral (a series of Xs or a noncolor

word) or congruent (the color word is the same as the stimulus color).

Cross-References

► Controlled Attention
► Orienting Response
► Reading Fluency
► Stroop Effect

References and Readings

MacLeod, C. M. (1992). The Stroop task: The "gold standard" of attentional measures. *Journal of Experimental Psychology: General, 121*, 12–14.
Stroop, J. R. (1935). Studies of interference in serial verbal reactions. *Journal of Experimental Psychology, 18*, 643–662.

Automatism

Douglas I. Katz
Department of Neurology, Boston University
School of Medicine, Braintree, MA, USA

Synonyms

Automatic behavior

Definition

This is a complex movement that occurs without conscious awareness or purposeful intent.

Current Knowledge

Automatisms may occur in the setting of complex-partial seizures. Typical simple movements include lip smacking, chewing, or finger rubbing. More complex automatisms include walking, running, undressing, and speaking. Emotional expressions, such as laughing or crying, may also occur as automatisms. Automatisms may occur during seizures or as postictal phenomena. Speech automatisms tend to lateralize to the left hemisphere, but lateralization is not predictable for other automatisms (Rasonyi et al. 2006). Responsiveness is usually lost when automatisms occur during seizures. Rarely, patients may have preserved responsiveness in the presence of seizure-induced automatisms and only with seizures that arise from right hemisphere foci (Ebner et al. 1995).

In addition to epileptic seizures, automatisms may also be observed in other situations including intoxication, sleep walking, hypoglycemia, and psychological disorders, such as dissociative fugue states. Forensic assessments aimed at determining culpability often center around the differential diagnosis of automatisms (Fenwick 1990).

Cross-References

► Complex Partial Seizure

References and Readings

Ebner, A., Dinner, D. S., Noachtar, S., & Luders, H. (1995). Automatisms with preserved responsiveness: A lateralizing sign in psychomotor seizures. *Neurology, 45*(1), 61–64.
Fenwick, P. (1990). Automatism, medicine and the law. *Psychological Medicine. Monograph Supplement, 17*, 1–27.
Rasonyi, G., Fogarasi, A., Kelemen, A., Janszky, J., & Halasz, P. (2006). Lateralizing value of postictal automatisms in temporal lobe epilepsy. *Epilepsy Research, 70*(2–3), 239–243.

Autonomic Nervous System

Scott Vota
Department of Neurology, Virginia
Commonwealth University, Richmond, VA, USA

Synonyms

Internal regulation system; Involuntary nervous system; Visceral nervous system

Definition

The autonomic nervous system is a complex and vital system that helps to maintain homeostasis and adaptation throughout the human body. It is composed of both central and peripheral components that provide thermoregulation, arterial blood pressure adaptation, as well as alterations in regional blood flow in response to metabolic demands, micturition, gastrointestinal motility, and sexual function.

Current Knowledge

Central Component
The central components of the autonomic nervous system are located within the cerebral cortex, thalamus, hypothalamus, hippocampus, and cerebellum. These components are integrally connected via a network of ascending and descending pathways (see Fig. 1). This provides a high level of control over autonomic function. These interconnections ultimately descend to specific cells within the brainstem and spinal cord. The thoracolumbar outflow consists of fibers that arise in the intermediolateral cell column of the thoracic and first two lumbar segments of the spinal cord. This is the origin of the sympathetic division of the autonomic nervous system. The cranial outflow, arising from the cranial nerve nuclei III, VII, IX, and X, and the sacral outflow, arising from cell bodies in the intermediate cell column of sacral segments 2 through 4, form the parasympathetic division of the autonomic nervous system.

Peripheral Component
The peripheral part of the autonomic nervous system is then composed of sympathetic and parasympathetic pathways. These pathways arise from two distinct anatomic portions of the brainstem and spinal cord. The parasympathetic fibers arise from the craniosacral portion, and the sympathetic fibers arise from the thoracolumbar region. Although anatomically separated, the two parts are complementary in maintaining a balance in the activities of many visceral structures and organs. The preganglionic neurons for both the

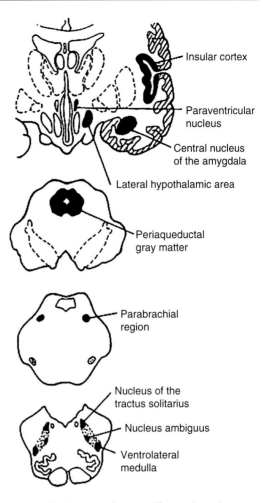

A

Autonomic Nervous System, Fig. 1 Central components of the autonomic nervous system (Benarroch et al. 1999)

parasympathetic and sympathetic divisions release acetylcholine, but the difference lies in the postganglionic neurotransmitter release. The parasympathetic postganglionic fibers release norepinephrine and epinephrine and thus are referred to as cholinergic. The sympathetic postganglionic fibers release norepinephrine and epinephrine and thus are classified as adrenergic. The terminals of sympathetic fibers on sweat glands, however, do not follow this pattern and are cholinergic (see Figs. 2 and 3).

Parasympathetic Nervous System
Parasympathetic outputs arise from the preganglionic neurons located in the nuclei of the brainstem

Autonomic Nervous System, Fig. 2 Autonomic nervous system. Parasympathetic nervous system (Benarroch et al. 1999)

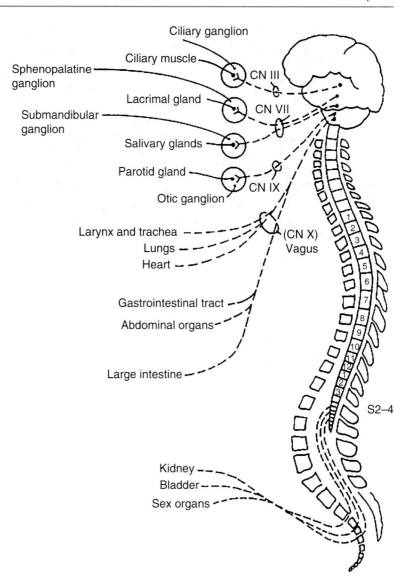

and sacral spinal cord. Preganglionic parasympathetic axons travel a long distance before eventually reaching their target ganglia, which are typically close to or within the target end organ.

The cranial preganglionic parasympathetic nuclei (Edinger-Westphal nuclei) project through the oculomotor nerve. These preganglionic axons synapse on neurons of the ciliary ganglion. The neurons innervate the iris and ciliary muscles, eliciting pupillary constriction and accommodation of the lens. The superior salivatory nucleus located in the pons projects via the facial nerve to the sphenopalatine ganglion. This innervates the lacrimal gland (producing lacrimation) and the cerebral and cranial blood vessels (eliciting vasodilatation). Axons also travel to the submandibular ganglion, providing secretomotor and vasodilator inputs to the corresponding salivary glands. The inferior salivatory nucleus sends axons via the glossopharyngeal nerve to ultimately synapse on the otic ganglion, stimulating parotid gland secretion. Most preganglionic parasympathetic output from the brainstem is mediated by the vagus nerve, which receives input from the dorsal motor nucleus of the vagus and the lateral portion of the nucleus ambiguus. The vagus nerve innervates the heart, respiratory tract, and

Autonomic Nervous System, Fig. 3 Autonomic nervous system. Sympathetic nervous system (Benarroch et al. 1999)

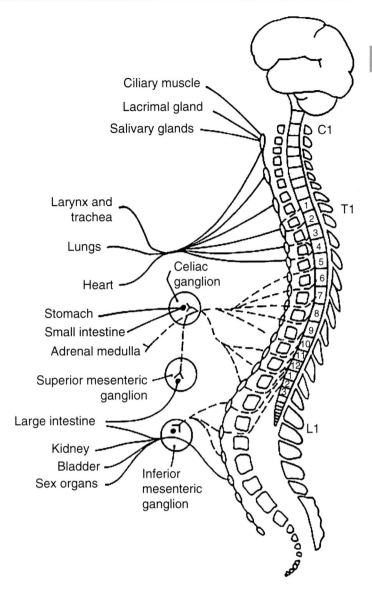

the entire gastrointestinal tract with the exception of the descending colon and rectum.

The sacral preganglionic output arises from neurons of the sacral preganglionic nucleus located in the lateral gray matter of the sacral spinal cord. These axons travel to the pelvic splanchnic nerves, which join the inferior hypogastric plexus to innervate the descending colon, bladder, and sexual organs. These outputs elicit contraction of the bladder detrusor muscle and circular smooth muscle of the rectum as well as regulating vasodilatation of the cavernous tissue of the penis required for erection.

Sympathetic Nervous System

The sympathetic preganglionic neurons are primarily located in the intermediolateral nucleus in the thoracic and upper lumbar regions of the spinal cord. The preganglionic sympathetic axons exit through the ventral roots and pass on to the corresponding spinal nerve to reach the paravertebral sympathetic chain. The majority of the presynaptic fibers branch and run rostrally or caudally along the sympathetic chain and synapse on the paravertebral ganglia. The remaining fibers pass through the paravertebral chain without synapsing. These form the splanchnic nerves which innervate prevertebral ganglia.

The paravertebral sympathetic ganglia are primarily a relay station for preganglionic inputs. They innervate all tissues and organs except those in the abdomen, pelvis, and perineum. For example, the superior cervical ganglion sends postganglionic axons to innervate the eye, facial sweat glands, salivary glands, and pineal, thyroid, and parathyroid glands. These outputs elicit pupil dilatation, contraction of the Muller muscle of the eyelid, facial sweating, and vasoconstriction in facial and cerebral circulation. The stellate ganglion, which receives preganglionic input from the mid-thoracic segment, sends postganglionic axons to innervate blood vessels and sweat glands in the upper limbs and trunk. These outputs produce either vasoconstriction or vasodilatation in the skin and muscle, sweating, or piloerection. Outputs from the stellate ganglion also elicit cardiac acceleration and bronchodilation. The lumbar paravertebral ganglia subsequently innervate the blood vessels and sweat glands in the lower limb.

The prevertebral ganglia are located anterior to the abdominal aorta. Preganglionic input from the lower thoracic segments is carried by the splanchnic nerves to the celiac and superior mesenteric ganglia and provides postganglionic fibers to the celiac plexus that innervates all abdominal viscera, with the exception of the descending colon. These outputs produce vasoconstriction and inhibition of the gastrointestinal tract motility. Preganglionic axons from the lumbar spinal segments travel via the lumbar splanchnic nerves to synapse in the inferior mesenteric ganglion. These axons innervate the descending colon, rectum, bladder, and sexual organs eliciting vasoconstriction, smooth muscle relaxation of the bladder and rectum, constriction of the internal sphincter of the bladder and rectum, and ejaculation.

Diagnosing Autonomic Dysfunction

Medical History
As the autonomic nervous system innervates all organ systems, a detailed medical history and physical examination is paramount. This will help develop a proper differential diagnosis and laboratory evaluation. The goals of the clinical evaluation are to identify the presence, location, and time course of autonomic dysfunction. This will help to determine which part(s) of the autonomic nervous system may be involved: sympathetic noradrenergic, sympathetic cholinergic, parasympathetic cholinergic, or adrenomedullary. Specific questions should be asked to determine if the patient may have symptoms of orthostatic hypotension, anhydrosis, weight change, constipation, sexual dysfunction, sialorrhea, or urinary retention. Questions related to aggravating and relieving factors need to be considered. Examples include relationship to meals, environmental temperature, and diurnal variation. A complete listing of all prescribed medications as well as over-the-counter herbal and dietary supplements need to be reviewed.

Examination
An exam should start with a general overview of the patient making note of facial expression, posture, and height. Vital signs should be checked in the supine, seated, and standing positions. A thorough skin examination making note of acrocyanosis, pallor, mottling, diaphoresis, alopecia, or erythema should be performed. An eye exam can also be valuable. Attention should be given to pupillary shape, size, and the response to light and accommodation.

Diagnostic Testing
A workup to uncover an etiology for autonomic dysfunction should begin with routine serologic testing. This includes serum electrolytes, glucose, hepatic function tests, protein electropheresis, and a complete blood count. Further serologic testing may include cortisol levels, paraneoplastic autoantibodies, and plasma catecholamines. An EKG and echocardiogram should also be performed.

A variety of more specialized tests, both invasive and noninvasive, may also need to be considered. These include but are not limited to the following: deep breathing and Valsalva ratio, isometric handgrip and cold pressor tests, thermoregulatory sweat and skin sympathetic tests, quantitative sudomotor axon reflex testing, power spectral analysis of heart rate variability, tilt table testing, and neuroimaging such as PET scanning.

Treatment

Both nonpharmacologic and pharmacologic treatments are available to treat patients with autonomic dysfunction. For certain disorders, surgical intervention may be needed. The goal is to ameliorate all symptoms while avoiding side effects.

Nonpharmacologic measurements start with patient education. Symptoms such as rising slowly from a seated position or modifying sodium intake may be enough in some autonomic disorders to provide patients with a symptom-free life.

Pharmacotherapy may include medications to increase central blood volume, such fludrocortisones, vasopressin analogues, acetylcholinesterase inhibition, or caffeine.

Cross-References

► Anticholinergic
► Arousal
► Cerebellum
► Cholinergic System
► Hippocampus
► Hypothalamus
► Thalamus

References and Readings

Benarroch, E. E., Westmoreland, B. F., Daube, J. R., Reagan, T. J., & Sandok, B. A. (1999). *Medical neurosciences: An approach to anatomy, pathology, and physiology by systems and levels* (4th ed.). Philadelphia: Lippincott Williams and Wilkins.
Bradley, W. G., Daroff, R. B., Fenichel, G., & Jankovic, J. (2004). *Neurology in clinical practice* (4th ed.). Boston: Butterworth-Heinemann.
Gilman, S., Newman, S. W., Manter, J. T., & Gatz, A. J. (2003). *Manter and Gatz's essentials of clinical neuroanatomy and neurophysiology* (10th ed.). Philadelphia: F.A. Davis Company.
Netter, F. H. (1991). *Nervous system, part 1: Anatomy and physiology* (Ciba collection of medical illustrations, Vol. 1). Summit: Ciba-Geigy Corporation.
Ropper, A. H., & Brown, R. H. (2005). *Adams and Victor's principles of neurology* (8th ed.). New York: McGraw-Hill.
Rowland, L. P. (2005). *Merritt's neurology* (11th ed.). Philadelphia: Lippincott Williams and Wilkins.

Autoreceptor

Maya Balamane[1], Beth Kuczynski[2] and Stephanie A. Kolakowsky-Hayner[3]
[1]Mount Sinai Brain Injury Research Center, San Francisco, CA, USA
[2]Imaging of Dementia and Aging (IDeA) Laboratory, Department of Neurology and Center for Neuroscience, University of California, Davis, CA, USA
[3]Department of Rehabilitation Medicine, Icahn School of Medicine at Mount Sinai, New York, NY, USA

Synonyms

Receptor

Definition

An autoreceptor is a receptor located on the neuron (terminals, soma, and/or dendrites), and the function is to bind a specific ligand (such as neurotransmitters or hormones) released by that same neuron. The autoreceptor is mainly used as a feedback mechanism to monitor neurotransmitter synthesis and/or release. In most cases, a negative feedback happens, inhibiting the release of the neurotransmitter. Dopaminergic neurons can have autoreceptors that regulate the release of dopamine. Autoreceptor regulation is very effective in modulating neurotransmission and is of interest for pharmacological intervention.

Cross-References

► Hormones
► Neurotransmitters

References and Readings

Carey, R., DePalma, G., Damianopoulos, E., Müller, C., & Huston, J. (2004). The 5-HT1A receptor and behavioral stimulation in the rat: Effects of 8-OHDPAT on spontaneous and cocaine-induced behavior. *Psychopharmacology, 177*(1/2), 46–54. https://doi.org/10.1007/s00213-004-1917-4.

Meltzer, H. (1980). Relevance of dopamine autoreceptors for psychiatry: Preclinical and clinical studies. *Schizophrenia Bulletin, 6*(3), 456–475.

Schilcker, E., & Feuerstein, F. (2016). Human presynaptic receptors. *Pharmacology and Therapeutics*. https://doi.org/10.1016/j.pharmthera.2016.11.005. (in press).

Autotopagnosia

John E. Mendoza
Department of Psychiatry and Neuroscience, Tulane Medical School and SE Louisiana Veterans Healthcare System, New Orleans, LA, USA

Definition

Disturbance of body schema involving the loss of ability to localize, recognize, or identify the specific parts of one's body.

Current Knowledge

While some reported cases exhibit impaired knowledge of most body parts, autotopagnosia is most frequently manifested as difficulty in identifying or naming specific fingers (*finger agnosia*), especially the three middle fingers. The problem extends to identifying comparable body parts on the examiner or graphic representations of body parts. The deficit usually involves both sides of the body, thus distinguishing it from unilateral neglect. While not typically classified as such, *right-left disorientation* likely reflects another form or subtype of autotopagnosia. In this condition, patients are unable to reliably identify the right and left sides of their bodies or those of others. Both finger agnosia and right-left disorientation are frequently present at the same time, particularly following lesions of the left angular gyrus and may be a part of what has been defined as Gerstmann's syndrome. The latter would also include deficits in writing (agraphia) and arithmetical operations (acalculia).

Cross-References

► Finger Agnosia
► Gerstmann's Syndrome
► Right Left Disorientation

References and Readings

Benton, A. L., & Sivan, A. B. (1993). Disturbances of the body schema. In K. M. Heilman & E. Valenstein (Eds.), *Clinical neuropsychology* (pp. 123–140). New York: Oxford University Press.

Denberg, N. L., & Tranel, D. (2003). Acalculia and disturbances of the body schema. In K. M. Heilman & E. Valenstein (Eds.), *Clinical neuropsychology* (pp. 161–184). New York: Oxford University Press.

Avoidant/Restrictive Food Intake Disorder

Kristin M. Graham
Department of Physical Medicine and Rehabilitation, Virginia Commonwealth University, Richmond, VA, USA

Synonyms

Feeding disorder of infancy or early childhood

Definition

Avoidant/restrictive food intake disorder (ARFID) is defined in the *Diagnostic and Statistical Manual of Mental Disorders* (5th ed.; *DSM-5*; American Psychiatric Association 2013) as a feeding and eating disorder characterized by avoidance or restriction of food intake. Symptoms often manifest as a lack of interest, sensory based avoidance (e.g., color, smell, texture), or concern of adverse consequences. Avoidance and/or restriction of food intake must also be accompanied by one or more key features, such as significant weight loss or nutritional deficiency, to meet diagnostic criteria.

Categorization

The disorder is classified with the feeding and eating disorders in DSM-5. The disorder replaces the DSM-IV diagnosis of feeding disorder of infancy or early childhood.

Current Knowledge

Development and Course
ARFID typically develops in infancy or early childhood but may continue into adulthood. The majority of individuals are female. In infants and young children, associated features may manifest as irritability, distress, or agitation during feeding, lack of engagement with caregiver, or lack of communication of hunger. Older children and adolescents may present with generalized emotional difficulties and failure to proceed along the expected developmental trajectory (e.g., growth delay). The condition can cause failure to thrive and nutritional deficiencies. In severe cases, malnutrition can be life-threatening and may require enteral feeding. Common comorbid conditions include anxiety disorders, obsessive-compulsive disorder, attention-deficit/hyperactivity disorder, and autism spectrum disorders.

Assessment and Treatment
Clinical assessment involves physical examination, laboratory testing, and evaluation of dietary intake to determine nutritional deficiency. Differential diagnoses include other medical conditions, reactive attachment disorder, autism spectrum disorder, anxiety disorders, mood disorders, and other eating disorders such as anorexia nervosa.

Because ARFID is a new diagnostic condition, effective treatment is still being researched. Treatment typically involves both medical and psychological interventions. Psychological interventions are guided by treatment of similar eating disorders such as anorexia nervosa.

See Also

▶ Anorexia Nervosa
▶ Feeding and Eating Disorders

References and Readings

American Psychiatric Association. (2013). *Diagnostic and statistical manual of mental disorders (DSM-5 ®).* Washington, DC: American Psychiatric Association.

Norris, M. L., & Katzman, D. K. (2015). Change is never easy, but it is possible: Reflections on avoidant/restrictive food intake disorder two years after its introduction in the DSM-5. *Journal of Adolescent Health, 57*(1), 8–9.

Williams, K. E., Hendy, H. M., Field, D. G., Belousov, Y., Riegel, K., & Harclerode, W. (2015). Implications of avoidant/restrictive food intake disorder (ARFID) on children with feeding problems. *Children's Health Care, 44*(4), 307–321.

Avolition

Irene Piryatinsky[1] and Paul Malloy[2]
[1]Butler Hospital and Alpert Medical School of Brown University, Providence, RI, USA
[2]Department of Psychiatry and Human Behavior, Brown University, Providence, RI, USA

Synonyms

Apathy

Definition

Avolition is a severe problem with initiation, volitional or willed action, and production of goal-directed behavior. It may reflect a general lack of motivation and drive. Avolition is commonly seen as one of the negative symptoms in patients with schizophrenia and is also common in frontal lobe disorders affecting medial frontal systems.

See Also

▶ Abulia
▶ Apathy
▶ Cingulate gyrus

Further Reading

Foussias, G., & Remington, G. (2008). Negative symptoms in schizophrenia: Avolition and Occam's Razor. *Schizophrenia Bulletin Advance Access.* 10. https://doi.org/10.1093/schbul/sbn094.

Liddle, P. F. (1994). Volition and schizophrenia. In A. S. David & J. C. Cutting (Eds.), *The neuropsychology of schizophrenia* (pp. 39–48). Psychology Press.

Rummel, C., Kissling, W., & Leucht, S. (2005). Antidepressants as add-on treatment to antipsychotics for people with schizophrenia and pronounced negative symptoms: A systematic review of randomized trials. *Schizophrenia Research, 80,* 85–97.

B

Babcock, Harriet (1807–1952)

Anthony Y. Stringer
Department of Rehabilitation Medicine, Emory
University, Atlanta, GA, USA

Major Appointments

- Manhattan State Hospital, New York, 1923–1925
- New York University, New York, 1931–1952

Major Honors and Awards

- Babcock was elected to the New York Academy of Science and was a Diplomate of the American Board of Examiners in Professional Psychology.

Landmark Clinical, Scientific, and Professional Contributions

- In the 1930s, Babcock began a longitudinal study of syphilitic patients, a project that was less notable for its outcomes (many of which were not subsequently replicated) than for its methodology. Classic neurological studies from the time of Paul Broca and Karl Wernicke were centered around clinical case observation. In a departure from this classic tradition, Babcock adopted the methods of scientific psychology to study the cognitive effects of neurological disease. Her research methods were well characterized and repeatable, she utilized standardized psychometric measures, and she incorporated normal control comparison groups in her research. Anticipating later batteries of neuropsychological tests, Babcock attempted to quantify deficits in discrete mental abilities and used an "efficiency index" to summarize the overall functioning of her patients.
- Babcock based her efficiency index on the idea that intellectual function varies over time. More specifically, people may exhibit a higher level of intellectual function while healthy and in the prime of life, than they do after suffering neurological or psychiatric disorders. Babcock believed that mental disorders do not affect tests of prior knowledge acquisition (e.g., vocabulary). She further identified a number of tests that she thought were sensitive to mental disorders, including tests familiar to contemporary neuropsychologists (e.g., reverse digit span and various reasoning tasks). Babcock quantified mental efficiency by contrasting performance on these two kinds of tests, a forerunner of the hold-don't hold test comparison (▶ Hold-Don't Hold Tests).
- Babcock's contemporary influence is also evident in her story memory format. In this format, a story is initially presented and recall is tested. The story is presented a second time followed by 10 min of interpolated activity

© Springer International Publishing AG, part of Springer Nature 2018
J. S. Kreutzer et al. (eds.), *Encyclopedia of Clinical Neuropsychology*,
https://doi.org/10.1007/978-3-319-57111-9

and a final recall test. This format has been adopted in some contemporary memory batteries and has the advantage of allowing the neuropsychologist to test both immediate and delayed recall, as well as learning with repetition. Although the original Babcock Story is rarely used today, some current memory batteries incorporate its format (▶ Wechsler Memory Scale All Versions). In this and other respects, Babcock's work continues to influence clinical and scientific neuropsychology.

Short Biography

Little has been written concerning Babcock's personal life. She was born in 1877 in Westerly, Rhode Island. She began her career late in life, earning her doctoral degree in her 50s. Prior to this, she lived a traditional life as a homemaker. She initially gained experience working in psychiatric facilities, but after earning her doctorate, she spent the balance of her career on the faculty at New York University. Despite her late beginning, Babcock's work was an important forerunner to the emergence of neuropsychology as a scientific field. Babcock died on December 12, 1952.

Cross-References

▶ Hold-Don't Hold Tests
▶ Intelligence
▶ Intelligence Quotient
▶ Wechsler Memory Scale All Versions

References and Readings

Hartman, D. E. (1991). Reply to reitan: Unexamined premises and the evolution of clinical neuropsychology. *Archives of Clinical Neuropsychology, 6,* 147–165.

Stringer, A. Y., & Cooley, E. L. (2002). Neuropsychology: A twentieth-century science. In A. Y. Stringer, E. L. Cooley, & A.-L. Christensen (Eds.), *Pathways to prominence in neuropsychology: Reflections of twentieth century pioneers* (pp. 3–26). New York: Psychology Press.

Babinski Reflex

Edison Wong[1] and Richard Kunz[2]
[1]Center for Pain and Medical Rehabilitation, Fitchburg, MA, USA
[2]Department of Physical Medicine and Rehabilitation, Virginia Commonwealth University, Richmond, VA, USA

Synonyms

Long tract sign; Plantar reflex; Upper motor neuron sign

Definition

The Babinski reflex is a component of the neurological exam, used to assess the adequacy of the pyramidal tract (upper motor neuron). This reflex is elicited by making contact along the lateral side of the plantar foot with a blunt implement and not causing pain, discomfort, or injury to the skin; the implement is run from the heel along a curve to the metatarsal pads. There are three responses possible:

- Extensor (positive or pathological): hallux (great toe) extension and the other toes abduct (fanning)
- Flexor (negative or normal): all toes flex and the foot everts
- Indifferent: no response

Current Knowledge

An extensor (positive) response signifies pathology in the upper motor neuron pathways, either in the spinal cord and/or brain, such as in multiple sclerosis, stroke, traumatic brain injury, or spinal cord injury. It may be the sole sign of upper motor neuron damage and is the most popular reflex for evaluation of these pathways for the lower limbs. All infants exhibit an extensor response from birth, which converts to a flexor response during ages 12–18 months as the nervous system matures given normal development; developmental delay may result in a persistent positive response. Indifferent responses may be found in normal individuals but may also indicate the presence of a lower motor neuron or other peripheral nervous system injury that interferes with the expression of a normal flexor response.

Cross-References

▶ Developmental Delay
▶ Multiple Sclerosis
▶ Spinal Cord Injury
▶ Stroke
▶ Traumatic Brain Injury (TBI)

References and Readings

Babinski, J. (1896). Sur le reflexe cutane plantaire dans certaines affections organiques du systeme nerveux central. *Comptes Rendus des Seances de la Societe de Biologie et de Ses Filiales, 48*, 207–208.
Larner, A. J. (2016). *A dictionary of neurological signs* (4th ed.). Basel: Springer.
Pearson, K., & Gordon, J. (2000). Spinal reflexes. In E. R. Kandel, J. H. Schwartz, & T. M. Jessell (Eds.), *Principles of neural science* (4th ed., pp. 713–736). New York: McGraw-Hill.

Backwards Masking

Eric S. Porges
Department of Clinical and Health Psychology, University of Florida, Gainesville, FL, USA
Center for Cognitive Aging and Memory, McKnight Brain Institute, University of Florida, Gainesville, FL, USA
Department of Neurology, University of Florida, Gainesville, FL, USA

Definition

Backward masking occurs when the perception of a stimulus is attenuated by the rapid presentation of a subsequent stimulus (the "mask"). Within the domains of neuropsychology and psychology, backward masking typically refers to visual phenomena. However, backward masking has been explored in other sensory domains such as ... (may want to list other domains here). In a typical backward masking paradigm, a visual stimulus (such as a letter) is rapidly presented and followed by a mask that encompasses the area of the visual field where the initial stimuli was presented (Breitmeyer and Ogmen 2000). The presentation of the initial stimulus, while rapid, is sufficiently long enough for a non-backward masked presentation to be perceptible. The mechanisms underlying backward masking are an active area of research; however, it is well established that central and likely cortical mechanisms are involved, given the time course of the effect as well as its ability to be produced with dichoptic presentation (stimulus and mask presented to separate eyes).

References and Readings

Breitmeyer, B. G., & Ogmen, H. (2000). Recent models and findings in visual backward masking: a comparison, review, and update. *Perception & Psychophysics, 62*(8), 1572–1595. Retrieved from http://www.ncbi.nlm.nih.gov/pubmed/11140180

Bacterial Ventriculitis

Courtney Murphy
Belmont Behavioral Hospital, Philadelphia, PA, USA

Synonyms

Intraventricular infection; Intraventricular inflammation; Ventriculomeningitis

Definition

Bacterial ventriculitis refers to inflammation of the cerebral ventricles, typically resulting from intraventricular infection or bacterial infection of cerebral spinal fluid.

Current Knowledge

Bacterial ventriculitis is a potential life-threatening condition that can result from the rupture of a cerebral abscess, an infection of an external ventriculostomy catheter, an infection of cerebral spinal fluid, and other infectious CNS conditions. Bacterial infection produces an immune response in the lining of the ventricles, resulting in inflammation.

Presenting symptoms can be headaches, dizziness, confusion, photophobia, and neck and upper back pain and nausea and vomiting in children. In infancy, it can cause unrecognized hydrocephalus. Ventriculitis must be confirmed by examination of the cerebrospinal fluid.

Cross-References

▶ Encephalitis (Viral)
▶ Meningitis

References and Readings

Agrawal, A. M., Cincu, R., & Jake, R. (2008). Current concepts and approach to ventriculitis. *Infectious Diseases in Clinical Practice, 16*(2), 100–104.

Centers for Disease Control and Prevention (CDC). (2017). CDC/NHSN surveillance definitions for specific types of infections. Retrieved from http://www.cdc.gov/nhsn/PDFs/pscManual/17pscNosInfDef_current.pdf.

Tabuchi, S., & Kadowaki, M. (2015). Neuroendoscopic surgery for ventriculitis and hydrocephalus after shunt infection and malfunction: Preliminary report of a new strategy. *Asian Journal Endoscopic Surgery, 8*, 180–184. https://doi.org/10.1111/ases.12162.

Weerakkody, Y., & Gaillard, F. (n.d.). Ventriculitis. Retrieved 9 Dec 2016, from https://radiopaedia.org/articles/ventriculitis.

Balance Disorders

Anna DePold Hohler[1] and Marcus Ponce de Leon[2]
[1]Boston University Medical Center, Boston, MA, USA
[2]Madigan Army Medical Center, Tacoma, WA, USA

Definition

Normal balance requires the integration of three sensory systems: visual, vestibular (found in the inner ear), and somatosensory (sensations from the skin, muscles, tendons, and joints) – in addition to muscle strength. When these systems are impaired, individuals may experience episodes of spinning, light headedness, trouble focusing their eyes, and/or poor balance or falls.

Categorization

Balance may be affected by disturbances of strength in the trunk or legs, sensation deficits, or difficulties with coordination. Multiple systems may be affected. A detailed history and neurological examination may help detect the affected area. Balance may be impaired after a focal event such as a stroke or may develop during the course of a neurodegenerative disease such as Parkinson's disease. Medications and infections of the brain or inner ear may also contribute to balance difficulties.

Epidemiology

Aging may also affect balance. Approximately 40% of people older than age 65 suffer falls each year. Vertigo is the most common form of dizziness.

Natural History

Balance disorders associated with neurodegenerative diseases tend to be progressive.

Neuropsychology and Psychology of Balance

Neurodegenerative disorders associated with balance that affect the cortex can also be associated with cognitive difficulties.

Evaluation

The history and physical examination often lead to a diagnosis. At times, laboratory tests and imaging are obtained for confirmation or to rule out harmful diagnoses. If a reversible cause is found and treated, significant recovery may occur. However, if the balance problem is due to a permanent or progressive neurological deficit, the patient may need training to manage their gait and balance difficulties.

Treatment

Physical therapy and vestibular rehabilitation may be useful in appropriate cases. They may improve current functioning and potentially decrease the potential for progression of deficits and complications from falls.

Cross-References

▶ Ataxia
▶ Parkinson's Disease

References and Readings

Ackley, S., Newell Decker, T., & Limb, C. J. (2007). *An essential guide to hearing and balance disorders*. Psychology Press.

Balint, R. (Rezso (Rudolf) Balint) (1874–1929)

Alyssa Eidson
Emory University/Rehabilitation Medicine, Atlanta, GA, USA

Major Appointments

• University of Budapest, Budapest, Hungary, 1910–1929

Major Honors and Awards

• Balint's work was honored by the later naming of his "triple-syndrome complex" as "Balint's Syndrome" by Hecaen and Ajuriaguerra (1954).

Landmark Clinical, Scientific, and Professional Contributions

• Hungarian physician Rezso Balint's first writings, published while he was still a medical student, were case studies examining muscular atrophy in hemiplegia. He went on to study tabes dorsalis and the treatment of epilepsy. In 1907, Dr. Balint recorded his observations of a patient who suffered from a unique constellation of neurologic symptoms including fixation of gaze, neglect of objects in his periphery, and misreaching for target objects. The patient was noted to first experience these symptoms following damage to the posterior parietal lobes. This "triple-syndrome complex" was later named "Balint's Syndrome."

Short Biography

Rezso Balint was born in 1874 to a German-Jewish family in Budapest, Hungary. He attended the University of Budapest, where he received his degree in medicine in 1897. Balint was a student of Friedrich von Koranyi. He was employed as a Lecturer at the University of Budapest in 1910 and was promoted to Professor of Internal Medicine in 1917.

At the onset of World War I, Dr. Balint turned his research focus from neurology to tuberculosis and metabolism and the treatment of diabetes. He is most well known in his home country of Hungary for the treatment of gastric ulcer with the use of alkali.

Rezso Balint died of thyroid cancer in 1929 at the age of 56.

Cross-References

▶ Neglect Syndrome
▶ Optic Ataxia

References and Readings

Hecaen, H., & Ajuriaguerra, J. (1954). Balint Syndrome (psychic paralysis of visual fixation) and its minor forms. *Brain, 77*, 373–400.

Husain, M., & Stein, J. (1988). Reszo Balint and his most celebrated case. *Archives of Neurology, 45*, 89–93.

Rezso Balint (physician). From Wikipedia. http://en. wikipedia.org/wiki/rezs. Retrieved 7 Jan 2009.

Balint's Syndrome

Uraina S. Clark
Department of Neurology, Icahn School of Medicine at Mount Sinai, New York, NY, USA

Short Description or Definition

Balint's syndrome was first described by Rezső Bálint in 1909. It consists of three visuospatial abnormalities: simultanagnosia, optic ataxia, and ocular motor apraxia. The syndrome typically occurs in the absence of visual field deficits. Individuals with Balint's syndrome experience significant perceptual limitations. Patients with this syndrome cannot perceive more than one object at a time. They experience great impairments in their ability to explore visual space: they have difficulty navigating through their environment; they get lost easily; and they experience difficulty reaching for or grasping items in need.

Balint's syndrome is usually associated with large bilateral lesions in the dorsal occipitoparietal region and is consequently rare. The most common causes of Balint's syndrome include ischemia (particularly watershed infarctions) and degenerative disorders (e.g., Alzheimer's disease, posterior cortical atrophy). Balint's syndrome can also result from trauma, tumors, leukoencephalopathies, and prion disorders. In individuals with HIV/AIDS, Balint's syndrome can develop secondary to HIV encephalitis or progressive multifocal leukoencephalopathy. Transient symptoms of Balint's syndrome have been reported in association with migraine onset.

Natural History, Prognostic Factors, and Outcomes

The prognosis for patients with Balint's syndrome varies depending on the etiology of the syndrome. Patients with posterior cortical atrophy usually experience a declining course, while some patients with acute infarction may demonstrate improved functioning with time.

Neuropsychology and Psychology of Balint's Syndrome

As noted above, individuals with Balint's syndrome display three classic symptoms, including simultanagnosia, optic ataxia, and ocular motor apraxia. Simultanagnosia is generally considered to be a disruption in spatial attention, which is associated with an inability to direct one's attention to more than one or a few objects at a time. It is not uncommon for patients with this syndrome to ignore or neglect all other objects once one object in the visual field has been fixated upon. Although patients can perceive and name individual objects regardless of the object's location within the visual field, they exhibit an inability to perceive and interpret the gestalt of the scene. The second symptom associated with Balint's syndrome is optic ataxia, which is defined as a deficit in reaching under visual guidance despite normal limb strength and position sense. As a result of this symptom, patients demonstrate an inability to manually respond to visual stimuli, and they often make location errors when pointing to or grasping for visual targets. Some of the impairments noted on tests of reaching abilities include increased action latency, poor control of hand trajectory, increased variability at the end of the reach, tendency to reach to one side, and dissociations of distance and direction control. The third symptom of Balint's syndrome includes ocular apraxia, which is manifested by an inability to voluntarily shift gaze toward a new visual target. The ability to make a saccade on command is significantly impaired and is next to impossible for patients with Balint's syndrome, whereas the ability to make reflexive saccades (e.g., those made to suddenly appearing visual objects or sudden noises) and random spontaneous saccades remains intact.

Evaluation

Before a diagnosis of Balint's syndrome can be made more general, cognitive dysfunction (e.g., hemineglect, visual impairments) should be ruled out. It is important that the patient's visual fields be assessed fully as some types of visual field abnormalities (e.g., extensive peripheral scotomata) can result in symptoms that are very similar to Balint's syndrome.

A typical method of assessing for simultanagnosia includes asking the patient to examine and describe the events depicted in a complex visual image (e.g., the Cookie Theft Picture from the Boston Diagnostic Aphasia Examination). In such a task, it is helpful if key elements of the image are presented in all four quadrants of the picture in order to assess visual attention more fully across the quadrants. Individuals with hemineglect may describe items on one side of the picture only. Patients with Balint's syndrome often are able to identify discrete items in the picture; however, they are frequently unable to integrate the various elements of the picture into a coherent story. Patients will also show impairments on visual search and counting tasks. Letter identification and reading abilities should be assessed for functional purposes.

In assessing for optic ataxia, one may place several items at different locations on a table and ask the patient to touch or grasp each of the items. It is important to assess whether the patient is able to grasp items within both hemifields with each hand independently. Patients with unilateral lesions typically demonstrate greater impairment when reaching for items located in the hemispace that is contralateral to the lesion, using the contralateral hand. Individuals with Balint's syndrome, by contrast, are typically impaired at reaching for visual targets for all locations within the visual field; however, it has been noted that some patients with Balint's syndrome do demonstrate reaching difficulties in which one arm is more affected than the other. Patients with this syndrome are noted to be clumsy when grasping for items, and they may often mislocate objects in space when reaching for or pointing to items. In contrast, reaching to somatosensory targets such as parts of the patient's own body (e.g., knee, shoulder) on command is frequently intact; however, patients with significant parietal spatial representation abnormalities may indeed demonstrate impairments in both reaching for objects as well as reaching to somatosensory targets.

In assessing for ocular motor apraxia, the patient's ability to make saccadic eye movements to targets on command can be compared to his/her ability to make reflexive saccades to targets that appear suddenly in their field of vision. The former can be tested by asking the patient to saccade between the clinician's left and right index fingers, spaced far apart and held at various locations across the patient's visual field. The latter can be tested in response to a person passing by or to a loud unexpected noise occurring in the periphery.

Treatment

Relatively little is known about treatment of patients with Balint's syndrome. Rehabilitation often utilizes a functional approach in which the patient's strengths are used to offset impairments. There is some evidence to suggest that cognitive and perceptual rehabilitation approaches using verbal cues and organizational search strategies can improve visual function and reaching abilities (see Perez et al. 1996). Case report studies, of which there are few, suggest that various rehabilitation strategies may be employed (see Rose et al. 2016; Zgaljardic et al. 2011), with minimal recovery of functional and physical abilities reported.

See Also

▶ Neglect Syndrome
▶ Simultanagnosia
▶ Visual Field Deficit

Further Reading

Perez, F. M., Tunkel, R. S., Lachmann, E. A., & Nagler, W. (1996). Balint's syndrome arising from bilateral posterior cortical atrophy or infarction: Rehabilitation strategies and their limitation. *Disability and Rehabilitation, 18*, 300–304.

Rose, A., Wilson, B. A., Manolov, R., & Florschutz, G. (2016). Seeing red: Relearning to read in a case of Balint's syndrome. *NeuroRehabilitation, 39*, 111–117.

Zgaljardic, D. J., Yancy, S., Levinson, J., Morales, G., & Masel, B. E. (2011). Balint's syndrome and post-acute brain injury rehabilitation: A case report. *Brain Injury, 25*, 909–917.

Barbiturates

JoAnn Tschanz
Department of Psychology, Utah State University, Logan, UT, USA
Center for Epidemiologic Studies, Utah State University, Logan, UT, USA

Synonyms

Central nervous system depressants; Sedative-hypnotics

Definition

Barbiturates belong to a class of medications known as sedative-hypnotics. Initially they were prescribed for their anxiolytic and relaxing properties. Later, they were also used as anticonvulsants, and shorter-acting forms were developed for use as anesthetics in surgery (Feldman et al. 1997).

Barbiturates affect a subtype of the receptors of the neurotransmitter, gamma aminobutyric acid (GABA), one of the most common inhibitory neurotransmitter systems in the brain. Their behavioral effects include relaxation, drowsiness, and feelings of euphoria. However, their widespread effects also result in the depression of reflexes and cardiovascular and respiratory functions, particularly at higher doses (Feldman et al. 1997).

The psychoactive effects of barbiturates increase their risk for drug dependence and abuse. Symptoms of tolerance and withdrawal develop with chronic use. Reportedly, tolerance develops to the psychoactive effects of barbiturates, but less to the respiratory depressant effects, thereby increasing the risk of a toxic overdose (Feldman et al. 1997). Cross-tolerance with other substances may also occur. For example, alcohol use may also increase tolerance to barbiturates, further increasing the risk of a toxic overdose.

Current Knowledge

The use of barbiturates has declined significantly with the development of other anxiolytic and anticonvulsant medications. Benzodiazepines, which are also anxiolytic compounds that interact with the $GABA_A$ receptor (although a different site than barbiturates), have a larger therapeutic window than barbiturates and have replaced their use as a safer alternative for the treatment of anxiety. Some studies suggest a potential role for barbiturates in alcohol withdrawal. A recent review reported potential benefit of barbiturates, most notably for severe withdrawal and for treating seizures (Martin and Katz 2016).

See Also

▶ Benzodiazepines

References and Readings

Feldman, R. S., Meyer, J. S., & Quenzer, L. F. (1997). Sedative-hypnotic and anxiolytic drugs. In *Principles of Neuropsychoparhmacology* (pp. 673–729). Sunderland, MA: Sinauer Associates.

Martin, K., & Katz, A. (2016). The role of barbiturates for alcohol withdrawal syndrome. *Psychosomatics*. Epub ahead of print. Mar 2. pii: S0033–3182(16)00041–4. https://doi.org/10.1016/j.psym.2016.02.011.

Barefoot v. Estelle (1983)

Robert L. Heilbronner
Chicago Neuropsychology Group, Chicago,
IL, USA

Synonyms

Prediction of future dangerousness

Historical Background

Thomas A. Barefoot burned down a bar and shot and killed a police officer who was investigating the arson. Barefoot was convicted by the jury of capital murder of a police officer. During the death penalty phase of the case, the state used psychiatric testimony to demonstrate that Barefoot posed a threat to society in the future. Specifically, the state had Drs. John Holbrook and James Grigson review a hypothetical fact situation based on evidence from the case and asked each of the doctors if the convicted individual would commit violent acts in the future or would pose a threat to society. Both doctors testified that the criminal would be a continued threat to society. In fact, Dr. Grigson concluded that there was a "one hundred percent and absolute" probability that Barefoot would commit violent acts in the future and thus pose a continued threat to society. The judge sentenced Thomas A. Barefoot to death. Barefoot appealed the decision and in the Court of Criminal Appeals raised several concerns about the way his trial was handled, most notably with respect to the probability that he would commit future violent acts. Barefoot argued that the psychiatrists testifying against him had not even examined him and were making determinations based on a hypothetical fact-based situation. Moreover, Barefoot called into question the ability of psychiatrists to predict future dangerousness. The Court of Criminal Appeals rejected all of Barefoot's arguments, and the US Supreme Court rejected Barefoot's suggestion that psychiatrists are not competent to make determinations regarding dangerousness in future. The US Supreme Court ruled that psychiatrists are no less reliable than laypersons and that laypersons' testimony of future dangerousness is indeed permissible. The Court upheld that the use of hypothetical questions to establish future dangerousness is just because such testimony is supported by the Federal Rules of Evidence (FRE) that death penalty cases do not present special evidentiary problems. Furthermore, there is evidence (e.g., Monahan 1992; Monohan and Steadman 1994; Mossman 1994) to suggest that mental health professionals do indeed predict violence significantly better than chance when "relevant" factors are included in the determination.

References and Readings

Denney, R. L. (2005). Criminal responsibility and other criminal forensic issues. In G. Larrabee (Ed.), *Forensic neuropsychology: A scientific approach*. New York: Oxford University Press.

Melton, G. B., Petrila, J., Poythress, N. G., & Slobogin, C. (1997). *Psychological evaluations for the courts: A handbook for mental health professionals and lawyers*. New York: Guilford.

Monahan, J. (1992). Mental disorder and violent behavior: Perceptions and evidence. *American Psychologist, 47*, 511–521.

Monahan, J., & Steadman, H. J. (1994). Toward a rejuvenation of risk assessment research. In J. Monahan & H. J. Steadman (Eds.), *Violence and mental disorder: Developments in risk assessment*. Chicago: University of Chicago Press.

Mossman, D. (1994). Assessing predictors of violence: Being accurate about accuracy. *Journal of Consulting and Clinical Psychology, 62*, 783–792.

Barona Index

Glen E. Getz
Department of Psychiatry, Allegheny General
Hospital, Pittsburgh, PA, USA
Neuropsychology Specialty Care, LLC,
Pittsburgh, PA, USA

Synonyms

Premorbid intelligence regression model

Definition

Barona Index is a demographically based regression method to estimate premorbid intelligence in terms of index scores on the Wechsler Adult Intelligence Scale-Revised (WAIS-R).

Historical Background

Attempts have long been made to estimate premorbid intellectual functioning. A frequent method in clinical practice is to estimate the level of premorbid cognitive skill by subjectively considering aspects of the individual's history such as education and occupation. Another common approach to estimate premorbid IQ is to use tests of present ability, which are thought to be relatively resistant to change even during the phases of a psychiatric disorder or those following a neurologically based disorder. A variant is the best performance method in which the highest score obtained by an individual is assumed to be the most likely premorbid level (▶ Best Performance Method). Research has been inconsistent as to the effectiveness of this approach. In an attempt to reduce the error in estimating intelligence based on current functioning and eliminate the subjectivity inherent in clinical judgment, demographically based regression equations were created to statistically predict intelligence test scores. A later method of combining demographic information and current performance on IQ has also been found to be relatively effective.

It is well established that demographic variables, such as education, social class and education, are correlated with measured IQ. Wilson et al. (1978) created a regression equation to predict WAIS IQ from demographic variables. They used regression modeling with WAIS Full Scale IQ, Verbal IQ, and Performance IQ as criteria and age, education, sex, race, and occupation as predictors. With the development of the WAIS-Revised (WAIS-R), further models were needed to estimate premorbid intelligence. Barona et al. (1984) generated demographic equations for the estimation of premorbid WAIS-R IQ. Subsequently, research demonstrated successful discrimination of neurologically based patients

from non-neurologically based patients utilizing the WAIS-R. As demonstrated in Fig. 1, the predictor variables incorporated into the model included those originally utilized by Wilson et al. (1978) as well as urban/rural residency, geographic location, and handedness. Although these equations resulted in less IQ variance and larger standard errors of estimate, cross validation studies were successful.

Current Knowledge

Currently, premorbid estimation of IQ functioning includes the WAIS-IV (Wechsler 2008). Algorithms derived from the WAIS-IV with demographic variables have been developed by the Advanced Clinical Solutions (ACS; Pearson 2009). Holdnack et al. (2013) discuss the clinical utility of the Test of Premorbid Functioning (TOPF) to determine if the a patient's current performance is expected or represents a decline from a previous estimated level of ability. The TOPF can be used alone or in conjunction with demographic characteristics to estimate premorbid level of functioning. Research consistently suggests that TOPF estimates from the ACS are reasonably effective in estimating premorbid intelligence.

Future Directions

As we are on the brink of the release and utilization of the Wechsler Adult Intelligence Scale-V, it is quite likely that future regression models to estimate premorbid functioning as indexed by scores on this test will be developed. It is necessary to continue to improve our methods of estimating premorbid abilities. Future models will most likely consider other variables and/or include more specific criteria for the existing models. For example, the expansion of technology along with fewer labor-based jobs and more technology-based jobs will very likely influence the occupations used for the equation. Similarly, as online education expands, an understanding of the type of education rather than amount of education may change the weighting of the model algorithms. As age expectancy increases, the role

WAIS-R VIQ = 54.23 + .49 (age) + 1.92 (sex) + 4.24 (race) + 5.25 (education) + 1.89 (occupation) + 1.24 (U-R residence.)

Standard Error of Estimate = 11.79; R^2= .38

WAIS-R PIQ = 61.58 + .31 (age) + 1.09 (sex) + 4.95 (race) + 3.75 (education) + 1.54 (occupation) + .82 (region)

Standard Error of Estimate = 13.23; R^2= .24

WAIS-R PIQ = 54.96 + .47 (age) + 1.76 (sex) + 4.71 (race) + 5.02 (education) + 1.89 (occupation) + .59 (region)

Standard Error of Estimate = 12.14; R^2= .36

Sex:	Female = 1.Male = 2
Race:	Black = 1, Other ethnicity = 2, White = 3
Education	0–7 years = 1,8 = 2,9–11 = 3, 12=4, 13–15 = 5, 16+ =6
Age:	16–17 years = 1,18–9 = 2, 20–24 = 3, 25–34 = 4, 35–44 = 5, 45–54 = 6, 55–64 = 7, 65–69 = 8, 70–74 = 9
Region:	Southern = 1, North Central = 2, Western = 3, Northeastern = 4.
Residence:	Rural = 1, Urban = 2
Occupation:	Farm Laborers, Farm Foremen & Laborers (unskilled) = 1
	Operatives, Service Workers, Farmers, & farm Managers (semiskilled) = 2
	Not in Labor Force = 3
	Craftsmen & Foremen (skilled workers) = 4
	Managers, Officials, Proprietors, Clerical & Sales Workers = 5
	Professional & Technical = 6

Barona Index, Fig. 1 Barona et al. (1984) regression formulas for pre-morbid IQ

of age on premorbid functioning will quite likely become a more important variable as well.

Cross-References

▶ Best Performance Method
▶ Intelligence
▶ Premorbid Estimate
▶ Premorbid Functioning

References and Readings

Advanced Clinical Solutions for WAIS-IV and WMS-IV. (2009). Administration and scoring manual.

Barona, A., & Chastin, R. L. (1986). An improved estimate of premorbid IQ for black and whites on the WAIS-R. *International Journal of Clinical Neuropsychology, 8*, 169–173.

Barona, A., Reynolds, C. R., & Chastain, R. (1984). A demographically based index of premorbid intelligence for the WAIS-R. *Journal of Consulting and Clinical Psychology, 52*, 885–887.

Schoenberg, M. R., Scott, J. G., Duff, K., & Adams, R. L. (2002). Estimation of WAIS-III intelligence from combined performance and demographic variables: Development of the OPIE-3. *The Clinical Neuropsychologist, 16*, 426–438.

Wilson, R. S., Rosenbuam, G., Broan, G., Rourke, D., Whitman, D., & Grisell, J. (1978). An index of premorbid intelligence. *Journal of Consulting and Clinical Psychology, 46*, 1554–1555.

Barrow Neuropsychological Screen

George P. Prigatano
Department of Clinical Neuropsychology, Barrow Neurological Institute, St. Joseph's Hospital and Medical Center, Phoenix, AZ, USA

Synonyms

BNIS

Description

The Barrow Neurological Institute (BNI) Screen for Higher Cerebral Functions (BNIS) was developed to rapidly, but reliably and validly, assess disturbances in higher integrative brain functions (Prigatano et al. 1995). In addition to sampling speech/language, orientation, attention/concentration, visual spatial, and visual problem-solving, and memory functions, it is unique as a neuropsychological screening instrument insofar as it also assesses affect expression and perception as well as the person's awareness of memory abilities. This provides for seven subtest scores and a possible total score of 50/50 points. The latter score can be converted to an age-adjusted T score. The test has been translated into eight different languages and typically takes between 10 and 15 to administer (Prigatano et al. 2013).

Historical Background

While several screening tests of higher cerebral or integrative brain functions exist (see Lezak et al. 2004), they do not assess both cognitive and affective functions. Various brain disorders affect both dimensions, but differentially. At the BNI, a wide variety of brain dysfunctional patients are evaluated and treated. This led Prigatano and colleagues to develop a screening test that assess, in brief fashion, cognitive and affective functions that could be negatively influenced by various brain disorders. In doing so, they attempted to provide the experienced clinician with both quantitative and qualitative information useful in patient evaluations, management, and research.

Psychometric Data

The initial standardization study (Prigatano et al. 1995) reported good test-retest reliability ($r = 0.94$) and good sensitivity for identifying brain dysfunctional patients (i.e., 92%). The specificity of the instrument was modest (48%). Specificity was increased if performance on memory tests was taken into account (83%). That is, good performance on memory items plus the total score on the BNIS successfully identified many normal functioning individuals.

Two doctoral dissertations have documented the reliability and validity of the BNIS. Wass (1997) demonstrated that performance on the BNIS correlated with independent and lengthier measures of neuropsychological test performance. BNIS subtest scores were also positively correlated with the Functional Independence Measure (FIM) and the adjunct of the Functional Assessment Measure (FIM + FAM of the Uniform Data Set for Medical Rehabilitation). Nearly 50% of the psychosocial-cognition score of the FIM-FAM was predicted by the seven independent subtests of the BNIS.

Denvall et al. (2002) administered a Swedish translation of the BNIS to 52 normal controls and 36 patients with well-documented brain disorders (the majority being those with traumatic brain injury and stroke). Swedish controls performed almost identically to American controls on this test. Swedish brain dysfunctional patients performed worst on the BNIS than Swedish controls. Hofgren (2009) further studied the Swedish version of the BNIS for her doctoral dissertation. The first study (Hofgren et al. 2007b) utilized 92 controls and 120 patients from a neurorehabilitation clinic. Significant differences were found between the control group and the patient group. Sensitivity was 88% and specificity was 78%. In a second study (see Hofgren 2009), the BNIS was compared to the Mini-Mental State Examination as well as to the FIM. Concordance between the BNIS total score and MMSE was good ($r = 0.744$). Both measures discriminated ADL-dependent from nondependent patients. A third study (Hofgren et al. 2007a) used the BNIS as a predictor of return to work and level of activities of daily living (ADL) in 58 stroke victims. At 1 year follow-up, the correlation of the BNIS total score and the psychosocial-cognitive scale of the FIM was $r = 0.376$ ($p = 0.001$). BNIS total score did not predict ability to return to work, but most of the patients studied did not return to work. In a fourth study, Hofgren et al. (2008) studied ADL, housing, and return to work 2 years after cardiac arrest in 22 patients. The BNIS total score was higher in patients living in their home and who were able to return to work (mean total score was 43/50 points, range 41–47). In contrast, the mean BNIS total score was notably lower in those living in their own home but not able to return to work (mean total score 37, range 35–42) and even lower for those living in sheltered accommodations (mean Total score was 24, range of 19–32).

A study from the Netherlands further supported the clinical utility and validity of the BNIS when measuring outcome after stroke (Boosman et al. 2013). The BNIS showed good internal consistency (alpha = 0.82) and no floor or ceiling effects in stroke patients described as having a good functional outcome using the Barthel Index. Selected subtests correlated with more time-consuming and extensive tests of different cognitive domains. For example, the Boston Naming Test scores correlated 0.538 ($p = 0.000$) with the speech/language subtest scores of the BNIS. Likewise, the memory subtest scores correlated with the total scores obtained from the Rey Auditory Verbal Learning Test ($r = 0.548$). These findings replicated the earlier observations of Wass (1997).

Recently, a normative study using the French translation of the BNIS also reported findings very similar to what was observed in the original American standardization study (see Prigatano et al. 2013).

Clinical Uses

Prigatano and Wong (1999) studied 95 heterogeneous brain dysfunctional patients treated on an inpatient neurorehabilitation unit who were classified as having achieved their rehabilitation goals or not. Patients who achieved their rehabilitation goals had higher BNIS total scores at admission compared to patients that did not achieve their rehabilitation goals. Impaired emotional functioning was equally important as impaired cognitive functioning when predicting goal attainment. Interestingly, both groups were equally impaired in their awareness of the memory functioning on admission. However, the group that eventually achieved their goals showed improved awareness after the rehabilitation experience.

Studies have also documented the potential value of the BNIS in cases of differential diagnosis.

Rosenstein et al. (1997) compared 41 patients with known cerebral dysfunction, with 22 psychiatric patients (some who were psychotic) and 22 medical inpatients. Psychiatric and medical patients scored significantly higher on the BNIS total score compared to the brain dysfunctional patients. Using the recommended cutoff score of 47/50 points, 40 of the 41 brain dysfunctional patients were correctly classified (97.5%). The specificity for medical controls was 68%. The specificity for psychiatric patients was much lower (40.9%). These findings suggest that multiple factors can influence the patient's BNIS total score, including the age, education, and psychiatric status of the patient.

In a French study, Prigatano et al. (2014a) demonstrated that patients with mild cognitive impairment of the amnestic type (MCI) had poorer scores on the BNI screen than age-matched patients who did not have MCI. MCI patients showed not only disturbance in memory functioning but impaired awareness and affect expression and perception. The study demonstrated the potential importance of assessing both cognitive and affective functions in cases of differential diagnosis.

Also, recent case studies have suggested that performance on the BNIS may help identify patients with anosognosia (e.g., Prigatano et al. 2014b).

References

Boosman, H., Visser-Meily, J. M. A., Post, M. W. M., Duits, A., & van Heugten, C. M. (2013). Validity of the Barrow Neurological Institute (BNI) screen for higher cerebral functions in stroke patients with good functional outcome. *The Clinical Neuropsychologist, 27*(4), 667–680.

Denvall, V., Elmstahl, S., & Prigatano, G. P. (2002). Replication and construct validation of the BNI Screen for higher cerebral function with the Swedish population. *Journal of Rehabilitative Medicine, 34*, 153–157.

Hofgren, C. (2009). Screening of cognitive functions: Evaluation of methods and their applicability in neurological rehabilitation (Doctoral Dissertation, University of Gothenburg, Gothenburg, Sweden).

Hofgren, C., Bjorkdahl, A., Esbjornsson, E., & Stibrant-Sunnerhagen, K. (2007a). Recovery after stroke: Cognition, ADL function and return to work. *Acta Neurologica, 115*, 73–80.

Hofgren, C., Esbjornsson, E., Aniansson, H., & Sunnerhagen, K. S. (2007b). Application and

B

validation of the Barrow Neurological Institute Screen for higher cerebral functions in a control population and in patient groups commonly seen in neurorehabilitation. *Journal of Rehabilitative Medicine, 39*, 547–553.

Hofgren, C., Lundgren-Nilsson, A., Esbjornsson, E., & Sunnerhagen, K. S. (2008). Two years after cardiac arrest; cognitive status, ADL function and living situation. *Brain Injury, 22*(12), 972–978.

Lezak, M. D., Howieson, D. B., & Loring, D. W. (2004). *Neuropsychological assessment* (4th ed.). New York: Oxford University Press.

Prigatano, G. P., & Wong, J. L. (1999). Cognitive and affective improvement in brain dysfunctional patients who achieve inpatient rehabilitation goals. *Archives of Physical Medicine and Rehabilitation, 80*, 77–84.

Prigatano, G. P., Amin, K., & Rosenstein, L. D. (1995). *Administration and scoring manual for the BNI Screen for higher cerebral functions*. Phoenix: Barrow Neurological Institute.

Prigatano, G. P., Tonini, A., Truelle, J. L., & Montreuil, M. (2013). Performance of a French sample on the French translation of the BNI Screen for higher cerebral functions. *Brain Injury, 27*(12), 1435–1440.

Prigatano, G. P., Montreuil, M., Chapple, K., Tonini, A., Toron, J., Paquet, C., Dumurgier, J., Hugon, J., & Truelle, J. L. (2014a). Screening for cognitive and affective dysfunction in patients suspected of mild cognitive impairment. *International Journal of Geriatric Psychiatry, 29*(9), 936–942.

Prigatano, G. P., Hendin, B. A., & Heiserman, J. E. (2014b). Denial or unawareness of cognitive deficit associated with multiple sclerosis? A case report. *Journal of Clinical and Experimental Neuropsychology, 36*(4), 335–341.

Rosenstein, L. D., Prigatano, G. P., & Nayak, M. (1997). Differentiating patients with higher cerebral dysfunction from patients with psychiatric or acute medical illness with the BNI Screen for higher cerebral functions. *Neuropsychiatry, Neuropsychology, and Behavioral Neurology, 10*(2), 113–119.

Wass, P. J. (1997). An analysis of the construct-related and ecological validity of the Barrow Neurological Institute Screen for higher cerebral functions (Doctoral Dissertation, University of Windsor, Windsor).

Barthel Index

Gavin Williams
Epworth Rehabilitation Centre Epworth Hospital, Richmond Melbourne, VIC, Australia

Synonyms

BI

Description

The Barthel Index (BI) measures ten functions that are important for independent living – feeding, bathing, grooming, dressing, bowel and bladder continence, toileting, transfers, mobility, and stair use. Items are weighted and scored according to their perceived importance. Higher scores indicate better performance. In the most commonly used version, the maximum score of 100 indicates full independence. Several versions of the Barthel Index and their associated scoring methods exist. Shah et al. (1989) expanded the scoring categories to improve the scale discriminability. Others have simplified the scoring system, while incorporating additional categories, to sum to a maximum of 20 points.

Historical Background

The BI evolved over a 10-year period from the mid-1950s until its publication in 1964. It was developed to permit nursing staff to assess the ability of patients with neuro-muscular and musculoskeletal disorders to care for themselves. It was one of the first measures of activities of daily living (ADL) to be developed. Since its initial publication, it has been modified to both expand and restrict the item scoring. The BI is widely used in rehabilitation centers, despite subsequent investigations identifying problems with the scaling and sum-scoring system. The BI remains popular as it includes the key physical and self-care items important for discharge planning and is simple to use.

Following the appearance of the BI, many other indices of function have been developed, underlining the importance of this type of tool in rehabilitation practice. The BI and the Functional Independence Measure (FIM) are the two most widely used measures of ADL in stroke research. The BI tends to be used more frequently in Europe, while the FIM is more likely to be used in North America.

Psychometric Data

The original version of the BI was developed without the investigation of content validity for item inclusion or validity of the scoring system. Many authors have questioned and subsequently suggested modifications to the scoring system. Most recently, de Morton et al. (2008) used Rasch analysis to investigate the validity of item score summation for the BI's original and modified versions. They found that score summation was not valid and although rescoring may improve the validity of the data collected at discharge, methods for rescoring outcome measures are not commonly used in rehabilitation.

Many studies have found the BI to have high inter-rater and retest reliability. The low number of scoring categories for some individual items means that the BI is less likely to be as discriminative or responsive to change as scales such as the Functional Independence Measure (FIM), which has seven scoring categories for each item.

Despite problems with some psychometric properties of the BI, it has good clinical utility in that it requires little staff training, is quick and easy to administer, and costs nothing.

Clinical Uses

The BI is widely used in inpatient rehabilitation settings. It encompasses most of the important physical aspects of daily function but does not directly address impairment to communication, cognition, or hearing and vision. The BI is simple and easy to use with well-defined categories; so minimal training or familiarization is required.

Cross-References

► Functional Independence Measure
► Rivermead Mobility Index

References and Readings

de Morton, N., Keating, J., & Davidson, M. (2008). Rasch analysis of the Barthel index in the assessment of hospitalized older patients after admission for an acute medical condition. *Archives of Physical Medicine and Rehabilitation, 89*(4), 641–647.

Mahoney, F., & Barthel, D. (1965). Functional evaluation: The Barthel index. *Maryland State Medical Journal, 14*, 61–65.

McDowell, I., & Newell, C. (1996). *Measuring health - a guide to rating scales and questionnaires* (2nd ed. pp. 56–63). New York: Oxford University Press.

Sangha, H., Lipson, D., Foley, N., Salter, K., Bhogal, S., Pohani, G., & Teasell, R. W. (2005). A comparison of the Barthel index and the functional independence measure as outcome measures in stroke rehabilitation: Patterns of disability scale usage in clinical trials. *International Journal of Rehabilitation Research, 28*(2), 135–139.

Shah, S., Vanclay, F., & Cooper, B. (1989). Improving the sensitivity of the Barthel index for stroke rehabilitation. *Journal of Clinical Epidemiology, 42*(8), 703–709.

Basal and Ceiling Rules

Matthew J. L. Page
Allegheny General Hospital, Pittsburgh, PA, USA
Psychology, Allegheny Health Network, Pittsburgh, PA, USA

Synonyms

Entry and discontinue rules

Definition

A basal and ceiling rule refers to the entry point and discontinue point of a psychometric test. The purpose of basal and ceiling rules is to reduce the number of items an examinee is required to attempt, by eliminating items that are too easy and too difficult. Doing so reduces administration time and burden on the examinee.

Although specific start and stop rules and administration procedures vary across tests, basal and ceiling rules are generally used for tests in which the items are ordered from easiest to most difficult. The most common basal procedure is to first start at an early, easier item based on the examinee's age. The examinee is then required to *establish a basal* by completing a predetermined number of consecutive items correctly (e.g., three correct items in a row). In general, items are administered in reverse order, so that they are increasingly easier, until the basal is established. In doing so, the examiner can refrain from administering easier items below the basal, assuming that the examinee would be able to answer them correctly. Once the basal has been established, items are then administered in forward order, becoming increasingly more difficult. The test continues in this fashion until a ceiling rule has been met. Ceiling rules typically require that an examinee answer a predetermined number of consecutive items incorrectly (e.g., three misses in a row). Some ceiling rules require a certain number of misses out of a larger number of consecutive items (e.g., four misses across five consecutive items). Once the ceiling rule has been met, the examiner discontinues the test under the assumption that the examinee would continue to answer the remaining, more difficult items incorrectly.

After administration is complete, some tests follow a *double basal* rule. In this situation, the examinee has established an initial basal (by completing a set number of consecutive items correctly) and then subsequently completed an additional string of correct items to meet a second basal. Depending on the test, some procedures allow for the examiner to count all items below the second basal as correct, even if the examinee actually responded to some of them incorrectly. Because of the wide variability across administration protocols, it is vital for the examiner to be familiar with basal and ceiling rules prior to administration.

Current Knowledge

Although many test companies do not publish details regarding the development of their basal and ceiling rules, the general goal of the rules is to reduce the number of administered items while minimizing the effects of these rules on raw and standard scores. The Wechsler tests (e.g., WAIS-IV, WMS-IV, WISC-V) describe one such development procedure that may be commonly used among other test publishers. For these tests, national tryout data are used to determine the difficulty of all test items, to order them from easiest to hardest based on how frequently they are answered correctly in the sample. Start points are then set

low and revised upward in the standardization procedure to ensure that a minimal number of examinee raw scores (commonly 5%) change by moving the start point forward. The ideal starting item has a high pass rate in the normative sample, to minimize the occurrence of reversal procedures. Discontinue rules in the standardization procedure are also initially conservative and then adjusted down to minimize changes in examinee raw and age-adjusted standard scores. Additionally, discontinue rules are developed to maintain a high rank-order correlation (e.g., 0.98) of total raw scores before and after the adjustment. This ensures that the standardization sample subjects maintain the same position in their rank order relative to others in their age group.

See Also

▶ Ceiling Effect
▶ Floor Effect
▶ Item Difficulty
▶ Standard Scores
▶ Test Construction
▶ Testing the Limits

References and Readings

Wechsler, D. (2008). *Wechsler adult intelligence scale* (4th ed.). Bloominton: Pearson.
Wechsler, D. (2009). *Wechsler memory scale* (4th ed.). Bloominton: Pearson.
Wechsler, D. (2014). *Wechsler intelligence scale for children* (5th ed.). Bloomington: Pearson.

Basal Forebrain

Randall E. Merchant
Department of Neurosurgery, Virginia
Commonwealth University, Richmond, VA, USA

Definition

The basal forebrain is a collection of nuclei and tracts that lie near the bottom and front of the brain. It includes the nucleus basalis, diagonal band of Broca, and medial septal nuclei. This area's neurons are major producers of acetylcholine which is then distributed throughout the brain and most importantly to the cerebral cortex and amygdala. The basal forebrain is most commonly damaged by an aneurysm of the anterior communicating artery. When this occurs, there is a reduction in the amount of acetylcholine in the brain, leading to impaired learning, amnesia, and confabulation. A decrease in cholinergic output by neurons of the basal forebrain is also known to occur in cases of Alzheimer's disease and senile dementia.

Cross-References

▶ Anterior Communicating Artery

Basal Ganglia

Christina R. Marmarou[1], Matthew R. Parry[1] and Ekaterina Dobryakova[2]
[1]Neurosurgery, Virginia Commonwealth University, Richmond, VA, USA
[2]Traumatic Brain Injury Research, Kessler Foundation, West Orange, NJ, USA

Synonyms

Basal nuclei

Definition

The basal ganglia refer specifically to a group of subcortical structures considered as extrapyramidal motor components. These components include caudate and putamen, substantia nigra, subthalamic nucleus, and globus pallidus (GP). Figure 1 depicts major circuitry within the basal ganglia.

Current Knowledge

Role in behavior and cognition. Rosvold demonstrated a topographical coupling between the prefrontal cortex and basal ganglia (Rosvold 1972; Johnson et al. 1968; Middleton and Strick 2000; Averbeck et al. 2014). Recent neuroimaging findings using functional magnetic resonance imaging (Arsalidou et al. 2013) and diffusion tensor imaging tools (Kotz et al. 2013) confirmed such topographical organization between the basal ganglia and the prefrontal cortex. Considering the major outflow of the basal ganglia to the thalamus (Haber and Calzavara 2009), it is not surprising that a substantial amount of research strongly supports the role of the basal ganglia in higher-order behavioral and cognitive tasks (Haber and Knutson 2010). Much of this research relies on striatal dopaminergic deficit and cortical lesion models in both human patients and animal models.

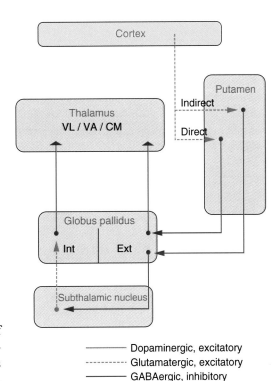

Basal Ganglia, Fig. 1 Basal ganglia circuitry. Diagram illustrates only major direct and indirect circuits. Significant cortical input is active at every level (not shown)

Studies in Parkinson's disease (PD) patients uncover the importance of the basal ganglia in attention – the behavior of target focusing in the presence of distractors (Brown et l. 1998). Levodopa therapy among PD patients improves motor behavior *and* attentional set-shifting; the absence of striatal dopamine has been shown to impair dual-task performance, self-monitoring (Brown and Marsden 1991; Brown et al. 1998; Taylor et al. 1986), and certain types of learning (Shohamy 2011). For example, PD patients demonstrate significant impairment in Petrides' self-ordered pointing task (Petrides and Milner 1982; West et al. 1998).

The basal ganglia have been shown to regulate temporal coupling and ordering of both motor and nonmotor sequences (Malapani et al. 1998; Kotz et al. 2009). Interestingly, a role in auditory rhythm detection and generation has been supported (Grahn and Brett 2007, 2008); this is analogous to the well-established role of the basal ganglia in motor timing and pattern generation, making the circuitry a "rhythm-pattern generator" both in executive (motor) and perceptual (cognitive) realms. The implications of this and similar work for the perceptual and executive aspects of language are well demonstrated (Kotz et al. 2009). For example, Smits-Bandstra et al. have described the basal ganglia in the setting of persons who stutter (Smits-Bandstra and De Nil 2007).

The basal ganglia are involved in a number of other higher-order cognitive functions. For instance, problem-solving tasks that activate the prefrontal cortex also activate the basal ganglia. Recent research has shown that the basal ganglia are significantly involved in learning, including motor skill learning, sequence learning, habit learning, automaticity, and category learning (Ashby et al. 2010; Seger 2008; Tricomi et al. 2009; Tricomi and Fiez 2008). Further, different subregions of the basal ganglia have been shown to process learning stimuli under different time scales and fulfill different roles during learning. For example, it has been shown that the anterior part of the basal ganglia (head of the caudate nucleus) is involved in learning through immediate feedback, while posterior regions of the basal ganglia (the putamen and GP) are involved in learning through feedback presented with a delay between action and outcome (Dobryakova and Tricomi 2013). The basal ganglia are also involved in a number of other cognitive functions including working memory (e.g., Baier et al. 2010), attentional systems (Sarter et al. 2006), and executive decision-making and control (Ino et al. 2010; Kim and Hikosaka 2013). While many of the behaviors engaged in seem simple and are taken for granted, these daily behaviors are really patterns of highly organized behaviors with very specific goals and purposes. As tasks are learned and practiced, they become automated and require little to no conscious control. The basal ganglia play a critical role in the smooth and efficient operation of such highly automated behaviors and as such are part of the complex "executive" system of the brain. Thus, the basal ganglia are critical in performing everyday practical tasks in an effortless and efficient manner (Koziol and Budding 2009).

Organization. The *striatal complex* is composed of the caudate nucleus and the putamen (Graybiel 2000). The caudate nucleus can be further subdivided into the head, body, and tail that play separable roles in cognition (Seger 2008). Embryologically the same, the caudate and putamen are separated by the internal capsule. Striosomes and matrix constitute a chemical and functional separation of the striatal complex: striosomes are areas of low acetylcholinesterase and high neuropeptide content, whereas matrix regions are rich in acetylcholinesterase (Bernacer et al. 2007). This difference in acetylcholinesterase content provides a convenient histochemical differentiation between neostriatal regions (DiFiglia et al. 1976).

Striatal function. The GABAergic cells of the striatum project to the internal segment of GP and substantia nigra (striosomes project mainly to pars compacta; matrix projects mainly to pars reticulata). These nuclei also receive substance-P and enkephalinergic input from the striatum (Menguala et al. 1999). The striatum tonically inhibits its pallidal and nigral targets.

The striatum itself receives inhibitory GABAergic projections from substantia nigra pars reticulata (Boyes and Bolam 2007). Major excitatory input is found in glutamatergic projections from thalamus (centromedian and parafascicular nuclei) and cortex (several motor areas), as well as dopaminergic input from substantia nigra pars compacta (Kubota et al. 1987). The latter dopaminergic input terminates in both D1 and D2 dopamine receptor subtypes, an important determinant in *excitation or inhibition* of striatal neurons (Surmeier et al. 2007).

The *substantia nigra* (*SN*) generally refers to two nuclei, pars compacta and pars reticulata (SNpc, SNpr, respectively). The SN lies within the midbrain, caudal to the crus cerebri and rostral to the red nucleus (Haines 2002). The SNpc contains dopaminergic neurons, while the SNpr contains mostly GABAergic neurons. Intra-nigral connections serve as modulatory loops: GABAergic input to SNpc decreases dopaminergic activity within the pars compacta; dopaminergic input to SNpr decreases GABAergic activity (Boyes and Bolam 2007; DeLong and Wichmann 2007).

Nigral function. The pars reticulata provides tonic inhibition of the thalamus, while the major function of the pars compacta is dopaminergic input to the striatum (Haines 2002).

The *subthalamic nucleus* (STN) is inferior to the thalamus and medial to the GP; a biconvex-shaped structure, the STN is surrounded by dense bundles of myelinated fibers. The internal capsule separates the STN from the GP (Haines 2004). Three major fiber tracts are associated with the STN: the subthalamic fasciculus (STF), the ansa lenticularis (AL), and the lenticular fasciculus (LF). The STF connects the STN and GP, crossing the internal capsule; the AL connects the GPi and the thalamus and differs from the STF in that it does not directly cross the internal capsule. Lastly, the LF crosses the internal capsule and ultimately joins the AL to form the thalamic fasciculus (or the H1 field of Forel).

Subthalamic function. The STN is thought to modulate the entire circuitry of the basal ganglia (Hamani et al. 2004).

The *GP* consists of two segments: internal (medial, GPi) and external (lateral, GPe). The nucleus is bounded medially by the internal capsule and laterally by the putamen (Haines 2004). Frequently, the term "lentiform nucleus" is used to refer to the GP and putamen together.

Pallidal function. The internal segment tonically inhibits the ventroanterior and ventrolateral nuclei of the thalamus. The external segment tonically inhibits the STN and provides transient inhibition to the internal segment (DeLong and Wichmann 2007). It is convenient to consider the GP as the "gateway" between the basal ganglia and the thalamus. The thalamus, in turn, relays to the motor areas of the cortex.

The basal ganglia have been described in terms of functionally opposing direct and indirect pathways. Broadly, the direct pathway promotes VA/VL thalamic relay to cortex, while the indirect pathway inhibits such traffic. The following description of direct and indirect pathways is a summary and integration of previous sources.

Direct pathway. The VA/VL thalamic complex is under tonic inhibition from both GPi and SNpr; transient inhibition of these nuclei is provided by the striatum. In this way, excitation of the striatum inhibits GPi output to the thalamus, and the net effect is *disinhibition* of the VA/VL thalamic complex. The activation of striatal GABAergic projections to SNpr and GPi has two sources: cortical glutamatergic stimulation and nigral dopaminergic stimulation acting upon D1 striatal receptors. In this way, the direct pathway is a case of thalamic disinhibition by suppression of GPi activity.

Indirect pathway. If the direct pathway is considered as a suppression of GPi activity leading to disinhibition of the thalamus, the indirect pathway is described as suppression of the GPe leading to disinhibition of STN. Tonic inhibition of STN comes from GPe (whereas tonic inhibition of thalamus comes from GPi). The striatum serves to transiently inhibit GPe (as well as inhibit GPi as previously described). The striatum contains both D1 and D2 dopamine receptors. While the direct pathway uses D1 receptors, the D2 subtype is the main striatal receptor of the indirect pathway. SNpc inhibits striatal output to GPe through these D2 receptors.

In general terms, activity through the direct pathway promotes thalamocortical activity by disinhibition of the thalamus; the indirect pathway suppresses thalamocortical activity. This opposing circuitry is thought to modulate the net effect of the basal ganglia on thalamic output.

Illness

Huntington disease, hyperkinetic, choreiform disease, autosomal dominant inheritance, and pathological CAG trinucleotide repeats (Shao and Diamond 2007). Mechanism of disease may include enhanced corticostriate activity and enhanced thalamic disinhibition (Centonze et al. 2007). The Unified Huntington's Disease Rating Scale is widely accepted to represent an array of disease signs and symptoms (Huntington Study Group 1996). Dopamine and glutamate antagonists as well as GABAergic therapy have been described (Bonelli et al. 2004). Speech and gait therapy are often employed. Depression is common among Huntington's disease patients, and antidepressant treatment has been described (Korenyi and Whittier 1967).

PD, late idiopathic onset, and early-onset signs include resting tremor, oculomotor disturbance, and loss of postural reflexes, among other dyskinesias. Pathology includes loss of nigral dopaminergic neurons, although the cause is multivariable (Nagatsu and Sawada 2007; Bergman et al. 1998). Treatment can involve levodopa therapy and decarboxylase antagonists, among a variety of other pharmacological agents (Pahwa 2006). Surgical intervention is a relatively recent development, often targeting STN and GPi (Kern and Kumar 2007).

Other basal ganglia disorders: Wilson disease, Sydenham chorea, and ballismus.

Summary of Major Components and Circuitry (See Fig. 1)

Striatum: Caudate, Putamen

Afferent
Thalamostriatal: glutamatergic, mainly from caudal intralaminar nuclei (centromedian and parafascicular nuclei); glutamatergic

Corticostriatal: glutamatergic, from primary-, pre-, supplementary-, and cingulate-motor areas

Nigrostriatal: dopaminergic from pars compacta, fibers terminate on two separate dopamine receptor types, also GABAergic from pars reticulata

Efferent
Striatopallidal: GABAergic and substance-P projections to internal segment, GABAergic and enkephalin projections to external segment of globus pallidus

Striatonigral: striosomal GABAergic projections to pars compacta, matrix GABAergic and enkephalinergic projections to pars reticulata

Globus Pallidus: Internal, External Segments

Afferent
Striatopallidal (see above)

Subthalamopallidal: glutamatergic mainly to internal segment

Nigropallidal: dopaminergic to external segment

Efferent
Pallidothalamic: GABAergic from internal segment mainly to ventral anterior nucleus of thalamus

Pallidonigral: GABAergic from external segment to pars reticulata

Pallidosubthalamic: GABAergic from external segment to subthalamic nucleus

Substantia Nigra: Pars Compacta, Pars Reticulata

Afferent
Striatonigral and pallidonigral (see above)

Subthalamonigral: glutamatergic to pars reticulata

Efferent
Nigrostriatal and nigropallidal (see above)

Nigrosubthalamic: dopaminergic from pars compacta to subthalamus

Nigrothalamic: GABAergic to ventromedian and ventrolateral nuclei of thalamus

Subthalamic Nucleus

Afferent
Pallidosubthalamic and nigrosubthalamic (see above)

Efferent
Subthalamopallidal and subthalamonigral (see above)

Cross-References

▶ Action Tremor
▶ Afferent
▶ Assisted Living
▶ Ataxia
▶ Bradykinesia
▶ Caudate Nucleus
▶ Cerebral Cortex
▶ Cholinesterase Inhibitors
▶ Chorea
▶ Cortical Motor Pathways
▶ Cortical-Subcortical Loop
▶ Corticobasal Degeneration
▶ Deep Brain Stimulator (Parkinson's)
▶ Diencephalon
▶ Dopamine-Related Dyskinesia
▶ Dystonia
▶ Efferent
▶ Essential Tremor
▶ Executive Functioning
▶ Gait Disorders
▶ Globus Pallidus
▶ Huntington's Disease
▶ Internal Capsule
▶ Masked Facies
▶ Mesolimbic Dopaminergic Projections
▶ Midbrain
▶ Movement Disorders
▶ Pallidotomy
▶ Pallidum
▶ Parkinson Plus Syndromes
▶ Parkinson's Disease
▶ Parkinson's Dementia
▶ Physiologic Tremor
▶ Putamen
▶ Pyramidal System

▶ Rigidity
▶ Striatum
▶ Substantia Nigra
▶ Supplementary Motor Area (SMA)
▶ Tardive Dyskinesia
▶ Thalamus
▶ Tremor

References and Readings

Arsalidou, M., Duerden, E. G., & Taylor, M. J. (2013). The centre of the brain: Topographical model of motor, cognitive, affective, and somatosensory functions of the basal ganglia. *Human Brain Mapping, 34*(11), 3031–3054. https://doi.org/10.1002/hbm.22124.

Ashby, F. G., Turner, B. O., & Horvitz, J. C. (2010). Cortical and basal ganglia contributions to habit learning and automaticity. *Trends in Cognitive Sciences, 14*(5), 208–215. https://doi.org/10.1016/j.tics.2010.02.001.

Averbeck, B. B., Lehman, J., Jacobson, M., & Haber, S. N. (2014). Estimates of projection overlap and zones of convergence within frontal-striatal circuits. *Journal of Neuroscience, 34*(29), 9497–9505. https://doi.org/10.1523/JNEUROSCI.5806-12.2014.

Baier, B., Karnath, H. O., & Dieterich, M. (2010). Keeping memory clear and stable-the contribution of human basal ganglia and prefrontal cortex to working memory. *The Journal of Neuroscience: The Official Journal of the Society for Neuroscience, 30*(29), 9788–9792.

Bergman, H., Feingold, A., Nini, A., Raz, A., Slovin, H., Abeles, M., et al. (1998). Physiological aspects of information processing in the basal ganglia of normal and parkinsonian primates. *Trends in Neurosciences, 21*(1), 32–38.

Bernacer, J., Prensa, L., & Gimenez-Amaya, J. M. (2007). Cholinergic interneurons are differentially distributed in the human striatum. *PloS One, 2*(11), e1174.

Bonelli, R. M., Wenning, G. K., & Kapfhammer, H. P. (2004). Huntington's disease: Present treatments and future therapeutic modalities. *International Clinical Psychopharmacology, 19*(2), 51–62.

Boyes, J., & Bolam, J. P. (2007). Localization of GABA receptors in the basal ganglia. *Progress in Brain Research, 160*, 229–243.

Brown, R., & Marsden, C. (1991). Dual task performance and processing resources in normal subjects and patients with Parkinson's disease. *Brain, 114*, 215–231.

Brown, R., Soliveri, P., & Jahanshahi, M. (1998). Executive process in Parkinson's disease – random number generation and response suppression. *Neuropsychologia, 36*, 1355–1362.

Centonze, D., Bernardi, G., & Koch, G. (2007). Mechanisms of disease: Basic-research-driven investigations in humans-the case of hyperkinetic disorders. *Nature Clinical Practical Neurology, 3*(10), 572–580.

Chang, H. T. (1988). Dopamine-acetylcholine interaction in the rat striatum: A dual-labeling immunocytochemical study. *Brain Research Bulletin, 21*, 295–304.

DeLong, M. R., & Wichmann, T. (2007). Circuits and circuit disorders of the basal ganglia. *Archives of Neurology, 64*, 20–24.

DiFiglia, M., Pasik, P., & Pasik, T. (1976). A Golgi study of neuronal types in the neostriatum of monkeys. *Brain Research, 114*, 245–256.

Dobryakova, E., & Tricomi, E. (2013). Basal ganglia engagement during feedback processing after a substantial delay. *Cognitive, Affective, & Behavioral Neuroscience, 13*(4), 725–736. https://doi.org/10.3758/s13415-013-0182-6.

Grahn, J., & Brett, M. (2007). Rhythm and beat perception in motor areas of the brain. *Journal of Cognitive Neuroscience, 19*, 893–906.

Grahn, J., & Brett, M. (2008). Impairment of beat-based rhythm discrimination in Parkinson's disease. *Cortex, 45*, 54–61.

Graybiel, A. M. (2000). The basal ganglia. *Current Biology, 10*(14), R509–R511. https://doi.org/10.1016/S0960-9822(00)00593-5.

Haber, S. N., & Calzavara, R. (2009). The cortico-basal ganglia integrative network: The role of the thalamus. *Brain Research Bulletin, 78*(2–3), 69–74. https://doi.org/10.1016/j.brainresbull.2008.09.013.

Haber, S. N., & Knutson, B. (2010). The reward circuit: Linking primate anatomy and human imaging. *Neuropsychopharmacology, 35*(1), 4–26. https://doi.org/10.1038/npp.2009.129.

Haines, D. (2002). *Fundamental neuroscience*. New York: Churchill Livingstone.

Hamani, C., Saint-Cyr, J., Fraser, J., Kaplitt, M., & Lozano, A. (2004). The subthalamic nucleus in the context of movement disorders. *Brain, 127*(Pt 1), 4–20.

Huntington Study Group. (1996). Unified Huntington's disease rating scale: Reliability and consistency. *Movement Disorders, 11*, 136–142.

Ino, T., Nakai, R., Azuma, T., Kimura, T., & Fukuyama, H. (2010). Differential activation of the striatum for decision making and outcomes in a monetary task with gain and loss. *Cortex, 46*(1), 2–14. https://doi.org/10.1016/j.cortex.2009.02.022.

Johnson, T., Rosvold, H., & Mishkin, M. (1968). Projections from behaviorally-defined sectors of the prefrontal cortex to the basal ganglia, septum, and diencephalons of the monkey. *Experimental Neurology, 21*, 20–34.

Kern, D., & Kumar, R. (2007). Deep brain stimulation. *The Neurologist, 13*(5), 237–252.

Kim, H. F., & Hikosaka, O. (2013). Distinct basal ganglia circuits controlling behaviors guided by flexible and stable values. *Neuron, 79*(5), 1001–1010. https://doi.org/10.1016/j.neuron.2013.06.044.

Korenyi, C., & Whittier, J. R. (1967). Drug treatment in 117 cases of Huntington's disease with special reference to fluphenazine (Prolixin). *Psychiatric Quarterly, 41*, 203–210.

Kotz, S., Schwartze, M., & Schmidt-Kassow, M. (2009). Non-motor basal ganglia functions: A review and proposal for a model of sensory predictability in auditory language perception. *Cortex, 45*, 982–990.

Kotz, S. A., Anwander, A., Axer, H., & Knösche, T. R. (2013). Beyond cytoarchitectonics: The internal and external connectivity structure of the caudate nucleus. *PloS One, 8*(7), e70141. https://doi.org/10.1371/journal.pone.0070141.

Koziol, L. F., & Budding, D. E. (2009). *Subcortical structures and cognition*. New York: Springer.

Kubota, Y., Inagaki, S., Shimada, S., Kito, S., Eckenstein, F., et al. (1987). Neostriatal cholinergic neurons receive direct synaptic inputs from dopaminergic axons. *Brain Research, 413*, 179–184.

Malapani, C., Rakitin, B., Levy, R., Meck, W., Deweer, B., Dubois, B., et al. (1998). Coupled temporal memories in Parkinson's disease: A dopamine-related dysfunction. *Journal of Cognitive Neuroscience, 10*, 316–331.

Menguala, E., de las Herasb, S., Erroa, E., Lanciegoa, J. L., & Gimenez-Amaya, J. M. (1999). Thalamic interaction between the input and the output systems of the basal ganglia. *Journal of Chemical Neuroanatomy, 16*(3), 185–197.

Middleton, F. A., & Strick, P. L. (2000). Basal ganglia and cerebellar loops: Motor and cognitive circuits. *Brain Research Reviews, 31*(2–3), 236–250.

Nagatsu, T., & Sawada, M. (2007). Biochemistry of postmortem brains in Parkinson's disease: Historical overview and future prospects. *Journal of Neural Transmission, Supplement, 72*, 113–120.

Pahwa, R. (2006). Understanding Parkinson's disease: An update on current diagnostic and treatment strategies. *Journal of the American Medical Directors Association, 7*(7 Suppl. 2), 4–10.

Petrides, M., & Milner, B. (1982). Deficits on subject-ordered tasks after frontal and temporal lobe lesions in man. *Neuropsychologia, 20*, 601–604.

Rosvold, H. (1972). The frontal lobe system: Cortical-subcortical interrelationships. *Acta Neurobiologica Experimentalis (Warsaw), 32*, 439–460.

Sarter, M., Gehring, W. J., & Kozak, R. (2006). More attention must be paid: The neurobiology of attentional effort. *Brain Research Reviews, 51*(2), 145–160. https://doi.org/10.1016/j.brainresrev.2005.11.002.

Seger, C. a. (2008). How do the basal ganglia contribute to categorization? Their roles in generalization, response selection, and learning via feedback. *Neuroscience and Biobehavioral Reviews, 32*(2), 265–278. https://doi.org/10.1016/j.neubiorev.2007.07.010.

Shao, J., & Diamond, M. I. (2007). Polyglutamine diseases: Emerging concepts in pathogenesis and therapy. *Human Molecular Genetics, 15*(16), R115–R123. Spec No 2.

Shohamy, D. (2011). Learning and motivation in the human striatum. *Current Opinion in Neurobiology, 21*(3), 408–414. https://doi.org/10.1016/j.conb.2011.05.009.

Smits-Bandstra, S., & De Nil, L. (2007). Sequence skill learning in persons who stutter: Implications for cortico- striato-thalamo-cortical dysfunction. *Journal of Fluency Disorders, 32*(4), 251–278.

Surmeier, D. J., Ding, J., Day, M., Wang, Z., & Shen, W. (2007). D1 and D2 dopamine-receptor modulation of striatal glutamatergic signaling in striatal medium spiny neurons. *Trends in Neurosciences, 30*(5), 228–235.

Taylor, A., Saint-Cyr, J., & Lang, A. (1986). Frontal lobe dysfunction in Parkinson's disease: The cortical focus of neostriatal outflow. *Brain, 109*, 845–883.

Tricomi, E., & Fiez, J. a. (2008). Feedback signals in the caudate reflect goal achievement on a declarative memory task. *NeuroImage, 41*(3), 1154–1167. https://doi.org/10.1016/j.neuroimage.2008.02.066.

Tricomi, E., Balleine, B. W., & O'Doherty, J. P. (2009). A specific role for posterior dorsolateral striatum in human habit learning. *The European Journal of Neuroscience, 29*(11), 2225–2232. https://doi.org/10.1111/j.1460-9568.2009.06796.x.

West, R., Ergis, A., Winocur, G., & Saint-Cyr, J. (1998). The contribution of impaired working memory monitoring to performance of the self-ordered pointing task in normal aging and Parkinson's disease. *Neuropsychology, 12*, 546–554.

BASC-3

Robert A. Altmann[1], Cecil R. Reynolds[2], Randy W. Kamphaus[3] and Kimberly J. Vannest[4]
[1]A-PsychEd Publication Services, Minneapolis, MN, USA
[2]Texas A&M University, College Station, TX, USA
[3]College of Education, The University of Oregon, Eugene, OR, USA
[4]Department of Educational Psychology, Texas A&M University, College Station, TX, USA

Description

The Behavior Assessment System for Children, Third Edition (BASC-3; Reynolds and Kamphaus 2015) is a multimethod, multidimensional system of related instruments that can be used to conduct a comprehensive assessment of behavioral and emotional functioning of children, adolescents, and young adults aged 2–25 years. The BASC-3 is a multimethod in that it has the following components, which may be used individually or in any combination:

1. A Teacher Rating Scale (TRS) and a Parent Rating Scale (PRS) that gather multiple perspectives of observable behavior across settings and raters, using age-appropriate forms
2. A Self-Report of Personality (SRP) that a child, adolescent, or young adult can use to describe his or her behaviors, emotions, and self-perceptions
3. A Structured Developmental History (SDH) form that provides information about the course of development and family history that are important to make accurate diagnosis
4. A Student Observation System (SOS) form that can be used for recording and classifying directly observed classroom behavior, using a smartphone, laptop computer, or paper form

The BASC-3 is multidimensional in that it measures numerous aspects of behavior and personality, including positive (adaptive) as well as negative (clinical) dimensions. Like its previous editions (BASC-2, Reynolds and Kamphaus 2004; BASC, Reynolds and Kamphaus 1992), the BASC-3 forms remain psychometrically strong instruments that are easy to complete and relevant to both school-based and clinically based settings. The norm samples are new and reflect the latest US Census estimates available at the time of the standardization project. In addition to new test items, the BASC-3 TRS, PRS, and SRP now offer Clinical Indexes and new Executive Functioning Indexes. The Clinical Indexes were developed based on items that discriminated between clinical and nonclinical samples and may be particularly useful for helping to rule in or rule out certain clinical diagnoses or educational classifications and for assessing the amount of functional impairment being experienced by the child or adolescent. The Executive Functioning Indexes found on the TRS and PRS provide insight into specific executive functioning domains that are important when working with deficits such as attention deficit hyperactivity disorder (ADHD), without the need for additional rating scales. The Self-Report of Personality Interview form, for ages 6–7, has been redesigned. Rather than simply reading a series of items to the child, a total of 14 items are read to the child. Responses are obtained using a semi-structured format that helps to elicit more natural responses by the child that can be used to supplement findings from the BASC-3 TRS and PRS and aid in treatment planning. The SDH form now offers an option for paired administration with the PRS. When both are administered digitally, additional items will be automatically included during the SDH administration based on PRS results, providing additional context that can be helpful for making accurate classification or diagnostic decisions.

While paper administration and hand scoring options are available for the TRS, PRS, SRP, SOS, and SDH forms, the primary way to administer and score BASC-3 forms is digitally using the Q-global web-based scoring and reporting platform. Forms can be administered locally on a laptop or web-enabled digital handheld device, or a web link can be emailed to a respondent to complete a form via a secured testing portal. Upon completion, forms can be immediately scored, and reports generated. Report options have been consolidated from previous editions. The basic report offered is the Interpretive Summary Report, which provides extensive score profiles, along with basic interpretive and clinical interpretive information, critical items, and item-by-scale listings. The most comprehensive report offered is the Interpretive Summary Report with Intervention Recommendations. This report provides intervention recommendations based on the obtained score profiles and is based on the BASC-3 Behavior Intervention Guide (Vannest et al. 2015a; see below for more detailed information).

Like its previous editions, the BASC-3 remains committed to a triangulated view of the child's behavioral and emotional functioning by examining behavior in multiple settings (at home and school) and evaluating the child's emotions, personality, and self-perceptions.

Key Features of the BASC-3

The BASC-3 has numerous features that make it one of the most sophisticated and reliable systems of behavior assessment available today. A hallmark of the BASC tools has been the comprehensiveness and breadth of behavioral and emotional problems covered. The number of problem areas included on the BASC-3 tools is useful for helping to rule in (and out) behavioral and emotional functioning deficits that can look similar in nature, providing a distinct advantage over more narrowband classification instruments. The information contained on the BASC-3 tools are directly relevant to behavioral disorders found in the *Diagnostic and Statistical Manual of Mental Disorders, Fifth Edition* (American Psychiatric Association 2013), as well as general categories of problems addressed in legislation such as the Individuals with Disabilities Education Act (e.g., the diagnosis of severe emotional disturbance). In addition, the inclusion of adaptive behaviors on the BASC-3 TRS, PRS, and SRP forms provides clinicians with information that can be used to help leverage a child's or adolescent's existing strengths when developing individualized intervention or treatment plans. Another key BASC-3 feature is a grounded development approach that emphasizes a balance of both theory and statistics, resulting in tools with strong psychometric properties and clinical utility. Finally, the BASC-3 tools promote ease of administration and scoring, and the inclusion of scales that can help detect threats to the validity and usefulness of obtained responses makes the BASC-3 applicable to numerous school, clinical, and forensic applications.

Historical Background

The original BASC (Reynolds and Kamphaus 1992) was published by American Guidance Service, following 7 years of development work. It was standardized for use with children and adolescents ages 4–18 years and was rapidly adopted as the most frequently administered behavior scales in the schools in the United States. Spanish versions were subsequently developed for international applications, as well as smaller research-only adaptations in several additional languages. The release of the second edition (BASC-2, Reynolds and Kamphaus 2004) continued to be well received by users in both the United States and a number of other countries. Several other tools in the BASC-2 family were released in subsequent years, including the Parenting Relationship Questionnaire (PRQ, Kamphaus and Reynolds 2006), the Behavioral and Emotional Screening System (BESS; Kamphaus and Reynolds 2007), the BASC-2 Intervention Guide (Vannest et al. 2008), and the BASC-2 Progress Monitor (Reynolds and Kamphaus 2010). These tools were consistent with the Response to Intervention movement in the US educational system that emphasized a screening, intervention, and monitoring approach to addressing a student's functional deficits. The BASC-3 continues the tradition of innovation with improvements to existing instruments and the development of the new components described below.

Psychometric Data

The scales included on the TRS, PRS, and SRP are designed to be highly interpretable and are built around clearly specified constructs with matching item content, developed through a balance of theory and empirical data. The ease of scale interpretation is partly attributable to the items which comprise them. The approach used to develop the original BASC items involved surveying teachers, parents, and students about behaviors that were the most difficult to manage or behaviors that were the most disruptive; in addition, respondents were asked to provide examples of positive behaviors that were observed. This survey process was repeated during the BASC-3 standardization project, helping to ensure that the items written during the development of the original BASC remain relevant and that new behaviors deemed important were also included on the BASC-3 edition. Factor-analytic evidence presented in the BASC-3 Manual provides support for the overall scale and composite structure used for reporting results.

The BASC-3 scales and composites have high internal consistency and test-retest reliability. Most alpha coefficients for the BASC-3 subscales and composites exceed 0.80 and are sufficiently

reliable for application to diagnostic and treatment issues. Additionally, the BASC-3 offers various types of validity checks to help the clinician detect careless or untruthful responding, misunderstanding, or other threats to validity. The BASC-3 Manual demonstrates validity evidence for the proposed applications of the BASC-3 scales that is extensive and covers both theoretical and actuarial bases. Correlations with numerous other rating scales and self-reports are given as well as studies of a large number of clinical groups.

BASC-3 Uses

Clinical Diagnosis

The BASC-3 aids in the clinical diagnosis of disorders that are usually first apparent in childhood or adolescence. It assesses a variety of symptoms that are noted in the DSM-5. Because the components of the BASC-3 can be used separately or in combination, the BASC-3 may be easily used in residential settings, in clinics, or by private practitioners. The PRS and SDH can be completed by a parent while the child is being evaluated by the practitioner, thus reducing the practitioner's time in the data collection process. The rating scales, the SRP, and the SOS can be repeated on a regular basis to monitor a child's progress and response to treatment. It is highly desirable that diagnosis be linked clearly to intervention. In this respect, treatment planning can also be facilitated by the BASC-3. Problem behaviors can be delineated and targeted in a program leading to their reduction. A similar strategy can be used with deficits in adaptive skills.

Educational Classification

Differential diagnosis is becoming an increasingly important issue in school settings. This is partly because the complexity of many children's problems requires an array of interventions that must be tailored to the individual child's needs. Consequently, the BASC-3 is designed to be sensitive to numerous presenting problems in the classroom, including deficiencies in social skills, study skills, or other adaptive skills. Academic difficulties are frequently linked to behavior problems.

Syndromes such as ADHD and depression have known academic consequences; learning disabilities and intellectual disability are often associated with adjustment problems such as low self-concept or anxiety. It is strongly suggested that every child experiencing academic difficulties receives a behavioral assessment. Additionally, research demonstrates that good behavioral assessment of constructs such as attitude to school, attitude to teachers, study skills, attention problems, and adaptability, in tandem with cognitive assessment, improves the prediction of both school performance and response to intervention.

Program Evaluation

Repeated use of the BASC-3 TRS, PRS, SRP, and SOS can aid in identifying a child's progress in specific programs. Improvement in designated areas of behavior and in affective states may be noted, and the strengths and weaknesses of programs thus identified. The original BASC was shown in a number of evaluation studies to be sensitive to the effects of various intervention programs for young children (including the evaluation component of Head Start's Project Mastery) and adolescents (e.g., the evaluation by the Civilian Health and Medical Program of the Uniformed Services, or CHAMPUS, of the effectiveness of residential treatment for adolescents). These and other applications of the BASC in program evaluation are reviewed in Reynolds and Kamphaus (2002).

Forensic Evaluation

The BASC-3 is appropriate for use in legal or forensic settings. According to several US Supreme Court rulings of the 1990s, evidence of the psychometric properties of tests used in a forensic setting is crucial for determining the admissibility of expert testimony based on test results. Reynolds and Kamphaus (2002) provide examples of uses of the original BASC in forensic situations such as child custody evaluations, personal injury litigation, and juvenile certification.

The BASC-3 Manual contains considerable information on the reliability of scale scores and associated standard errors of measurement, on the normative samples, and on validation studies, all of which are considered by judges in determining admissibility of testimony based partially or wholly on test data. Also presented are additional crucial data on the ability of the BASC-3 scale scores to measure child and adolescent psychopathology and to discriminate among various diagnostic groups, capabilities that also are included in the consideration of admissible evidence. The BASC-3 is well established in clinical environments such as schools, child guidance centers, university clinics, and private practice settings in the United States and abroad. The use of tests in a wide variety of settings is important in establishing credibility and admissibility in various legal proceedings.

When choosing instruments for forensic evaluations, it is also important for clinicians to evaluate the instruments' ability to detect dissimulation (Reynolds and Kamphaus 2002). In court proceedings, individuals may have much to gain by appearing to have more or fewer problems than what actually exist. Because nearly any behavioral or emotional problem or disorder can be minimized or exaggerated, objective methods are needed to determine whether dissimulation has occurred. The BASC-3 has scales designed and tested for the detection of dissimulation in responding by parents, teachers, and children. In particular, the BASC-3 validity scales can identify exaggerated responding, minimization of problem reporting, inconsistencies, random answering patterns, and other response methods that lead to inaccurate depictions of the child's or adolescent's behavior.

Additional BASC-3 Components

The BASC-3 includes a variety of other instruments that can be used to help identify and improve behavioral and emotional functioning. Each of these instruments is described briefly below.

BASC-3 Behavioral and Emotional Screening System (BESS)

The BASC-3 BESS (Kamphaus and Reynolds 2015b) is designed to quickly and efficiently identify risk for behavioral or emotional problems and predict mental health and educational outcomes.

The BASC-3 BESS consists of two teacher forms (ages 3–5 and ages 6–18), two parent forms (ages 3–5 and ages 6–18), and one self-report form (ages 8–18). Each form of the BASC-3 BESS is brief and requires no prior training and coaching of the informant.

Each BASC-3 BESS form provides a Behavioral and Emotional Risk Index (BERI), which indicates the amount of risk a child or adolescent has of having or developing a behavioral or emotional problem. The teacher and parent forms offer additional subindex scores, including an Externalizing Risk Index, Internalizing Risk Index, and Adaptive Skills Risk Index. In addition to the BERI, the self-report form also provides subindex scores for an Internalizing Risk Index, a Self-Regulation Risk Index, and a Personal Adjustment Risk Index.

Using the same item response formats as the BASC-3 TRS and PRS, each BASC-3 BESS form produces a single score indicating "normal risk" (T = 20–60), "elevated risk" (61–70), or "extremely elevated risk" (T = 71 or higher). Validity indexes are provided for each form, and Spanish adaptations and translations are available for parent and student forms. Administration, scoring, and reporting (both individual- and group-level reports) are available on the Q-global testing platform.

The BASC-3 BESS manual includes a detailed discussion of development procedures and a separate chapter devoted to validity and reliability evidence collected to date. All BERI reliability coefficients exceed 0.90, and test-retest correlations are in the upper .80s or higher. A variety of correlational studies are presented, including the BASC-3 TRS, PRS, and SRP, along with other behavioral/emotional functioning tests. The BASC-3 BESS manual also provides a detailed discussion of promising screening practices, including the use of multiple "gates" (i.e., assessment stages that range from broad-based screening on all students to more detailed assessment/ evaluation on students identified at previous gates). In addition, the Manual discusses linking screening results with early intervention strategies aimed at preventing the onset of mental health disorders or unsuccessful educational outcomes.

BASC-3 Parenting Relationship Questionnaire (PRQ)

The BASC-3 Parenting Relationship Questionnaire (PRQ; Kamphaus and Reynolds 2015a) is designed to capture a parent's perspective of the parent-child relationship (or the perspective of a person serving a similar role). It assesses traditional parent-child dimensions such as attachment and involvement and also provides information on parenting style, parenting confidence, stress, and satisfaction with the child's school. The BASC-3 PRQ is used in clinical, pediatric, counseling, school, and other settings where there is a need to understand the nature of the parent-child relationship. It is particularly important when implementing home-based intervention strategies and/or treatment monitoring. The BASC-3 PRQ can be completed in approximately 15 minutes and is available in English and Spanish. It should be administered to mothers and fathers (or caregivers) of children ages 2–18 years. Administration, scoring, and reporting are available on the Q-global platform. The BASC-3 PRQ Manual provides information about the reliability and validity of evidence collected during the standardization stage of development. Internal consistency reliability coefficients for each scale were typically in the mid-.80s or higher. A variety of correlational studies are also presented.

BASC-3 Flex Monitor

The BASC-3 Flex Monitor (Reynolds and Kamphaus 2016) is used to monitor and track the effect of behavioral interventions implemented by a psychologist or other professionals in a school or clinical environment. Available via Q-global, the BASC-3 Flex Monitor provides a bank of over 700 behaviorally or emotionally based items that can be selected to create a customized monitoring form for teachers, parents, or students (via a self-report form) that enable score comparisons to a nationally representative population sample. While creating forms, users can automatically calculate reliability estimates that are based on a normative sample. In addition, the BASC-3 Flex Monitor offers a variety of standard forms that are available for immediate use, including inattention/hyperactivity, internalizing problems, disruptive behaviors, developmental social disorders, and school problems. Parent and self-report forms are available in both English and Spanish. Individual reports tracking progress on up to ten administrations of a form or aggregated group-based reports can be easily generated on the Q-global platform.

BASC-3 Behavior Intervention Guide

The BASC-3 Behavior Intervention Guide (Vannest et al. 2015a) provides evidence-based intervention strategies for 11 common types of emotional and behavioral problems: aggression, conduct problems, hyperactivity, attention problems, academic problems, anxiety, depression, somatization, functional communication, adaptability, and social skills. These interventions represent a compendium of the most effective strategies that have been published in empirically based research studies.

In addition to providing background characteristics and conditions of each behavioral or emotional problem area, each chapter provides a number of intervention strategies that are presented in a preparation, implementation, and evaluation format. The intervention steps that are provided can be easily used by behavior experts (e.g., psychologists, counselors, behavioral specialists) to promote more desirable behavior and reduce problem behaviors. The BASC-3 Behavior Intervention Guide also offers accompanying tools that are designed to promote intervention fidelity and positive outcomes, including parent tip sheets that promote and provide structured involvement by parents or caregivers, supplemental forms that accompany the intervention strategies (e.g., daily log journals, activities, sample forms, etc.), and a fidelity documentation checklist.

For small group or classroom-based solutions, the BASC-3 Behavioral and Emotional Skill Building Guide (Vannest et al. 2015b) can be used in general or special education settings to help promote positive behavioral and emotional functioning. Based on the foundations established in the BASC-3 Behavior Intervention Guide, this guide provides tier one and tier two intervention strategies in a classroom curriculum format, as well as additional strategies that are targeted for small group settings. Teachers can follow the lesson plans provided in the guide to teach schoolwide expectations using activities that are fast-paced and brief, lasting around 5 minutes each. Additional instructional strategies for classrooms and small groups are also available for the behavioral and emotional problems included in the BASC-3 Behavior Intervention Guide.

References and Readings

American Psychiatric Association. (2013). *Diagnostic and statistical manual of mental disorders* (5th ed.). Washington, DC: American Psychiatric Association.

Kamphaus, R. W., & Reynolds, C. R. (2006). *Parenting relationship questionnaire*. Minneapolis: Pearson.

Kamphaus, R. W., & Reynolds, C. R. (2007). *Behavioral and emotional screening system*. Minneapolis: Pearson.

Kamphaus, R. W., & Reynolds, C. R. (2015a). *BASC-3 parenting relationship questionnaire*. Bloomington: NCS Pearson Inc.

Kamphaus, R. W., & Reynolds, C. R. (2015b). *BASC-3 behavioral and emotional screening system*. Bloomington: NCS Pearson Inc.

Reynolds, C. R., & Kamphaus, R. W. (1992). *Behavior assessment system for children*. Bloomington: Pearson Assessments.

Reynolds, C. R., & Kamphaus, R. W. (2002). *The clinician's guide to the behavior assessment system for children*. New York: Guilford.

Reynolds, C. R., & Kamphaus, R. W. (2004). *Behavior assessment system for children* (2nd ed.). Bloomington: Pearson Assessments.

Reynolds, C. R., & Kamphaus, R. W. (2010). *BASC–2 progress monitor*. Bloomington: NCS Pearson Inc.

Reynolds, C. R., & Kamphaus, R. W. (2015). *Behavior assessment system for children* (3rd ed.). Bloomington: NCS Pearson, Inc. (BASC–3).

Reynolds, C. R., & Kamphaus, R. W. (2016). *BASC–3 Flex Monitor*. Bloomington: NCS Pearson, Inc.

Vannest, K. J., Reynolds, C. R., & Kamphaus, R. W. (2008). *Behavior assessment system for children – second edition (BASC-2) intervention guide for emotional and behavioral problems*. Bloomington: Pearson.

Vannest, K. J., Reynolds, C. R., & Kamphaus, R. W. (2015a). *BASC-3 behavior intervention guide*. Bloomington: Pearson.

Vannest, K. J., Reynolds, C. R., & Kamphaus, R. W. (2015b). *BASC-3 behavioral and emotional skill building guide*. Bloomington: Pearson.

Base Rate (Population)

Molly E. Zimmerman
Department of Psychology, Fordham University,
Bronx, NY, USA

Definition

The population prevalence of a variable of interest is known as the base rate.

Current Knowledge

Base rates can be calculated using the following formula (Gouvier 1999):

$$\text{Base rate} = \#\text{cases with condition of interest}/\#\text{cases in a population}$$

In neuropsychological settings, base rates are often used to characterize diagnostic accuracy and interpret the sensitivity and specificity of a clinical assessment. The sensitivity of a test is the probability of correctly identifying an individual with impaired functioning as actually being impaired, while the specificity of a test is the probability of correctly identifying an individual with normal functioning as actually being normal (Lezak et al. 2012). When the base rates of a condition are low, the sensitivity of a test may be misleading. When the base rates of a condition are high, the specificity of a test may be misleading (Podell et al. 2003). The neuropsychologist should consider base rates of a disorder when selecting tests for use in a specific population. Knowledge of base rates may also indicate that impairment cutoff scores should be adjusted to interpret diagnostic accuracy. Assessments of malingering or suboptimal effort should also be conducted with consideration of base rates for a particular condition of interest (Gouvier 1999).

Cross-References

▶ Sensitivity

References and Readings

Gouvier, W. D. (1999). Base rates and clinical decision making in neuropsychology. In J. J. Sweet (Ed.), *Forensic neuropsychology* (pp. 27–38). New York: Taylor & Francis.

Lezak, M. D., Howieson, D. B., Bigler, E. D., & Tranel, D. (2012). *Neuropsychological assessment*. Oxford: Oxford University Press.

Podell, K., Defina, P. A., Barrett, P., McCullen, A., & Goldberg, E. (2003). Assessment of neuropsychological functioning. In I. B. Weiner, D. K. Freedheim, J. A. Schinka, & W. F. Velicer (Eds.), *Handbook of psychology* (pp. 443–466). New York: Wiley.

Basic Achievement Skills Inventory

Kelly Broxterman[1], Doris S. Mok[2] and Alyssa Beukema[1]
[1]School Psychology, The Chicago School of Professional Psychology, Chicago, IL, USA
[2]Department of Psychology, Faculty of Social Sciences and Humanities University of Macau, Taipa, Macau SAR, China

Synonyms

BASI

Description

The Basic Achievement Skills Inventory (BASI) is a commercially published, norm-referenced achievement test that assesses math, reading, and language skills for children and adults. It is published by Pearson and was first made available in 2004. Information on the test is easily accessible through the publishers' webpage (http://www.pearsonassessments.com/basi.aspx), which includes relevant excerpts from the manual, a flash demonstration, training modules, sample reports, and others.

Forms

There are two forms: a comprehensive form and a survey form. The comprehensive form comprises six timed subtests: vocabulary, spelling, language mechanics, reading comprehension, math computation, and math application. The subtests can be administered independently to measure specific skills or in any combination. There are four grade levels (I–IV), 3rd–4th grade, 5th–6th grade, 7th–8th, and 9th–12th. The survey form is a screening tool comprising two subtests: verbal skills and math skills. Verbal skills are assessed using vocabulary, language mechanics, and reading comprehension questions, and math skills are assessed using math computation and math application questions. Student progress can be assessed through Form A with Fall norms (August to December) and Form B with Spring norms (January to July). A growth scale value (GSV) is made available to measure the progress of students.

Administration

The tests can be administered individually or in groups, timed or untimed; the comprehensive form takes about 2 h, and the survey form takes about 50 min to complete.

Scoring and Report

Scoring for the comprehensive form is available through Q-global web-based administration, Q local software, or mail-in scoring. The student summary report is a one-page report that summarizes the student's performance by skills composite, subtest, and learning objectives. The student summary report includes standard scores, percentile scores, age equivalents, and grade equivalents as well as a performance classification (low average, average to above average) by achievement area. A parent's report is included with each student report. The parent's report graphs percentile scores and includes a space for written comments. There is also an optional report available for level 4 of the BASI comprehensive version, titled the BASI college report. The college report shows how a student's BASI scores compared to the scores of a census-matched national sample at the student's grade level.

The adult summary report is a one-page report that summarizes an adult's performance by skills composite, subtest, and learning objectives. It includes percent correct, grade equivalent, and classification by achievement area.

Historical Background

Achilles N. Bardos, PhD, is the author of the test (http://www.unco.edu/cebs/SchoolPsych/faculty/BASI/index.html). The BASI was published in 2004. Content was based on curriculum standards from The Model Curriculum and Assessment Database (MCAD), a database used by educators to align with district, state, and national curriculum requirements and standards.

Psychometric Data

Standardization is reportedly based on stratified random sampling to match closely with the US Census 2000. For the comprehensive form, a grade-appropriate sample was stratified according to gender, race, parental education, and region. Standardization of Form A was based on 2,439 students tested during Fall 2002, and standardization of Form B was based on 2,130 students tested in Spring 2003. The survey form included a school-age standardization sample of 2,518 students (aged 8–18) tested in school settings and an adult sample of 2,452 adults (aged 19–80) recruited in a variety of settings.

Buros Institute test reviewers (Rhoades 2007; Trevisan 2007) reported the test-retest stability, internal consistency, and alternate-forms reliability to be fairly strong, with estimates ranging from 0.54 to 0.96 for individual subtest scores and 0.67–0.98 for composite scores. Test validity is established through the Iowa Tests of Basic Skills (ITBS), the Iowa Tests of Education Development (ITED), the Tests of Adult Basic Education (TABE), the Wechsler Individual Achievement Test Second Edition (WIAT-II), and the Woodcock Johnson Psychoeducational Battery III (WJ-III).

Clinical Uses

The author proposes that the comprehensive form provides a complete evaluation of academic skills to "(1) determine academic strengths and weaknesses; (2) screen for and assist in diagnosing learning disabilities in reading, writing and math; (3) place for college students; (4) make placement decisions for ESL, GED, and program placement; (5) track academic progress, (6) efficiently complete triennial evaluations for students with an IEPs or 504 plans; and (7) practice for or predict performance on high-stakes tests." Specific applications in four settings are proposed in the BASI Flash demonstration (http://www.pearsonassessments.com/basidemo/basi.swf): (1) K-12 school/educational setting, (2) corrections setting for intake and evaluation of offenders for placement in programs, (3) public safety for employment screening, and (4) adult and child clinical setting. In adult and child clinical settings, the BASI Comprehensive Form is recommended to be used as a time- and cost-effective screening, providing an overview of achievement or alternative for individually administered achievement test when detailed information is not needed.

Cross-References

▶ Academic Skills

References and Readings

Griffith, R. (2006). An examination of factors influencing differences in academic performance among active duty military students and naval reserve officer training corps scholarship students in a university setting. *Dissertation Abstracts International Section A 67*, 2071. Retrieved from PsycINFO database.

Rhoades, E. K. (2007). Test review of the basic achievement skills inventory. In K. F. Geisinger, R. A. Spies, J. F. Carlson, & B. S. Plake (Eds.), *The seventeenth mental measurements yearbook* [Electronic Version]. Retrieved 17 Feb 2009 from the Buros Institute's Test Reviews Online website: http://unl.edu/buros

Trevisan, M. S. (2007). Test review of the basic achievement skills inventory. In K. F. Geisinger, R. A. Spies, J. F. Carlson, & B. S. Plake (Eds.), *The seventeenth mental measurements yearbook* [Electronic Version]. Retrieved 17 Feb 2009 from the Buros Institute's Test Reviews Online website: http://unl.edu/buros

Basilar Artery

Elliot J. Roth
Department of Physical Medicine and Rehabilitation, Northwestern University, Feinberg School of Medicine, Chicago, IL, USA

Definition

The *basilar artery* provides blood to the brain. This artery and the two vertebral arteries comprise the *vertebrobasilar system*, which supplies blood to the posterior part of circle of Willis and connects ("anastomoses") with blood supplied to the anterior part of the circle of Willis from the carotid arteries. It arises from the confluence of the two vertebral arteries, next to the lower brain stem, ascends parallel to the brain stem, and gives rise to the anterior inferior cerebellar artery, which supplies part of the cerebellum, some smaller branches that supply the brain stem, and the superior cerebellar artery. It finally divides into the two posterior cerebral arteries (PCA). These supply the upper brain stem, the occipital lobe, and the posterior portion of the temporal lobes.

Current Knowledge

The clinical manifestations of basilar artery occlusion depend on the location of the occlusion, the extent of thrombus, and the collateral flow. Normally, the blood flows in an anterograde fashion from the vertebral arteries to the basilar artery up to its terminal branches. This pattern of flow may vary. If the proximal segment of the basilar artery is occluded and the occlusion resulted from a slowly progressive stenosis, collateralization occurs within the cerebellum into the circumferential branches of the basilar artery. In addition, flow can be reversed from the PCAs into the distal basilar artery. Thrombosis of the basilar artery causes various clinical syndromes that result from brainstem ischemia, including cranial nerve dysfunction, difficulty in swallowing and breathing, and at its most severe, locked-in syndrome. Basilar artery thrombosis is the most common cause of locked-in syndrome. Mortality rate of basilar artery occlusion is 70%, but this can be reduced substantially through the use of anti-thrombotic agents.

Cross-References

▶ Circle of Willis
▶ Posterior Cerebral Artery
▶ Vertebrobasilar System

Battery Approach

Molly E. Zimmerman
Department of Psychology, Fordham University, Bronx, NY, USA

Definition

A battery approach to neuropsychological assessment is the administration of multiple measures that cover a wide range of cognitive abilities to fully characterize an individual's neuropsychological strengths and weaknesses.

Current Knowledge

The battery approach is predicated on the existence of a variety of instruments that have been empirically developed to measure myriad aspects of neuropsychological function. Neuropsychological batteries generally contain a measure of general intellectual functioning or premorbid functioning as well as assessments of basic neuropsychological functions that may include attention, executive function, language, memory, visuospatial perception and construction, and psychomotor function. Performance on a test of general intellectual function serves as a context in which performance across neuropsychological domains can be considered. Selection of individual tests that comprise a neuropsychological

battery is very likely to depend on the assessment setting, nature of the presenting problem and differential diagnosis, and the theoretical orientation of the clinician.

One of the first battery approaches was what is commonly referred to today as the "fixed battery." In the fixed battery approach, test selection is predetermined irrespective of the patient's presenting problem. A comprehensive battery of tests is administered to all patients in the same standardized manner. Collection of collateral medical and social history is obtained following administration and scoring of the neuropsychological data to avoid response bias on the part of the test administrator. Examples of this psychometrically oriented, data-driven approach include the Luria-Nebraska Battery and the Halstead-Reitan Battery. An advantage of the fixed battery approach is that it facilitates comparison of test scores across patient groups and assessment settings. Another advantage of the battery approach, when using standardized tests, is that this approach facilitates the use of technicians in the administration of the tests. This approach can also facilitate the development of data banks for research purposes. A disadvantage, however, is that it is often time-consuming, cost-prohibitive, and may produce excessive testing sessions that are poorly tolerated by patients (Mitrushina et al. 2005).

An alternative neuropsychological assessment method is the "flexible battery" approach. In this hypothesis-driven approach, initial test selection is guided by the patient referral question, presenting problem, and the clinical interview. A modest range of measures that survey a broad range of cognitive functions is specifically chosen to probe and characterize the patient's presumed strengths and weaknesses. Following this initial assessment, which is sometimes referred to as a "core" or "screening" battery, the clinician will then select additional tests based on the patient's performance on the core battery and reported cognitive concerns (Strauss et al. 2006). The flexible battery approach is more focused on each individual patient's presenting problem and differential diagnosis than the fixed battery approach. As a result, the total assessment period is restricted and may be more cost-effective. However, inherent in the flexible battery approach is the inconsistent administration of tests across patient groups. That is, not all of a neuropsychologist's patients will receive the same tests, thereby limiting comparisons of findings across patient groups or settings (Mitrushina et al. 2005).

A variant of the flexible battery approach is the "process" approach, also known as the Boston process approach (Lezak et al. 2012). This method entails emphasis on the more qualitative aspects of neuropsychological performance. When completing a task, patients are closely observed for strategy formation and execution. Atypical performances will be further probed by the clinician with direct questioning or modified re-administration of the task to more fully examine the nature of the behavioral dysfunction. This approach affords a more in-depth characterization of the patient's neuropsychological abilities. However, it has been criticized for its lack of normative data and standards for the reliability and validity of its methods (Strauss et al. 2006).

Future Directions

Although all battery approaches to neuropsychological assessment have advantages and disadvantages, results from a survey from Sweet et al. (2011) suggest that the flexible battery approach is the method that is most preferred by clinicians. According to this report, the percentage of clinicians who endorsed the flexible battery approach increased from 54% in 1989 to 78% in 2010. These data reflect the relative popularity of this approach and suggest that it is likely to remain in favor in the coming years.

Cross-References

▶ Boston Process Approach
▶ Fixed Battery
▶ Flexible Battery

References and Readings

Lezak, M. D., Howieson, D. B., Bigler, E. D., & Tranel, D. (2012). *Neuropsychological assessment.* Oxford: Oxford University Press.

Mitrushina, M., Boone, K. B., Razani, J., & D'Elia, L. F. (2005). *Handbook of normative data for neuropsychological assessment.* Oxford: Oxford University Press.

Strauss, E., Sherman, E. M. S., & Spreen, O. (2006). *A compendium of neuropsychological tests: Administration, norms, and commentary.* Oxford: Oxford University Press.

Sweet, J. J., Meyer, D. G., Nelson, N. W., & Moberg, P. J. (2011). The TCN/AACN 2010 "salary survey": Professional practices, beliefs, and incomes of U.-S. neuropsychologists. *The Clinical Neuropsychologist, 25,* 12–61.

Battle's Sign

Beth Rush
Psychiatry and Psychology, Mayo Clinic, Jacksonville, FL, USA

Synonyms

Periauricular or mastoid ecchymosis

Definition

Named after English surgeon, Dr. William Henry Battle, this is a clinical symptom suggestive of basilar skull/middle cranial fossa fracture. After blunt force head trauma, leaking of blood from the blood vessels in the skull, typically the posterior auricular artery, leads to a crescent-shaped bruise wrapping behind the base of the earlobe and extending posteriorly toward the point of the neck where the base of the skull meets the neck. A patient with this symptom may present with acute bloody discharge of the ear and/or nose. Battle's sign may occur a few days following the onset of the skull fracture.

Cross-References

▶ Depressed Skull Fracture

References and Readings

Victor, M., & Ropper, A. H. (2001). *Principles of neurology* (7th ed.pp. 925–953). New York: McGraw-Hill.

Battlefield Assessment

Tamara McKenzie-Hartman
Defense and Veterans Brain Injury Center, James A. Haley, VA Hospital, Tampa, FL, USA

Description

Researchers report that "Due to enemy tactics and the frequency of operational missions, many service members are at risk of sustaining more than one concussion during deployment" (Barth et al. 2010). It is further noted that as numerous service members go on multiple deployments, the opportunity for injury is increased. According to the Defense and Veterans Brain Injury Center (DVBIC), 40% of all blast injuries in the Operation Enduring Freedom/Operation Iraqi Freedom (OEF/OIF) conflicts involve traumatic brain injury (TBI). Furthermore, many mild and moderate head injuries are reportedly overlooked due to more imminent medical treatments focused on polytrauma injuries including amputation and burns (Martin et al. 2008).

DoD instructional policy (DoDi 6490.11), entitled "Guidance for Management of Mild Traumatic Brain Injury/Concussion in the Deployed Setting," is intended to protect service members involved in potentially concussive events, direct leaders on mandated screening and reporting requirements, guide medical evaluation and treatments, and outline minimum mandatory rest periods. Specifically, the policy mandates that a service member be medically evaluated if exposed to a potentially concussive event such as (1) involvement in a vehicle blast, collision, or rollover, (2) a direct blow to the head or witnessed loss of consciousness, (3) presence within 50 m of a blast (inside or outside), and/or (4) exposure to

more than one blast event (the service member's commander shall direct a medical evaluation). Beginning with recognition, the policy outlines additional steps including, refer, report, rest, and return to duty.

Command Guidance

Recognize
Military leadership is required to recognize all personnel involved in any potentially concussive event, including those without apparent injuries, as soon as safely possible using the IED/HEADS checklist (Table 1).

Refer
Leaders refer any service member involved in a potentially concussive event to be evaluated by a medic or health care provider and if applicable, be re-evaluated and medically cleared before returning to duty.

Report
Military leaders are required to report all service members involved in a potentially concussive event by completing the significant activities (SIGACT) report within 24 h of the injury. Depending on the command, reports may be required using the Blast Exposure and Concussion Incident Report (BECIR) module, located

Battlefield Assessment, Table 1: IED/HEADS checklist

I-Injury	Was the service member injured during the event?	Yes/no
E-evaluation	Are any of the "HEADS" symptoms present? H-headaches and/or vomiting? (yes/no) E-ears ringing? (yes/no) A-amnesia, altered/loss of consciousness? (yes/no) D-double vision and/or dizziness? (yes/no) S-something feels wrong or is not right? (yes/no)	Yes/no
D-distance/proximity	Was the service member within 50 m of the blast? Record distance from blast	Yes/no

within the Combined Information Data Network Exchange (CIDNE).

Medical Guidance

Medical requirements include (1) utilization of the Military Acute Concussion Evaluation (MACE) for screening of a potentially concussive event, (2) documentation and appropriate International Classification of Diseases (ICD) coding of the medical encounter within the electronic health record, (3) and utilization of the "Concussion Management in Deployed Settings" algorithm (DCoE 2011; Fig. 1). The algorithm outlines three levels of intervention: (1) Level I: Combat Medic/Corpsman Concussion Triage, (2) Level II: Initial Management of Concussion in Deployed Setting, and (3) Level III: Comprehensive Concussion Evaluation.

Medical personnel are instructed to use section one of the MACE (Fig. 2), which is used to assess the service member's potential concussion/mild traumatic brain injury (mTBI). Questions on the MACE guide the provider to obtain a description of the incident, as well as assess of any alterations or losses of consciousness (AOC/LOC), and/or post-traumatic amnesia (PTA). Assessments are to be completed as close to the time of injury as feasible. The MACE is currently the primary instrument, used mostly by corpsmen/medics, to assess in-theater concussive events and determine the need for additional levels of care.

Rest

Service members must receive a minimum of 24 h of rest/downtime after a potentially concussive event. The 24-h clock starts at the time of the event, not at the time of the evaluation. Recovery care is to include sleep and pain management. As current research supports the return to neurocognitive baseline as soon as a few days post-injury, and many times without formal intervention (Mittenberg and Strauman 2000), the service member should remain in place for several days to allow for this recovery (Barth et al. 2010).

If the service member has been diagnosed with two concussions within the prior 12 months, the service member should receive seven additional days of rest after symptoms resolve. If three or more concussions have been diagnosed within the previous 12 months, the service member is mandated to receive a recurrent concussion evaluation before returning to duty. Of note, commanders may determine that mission requirements supersede an individual's welfare in certain circumstances and can waive or postpone the mandatory rest period.

The recurrent concussion evaluation can be initiated at any time that it is clinically warranted and should be used to inform treatment and return-to-duty (RTD) decisions. Recurrent concussion evaluations are to include (1) neurological examination, including completion of the Neurobehavioral Symptom Inventory (NSI), a validated acute stress reaction assessment, and a vestibular assessment; (2) neuroimaging; (3) neuropsychological assessment; (4) functional assessment, including evaluation of cognitive, sensorimotor, and physical endurance; (5) and a duty status determination by a neurologist or other qualified licensed independent practitioner trained according to service policies in the care of mTBI/concussion.

Regarding neuropsychological assessment, the Clinical Recommendation (DCoE 2011) indicates that a neurocognitive assessment tool (NCAT) should be considered if symptoms persist. In accordance with the National Defense Authorization Act (NDAA HR 4986), the DoD selected the Automated Neuropsychological Assessment Metrics (ANAM) as the NCAT to be utilized for predeployment baseline assessments and for post-concussion testing in theater.

In theater, clinical guidelines indicate that the ANAM test battery be administered if symptoms of concussion are present 24-h post-injury. The first administration of the test should be within 24–72 h from injury, and the test can be readministered on a regular basis to assess for cognitive deficits and symptom resolution (Kelly et al. 2012). To this end, the service member's post-injury test scores can be compared to his/her own baseline data, if possible, or to the normative database to determine recovery (DCoE 2011).

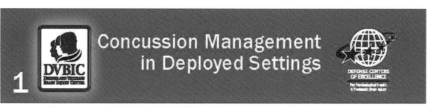

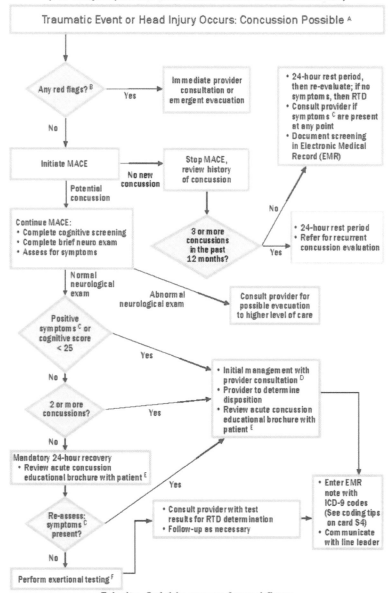

Battlefield Assessment, Fig. 1 (continued)

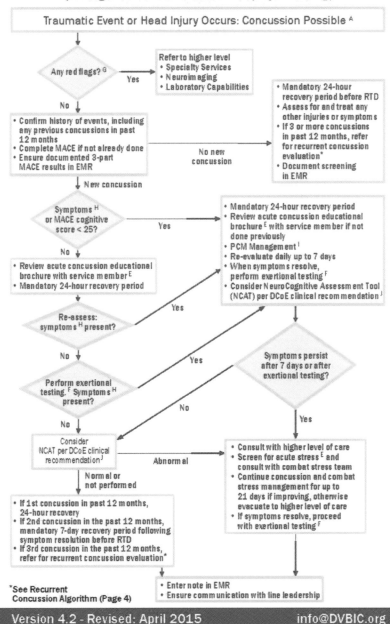

B

Battlefield Assessment, Fig. 1 (continued)

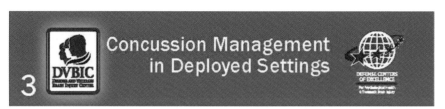

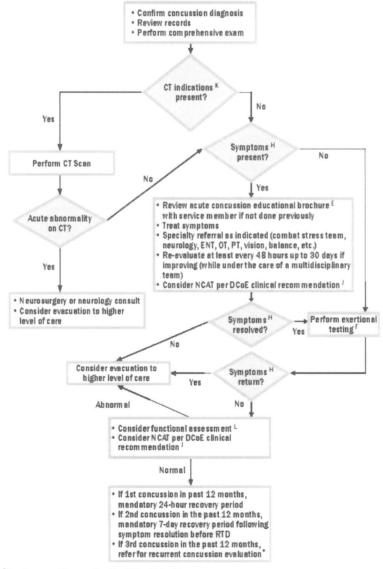

Battlefield Assessment, Fig. 1 (continued)

Concussion Management
in Deployed Settings

4

B

RECURRENT CONCUSSION EVALUATION
(three or more documented in 12-month span)

1. Comprehensive neurological evaluation by neurologist or
   otherwise qualified provider
   * Review of prior concussion history with focus on timeline
     or resolution of symptoms
   * Assessment of symptoms (face-to-face interview by provider)
     Consider:
     ▶ Neurobehavioral Symptom Inventory [E]
     ▶ Acute Stress Reaction questionnaire [E]
   * Balance assessment [M]

2. Neuroimaging per provider judgement

3. Neuropsychological assessment by psychologist
   * Evaluate: attention, memory, processing speed and
     executive function
   * Perform a psychosocial and behavioral assessment
   * Include measure of effort
   * Consider NCAT per DCoE clinical recommendation [J]

4. Functional assessment [L] completed by occupational therapy/
   physical therapy

5. Neurologist (or qualified provider) determines RTD status

Version 4.2 - Revised: April 2015   info@DVBIC.org

Battlefield Assessment, Fig. 1 (continued)

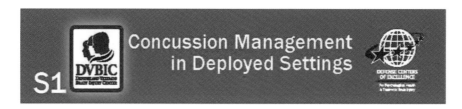

Traumatic Event or Head Injury Occurs: Concussion Possible

A Mandatory Events Requiring Concussion Evaluation:

1. Any service member in a vehicle associated with a blast event, collision or rollover
2. Any service member within 50 meters of a blast (inside or outside)
3. Anyone who sustains a direct blow to the head
4. Command directed—such as, but not limited to, repeated exposures

B Medic/Corpsman Algorithm Red Flags:

1. Witnessed loss of consciousness (LOC)
2. Two or more blast exposures within 72 hrs
3. Unusual behavior/combative
4. Unequal pupils
5. Seizures
6. Repeated vomiting
7. Double vision/loss of vision
8. Worsening headache
9. Weakness on one side of the body
10. Cannot recognize people or disoriented to place
11. Abnormal speech

C Medic/Corpsman Algorithm Symptoms:

(Persisting beyond initial traumatic event)

1. Headache
2. Dizziness
3. Memory problems
4. Balance problems
5. Nausea/vomiting
6. Difficulty concentrating
7. Irritability
8. Visual disturbances
9. Ringing in the ears
10. Other_____

D Medic/Corpsman Initial Management of Concussion:

1. Give acute concussion educational brochure to all concussion patients, available at: dvbic.dcoe.mil
2. Reduce environmental stimuli
3. Mandatory 24-hour recovery period
4. Aggressive headache management
   - Use acetaminophen q 6 hrs x 48 hrs After 48 hours may use naproxen pm
5. Avoid tramadol, Fioricet, excessive triptans and narcotics

E Available Resources (dvbic.dcoe.mil):

- Acute Stress Reaction Questionnaire
- Acute Concussion Educational Brochure
- Neurobehavioral Symptom Inventory
- Line Leader Fact Sheet
- Coding Guidance
- DCoE NeuroCognitive Assessment Tool (NCAT) Recommendation

Version 4.2 - Revised: April 2015   info@DVBIC.org

Battlefield Assessment, Fig. 1 (continued)

Concussion Management in Deployed Settings — S2

F Exertional Testing:

1. Exert to 65-85% of target heart rate (THR=220-age) using push-ups, sit-ups, running in place, step aerobic, stationary bike, treadmill and/or hand crank
2. Maintain this level of exertion for approximately 2 minutes
3. Assess for symptoms (headache, vertigo, photophobia, balance, dizziness, nausea, visual changes, etc.)
4. If symptoms/red flags exist with exertional testing, stop testing, and consult with provider

G Provider Algorithm Red Flags:

1. Progressively declining level of consciousness
2. Progressively declining neurological exam
3. Pupillary asymmetry
4. Seizures
5. Repeated vomiting
6. Clinically verified GCS < 15
7. Neurological deficit: motor or sensory
8. LOC > 5 minutes
9. Double vision
10. Worsening headache
11. Cannot recognize people or disoriented to place
12. Slurred speech
13. Unusual behavior

H Provider Algorithm Symptoms:

1. Confusion (24 hours)
2. Irritability
3. Unsteady on feet
4. Vertigo/dizziness
5. Headache
6. Photophobia
7. Phonophobia
8. Sleep issues

I Primary Care Management (PCM):

1. Give acute concussion educational brochure to all concussion patients, available at: **dvbic.dcoe.mil**
2. Reduce environmental stimuli
3. Mandatory 24-hour recovery period
4. Aggressive headache management
   - Use acetaminophen q 6 hrs x 48 hrs After 48 hours may use naproxen prn
5. Avoid tramadol, Fioricet, excessive triptans and narcotics
6. Consider nortriptyline q HS or amitriptyline q HS for persistent headache (> 7 days). Prescribe no more than 10 pills.
7. Implement duty restrictions
8. Review current medications and sleep hygiene (Healthy Sleep fact sheet available at dvbic.dcoe.mil) and consider short-term low dose non-benzodiazepine hypnotic (e.g., zolpidem 5mg)
9. Pain management if applicable
10. Send consult to med.consult.army@mail.mil for further guidance if needed
11. Consider evacuation to higher level of care if clinically indicated
12. Document concussion diagnosis in EMR

> **med.consult.army@mail.mil** is a Department of Defense email consultation service provided by the Army OTSG Telemedicine Teleconsultation Programs to assist deployed clinicians with the treatment of TBI and RTD decisions.

Version 4.2 - Revised: April 2015   info@DVBIC.org

Battlefield Assessment, Fig. 1 (continued)

Concussion Management in Deployed Settings

S3

^J DCoE NeuroCognitive Assessment Tool (NCAT) Recommendation:
Current DoD policy is that all service members must be tested with a neurocognitive assessment tool (NCAT) prior to deployment. Among several tests that are available, the DoD has selected the Automated Neuropsychological Assessment Metrics (ANAM) as the NCAT to use for both pre-deployment baseline testing and for post-concussion assessment in theater. Detailed instructions for administering a post-injury ANAM are provided at **dvbic.dcoe.mil**.

For ANAM baseline results send requests to:
usarmy.jbsa.medcom.mbx.otsg--anam-baselines@mail.mil

^K CT Indications:*

1. Physical evidence of trauma above the clavicles
2. Seizures
3. Vomiting
4. Headache

5. Age > 60
6. Drug or alcohol intoxication
7. Coagulopathy
8. Focal neurologic deficits

* Haydel MJ, Preston CA, Mills TJ, Luber S, Blaudeau E, DeBlieux PM. Indications for computed tomography in patients with minor head injury. N Engl J Med. 2000 Jul 13;343(2):100-5.

^L Functional Assessment:
Assess the service member's performance of military-relevant activities that simulate the multi-system demands of duty in a functional context. Selected assessment activities should concurrently challenge specific vulnerabilities associated with mTBI including cognitive (such as executive function), sensorimotor (such as balance and gaze stability), and physical endurance. Rehabilitation providers should not only evaluate the service member's performance but also monitor symptoms before, during and after functional assessment.

^M The Balance Error Scoring System (BESS - Modified):**
Stand on flat surface, eyes closed, hands on hips in 3 positions:
1. On both feet (20 seconds)
2. On one foot (20 seconds)
3. Heel-to-toe stance (20 seconds)
For each position, score 1 point for any of the following errors:

1. Stepping, stumbling or falling
2. Opening eyes
3. Hands lifted above the iliac crests

4. Forefoot or heel lifted
5. Hip moved > 30 degrees flexion or abduction
6. Out of test position > 5 seconds

Score 10 points if unable to complete

Total Balance Score_____

** Guskiewicz KM, Ross SE, Marshall SW. Postural Stability and Neuropsychological Deficits After Concussion in Collegiate Athletes. J Athl Train. 2001 Sep;36(3):263-273.

Version 4.2 - Revised: April 2015   info@DVBIC.org

Battlefield Assessment, Fig. 1 (continued)

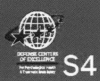

Concussion Management in Deployed Settings · S4

2015 DoD Definition of Traumatic Brain Injury:

A traumatically induced structural injury or physiological disruption of brain function, as a result of an external force, that is indicated by new onset or worsening of at least one of the following clinical signs immediately following the event:

- Any alteration in mental status (e.g., confusion, disorientation, slowed thinking, etc.).
- Any loss of memory for events immediately before or after the injury.
- Any period of loss of or a decreased level of consciousness, observed or self-reported.

Coding Tips:

1. Primary code (corpsman/medics require co-sign)
   - 850.0 - Concussion without LOC
   - 850.11 - Concussion with LOC ≤ 30 min.
2. Personal history of TBI in Global War on Terror (GWOT)
   - V15.52_2 - Injury related to GWOT, mild TBI
3. Symptom codes
   - As appropriate
4. Deployment status code
   - V70.5_5 - During deployment encounter
5. Screening code for TBI
   - V80.01
6. External cause of injury code (E-code)
   - E979.2 (if applicable) - Terrorism involving explosions and fragments

Key Algorithm Directives:

- Personnel are required to use the algorithms to treat concussion in the deployed setting
- Mandatory event-driven protocols for exposure to potentially concussive events
   - Requires a medical evaluation and minimum 24-hour rest period
- All sports and activities with risk of concussion are prohibited until after a 24-hour rest period
- Military Acute Concussion Evaluation (MACE) documentation will address all 3 MACE parts
- Service members diagnosed with concussion will be given the acute concussion educational brochure available at: dvbic.dcoe.mil
- Specific protocols for anyone sustaining ≥ 2 concussions within 12 months

MACE Documentation

Document using the mnemonic "CNS"
   (1) C – Cognitive score
   (2) N – Neurological exam reported as normal or abnormal
   (3) S – Symptoms reported as present or absent

If a head injury event or AOC/LOC/PTA is not reported, then a concussion has not occurred. The MACE is stopped because the cognitive portion is not valid in non-concussed patients. Evaluate and treat any other symptoms or injuries, and document the event in the EMR. The MACE score should be reported as N/A.

Repeat MACE Tips:

Repeating the MACE's Cognitive Exam with a different version (A-F) may be used to evaluate acute concussion recovery; however, a physical exam and symptom assessment must accompany any repeated cognitive exam. Providers should be mindful of other factors affecting the MACE cognitive score such as sleep deprivation, medications or pain.

For additional copies or information call 1.866.966.1020 or email info@DVBIC.org

Version 4.2 - Revised: April 2015   info@DVBIC.org

Battlefield Assessment, Fig. 1 DVBIC concussion-management-algorithm pocket-cards version-4.2

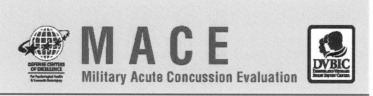

Patient Name: _____

Service Member ID#: _____ Unit: _____

Date of Injury: _____ Time of Injury: _____

Examiner: _____

Date of Evaluation: _____ Time of Evaluation: _____

CONCUSSION SCREENING

Complete this section to determine if there was both an injury event AND an alteration of consciousness.

1. Description of Incident

A. Record the event as described by the service member or witness.
Use open-ended questions to get as much detail as possible.

_____   Key questions:
_____   • Can you tell me what
_____   you remember?
_____   • What happened?

B. Record the type of event.
Check all that apply:

☐ Explosion/Blast   ☐ Fragment   ☐ Motor Vehicle Crash

☐ Blunt Object   ☐ Sports Injury   ☐ Gunshot Wound

☐ Fall   ☐ Other _____

C. Was there a head injury event?   Key questions:

☐ YES   ☐ NO   • Did your head hit any objects?
                                            • Did any objects strike your head?
                                            • Did you feel a blast wave?
                                               (A blast wave that is felt striking
                                               the body/head is considered
                                               a blow to the head.)

Battlefield Assessment, Fig. 2 (continued)

MACE - Military Acute Concussion Evaluation

CONCUSSION SCREENING – continued

2. Alteration of Consciousness or Memory (AOC/LOC/PTA)

A. Was there Alteration of Consciousness (AOC)?
AOC is temporary confusion or "having your bell rung."

☐ YES ☐ NO

If yes, for how long? _____ minutes

Key question:
- Were you dazed, confused, or did you "see stars" immediately after the injury?

B. Was there Loss of Consciousness (LOC)?
LOC is temporarily passing out or blacking out.

☐ YES ☐ NO

If yes, for how long? _____ minutes

Key question:
- Did you pass out or black out?

C. Was there any Post Traumatic Amnesia (PTA)?
PTA is a problem remembering part or all of the injury events.

☐ YES ☐ NO

If yes, for how long? _____ minutes

Key questions:
- What is the last thing you remember before the event?
- What is the first thing you remember after the event?

D. Was there a witness?

☐ YES ☐ NO

If yes, name of witness:
_____

Tips for assessment:
- Ask witness to verify AOC/LOC/PTA and estimate duration.

CONCUSSION SCREENING RESULTS (Possible Concussion?)

YES to 1C	NO to 1C
AND	**OR**
YES to 2A, 2B or 2C	NO to 2A, 2B and 2C

CONTINUE the MACE:	STOP the MACE:
• Complete the Cognitive, Neurological and Symptoms portions of the MACE	• Evaluate and treat any other injuries or symptoms • Enter negative screening result into electronic medical record (V80.01) • Communicate results with provider and line commanders • Check for history of previous concussions and refer to Concussion Management Algorithm for appropriate rest period

Battlefield Assessment, Fig. 2 (continued)

MACE - Military Acute Concussion Evaluation

COGNITIVE EXAM[a]

3. Orientation
Score 1 point for each correct response.

Ask This Question	Incorrect	Correct
"What month is this?"	0	1
"What is the date or day of the month?"	0	1
"What day of the week is it?"	0	1
"What year is it?"	0	1
"What time do you think it is?"	0	1
Correct response must be within 1 hour of actual time.		

ORIENTATION TOTAL SCORE   /5

4. Immediate Memory
Choose one list (A-F below) and use that list for the remainder of the MACE.
Read the script for each trial and then read all 5 words. Circle the response for each word for each trial. Repeat the trial 3 times, even if the service member scores perfectly on any of the trials.

Trial 1 Script:
- "I am going to test your memory. I will read you a list of words and when I am done, repeat back to me as many words as you can remember, in any order."

Trials 2 and 3 Script:
- "I am going to repeat that list again. Repeat back to me as many words as you can remember, in any order, even if you said them before."

List F	Trial 1		Trial 2		Trial 3	
	Incorrect	Correct	Incorrect	Correct	Incorrect	Correct
Dollar	0	1	0	1	0	1
Honey	0	1	0	1	0	1
Mirror	0	1	0	1	0	1
Saddle	0	1	0	1	0	1
Anchor	0	1	0	1	0	1

IMMEDIATE MEMORY TOTAL SCORE   /15

Immediate Memory Alternate Word Lists

List E	List D	List C	List B	List A
Jacket	Finger	Baby	Candle	Elbow
Arrow	Penny	Monkey	Paper	Apple
Pepper	Blanket	Perfume	Sugar	Carpet
Cotton	Lemon	Sunset	Sandwich	Saddle
Movie	Insect	Iron	Wagon	Bubble

Battlefield Assessment, Fig. 2 (continued)

MACE - Military Acute Concussion Evaluation

NEUROLOGICAL EXAM

5. Eyes
Test pupil response to light, tracking

☐ Normal

☐ Abnormal

Tips for assessment:
- Pupils should be round, equal in size and briskly constrict to a direct, bright light.
- Both eyes should smoothly track your finger side-to-side and up and down.

6. Speech
Test speech fluency and word finding

☐ Normal

☐ Abnormal

Tips for assessment:
- Speech should be fluid and effortless – no pauses or unnatural breaks.
- Assess difficulties with word finding:
  - Does service member have trouble coming up with the name of a common object?

7. Motor
Test grip strength and pronator drift

☐ Normal

☐ Abnormal

Tips for assessment:
- Assess grip strength.
- Assess for pronator drift for 5-10 seconds by directing patient to close eyes and extend arms forward, parallel to the ground with palms up:
  - Does either palm turn inward?
  - Does either arm drift down?

8. Balance
Tandem Romberg Test

☐ Normal

☐ Abnormal

Tips for assessment:
- Have patient stand with eyes closed, one foot in front of the other heel-to-toe, arms extended forward, palms up. Observe for 5-10 seconds:
  - Does the service member stumble or shift feet?

NEUROLOGICAL EXAM RESULTS

☐ All Normal
Green

☐ Any Abnormal
Red

Battlefield Assessment, Fig. 2 (continued)

MACE - Military Acute Concussion Evaluation

COGNITIVE EXAM² - Continued

9. Concentration
A. Reverse Digits
Read the script and begin the trial by reading the first string of numbers in Trial 1.

Script:
- "I am going to read you a string of numbers. When I am finished, repeat them back to me backward. That is, in reverse order of how I read them to you. For example, if I said 7 - 1 - 9, then you would say 9 - 1 - 7."

Circle the response for each string.
- If correct on string length of Trial 1, proceed to the next longer string length in the same column.
- If incorrect on string length of Trial 1, move to the same string length of Trial 2.
- If incorrect on both string lengths in Trials 1 and 2, **STOP** and record score as zero for that string length. Record total score as sum of previous correct trials.

List F

Trial 1	Trial 2 (if Trial 1 is incorrect)	Incorrect	Correct
2-7-1	4-7-9	0	1
1-6-8-3	3-9-2-4	0	1
2-4-7-5-8	8-3-9-6-4	0	1
5-8-6-2-4-9	3-1-7-8-2-6	0	1

REVERSE DIGITS SCORE (9A) ___/4

Concentration Alternate Number Lists
Note: Use the same list (A-F) that was used in Question 4.

List E Trial 1	Trial 2	List D Trial 1	Trial 2
3-8-2	5-1-8	7-8-2	9-2-6
2-7-9-3	2-1-6-9	4-1-8-3	9-7-2-3
4-1-8-6-9	9-4-1-7-5	1-7-9-2-6	4-1-7-5-2
6-9-7-3-8-2	4-2-7-9-3-8	2-6-4-8-1-7	8-4-1-9-3-5

List C Trial 1	Trial 2	List B Trial 1	Trial 2	List A Trial 1	Trial 2
1-4-2	6-5-8	5-2-6	4-1-5	4-9-3	6-2-9
6-8-3-1	3-4-8-1	1-7-9-5	4-9-6-8	3-8-1-4	3-2-7-9
4-9-1-5-3	6-8-2-5-1	4-8-5-2-7	6-1-8-4-3	6-2-9-7-1	1-5-2-8-5
3-7-6-5-1-9	9-2-6-5-1-4	8-3-1-9-6-4	7-2-7-8-5-6	7-1-8-4-6-3	5-3-9-1-4-8

Battlefield Assessment, Fig. 2 (continued)

MACE - Military Acute Concussion Evaluation

COGNITIVE EXAM[a] - Continued

9. Concentration - Continued
B. Months in Reverse Order
Script:
- "Now tell me the months of the year in reverse order. Start with the last month and go backward. So you'll say: December, November...Go ahead."

Correct Response:
Dec – Nov – Oct – Sep – Aug – Jul – Jun – May – Apr – Mar – Feb – Jan

	Incorrect	Correct
ALL months in reverse order	0	1

MONTHS IN REVERSE ORDER (9B) /1

CONCENTRATION TOTAL SCORE
Sum of scores:
9A (0-4 points) and 9B (0 or 1 point) /5

10. Delayed Recall
Read the script and circle the response for each word.
Do NOT repeat the word list.

Note: Use the same list (A-F) that was used in Question 4.

Script:
- "Do you remember that list of words I read a few minutes earlier? I want you to tell me as many words from that list as you can remember. You can say them in any order."

List F	Incorrect	Correct
Dollar	0	1
Honey	0	1
Mirror	0	1
Saddle	0	1
Anchor	0	1

DELAYED RECALL TOTAL SCORE /5

Delayed Recall Alternate Word Lists

List E	List D	List C	List B	List A
Jacket	Finger	Baby	Candle	Elbow
Arrow	Penny	Monkey	Paper	Apple
Pepper	Blanket	Perfume	Sugar	Carpet
Cotton	Lemon	Sunset	Sandwich	Saddle
Movie	Insect	Iron	Wagon	Bubble

Battlefield Assessment, Fig. 2 (continued)

MACE - Military Acute Concussion Evaluation

SYMPTOM SCREENING

11. Symptoms — Check all that apply:

☐ Headache ☐ Balance Problems ☐ Irritability

☐ Dizziness ☐ Nausea/Vomiting ☐ Visual Disturbances

☐ Memory Problems ☐ Difficulty Concentrating ☐ Ringing in the Ears

☐ Other _____

SUMMARY
Record the data for correct MACE documentation.

Cognitive Summary

Orientation Total Score - Q3   /5

Immediate Memory Total Score (all 3 trials) **- Q4**   /15

Concentration Total Score (Sections A and B) **- Q9**   /5

Delayed Recall Total Score - Q10   /5

COGNITIVE RESULTS   /30

NEUROLOGICAL RESULTS
(Page 4)

☐ Normal (Green)   ☐ Abnormal (Red)

SYMPTOM RESULTS

☐ No symptoms (A)   ☐ 1 or more symptoms (B)

MACE RESULTS (Report all 3 parts.) Example: 24/Red/B
Abnormality in any area should be discussed with provider.

C _____ / N _____ / S _____
   Cognitive   Neurological   Symptoms

CONCUSSION HISTORY IN PAST 12 MONTHS

12. During the past 12 months have you been diagnosed with a concussion, not counting this event?

☐ YES   ☐ NO
If yes, how many? _____

Refer to Concussion Management Algorithm for clinical care guidance.

Release 02/2012   dvbic.dcoe.mil   Page 7 of 8

Battlefield Assessment, Fig. 2 (continued)

MACE - Military Acute Concussion Evaluation

ADDITIONAL INFORMATION ABOUT MACE COGNITIVE SCORES

Although cognitive is listed first in the summary of MACE results, this should not suggest that any one of the three screening categories is more or less important than the others. Each area (Cognitive, Neurological, Symptoms) must be evaluated carefully. The results of all three evaluations must be included in any MACE report for it to be considered complete.

Regarding cognitive scores, in studies of non-concussed subjects, the mean total cognitive score was 28. Therefore, a score of < 30 does not imply that a concussion has occurred. Definitive normative data for a cut-off score are not available. The Concussion Management Algorithm stipulates that a cognitive score of < 25 or the presence of symptoms requires consultation with a provider.

Repeating the MACE cognitive exam with a different version (A-F) may be used to evaluate acute concussion recovery; however, a physical exam and symptom assessment must accompany any repeated cognitive exam. Providers should be mindful of other factors affecting the MACE cognitive score such as sleep deprivation, medications or pain.

Coding Tips for Concussion:
1. Primary code (corpsmen/medics require co-sign)
   - 850.0 – Concussion without LOC
   - 850.11 – Concussion with LOC ≤ 30 min.
2. Personal history of TBI in Global War on Terror (GWOT)
   - V15.52_2 – Injury related to GWOT, mild TBI
3. Symptom codes
   - As appropriate
4. Deployment status code
   - V70.5_5 – During deployment encounter
5. Screening code
   - V80.01 – Special screening for TBI code
6. E-code (external cause of injury)
   - E979.2 (if applicable) – Terrorism involving explosions and fragments

References
a. McCrea, M. Standardized Mental Status Testing on the Sideline After Sport-Related Concussion. J Athl Train. 2001 Sep;36(3):274-279.

THIS TOOL MAY BE COPIED FOR CLINICAL USE.

DVBIC is proud to partner with the Army, Navy, Air Force, Marine Corps and Coast Guard on this product.

For additional copies or information call 1.866.966.1020 or visit dvbic.dcoe.mil

Release 02/2012   dvbic.dcoe.mil   Page 8 of 8

Battlefield Assessment, Fig. 2   DVBIC military-acute-concussion-evaluation pocket-card

When the concussed service member is no longer reporting symptoms, physical exertion testing is recommended. Exertional testing is typically conducted by having the service member exert 65–85% of their target heart rate by engaging in aerobic activities (i.e., treadmill running, push-ups, or stationary biking), which is theorized to increase intracranial pressure and activate dormant symptoms (Barth et al. 2010). Immediately after exertion (after approximately 2 min), the medical provider assesses for the presence of any symptoms (i.e., headache, dizziness, vision changes, vertigo, etc.). If symptoms are present, then continued rest and observation is recommended, while those who remain asymptomatic may be considered for RTD.

Service members exhibiting symptoms of concussion for extended periods of time post-injury may require referral to a higher-level facility, where neuropsychological assessment in conjunction with a clinical examination and input from various disciplines (e.g., physical and occupational therapies) is strongly encouraged to determine return-to-duty (RTD) recommendations. After treatment in theater and/or via combat support hospital, the wounded service member requiring greater intensity of care is transported to Landstuhl Regional Medical Center (LRMC) in Germany, and then later to Walter Reed National Military Medical Center (WRNMMC) in Washington, D.C. From there, service members are assessed, treated, and transferred to other military and Veterans Administration (VA) facilities as needed (French et al. 2012).

Return to Duty

While recovering from TBI, service members should not return to duty or engage in other activities that place them at risk for concussion (i.e., sports, combatives, etc.). Military leaders are instructed to consult with medical personnel for RTD recommendations.

While service members may need to be removed from combat to ensure safety of the individual as well as of others, Barth et al. (2010) caution that clinicians must also take into consideration mission goals and iatrogenic effects of imposed rest:

> Unit cohesion is an important component of military life, lengthy separations can reduce expectations of return to duty, and service members may become less likely to recover and return to full duty. Keeping people out of action or evacuating them so they can recover must be balanced with the negative expectations about not returning to duty that may arise when they are removed from their units. (Barth et al. 2010, pp. 135)

Historical Background

The assessment of mTBI can be challenging to diagnose as symptoms can vary from person to person and may not seem sufficiently "bad enough" for a service member or their command to discern that an injury has occurred. The Army Research Laboratory's report on the use of the ANAM for TBI assessment highlighted the importance of assessment:

> Some service members who are determined to accomplish their mission and feel a strong desire to remain in-country and support their unit, may mask their symptoms (e.g., cognitive deficiency, chronic daily headaches) by simply not seeking care. The motivation not to leave one's fellow service members behind is strong, even when an individual has been injured, and perhaps even more so when the injured service member is uncertain whether their injury is real or an imagined set of symptoms related to stress. Undiagnosed mTBI can endanger not only the individual, but also the entire unit. A soldier's cognitive as well as physical and emotional deficits may not be evident until a mistake is made that could put both the service member and his or her team in jeopardy. (Rice et al. 2011, pp. 1)

In 2006, the Defense and Veterans Brain Injury Center and Brain Trauma Foundation in collaboration with academic experts developed Guidelines for the Field Management of Combat-Related Head Trauma. This guideline included the development of the Military Acute Concussion Evaluation (MACE) tool (French et al. 2008) and a decision tree for determining additional evaluation and treatment.

In 2007, mandatory concussion screening protocols (i.e., MACE) were implemented throughout the DoD. Consequently, this led to abrupt increases in the reporting of TBI in the deployed setting as well as across military installations, both before and after deployment (Helmick et al. 2015). Research has also consistently shown the majority of TBI occurs in non-deployed settings secondary to military training accidents, auto accident (private and military vehicles), falls, sports, and recreational activities. However, many of those injuries diagnosed post-deployment have been found to be deployment-related events that were diagnosed weeks or months after return from deployment (Scholten et al. 2012). Prior to DoD instruction on concussion management in the deployed setting, the identification of concussion was somewhat challenging as the military culture traditionally discouraged admitting to being injured, so that the service member could "get back to the fight."

In 2010, the DoD responded to this trend by implementing an incident-based system of reporting (DoDi 6490.11) in which command leaders were required to remove service members from combat and report all service members who had been exposed to a potentially concussive event (DoD 2012). This policy, as described in the description in the above section, has reportedly increased awareness of mTBI and consequently decreased the stigma, which will optimistically mitigate any potential long-term effects of secondary to mTBI (Helmick et al. 2015).

See Also

► Automated Neuropsychological Assessment Metrics (ANAM)
► Blast Effects
► Concussion
► Defense and Veterans Brain Injury Center
► Mild Traumatic Brain Injury
► Military Acute Concussion Evaluation

References and Readings

Barth, J., Isler, W., Helmick, K., Wingler, I., & Jaffee, M. (2010). Acute battlefield assessment of concussion/mild TBI and return-to-duty evaluations. In C. H. Kennedy & J. Moore (Eds.), *Military neuropsychology* (pp. 127–174). New York: Springer.

Bryan, C., & Hernandez, A. M. (2012). Magnitudes of decline on automated neuropsychological assessment metrics subtest scores relative to predeployment baseline performance among service members evaluated for traumatic brain injury in Iraq. *The Journal of Head Trauma Rehabilitation, 27*(1), 45–54. https://doi.org/10.1097/HTR.0b013e318238f146.

Defense and Veterans Brain Injury Center. In *DoD world-wide numbers for TBI*. Retrieved from http://Dvbic.Dcoe.Mil/Dod-Worldwide-Numbers-TBi

Defense and Veterans Brain Injury Center. (2012, November). *Policy guidance for management of mild traumatic brain injury/concussion in the deployed setting* (line leader fact sheet). Retrieved from http://dvbic.Dcoe.Mil/files/line-leader-fact-sheet-2012_V3_Final.Pdf

Defense Centers of Excellence (DCoE) for Psychological Health and Traumatic Brain Injury. (2011, May). *Indications and conditions for in-theater post-injury neurocognitive assessment tool (NCAT) testing* (DCoE clinical recommendation). Retrieved from http://dvbic.Dcoe.Mil/files/resources/DCoE_clinical_Recommendations_post_injury_NCAT_05-31-2011_f.Pdf

Department of Defense. (2008). *National defense authorization act for fiscal year 2008 (HR 4986, section 1673)*. Retrieved from https://www.Congress.Gov/Bill/110th-congress/house-bill/4986

Department of Defense. (2012, September). *DoD policy guidance for management of mild traumatic brain injury/concussion in the deployed setting* (DoDi 6490.11). Retrieved from http://www.Dtic.Mil/whs/directives/corres/pdf/649011p.Pdf

Eckner, J. T., Kutcher, J. S., Broglio, S. P., & Richardson, J. K. (2014). Effect of sport-related concussion on clinically measured simple reaction time. *British Journal of Sports Medicine, 48*(2), 112–118. https://doi.org/10.1136/bjsports-2012-091579.

French, L., McCrea, M., & Baggett, M. (2008). The military acute concussion evaluation (MACE). *Journal of Special Operations Medicine, 8*(1), 68–77.

French, L. M., Anderson-Barnes, V., Ryan, L. M., Zazeckis, T. M., & Harvey, S. (2012). Neuropsychological practice in the military. In C. H. Kennedy & E. A. Zillmer (Eds.), *Military psychology: Clinical and operational applications* (2nd ed., pp. 185–210). New York: Guilford Press.

Helmick, K. M., Spells, C. A., Malik, S. Z., Davies, C. A., Marion, D. W., & Hinds, S. R. (2015). Traumatic brain injury in the US military: Epidemiology and key clinical and research programs. *Brain Imaging and Behavior, 9*, 358–366. https://doi.org/10.1007/s11682-015-9399-z.

Joint Mental Health Advisory Team 7 (J-MHAT 7). (2011). Report of the advisory team on *Operation Enduring Freedom 2010 Afghanistan*. Retrieved from http://armymedicine.Mil/documents/J_MHAT_7.pdf

Kelly, M. P., Coldren, R. L., Parish, R. V., Dretsch, M. N., & Russell, M. L. (2012). Assessment of acute concussion in the combat environment. *Archives of Clinical Neuropsychology, 27*(4), 375–388. https://doi.org/10.1093/arclin/acs036.

Martin, E. M., Lu, W. C., Helmick, K., French, L., & Warden, D. (2008). Traumatic brain injuries sustained in the Afghanistan and Iraq wars. *American Journal of Nursing, 108*(4), 40–47. https://doi.org/10.1097/01.NAJ.0000315260.92070.3f.

Mittenberg, W., & Strauman, S. (2000). Diagnosis of mild head injury and the postconcussion syndrome. *The Journal of Head Trauma Rehabilitation, 15*(2), 783–791. Retrieved from http://journals.Lww.Com/headtraumarehab/abstract/2000/04000/Diagnosis_of_mild_Head_injury_and_the.3.Aspx.

Norris, J. N., Carr, W., Herzig, T., Labrie, D. W., & Sams, R. (2013). ANAM4 TBI reaction time-based tests have prognostic utility for acute concussion. *Military Medicine, 178*(7), 767–774. https://doi.org/10.7205/MILMED-D-12-00493.

Rice, V. J., Lindsay, G., Overby, C., Jeter, A., Alfred, P. E., Boykin, G. L., & Bateman. R. (2011, July). *Automated neuropsychological assessment metrics (ANAM) traumatic brain injury (TBI): Human factors assessment* (Army Research lab report ARL-TN-0440). Retrieved from http://www.Dtic.Mil/Cgi-bin/GetTRDoc?AD=ADA549141

Scholten, J. D., Sayer, N. A., Vanderploeg, R. D., Bidelspach, D. E., & Cifu, D. X. (2012). Analysis of US veterans health administration comprehensive evaluations for traumatic brain injury in operation enduring freedom and operation Iraqi freedom veterans. *Brain Injury, 26*(10), 1177–1184. https://doi.org/10.3109/02699052.2012.661914.

Baxter v. Temple (2005)

Robert L. Heilbronner
Chicago Neuropsychology Group, Chicago, IL, USA

Synonyms

Admissibility of psychological/neuropsychological evidence

Historical Background

One of the first decisions to address the admissibility of expert testimony by a psychologist or neuropsychologist as to the existence of a brain injury or mental defect was *Jenkins v. United States* (1962). This was a criminal trial in which the jury was instructed to disregard the testimony of the psychologists on the grounds that they could not give a medical opinion as to mental disease or defect because they did not have medical training. The appellate court reversed the decision holding that the expert did not need to be a medical practitioner. A later opinion, in *United States v. Riggleman* (1969) supported the position that psychologists were not excluded from testifying about criminal sanity solely because they lacked medical training. *Simmons v. Mullins* (1975) was an early appellate court decision that essentially reversed a trial court opinion that neuropsychologists were not competent to offer expert testimony on brain malfunctions from motor vehicle accidents. The appellate court held that to exclude such testimony on physical matters by psychologists would be to ignore present medical and psychological practice. Most states allow neuropsychological testimony about brain damage (Richardson and Adams 1992) while there is a greater diversity of opinion as to testimony about causation.

Current Knowledge

In *Baxter v. Temple* (2005), defense filed a motion in limine to exclude the testimony of a neuropsychologist in a case of lead exposure as insufficiently unreliable because opinions were based on results from a flexible neuropsychological test battery. The defense argued successfully that the neuropsychologist's testimony should be excluded because the Boston approach had not been subject to peer review and publication, has no known or potential error rate, and is not generally accepted in the appropriate scientific literature. In other words, Daubert factors were used by the trial judge to exclude expert neuropsychological evidence. Furthermore, the court made an important distinction between the roles of a clinical provider and forensic examiner, emphasizing that neuropsychologists in forensic practice must employ objective methods that allow them to be unbiased truth seekers. The defendant motion in limine was granted. Some (Reed 1996) have argued that Daubert challenges of idiosyncratic (flexible) test combinations will eliminate the use of flexible neuropsychological batteries in forensic consulting. However, recent surveys of neuropsychologists show that the majority of neuropsychologist practitioners use a carefully constructed battery approach specifically tailored to the patient/examinee's specific issues. In 2008, the New Hampshire Supreme Court reviewed the neuropsychological literature and practices of neuropsychologists, considered relevant Daubert standards and various amicus briefs, and concluded that the exclusion of the neuropsychological testimony in *Baxter v. Temple* (2005) was in error.

Cross-References

▶ Admissibility
▶ Daubert v. Merrell Dow Pharmaceuticals (1993)
▶ *Expert v. Treater Role*
▶ Federal Rules of Evidence
▶ *Kumho Tire v. Carmichael*

References and Readings

Chapple v. Ganger, 851 F. Suppl. 1481 (E. D. Wash, 1994).

Greiffenstein, M. F. (2009). Basics of forensic neuropsychology. In J. Morgan & J. Ricker (Eds.), *Textbook of clinical neuropsychology*. New York: Taylor & Francis.

Greiffenstein, M. F., & Cohen, L. (2005). Neuropsychology and the law: Principles of productive attorney-neuropsychologists relations. In G. Larrabee (Ed.), *Forensic neuropsychology: A scientific approach*. New York: Oxford University Press.

Jenkins v. United States (1962). 307 F. 2d 637.

Kaufmann, P. M. (2008). Admissibility of neuropsychological evidence in criminal cases: Competency, insanity, culpability, and mitigation. In R. Denney & J. Sullivan (Eds.), *Clinical neuropsychology in the criminal forensic setting*. New York: Guilford Press.

Richardson, R. E. L., & Adams, R. L. (1992). Neuropsychologists as expert witnesses: Issues of admissibility. *The Clinical Neuropsychologist, 6*, 295–308.

Simmons v. Mullins (Pa. Super Ct. 1975). 331 A2D 892, 897.

United States v. Riggleman (4th Cir. 1969). 411 F.2d 1190.

Bayley Scales of Infant and Toddler Development

Glen P. Aylward
SIU School of Medicine- Developmental-Behavioral Pediatrics, Springfield, IL, USA

Synonyms

Bayley; BSID-III

Description

The Bayley Scales of Infant and Toddler Development-Third Edition (BSID-III; 2006) is considered to be the reference standard for developmental assessment. It is an individually administered test, applicable from 1 to 42 months of age. The primary purpose of the BSID-III is to identify children with developmental delay and to provide information for interventions.

The BSID-III was normed on 1700 children (divided into 17 age groups) and development is assessed across five domains: Cognitive (91 items), Language (49 receptive and 48 expressive), Motor (66 fine motor and 72 gross motor), Social-Emotional, and Adaptive. Like its predecessors, the BSID-III is a modified power test. Assessment of the first three domains is accomplished by item administration, while the latter two are completed using caregiver response to a questionnaire. A Behavior Observation Inventory can be completed by both the examiner and the caregiver and allows assessment of the child's behavior during testing and at home. The Language scale includes Receptive Communication and Expressive Communication subtests; the Motor scale includes a Fine Motor and a Gross Motor subtest. The BSID-III Social-Emotional scale is an adaptation of the Greenspan Social-Emotional Growth Chart: A Screening Questionnaire for Infants and Young Children (Greenspan 2004). The first eight items yield a Sensory Processing Score. The Adaptive Behavior scale is composed of items from the Parent/Primary

Caregiver Form of the Adaptive Behavior Assessment System-Second Edition (Harrison and Oakland 2003). This scale measures areas such as communication, community use, health and safety, leisure, self-care, self-direction, functional pre-academics, home living, social and motor, and yields a General Adaptive Composite (GAC). Discrepancies between scaled scores can be reviewed to determine whether the differences between subtests are statistically significant.

Historical Background

The original BSID (Bayley 1969) evolved from versions of developmental tests such as the California Scales that were administered to infants enrolled in the landmark National Collaborative Perinatal Project. It was considered the reference standard for the assessment of infant development, administered to infants over the first 2½ years. The BSID was theoretically eclectic and borrowed from different research and test instruments. The test contained three components: the Mental Developmental Index (MDI), the Psychomotor Developmental Index (PDI) (M = 100, SD = 16) and the Infant Behavior Record, and was applicable from 2 to 30 months.

The BSID subsequently was revised into the BSID-II (Bayley 1993), this due in part to the upward drift of approximately 11 points on the MDI and 10 points on the PDI, reflecting the Flynn effect. Although the mean remained the same (100), the SD was now 15. When compared to the original BSID, the BSID-II MDI scores were 12 points lower and the PDI was 10 points lower. The Behavior Rating Scale was developed to enable the assessment of state, reactions to the environment, motivation, and interaction with people. The age range of the BSID-II was expanded to span 1–42 months. The instrument contained 22 item sets and basal and ceiling rules that differed from the original BSID. These rules were controversial because if correction for prematurity was used to determine the item set to begin administration, or if an earlier item set was employed because of developmental problems, scores tended to be somewhat lower, because the child was not automatically given credit for passing the lower item set. The BSID-II was also criticized because it did not provide area scores compatible with IDEA Part C requirements for estimates of cognitive, motor, communication, social, and adaptive function.

Psychometric Data

On the BSID-III, norm-referenced scaled scores (M = 10, SD = 3), composite scores (M = 100, SD = 15), percentile ranks, and growth scores are provided, in addition to confidence intervals for the scales and developmental age equivalents. Composite scores range from 55 to 155, depending on the scale. Internal consistency of the subtests range from 0.86 to 0.93; the intercorrelation between Cognitive and Language composites is 0.52, for Cognitive and Motor composites, 0.50, and the intercorrelation between Language and Motor composites is 0.49. Growth scores are provided and are used to longitudinally plot the child's growth over time for each subscale. This metric is calculated based on the subtest total raw score and ranges from 200 to 800 (M = 500, SD = 100). Similar to the original BSID, there are basal rules (passing the first three items at the appropriate age start-point) and ceiling or discontinue rules (a score of 0 for five consecutive items).

The correlation between the BSID-III Language Composite and the previous BSID-II MDI is 0.71, the Motor Composite and the BSID-II PDI = 0.60, and the Cognitive Composite and the BSID-II MDI = 0.60. However, in contrast to the expected Flynn effect, the Bayley-III Mental and Motor composite scores, on average, are approximately seven points *higher* than the corresponding BSID-II MDI and PDI. This phenomenon has also been reported with other developmental tests and has been termed the "reverse Flynn effect."

The increase in scores may be due to inclusion of infants at risk for developmental delay in the standardization sample (10%). These "mixed norms" inflate scores and decrease diagnostic accuracy. In addition, there are concerns regarding a weak test floor. However, despite at-risk infants receiving "normal" scores, these still are below comparison group scores, which typically are higher than the standardization mean (as seen in comparison of preterm infants and term controls). This conundrum becomes further complicated by the possibility that the Bayley-II was too conservative and underestimated development.

Clinical Uses

Administration of the BSID-III yields quantitative and qualitative data that provide insight into the child's current levels of development. Repeated administration can document the effects of an intervention program. However, changes in test content and alteration of scales in conjunction with the Flynn effect and the more recent increase in mean scores (in comparison to the previous version) make longitudinal comparisons of scores difficult in individual children or cohorts. There also are concerns that the Bayley-III under-identifies children who could qualify for intervention services. Extracting language items from the cognitive scale also affects comparability with the MDI found in previous versions. Conversely, the five domains now allow the BSID-III to be more compatible with early intervention requirements (IDEA; PL 108–446, Part C). A criticism of the test is that it can take an exceptionally long time to administer (e.g., >90 min at 13 months) and this is problematic when testing infants and toddlers. The BSID-III can be used in multidisciplinary clinics, NICU follow-up programs, or as a follow-up evaluation after a child has been identified by the use of a screening test.

References and Readings

Aylward, G. P. (2013). Continuing issues with the Bayley-III: Where to go from here. *Journal of Developmental and Behavioral Pediatrics, 9*, 697–701.

Bayley, N. (1969). *The Bayley scales of infant development*. San Antonio: The Psychological Corporation.

Bayley, N. (1993). *The Bayley scales of infant development* (2nd ed.). San Antonio: The Psychological Corporation.

Bayley, N. (2006). *Bayley scales of infant and toddler development* (3rd ed.). San Antonio: The Psychological Corporation.

Greenspan, S. I. (2004). *Greenspan social-emotional growth chart. A screening questionnaire for infants and young children*. San Antonio: Harcourt Assessment.

Harrison, P. L., & Oakland, T. (2003). *Adaptive behavior assessment system* (2nd ed.). San Antonio: The Psychological Corporation.

Weiss, L. G., Oakland, T., & Aylward, G. P. (Eds.). (2010). *Bayley III: Clinical use and interpretation*. Boston: Elsevier.

Beck Anxiety Inventory

Amy J. Starosta[1] and Lisa A. Brenner[2,3]
[1]Departments of Psychiatry and Physical Medicine and Rehabilitation, University of Colorado Denver, Aurora, CO, USA
[2]Rocky Mountain Mental Illness Research Education and Clinical Center, Denver, CO, USA
[3]University of Colorado, Anschutz Medical Campus, Aurora, CO, USA

Description

The Beck Anxiety Inventory (BAI) (Beck et al. 1988; Beck and Steer 1993) is a 21-item inventory which identifies anxiety symptoms and quantifies their intensity. Respondents are asked to rate how much they have been bothered by each item over the past week, including today, on a four-point scale ranging from 0 ("not at all") to 3 ("severely – I could barely stand it"). Items are summed, resulting in a total score ranging from 0 to 63, with higher scores representing greater levels of anxiousness (Table 1).

This assessment generally takes adults 5–10 min to complete. It can be self-report or interviewer administered. Traditionally, this assessment is administered in a paper-and-pencil or interview formats, but it is also increasingly given via the computer.

Beck Anxiety Inventory, Table 1 Anxiety categorization by score (Beck and Steer 1993)

Anxiety level	Minimal	Mild	Moderate	Severe
BAI score	0–7	8–15	16–25	26–63

Historical Background

The BAI was designed to assess anxiety symptoms independent of depressive symptoms. Authors compiled a pool of 86 items from three preexisting anxiety symptom checklists (the Anxiety Checklist (Beck et al. 1985), the Physician's Desk Reference Checklist (Beck 1978), and the Situational Anxiety Checklist (Beck 1982)). They eliminated repetitive items, conducted successive iterative principal factor analyses, and completed a series of validity analyses to whittle the item list down to 21. This final 21-item BAI was found to have high internal consistency. It also demonstrated both convergent validity with non-symptom constructs theoretically associated with anxiety and discriminant validity with those constructs associated with depression among a psychiatric outpatient population.

Psychometric Data

In the years since its original publication, the BAI has consistently shown good reliability in a variety of both clinical and nonclinical populations. A meta-analysis by de Ayala et al. (2005) found the average coefficient alpha to be 0.91. Test-retest values showed significantly more heterogeneity, ranging from 0.35 to 0.83, with the greatest variability among nonpsychiatric noncollege populations. Given increasing use of computer-based assessment administration, it is critical to consider the impact of the mode of administration on the psychometrics of questionnaires. Preliminary studies evaluating effect of administration mode found comparable internal consistencies but lower mean scores when the BAI was administered via the internet compared to paper-and-pencil versions (Carlbring et al. 2007). This suggests that it may be necessary to use "internet norms" when administering the BAI in a computer format.

The BAI shows strong convergent validity with anxiety symptom self-report instruments, clinical ratings, and diaries. It has also shown moderate discriminant validity with measures of other types of psychopathology in both clinical and nonclinical samples (Steer 2009). Discriminant validity with depression symptoms is more variable based on populations, with lower discriminant validity among older adults (Morin et al. 1999; Wetherell and Gatz 2005) and nonclinical Spanish speakers (Magán et al. 2008). Scores on the BAI are linearly related to depression scales; however, individual items from these assessments have a strong tendency to load onto different factors (Beck et al. 1988).

Among clinical populations, factor analytic studies generally support a two-factor structure, with one factor representing cognitive symptoms of anxiety and the other representing somatic symptoms (Wilson et al. 1999). Among nonclinical populations, the factor structure is more varied, with evidence to support four (subjective, neurophysiological, autonomic, and panic (Osman et al. 1993)), five (subjective fear, somatic nervousness, neurophysiological, muscular/motoric, respiration (Borden et al. 1991)), and six (somatic, fear, autonomic hyperactivity, panic, nervousness, and motor tension (Morin et al. 1999)) factor models. The broad categories of subjective and physiological symptoms still apply, but findings suggest that at nonclinical levels of anxiety, respondents may experience more nuanced physiological symptoms of anxiety. Given the lack of consensus in the literature regarding factor structure, the use of the total score remains the recommended approach for measuring anxiety symptoms with this scale (Steer 2009).

Clinical Uses

Overall, the BAI's strongest qualities are its ability to assess panic symptomology and distinguish between panic disorder and non-panic disorder symptom profiles (Leyfer et al. 2006). It is sensitive to changes in anxiety symptoms both in psychiatric (Brown et al. 1997) and medical populations (Lee et al. 2010). Because of its brevity and ease of administration, the BAI is commonly used as an anxiety screening instrument.

However, the BAI is not a diagnostic measure, and research suggests it has limited utility when used in isolation as a measure of anxiety (Manne et al. 2001; Hoyer et al. 2002).

In addition to its use with general clinical populations, the BAI has demonstrated utility in neuropsychological populations as well. The BAI has been used in clinical trials of psychotropic interventions for depression following traumatic brain injury (TBI) (Ashman et al. 2009) and as a measure of anxiety following TBI (Zhou et al. 2013; Cantor et al. 2005). The BAI has been used to assess anxiety among Veterans with a history of TBI and was found to be associated with increased neuropsychiatric symptoms (King et al. 2012). It has also been used to assess anxiety poststroke (Baker-Collo 2007).

While the BAI has been used often with medical and neuropsychiatric populations, research suggests that there may be some overlap with somatic symptoms, which would be potentially problematic in a medical setting. As the BAI was developed to assess anxiety independent of depression, it excludes many anxiety symptoms which overlap with depression. It has been criticized for placing too heavy emphasis on somatic symptoms of anxiety, which may be more characteristic of panic as opposed to the overall construct of anxiety. Of the 21 items, 14 assess somatic symptoms, and patients with panic disorder have been shown to score higher on the BAI (Leyfer et al. 2006). Because of its emphasis on somatic symptoms, the BAI has less utility in populations with greater medical illnesses (such as older adults Wetherell and Gatz 2005). These populations endorse more physical complaints, which results in inflated scores on the BAI. Providers should use caution when using the BAI as a broad anxiety screening tool, particularly with populations with increased medical complications.

Diversity Considerations

Internal reliability is comparable between the genders; however, women consistently score higher on the BAI than men (Beck and Steer 1993; Hewitt and Norton 1993; Osman et al. 1993; Morin et al. 1999; Vázquez-Morejón et al. 2014). This gender difference remains even after differential item analysis identified and removed potentially biased items (Magán et al. 2008). These findings are consistent with lifetime prevalence data, which suggests that women have higher rates of anxiety (Kessler et al. 2005).

While the BAI is one of the most widely used tool for measuring anxiety symptomology, there is little research regarding its use in ethnic minority populations. An initial study examining the factor structure of the BAI for African Americans (Chapman et al. 2009) found that the originally proposed two factor structure did not hold for an African American nonclinical sample. Rather, they proposed an alternative two factor model with more items loading onto the somatic factor. Examination of the psychometric properties of the BAI in Latino populations (Contreras et al. 2004) supported the original factor structure and found that the BAI had strong internal reliability. Of note, nonclinical Latino participants' average scores were within normal ranges but significantly higher than Caucasian American populations.

The BAI has been translated and validated in several other languages, including Spanish (Fernández and Navarro 2003), French (Freeston et al. 1994), Turkish (Ulusoy et al. 1998), Norwegian (Nordhagen 2001), and Icelandic (Sæmundsson et al. 2015). While there are some reported differences in factor structures, the overall findings suggest comparable psychometric properties to the English version of the BAI. Findings from studies examining the utility of the BAI in the international community have varied, with some finding comparable normative values and others showing significant variability between cultures (Pillay et al. 2001; Hoge et al. 2006). The BAI has demonstrated some cross-cultural utility, but it should continue to be used with caution in diverse settings.

See Also

▶ Anxiety

References

Ashman, T. A., Cantor, J. B., Gordon, W. A., Spielman, L., Flanagan, S., Ginsberg, A., Engmann, C., Egan, M., Ambrose, F., & Greenwald, B. (2009). A randomized controlled trial of sertraline for the treatment of depression in persons with traumatic brain injury. *Archives of Physical Medicine and Rehabilitation, 90*(5), 733–740.

Barker-Collo, S. L. (2007). Depression and anxiety 3 months post stroke: Prevalence and correlates. *Archives of Clinical Neuropsychology, 22*(4), 519–531.

Beck, A. T. (1978). *PDR checklist*. Philadelphia: University of Pennsylvania, Center for Cognitive Therapy.

Beck, A. T. (1982). *Situational anxiety checklist (SAC)*. Philadelphia: University of Pennsylvania, Center for Cognitive Therapy.

Beck, A. T., & Steer, R. A. (1993). *Beck anxiety inventory manual*. San Antonio: Psychological Corporation.

Beck, A. T., Steer, R. A., & Brown, G. (1985). *Beck anxiety checklist*. Unpublished manuscript, University of Pennsylvania.

Beck, A. T., Epstein, N., Brown, G., & Steer, R. A. (1988). An inventory for measuring clinical anxiety: Psychometric properties. *Journal of Consulting and Clinical Psychology, 56*(6), 893.

Borden, J. W., Peterson, D. R., & Jackson, E. A. (1991). The Beck anxiety inventory in nonclinical samples: Initial psychometric properties. *Journal of Psychopathology and Behavioral Assessment, 13*(4), 345–356.

Brown, G. K., Beck, A. T., Newman, C. F., Beck, J. S., & Tran, G. Q. (1997). A comparison of focused and standard cognitive therapy for panic disorder. *Journal of Anxiety Disorders, 11*(3), 329–345.

Cantor, J. B., Ashman, T. A., Schwartz, M. E., Gordon, W. A., Hibbard, M. R., Brown, M., Spielman, L., Charatz, H. J., & Cheng, Z. (2005). The role of self-discrepancy theory in understanding post-traumatic brain injury affective disorders: A pilot study. *The Journal of Head Trauma Rehabilitation, 20*(6), 527–543.

Carlbring, P., Brunt, S., Bohman, S., Austin, D., Richards, J., Öst, L. G., & Andersson, G. (2007). Internet vs. paper and pencil administration of questionnaires commonly used in panic/agoraphobia research. *Computers in Human Behavior, 23*(3), 1421–1434.

Chapman, L. K., Williams, S. R., Mast, B. T., & Woodruff-Borden, J. (2009). A confirmatory factor analysis of the Beck anxiety inventory in African American and European American young adults. *Journal of Anxiety Disorders, 23*(3), 387–392.

Contreras, S., Fernandez, S., Malcarne, V. L., Ingram, R. E., & Vaccarino, V. R. (2004). Reliability and validity of the Beck depression and anxiety inventories in Caucasian Americans and Latinos. *Hispanic Journal of Behavioral Sciences, 26*(4), 446–462.

de Ayala, R. J., Vonderharr-Carlson, D. J., & Kim, D. (2005). Assessing the reliability of the Beck anxiety inventory scores. *Educational and Psychological Measurement, 65*(5), 742–756.

Fernández, J. S., & Navarro, M. E. (2003). Propiedades psicométricas de una versión española del Inventario de Ansiedad de Beck (BAI) en estudiantes universitarios. *Ansiedad y Estrés, 9*(1), 59–84.

Freeston, M. H., Ladouceur, R., Thibodeau, N., & Gagnon, F. (1994). L'inventaire d'anxiété de Beck. Propriétés psychométriques d'une traduction française. *L'Encéphale: Revue de psychiatrie clinique biologique et thérapeutique*.

Hewitt, P. L., & Norton, G. R. (1993). The Beck anxiety inventory: A psychometric analysis. *Psychological Assessment, 5*(4), 408.

Hoge, E. A., Tamrakar, S. M., Christian, K. M., Mahara, N., Nepal, M. K., Pollack, M. H., & Simon, N. M. (2006). Cross-cultural differences in somatic presentation in patients with generalized anxiety disorder. *The Journal of Nervous and Mental Disease, 194*(12), 962–966.

Hoyer, J., Becker, E. S., Neumer, S., Soeder, U., & Margraf, J. (2002). Screening for anxiety in an epidemiological sample: Predictive accuracy of questionnaires. *Journal of Anxiety Disorders, 16*(2), 113–134.

Kessler, R. C., Berglund, P., Demler, O., Jin, R., Merikangas, K. R., & Walters, E. E. (2005). Lifetime prevalence and age-of-onset distributions of DSM-IV disorders in the National Comorbidity Survey Replication. *Archives of General Psychiatry, 62*(6), 593–602.

King, P. R., Donnelly, K. T., Donnelly, J. P., Dunnam, M., Warner, G., Kittleson, C. J., Bradshaw, C. B., Alt, M., & Meier, S. T. (2012). Psychometric study of the neurobehavioral symptom inventory. *Journal of Rehabilitation Research and Development, 49*(6), 879.

Lee, Y. W., Park, E. J., Kwon, I. H., Kim, K. H., & Kim, K. J. (2010). Impact of psoriasis on quality of life: Relationship between clinical response to therapy and change in health-related quality of life. *Annals of Dermatology, 22*(4), 389–396.

Leyfer, O. T., Ruberg, J. L., & Woodruff-Borden, J. (2006). Examination of the utility of the Beck anxiety inventory and its factors as a screener for anxiety disorders. *Journal of Anxiety Disorders, 20*(4), 444–458.

Magán, I., Sanz, J., & García-Vera, M. P. (2008). Psychometric properties of a Spanish version of the Beck Anxiety Inventory (BAI) in general population. *The Spanish Journal of Psychology, 11*(02), 626–640.

Manne, S., Nereo, N., DuHamel, K., Ostroff, J., Parsons, S., Martini, R., Williams, S., Mee, L., Sexson, S., Lewis, J., Vickberg, S. J., & Redd, W. H. (2001). Anxiety and depression in mothers of children undergoing bone marrow transplant: Symptom prevalence and use of the Beck Depression and Beck anxiety inventories as screening instruments. *Journal of Consulting and Clinical Psychology, 69*(6), 1037.

Morin, C. M., Landreville, P., Colecchi, C., McDonald, K., Stone, J., & Ling, W. (1999). The Beck anxiety inventory: Psychometric properties with older adults. *Journal of Clinical Geropsychology, 5*(1), 19–29.

Nordhagen, T. (2001). Beck anxiety inventory: Translation and validation of a Norwegian version (Master's thesis, The University of Bergen).

Osman, A., Barrios, F. X., Aukes, D., Osman, J. R., & Markway, K. (1993). The Beck anxiety inventory: Psychometric properties in a community population. *Journal of Psychopathology and Behavioral Assessment, 15* (4), 287–297.

Pillay, A. L., Edwards, S. D., Sargent, C., & Dhlomo, R. M. (2001). Anxiety among university students in South Africa. *Psychological Reports, 88*(3c), 1182–1186.

Sæmundsson, B. R., Þórsdóttir, F., Kristjánsdóttir, H., Ólason, D. Þ., Smári, J., & Sigurðsson, J. F. (2015). Psychometric properties of the Icelandic version of the Beck anxiety inventory in a clinical and a student population. *European Journal of Psychological Assessment, 27*, 133–141.

Steer, R. A. (2009). Amount of general factor saturation in the Beck anxiety inventory responses of outpatients with anxiety disorders. *Journal of Psychopathology and Behavioral Assessment, 31*(2), 112–118.

Ulusoy, M., Sahin, N. H., & Erkmen, H. (1998). Turkish version of the Beck anxiety inventory: Psychometric properties. *Journal of Cognitive Psychotherapy, 12*(2), 163–172.

Vázquez Morejón, A. J., Vázquez-Morejón Jiménez, R., & Zanin, G. B. (2014). Beck anxiety inventory: Psychometric characteristics in a sample from the clinical Spanish population. *The Spanish Journal of Psychology, 17*, E76.

Wetherell, J. L., & Gatz, M. (2005). The Beck anxiety inventory in older adults with generalized anxiety disorder. *Journal of Psychopathology and Behavioral Assessment, 27*(1), 17–24.

Wilson, K. A., De Beurs, E., Palmer, C., & Chambless, D. (1999). Beck anxiety inventory. *The use of psychological testing for treatment planning and outcomes assessment, 2*, 971–992.

Zhou, Y., Kierans, A., Kenul, D., Ge, Y., Rath, J., Reaume, J., Grossman, R. I., & Lui, Y. W. (2013). Mild traumatic brain injury: Longitudinal regional brain volume changes. *Radiology, 267*(3), 880–890.

Beck Depression Inventory

Joyce Suh and Jennifer Linton Reesman
Kennedy Krieger Institute/Johns Hopkins
University School of Medicine, Baltimore,
MD, USA

Synonyms

BDI; BDI-II

Description

The Beck Depression Inventory (BDI; Beck et al. 1961) is one of the most widely used self-report measures to assess depressive symptom severity in adolescents and adults. It was amended in 1979 to allow for simpler administration and scoring (BDI-IA; Beck et al. 1979). In 1996, a more substantial revision was made so it would correspond to the Diagnostic and Statistical Manual of Mental Disorders – Fourth Edition (DSM-IV; American Psychiatric Association 1994) criteria for clinical depression (BDI-II; Beck et al. 1996b).

The BDI-II is a self-report measure comprised of 21 items reflecting specific cognitive, affective, and physical symptoms of depression. Scores range from 0 to 3, with higher numbers indicating greater symptom severity. If more than one statement from a given item is chosen by the patient, the statement of greatest severity is scored. The maximum total score is 63.

The BDI-II takes approximately 5–10 min to complete and can be administered to individuals 13–80 years old. It is typically self-administered, although if clinically indicated, the examiner may read the items to the individual.

Historical Background

The original BDI (Beck et al. 1961) was developed with the use of descriptors provided by clinicians and patients with depression. These descriptors were then consolidated into 21 items. Directions for the assessment instructed the individual to choose the descriptor that best described how they felt *at the moment*. Originally, it was a measure administered by the examiner reading the statements to the examinee. Revisions on the BDI-IA (1979) turned it into a self-report, pencil-and-paper measure, and made the instrument easier to understand, such as by removing double negatives. In total, 15 of the original 21 items were modified. Additionally, directions were revised to instruct the individual to choose the descriptor that best described how they have felt *in the past week, including the current day*. A criticism of the BDI-IA, however, was that it only addressed six out of the nine DSM-III criteria for depression (e.g., Moran and Lambert 1983). Also, inconsistent with DSM-III criteria for clinical depression, the BDI-IA did not address symptoms such as agitation and feelings of worthlessness, and it only addressed decreases (not increases) in appetite and sleep.

Therefore, the measure was again revised. The BDI-II reworded select statements and introduced items to assess agitation, worthlessness, concentration difficulties, and loss of energy. It also included questions to reflect *increases* in sleep and appetite. Furthermore, items assessing body image, work difficulty, weight loss, and somatic preoccupations were removed, and the directions were modified so that the individual was instructed to choose the descriptor that best described how they have felt *in the past 2 weeks*. These changes improved correspondence to DSM-III-R (1987) and-DSM-IV (1994) criteria for clinical depression.

Psychometric Data

Standardization data for the BDI-II was obtained from 500 psychiatric outpatients and 120 undergraduates. Internal consistency was high for each sample ($\alpha = 0.92$ and 0.93, respectively). This is consistent with later independent study samples, which have found alphas ranging from 0.86 to 0.93 when assessing nonclinical populations, including high school-aged students (ages 14–18 years; Osman et al. 2008), undergraduates (ages 17–39 years; Storch et al. 2004), and older adults (ages 59–90 years; Segal et al. 2008), as well as clinical samples, including adolescents (ages 13–17 years; Osman et al. 2004) and adults (mean age = 37.6 years; Beck et al. 1996a).

Test-retest reliability of the BDI-II was assessed by Beck and colleagues (1996b), yielding correlation coefficients of 0.92 in a sample of 26 psychiatric outpatients, and 0.93 for their sample of college students.

Convergent and discriminant validity of the BDI-II was demonstrated by Beck and colleagues (1996b), who assessed 87 psychiatric outpatients with the BDI-II, Hamilton Rating Scale for

Depression (HRSD; Hamilton 1960), and Hamilton Rating Scale for Anxiety (HAM-A; Hamilton 1959). The BDI-II was more positively correlated with the HRSD ($r = 0.71$) than the HAM-A ($r = 0.47$).

Factor validity of the BDI-II was also assessed by Beck and colleagues (1996b), who found a two-factor solution using their outpatient standardization sample. Dozois et al. (1998) suggested that, overall, "somatic-affective" and "cognitive" are the two factors that tend to emerge in clinical samples, whereas "cognitive-affective" and "somatic" are the two factors that tend to emerge in nonclinical samples.

Overall, the BDI-II has demonstrated good internal consistency, test-retest reliability, convergent and discriminant validity, and factor validity.

Clinical Uses

The purpose of the BDI-II is to measure depression symptom severity. It can be used as part of a diagnostic battery or as a repeated measure to track treatment efficacy. Additionally, clinicians are advised to be aware that a score of "2" or "3" on item 2 (pessimism) or 9 (suicidal thoughts or wishes) is associated with greater risk for suicide (Beck et al. 1996b). Overall, the manual designates the following total raw score classifications for depression severity: 0–13 = *minimal*, 14–19 = *mild*, 20–28 = *moderate*, and ≥ 29 = *severe*. However, the instrument's developers suggest that different cutoff scores may be required depending on the characteristics of the sample and the purpose for using the instrument (e.g., lower thresholds for greater sensitivity in identifying depression, greater thresholds for greater specificity, such as in research). Other factors to consider when interpreting the BDI-II include individual characteristics, such as ethnic and cultural background, gender, age, and presence of additional medical conditions.

Given the ethnic and cultural diversity of psychiatric and neurological patient populations, there is a need for linguistically diverse and culturally sensitive psychiatric inventories. The BDI-II has been translated into numerous languages including Arabic (e.g., Hamdi et al. 1988), Chinese (e.g., Wu and Chang 2008), Dutch (e.g., Roelofs et al. 2013), Japanese (e.g., Kojima et al. 2002), Korean (e.g., Hong and Wong 2005), Portuguese (e.g., Gomes-Oliveira et al. 2012), Spanish (e.g., Gonzalez et al. 2015; Wiebe and Penley 2005), Turkish (e.g., Canel-Çınarbaş et al. 2011), and Xhosa (e.g., Edwards and Steele 2008). Some studies have suggested that BDI-II responding in different languages and cultures may have different psychometric properties. For example, studies have found that a three-factor model (instead of a two-factor model) may emerge among some ethnic groups (e.g., Mexicans: Gonzalez et al. 2015) or more ethnically diverse groups (e.g., ethnically diverse group of college students: Carmody 2005; Whisman et al. 2013); other studies, however, have confirmed the two-factor model (e.g., Chinese-heritage and European-heritage college students in Canada: Dere et al. 2015; Japanese: Kojima et al. 2002). Nevertheless, overall, studies have shown that the psychometric properties of the BDI-II in other languages and cultures are often comparable to that of the English version. Clinicians utilizing a translated measure should be aware of the different ways diverse groups may describe and experience symptoms of depression. For example, although Canel-Çınarbaş et al. (2011) found many of the psychometric properties of the Turkish version of the BDI-II to be comparable to its English counterpart, they noted that the Turkish word for depression connotes somatic symptoms such as "bodily tightness"; consistent with this, somatic symptoms were more likely be endorsed in this population.

Some studies have found gender differences in reporting on the BDI-II. Beck and colleagues (1996b) found that, among their sample of 500 outpatients, there was a significant mean difference among sexes, with women having higher overall scores than men (23.61 (SD = 12.31) for females, 20.44 (SD = 13.28) for males). The same pattern was found among their sample of 120 college students. Other studies have also found higher overall scores for women (e.g., Kojima et al. 2002; Roelofs et al. 2013). Additionally, Wagener et al. (2016) found that, in terms of specific symptom endorsements, women are more likely to score higher on sadness and self-criticalness, while men are more likely to endorse past failure and loss of pleasure. However, studies with other populations have not found similar gender differences (e.g., chronic pain; Harris and D'Eon 2008). Likewise, among US college students, the BDI-II provided an assessment of the severity of depression symptoms that was equivalent across gender, race, and ethnicity (Whisman et al. 2013). Consistent with this finding, in terms of BDI-II reporting by patients of different ages, studies have found it to also have strong psychometric support among geriatric patients (Segal et al. 2008; Steer et al. 2000).

It is also important to consider the possible differences in items endorsed among individuals with specific medical conditions. Physical sequelae of certain conditions may mimic somatic symptoms of depression, resulting in false classifications of depressive symptomatology. Despite this possibility, overall, the BDI-II has been found to be useful across medical populations, including individuals with chronic pain (Harris and D'Eon 2008), multiple sclerosis (Sacco et al. 2016), myocardial infarction (Huffman et al. 2010), and traumatic brain injury (Rowland et al. 2005). Some studies have suggested, however, that there may be different optimal cutoff scores for different populations (e.g., Huffman et al. (2010) found $>=16$ to be the optimal cutoff for patients with a history of myocardial infarction). Patterson et al. (2011) found that, among patients with hepatitis C, questions targeting cognitive and affective symptoms (rather than somatic symptoms) may be a more valid measurement of depression.

While the reading level requirement for the BDI-II is reported at a fifth to sixth grade level, examination of the cognitive complexity of this measure may require more scrutiny with certain clinical populations. The presence of multiple response options increases the complexity of this self-administered measure, which may impact its appropriateness for specific populations or settings in which motivation to respond may be low, even when the individual possesses the literacy skills necessary for response (Shumway et al. 2004).

The BDI-II was developed to correspond with depressive disorder criteria set forth by the

DSM-IV. The reliability and validity of the instrument have been established across several studies including psychiatric and neurological patients as well as nonclinical community-dwelling individuals. This generally appears to extend to ethnic and culturally diverse populations as well, although research is ongoing. Of note, the BDI-II is not intended to be used for the sole purpose of "specifying a clinical diagnosis," but as an indicator of the severity of depressive symptoms (Beck et al. 1996b). Therefore, it is important for clinicians to use clinical judgment, consider the demographic characteristics and medical condition of their patients, and consult current research when evaluating a patient for depression and interpreting BDI-II results.

Cross-References

▶ Center for Epidemiological Studies: Depression
▶ Geriatric Depression Scale
▶ Hamilton Depression Rating Scale
▶ Self-Report Measures
▶ Zung Self-Rating Depression Scale

References and Readings

American Psychiatric Association. (1987). *Diagnostic and statistical manual of mental disorders* (3rd ed.). Washington, DC: American Psychiatric Association.
American Psychiatric Association. (1994). *Diagnostic and statistical manual of mental disorders* (4th ed.). Washington, DC: American Psychiatric Association.
Beck, A. T., & Steer, R. A. (1987). *Manual for the Beck Depression Inventory*. San Antonio: The Psychological Corporation.
Beck, A., Ward, C. H., Mendelson, L., Mock, J., & Erbaugh, J. (1961). An inventory for measuring depression. *Archives of General Psychiatry, 4*, 561–571.
Beck, A. T., Rush, A. J., Shaw, B. F., & Emery, G. (1979). *Cognitive therapy of depression*. New York: Guilford Press.
Beck, A. T., Steer, R. A., Ball, R., & Ranieri, W. (1996a). Comparison of Beck Depression Inventories-IA and -II in psychiatric outpatients. *Journal of Personality Assessment, 67*(3), 588–597.
Beck, A. T., Steer, R. A., & Brown, G. K. (1996b). *Beck Depression Inventory manual* (2nd ed.). San Antonio: The Psychological Corporation.
Beck, A. T., Guth, D., Steer, R. A., & Ball, R. (1997). Screening for major depression disorders in medical inpatients with the Beck Depression Inventory for primary care. *Behavior Research and Therapy, 35*, 785–791.
Canel-Çınarbaş, D., Cui, Y., & Lauridsen, E. (2011). Cross-cultural validation of the Beck Depression Inventory–II across U.S. and Turkish samples. *Measurement and Evaluation in Counseling and Development, 44*(2), 77–91.
Carmody, D. P. (2005). Psychometric characteristics of the Beck Depression Inventory-II with college students of diverse ethnicity. *International Journal of Psychiatry in Clinical Practice, 9*(1), 22–28.
Dere, J., Watters, C. A., Yu, S. C., Bagby, R. M., Ryder, A. G., & Harkness, K. L. (2015). Cross-cultural examination of measurement invariance of the Beck Depression Inventory–II. *Psychological Assessment, 27*(1), 68–81.
Dozois, D. J. A., Dobson, K. S., & Ahnberg, J. L. (1998). A psychometric evaluation of the Beck Depression Inventory–II. *Psychological Assessment, 10*, 83–89.
Edwards, D. A., & Steele, G. I. (2008). Development and validation of the Xhosa translations of the Beck inventories: 3. Concurrent and convergent validity. *Journal of Psychology in Africa, 18*(2), 227–236.
Gomes-Oliveira, M. H., Gorenstein, C., Neto, F. L., Andrade, L. H., & Wang, Y. P. (2012). Validation of the Brazilian Portuguese version of the Beck Depression Inventory-II in a community sample. *Revista Brasileira de Psiquiatria, 34*(4), 389–394.
González, D. A., Rodríguez, A. R., & Reyes-Lagunes, I. (2015). Adaptation of the BDI–II in Mexico. *Salud Mental, 38*(4), 237–244.
Hamdi, N., Abu-Hajlah, N., & Abu-Talib, S. (1988). The factorial structure, reliability, and validity of an Arabic version of the Beck Depression Inventory. *Dirasat, 15*(1), 30–40.
Hamilton, M. (1959). The assessment of anxiety states by rating. *British Journal of Medical Psychology, 32*, 50–55.
Hamilton, M. (1960). A rating scale for depression. *Journal of Neurology and Neurosurgical Psychiatry, 23*, 56–62.
Harris, C. A., & D'Eon, J. L. (2008). Psychometric properties of the Beck Depression Inventory-Second Edition (BDI-II) in individuals with chronic pain. *Pain, 137*(3), 609–622.
Hong, S., & Wong, E. C. (2005). Rasch rating scale modeling of the Korean version of the Beck Depression Inventory. *Educational and Psychological Measurement, 65*(1), 124–139.
Huffman, J. C., Doughty, C. T., Januzzi, J. L., Pirl, W. F., Smith, F. A., & Fricchione, G. L. (2010). Screening for major depression in post-myocardial infarction patients: Operating characteristics of the Beck-Depression Inventory-II. *International Journal of Psychiatry in Medicine, 40*(2), 187–197.
Kojima, M., Furukawa, T. A., Takahashi, H., Kawai, M., Nagaya, T., & Tokudome, S. (2002). Cross-cultural validation of the Beck Depression Inventory-II in Japan. *Psychiatry Research, 110*(3), 291–299.
Moran, P. W., & Lambert, M. J. (1983). A review of current assessment tools for monitoring changes in depression. In J. S. Lambert, E. R. Christensen, & S. DeJulio (Eds.), *The assessment of psychotherapy outcome* (pp. 263–303). New York: Wiley.

Osman, A., Kopper, B. A., Barrios, F., Gutierrez, P. M., & Bagge, C. L. (2004). Reliability and validity of the Beck Depression Inventory-II with adolescent psychiatric inpatients. *Psychological Assessment, 16*(2), 120–132.

Osman, A., Barrios, F. X., Gutierrez, P. M., Williams, J. E., & Bailey, J. (2008). Psychometric properties of the Beck Depression Inventory-II in nonclinical adolescent samples. *Journal of Clinical Psychology, 64*(1), 83–102.

Patterson, A. L., Morasco, B. J., Fuller, B. E., Indest, D. W., Loftis, J. M., & Hauser, P. (2011). Screening for depression in patients with hepatitis C using the Beck Depression Inventory-II: Do somatic symptoms compromise validity? *General Hospital Psychiatry, 33*(4), 354–362.

Roelofs, J., van Breukelen, G., de Graaf, L. E., Beck, A. T., Arntz, A., & Huibers, M. H. (2013). Norms for the Beck Depression Inventory (BDI-II) in a large Dutch community sample. *Journal of Psychopathology and Behavioral Assessment, 35*(1), 93–98.

Rowland, S. M., Lam, C. S., & Leahy, B. (2005). Use of the Beck Depression Inventory-II (BDI-II) with persons with traumatic brain injury: Analysis of factorial structure. *Brain Injury, 19*(2), 77–83.

Sacco, R., Santangelo, G., Stamenova, S., Bisecco, A., Bonavita, S., Lavorgna, L., …, & Gallo, A. (2016). Psychometric properties and validity of Beck Depression Inventory II in multiple sclerosis. *European Journal of Neurology, 23*(4), 744–750.

Segal, D. L., Coolidge, F. L., Cahill, B. S., & O'Riley, A. A. (2008). Psychometric properties of the Beck Depression Inventory II (BDI-II) among community-dwelling older adults. *Behavior Modification, 32*(1), 3–20.

Shumway, M., Sentell, T., Unick, G., & Bamberg, W. (2004). Cognitive complexity of self-administered depression measures. *Journal of Affective Disorders, 83*(2–3), 191–198.

Steer, R. A., Rissmiller, D. J., & Beck, A. T. (2000). Use of Beck Depression Inventory-II with depressed geriatric inpatients. *Behaviour Research and Therapy, 38*(3), 311–331.

Storch, E. A., Roberti, J. W., & Roth, D. A. (2004). Factor structure, concurrent validity, and internal consistency of the Beck Depression Inventory-Second Edition in a sample of college students. *Depression and Anxiety, 19*(3), 187–189.

Wagener, A., Baeyens, C., & Blairy, S. (2016). Depressive symptomatology and the influence of the behavioral avoidance and activation: A gender-specific investigation. *Journal of Affective Disorders, 193*, 123–129.

Whisman, M. A., Judd, C. M., Whiteford, N. T., & Gelhorn, H. L. (2013). Measurement invariance of the Beck Depression Inventory–Second Edition (BDI-II) across gender, race, and ethnicity in college students. *Assessment, 20*(4), 419–428.

Wiebe, J. S., & Penley, J. A. (2005). A psychometric comparison of the Beck Depression Inventory-II in English and Spanish. *Psychological Assessment, 17*(4), 481–485.

Wu, P., & Chang, L. (2008). Psychometric properties of the Chinese version of the Beck Depression Inventory-II using the Rasch model. *Measurement and Evaluation in Counseling and Development, 41*(1), 13–31.

Beery Developmental Test of Visual-Motor Integration (VMI), Sixth Edition

Kelly Teresa Macdonald[1] and Ida Sue Baron[2]
[1]Department of Psychology, University of Houston, Houston, TX, USA
[2]Potomac, MD, USA

Synonyms

Beery VMI; Developmental test of visual-motor integration

Description

The Beery-Buktenica Developmental Test of Visual-Motor Integration (VMI; Beery et al. 2004), typically referred to as the Beery VMI, is designed to assess the integration of visual and motor abilities. The current version includes two forms for the Beery VMI and two supplemental subsections, motor coordination and visual perception. The supplemental tests may be administered after results from the VMI test indicate the need for further assessment in order to separate an individual's pure motor and visual abilities. For the VMI, examinees are administered either a 21-item short form or a 30-item long form; each requires copying geometric forms that become increasingly complex. The short form is designed for use with children aged 2–7 years, and the long form for individuals up to age 100. The long form takes approximately 10–15 min to administer, and the short form takes approximately 10 min. The test may also be administered to a group; however, the authors recommend individual testing for children who have developmental delays or neurological impairments. For children at or over the functional age of 5, administration begins with item 7. If the examinee is unable to complete item 7 correctly, the manual provides instructions for how to proceed. The examinees use a pen or pencil to complete the geometric forms. One point is given for each correctly drawn figure, and testing is discontinued after three consecutive failures. A composite standard score is obtained.

Background

The first edition of the Beery VMI was published in 1967 (Beery, Buktenica, and Beery). While other measures of visual-motor integration were available at the time, none involved a sequence of increasingly complex geometric forms. Although the Beery VMI is currently in its sixth edition, the test items found in the current edition are almost identical to the original stimuli. The 1997 edition added the two supplemental forms so that visual-motor integration could be compared to pure visual or pure motor performance. The sixth and most recent edition includes suggestions for teaching and improving visual-motor integration.

Psychometric Data

The Beery VMI manual reports internal consistency reliabilities averaging 0.92 for visual-motor integration, 0.91 for visual perception, and 0.90 for motor coordination. Analyses of convergent validity found the Beery VMI correlates 0.52 with the drawing subtest of the Wide Range Assessment of Visual Motor Abilities (WRAVMA) and 0.75 with the copying subtest of the Developmental Test of Visual Perception (DTVP-2).

Normative data for the Beery VMI were updated in the sixth edition (2010) with a sample of 1,700 individuals with demographic characteristics closely matching those from the 2010 US Census. From ages 2–13, standard scores are provided in 2-month intervals for the Beery VMI, and in 3-month intervals for the two supplemental tests. For ages 13–19, Beery VMI norms are by year, and the supplemental tests are by 2-year periods. For adults, norms are by decade. Standard scores have a mean of 100 and standard deviation of 15, and scores may be converted to other scales (e.g., scaled scores, percentiles).

Clinical Use

The Beery VMI is a useful early screening tool for psychologists, learning disability specialists, school counselors, teachers, and other professionals to identify children with visual-motor impairments. Test results assist in making appropriate referrals for services, or to test the effectiveness of educational and other intervention programs. Researchers use the test to examine deficits in visual-motor integration in specific neurodevelopmental disorders. In one study, the Beery VMI was used to compare visual-motor integration in children diagnosed with ADHD and those with comorbid ADHD and reading disability, and/or oppositional defiant disorder (Kooistra et al. 2005). This study found increases in motor impairments among children with ADHD as a function of comorbid diagnoses, particularly reading disability. Another study examined differences in VMI performance between children with traumatic brain injury and ADHD in order to examine the instrument's validity, and found support for the use of the VMI in children with both developmental and acquired brain dysfunction (Sutton et al. 2011). The Beery VMI has also been used in research studies of the neuropsychological outcomes for children born preterm (Baron et al. 2009), and individuals with Autism Spectrum Disorder (Green et al. 2015). Performance on the Beery VMI can inform diagnostic decisions across a wide spectrum of disorders.

Cross-References

► Rey Complex Figure Test

References and Further Readings

Baron, I. S., Erickson, K., Ahronovich, M., Coulehan, K., Baker, R., & Litman, F. (2009). Visuospatial and verbal fluency relative deficits in 'complicated' late-preterm preschool children. *Early Human Development, 85,* 751–754.

Beery, K. E., Buktenica, N. A., & Beery, N. A. (2004). *The Beery-Buktenica developmental test of visual-motor* integration: Administration, scoring, and teaching manual (5th ed.). Minneapolis: NCS Pearson, Inc..

Beery, K. E., Buktenica, N. A., & Beery, N. A. (2010). The Beery-Buktenica developmental test of visual-motor integration: Administration, scoring, and teaching manual (6th ed.). Minneapolis: NCS Pearson, Inc..

Green, R. R., Bigler, E. D., Froehlich, A., Prigge, M. B., Travers, B. G., Cariello, A. N., & Lainhart, J. E. (2015). Beery VMI performance in autism spectrum disorder. Child Neuropsychology. https://doi.org/10.1080/09297049.2015.1056131.

Kooistra, L., Crawford, S., Dewey, D., Cantell, M., & Kaplan, B. J. (2005). Motor correlates of ADHD contribution of reading disability and oppositional defiant disorder. Journal of Learning Disabilities, 38, 195–206.

Sutton, G. P., Barchard, K. A., Bello, D. T., Thaler, N. S., Ringdahl, E., Mayfield, J., & Allen, D. N. (2011). Beery-Buktenica developmental test of visual-motor integration performance in children with traumatic brain injury and attention-deficit/hyperactivity disorder. Psychological Assessment, 23, 805.

Behavior Management

Glenn S. Ashkanazi
Department of Clinical and Health Psychology, Clinical and Health Psychology Clinic, College of Public Health and Health Professions, University of Florida, Gainesville, FL, USA

Definition

Techniques used to control or modify an action or performance of a subject. This is a less-intensive version of behavior modification in which the goal is to develop, strengthen, maintain, decrease, or eliminate behaviors in a planned or systematic way. Behavior management skills are particularly important to enhance the probability that individuals, or groups, choose behaviors that are prosocial. Prosocial behaviors are typically seen as personally fulfilling, productive, and socially acceptable. The process typically includes identifying negative behaviors, raising awareness about alternative behaviors, and changing the environment by modifying antecedents to behaviors or the consequences. Persons surviving a traumatic brain injury (TBI) often have behavioral disturbances such as disinhibition and/or agitation. Due to learning impairments

as a result of their TBI, the traditional behavior management approaches, which are based on learning theory principles, are modified. For example, behavior management approaches with TBI survivors may focus more on stimulus control (e.g., controlling environmental (antecedent) cues) than operant conditioning (e.g., recalling the contingency between behaviors and the resulting consequences).

Cross-References

▶ Applied Behavior Analysis
▶ Behavior Modification
▶ Behavioral Therapy

References and Readings

Jacobs, H. E. (1993). Behavior analysis guidelines and brain injury rehabilitation: People, principles and programs. Gaithersburg: Aspen.

Karol, R. L. (2003). Neuropsychological intervention: The practical treatment of severe behavioural dyscontrol after acquired brain injury. Boca Raton: CRC Press.

Novack, T., PhD. (n.d.). Management of behavioral problems during acute rehabilitation of individuals with TBI. Retrieved 30 Nov 2016, from http://www.brainline.org/content/2008/07/management-behavioral-problems-during-acute-rehabilitation-individuals-tbi_pageall.html

Behavior Modification

Chava Creque[1] and Stephanie A. Kolakowsky-Hayner[2]
[1]Department of Psychology and Neuroscience, University of Colorado Boulder, Boulder, CO, USA
[2]Department of Rehabilitation Medicine, Icahn School of Medicine at Mount Sinai, New York, NY, USA

Synonyms

Applied behavioral analysis; Behavior therapy; Cognitive-behavioral modification

Definition

Behavior modification is the use of basic learning techniques, such as conditioning, biofeedback, assertiveness training, positive or negative reinforcement, hypnosis, or aversion therapy, to change unwanted individual or group behavior and improve daily functioning. These techniques are typically based on functional assessment and used to reinforce adaptive behaviors while diminishing or extinguishing maladaptive behaviors. Behavioral modification techniques can be used to address learning issues as well as social, emotional, behavioral, or psychiatric problems. Seven characteristics of behavior modification, identified by Martin and Pear (2015), include:

- A strong emphasis on defining problems in terms of measurable behavior
- Making environmental adjustments to improve functioning
- Precise methods and rationales
- Dynamic real-life application of techniques
- Techniques grounded in learning and behavior theory
- Scientific demonstration linking the imposed technique with behavior change
- Strong emphasis on accountability

Cross-References

▶ Applied Behavior Analysis
▶ Behavioral Assessment
▶ Behavior Management
▶ Behavioral Therapy

References and Readings

Crum, C. (2004). Using a cognitive-behavioral modification strategy to increase on-task behavior of a student with a behavior disorder. *Intervention in School and Clinic, 39*(5), 305.
Hicinbothem, J., Gonsalves, S., & Lester, D. (2006). Body modification and suicidal behavior. *Death Studies, 30*(4), 351.
Kazdi, A. E. (2012). *Behavior modification in applied settings*. Long Grove: Waveland Press.
Lindsey, N., Reif, J., Bachand, A., & Seys, S. (2005). Behavior modification following a diagnosis of hepatitis C infection. *American Journal of Health Behavior, 29*(6), 512–519.
Martin, G. L., & Pear,J.J. (2015). *Behavior modification: What it is and how to do it* (10th ed.). New York, NY: Routledge Psychology Press.
Ntinas, K. (2007). Behavior modification and the principle of normalization: Clash or synthesis? *Behavioral Interventions, 22*(2), 165–177.

Behavior Rating Inventory for Executive Function

Gerard A. Gioia[1], Peter K. Isquith[2] and Robert M. Roth[3]
[1]Children's National Medical Center, Rockville, MD, USA
[2]Dartmouth Medical School, Lebanon, NH, USA
[3]Geisel School of Medicine at Dartmouth / DHMC, Lebanon, NH, USA

Synonyms

BRIEF; BRIEF2; BRIEF-A; BRIEF-P; BRIEF-SR

Description

The Behavior Rating Inventory of Executive Function (BRIEF) family of measures are rating scales designed to facilitate assessment of the behavioral manifestations of executive dysfunction in everyday environments such as home, school, and work. First published in 2000 as parent and teacher rating scales of executive function in children and adolescents, the family of measures has grown to include versions for assessing preschool children, adolescents' self-report, and adults.

The original BRIEF consists of two forms, a parent questionnaire and a teacher questionnaire, designed to assess executive function behaviors in children and adolescents aged 5–18 years in home and school environments. It includes 86 items with 8 theoretically and empirically derived clinical scales measuring Inhibit, Shift, Emotional Control, Initiate,

Working Memory, Plan/Organize, Monitor, and Organization of Materials. The BRIEF also includes two validity scales, Inconsistency and Negativity. The eight scales form two broader indexes based on the factor structure, Behavioral Regulation and Metacognition, as well as an overall score, the Global Executive Composite (GEC).

In 2015, the first revision of the BRIEF, the BRIEF2, was published, reducing the length of the measure by approximately one quarter while adding numerous enhancements. These were informed by the hundreds of peer-reviewed papers that have employed the measure in a wide range of clinical and normative groups in multiple languages on six continents; tested the factor structure; explored relationships with academic, behavioral, emotional, social, and adaptive functioning; documented associations with biological factors including brain structure and function; and demonstrated sensitivity to change with recovery or treatment. The BRIEF2 includes parallel Parent and Teacher forms and incorporates the previously separate adolescent self-report form. Parent and Teacher forms are composed of 63 items within 9 theoretically and empirically derived clinical scales that are largely consistent with those of the BRIEF, with the exception that the Monitor scale was separated into Self-Monitor and Task Monitor scales. The BRIEF2 includes three validity scales, Inconsistency, Negativity, and a new Infrequency scale. Finally, the nine scales form three broader indexes based on the factor structure, Behavior Regulation, Emotion Regulation, and Cognitive Regulation (similar to the metacognition index on the BRIEF), as well as a Global Executive Composite score, or the GEC.

The BRIEF2 also includes a revised and co-normed version of the BRIEF Adolescent Self-Report. This is a 55-item Self-Report form designed to complement the BRIEF2 Parent and Teacher forms. It is appropriate for older children and adolescents ages 11–18 years with a fifth-grade or higher reading ability. The items yield information for seven clinical scales: Inhibit, Self-Monitor, Shift, Emotional Control, Task Completion, Working Memory, and Plan/Organize. The clinical scales form three indexes, the Behavior Regulation Index (BRI), Emotion Regulation Index (ERI), and Cognitive Regulation Index (CRI), and an overall summary score, the Global Executive Composite (GEC). The BRIEF2 Self-Report also includes three validity scales – Infrequency, Inconsistency, and Negativity.

An important enhancement in the BRIEF2 is the inclusion of three 12-item screening forms for parents, teachers, and adolescents. These concise forms were created to meet the needs of large-scale assessment in education, health, and research settings. Each correlates strongly with the BRIEF2 Global Executive Composite score (r > 90) and discriminates between typically developing children and those with executive function deficits with large effect sizes. Reliabilities are strong, there are multiple lines of evidence for validity, and the standardization sample was large and stratified by gender, race/ethnicity, parent education, and geographic region. Classification statistics including sensitivity/specificity and likelihood ratios are used to identify children at risk for executive function problems who should be more fully assessed.

The BRIEF-Preschool Version (BRIEF-P) measures the behavioral manifestations of executive function in preschool-aged children, ages 2–5. It consists of a single form completed by parents and/or teachers/caregivers to rate the child's executive functions within the home and preschool settings. The questionnaire consists of 63 items comprising 5 theoretically and empirically derived clinical scales measuring Inhibit, Shift, Emotional Control, Working Memory, and Plan/Organize. These scales form three factor-derived indexes, Inhibitory Self-Control, Flexibility, and Emergent Metacognition, and one composite score, the GEC. The BRIEF–P also includes two validity scale, Inconsistency and Negativity.

The BRIEF-A measures an adult's executive functions in his or her everyday home and work environment. Two forms are available, a Self-Report and an Informant Report. The Self-Report form is designed to be completed by adults

18–90 years of age, while the Informant Report form is administered to an adult who is familiar with the rated individual's everyday functioning. The latter form can be used alone when the rated individual is unable to complete the Self-Report form or has limited awareness of his or her own difficulties or with the Self-Report form to gain multiple perspectives on the individual's functioning. The BRIEF-A is composed of 75 items within 9 clinical scales measuring: Inhibit, Self-Monitor, Shift, Emotional Control, Initiate, Working Memory, Plan/Organize, Task-Monitor, and Organization of Materials. The clinical scales form two broader factor-based indexes: Behavioral Regulation (BRI) and Metacognition (MI), and these indexes form the overall summary score, the GEC. The BRIEF-A also includes three validity scales: Negativity, Inconsistency, and Infrequency.

Historical Background

Executive functions have been historically evaluated using laboratory-based performance tests. While these types of measures offer the advantages of control over extraneous variables and potential to fractionate and examine components of executive function separately such as planning versus working memory, they are limited in ecological validity or ability to predict functioning in the everyday environment. Fundamentally, executive functions are necessary for organization of goal-directed behavior in the everyday, "real-world" environment. Thus, in addition to assessing these functions with clinical performance measures, it is important to also capture behavioral manifestations of executive function or dysfunction. The BRIEF was developed to measure executive functions through the assessment of an individuals' behavior in their everyday environments. Given the challenges of executive function assessment in the laboratory and inherent limitations to applicability in the everyday environment and to treatment, attention has increasingly turned to alternative methods of evaluation that offer enhanced ecological validity. Assessment methods that reliably tap the individual's

everyday executive problem-solving in natural settings offer a complementary approach to clinical performance-based assessment.

Executive function is generally viewed as a broad umbrella term that encompasses a set of interrelated subdomains. Although authors vary with respect to which cognitive and behavioral processes are viewed as part of the executive function domain, they typically include initiation of goal-directed behavior, inhibition of competing actions or stimuli, planning and selection of relevant task goals, organization of behavior to solve novel and/or complex problems, flexible shifting of behavior and problem-solving strategies when necessary, monitoring and evaluation of problem-solving behavior and task performance more generally, as well as monitoring the effects of one's own behavior on others. In support of these behaviors, working memory capacity plays a fundamental role in holding information actively "online" in the service of problem-solving, including planning and organization. Importantly, the executive functions are not exclusive to cognition; emotional control is also relevant to effective problem-solving activity and should be considered in any definition. Historically, executive functions have been closely associated with the integrity of the frontal lobes of the brain. Much of the evidence supporting a role for the frontal lobes in executive functions has come from studies of individuals with acquired focal damage to this region, as well as studies using advanced brain imaging techniques such as positron emission tomography (PET) and functional magnetic resonance imaging (fMRI). However, these same studies have also clearly shown that executive functions are not subserved by the frontal lobes alone, but rather by distributed neural circuitry that includes other cortical regions and subcortical structures as well as the cerebellum. Damage to any given component of this circuitry may result in executive dysfunction.

The BRIEF was originally developed beginning in 1994 following a commonly accepted developmental model of executive function (Welsh and Pennington 1988; Holmes-Bernstein and Waber 1990). The impetus arose from the authors' frequent observations in clinical practice that parent and teacher reports of a child's functioning in the everyday environment did not always, or even often, fit with the same child's test performance on putative executive function performance tests. The measure found acceptance initially within the field of pediatric neuropsychology and was published first in 2000. Since then, the several versions of the BRIEF have become widely used across the age spectrum and across clinical, school, and research settings. Since publication, a substantial body of literature has developed examining BRIEF profiles with a wide range of clinical groups (Roth et al. 2014; Strauss et al. 2006).

Psychometric Data

BRIEF2 (Ages 5–18 Years: Parent and Teacher Forms)

Standardization: Normative data are based on 1,400 parents and 1,400 teachers from rural, suburban, and urban areas. The samples were diverse to match proportions of race/ethnicity, parental education level, geographic region, and gender across all 50 states, based on the US population data from the Current Population Survey, March 2013 by the US Census Bureau, 2012, Washington, DC. Separate normative tables, including T scores, percentiles, and confidence intervals, are provided for four age groups for boys and girls separately, with norms for both the Parent and Teacher forms. Clinical data are based on 2,892 parents and 1,889 teachers rating children with developmental disorders or acquired neurological disorders (e.g., learning disabilities, ADHD, TBI, Tourette's syndrome, mental retardation, epilepsy, and language disorders).

Reliability: High internal consistency (Cronbach's alpha >0.90 for Parent and Teacher Index Scores). Test-retest reliability for composites was $r = 0.82$–0.89 for parent normative ratings and $r = 0.83$–0.90 for teacher normative ratings. Interobserver reliability reflected moderate to high correlations for parent-parent ratings (mean $r = 0.77$ for normative sample, 0.59 for clinical sample), moderate correlations for parent-teacher (mean $r = 0.30$–0.50), teacher-teacher

ratings (mean $r = 0.39$ for normative sample, mean $r = 0.56$ for clinical sample).

Validity: Evidence of validity is demonstrated by several lines of evidence including high inter-rater agreement for item-scale assignments by expert panel, factor analytic studies, and structural equation modeling. Convergent and divergent validity evidence is demonstrated by convergence with scales of inattention and impulsivity and divergence of behavioral/emotional functioning from executive functioning using the ADHD-IV, BASC, CBCL, and CRS. Exploratory and confirmatory factor analysis of the BRIEF2 Parent, Teacher, and Self-Report forms yielded a consistent three-factor solution (i.e., Behavior Regulation, Emotion Regulation, Cognitive Regulation) for normative and clinical samples. Two of the scales, Working Memory and Inhibit, are clinically useful in detecting and predicting the diagnosis of attention-deficit/hyperactivity disorder (ADHD).

BRIEF2 Self-Report (BRIEF2-SR)

Standardization: The BRIEF2-SR was standardized and validated for use with children and adolescents aged 11–18 years. The normative sample includes 803 participants using the same comprehensive sampling as the Parent and Teacher forms matched to the US Census data. Clinical data are based on 473 children and adolescents with a variety of developmental disorders or acquired neurological disorders (e.g., learning disabilities, ADHD, TBI, Tourette's syndrome, autism spectrum disorders, epilepsy, and brain tumor disorders).

Reliability: The BRIEF2-SR scales demonstrate appropriate reliability. Internal consistency is high for the GEC ($\alpha = 0.97$) and moderate to high for the clinical scales ($\alpha = 0.81$–0.88). Temporal stability is strong ($\underline{r} = 0.85$ for the GEC over a period of 3.7 weeks), and there is strong inter-rater agreement for the GEC with parent ratings on the BRIEF ($r = 0.71$). Teacher ratings on the BRIEF2-SR correlated moderately with adolescent ratings on the BRIEF-SR (GEC $r = 0.57$).

Validity: Principal factor analysis of the BRIEF2-SR yielded a three-factor solution (i.e., Behavior Regulation, Emotion Regulation,

Cognitive Regulation) for normative and clinical samples. Correlational analyses with other self-report behavior rating scales (i.e., Child Behavior Checklist/Youth Self-Report [CBSL/YSR], Behavior Assessment System for Children Self-Report of Personality [BASC-SRP], Child Health Questionnaire [CHQ], Profile of Mood States-Short Form [POMS-SF]) provide evidence of convergent and divergent validity for the BRIEF-SR. Examination of BRIEF2-SR profiles in a variety of clinical groups provides further evidence of validity based on clinical utility. BRIEF2-SR ratings for groups of adolescents with ADHD-I, ADHD-C, insulin-dependent diabetes mellitus, autism spectrum disorders, and anxiety and depressive disorders showed different patterns of scale elevations for each group compared to matched control groups. Correlations between adolescent and parent ratings for the clinical groups were low to moderate (r = 0.25–0.35), suggesting agreement yet different perspectives as well.

BRIEF-Preschool (BRIEF-P: Ages 2–5 Years, Parent and Caretaker Forms)

Standardization: Normative data based on child ratings from 460 parents and 302 teachers from urban, suburban, and rural areas, reflecting 1999 US Census estimates for race/ethnicity, gender, socioeconomic status, and age. Clinical samples included children in the following diagnostic/clinical groups: ADHD, low birth weight/prematurity, language disorders, autism spectrum disorders, and a mixed clinical group.

Reliability: High internal consistency (α = 0.80–0.95 for parent sample and α = 0.90–0.97 for teacher sample), test-retest reliability (r = 0.78–0.90 for parents and 0.64–0.94 for teachers), and modest correlations between parent and teacher ratings (r = 0.14–0.28).

Validity: Convergent and discriminant validity evidence established with other measures of inattention, hyperactivity-impulsivity, depression, atypicality, anxiety, and somatic complaints (ADHD-IV-P, CBCL/1½–5, BASC–PRS). Factor analytic studies provide support for a three-factor model of executive functioning embodied by the three indexes in the parent and teacher normative groups, respectively. The Working Memory and the Plan/Organize scales define the first component, the Shift and Emotional Control scales comprise the second component, and the Inhibit and Emotional Control scales define the third component.

BRIEF-Adult (BRIEF-A: Self-Report and Informant Report)

Standardization: The BRIEF-A was standardized and validated for use with men and women from ages 18–90 years. The normative sample includes 1,050 adult self-reports and 1,200 informant reports from a wide range of racial/ethnic backgrounds, educational backgrounds, as well as geographic regions that are matched to US Census data.

Reliability: The BRIEF-A has demonstrated multiple lines of evidence for reliability. Internal consistency was moderate to high for the Self-Report normative sample (α = 0.73–0.90 for clinical scales; 0.93–0.96 for indexes and GEC) and high for the Informant Report normative sample (α = 0.80–0.93 for clinical scales; 0.95–0.98 for indexes and GEC). Using a mixed sample of clinical or healthy adults who were seen for clinical evaluation or research study participation, internal consistency was high for the Self-Report form (α = 0.80–0.94 for clinical scales; 0.96–0.98 for indexes and GEC) and the Informant Report form (α = 0.85–0.95 for clinical scales; 0.96–0.98 for indexes and GEC). Test-retest correlations over a 4-week period across the clinical scales ranged from r = 0.82–0.93 for the Self-Report form (n = 0.50) and from r = 0.91–0.94 for the Informant Report Form (n = 0.44). Correlations between Self-Report ratings and Informant Report ratings were moderate, ranging from r = 0.44–0.68 for the clinical scales and from 0.61–0.63 for the indexes and the GEC.

Validity: The BRIEF-A exhibits multiple lines of validity evidence as an ecologically sensitive measure of executive functioning in individuals with a range of conditions across a wide age range. In terms of convergent validity evidence, the Self- and Informant Report Form of the BRIEF-A scales, indexes, and GEC demonstrated significant correlations in the expected direction with Self-Report and Informant Report on the

Frontal Systems Behavior Scale, Dysexecutive Questionnaire, and Cognitive Failures Questionnaire. Validity has been further demonstrated via studies of clinical populations. Factor analysis of Self-Report form data yielded a two-factor solution (i.e., Behavioral Regulation, Metacognition) for normative and mixed clinical/healthy adult samples, accounting for 73% and 76% of the variance, respectively. Factor analysis of Informant Report form data also yielded a similar two-factor solution for the normative and mixed clinical/healthy adult samples, accounting for 81% and 78% of the variance, respectively.

Clinical Uses

Given the central importance of the executive functions to the direction and control of dynamic "real-world" behavior, the BRIEF family of instruments was designed for a broad range of individuals with developmental, neurological, psychiatric, and medical conditions. Deficits in various subdomains of the executive functions are central characteristics of many developmental and acquired neurological disorders across the life span. Executive function deficits measured via the BRIEF have been demonstrated in a variety of populations such as ADHD, traumatic brain injury, lesions of the frontal lobes, type 1 diabetes mellitus, autism spectrum disorders, learning disabilities, myelomeningocele and hydrocephalus, Tourette's syndrome, phenylketonuria, bipolar disorder, obstructive sleep apnea, 22q11 deletion syndrome, galactosemia, sickle cell disease, and prenatal alcohol exposure. The BRIEF-A has been examined in clinical populations such as mild cognitive impairment, ADHD, epilepsy, traumatic brain injury, schizophrenia, and cancer survivors.

The measures also show promise for veridicality, that is, predicting behavior in the natural environment. For example, correlational analyses suggest strong, logical relationships between the Inhibit scale and aggression and the Working Memory scale with attention problems. Correlations have also been reported between BRIEF and aspects of real-world functioning such as adaptive functioning in individuals with developmental disabilities, scholastic achievement and performance on high-stakes testing in children, as well as college adjustment and academic procrastination in young adults. While there are modest correlations between the BRIEF and performance tests that tap aspects of executive functions, the BRIEF shows significant associations with biological markers such as lead levels, structural and functional neuroimaging (e.g., frontal lobe volume, white matter integrity), and genetic markers (e.g., polymorphisms of the monoamine oxidase A gene). Finally, certain BRIEF profiles of executive function in the everyday environment can help predict diagnoses such as ADHD and autism spectrum disorder.

Data from the BRIEF can help the clinician focus on potentially problematic areas requiring further assessment. The same data may inform decisions about targets for treatment and types of interventions based on the potential for ameliorating real-world problems. An understanding of the individual's profile of executive function strengths and weaknesses can lead to targeted pharmacological, behavioral, cognitive, or other therapeutic interventions. Such strategies may be specifically targeted toward one area of executive functions, such as antecedent management for children with inhibitory control deficits, or may be more programmatic, such as the comprehensive cognitive rehabilitation programs. For example, an individual who is described as disinhibited in the everyday world might have treatments and supports targeted specifically toward boosting inhibitory control or limiting opportunity for impulsive behavior. A child with difficulties shifting set might benefit from teaching and intervention strategies that incorporate use of routines and schedules to reduce agitation and anxiety when change is needed.

Finally, assessment of executive function with the BRIEF can inform clinical treatment design, monitoring, and outcome evaluation. Given the inherent difficulty in administering performance measures of executive function in a repeated fashion, behaviorally anchored measures may be well suited to such within-subject methods. For example, a patient concerned about attentional difficulties might reveal problems with inhibitory control and working memory on the BRIEF. After appropriate interview and clinical diagnosis, treatment methods might include medication and cognitive behavior therapy. To evaluate effectiveness of treatment, the measure may be administered again after starting medication and again after a longer period to determine whether the effects of treatment are maintained. Ratings can be provided by the individual themselves or an informant in their environment who has the opportunity to regularly observe their behavior (e.g., parent, teacher, spouse). More frequent monitoring might also be appropriate in some cases, such as for individuals who sustain a mild TBI, where full neuropsychological evaluation may not be feasible or appropriate at the time, but rapid, timely assessment of functioning is important for determining when the individual may return to normal activities (Ransom et al. 2016). The BRIEF2 monitoring form may be especially useful for such situations where frequent reassessment is needed in a time- and resource-sensitive manner.

See Also

▶ Attention Deficit Hyperactivity Disorder
▶ Concussion
▶ Executive Functioning
▶ Traumatic Brain Injury (TBI)

Further Reading

Gioia, G. A., Isquith, P. K., & Guy, S. C. (2001). Assessment of executive functions in children with neurologic impairment. In R. J. Simeonsson & S. Rosenthal (Eds.), *Psychological and developmental assessment: Children with disabilities and chronic conditions*. New York: Guilford Press.

Gioia, G. A., Isquith, P. K., Kenworthy, L., & Barton, R. M. (2002). Profiles of everyday executive function in acquired and developmental disorders. *Child Neuropsychology, 8*, 121–137.

Gioia, G. A., Isquith, P. K., & Kenealy, L. (2008). Assessment of behavioral aspects of executive function. In V. Anderson, R. Jacobs, & P. Anderson (Eds.), *Executive functions and the frontal lobes: A life span approach*. Sussex: Psychology Press.

Gioia, G. A., Kenworthy, L., & Isquith, P. K. (2010). Executive function in the real world: BRIEF lessons from mark Ylvisaker. *The Journal of Head Trauma Rehabilitation, 25*(6), 433–439.

Holmes-Bernstein, J., & Waber, D. (1990). Developmental neuropsychological assessment: A systemic approach. *NeuroMethods, 17*, 311–372.

Isquith, P. K., Crawford, J. S., Espy, K. A., & Gioia, G. A. (2005). Assessment of executive function in preschool children. *Mental Retardation and Developmental Disability Research Review, 11*, 209–215.

Isquith, P. K., Roth, R. M., & Gioia, G. (2013). Contribution of rating scales to the assessment of executive functions. *Applied Neuropsychology: Child, 2*(2), 125–132.

Isquith, P. K., Roth, R. M., Kenworthy, L., & Gioia, G. (2014). Contribution of rating scales to intervention for executive dysfunction. *Applied Neuropsychology: Child, 3*(3), 197–204.

Malloy, P., & Grace, J. (2005). A review of rating scales for measuring behavior change due to frontal systems damage. *Cognitive and Behavioral Neurology, 18*, 18–27.

Ransom, D. M., Burns, A., Youngstrom, E. A., Sady, M. D., Vaughan, C. G., & Gioia, G. A. (2016). Applying an evidence-based assessment model to identify students at risk for perceived academic problems following concussion. *Journal of the International Neuropsychological Society, 22*(10), 1038–1049.

Roth, R. M., Isquith, P. K., & Gioia, G. A. (2014). Assessment of executive functioning using the behavior rating inventory of executive function (BRIEF). In S. Goldstein & J. A. Naglieri (Eds.), *Handbook of executive functioning* (2nd ed., pp. 301–331). New York: Springer.

Strauss, E., Sherman, E. M. S., & Spreen, O. (2006). Behavior rating inventory of executive function (BRIEF). In *A compendium of neuropsychological tests, administration, norms, and commentary* (3rd ed., pp. 1090–1099). Oxford: Oxford University Press.

Behavioral Assessment

Dawn E. Bouman
Neuropsychology and Medical Psychology, University of Cincinnati, Department of Neurology and Rehabilitation Medicine, Cincinnati, OH, USA

Synonyms

Behavior/behavioral analysis; Behavior/behavioral observation

Definition

Behavioral assessment is a systematic collection of data, obtained through direct observation, often in natural settings, rather than sole administration of standardized tests. Behavior assessment can be informal or formal and standardized. Based on learning theory, behavioral assessment considers the context of a person's actions, including antecedents that precede and might trigger the action, as well as consequences that follow the behavior which might reinforce the behavior. Behavior assessment can be used to describe a person's functioning (i.e., arousal, initiation, or agitation) and evaluate effectiveness of therapy interventions or medications. In persons who have behavioral disorders due to neurological causes, behavior assessment is the first step for evaluating the situation so that remediation recommendations can be made. Patients are often directly observed in physical or occupational therapy sessions and in the home or classroom.

Cross-References

▶ Applied Behavior Analysis
▶ Behavior Management
▶ Behavior Modification
▶ Behavior Rating Inventory for Executive Function
▶ Behavioral Assessment of the Dysexecutive Syndrome
▶ Behavioral Therapy
▶ Conners Comprehensive Behavior Rating Scales™
▶ Functional Assessment
▶ Functional Assessment Measure

References and Readings

Jacobs, H. E. (1993). *Behavior analysis guidelines and brain injury rehabilitation*. Gaithersburg: Aspen.

Behavioral Assessment of the Dysexecutive Syndrome

Shahal Rozenblatt
Advanced Psychological Assessment P. C., Smithtown, NY, USA

Synonyms

BADS

Description

The BADS (Wilson et al. 1996) is a test battery aimed at predicting everyday difficulties that arise as a result of the Dysexecutive Syndrome (DES). It consists of six subtests and a 20-item questionnaire that tap executive functioning in an ecologically valid way. The subtests are as follows: The Rule Shift Cards Test is a measure of cognitive flexibility that consists of 21 spiral-bound cards that are used to assess the individual's ability to respond correctly to a rule and to shift from one rule to another. It is scored based on the time taken and number of errors made. In the first part, the individual is asked to respond "Yes" to a red card and "No" to a black card. This component establishes a pattern of behavior that is geared to increase the probability of perseverative errors in the second part, when the rules are changed. In the second part, the individual is asked to respond "Yes" if the card just turned over is the same color as a previously turned card and "No" if it is different.

The Action Program Test involves five steps that require simple skills that are typically part of most people's repertoires. It requires the individual to determine what needs to be done prior to concentrating on how that end is to be achieved. The test consists of a rectangular stand with a thin transparent tube with a removable lid and a cork on the bottom, while at the other end there is a beaker that is two-thirds full of water. An L-shaped rod that is not long enough to reach the cork is to the left of the stand. The individual is asked to get the cork out of the tube using any of the objects around without lifting the stand, the, tube or the beaker and without touching the lid with their fingers.

In the Key Search Test, the individual is presented with an A4-sized piece of paper with a 100 mm square in the middle and a small black dot 50 mm below it. The individual is told to pretend that the square is a field in which they lost their keys and are asked to draw a line, starting at the black dot, demonstrating how they would go about searching the field. The individual is scored based on how efficient the search process is.

The Temporal Judgment Test comprises four questions concerning everyday events which range from requiring a few seconds to several years. The individual is asked to make a sensible guess as to how long an event will take (e.g., How long do most dogs live?).

In the Zoo Map Test, subjects are asked to show how they would visit a series of designated locations on a map of a zoo while following certain rules. In the high demand component, the individual will incur a high number of errors by simply visiting the locations in the order given in the instructions. In the low demand component, the individual is simply required to follow the instructions to produce an error-free performance. The goal of the test is to assess the individual's spontaneous planning abilities.

The Modified Six Elements Test requires the completion of three tasks (i.e., dictation, arithmetic, and picture naming), each of which is divided into parts A and B. The individual is required to attempt at least a part from each of the six subtests within a 10-minute period and is instructed not to do the two parts of the same task consecutively. The goal of this component is to determine the person's ability to plan, organize, and monitor their behavior.

The Dysexecutive Questionnaire (DEQ) consists of 21 items that sample the range of problems commonly associated with the Dysexecutive Syndrome. Four broad areas are sampled: emotional or personality changes, motivational changes, behavioral changes, and cognitive changes. Items are scored on a 5-point (0–4) Likert scale, ranging from "Never" to "Very Often." Two versions are available, one completed by the individual and the other by an informant.

Historical Background

The BADS is designed to evaluate the pattern of deficits that are typically subsumed under the functions of the frontal lobes. Rylander (1939) enumerated the deficits as involving disturbances in attention, increased distractibility, impaired ability to learn new tasks, and deficits contending with complex information. Shallice (1982) described this pattern of deficits as comprising impairment in attentional control, which he termed the supervisory system. Baddeley (1986) analogized the supervisory system to the central executive component of working memory and suggested the term Dysexecutive Syndrome as a way of characterizing patients with this pattern of impairment. Such patients are likely to present as impulsive, distractible, and unable to use feedback to modify their responses and behave inappropriately in social situations.

The BADS was developed due to the fact that patients with impaired executive functioning often performed adequately on tests such as the Wisconsin Card Sorting Test or the Stroop Test. These same individuals, however, exhibited obvious impairment in their day-to-day functioning. To this end, Shallice and Burgess (1991) developed the Six Elements Test, which required the individual to carry out six tasks in a limited time frame without violating certain rules. It was tailored to a difficulty level that was in line with the high level of functioning of Shallice and Burgess' patients. Wilson et al. (1996) modified the Six Elements Test, simplifying it for more severely impaired and less intellectually able patients that are often seen by neuropsychologists. This evolved into the BADS.

Psychometric Data

Multiple studies attest to the psychometric properties of the BADS. Wilson et al. (1996) found that inter-rater reliability was high, ranging from 0.88 to 1.00. Test-retest reliability was also examined with subjects generally performing slightly higher after the second administration, but the differences were not statistically significant. Correlations between the first and second test administrations were moderate, with the exception of the Zoo Map Test, where virtually no correlation was found. This was attributed to the presence of outliers and small sample size ($n = 25$). The test-retest reliability of the BADS was similar in pattern to other tests of frontal lobe functioning administered at the same time (e.g., Modified Card Sorting Test; Nelson 1976).

The validity of the BADS was assessed across varied populations. Bennett et al. (2005) investigated the sensitivity of the BADS to executive dysfunction in a sample of 64 Australian patients who were involved in motor vehicle or workplace accidents. All experienced loss of consciousness and varying degrees of post-traumatic amnesia (PTA). Based on their findings, the authors concluded that scores derived from the BADS and other measures used in their study were only moderately useful in assessing executive dysfunction. On the other hand, several studies have found the BADS to discriminate between patients and controls. Krabbendam et al. (1999) were able to discriminate between schizophrenic patients and controls, while Katz et al. (2007) were able to discriminate between acute and chronic schizophrenics, the latter evidencing greater executive dysfunction. Verdejo-Garcia and Perez-Garcia (2007) examined the usefulness of the BADS in determining executive dysfunction in a Spanish sample of substance-dependent individuals (SDI). They concluded that the BADS yielded greater effect sizes for differences between SDI and controls than traditional measures of executive function. SDI performance on the BADS was also useful as a predictor of problems in daily activities. Third, deficits in BADS scores persisted following protracted abstinence, even when other neuropsychological indices showed recovery.

Canali et al. (2011) examined the reliability of the BADS in its ability to discriminate Brazilian older adults with and without mild Alzheimer's disease. Intergroup differences were reported on

most components of the measure, including task switching, time monitoring, and rule-shifting subtests. The highest level of discrimination between controls and patients was found on the Modified Six Elements, with a sensitivity index of 80% and specificity index of 90%.

Clinical Uses

Wilson et al. (1996) developed the BADS to aid those involved in the assessment of individuals with brain injury to determine the extent of executive dysfunction that is present and the likelihood that it will interfere with everyday life. It can also be used to determine the presence of executive dysfunction in other patient groups, such as schizophrenics and substance abusers. The BADS can be a useful part of the rehabilitation process as a tool that can pick up subtle difficulties with planning and organization, which are then amenable to intervention. For example, Baba et al. (2010) found that the executive functioning of 20 Japanese adults with remitted major depressive disorder were more impaired on the Modified Six Elements subtest relative to 29 healthy comparison subjects.

See Also

▶ Frontal Lobe

Further Reading

Baba, K., Baba, H., Noguchi, I., Arai, R., Suzuki, T., & Mimura, M. (2010). Executive dysfunction in remitted late-life depression: Juntendo University mood disorder projects (JUMP). *The Journal of Neuropsychiatry and Clinical Neurosciences, 22*, 70–74.

Baddeley, A. D. (1986). *Working memory*. Oxford: Clarendon Press.

Bennett, P. C., Ong, B., & Ponsford, J. (2005). Assessment of executive dysfunction following traumatic brain injury: Comparison of the BADS with other clinical neuropsychological measures. *Journal of the International Neuropsychological Society, 11*, 606–613.

Canali, F., Brucki, S. M. D., Bertolucci, P. H. F., & Bueno, O. F. A. (2011). Reliability study of the behavioral assessment of the dysexecutive syndrome adapted for a Brazilian sample of older-adult controls and probable early Alzheimer's disease patients. *Revista Brasileira de Psiquiatria, 33*, 338–346.

Katz, N., Tadmor, I., Felzen, B., & Hartman-Maeir, A. (2007). The behavioural assessment of the dysexecutive syndrome (BADS) in schizophrenia and its relation to functional outcomes. *Neuropsychological Rehabilitation, 17*, 192–205.

Krabbendam, L., de Vugt, M. E., Derix, M. M. A., & Jolles, J. (1999). The behavioural assessment of the dysexecutive syndrome as a tool to assess executive functions in schizophrenia. *The Clinical Neuropsychologist, 13*, 370–375.

Nelson, H. E. (1976). A modified card sorting test sensitive to frontal lobe defects. *Cortex, 12*, 313–324.

Rylander, G. (1939). Personality changes after operation on the frontal lobes. *Acta Psychiatrica Neurologica*, (30).

Shallice, T. (1982). Specific impairments of planning. *Philosophical Transactions of the Royal Society of London. Series B, Biological Sciences, 298*, 199-209.

Shallice, T., & Burgess, P. (1991). Deficits in strategy application following frontal lobe damage in man. *Brain, 114*, 727–741.

Verdejo-Garcia, A., & Perez-Garcia, M. (2007). Ecological assessment of executive functions in substance dependent individuals. *Drug and Alcohol Dependence, 90*, 48–55.

Wilson, B. A., Alderman, N., Burgess, P. W., Emslie, H., & Evans, J. J. (1996). *Behavioural assessment of the dysexecutive syndrome*. London: Harcourt Assessment.

Behavioral Inattention Test (BIT)

Elena Polejaeva[1] and Adam J. Woods[2,3,4]
[1]Department of Clinical and Health Psychology, University of Florida, Gainesville, FL, USA
[2]Department of Clinical and Health Psychology, College of Public Health and Health Professions, University of Florida, Gainesville, FL, USA
[3]Center for Cognitive Aging and Memory, McKnight Brain Institute, University of Florida, Gainesville, FL, USA
[4]Department of Neuroscience, University of Florida, Gainesville, FL, USA

The Behavioral Inattention Test (BIT) was developed in the United Kingdom in 1987 to assess hemi-inattention and has predominantly been used with stroke patients to assess unilateral spatial neglect (Wilson et al. 1987b; Halligan et al. 1991). Unilateral spatial neglect is commonly defined as an inability to respond to or notice stimuli that is present on the side opposite of the brain lesion location. This spatial neglect is not attributed to motor or sensory deficits (Heilman et al. 1993). In an attempt to improve ecological validity, the BIT incorporated nine behavioral subtests in addition to six conventional subtests. The behavioral subtests aim to assess unilateral spatial neglect as well as an individual's functioning on activities of daily living.

The BIT takes approximately 40 min to complete and can be administered to individuals ages 19–83. The conventional subtests consist of line crossing, star cancellation, letter cancellation, line bisection, figure/ shape copying, and representation drawing. Line crossing and the cancellation subtests require the examinee to cross out the target items, where the cancellation subtests add a level of difficulty with the presence of various nontarget items. Line bisection requires the examinee to estimate and mark the center of three horizontal lines. In the figure copying portion of the subtest, the examinee is presented with a drawing of a four-pointed star, a cube, and a daisy in a vertical orientation where each of the items are pointed out to the examinee prior to asking the examinee to draw the items. The shape copying portion of the same subtests consists of the examinee drawing three geometric shapes that are presented but not distinctly pointed out to the examinee. The representation drawing subtest requires the examinee to draw a clock face with numbers, a man or woman, and a butterfly. Both of the drawing subtests include images that tend to be bilaterally symmetric (Halligan et al. 1991).

The behavioral subtests of the BIT are comprised of: menu reading, article reading, address/ sentence copying, telling/setting the time, telephone dialing, picture scanning, coin sorting, card sorting, and map navigation. Menu reading consists of a list of common food items presented in columns. The article reading subtest contains three columns of text that are to be read by the examinee. Address/Sentence copying asks the examinee to copy four lines of an address and three lines of sentences. Telling/setting time requires the examinee to read the time on a digital clock as well as analogue clock and to set time on an analogue clock with moveable hands based on the examiner's verbal instructions. Telephone dialing utilizes a disconnected telephone and requires the examinee to dial three numbers presented in large print on separate cards. The picture scanning subtest presents the examinee with three large color photographs of a plate of food, a bathroom, and a hospital room. The examinee is asked to look at each of the photos one at a time and to point as well as name the major items in each of the photos. Coin sorting presents three rows of coins with six different denominations where the examinee is asked to identify and locate the coins as the examiner names various coins. The card sorting subtest involves the examiner pointing out each of the 16 cards to the examinee and then asking the examinee to point to the card being named by the examiner. Map navigation contains a grid of different paths marked by a letter and as the examiner says letter pairs the examinee is asked to follow the path using their finger (Halligan et al. 1991; Lezak et al. 2012).

The reliability of the BIT was initially based on a small sample size but contained excellent test-retest reliability with the behavioral subtest at $r = 0.97$ and the conventional subtests at $r = 0.89$. The conventional and behavioral subtests are also highly correlated with each other at $r = 0.75$. In terms of inter-rater reliability, the BIT is also highly reliable with both the behavioral and conventional subtests being $r = 0.99$ (Halligan et al. 1991). Thus, the BIT has been a common neuropsychological measure used to assess unilateral neglect postinjury and throughout recovery (Azouvi 2016). Maximum total score for the conventional subtests is 146 with a clinical cutoff of 129. While the behavioral subtests total maximum score is 81 with a clinical cutoff score of 67. When an individual scores lower on either one of these they are classified as having unilateral spatial neglect via BIT (Wilson et al. 1987a).

Using the BIT to predict functional outcomes, one study found BIT scores to be significantly correlated with Functional Independence Measure (FIM) scores at the time of discharge from rehabilitation, 0.385 ($P = 0.004$) for the conventional BIT and 0.396 ($P = 0.003$) for the behavioral BIT subtests (Di Monaco et al. 2011). These results indicate that the severity of unilateral spatial neglect should be accounted for when estimating functional outcome poststroke and is consistent with prior findings (Buxbaum et al. 2004; Cherney et al. 2001). In general, studies have found that unilateral spatial neglect contributes to worse functional outcomes and longer rehabilitation durations (Gillen et al. 2005; Franceschini et al. 2010). In fact, having unilateral spatial neglect was indicative of poorer functional outcomes in 25 out of 26 studies examined and the BIT has been shown to be the greatest predictor of function poststroke at 3, 6, and 12 months postinjury (Jehkonen et al. 2006; Jehkonen et al. 2000). To examine the ecological validity of the BIT, the behavioral subtests have been compared to task performance as well as to Activities of Daily Living (ADLs) checklist in patient samples. The results found that six out of the nine subtests correlated with task performance and ADLs. Additionally, seven out of the nine behavioral subtests were able to differentiate between individuals with and without spatial neglect (Hartman-Maeir and Katz 1995).

Research studies often implement one or several of the BIT subtests but this may not be an accurate way to distinguish unilateral neglect (Lopes et al. 2007). In cases where only one subtest is administered, the sensitivity of the measure may be lost. Lopes and colleagues found that all of the patients with hemi-neglect were properly identified using figure and shape copying as well as the representational drawing subtests. However, this was not the case with other subtests of the BIT when examined in a stand-alone manner. Ultimately, the full BIT test administration is still recommended for greater sensitivity.

References

Azouvi, P. (2016). The ecological assessment of unilateral neglect. *Annals of Physical and Rehabilitation Medicine.* https://doi.org/10.1016/j.rehab.2015.12.005.

Buxbaum, L. J., Ferraro, M. K., Veramonti, T., Farne, A., Whyte, J., Ladavas, E., et al. (2004). Hemispatial neglect: Subtypes, neuroanatomy, and disability. *Neurology, 62*, 749–756.

Cherney, L. R., Halper, A. S., Kwasnica, C. M., Harvey, R. L., & Zhang, M. (2001). Recovery of functional status after right hemisphere stroke: Relationship with unilateral neglect. *Archives of Physical Medicine and Rehabilitation, 82*, 322–328.

Di Monaco, M., Schintu, S., Dotta, M., Barba, S., Tappero, R., & Gindri, P. (2011). Severity of unilateral spatial neglect is an independent predictor of functional outcome after acute inpatient rehabilitation in individuals with right hemispheric stroke. *Archives of Physical Medicine and Rehabilitation, 92*, 1250–1255.

Franceschini, M., La Porta, F., Agosti, M., & Massucci, M. (2010). Is health-related-quality of life of stroke patients influenced by neurological impairments at one year after stroke? *European Journal of Physical and Rehabilitation Medicine, 46*, 389–399.

Gillen, R., Tennen, H., & McKee, T. (2005). Unilateral spatial neglect: Relation to rehabilitation outcomes in patients with right hemisphere stroke. *Archives of Physical Medicine and Rehabilitation, 86*, 763–767.

Halligan, P. W., Cockburn, J., & Wilson, B. (1991). The behavioural assessment of visual neglect. *Neuropsychological Rehabilitation, 1*, 5–32.

Hartman-Maeir, A., & Katz, N. (1995). Validity of the behavioral inattention test (BIT): Relationships with functional tasks. *American Journal of Occupational Therapy, 49*, 507–516.

Heilman, K. M., Watson, R. T., & Walenstein, E. (1993). Neglect and related disorders. In K. M. Heilman & E. Valenstein (Eds.), *Clinical neuropsychology* (pp. 279–336). New York: Oxford University Press.

Jehkonen, M., Ahonen, J. P., Dastidar, P., Koivisto, A. M., Laippala, P., Vilkki, J., & Molnar, G. (2000). Visual neglect as a predictor of functional outcome one year after stroke. *Acta Neurologica Scandinavica, 101*, 195–201.

Jehkonen, M., Laihosalo, M., & Kettunen, J. E. (2006). Impact of neglect on functional outcome after stroke: A review of methodological issues and recent research findings. *Restorative Neurology and Neuroscience, 24*, 209–215.

Lezak, M. D., Howieson, D. B., Bigler, E. D., & Tranel, D. (2012). *Neuropsychological assessment* (5th ed.pp. 428–439). New York: Oxford University Press.

Lopes, M. A., Ferreira, H. P., Carvalho, J. C., Cardoso, L., & Andre, C. (2007). Screening tests are not enough to detect hemineglect. *Arquivos de Neuro-Psiquiatria, 65*, 1192–1195.

Wilson, B., Cockburn, J., & Halligan, P. W. (1987a). *Behavioural inattention test manual*. Hants/Los Angeles: Thames Valley Test Company/Western Psychological Services.

Wilson, B., Cockburn, J., & Halligan, P. W. (1987b). Development of a behavioural test of visuospatial neglect. *Archives of Physical Medicine and Rehabilitation, 68*, 98–102.

Behavioral Therapy

Glenn S. Ashkanazi
Department of Clinical and Health Psychology, Clinical and Health Psychology Clinic, College of Public Health and Health Professions, University of Florida, Gainesville, FL, USA

Synonyms

Behavior management; Behavior modification

Definition

Behavioral therapy is a type of psychotherapy that focuses on changing and gaining control over unwanted behaviors based upon the principles of classical and operant conditioning. It is useful in the treatment of depression, anxiety disorders, phobias, smoking cessation, weight loss, stuttering, enuresis, tics, and other medical conditions.

Historical Background

Attempts to help people solve behavioral problems through attempts that closely mirror today's "behavioral therapy" have a very long history. It is based on the idea that all behaviors are learned and in the case of psychotherapy, these unhealthy behaviors can be changed.

Nineteenth-century British penal colonies used "token economies" to reinforce inmates for obeying prison rules. The early Romans used "aversive conditioning" (e.g., placement of "putrid" spiders in the glasses of alcohol abusers) in order to decrease problem drinking. Seventeenth-century French physicians were using "thought stopping" to treat cases of obsessional thinking.

Behavioral therapy's philosophical roots are from the school of behaviorism, which posits that psychological matters can be studied scientifically by observing overt behaviors and without reference to internal mental states. Some of the early behavior therapists included Joseph Wolpe

(South Africa) and Hans Eysenck (United Kingdom). Perhaps the most well-known contributors to the early development of behavioral therapy are Ivan Pavlov and B. F. Skinner.

Ivan Pavlov (1849–1936) was a Russian physician and physiologist who published extensively in the early part of the twentieth century on his conditioned learning experiments, later to be termed "classical conditioning." In classical conditioning, also called respondent conditioning, Pavlov found that dogs would naturally salivate ("unconditioned response") when presented with food ("unconditioned stimulus"). If he paired the presentation of the unconditioned stimulus with a previously neutral stimulus, like a bell ("conditioned stimulus"), the previously neutral stimulus produced the same unconditioned response as the unconditioned stimulus, even if the unconditioned stimulus was absent. The unconditioned response thus became the "conditioned response" to the newly acquired conditioned stimulus. In other words, Pavlov found that if he rang a bell before feeding the dogs (who naturally salivated when the food was presented), eventually the bell ringing alone would make the dogs salivate whether or not the food appeared. An important behavioral therapy principle derived from this work is that if the conditioned stimulus (bell) is repeatedly presented without the unconditioned stimulus (food), the conditioned response (salivation) decreases in intensity. This process is termed "extinction" and can be found in human behavioral therapy in the treatment of phobias. For example, Wolpe treated phobic patients with a technique he named "systematic desensitization," which involves gradually exposing a patient to an anxiety-provoking stimulus until the anxiety reaction is extinguished.

Burrhus Frederic (B. F.) Skinner (1904–1990) expanded on the work of Pavlov with his concept of "operant conditioning," which postulates that behavior can be affected by rewards and punishments. In a famous operant conditioning experiment, a rat is in a box equipped with an automatic food dispenser. When the rat hears the dispenser releases food pellets, it moves to the food tray and eats. Next, a lever is placed in the box that dispenses a few pellets of food when pressed. When the rat touches the lever, food is dispensed. Soon the rat is pressing the lever repeatedly to obtain the food. Through "operant conditioning," the rat's behavior of pressing the lever is reinforced as the rat learns to pair the pressing of the lever with the reward.

In terms of behavioral therapy, human behavior can be affected by reinforcement in that desired behaviors can be rewarded (reinforced) and thereby increase in frequency while undesired behaviors can be cut off from their reinforcement and extinguished. Skinner found that the frequency and timing of the rewards given also affected how fast the new behaviors were acquired and how hard it was to extinguish them. These became known as "schedules of reinforcement." The work of Skinner also led to what is called "shaping," in which the desired behavior (e.g., training a chicken to peck a piano) could be gradually acquired by rewarding approximations to the behavior.

Current Knowledge

Behavioral therapy has been successfully used for a variety of problem behaviors including, but not limited to, chronic pain, substance abuse, depression, phobias, autism, obesity, managing stress, smoking cessation, anorexia, obsessive-compulsive disorder, and attention deficit/hyperactivity disorder. It has been extensively used in patients with developmental disabilities, severely disturbed psychotic patients, survivors of brain injury, and others where insight-oriented or cognitive therapies may not be effective. There are a myriad of methods involved including (but not limited to):

- Self-monitoring
- Systematic desensitization (SD)
- Exposure and response prevention
- Contingency management
- Flooding
- Modeling
- Applied behavior analysis
- Operant conditioning
- Respondent conditioning
- Role-playing

Some of these techniques are used in everyday life. For example, parents and teachers place stars on a refrigerator chart or bulletin board to reward desirable behavior by children. Some techniques involve accumulating points for performing a desired behavior, points that can later be exchanged for some desirable reinforcer. These "token economies" are a variation of operant conditioning and are used in a variety of settings. In addition, extinction of undesired behavior has penetrated the mainstream as seen by the use of "time-out," a technique involving the removal of a child from reinforcement, seen by the child as somewhat aversive, or punishing, with the hope of decreasing the unwanted behavior.

Behavioral therapy is based on the concepts that (1) targeted behaviors can be modified by a variety of behavioral techniques and (2) that the newly acquired behaviors will be more adaptive than the undesired ones. These techniques tend to be empirical (data-driven) and observable. They do not rely for their effectiveness on any mental (cognitive) constructs like unconscious motivations. They simply identify a behavior to change and change it rather than trying to understand why the individual was performing that behavior. An example of one of these techniques is the use of systematic desensitization.

This technique is often used with people who have a specific phobia (e.g., fear of snakes, fear of closed spaces, fear of heights, etc.). The phobic behavior can be defined as avoidance of, or escape from, the phobic stimulus (e.g., escaping/running away from a spider or avoiding situations involving public speaking). By escaping from the phobic stimulus, patients can reduce their anxiety. The behavior of escape/avoidance is reinforced since the reduction of the anxiety is reinforcing for the individual (negative reinforcement is a concept derived from operant conditioning). In SD, patients are gradually exposed to the phobic stimuli, allowing them to acclimate themselves to it, until they are able to tolerate it. Patients create a hierarchy of fear steps that they must overcome to reach the last step, the phobic stimulus. These hierarchies can be imaginable pictures or actual exposure. Patients deal with each successive step until the hierarchy is completed. Typically, patients are taught relaxation skills to control fear responses during exposure to the hierarchy.

Behavioral therapy treatment tends to be of shorter duration than more traditional (e.g., insight oriented) modes of psychotherapy (e.g., psychodynamic). Initial sessions are dedicated to the explanation of the basic tenets of behavioral change (e.g., reinforcement, extinction, punishment, etc.). Once established, a variety of techniques may be utilized including:

- *Role-playing* – therapist models desired behaviors or reactions.
- *Skills training* – patient is taught new desired behaviors to replace undesired ones for parenting, social situations, public speaking, etc.
- *Flooding* – form of systematic desensitization where the patient is exposed directly to the feared stimulus to extinguish the fear response.
- *Modeling* – patients learn responses simply by observing other individuals and repeating their behavior.
- *Homework* – patients are to try out new behaviors learned in therapy in real-life situations.
- *Conditioning* – application of reinforcement to increase a desired behavior or the removal of reinforcement to decrease an unwanted behavior (e.g., token economies).
- *Relaxation training* – used to help patients relieve anxiety/tension, an important component of systematic desensitization.

The use of behavioral therapy in the treatment of survivors of severe traumatic brain injury (TBI) can be problematic. These problems can range from aggression to agitation and from depression to nonadherence. Those who demonstrate severe behavioral dyscontrol as a result of their TBI also likely possess cognitive sequelae that hinder the successful therapeutic use of these techniques. Persons with severe memory deficits may not be able to recall the behavior they performed to earn a reinforcer in a contingency management system. Memory problems may also interfere with a survivor's ability to recall that a particular behavior led to a particular consequence. Without this ability to recall contingencies, survivors are likely to not be able to make different choices (i.e., make behavior changes) for which behavior they exhibit in given situations. Therefore, behavior management strategies place special emphasis on controlling environmental stimuli in order to reduce problem behaviors (e.g., disinhibition and agitation). One approach to examining these behaviors sees behavioral dysfunction as more of a signal that a person is beyond their personal capacities to manage presenting challenges and thus requiring support that is contextually relevant. In this paradigm, "behavior" is seen as both a person's competencies and incompetencies in managing their environment, personal functioning, emotional/behavioral stability, and independence.

The goal of behavior therapy with moderate or mild TBI survivors is to provide the patient with a behavioral repertoire that they can use to solve daily life problems as a result of cognitive deficits (i.e., compensatory approaches). Critical behavioral therapy techniques utilized include self-monitoring, scheduling of activities, role-playing, modeling, and contingency contracting.

Future Directions

Chronic diseases have replaced acute illness as the leading cause of premature death. These chronic conditions often have unhealthy behaviors at their root cause. Examples include cigarette smoking, obesity, lack of exercise, poor nutritional habits, substance abuse, and medical noncompliance. For this reason, behavioral therapy has demonstrated great clinical value in the treatment and prevention of chronic health problems. An example of behavioral therapy's potential can be seen in the work of Carl Simonton in the treatment of cancer patients. His results confirm that patients who have received behavioral treatment plus conventional oncology treatment live twice as long as patients who had received conventional cancer treatment alone. Mark and Linda Sobell view alcoholic drinking as a discriminated, operant response that can be treated through aversive conditioning (electric shocks). Their research has important implications for future treatments since the experimental subjects functioned significantly better than controls post-intervention.

Cross-References

▶ Applied Behavior Analysis
▶ Behavioral Assessment
▶ Behaviorism
▶ Cognitive Behavioral Therapy
▶ Homework
▶ Psychotherapy
▶ Relaxation Training
▶ Social Skills Training

References and Readings

Gelder, M. (1997). The future of behavior therapy. *Journal of Psychotherapy Practice, 6*(4), 285–293.

Jacobs, H. (1993). *Behavior analysis guidelines and brain injury rehabilitation: People, principles and programs.* Gaithersburg: Aspen Publishing Company.

Jacobs, H. (2014). Perspectives on behavior and acquired brain injury. *NeuroRehabilitation, 34,* 597–599.

Kazdin, A., & Hersen, M. (1980). The current status of behavior therapy. *Behavior Modification, 4*(3), 283–302.

Masters, J., Burish, T., Holton, S., & Rimm, D. (1987). *Behavior therapy: Techniques and empirical findings.* San Diego: Harcourt Press Jovanovich.

Sobell, L., & Sobell, M. (2016). Individualized behavior therapy for alcoholics. *Behavior Therapy, 47*(6), 937–949.

Wilson, K. (1997). Science and treatment development: Lessons from the history of behavior therapy. *Behavior Therapy, 28,* 547–558.

Behaviorism

Anthony Y. Stringer
Department of Rehabilitation Medicine, Emory University, Atlanta, GA, USA

Synonyms

Behavioral psychology; Cognitive behaviorism

Definition

Behaviorism is a psychological theory (and branch of psychology), focusing on observable behavior rather than mental phenomena, that attempts to explain behavior by learning principles such as classical and operant conditioning. In classical conditioning, an unconditioned stimulus already eliciting a response is paired with a neutral stimulus. With repeated pairing, the neutral (conditioned) stimulus begins to elicit the same response as the unconditioned stimulus. Operant conditioning focuses on environmental consequences that increase (positive reinforcement) or decrease (negative reinforcement) the frequency of behavior. Early behaviorists focused exclusively on observable behavior, while more recent cognitive behaviorists have applied learning principles to patterns of thought. As behaviorism historically attempted to account for behavior solely in terms of environmental factors, neuropsychology has had limited impact on the development of this approach to psychology. In contrast, neuropsychologists have attempted to understand the neural mechanisms of learning, a notable example being Donald Hebb's seminal postulate that concordant firing in synaptically coupled neurons increases the strength of the connection between the two neurons. Despite behaviorism's historical avoidance of physiological explanations of behavior (Skinner 1950), those clinical neuropsychologists who include psychotherapy as part of their professional practice make use of classic and cognitive behavioral approaches in their work with brain injury survivors.

Cross-References

▶ Behavior Modification
▶ Cognitive Behavioral Therapy
▶ Learning

References and Readings

Beggs, J. M., Brown, T. Y., Byrne, J. H., Crow, T., LeDoux, J. E., & LeBar, K. (1999). Learning and memory: Basic mechanisms. In M. J. Zigmond, F. E. Bloom, S. C. Landis, J. L. Roberts, & L. R. Squire (Eds.), *Fundamental neuroscience* (pp. 1411–1454). San Diego: Academic.
Mills, J. A. (1998). *Control: A history of behavioural psychology.* New York: New York University Press.
O'Donohue, W. T. (2001). *The psychology of B.F. Skinner.* Thousand Oaks: Sage.
Skinner, B. F. (1950). Are theories of learning necessary? *Psychological Review, 57*(4), 193–216.
Staddon, J. E. R. (2000). *The new behaviorism: Mind, mechanism, and society.* Philadelphia: Psychology Press.

Bell Curve

Ericka L. Wodka
Center for Autism and Related Disorders, Kennedy Krieger Institute and The Johns Hopkins University School of Medicine, Baltimore, MD, USA

Synonyms

Gaussian distribution; Normal curve; Normal distribution

Definition

A normal distribution of observations/scores is shaped like a "bell," with the majority of observations/scores occurring around the mean and increasingly fewer observations/scores occurring farther (above/below) from the mean (68.26% of observations/scores fall within one standard deviation of the mean; 95.44% fall within two standard deviations of the mean). A normal distribution of observations is typical in large samples acting additively and independently and is assumed in parametric statistics (e.g., t-tests, ANOVA). Standardized scores derived from neuropsychological measures are based upon (assume) normal distribution of the standardization sample. While this assumption provides a common metric that allows for direct comparison of performance between different measures, it is important to note that score distributions for a number of neuropsychological tests are non-normal (e.g., Boston Naming Test, Wisconsin Card Sorting Test, Mini-Mental Status Exam, Test of Memory Malingering). For this reason, selection of measures and interpretation of test findings must include consideration of score distributions (Strauss et al. 2006).

Cross-References

▶ Base Rate (Population)
▶ Cutoff Scores, Cutting Scores
▶ Intelligence Quotient
▶ Mental Age
▶ Percentiles
▶ Standard Scores

References and Readings

Lezak, M. D., Howieson, D. B., Bigler, E. D., & Tranel, D. (2012). *Neuropsychological assessment* (5th ed.). New York: Oxford University Press.
Sattler, J. M. (2001). *Assessment of children: Cognitive foundations* (5th ed.). La Mesa: Jerome M. Sattler.
Strauss, E., Sherman, E. M. S., & Spreen, O. (2006). *A compendium of neuropsychological tests: Administration, norms, and commentary* (3rd ed., pp. 3–43). New York: Oxford University Press.

Bell's Palsy

Theslee Joy DePiero
Braintree Rehabilitation Hospital, Boston University School of Medicine, Boston, MA, USA

Synonyms

Idiopathic facial paralysis

Definition

Bell's palsy is the acute onset of paralysis of the muscles innervated by the facial nerve, not due to obvious causes such as trauma, stroke, or local infection.

Current Knowledge

Anatomy

The facial nerve innervates the muscles that control the forehead and eyebrow, close the eyelids, and move the cheeks and lips. It also supplies taste to the anterior two thirds of the tongue and innervates the stapedius muscle (a small muscle in the middle ear, connecting the tympanic membrane to the stapes, that dampens excessive vibration in the tympanic membrane due to loud noises).

Clinical Presentation

The onset of paralysis may be preceded by pain behind the ear for 1 or 2 days. The paralysis is complete in 2 days in half the patients and by 5 days in almost all the patients. If the stapedius muscle is involved, there may be sensitivity to noise. Taste is impaired in almost all patients. Clinically, the forehead is unfurrowed, the eye cannot close fully, the lower eyelid droops, and tears may run down the cheek. Due to weakness of the oral muscles, saliva may drip from the corner of the mouth on the effected side.

This is distinguished from a central facial palsy (e.g., due to stroke), by forehead weakness and weakness of eye closure. In a central facial weakness, there is little or no forehead involvement. In the Bell's palsy, the forehead is unfurrowed and the eyebrow is lower than on the uninvolved side and cannot be voluntarily raised. In a central facial weakness, the eyelid closes fully, though closure may be weaker than on the uninvolved side. In Bell's palsy, eye closure is incomplete, and the lower sclera and cornea may be reddened due to exposure to air without lubrication from tears.

Epidemiology

- Incidence: 23/100,000 annually.
- Cases in women and men are equal.
- Season: no seasonal preference.
- Age: occurs equally in all age groups.

Etiology

The etiology of Bell's palsy is thought to be viral. The genome of herpes simplex virus type 1 has been identified in the fluid surrounding the facial nerve in several cases, but there is no convincing evidence that this is the case in the majority of cases.

Lyme disease can also cause Bell's palsy. In endemic areas, Lyme disease antibody tests should be done.

Ramsay-Hunt syndrome refers to Bell's palsy caused by varicella zoster (the virus that causes chicken pox and shingles). The distinguishing characteristic of Ramsay-Hunt is the presence of vesicles (small fluid filled blisters) in the eternal auditory canal or on the eternal ear.

Treatment

Antiviral agents are not effective in idiopathic cases. Steroids (prednisone is most common) decrease the probability of permanent paralysis or aberrant reinnervation. Because of the paralysis of the muscles that close the eye, the cornea must be protected, especially at night. Artificial tears, liquid or ointment, and taping the eye shut are common treatments.

Antiviral treatment is indicated in Ramsay-Hunt, as is antimicrobial treatment in Lyme-positive patients.

Prognosis

Eighty percent recover within a few weeks to 2 months. Recovery of some motor function in the first week is a good prognostic sign.

Cross-References

▶ Lyme Disease

References and Readings

Gilden, D. (2004). Clinical practice. Bell's palsy. *New England Journal of Medicine, 351*, 1323–1331.
Hazin, R., Azizzadeh, B., & Bhatti, M. (2009). Medical and surgical management of facial nerve palsy. *Current Opinion in Opthalmology, 20*(6), 440–450.

Bender Visual-Motor Gestalt Test II

Scott L. Decker and Rachel M. Bridges
Department of Psychology, University of South Carolina, Columbia, SC, USA

Synonyms

Bender-Gestalt, Second Edition; BG-II

Description

The Bender-Gestalt test was first published in 1938, as a brief measure of visual-motor functioning. As with any measure, research identifies various measurement, scoring, and standardization issues. Recent research culminated in the revision of the test, the Bender-Gestalt, Second Edition (BG-II), which was revised by Brannigan and Decker in 2003. The BG-II maintains many historical properties that appealed to clinicians, while improving the psychometric adequacy of the test. The BG-II is divided into two phases: copy and recall. The copy phase requires the duplication of 16 geometric images, shown sequentially on separate 3×5 cards, onto a blank piece of paper with a No. 2 pencil. The recall phase involves drawing these images from memory on a new sheet of paper. Using the Global Scoring System, the drawing productions are rated on a 5-point scale based on the similarity to the original image and yield percentile ranks, scaled scores, T-scores, and confidence intervals. Additionally, the BG-II also contains two supplemental measures to screen for specific difficulties and can be used to better understand low performance.

Like the original, the BG-II has high reliability and validity and discriminates performance in individuals with a variety of learning and psychological problems. It is this latter finding – that individuals from a wide variety of clinical conditions show poor performance on line copy tasks – that contributes to the test's clinical utility. Unfortunately, theoretical explanations for poor performance as well as explanations for qualitative errors, such as figure rotations and perseverations, are still lacking. Although previous research incorporated the use of psychodynamic and personality paradigms, the most evidence-based supported inference of performance on the BG-II is as a measure of visual/perceptual-motor integration. Although many subcomponents are required in performance such as visual acuity and graphomotor skills, the integration of a visual percept with a motor programming controlling seems to be the largest source of variance on test performance (Decker et al. 2006). Additionally, research with the BG-II has shed insight on the development of visual-motor abilities across the life-span(-Decker 2008). Specifically, using this measure it has been demonstrated that visual-motor integration rapidly matures into adolescence, gradually declines through adulthood, and rapidly decreases in late adulthood.

Historical Background

The Bender-Gestalt has historically been one of the most used measures in psychology. The Bender-Gestalt originated from Lauretta Bender's research in perception and psychopathology. She adapted designs used by Wertheimer (1923) to be used as a measure of development and psychopathology. Initially, performance was qualitatively interpreted, but eventually the need for standardized scoring systems emerged. Numerous scoring systems have been developed, with the most notable being the Pascal and Suttell (1951) method, the Koppitz (1963) developmental scoring system, and Lacks (1999) scoring system for screening for brain dysfunction. The various scoring techniques and the multifaceted use of the Bender-Gestalt test, whether used as a "warm-up" prior to more intellectually challenging tasks or to screen for brain injury, have contributed to the long-standing and sustained use of the measure.

Clinical Uses

The Bender-Gestalt was initially utilized by Lauretta Bender as a measure of perception and psychopathology.

The BG-II is appropriate for use with children as young as 4 years old to individuals over the age of 85 years old and typically takes no longer than 15 min to administer. It has been used extensively for educational, medical, and other purposes, particularly in education as a determinant of fine motor or visual-spatial difficulties.

References and Readings

Bender, L. (1938). *A visual motor Gestalt test and its clinical use*. New York: American Orthopsychiatric Association.

Decker, S. L. (2008). Measuring growth and decline in visual motor processes with the Bender-Gestalt, Second Edition. *Journal of Psychoeducational Assessment, 26*, 3–15.

Decker, S. L., Allen, R., & Choca, J. P. (2006). Construct validity of the Bender-Gestalt II: Comparison with Wechsler intelligence scale for children III. *Perceptual and Motor Skills, 102*, 113–141.

Koppitz, E. M. (1963). *The Bender Gestalt test for young children*. New York: Grune and Stratton.

Lacks, P. (1999). *Bender Gestalt screening for brain dysfunction* (2nd ed.). New York: Wiley.

Pascal, G. R., & Suttell, B. J. (1951). *The Bender Gestalt test*. New York: Grune & Stratton.

Wertheimer, M. (1923). Studies in the theory of Gestalt psychology. *Psychologische Forschung, 4*, 301–350.

Benign Senescent Forgetfulness

Richard F. Kaplan and Joshua Johnson
Department of Psychiatry (MC-2103), UConn
Health Center, Farmington, CT, USA

Synonyms

Age-associated memory impairment (AAMI); Late-life forgetfulness

Definition

The term "benign senescent forgetting" was coined by V.A. Kral (see Kral 1962) to describe an age-related memory decline that is distinct from memory impairment due to known neurological damage or disease.

Current Knowledge

Changes in cognitive functioning are prevalent in aging populations. It has become clear that there is most likely a continuum between normal and abnormal mental function in those individuals who will ultimately develop dementia. Recent studies focusing on the characterization of the earliest stages of cognitive impairment have identified an intermediate period between the cognitive changes of normal aging and dementia (see Petersen et al. 2001). This transitional zone has been described using a variety of terms, including benign senescent forgetfulness (BSF), age-associated memory impairment (AAMI), age-associated cognitive decline (ACCD), cognitive impairment-no dementia (CIND), and, most recently, mild cognitive impairment (MCI). AAMI differs from BSF in that it includes specific memory test performance criteria of 1 SD below young-adult levels (see Larrabee and Crook 1994). AACD expands the definition to decrements in performance in other cognitive domains. MCI further refined the definition to include the presence of memory complaints, normal activities of daily living, normal global cognitive functioning, but abnormal memory performance compared to age- and education-matched controls (see Smith and Rush 2006). The clinical concept of MCI is important because it is a significant risk factor for dementia. While conversion rates vary widely, most researchers estimate that individuals with MCI develop dementia at a rate of 10–15% per year, in contrast to the rate of 1–2% per year for age-matched controls.

Cross-References

▶ Age Decrements
▶ Mild Cognitive Impairment
▶ Normal Aging

References and Readings

Kral, V. A. (1962). Senescent forgetfulness: Benign and malignant. *Journal of the Canadian Medical Association, 86,* 257–260.

Larrabee, G. J., & Crook, T. H. (1994). Estimated prevalence of age-associated memory impairment derived from standardized tests of memory function. *International Psychgeriatrics, 6,* 95–104.

Petersen, R. C., Stevens, J. C., Ganguli, M., Tangalos, E. G., Cummings, J. L., & DeKosky, S. T. (2001).

Practice parameter: Early detection of dementia: Mild cognitive impairment (an evidence-based review) report of the quality standards Subcommittee of the American Academy of neurology. *Neurology, 56,* 1133–1142.

Smith, G., & Rush, B. K. (2006). Normal aging and mild cognitive impairment. In D. K. Attix & K. A. Welch-Bohmer (Eds.), *Geriatric neuropsychology assessment and intervention* (pp. 27–56). New York: Guilford.

Benton Visual Retention Test

Carlye B. G. Manna[1], Carole M. Filangieri[2], Joan C. Borod[3,4], Karin Alterescu[1] and H. Allison Bender[4]

[1]Department of Psychology, Queens College of the City University of New York (CUNY), Flushing, NY, USA

[2]Department of Behavioral Health, NYU Winthrop Hospital, Mineola, NY, USA

[3]Department of Psychology, Queens College and The Graduate Center of the City University of New York (CUNY), Flushing, NY, USA

[4]Department of Neurology, Icahn School of Medicine at Mount Sinai, New York, NY, USA

Synonyms

Benton test; BVRT

Description

The Benton Visual Retention Test (BVRT) is a widely used test of visual memory, visual perception, and/or visual construction. Now in its fifth edition (Sivan 1992), the test consists of three equivalent forms (Forms C, D, and E), each composed of ten items of visual stimuli. Most items include three geometric forms presented along a horizontal plane, making the test particularly sensitive to visual neglect (Sivan 1992).

The following description of the BVRT was adapted from Strauss et al. (2006). The test includes four alternative methods of administration (A, B, C, and D) that assess different aspects of functioning. The most common administration (A) assesses immediate recall of a visual display. After presenting a stimulus card for 10 s, the card is removed, and the examinee is asked to draw the design from memory. Administration B follows the same procedure as A, but with a 5-s exposure interval. Administration C allows the examiner to dissociate memory functioning from perceptual and motor aspects of the task by asking the examinee to reproduce the designs while each item is in plain view. There is no time limit, but individuals who work very slowly should be encouraged to increase their speed. In Administration D, a 15-s interval is inserted between the 10-s encoding phase and the figure reproduction, allowing the examiner to assess short-term retention of visual information. Scoring consists of both the number of correct designs and the number of six different types of errors: omissions, distortions, perseverations, rotations, misplacements, and size errors. Administration time for each form is approximately 5 min. Several sets of norms are available and reflect different demographic characteristics, including age ranges and education levels (Mitrushina et al. 2005; Strauss et al. 2006). A multiple-choice recognition administration (Administration M, with alternate forms F and G) is also sometimes used to assess visual memory without visuoconstructional or motor coordination demands (Amieva et al. 2006). For Administration M, the examinee views a target stimulus for 10 s and, after it has been removed, is required to identify it from among four choices. Although not part of the English-language version, materials for this special administration are available in the German (Sivan and Spreen 1996) and French (Benton 1965) editions.

Historical Background

Dr. Arthur L. Benton developed the Visual Retention Test as a brief measure of immediate nonverbal memory to supplement the popular auditory digit span test in neuropsychological evaluations (Benton 1945). It was first published in 1946. Memory-for-designs tasks had appeared earlier in the century as part of larger intelligence tests but included only a few designs and did not have separate normative data. As an addition to the digit span test, the BVRT was intended to provide a broader assessment of short-term memory, and its format was selected for its resistance to emotional influence, employment of different sensorimotor components (graphomotor versus auditory-vocal), and minimal examiner-subject interaction (freedom from interpersonal demands). The initial version included seven cards and two parallel forms. A 1955 revision increased the number of designs and alternate forms and added norms for children aged 8–16. Later editions included a design copy administration and updated norms. The most recent revision was authored by Abigail Benton Sivan (Sivan 1992) and is available from its publisher, Pearson Assessments (http://pearsonassess.com).

Psychometric Data

Information on reliability and validity may be found in the manual. Test-retest reliability is 0.85. Alternate form reliability ranges from 0.79 to 0.84. There is evidence that Form C is slightly less difficult than Forms D and E under Administration A. Correlations between immediate (Administration A) and delayed (Administration D) recall are positive and range from 0.40 to 0.83, depending on the combination of forms used. Construct validity has been demonstrated through moderate correlations (0.46–0.62) of the BVRT with nonverbal subtests from the Wechsler Adult Intelligence Scales.

Child and adolescent normative data are included for Administrations A and C. The normative data for each method of administration are based on different standardization samples, and sample characteristics are provided for Administrations A, B, and C. (Normative data for Administration D are not included in the manual.) The standardization sample for Administration A is based on a compilation of three separate studies totaling over 1,300 participants, ranging in age from 8 to 69. (See manual for discussion of participant inclusion criteria for each of these studies.) The standardization sample for Administration B is based on 103 medical inpatients and outpatients, aged 16–60 years, with no evidence or history of brain disease. The standardization samples for Administration C are 200 medical patients with no history of brain disease for the adult norms and 236 children, aged 6–13 years, enrolled in public schools in Iowa and Wisconsin for the child and adolescent norms.

Clinical Uses

As it recruits a number of different cognitive functions, the BVRT is sensitive to many forms of brain damage and disease; however, its ability to discriminate among diagnoses is low (for a review, see Mitrushina et al. 2005). An individual's global performance, quantified as either the number correct score or error score, provides the best indicator of impairment. According to the manual, measures of specific error types, such as omissions, perseverations, and distortions, are not by themselves diagnostic but may raise hypotheses for further testing. For example, a high number of perseverative errors suggests possible frontal lobe damage, particularly if supported by other test and behavioral data. Omission of peripheral figures may raise suspicion of brain damage and is most frequently associated with left hemispatial neglect as a result of damage to right parietal lobe regions. In contrast, global performance has not been found to consistently distinguish between patients with unilateral right and left brain damage. Though the BVRT is sensitive to visuospatial disturbance often observed in patients with right hemisphere damage, studies have shown that individuals with unilateral left hemisphere damage can exhibit similarly poor results on Administration A (Vakil et al. 1989), as well as on copy and multiple-choice administrations (Arena and Gainotti 1978). This indicates that memory for the BVRT designs, many of which can be verbalized, is mediated by both hemispheres. However, the presence of a delay interval may differentially affect verbally and visually encoded material. Participants with right hemisphere damage achieved a lower total correct score on Administration D than Administration A, whereas individuals with left hemisphere damage had the opposite pattern of performance, benefitting from the delay. In contrast, scores from healthy participants

did not differ between the two administrations (Vakil et al. 1989).

Both copy and memory administrations are highly sensitive to early dementia and may also help to identify individuals who are at risk for developing dementia in the future. In one such study, participants with six or more errors on Administration A were nearly twice as likely to develop Alzheimer's disease 10–15 years later, when compared to participants who had fewer errors (Kawas et al. 2003). The BVRT also aids in identifying children with a learning disability and discriminating among types of learning disabilities, with reading deficits associated with the lowest levels of performance (Snow 1998). Poorer performance on the BVRT in learning disabilities has been linked with deficits in the identification of facial emotional expression (Dimitrovsky et al. 1998). Children with attention-deficit/ hyperactivity disorder receiving stimulant medication have also been shown to perform more poorly on the BVRT than healthy participants (Risser and Bowers 1993). Poorer performance is also evident in a subset of patients with schizophrenia and may result from abnormal patterns of visual scanning and fixation related to deficient attention (Obayashi et al. 2003) or be related to poor executive functions (Egan et al. 2011). Another clinical application is the inclusion of the BVRT in a neuropsychological battery for the prediction of driving safety in patients with early dementia (Dawson et al. 2009). The BVRT may also be useful in detecting malingering, which has been characterized by a greater number of errors, particularly distortion errors, than seen in neuropsychologically impaired patients (Suhr et al. 1997).

In evaluating results, it is important to consider that the BVRT may also be sensitive to individual differences that do not reflect neuropathology. Stratified normative data confirm that age is negatively correlated and that baseline intellectual functioning is positively correlated with the BVRT number correct score. The association with baseline intellect is strongest in the lower than average IQ ranges. Education-stratified norms are also available and indicate a positive relationship between years of education and the number correct score (Strauss et al. 2006). Declines in executive function and attention with normal aging have been associated with lower BVRT scores and may be related to educational level or "cognitive reserve." In a large sample of healthy elderly adults, those with higher education performed better by using a more exhaustive search strategy in the multiple choice administration (Le Carret et al. 2003). The BVRT is used worldwide, and normative data have been published from more than a dozen countries (Mitrushina et al. 2005). Most studies have shown no gender differences. While relatively few in number, studies involving direct cross-cultural comparisons demonstrate generally good consistency; however, caution is recommended when testing individuals with very low levels of education (Mitrushina et al. 2005). Results from a large Columbian sample of school-aged children did not differ from North American norms (Rosselli et al. 2001), suggesting that when educational quality is similar, as is increasingly more common in developed countries, cross-cultural differences, if present, are relatively small.

See Also

▶ Short-Term Memory
▶ Visual-Motor Function
▶ Visuoperceptual
▶ Wechsler Memory Scale All Versions

Further Reading

Amieva, H., Gaestel, Y., & Dartigues, J. (2006). The multiple-choice formats (forms F and G) of the Benton visual retention test as a tool to detect age-related memory changes in population-based studies and clinical settings. *Nature Protocols, 1*, 1936–1938.

Arena, R., & Gainotti, G. (1978). Constructional apraxia and visuoperceptive disabilities in relation to laterality of lesions. *Cortex, 14*, 463–473.

Benton, A. L. (1945). A visual retention test for clinical use. *Archives of Neurology and Psychiatry, 54*, 212–216.

Benton, A. L. (1965). *Manuel pour l'application du test de rétention visuelle (1965).* Paris: Les Editions du Centre de Psychologie Applique.

Benton, A. L. (1974). *Revised visual retention test: Clinical and experimental applications* (4th ed.). New York: Psychological Corporation.

Dawson, J. D., Anderson, S. W., Uc, E. Y., Dastrup, E., & Rizzo, M. (2009). Predictors of driving safety in early Alzheimer disease. *Neurology, 72*, 521–527.

Dimitrovsky, L., Spector, H., Levy-Shiff, R., & Vakil, E. (1998). Interpretation of facial expressions of affect in children with learning disabilities with verbal or nonverbal deficits. *Journal of Learning Disabilities, 31*, 286–292.

Egan, G. J., Hasenkamp, W., Wilcox, L., Green, A., Hsu, N., Boshoven, W., Lewison, B., Keyes, M. D., & Duncan, E. (2011). Declarative memory and WCST-64 performance in subjects with schizophrenia and healthy controls. *Psychiatry Research, 188*, 191–196.

Kawas, C. H., Corrada, M. M., Brookmeyer, R., Morrison, A., Resnick, S. M., Zonderman, A. B., & Arenberg, D. (2003). Visual memory predicts Alzheimer's disease more than a decade before diagnosis. *Neurology, 60*, 1089–1093.

Le Carret, N., Rainville, C., Lechevailler, N., Lafont, S., Letenneur, L., & Fabrigoule, C. (2003). Influence of education on the Benton visual retention test performance as mediated by a strategic search component. *Brain and Cognition, 53*, 408–411.

Mitrushina, M. N., Boone, K. B., Razani, J., & D'Elia, L. F. (2005). *Handbook of normative data for neuropsychological assessment* (2nd ed.). New York: Oxford University Press.

Obayashi, S., Matsushima, E., Ando, H., Ando, K., & Kojima, T. (2003). Exploratory eye movements during the Benton visual retention test: Characteristics of visual behavior in schizophrenia. *Psychiatry and Clinical Neurosciences, 57*, 409–415.

Risser, M. G., & Bowers, T. G. (1993). Cognitive and neuropsychological characteristics of attention deficit hyperactivity disorder children receiving stimulant medications. *Perceptual and Motor Skills, 77*, 1023–1031.

Rosselli, M., Ardila, A., Bateman, J. R., & Guzman, M. (2001). Neuropsychological test scores, academic performance, and developmental disorders in Spanish-speaking children. *Developmental Neuropsychology, 20*, 355–373.

Sivan, A. B. (1992). *Benton visual retention test* (5th ed.). San Antonio: Psychological Corporation.

Sivan, A. B., & Spreen, O. (1996). *Der Benton-Test* (7th ed.). Bern: Verlag Hans Huber.

Snow, J. H. (1998). Clinical use of the Benton visual retention test for children and adolescents with learning disabilities. *Archives of Clinical Neuropsychology, 13*, 629–636.

Strauss, E., Sherman, E. M. S., & Spreen, O. (2006). *A compendium of neuropsychological tests: Administration, norms, and commentary* (2nd ed.). New York: Oxford University Press.

Suhr, J., Tranel, D., Wefel, J., & Barrash, J. (1997). Memory performance after head injury: Contributions of malingering, litigation status, psychological factors, and medication use. *Journal of Clinical and Experimental Neuropsychology, 19*, 500–514.

Vakil, E., Blachstein, H., Sheleff, P., & Grossman, S. (1989). BVRT-scoring system and time delay in the differentiation of lateralized hemispheric damage. *International Journal of Clinical Neuropsychology, 11*, 125–128.

Benton, Arthur (1909–2006)

Steven W. Anderson
University of Iowa Hospitals and Clinics, Iowa
City, Iowa, USA

Landmark Clinical, Scientific, and Professional Contributions

- Arthur Benton was one of the pioneering figures in clinical neuropsychology. Beginning in the 1940s, he introduced and applied novel and objective assessment techniques that provided a basis for fundamental brain-behavior studies in aphasia, visuospatial abilities, hemispheric specialization, and other cognitive processes. Through the development of standardized tasks that stressed specific abilities, together with the collection of data from neurological patients and normal comparison subjects, he was able to bring increased reliability and sensitivity to the mental status exam, helping to establish neuropsychology as a valuable clinical entity. He developed a number of neuropsychological tests that have been in wide use in clinical and research settings worldwide for several decades, including the Visual Retention Test, Judgment of Line Orientation, Three-Dimensional Block Construction, and Facial Recognition. He advocated a flexible approach to clinical assessment, with the content and scope of testing determined by the referral question, context, and patient abilities.

Education and Training

He received his B.A. and M.A. degrees from Oberlin College and completed his Ph.D. at Columbia University in 1935 under the mentorship of Carney Landis, followed by clinical training at the Payne Whitney Psychiatric Clinic of New York Hospital.

Major Appointments

- Dr. Benton volunteered for military service in the US Navy in 1941 and was commissioned as a lieutenant in the medical department. His active duty ended in 1945, but he continued to serve in the US Navy Reserve for many years, eventually retiring at the rank of captain. In 1946, he accepted a position in the Psychology Department at the University of Louisville. In 1948, he became a professor at the University of Iowa, where he would remain for over 50 years. He initially was appointed Professor and Director of Graduate Training in Clinical Psychology and then accepted a joint appointment in the Departments of Psychology and Neurology in 1958. He officially retired in 1978 but remained active in research, teaching, and other professional activities for another 20 years.

Major Honors and Awards

- President, American Orthopsychiatric Association, 1965
- President, International Neuropsychological Society, 1970
- Secretary-General, Research Group on Aphasia of the World Federation of Neurology, 1971–1978
- Distinguished Professional Contribution Award, American Psychological Association, 1978
- Outstanding Scientific Contribution Award, International Neuropsychological Society, 1981
- Samuel Torrey Orton Award, Orton Dyslexia Society, 1982
- Distinguished Service and Outstanding Contribution Award, American Board of Professional Psychology, 1985
- Distinguished Clinical Neuropsychologist Award, National Academy of Neuropsychology, 1989
- Gold Medal Award for Life Achievement in the Application of Psychology, American Psychological Foundation, 1992 (Fig. 1)

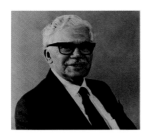

Benton, Arthur (1909–2006), Fig. 1 Benton, Arthur
(1909–2006)

Biography

Arthur Benton was born in New York City on
October 16, 1909. Educated at Oberlin and
Columbia, he was a great historian who could
trace his academic lineage to the earliest psychologists. During his military assignment to the San
Diego Naval Hospital prior to beginning his academic career, he worked with neurologist Morris
Bender and examined servicemen with traumatic
brain injury. This experience helped convince
him of the value of standardized clinical tests
and led to the development of the Benton Visual
Retention Test.

During his first academic appointment at the
University of Louisville, Benton cowrote with
Spafford Ackerly the seminal paper on childhood-
onset damage to the prefrontal cortex. This detailed
neuropsychological and neuroanatomical study of
a single patient dispelled the notion that early damage to the brain was always followed by good
recovery and presaged later work illuminating the
prefrontal cortex as a critical region underlying
social and emotional behavior.

In 1948, Benton began his long career at the
University of Iowa when he took the position of
Professor and Director of Graduate Training in
Clinical Psychology. Two years later, A.L. Sahs,
Chairman of the Department of Neurology at the
University of Iowa Hospitals and Clinics, invited
him to set up a laboratory in the hospital for the
purpose of studying behavioral impairments
related to brain disease, a move strongly
supported by Dr. Russell Meyers (Chairman of

the Division of Neurosurgery) and Dr. Maurice
Van Allen (Iowa City VA Hospital). From its
inception, his neuropsychology program was
dedicated to the tripartite goals of scientific
investigation, patient care, and student training,
united by a focus on developing objective psychological measures for the impairments
resulting from brain dysfunction. The beginnings
of the program were quite humble, with the original neuropsychology unit being housed in a
windowless $5 \times 6'$ room shared with the Department of Urology, which utilized it for "special
purposes."

The laboratory rapidly expanded, and with
access to the high volume of neurological
patients at the University Hospitals and other
nearby institutions, Benton and his students systematically approached each of the primary
domains of cognition, devising and validating
tests of language, memory, attention, visual perception, visuomotor abilities, auditory recognition, tactile perception, body schema, and more.
The enduring value of their empirical approach is
reflected in the fact that several of these tests
remain in the batteries of most neuropsychologists today.

Benton advocated a hypothesis-testing
approach to neuropsychological evaluation.
According to this flexible approach, hypotheses
regarding the patient's condition would arise from
behavioral observations, the patient's history, and
performances on an initial brief battery of tests.
These hypotheses would then be tested with subsequent targeted behavioral tests. "I think that we
should regard neuropsychological assessment in
the same way as we view the physical or neurological examination, i.e., as a logical, sequential
decision-making process rather than as simply
the administration of a fixed battery of tests"
(Benton 1985). He was a strict empiricist and
did not hesitate to challenge popular beliefs if
his data indicated otherwise. Perhaps the best
known was his characterization of the
Gerstmann syndrome as "… a fiction; it is simply an artifact of defective and biased observations" (1961), based on his systematic
observation that the components of the

Gerstmann syndrome did not co-occur with one another anymore than with deficits not considered part of the syndrome.

Benton was instrumental in bringing together the international neuropsychological community. He used his knowledge of French, German, and Italian to translate and bring to attention reports of neurological syndromes that had been largely overlooked because they were published in languages other than English. He was a visiting scholar at the University of Milan (1964); the Neurosurgical Clinic, Hospital Sainte-Anne, Paris (1968); the Hebrew University Medical School, Jerusalem (1969); the Free University of Amsterdam (1971); the University of Helsinki (1974); the Tokyo Metropolitan Institute of Gerontology (1974); the University of Melbourne (1977); L'Ecole des Hautes Etudes, Paris (1979); the University of Victoria, British Columbia (1980); the University of Minnesota Medical School (1980); and the University of Michigan (1986).

In the context of all of his professional accomplishments, Dr. Benton's dedication to education in neuropsychology was perhaps his greatest contribution. During neuropsychology's formative years, he was instrumental in developing training standards for the field. At the first scientific session of the INS, held in Washington, D.C., in 1967, he moderated an afternoon symposium on the development of a comprehensive training program in neuropsychology, and he remained active in refining these standards over the years. At the University of Iowa, he supervised 46 doctoral dissertations and 24 master's theses, and he provided consultation to leading neuropsychology centers around the world. He was known for supervision characterized by frankly honest feedback, often bruising to the student's ego, but always accompanied by sage guidance for improving the situation.

Dr. Benton officially retired in 1978, at which time the Benton Laboratory of Neuropsychology in the Department of Neurology was dedicated. His retirement was incomplete, however, as he continued to provide guidance for the neuropsychologists at Iowa and elsewhere and continued writing for more than another two decades. Today, the Benton Neuropsychology Laboratory at the University of Iowa Department of Neurology remains a vital program for research, training, and patient care, in the tradition established by Dr. Benton more than a half century ago.

Benton's wife, Rita, was a professor of musicology at the University of Iowa, where she was the first head of the Music Library in 1957. Arthur and Rita met in 1939 while they both were vacationing in Paris, and they married later that year. Upon Rita Benton's death in 1980, the Music Library was named in her honor. They had three children: Raymond, Abigail, and Daniel. Arthur Benton died in Glenview, Illinois, on December 27, 2006, from complications of emphysema, at the age of 97.

Cross-References

▶ American Board of Professional Psychology (ABPP)
▶ American Psychological Association (APA)
▶ Aphasia
▶ Benton Visual Retention Test
▶ Clinical Neuropsychology
▶ Facial Recognition Test
▶ Flexible Battery
▶ Frontal Lobe
▶ Gerstmann's Syndrome
▶ Hemispheric Specialization
▶ Hypothesis Testing Approach to Evaluation
▶ Judgment of Line Orientation
▶ Mental Status Examination
▶ Multilingual Aphasia Examination
▶ National Academy of Neuropsychology (NAN)
▶ Standardized Tests

References

Ackerly, S. S., & Benton, A. L. (1948). Report of a case of bilateral frontal lobe defect. In *The frontal lobes; proceedings of the Association for Research in Nervous and Mental Disease 1947, 27* (pp. 479–504). Baltimore: Williams and Wilkins.

Benton, A. L. (1945). A visual retention test for clinical use. *Archives of Neurology and Psychiatry, 54,* 212–216.

Benton, A. L. (1955). Right-left discrimination and finger-localization in defective children. *Archives of Neurology and Psychiatry, 74,* 383–389.

B

Benton, A. L. (1956). The concept of pseudo-feeblemindedness. *Archives of Neurology and Psychiatry, 75*, 379–388.

Benton, A. L. (1960). Motivational influences on performances in brain-damaged patients. *American Journal of Orthopsychiatry, 30*, 313–321.

Benton, A. L. (1961). The fiction of the "Gerstmann syndrome". *Journal of Neurology, Neurosurgery, and Psychiatry, 24*, 176–181.

Benton, A. L. (1962). Behavioral indices of brain injury in school children. *Child Development, 33*, 199–208.

Benton, A. L. (1964a). Contributions to aphasia before Broca. *Cortex, 1*, 314–327.

Benton, A. L. (1964b). Developmental aphasia and brain damage. *Cortex, 1*, 40–52.

Benton, A. L. (1967). Problems of test construction in the field of aphasia. *Cortex, 3*, 32–58.

Benton, A. L. (1969). Development of a multilingual aphasia battery: Progress and problems. *Journal of Neurological Sciences, 9*, 39–48.

Benton, A. L. (1977). Interactive effects of age and brain disease on reaction time. *Archives of Neurology, 34*, 369–370.

Benton, A. L. (1985). Some problems associated with neuropsychological assessment. *Bulletin of Clinical Neurosciences, 50*, 11–15.

Benton, A. L., & Fogel, M. L. (1962). Three-dimensional constructional praxis. *Archives of Neurology, 7*, 347–354.

Benton, A. L., & Howell, I. L. (1941). The use of psychological tests in the evaluation of intellectual function following head injury. *Psychosomatic Medicine, 3*, 138–151.

Benton, A. L., & Van Allen, M. W. (1968). Impairment in facial recognition in patients with unilateral cerebral disease. *Cortex, 4*, 344–358.

Benton, A. L., Hamsher, K. deS., Varney, N. R., & Spreen, O. (1983). Contributions to neuropsychological assessment. New York: Oxford University Press.

Levin, H. S., & Benton, A. L. (1975). Temporal orientation in patients with brain disease. *Applied Neurophysiology, 38*, 56–60.

Ben-Yishay, Yehuda (1933–)

Amy Alderson[1] and Christine Mullen[2]
[1]Department of Rehabilitation Medicine, Emory University, Atlanta, GA, USA
[2]Emory Health Care, Atlanta, GA, USA

Major Appointments

- 1964–1966 Assistant Professor of Clinical Rehabilitation Medicine, New York University School of Medicine
- 1967–1974 Associate Professor of Clinical Rehabilitation Medicine, New York University School of Medicine
- 1975–2011 Tenured Professor of Clinical Rehabilitation Medicine, New York University School of Medicine
- 1975–1976 Visiting Professor, Tel Aviv University, Department of Psychology
- 1974–1976 Clinical Director of Israel Head Trauma Project, New York University Medical Center, Rusk Institute, and Israel Ministry of Defense Joint Research Project, Afeka, Israel
- 1976–1983 Visiting Clinical Director, New York University Medical Center, Rusk Institute, and Israel Ministry of Defense Joint Research Project, Afeka, Israel
- 1995–1997 Clinical Director, Kurt Goldstein Institute for Holistic Neuropsychological Rehabilitation Steinach, Germany
- 1996–2011 Assistant Chief of Behavioral Sciences, Rusk Institute of Rehabilitation
- 1975–2011 Tenured Professor of Clinical Rehabilitation Medicine, New York University of School of Medicine

Major Honors and Awards

- 1976 Howard A. Rusk Award for Outstanding Accomplishments in Rehabilitation
- 1982 William F. Caveness Award for Distinguished Contributions in the field of Head Injury, National Head Injury Foundation
- 1988 Thomas J. Dean Award of Excellence in Head Injury Rehabilitation, Dallas, Rehabilitation Foundation
- 1991 Distinguished Career Achievement Award, American Board of Medical Psychotherapists
- 2006 Outstanding Lifetime Scientific Contributions to Rehabilitation Psychology. American Psychological Association, Division 22

Landmark Clinical, Scientific, and Professional Contributions

- Dr. Ben-Yishay is the father of holistic brain injury rehabilitation. Initially developed in

Israel for war veterans with head injuries and later transitioned to the New York University School of Medicine at the Rusk Institute, Dr. Ben-Yishay's treatment interventions with individuals with brain injuries combined contributions from neuropsychology, behavioral psychology, cognitive-behavioral psychotherapy, special education, social psychology, and psychodrama. He adapted these modalities to the needs and capabilities of his patients, systematically applying them in therapeutic community settings to reach maximal effectiveness. Through his holistic approach to the treatment of brain injury, a foundation for cognitive and neuropsychological rehabilitation was established.

• The holistic rehabilitation approach developed by Dr. Ben-Yishay includes a number of components in addition to traditional cognitive retraining: development of a therapeutic milieu or community, psychotherapy, regular involvement of family and caregivers, psychoeducation, and transitional work opportunities. Within the therapeutic milieu or community, persons with brain injury not only participate in activities aimed at adaptation to and compensation for their deficits but also meet regularly with staff members to monitor their progress. Interaction with other individuals with brain injury is also an important part of the therapeutic milieu. During individual and group psychotherapy, persons with brain injury address the many adjustment issues associated with their deficits. In addition, the involvement of family and caregivers in the rehabilitation process not only provides additional support for the person with a brain injury as they complete therapies but also assists with the transition back to the community by providing realistic education and information regarding the person's progress and injury. Finally, transitional work opportunities provide important information regarding individuals' abilities outside of structured settings and help to provide additional functional goals for rehabilitation therapies.

• Dr. Ben-Yishay's work has been researched and applied both within the United States and abroad, and premiere rehabilitation institutes around the world utilize his model of cognitive rehabilitation as the foundation for their own brain injury programs. His teaching methods are studied by students and professionals from all over the world, and he is internationally known as a clinician, teacher, researcher, and expert in the field of holistic rehabilitation.

Short Biography

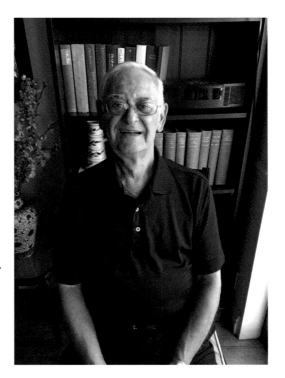

Yehuda Bin-Yishay was born on February 11, 1933, in Cluj, Romania. He grew up in Israel and served in the Israeli army. In 1957, he received a B.A. degree in Sociology and Special Education from Hebrew University in Jerusalem, Israel. Then, in 1958, he came to the United States on a scholarship from the New School University in New York City. There, he studied under Kurt Goldstein. He completed an internship in Clinical Psychology in 1960 at Trenton State Hospital in Trenton,

NJ. His master's degree in Personality Psychology was completed in 1961.

After completing his master's degree, Dr. Ben-Yishay served as the psychologist for a research project in the Department of Rehabilitation at the Albert Einstein College of Medicine in New York. The study tested the effectiveness of a "therapeutic community" model of rehabilitation.

Ben-Yishay obtained his Ph.D. from New York University, following the completion of studies investigating the effects of normobaric oxygen on stroke patients' performances on neurologic, sensory-motor, and cognitive measures. In 1964, Dr. Ben-Yishay joined the faculty at New York University. While at New York University, Dr. Ben-Yishay's research over the next several years focused on three key areas: (1) rehabilitation outcome prediction studies, (2) comparisons between normal controls and brain-injured individuals across a variety of measures, and (3) development and efficacy studies of cognitive rehabilitation modules. From 1974 to 1977, Dr. Ben-Yishay conducted a pilot study in Israel to investigate the effects of holistic brain injury rehabilitation on Israeli war veterans. The results of the study were impressive and were followed in September of 1978 by a 5-year research grant on brain injury rehabilitation at New York University (NYU) Rusk Rehabilitation Head Trauma Program.

Throughout his career, Dr. Ben-Yishay trained numerous rehabilitation neuropsychologists, who have gone on to institute his model of cognitive rehabilitation. Individuals such as Anne-Lise Christensen, Ph.D., and George Prigatano, Ph.D., have been greatly influenced by Ben-Yishay's work and established programs built upon principles learned under his tutelage. Ben-Yishay maintains that the objective of all neurorehabilitation interventions is to optimize the person's compensatory repertoire, including helping the individual in mastering and reliably applying learned compensatory skills in his or her post-rehabilitation life.

Dr. Ben-Yishay's work in the area of holistic brain injury rehabilitation continues to the present day, and he has earned worldwide recognition for his work. He has received numerous awards and honors, including the 2006 Lifetime Scientific Contributions to Rehabilitation Psychology Award from Division 22 of the American Psychological Association. In addition to his many international committee and consultant positions, Dr. Ben-Yishay has served on a number of important editorial boards, including *Archives of Physical Medicine and Rehabilitation*, *Journal of Head Trauma Rehabilitation*, *Brain Injury, and Neuropsychological Rehabilitation*.

Of all of his achievements, Dr. Ben-Yishay greatest satisfaction stems from the programs all over the world that subscribe to his philosophy of brain injury rehabilitation and the many acknowledgments of his influence on clinical practice (personal communication, July 15, 2016).

Dr. Ben-Yishay formally retired in 2009 and has since volunteered at the NYU Rusk Rehabilitation Day Program. He continues to work on several publications, including work identifying the major predictors of successful outcomes of intensive neuropsychological rehabilitation and patient acceptance of the limitations imposed by brain injury. In regard to the future of the field, Dr. Ben-Yishay believes the "therapeutic community" portion of the holistic approach merits a wider application in order to improve outcomes (personal communication, July 15, 2016).

Cross-References

► Christensen, Anne-Lise (1926–)
► Cognitive Rehabilitation
► Goldstein, Kurt (1878–1965)

References and Readings

Ben-Yishay, Y. (1996). Reflections on the evolution of the therapeutic milieu concept. *Neuropsychological Rehabilitation, 6*(4), 327–343.
Ben-Yishay, Y. (2000). Postacute neuropsychological rehabilitation: A holistic perspective. In A. Christensen & B. P. Uzzell (Eds.), *International*

handbook of neuropsychological rehabilitation (pp. 127–135). Dordrecht: Kluwer Academic/Plenum Publishers.

Ben-Yishay, Y. (2008). Foreword. In F. Gracey and T. Ownsworth (Eds). The self and identity in rehabilitation: A special issue of the journal *Neuropsychological Rehabilitation*,18(5), 513–521.

Ben-Yishay, Y., & Diller, L. (1993). Cognitive remediation in traumatic brain injury: Update and issues. *Archives of Physical Medicine and Rehabilitation, 74*(2), 204–213.

Ben-Yishay, Y., & Diller, L. (2008). Kurt Goldstein's holistic ideas: An alternative, or complementary, approach to the management of traumatically brain injured individuals. *US Neurology, 4*(1), 79–80.

Ben-Yishay, Y., & Diller, L. (2016). *Turning points: Positive outcomes of insensitive psychotherapeutic interventions in holistic neuropsychological rehabilitation settings*. Youngsville: Lash and Associates Publishing.

Ben-Yishay, Y., & Gold, J. (1990). Therapeutic milieu approach to neuropsychological rehabilitation. In R. L. Wood (Ed.), *Neurobehavioral sequelae of traumatic brain injury* (pp. 194–215). London: Taylor and Francis.

Ben-Yishay, Y., & Lakin, P. (1989). Structured group treatment for brain-injury survivors. In D. Ellis & A. L. Christensen (Eds.), *Neuropsychological treatment after brain injury* (pp. 271–295). Boston: Kluwer Academic.

Ben-Yishay, Y., Ben-Nachum, Z., Cohen, A., Gross, Y., Hoofien, D., Rattok, J., & Diller, L. (1978). Digest of a two-year comprehensive clinical research program for out-patient head injured Israeli veterans. *NYU Rehabilitation Monograph, 60*, 1–61.

Ben-Yishay, Y., Rattok, J., Lakin, P., Piasetsky, E. B., Ross, B., Silver, S., ... & Ezrachi, O. (1985). Neuropsychologic rehabilitation: Quest for a holistic approach. *Seminars in Neurology*, 5(3), 252–259.

Ben-Yishay, Y., Silver, S. M., Piasetsky, E., & Rattok, J. (1987). Relationship between employability and vocational outcome after intensive holistic cognitive rehabilitation. *The Journal of Head Trauma Rehabilitation, 2*(1), 35–48.

Ezrachi, O., Ben-Yishay, Y., Kay, T., Diller, L., & Rattok, J. (1991). Predicting employment in traumatic brain injury following neuropsychological rehabilitation. *The Journal of Head Trauma Rehabilitation, 6*(3), 71–84.

Prigatano, G. P., & Ben-Yishay, Y. (1999). Psychotherapy and psychotherapeutic interventions in brain injury rehabilitation. In M. Rosenthal, E. R. Griffith, J. Korutzer, & B. Pentland (Eds.), *Rehabilitation of the adult and child with traumatic brain injury* (3rd ed.). Philadelphia: F.A. Davis.

Rattok, J., Ross, B., Ben-Yishay, Y., Ezrachi, O., Silver, S., Lakin, P., & ... Diller, L. (1992). Outcome of different treatment mixes in a multidimensional neuropsychological rehabilitation program. *Neuropsychology*, 6(4), 395–415.

Benzodiazepines

JoAnn Tschanz
Department of Psychology, Utah State University, Logan, UT, USA
Center for Epidemiologic Studies, Utah State University, Logan, UT, USA

Synonyms

Anxiolytics; Sedative-hypnotics

Definition

Benzodiazepines belong to a class of medications known as sedative-hypnotics. The benzodiazepine molecule binds to the subtype A portion of the protein receptor of the primary inhibitory neurotransmitter substance in the brain, gamma aminobutyric acid (GABA). The simultaneous binding of the endogenous neurotransmitter GABA on the GABA-A postsynaptic receptor increases the frequency of the opening of the chloride channel, allowing greater amounts of this negatively charged anion, chloride, to rapidly enter the cell due to the concentration gradient. The additional entry of chloride into the cytoplasm hyperpolarizes the cell, which reduces depolarization, or firing, of the cell. Hence, greater stimulation is required for cell firing. This is known as the GABA-benzodiazepine receptor complex (Stahl 2004).

Benzodiazepines have wide-ranging effects. Their popular use is reflected in their anxiolytic, muscle relaxant, sedative, anesthetic, and anticonvulsant properties. Due to their safety profile, benzodiazepines became very popular in the 1970s, replacing older drugs such as barbiturates and meprobamate for the treatment of anxiety symptoms, insomnia and other sleep disorders (Iversen et al. 2009), and alcohol withdrawal syndrome (Ntais et al. 2005). However, negative effects of benzodiazepine use have also been reported. Although these "side effects" vary depending upon the original indication for benzodiazepine use, some of the unwanted effects include drowsiness, decreased concentration, memory impairment, psychomotor slowing (Buffett-Jerrott and Stewart 2002), and postural instability (with increased risk of falls) among the elderly (Allain et al. 2005). Chronic use also carries the risk of substance dependence and abuse and cognitive impairment with prolonged use at high doses (Stewart 2005; Barker et al. 2004). For these and other reasons, medications in this class are now more commonly used on a short-term rather than a long-term basis (Iversen et al.).

Current Knowledge

Current uses of benzodiazepines include the treatment of spasticity (Gold and Oreja-Guevara 2013) and tremor (Meador et al. 2016) in patients with multiple sclerosis. As reported above, chronic use of benzodiazepines has declined, particularly for the treatment of anxiety disorders and insomnia. Tricyclic antidepressants (TCAs) and selective serotonergic agents are increasingly being prescribed over benzodiazepines for the treatment of anxiety disorders. For example, selective TCAs are reportedly as effective as benzodiazepines in the treatment of generalized anxiety disorder, and certain selective serotonin reuptake inhibitors and TCAs are effective in the treatment of panic and obsessive compulsive disorder (Bourin and Lambert 2002).

With respect to insomnia, benzodiazepines were the treatment of choice over barbiturates. However, negative effects such as the development of tolerance, residual daytime sleepiness, aggravation of respiratory conditions, and reduced duration of slow-wave (restorative) and REM sleep were also reported. Newer, non-benzodiazepine hypnotic compounds such as zopiclone and zaleplon are also effective in treating insomnia yet have fewer side effects than those of benzodiazepines (Montplaisir et al. 2003).

See Also

▶ Anxiolytics
▶ Barbiturates

References

Allain, H., Bentu'e-Ferrer, D., Polard, E., Akwa, Y., & Patat, A. (2005). Postural instability and consequent falls and hip fractures associated with use of hypnotics in the elderly. A comparative review. *Drugs in Aging, 22*, 749–765.

Barker, M. J., Greenwood, K. M., Jackson, M., & Crowe, S. F. (2004). Cognitive effects of long-term benzodiazepine use. A meta-analysis. *CNS Drugs, 18*, 37–48.

Bourin, M., & Lambert, O. (2002). Pharmacotherapy of anxious disorders. *Human Psychopharmacology: Clinical and Experimental, 17*, 383–400.

Buffett-Jerrott, S. E., & Stewart, S. H. (2002). Cognitive and sedative effects of benzodiazepine use. *Current Pharmaceutical Design, 8*, 45–58.

Gold, R., & Oreja-Guevara, C. (2013). Advances in the management of multiple sclerosis spasticity: Multiple sclerosis spasticity guidelines. *Expert Review of Neurotherapeutics, 13*(12 Suppl), 55–59.

Iversen, L. L., Iversen, S. D., Bloom, F. E., & Roth, R. H. (2009). Antidepressants and anxiolytics. In *Introduction to neuropsychopharmacology* (pp. 306–335). New York: Oxford University Press.

Meador, W., Salter, A. R., & Rinker, J. R., 2nd. (2016). Symptomatic management of multiple sclerosis-associated tremor among participants in the NARCOMS registry. *International Journal of MS Care, 18*, 147–153.

Montplaisir, J., Hawa, R., Moller, H., Morin, C., Fortin, M., Matte, J., Reinish, L., & Shapiro, C. M. (2003). Zopiclone and zaleplon vs benzodiazepines in the treatment of insomnia: Canadian consensus statement. *Human Psychopharmacology: Clinical and Experimental, 18*, 29–38.

Ntais, C., Pakos, E., Kyzas, P., & Ioannidis, J. P. (2005). Benzodiazepines for alcohol withdrawal. *Cochrane Database of Systematic Reviews, 20*, CD005063.

Stahl, S. M. (2013). Anxiolytics and sedative hypnotics. In *Essential psychopharmacology: Neuroscientific basis and practical applications* (pp. 297–333). New York: Cambridge University Press.

Berg Balance Scale

Kari Dunning
Department of Rehabilitation Sciences,
University of Cincinnati, Cincinnati, OH, USA

Synonyms

7-item BBS-3P; BBS

Description

The Berg Balance Scale (BBS) is a 14-item performance observation measure that assesses balance on a scale from 0 to 4 for each item, yielding a total score range of 0–56, where higher scores indicate better balance. The BBS tests both static and dynamic balance with items meant to mimic balance challenges encountered in daily life.

Historical Background

In 1989, Berg developed the BBS to fill the need for a quantitative balance assessment tool to screen older adults for fall risk. The BBS has subsequently become the best known clinical balance instrument. Shorter versions of the BBS, such as the seven-item BBS-3P (which also has a condensed rating scale), have also been developed and validated.

Psychometric Data

The high reliability, validity, and sensitivity of the BBS, including predictive validity for fall risk, are well documented in the literature. Some authors initially dichotomized the scale, using the threshold value <45 points as an indication of fall risk. However, more rigorous study has determined that a gradient of fall risk exists over the entire scale. A retrospective study of community-dwelling persons with stroke demonstrated that changing from 3 to 4 for the "standing on one leg" item had a sensitivity of 0.90 and a specificity of 0.50 for predicting the history of multiple falls.

Clinical Uses

The BBS is available online (Internet Stroke Center 2007). Administration requires 10–20 min, a chair, a step, a ruler, and a stopwatch. Balance ability is sometimes grossly categorized as good, fair, or poor for score ranges from 56 to 41, 40 to 21, and 20 to 0, respectively. As stated above, a gradient of fall risk exists over the entire scale.

BBS scores are used when prescribing mobility aids and treatment interventions, identifying safe and unsafe activities, and to measure treatment effect. When assessing the treatment effect for individual patients with stroke, a score change of 6 points has been shown to represent real change, beyond measurement error, with 90% confidence. For individuals with multiple sclerosis, the minimal clinically important difference has been determined to be 3 points.

Although originally designed to screen older adults for fall risk, the BBS has subsequently been validated for persons with stroke, multiple sclerosis, Parkinson's disease, and chronic obstructive pulmonary disease (COPD).

Cross-References

▶ Balance Disorders
▶ Multiple Sclerosis
▶ Parkinson's Disease
▶ Sensitivity
▶ Specificity
▶ Stroke

References and Readings

Alzayer, L., Beninato, M., & Portney, L. G. (2009). The accuracy of individual berg balance scale items compared with the total berg score for classifying people with chronic stroke according to fall history. *Journal of Neurologic Physical Therapy: JNPT, 33*(3), 136–143.

Berg, K., Wood-Dauphinee, S., Williams, J. I., & Gayton, D. (1989). Measuring balance in the elderly: Preliminary development of an instrument. *Physiotherapy Canada, 41*, 304–311.

Berg, K., Wood-Dauphinee, S., & Williams, J. I. (1995). The balance scale: Reliability assessment with elderly residents and patients with an acute stroke. *Scandinavian Journal of Rehabilitation Medicine, 27*(1), 27–36.

Blum, L., & Korner-Bitensky, N. (2008). Usefulness of the berg balance scale in stroke rehabilitation: A systematic review. *Physical Therapy, 88*(5), 559–566.

Chou, C. Y., Chien, C. W., Hsueh, I. P., Sheu, C. F., Wang, C. H., & Hsieh, C. L. (2006). Developing a short form of the berg balance scale for people with stroke. *Physical Therapy, 86*(2), 195–204.

Gervasoni, E., Jonsdottir, J., Montesano, A., & Cattaneo, D. (2016). Minimal clinically important difference of berg balance scale in people with multiple sclerosis.

Archives of Physical Medicine and Rehabilitation, epub.

Internet Stroke Center. (2007). *Berg balance scale*. http://www.strokecenter.org/Trials/scales/berg.html. Accessed 19 May 2010.

Jacome, C., Cruz, J., Olivera, A., & Marques, A. (2016). Validity, reliability, and ability to identify fall status of the berg balance scale, BESTest, Mini-BESTest, and Brief-BESTest in patients with copd. *Physical Therapy, 96*, 1807–1815.

Mao, H., Hsueh, I., Tang, P., Sheu, C., & Hsieh, C. (2002). Analysis and comparison of the psychometric properties of three balance measures for stroke patients. *Stroke, 33*(4), 1022–1027.

Muir, S. W., Berg, K., Chesworth, B., & Speechley, M. (2008). Use of the berg balance scale for predicting multiple falls in community-dwelling elderly people: A prospective study. *Physical Therapy, 88*(4), 449–459.

Stevenson, T. J. (2001). Detecting change in patients with stroke using the berg balance scale. *The Australian Journal of Physiotherapy, 47*, 29–38.

Tyson, S. F., & Connell, L. A. (2009). How to measure balance in clinical practice. A systematic review of the psychometrics and clinical utility of measures of balance activity for neurological conditions. *Clinical Rehabilitation, 23*(9), 824–840.

Best Performance Method

Glen E. Getz
Department of Psychiatry, Allegheny General Hospital, Pittsburgh, PA, USA
Neuropsychology Specialty Care, LLC, Pittsburgh, PA, USA

Synonyms

Cognitive potential

Definition

Neuropsychologists typically do not have an opportunity to evaluate patients before the onset of neurological illness or injury. Judgments about impairment are often made by comparing obtained test scores with estimates of premorbid ability. There are several approaches to estimating premorbid level of ability. One such approach is the Best Performance Method. Using this method, data are collected from multiple sources, including, but not limited to, test scores, observations, interviews, reports from family, and historical data. After the data are collected, the data source that yields the highest level of functioning is the set standard to which all other aspects of functioning are compared. The Best Performance Method assumes that one performance level exists for each person's cognitive abilities. A notable discrepancy between a patient's best and other performances is indicative of neuropsychological impairment. The Best Performance Method also assumes that performance should be consistent across all areas of functioning. For example, very superior intellectual and other abilities would be expected from a patient who has earned a doctoral degree in engineering. The method has been criticized by some who believe that there is a high likelihood of overestimating premorbid ability, and research does not support that performance on cognitive testing is uniform across different tests or cognitive domains. In fact, abnormal performance on some proportion of neuropsychological testing has proven to be psychometrically normal (Binder et al. 2009).

Cross-References

▶ Deficit Measurement
▶ Premorbid Estimate
▶ Premorbid Functioning
▶ Premorbid Intelligence

References and Readings

Binder, L. M., Iverson, G. L., & Brooks, B. L. (2009). TO err is human: "Abnormal" neuropsychological scores and variability are common in healthy adults. *Archives of Clinical Neuropsychology, 24*, 31–46.

Lezak, M. D., Howieson, D. B., Bigler, E. D., & Tranel, D. (2012). The rationale of deficit measurement. In *Neuropsychological assessment* (5th ed.). New York: Oxford University Press.

Mortensen, E. L., Gade, A., & Reinisch, J. M. (1991). "Best performance method" in clinical neuropsychology. *Journal of Clinical and Experimental Neuropsychology, 13*, 361–371.

Beta-Interferons

Kathleen L. Fuchs
Department of Neurology, University of Virginia
Health System, Charlottesville, VA, USA

Synonyms

Avonex®; Betaseron®; Rebif®

Definition

Interferon β is a disease-modifying drug currently indicated for treatment of relapsing forms of multiple sclerosis. Its mechanism of action is complex and is presumed to inhibit immune system T-cell activation and migration into the central nervous system as well as modulate the action of some pro-inflammatory proteins (cytokines). There are three FDA approved beta interferons available in the US - Avonex® (INF-β1a), Betaseron® (INF-β1b), and Rebif® (INF-β1a). These medications are administered via injection, and each has been shown to reduce the frequency of MS relapses, reduce MRI evidence of brain lesions, and possibly reduce disability progression.

Cross-References

► Multiple Sclerosis

References and Readings

National Clinical Advisory Board of the National Multiple Sclerosis Society. (2007). Disease management consensus statement. Retrieved 15 Feb 2010, from http://www.nationalmssociety.org/download.aspx?id=8.

Noseworthy, J., Miller, D., & Compston, A. (2006). Disease-modifying treatments in multiple sclerosis. In A. Compston, C. Confavreux, H. Lassman, I. McDonald, D. Miller, J. Noseworthy, et al. (Eds.), McAlpine's multiple sclerosis (4th ed., pp. 729–802). Philadelphia: Elsevier.

Zhang, J., Hutton, G., & Zang, Y. (2002). A comparison of the mechanisms of action of interferon beta and glatiramer acetate in the treatment of multiple sclerosis. Clinical Therapeutics, 24, 1998–2021.

Beyond a Reasonable Doubt

Robert L. Heilbronner
Chicago Neuropsychology Group, Chicago, IL, USA

Definition

Beyond a reasonable doubt is the standard of proof required in most criminal cases within an adversarial system. Generally, the prosecution bears the burden of proof and is required to prove their version of events to this standard. This means that the proposition being presented by the prosecution must be proven to the extent that there is no "reasonable doubt" in the mind of a reasonable person that the defendant is guilty. There can still be a doubt but only to the extent that it would not affect a "reasonable person's" belief regarding whether or not the defendant is guilty. The "shadow of a doubt" is sometimes used interchangeably with reasonable doubt, but this extends beyond the latter to the extent many believe is an impossible standard. Reasonable doubt is therefore used. If doubt affects a "reasonable person's" belief that the defendant is guilty, the jury is not satisfied beyond a "reasonable doubt." The precise meaning of words such as "reasonable" and "doubt" is usually defined within jurisprudence of the applicable country.

The standard that must be met by the prosecution's evidence in a criminal prosecution is that no other logical explanation can be derived from the facts except that the defendant committed the crime, thereby overcoming the presumption that a person is innocent until proven guilty. If the jurors or judge have no doubt as to the defendant's guilt or if their only doubts are unreasonable doubts, then the prosecutor has proven the defendant's guilt beyond a reasonable doubt, and the defendant should be pronounced guilty. The term "reasonable doubt" connotes that evidence establishes a particular point to a moral certainty and that it is beyond dispute that any reasonable alternative is possible. It does not mean that no doubt exists as to the accused's guilt, but only that no reasonable doubt is possible from the evidence presented.

Beyond a reasonable doubt is the highest standard of proof that must be met in any trial. In civil litigation, the standard of proof is either proof by a "preponderance of the evidence" or proof by "clear and convincing evidence." These are lower burdens of proof. A preponderance of the evidence simply means that one side has more evidence in its favor than the other, even by the smallest degree. Clear and convincing proof is evidence that establishes a high probability that the fact sought to be proven is true. The main reason that the high-proof standard of reasonable doubt is used in criminal trials is that such proceedings can result in the deprivation of a defendant's liberty or even in his or her death. These outcomes are far more severe than in civil trials, in which money damages are the common remedy.

Cross-References

▶ Burden of Proof
▶ Clear and Convincing Evidence
▶ Preponderance of the Evidence

References and Readings

Denney, R. L. (2005). Criminal forensic neuropsychology and assessment of competency. In G. Larrabee (Ed.), *Forensic neuropsychology: A scientific approach.* New York: Oxford University Press.
Melton, G. B., Petrila, J., Poythress, N. G., & Slobogin, C. (2007). *Psychological evaluations for the courts: A handbook for mental health professionals and lawyers* (3rd ed.). New York: Guilford.

Bias

Robert L. Heilbronner
Chicago Neuropsychology Group, Chicago, IL, USA

Synonyms

Partiality; Prejudice

Definition

Faust et al. (1991) and Wedding and Faust (1989) explain chief forms of bias related to clinical judgment and decision-making in neuropsychology. First, *hindsight bias* is the tendency to believe, after the outcome of an incident is determined, that the outcome could have been more reliably predicted than is actually true. This form of bias suggests that being aware of an event via a client's clinical history may lead the clinician to conclude that they can determine the outcome of the event and make diagnostic determinations. *Confirmation bias* refers to the tendency to seek confirming evidence while failing to consider disconfirming evidence when generating diagnostic impressions. Thus, a clinician seeks to confirm initial hypotheses while failing to gather information related to alternative hypotheses. Moreover, it has been demonstrated that clinicians tend to stop hypothesis evaluation once information in support of an initial hypothesis has been gathered, thus potentially terminating the evaluation prior to adequate consideration of competing hypotheses.

To combat against bias in neuropsychological assessment and testimony, Wedding and Faust (1989) and Sweet and Moulthrop (1999) provided a number of strategies for clinicians to consider when testifying and preparing reports. First and foremost, they recommended that clinicians be familiar with the scientific literature regarding human judgment and decision-making. Moreover, they recommend that clinicians begin with consideration of the most valid information, generating alternative diagnostic hypotheses and then gathering and considering evidence for each and providing an outline of disconfirmatory information. Thus, in the context of a neuropsychological evaluation, it is recommended that clinicians generate a list of test findings that support specific hypotheses but also list data that disputes such hypotheses. Larrabee (2000) suggests a four-component consistency analysis for neuropsychological decision-making, including asking the following four questions: (a) Are the data consistent within and between neuropsychological domains? (b) Is the neuropsychological profile consistent with the suspected etiologic condition? (c) Are the neuropsychological data consistent with the documented severity of injury? and (d) Are the neuropsychological data consistent with the subject's behavioral presentation? Several pieces of data must be analyzed in order to address the aforementioned questions: comprehensive interview, meticulous record review, and comprehensive and redundant neuropsychological tests within each domain (language, perception, sensorimotor functioning, attention/information processing, psychomotor speed, verbal and visual learning and memory, intelligence, problem solving, motivation, and personality).

References and Readings

Faust, D., Ziskin, J., & Hiers Jr., J. B. (1991). *Brain damage claims: Coping with neuropsychological evidence*. Marina del Rey: Law & Psychology Press.

Larrabee, G. J. (2000). Forensic neuropsychological assessment. In R. D. Vanderploeg (Ed.), *Clinicians guide to neuropsychological assessment* (2nd ed., pp. 301–335). Mahwah: Lawrence Erlbaum.

Sweet, J. J., & Moulthrop, M. A. (1999). Self-examination questions as a means of identifying bias in adversarial assessments. *Journal of Forensic Neuropsychology, 1,* 73–88.

Van Gorp, W., & McMullen, W. (1997). Potential sources of bias in forensic neuropsychological evaluations. *The Clinical Neuropsychologist, 11,* 180–187.

Wedding, D., & Faust, D. (1989). Clinical judgment and decision-making in neuropsychology. *Archives of Clinical Neuropsychology, 4,* 233–265.

Bicycle Drawing Test

Ronald A. Cohen
Department of Clinical and Health Psychology, College of Public Health and Health Professions, University of Florida, Gainesville, FL, USA
Center for Cognitive Aging and Memory, McKnight Brain Institute, University of Florida, Gainesville, FL, USA

Definition

As the name suggests, the bicycle drawing test requires patients to draw a picture of a bicycle in freehand using a pencil. It can be a useful measure of visual-spatial and visual-motor impairments and also has been used in the assessment of hemi-neglect syndromes. Typically, the patient is asked to draw a copy of a simple line drawn picture of a bicycle. Many clinicians first ask the patient to draw a bicycle in freehand from their own memory, to assess their constructional ability in the absence of a model.

History and Clinical Evidence

The bicycle drawing test is widely associated with Piaget's (1955) investigations of cognitive development, though similar tests seem to have been employed earlier (Poppelreuter 1990; Veiders 1934). Neuropsychological investigations of focal unilateral lesions (Hecaen and Assal 1970) have demonstrated differences in performance between patients with left- and right-sided posterior brain lesions. Such comparisons have also suggested qualitative differences in the types of errors made among patients with left- and right-sided lesions (Angenent 1971). Such findings led to the inclusion of this test as a measure of constructional ability. One study compared the bicycle drawing test to the Bender-Gestalt test (Greenberg et al. 1994) and found bicycle drawing to be more sensitive to brain dysfunction in children with visual-spatial problems than the Bender-Gestalt test. Interestingly, improvements in bicycle drawing performance have been described in studies of patients with Parkinson's disease, multiple sclerosis, and Tourette's syndrome (Sandyk 1994, 1997a, b), with reversal of spatial orientation in Parkinson's patients when they received electromagnetic pulses to their brain (Sandyk 1998). The quality and complexity of the drawing produced by children and adults has also been linked to their intellectual ability (Sharma 1972).

Current Clinical Use

Formal scoring systems exist for the bicycle drawing test (Greenberg et al. 1994) providing a means for deriving quantitative results when using this test. Studies comparing the drawings of amateurs with artists have also shown that observational, experimental, and neuropsychological methods for scoring drawings can provide systemic differences in cognitive skills among individuals (van Sommers et al. 1995). Yet, most clinicians currently use the bicycle drawing test in conjunction with other constructional tests, including coping or freehand drawing tasks (e.g., cube, house), and examine results qualitatively for gross spatial distortion or omissions. Other tests, such as copying of the Rey complex figure, are now more widely used for visual-motor assessment. Yet, the bicycle drawing test is an easy-to-administer task that can yield valuable information about the visual-spatial and constructional abilities of patients. It can also detect hemi-neglect syndrome, as some patients may omit one side of the bicycle. It can yield information about additional information on intellectual development when used in the assessment of children. Generally, it should not be used as a stand-alone test but should rather be used in conjunction with other tests of visual constructional functioning.

Cross-References

▶ Bender Visual-Motor Gestalt Test II
▶ Block Design
▶ Clock Drawing
▶ Rey Complex Figure Test

References and Readings

Angenent, H. L. (1971). The development of thought structure among normal and mentally retarded children. *Nederlands Tijdschrift voor de Psychologie en haar Grensgebieden, 26*(4), 215–232.

Greenberg, G. D., Rodriguez, N. M., & Sesta, J. J. (1994). Revised scoring, reliability, and validity investigations of Piaget's bicycle drawing test. *Assessment, 1*(1), 89–101.

Hecaen, H., & Assal, G. (1970). A comparison of constructive deficits following right and left hemispheric lesions. *Neuropsychologia, 8*(3), 289–303.

Piaget, J. (1955). Perceptual and cognitive (or operational) structures in the development of the concept of space in the child. *Acta Psychologica, 11*, 41–46.

Poppelreuter, W. (1990). *Disturbances of lower and higher visual capacities caused by occipital damage: With special reference to the psychopathological, pedagogical, industrial, and social implications.* Oxford: Clarendon Press/Oxford University Press.

Sandyk, R. (1994). Reversal of a visuoconstructional deficit in Parkinson's disease by application of external magnetic fields: A report of five cases. *International Journal of Neuroscience, 75*(3–4), 213–228.

Sandyk, R. (1997a). Progressive cognitive improvement in multiple sclerosis from treatment with electromagnetic fields. *International Journal of Neuroscience, 89*(1–2), 39–51.

Sandyk, R. (1997b). Reversal of a visuoconstructional disorder by weak electromagnetic fields in a child with Tourette's syndrome. *International Journal of Neuroscience, 90*(3–4), 159–167.

Sandyk, R. (1998). Reversal of the bicycle drawing direction in Parkinson's disease by AC pulsed electromagnetic fields. *International Journal of Neuroscience, 95* (3–4), 255–269.

Sharma, T. R. (1972). Measuring intelligence through bicycle drawings. *Indian Educational Review, 7*(1), 1–30.

van Sommers, P. (1995). Observational, experimental and neuropsychological studies of drawing. In C. Lange-Küttner & G. V. Thomas (Eds.), *Drawing and looking: Theoretical approaches to pictorial representation in children* (pp. 44–61). Hertfordshire: Harvester Wheatsheaf.

Veiders, E. (1934). Analyse der Fähigkeit zum räumlichen Denken. Analysis of the ability for spatial thinking. *Psychotechnisches Zeitschrift, 9*, 52–60.

B

Bilingual Aphasia

Margarita Kaushanskaya[1] and Henrike K. Blumenfeld[2]
[1]University of Wisconsin-Madison, Madison, WI, USA
[2]School of Speech, Language and Hearing Sciences, San Diego State University, San Diego, CA, USA

Definition

Bilingual aphasia is a term referring to aphasia in an individual who is bilingual or multilingual. The degree and nature of impairment vary widely, and depend on the interplay among a number of factors, including site and size of the lesion, the individual's premorbid language learning and experience history, and proficiency and immersion in each language. Current evidence suggests that the same classification/diagnosis of aphasia (e.g., fluent, nonfluent) tends to hold across both languages, with varying degrees of impairment and recovery trajectories (Paradis 1998). In the USA, 45,000 new cases of bilingual aphasia are expected each year (Paradis 2001).

Historical Background

Knowledge of bilingual aphasia is primarily based on a history of case studies (for reviews, see Ansaldo and Ghazi Saidi 2014; Lorenzen and Murray 2008; Pearce 2005), including documented cases as early and varied as a patient who could read Latin but not German (Gesner 1770); a patient in Southern France who, after brain damage, showed a selective deficit in French but not Occitan (Lordat 1843); and a trilingual patient who recovered French and Spanish, but lost the ability to even understand Italian (Pitres 1895). Based on early case studies, a number of predictions have been made about patterns of impairment and recovery in bilingual individuals with aphasia, including better recovery of the mother tongue (Ribot's Law 1882), the most familiar language (Pitres' Rule 1895), the language dominant in the environment (Bychowsky 1919), and the language "closest to our heart" (Minkowski 1927).

Current Knowledge

A systematic and theoretical understanding of bilingual aphasia relies on an understanding of the bilingual language system and its neural correlates. While more similarities than differences have been observed with regard to linguistic processing and neuroanatomical correlates of language for bilinguals and monolinguals, language function of a bilingual speaker is not equivalent to that of a monolingual speaker. With two language systems instead of one, bilinguals have been shown to activate their two languages in parallel

and experience interaction and interference between them. In addition, bilinguals frequently switch and translate between languages.

There is still considerable debate regarding the functional localization of language in bilinguals. The evidence to date indicates that the extent of overlap in representation of languages depends on the speaker's language proficiency and the age at which the second language was acquired. Neuroimaging research suggests that different languages are most likely to share the same brain regions when the second language is acquired earlier, with age of second-language acquisition treated as a continuous variable (Nichols and Joanisse 2016) or as a categorical variable where a late age of acquisition is defined as 10 years or older (e.g., Wartenburger et al. 2003). Bilinguals' languages also show more overlap when both are highly proficient (e.g., Abutalebi and Green 2007; Chee et al. 1999; Golestani et al. 2006; Klein et al. 1999; Perani et al. 2003). Even in languages that are structurally different from each other, at least partially shared representations have been identified (e.g., English/Chinese; English/ASL, Chee et al. 1999; Emmorey et al. 2007).

Additional brain areas have also been identified during bilingual language processing, pointing to a complex neural network involved in the cognitive control of bilinguals' two languages (e.g., Green and Abutalebi 2013). For example, bilinguals may engage the prefrontal cortex to a larger extent when they process a less proficient language than when they process a more proficient language (e.g., Golestani et al. 2006; Indefrey 2006; Marian et al. 2007; Perani et al. 2003; Sakai et al. 2004). Increased activation in dorsolateral prefrontal cortex, anterior cingulate gyrus, and supramarginal gyrus has been observed during language switching (Hernandez et al. 2000; Price et al. 1999; Wang et al. 2007), while increased activation in anterior cingulate gyrus and basal ganglia has been noted during translation (Price et al. 1999). Finally, bilinguals show activation of the left caudate nucleus and anterior cingulate gyrus for naming tasks in a bilingual context (Abutalebi et al. 2007). Altogether, the neural network that supports language control in bilinguals likely includes anterior cingulate cortex, presupplementary motor area, prefrontal and inferior frontal cortex, caudate nucleus/putamen/thalamus, left inferior parietal lobule, and the cerebellum (Green and Abutalebi 2013).

Bilingual individuals with aphasia typically go through a variety of changes in their language abilities, where their languages are available to different degrees during the acute phase of recovery (up to 4 weeks postonset). During this phase, availability of representations may vary because of diaschisis. As impairment patterns stabilize during the postacute phase (up to 5 months postonset), language impairment becomes more directly related to site of lesion and damage to specific linguistic and cognitive representations.

Clinical Variants and Recovery Patterns

Bilingual individuals with aphasia show great variability in impairment and recovery patterns. Paradis (2001), in a review of 132 cases of bilingual aphasia, found that 61% showed parallel recovery of their two languages, 18% showed differential recovery of their two languages, 7% showed blended recovery, and 5% showed selective recovery (for similar distributions on a sample of 20 Italian–Friulian patients, see Fabbro 2001). Reports of atypical and pragmatically inappropriate language switching behaviors in bilingual individuals with aphasia have also appeared (Muñoz et al. 1999).

Parallel impairment and recovery is the most prevalent pattern observed in bilingual aphasia (e.g., Paradis 2001), *Parallel impairment* refers to aphasia of the same type and severity in both languages. The two languages are impaired and recover simultaneously (relative to premorbid language proficiency). *Differential impairment* refers to aphasia of the same type in both languages (e.g., fluent vs. nonfluent) with crosslinguistic differences in severity levels. In contrast, *differential aphasia* refers to different aphasia symptoms in each language. *Differential recovery* refers to one language recovering better than the other (relative to premorbid levels). *Blended impairment* refers to the inappropriate combination of two or more languages (e.g., the patient may lose the ability to discriminate between languages). *Pathological mixing*, characterized by inadvertent and uncontrolled language switches, is typically associated with blended impairment. In contrast, *pathological fixation* is an inability to switch languages. *Antagonistic recovery* refers to a pattern where one language recovers first and starts regressing when the other language starts to recover. *Alternating antagonism* refers to repetition of the antagonistic pattern, with the two languages alternating in availability (cycles may range from hours to months). *Selective impairment* refers to aphasia in only one language, while the other language remains intact (relative to premorbid language proficiency). In addition, a variety of deficits have been identified in bilingual aphasics' ability to translate from one of their languages to the other. An *inability to translate* is reflected in bilinguals' inability to translate either forward (from their native language to their second language) or backward (from their second language to their native language). *Paradoxical translation* is an ability to translate from one language to the other, but not the other way around. *Translation without comprehension* is a preserved ability to translate without an ability to comprehend the meaning of either translation. Finally, *spontaneous translation* is the involuntarily production of translations that cannot be inhibited.

The heterogeneity of the bilingual population makes it difficult to link language profiles and lesion site/size with specific impairment and recovery patterns in individuals with bilingual aphasia. However, a number of *linguistic factors* in impairment and recovery patterns have been identified. Naming and translation of cognate words (that share sound and meaning in the two languages, e.g., *lamp-lámpara*) is frequently less impaired in bilingual individuals with aphasia than naming and translation of noncognate words (*key – llave*, Goral et al. 2006; Kohnert 2004; Roberts and Deslauriers 1999). However, variability in such cognate effects has been demonstrated across individuals with aphasia, ranging from facilitation to interference effects (Hughes and Tainturier 2015). In general, aspects of bilinguals' languages that are more shared are also more resistant to impairment (e.g., Kiran and

Tuctenhagen 2005). Linguistic features that differ between languages (e.g., different grammatical systems) may result in differences in how symptoms of aphasia are expressed even if the same underlying deficit exists. For example, a morphologically rich language can theoretically undergo greater morphological breakdown, and morphological deficits may look more severe. Therefore, cross-linguistic differences in the symptoms and recovery patterns of bilingual aphasia frequently occur at points where the two linguistic systems diverge.

Another explanation for divergent recovery patterns in bilingual aphasia is the Cue Strength hypothesis (e.g., Wulfeck et al. 1991). According to this hypothesis, the linguistic importance of a grammatical structure or the contribution it makes to the linguistic message may account for crosslinguistic differences in syntactic deficits, with higher-ranked cues more likely to be preserved. For example, English-speaking individuals with aphasia were found to be more sensitive to word-order errors during grammaticality judgments while Italian-speaking individuals with aphasia were more sensitive to morphological errors. Similarly, differences in reading impairments have been found across languages with different orthographies. Readers are referred to reviews of bilingual aphasia by Lorenzen and Murray (2008) and Ansaldo and Ghazi Saidi (2014).

Assessment

An important part of assessment in bilingual aphasia consists of establishing premorbid proficiency levels as accurately as possible and determining the nature and extent of impairment in each language relative to these premorbid proficiency levels. Self-reports, questionnaires about the history of language use (e.g., code-switching), reports from family members or friends, and written or recorded samples of patients' language abilities are typically used to establish premorbid proficiency levels. Once premorbid proficiency levels have been established, it is important to assess both of the patients' languages in order to gauge their full linguistic capacity and impairments across languages.

There are currently no assessment measures for bilingual aphasia that meet *all* standards for measurement validity. The bilingual aphasia test (BAT, Paradis 1987) is the most comprehensive tool available, providing systematic ways to assess aphasia in more than 59 languages, including cross-linguistic interactions in an even larger combination of language pairs. Tasks on the BAT are equivalent in linguistic complexity across languages and cover assessment of multiple linguistic levels (phonological, lexical-semantic, morphological, syntactic), linguistic skills (comprehension, formulation, repetition, judgment, lexical access), and linguistic units (words, sentences, paragraphs). The BAT assumes that the test-taker has premorbid proficiency in each language that is equivalent to at least 400 language-learning hours. The test is administered in each language on different days. Where it is not feasible to obtain all language versions of the BAT, its principles may be followed during assessment.

Additional tasks that may be useful in examining bilingual individuals' language impairments include the type-token ratio in each language based on comparable language samples, number of verbs and grammatical clauses per utterance, semantic acceptability, confabulation, and total number of words or utterances within a set time window (fluency measures). Preservation of links between languages may be assessed by testing participants' translation abilities from the native language to the second language and vice versa. As part of cognitive assessment, language switching behaviors may be examined. It may be possible to distinguish pathological mixing from nonpathological mixing, although such an analysis should be embedded within a careful documentation of code-switching practices characterizing the patient's community.

If, due to limitations in resources, assessment and treatment are done only in English, the clinician may obtain information on the structure of the clients' other language in order to identify cross-linguistic influences in the clients' English output. This may allow the clinician to distinguish low premorbid proficiency in English from a disorder. The *dynamic assessment* approach provides an alternative method for examining deficits in situations of low premorbid language proficiency. Dynamic assessment focuses on the ability to learn new information, rather than the ability to retrieve known information. A clinician may explain a new grammatical rule and test the client's ability to generalize it. If the client generalizes the rule easily, then weak linguistic performance is likely due to the influence of the nontarget language or low proficiency in the target language, rather than aphasia.

Treatment

Assessment of both languages, together with the social communication needs of the client, will inform choice of therapy language and specific therapy goals. A primary goal in the treatment of bilingual individuals with aphasia is to maximally benefit both languages even if treatment occurs in only one language.

Treatment may be conducted to target both languages directly. During bilingual treatment, language-switching may be encouraged as a compensatory strategy to allow the client to use his/her full linguistic capacity. Translation may be used in a similar manner to aid lexical access. For example, switch-back through translation (SBT) treatment (Ansaldo and Marcotte 2007) is a procedure where the client is cued to translate the word back into the other language whenever an inadvertent switch occurs.

If resources are only available to treat in English, the speech-language pathologist may work to identify outside resources in helping to rehabilitate the clients' other languages. Such linguistic resources may include language-specific community groups, or guidance of family members. Cross-linguistic generalization is most likely to occur when shared representations are targeted for treatment, cross-linguistic associative links are used, or similar cognitive processes are a focus of intervention (e.g., reading in alphabetic languages). Current evidence suggests that treatment in a patient's weaker or equally dominant language may generalize to their other language, especially when treatment targets are similar across languages (e.g., Edmonds and Kiran 2004). Generalization of treatment effects across languages has been shown when cognate words

are used in treatment (Kohnert 2004, but see Kurland & Falcon for cognate interference during treatment 2011), when semantic features are treated (Edmonds and Kiran 2004, 2006; Knoph et al. 2015), when general cognitive function is treated (Kohnert 2004), and may be more likely when languages are structurally similar to each other (e.g., Ansaldo and Ghazi Saidi 2014; Knoph et al. 2015). However, generalization from a stronger to a weaker language is less likely and, in general, cross-linguistic generalization does not always occur (e.g., Galvez and Hinckley 2003). In contrast, *within*-language generalization of treatment effects has been shown to be more substantial in the more proficient language (Edmonds and Kiran 2006; Kurland and Falcon 2011), a result that must also be considered when selecting treatment languages. Although language dominance patterns are frequently the same pre- and postmorbidly, this is not always the case. While much of the current treatment literature suggests that premorbid proficiency levels influence cross-linguistic generalization of treatment, others have argued that generalization patterns may also be determined by postmorbid proficiency levels (for a review, see Ansaldo and Ghazi Saidi 2014).

Future Directions

In 2011, 21% of the population older than 5 years of age (more than 60 million people) spoke a language other than English at home, up from 18% in 2000, 14% in 1990, and 11% in 1980 (Ryan 2013). As the bilingual population grows, with special growth in older adults, the need for accommodation of bilingual individuals with aphasia will increase. Among Mexican Americans, stroke incidence is slightly higher (1.63%) than in non-Latino white peers (1.36%), and transient ischemic attacks are more frequent at younger ages (Lorenzen and Murray 2008). The US Department of Health and Human Services found that individuals of Latino origin were 33% less likely to receive necessary health-care services, compared to non-Latino white peers (Lorenzen and Murray 2008). With these changes in population dynamics, systematic evidence-based research on the efficacy of various treatment approaches for bilingual aphasia has become increasingly necessary.

One avenue of research in bilingual aphasia that has been virtually unexplored is in the area of cognitive control, and more broadly, in attention and executive function skills. There exists a significant body of literature attempting to link language and communication outcomes in people with aphasia to deficits in nonverbal cognitive domains of attention and executive function (Erickson et al. 1996; Fridriksson et al. 2006; Helm-Estabrooks 2002; Hula and McNeil 2008; Keil and Kaszniak 2002; Murray 2012; Ramsberger 2005; Zinn et al. 2007). These nonverbal cognitive skills may be honed with bilingual experience, as bilinguals must suppress one language in favor of another language every time they speak. Although the evidence for bilingual effects on cognitive control abilities remains divided (e.g., Hilchey and Klein 2011; Paap and Greenberg 2013), balanced bilinguals have been shown to have cognitive advantages over monolinguals on nonlinguistic executive function tasks, especially as they age (Bialystok et al. 2004; Kave et al. 2008; Zied et al. 2004). Examination of the relation between cognitive control and language skills in bilinguals with aphasia will extend current understanding of the cognitive foundations of bilingual language processing (e.g., Dash and Kar 2014). Furthermore, given the important role of the executive control system in both aphasia and in bilinguals' ability to appropriately maintain and switch between languages, it is important to examine the integrity of the cognitive control system in bilingual individuals with aphasia. Recent evidence suggests that bilingualism may influence cognitive outcomes after stroke. In a study of 608 patients with ischemic stroke, Alladi et al. (2016) found that a larger proportion of bilinguals had normal cognition compared with monolinguals, although there were no differences in the frequency of aphasia for bilinguals and monolinguals. It is also possible that cognitive-control advantages may support language recovery and responsiveness to treatment in bilingual patients with aphasia.

Cross-References

▶ Aphasia
▶ Aphasia Tests
▶ Multilingual Aphasia Examination
▶ Speech-Language Pathology
▶ Speech-Language Therapy

References and Readings

Abutalebi, J., & Green, D. (2007). Bilingual language production: The neurocognition of language representation and control. *Journal of Neurolinguistics, 20*, 242–275.

Abutalebi, J., Brambati, S. M., Annoni, J. M., Moro, A., Cappa, S. F., & Perani, D. (2007). The neural cost of the auditory perception of language switches: An event-related fMRI study in bilinguals. *Journal of Neuroscience, 27*, 13762–13769.

Alladi, S., Bak, T. H., Mekala, S., Rajan, A., Chaudhuri, J. R., Mioshi, E., Krovvidi, R., Surampudi, B., Duggirala, V., & Kaul, S. (2016). Impact of bilingualism on cognitive outcome after stroke. *Stroke, 47*, 1–4.

Ansaldo, A. I., & Ghazi Saidi, L. (2014). Aphasia therapy in the age of globalization: Cross-linguistic therapy effects in bilingual aphasia. *Behavioral Neurology, 2014*, 1–10.

Ansaldo, A. I., & Marcotte, K. (2007). Language switching and mixing in the context of bilingual aphasia. In J. G. Centeno, L. K. Obler, & R. T. Anderson (Eds.), *Studying communication disorders in Spanish speakers: Theoretical, research, and clinical aspects*. Clevedon: Multilingual Matters.

Bialystok, E., Craik, F. I. M., Klein, R., & Viswanathan, M. (2004). Bilingualism, aging, and cognitive control: Evidence from the Simon task. *Psychology and Aging, 19*, 290–303.

Bychowsky, Z. (1919). Concerning the restitution of language loss subsequent to a cranial gunshot wound in a polyglot aphasic. In M. Paradis (Ed.), *Readings on aphasia in bilinguals and polyglots* (pp. 130–144). Montreal: Didier.

Chee, M. W., Caplan, D., Soon, C. S., Sriram, N., Tan, E. W., Thiel, T., et al. (1999). Processing of visually presented sentences in Mandarin and English studied with fMRI. *Neuron, 23*, 127–137.

Dash, T., & Kar, B. R. (2014). Bilingual language control and general purpose cognitive control among individuals with bilingual aphasia: Evidence based on negative priming and flanker tasks. *Behavioral Neurology, 2014*, 1–20.

Edmonds, L., & Kiran, S. (2004). Confrontation naming and semantic relatedness judgments in Spanish/English bilinguals. *Aphasiology, 18*, 567–579.

Edmonds, L., & Kiran, S. (2006). Effect of semantic naming treatment on crosslinguistic generalization in bilingual aphasia. *Journal of Speech, Language, and Hearing Research, 49*(4), 729–748.

Emmorey, K., Mehta, S., & Grabowski, T. (2007). The neural correlates of sign versus word production. *NeuroImage, 36*, 202–208.

Erickson, R. J., Goldinger, S. D., & LaPointe, L. L. (1996). Auditory vigilance in aphasic individuals: Detecting nonlinguistic stimuli with full or divided attention. *Brain and Cognition, 30*, 244–253.

Fabbro, F. (2001). The bilingual brain: Bilingual aphasia. *Brain and Language, 79*, 201–210.

Fridriksson, J., Nettles, C., Davis, M., Morrow, L., & Montgomery, A. (2006). Functional communication and executive function in aphasia. *Clinical Linguistics & Phonetics, 20*, 401–410.

Galvez, A., & Hinckley, J. J. (2003). Transfer patterns of naming treatment in a case of bilingual aphasia. *Brain and Language, 87*, 173–174.

Gesner, J. A. P. (1770). *Sammlung von Beobachtungen aus der Arzneygelehrtheit und Naturkunde* (pp. 1769–1776). Nördlingen: CG Beck.

Golestani, N., Alario, F. X., Meriaux, S., Le Bihan, D., Dehaene, S., & Pallier, C. (2006). Syntax production in bilinguals. *Neuropsychologia, 44*(7), 1029–1040.

Goral, M., Levy, E. S., & Obler, L. K. (2006). Neurolinguistic aspects of bilingualism. *International Journal of Bilingualism, 6*, 411–440.

Green, D. W., & Abutalebi, J. (2013). Language control in bilinguals: The adaptive control hypothesis. *Journal of Cognitive Psychology, 25*, 515–530.

Helm-Estabrooks, N. (2002). Cognition and aphasia: A discussion and a study. *Journal of Communication Disorders, 35*, 171–186.

Hernandez, A. E., Martinez, A., & Kohnert, K. (2000). In search of the language switch: An fMRI study of picture naming in Spanish-English bilinguals. *Brain and Language, 73*, 421–431.

Hilchey, M. D., & Klein, R. M. (2011). Are there bilingual advantages on nonlinguistic interference tasks? Implications for the plasticity of executive control processes. *Psychonomic Bulletin & Review, 18*, 625–658.

Hughes, E., & Tainturier, M.-J. (2015). The cognate advantage in bilingual aphasia: Now you see it, now you don't. *Frontiers in Psychology, 6, Conference Abstract: Academy of Aphasia 53rd Annual Meeting.* https://doi.org/10.3389/conf.fpsyg.2015.65.00086.

Hula, W. D., & McNeil, M. R. (2008). Models of attention and dual-task performance as explanatory constructs in aphasia. *Seminars in Speech and Language, 29*, 169–187.

Indefrey, P. (2006). A meta-analysis of hemodynamic studies on first and second language processing: Which suggested differences can we trust and what do they mean? In M. Gullberg & P. Indefrey (Eds.), *The cognitive neuroscience of second language acquisition* (pp. 279–304). Malden: Blackwell.

Kave, G., Eyal, N., Shorek, A., & Cohen-Mansfield, J. (2008). Multilingualism and cognitive state in the oldest old. *Psychology and Aging, 23*, 70–78.

Keil, K., & Kaszniak, A. W. (2002). Examining executive function in individuals with brain injury: A review. *Aphasiology, 16*, 305–335.

Kiran, S., & Tuctenhagen, J. (2005). Imageability effects in normal bilingual adults and in aphasia: Evidence from naming to definition and semantic priming tasks. *Aphasiology, 19*, 315–325.

Klein, D., Milner, B., Zatorre, R. J., Zhao, V., & Nikelski, J. (1999). Cerebral organization in bilinguals: A PET study of Chinese–English verb generation. *NeuroReport, 10*, 2841–2846.

Knoph, M. I. N., Lind, M., & Simonsen, H. G. (2015). Semantic feature analysis targeting verbs in a quadrilingual speaker with aphasia. *Aphasiology, 29*, 1473–1496.

Kohnert, K. (2004). Cognitive and cognate-based treatments for bilingual aphasia: A case study. *Brain and Language, 91*, 294–302.

Kurland, J., & Falcon, M. (2011). Effects of cognate status and language of therapy during intensive semantic naming treatment in a case of severe nonfluent bilingual aphasia. *Clinical Linguistics & Phonetics, 25*, 584–600.

Lordat, J. (1843). Leçons tirées du cours de physiologie de l'année scolaire 1842–1843. *Journal de la Société de Médecine Pratique de Montpellier, 7*, 333–353.

Lorenzen, B., & Murray, L. (2008). Bilingual aphasia: A theoretical and clinical review. *American Journal of Speech-Language Pathology, 17*, 299–317.

Marian, V., Shildkrot, Y., Blumenfeld, H. K., Kaushanskaya, M., Faroqui-Shah, Y., & Hirsch, J. (2007). Cortical activation during word processing in late bilinguals: Similarities and differences as revealed by fMRI. *Journal of Clinical and Experimental Neuropsychology, 29*, 247–265.

Marrero, M. Z., Golden, C. J., & Espe-Pfeifer, P. (2002). Bilingualism, brain injury, and recovery: Implications for understanding the bilingual and for therapy. *Clinical Psychology Review, 22*, 465–480.

Minkowski, E. (1927). *La Schizophrénie*. Paris: Payot.

Muñoz, M. L., Marquardt, T., & Copeland, G. (1999). A comparison of the code-switching patterns of speakers with aphasia and neurologically normal bilingual speakers of English and Spanish. *Brain and Language, 66*, 249–274.

Murray, L. (2012). Attention and other cognitive deficits in aphasia: Present and relation to language and communication measures. *American Journal of Speech-Language Pathology, 21*, S51–S64.

Nichols, E. S., & Joanisse, M. F. (2016). Functional activity and white matter microstructure reveal the independent effects of age of acquisition and proficiency on second-language learning. *NeuroImage, 143*, 15–25.

Paap, K. R., & Greenberg, Z. I. (2013). There is no coherent evidence for a bilingual advantage in executive processing. *Cognitive Psychology, 66*, 232–258.

B

Paradis, M. (1987). *The assessment of bilingual aphasia*. Hillsdale: Erlbaum.

Paradis, M. (Ed.). (1995). *Aspects of bilingual aphasia*. Oxford: Pergamon.

Paradis, M. (1998). Aphasia in bilinguals: What is atypical? In P. Coppens, Y. Lebrun, & A. Basso (Eds.), *Aphasia in atypical populations* (pp. 35–66). Hillsdale: Erlbaum.

Paradis, M. (2001). Bilingual and polyglot aphasia. In R. S. Berndt (Ed.), *Handbook of neuropsychology* (2nd ed., pp. 69–91). Oxford: Elsevier Science.

Pearce, J. M. S. (2005). A note on aphasia in bilingual patients: Pitres' and Ribot's laws. *European Neurology, 54*, 27–31.

Perani, D., Abutalebi, J., Paulesu, E., Brambati, S., Scifo, P., Cappa, S. F., et al. (2003). The role of age of acquisition and language usage in early, high-proficient bilinguals: A fMRI study during verbal fluency. *Human Brain Mapping, 19*, 170–182.

Pitres, A. (1895). Etude sur l'aphasie chez les polyglottes. *Revue de Medicine, 15*, 873–899.

Price, C. J., Green, D. W., & von Studnitz, R. (1999). A functional imaging study of translation and language switching. *Brain, 122*, 2221–2235.

Ramsberger, G. (2005). Achieving conversational success in aphasia by focusing on non-linguistic cognitive skills: A potentially promising new approach. *Aphasiology, 19*, 1066–1073.

Roberts, P. M., & Deslauriers, L. (1999). Picture naming of cognate and non-cognate nouns in bilingual aphasia. *Journal of Communication Disorders, 32*, 1–22.

Ryan, C. (2013). Language use in the United States: 2011. http://www.census.gov/content/dam/Census/library/publications/2013/acs/acs-22.pdf. Retrieved 11 Mar 2016.

Sakai, K. L., Miura, K., Narafu, N., & Muraishi, Y. (2004). Correlated functional changes of the prefrontal cortex in twins induced by classroom education of second language. *Cerebral Cortex, 14*, 1233–1239.

Wang, Y., Xue, G., Chen, C., Xue, F., & Donga, Q. (2007). Neural bases of asymmetric language switching in second-language learners: An ER-fMRI study. *NeuroImage, 35*, 862–870.

Wartenburger, I., Heekeren, H. R., Abutalebi, J., Cappa, S. F., Villringer, A., & Perani, D. (2003). Early setting of grammatical processing in the bilingual brain. *Neuron, 37*, 159–170.

Wulfeck, B., Bates, E., & Capasso, R. (1991). A cross-linguistic study of grammaticality judgments in Broca's aphasia. *Brain and Language, 41*, 311–336.

Zied, K. M., Phillipe, A., Karine, P., Valerie, H. T., Ghislaine, A., Arnaud, R., et al. (2004). Bilingualism and adult differences in inhibitory mechanisms: Evidence from a bilingual stroop task. *Brain and Cognition, 54*, 254–256.

Zinn, S., Bosworth, H. B., Hoenig, H. M., & Swartwelder, H. S. (2007). Executive function deficits in acute stroke. *Archives of Physical Medicine and Rehabilitation, 88*, 173–180.

Binge-Eating Disorder

Kristin M. Graham
Department of Physical Medicine and Rehabilitation, Virginia Commonwealth University, Richmond, VA, USA

Synonyms

Compulsive eating

Definition

Binge-eating disorder is defined in the *Diagnostic and Statistical Manual of Mental Disorders* (5th ed.; *DSM-5*; American Psychiatric Association 2013) as a feeding and eating disorder characterized by repeated instances of binge eating in which the individual consumes an amount of food during a limited time period that is proportionally larger than what would be typically eaten during a similar time period. Binge-eating episodes are accompanied by a sense of lack of control. While a binge-eating episode may occur in one setting, it may also begin in one setting, such as a restaurant, and continue upon returning home. Binge-eating episodes are characterized by the amount of food consumed, and by marked distress. Individuals may report eating very quickly and eating until uncomfortably full. These episodes typically occur in secrecy or social isolation and individuals report negative affect.

Categorization

The disorder is classified with the feeding and eating disorders in DSM-5.

Current Knowledge

Development and Course
The development of binge-eating disorder is common in adolescents and young adults but can

occur later in life. Individuals typically fall within a normal to obese weight range; however, binge-eating disorder is distinct from obesity. The disorder is slightly more common in females (1.6%) than in males (0.8%; APA 2013). Binge-eating disorder is persistent, but remission rates are higher for than for anorexia nervosa or bulimia nervosa. The condition is associated with social maladjustment, poor quality of life, obesity, and increased mortality. Mood disorders and anxiety disorders commonly co-occur, as do substance abuse disorders to a lesser extent.

Assessment and Treatment

Diagnosis typically involves medical and psychiatric evaluation. Individuals seeking treatment for binge-eating disorder are typically older than those seeking treatment for bulimia nervosa or anorexia nervosa. Treatment typically involves pharmacotherapy and psychotherapy. Medications with some empirical evidence include selective serotonin reuptake inhibitors, tricyclic antidepressants, anticonvulsants, and antiobesity medications (Bulik et al. 2007). Empirically supported psychotherapeutic interventions include cognitive-behavioral therapy and dialectical behavior therapy.

See Also

▶ Anorexia Nervosa
▶ Bulimia Nervosa
▶ Feeding and Eating Disorders

References and Readings

American Psychiatric Association. (2013). *Diagnostic and statistical manual of mental disorders (DSM-5 ®)*. Washington, DC: American Psychiatric Association.
Berkman, N. D., Brownley, K. A., Peat, C. M., Lohr, K. N., Cullen, K. E., Morgan, L. C., ..., Bulik, C. M. (2015). Management and outcomes of binge-eating disorder. Comparative Effectiveness Review No. 160. (Prepared by the RTI International-University of North Carolina Evidenced-based Practice Center under Contract No. 290-2012-00008-I.) AHRQ Publication No. 15(16)-EHC030-EF. Rockville, MD: Agency for Healthcare Research and Quality; December 2015. www.effective-healthcare.ahrq.gov/reports/final.cfm.
Bulik, C., Brownley, K., & Shapiro, J. (2007). Diagnosis and management of binge eating disorder. *World Psychiatry, 6*(3), 142–148.
Cossrow, N., Pawaskar, M., Witt, E. A., Ming, E. E., Victor, T. W., Herman, B. K., ..., Erder, M. H. (2016). Estimating the prevalence of binge eating disorder in a community sample from the United States: Comparing DSM-IV-TR and DSM-5 criteria. *The Journal of Clinical Psychiatry, 77*(8), e968–e974.

Binocular Disparity

Sarah M. Szymkowicz[1] and Adam J. Woods[1,2,3]
[1]Department of Clinical and Health Psychology, College of Public Health and Health Professions, University of Florida, Gainesville, FL, USA
[2]Center for Cognitive Aging and Memory, McKnight Brain Institute, University of Florida, Gainesville, FL, USA
[3]Department of Neuroscience, University of Florida, Gainesville, FL, USA

Human eyes are separated by about 50–75 mm between pupils (Dodgson 2004). Therefore, each eye views the world in a slightly different way. The difference between these images is referred to as binocular disparity and provides important information that is not available from either image alone. The amount of disparity depends on the difference in the distance of the two objects and the distance of the fixation point. The greater the disparity, or distance, between the two images, the closer the object is to the fixation point. Binocular disparity is a necessary condition for stereopsis, which is the sense of depth the brain generates from information obtained by the left and right eye. This helps us to see the world in three dimensions, rather than two dimensions.

The idea that binocular disparity contributes to depth perception was first described by Sir Charles Wheatstone in the nineteenth century after he invented the stereoscope, a device used for observing pictures in three dimensions (Qian 1997). Since then, much research has focused on unraveling how the brain processes these disparities, particularly in animal models. A seminal study by Barlow et al. (1967) conducted in the cat's primary visual cortex found that neurons are tuned, or excited, at different distances. A subsequent study by Poggio and Fischer (1977) described four types of depth cells in the striate and prestriate cortex of the rhesus monkey: (1) "tuned excitatory neurons," which respond to a narrow range of depth around the fixation point, (2) "tuned inhibitory neurons," whose responses are suppressed by stimuli at or close to the fixation point, (3) "near neurons," which respond to stimuli near the fixation point and suppress information behind it, and (4) "far neurons," which respond to information behind the fixation point and suppress information near it. While Poggio and collaborators classified cells into these discrete categories, additional research suggests there is a continuous distribution of these cells (LeVay and Voigt 1988). Nevertheless, recordings indicate that disparity neurons are primarily located in V2, V3/V3A, and MT/V5, with weak clustering shown in V1 (Parker 2007).

In humans, the architecture of disparity is less understood. This is partially due to differences in neuronal firing for absolute versus relative disparities (Neri 2005). When looking at a pair of objects that are different distances apart, absolute disparity refers to the differences between the two retinal images generated by the object alone with respect to the fixation point and relative disparity refers to the difference between the two absolute disparities (Neri 2005; Parker 2007). Humans are more sensitive to relative, compared to absolute, disparities (Westheimer 1979). Both the dorsal and ventral streams process binocular cues; however, each stream carries out different types of processing. In animals, the dorsal stream is involved in processing relative disparity, particularly as it relates to spatially extended surfaces (Roy et al. 1992; Upadhyay et al. 2000). In contrast, the ventral stream is also sensitive to relative disparity but appears to be selectivity involved in the relative depth of objects and their three-dimensional configurations (Janssen et al. 2000, 2001; Uka et al. 2005; Umeda et al. 2007). Neurons in the dorsal and ventral streams do fire for both relative and absolute disparities, but, to date, no single cortical region in humans has been found to

be solely involved in relative disparity (Parker 2007), though a recent functional magnetic resonance imaging study showed that disparity preferences for depth perception were clustered in dorsal visual areas, including V3A and V3B/KO (Goncalves et al. 2015).

References

Barlow, H. B., Blakemore, C., & Pettigrew, J. D. (1967). The neural mechanism of binocular depth discrimination. *The Journal of Physiology, 193*(2), 327–342.

Dodgson, N. A. (2004). Variation and extrema of human interpupillary distance. In M. T. Bolas, A. J. Woods, J. O. Merritt, & S. A. Benton (Eds.), *Proceedings of SPIE: Stereoscopic displays and virtual reality systems XI* (Vol. 5291, pp. 36–46). San Jose. https://doi.org/10.1117/12.529999

Goncalves, N. R., Ban, H., Sanchez-Panchuelo, R. M., Francis, S. T., Schluppeck, D., & Welchman, A. E. (2015). 7 tesla FMRI reveals systematic functional organization for binocular disparity in dorsal visual cortex. *The Journal of Neuroscience, 35*(7), 3056–3072.

Janssen, P., Vogels, R., & Orban, G. A. (2000). Three-dimensional shape coding in inferior temporal cortex. *Neuron, 27*(2), 385–397.

Janssen, P., Vogels, R., Liu, Y., & Orban, G. A. (2001). Macaque inferior temporal neurons are selective for three-dimensional boundaries and surfaces. *The Journal of Neuroscience, 21*(23), 9419–9429.

LeVay, S., & Voigt, T. (1988). Ocular dominance and disparity coding in cat visual cortex. *Visual Neuroscience, 1*(4), 395–414.

Neri, P. (2005). A stereoscopic look at visual cortex. *Journal of Neurophysiology, 93*(4), 1823–1826.

Parker, A. J. (2007). Binocular depth perception and the cerebral cortex. *Nature Reviews. Neuroscience, 8*(5), 379–391.

Poggio, G. F., & Fischer, B. (1977). Binocular interaction and depth sensitivity in striate and prestriate cortex of behaving rhesus monkey. *Journal of Neurophysiology, 40*(6), 1392–1405.

Qian, N. (1997). Binocular disparity and the perception of depth. *Neuron, 18*(3), 359–368.

Roy, J. P., Komatsu, H., & Wurtz, R. H. (1992). Disparity sensitivity of neurons in monkey extrastriate area MST. *The Journal of Neuroscience, 12*(7), 2478–2492.

Uka, T., Tanabe, S., Watanabe, M., & Fujita, I. (2005). Neural correlates of fine depth discrimination in monkey inferior temporal cortex. *The Journal of Neuroscience, 25*(46), 10796–10802.

Umeda, K., Tanabe, S., & Fujita, I. (2007). Representation of stereoscopic depth based on relative disparity in macaque area V4. *Journal of Neurophysiology, 98*(1), 241–252.

Upadhyay, U. D., Page, W. K., & Duffy, C. J. (2000). MST responses to pursuit across optic flow with motion parallax. *Journal of Neurophysiology, 84*(2), 818–826.
Westheimer, G. (1979). Cooperative neural processes involved in stereoscopic acuity. *Experimental Brain Research, 36*(3), 585–597.

Binswanger's Disease

Matthew Kraybill[1] and Yana Suchy[2]
[1]Neuropsychology, Cottage Rehabilitation Hospital, Santa Barbara, CA, USA
[2]Department of Psychology, The University of Utah, Salt Lake City, UT, USA

Synonyms

CADASIL; Multi-infarct dementia; Subcortical leukoencephalopathy; Subcortical vascular dementia

Definition

Binswanger's disease (BD) is a type of subcortical vascular dementia caused by widespread, microscopic damage to cerebral white matter. The damage is usually the result of atherosclerosis (i.e., narrowing of arterial blood vessels) that reduces the supply of blood to subcortical areas of the brain, causing tissue to die. The characteristic pattern of BD-damaged brain tissue can be seen using brain imaging techniques such as computed tomography (CT) or magnetic resonance imaging (MRI). CT imaging of BD often reveals symmetric, noncontrasting hypodensities also called "leukoaraiosis," and more sensitive MRI imaging reveals diffuse white matter lesions and scattered multiple lacunes (Akiguchi et al. 2014).

There is some controversy in the literature about whether BD constitutes a distinct clinical entity or simply describes the result of different neuropathologies that affect subcortical white matter (Akiguchi et al. 2014; Caplan 1995; Hachinski et al. 2006; Olsen and Clasen 1998; Pantoni and Garcia 1995; Rosenberg et al.

2015). Although the precise cause of BD is unclear, it is frequently associated with diabetes, cardiovascular disease, previous cerebrovascular accident, malnutrition, and, most notably, hypertension. The age of onset for BD is typically between ages 60 and 79 years, with men and women equally affected. Estimates about the incidence of BD range from 3% to 12% (Babikian and Ropper 1987).

Current Knowledge

Neuropathology

Gross pathology of brain tissue affected by BD is characterized by gyral atrophy and widening of the sulci resulting from the loss of cerebral white matter. Lateral ventricles are also typically enlarged. Lacunar infarctions can be found in the white matter, pons, and basal ganglia as well as occasionally in the cerebellum. Microscopic pathology of BD is marked by diffuse and patchy white matter demyelination with areas of reactive gliosis and decreased nerve fibers. The small arteries of the white matter also show fibrous thickening, which is associated with hypertension and cardiovascular disease. There is growing evidence that white matter pathology in BD is related to endothelial dysfunction and neuroinflammation (Huisa and Rosenberg 2014).

Clinical Symptoms

BD typically has a slow, insidious onset that eventually manifests in cognitive and motor dysfunctions related to the disruption of subcortical neural circuits. Specifically, patients exhibit executive dysfunction (e.g., impaired initiation, inhibition, monitoring of goal-directed behavior, and verbal fluency), psychomotor slowing, inattention, and short-term memory loss with poor retrieval but intact recognition (Roman 2003). Other symptoms include changes in speech, an unsteady gait, postural instability, changes in personality or mood (including apathy, irritability, and depression), as well as urinary incontinence (Babikian and Ropper 1987; Caplan 1995; Lezak et al. 2004; Roman 2003).

Treatment

Treatment of BD is often targeted at specific symptoms. For example, medications such as donepezil and memantine may be used to treat the cognitive symptoms associated with BD. Individuals with depression may be treated with antidepressant medications (e.g., selective serotonin reuptake inhibitors (SSRIs) such as sertraline or citalopram) and individuals with agitation or disruptive behavior can be treated with atypical antipsychotic medications such as risperidone or olanzapine (Sink et al. 2005). Antiplatelet therapy and statins have also been recommended for stroke prevention in BD (Huisa and Rosenberg 2014). Other treatment interventions are often focused on reducing cardiovascular risk factors by eating a healthy diet, exercising, and not smoking or drinking too much alcohol. Controlling vascular risk factors can help improve cognition and may even help prevent the development of dementia (Roman 2005).

Prognosis

BD is a progressive disease and there is currently no cure. The course of BD can be variable and deterioration can occur suddenly or gradually and then progress in a stepwise manner (Santamaria Ortiz and Knight 1994).

Cross-References

▶ Leukoaraiosis

References and Readings

Akiguchi, I., Budka, H., Shirakashi, Y., Woehrer, A., Watanabe, T., Shiino, A., Yamamoto, Y., Kawamoto, Y., Krampla, W., Jungwirth, S., & Fischer, P. (2014). MRI features of Binswanger's disease predict prognosis and associated pathology. *Annals of Clinical and Translational Neurology, 1*(10), 813–821.

Babikian, V., & Ropper, A. H. (1987). Binswanger's disease: A review. *Stroke, 18*(1), 2–12.

Caplan, L. R. (1995). Binswanger's disease – Revisited. *Neurology, 45*(4), 626–633.

Hachinski, V., Iadecola, C., Petersen, R. C., Breteler, M. M., Nyenhuis, D. L., Black, S. E., et al. (2006). National Institute of Neurological Disorders and Stroke-Canadian Stroke Network vascular cognitive impairment harmonization standards. *Stroke, 37*(9), 2220–2241.

Huisa, B. N., & Rosenberg, G. A. (2014). Binswanger's disease: Toward a diagnosis agreement and therapeutic approach. *Expert Review of Neurotherapeutics, 14*(10), 1203–1213.

Lezak, M. D., Howieson, D. B., & Loring, D. (2004). *Neuropsychological assessment* (4th ed.p. 1016). New York: Oxford University Press.

Olsen, C. G., & Clasen, M. E. (1998). Senile dementia of the Binswanger's type. *American Family Physician, 58*(9), 2068–2074.

Pantoni, L., & Garcia, J. H. (1995). The significance of cerebral white matter abnormalities 100 years after Binswanger's report. A review. *Stroke, 26*(7), 1293–1301.

Roman, G. C. (2003). Neurological aspects of vascular dementia: Basic concepts, diagnosis, and management. In P. A. Lichtenberg, D. L. Murman, & A. M. Mellow (Eds.), *Handbook of dementia – Psychological, neurological, and psychiatric perspectives* (pp. 149–171). Hoboken: Wiley.

Roman, G. C. (2005). Vascular dementia prevention: A risk factor analysis. *Cerebrovascular Diseases, 20*(Suppl. 2), 91–100.

Rosenberg, G. A., Wallin, A., Wardlaw, J. M., Markus, H. S., Montaner, J., Wolfson, L., Costantino, I., Zlokovic, B. V., Joutel, A., Dichgans, M., Duering, M., Schmidt, R., Korczyn, A. D., Grinberg, L. T., & Hachinski, V. (2015). Consensus statement for diagnosis of subcortical small vessel disease. *Journal of Cerebral Blood Flow and Metabolism, 36*(1). 1–13.

Santamaria Ortiz, J., & Knight, P. V. (1994). Review: Binswanger's disease, leukoaraiosis and dementia. *Age and Ageing, 23*(1), 75–81.

Sink, K. M., Holden, K. F., & Yaffe, K. (2005). Pharmacological treatment of neuropsychiatric symptoms of dementia: A review of the evidence. *JAMA, 293*(5), 596–608.

Biomechanics of Injury

Beth Rush
Psychiatry and Psychology, Mayo Clinic, Jacksonville, FL, USA

Definition

An inclusive term to explore and describe the mechanical and physical factors that result in traumatic brain injury.

Current Knowledge

Biomechanical injuries typically occur without the direct impact of an outside object on the skull or brain, but rather in the context of acceleration-deceleration injuries or blast injuries. High-speed situations such as motor vehicle accidents and sports provide mediums for these inertia-based injuries. The structure of the skull includes sinuses and bony protective regions. Underlying brain tissue is held in suspension underneath the skull not only by the meninges, but also by a cushion of cerebral spinal fluid. Different inertial forces such as linear acceleration, rotation of the head, or massive vibration or air pressure changes in the environment can result in a wide range of potential damage to these underlying substances. These disruptions may include skull fracture, linear acceleration injury, rotational injury, and the effects of vibration of the skull and brain against one another.

Superficial or deep lesions may result in parenchymal injury depending on the type of mechanical force that occurred at the time of head trauma. Linear acceleration injuries are most often associated with superficial brain injuries such as cerebral contusions, while rotational injuries are most often associated with disruptions to deep white matter tracts and projections, and centrally located brain structures and neural networks. Consequently, rotational injuries may be more severe with regard to effects on cognition, motor skills, and functional status. Concussion with or without loss of consciousness is also a consequence of biomechanical forces and the subsequent effects on underlying brain tissue.

The biomechanics of injury differentially affect initial and long-term recovery from acquired brain injury. Understanding these different mechanical forces may help one to improve understanding of injury severity. Increased understanding of the biomechanics underlying brain injury has led to the development of protective headgear in high-speed or direct-impact sports such as biking, motor racing, football, and hockey.

Cross-References

▶ Acceleration Injury
▶ Deceleration Injury
▶ Diffuse Axonal Injury
▶ Rotational Acceleration
▶ Traumatic Brain Injury (TBI)

References and Readings

Bayly, P. V., Cohen, T. S., Leister, E. P., Ajo, D., Leuthardt, E. C., & Genin, G. M. (2005). Acceleration-induced deformation of the human brain. *Journal of Neurotrauma, 22,* 845–856.

Goriely, A., Geers, M. G., Holzapfel, G. A., Jayamohan, J., Jerusalem, A., Sivaloganathan, S., Squier, W., van Dommelen, J. A., Waters, S., & Kuhl, E. (2015). Mechanics of the brain: Perspectives, challenges, and opportunities. *Biomechanical Models of Mechanobiology, 14*(5), 931–965.

Oeur, R. A., Karton, C., Post, A., Rousseau, P., Hoshizaki, T. B., Marshall, S., Brien, S. E., Smith, A., Cusimano, M. D., & Gilchrist, M. D. (2015). A comparison of head dynamic response and brain tissue stress and strain using accident reconstructions for concussion, concussion with persistent postconcussive symptoms, and subdural hematoma. *Journal of Neurosurgery, 123*(2), 415–422.

Ommaya, A. K., Goldsmith, W., & Thibault, L. (2002). Biomechanics and neuropathology of adult and pediatric head injury. *British Journal of Neurosurgery, 16,* 220–242.

Biopsy

Bram Goldstein
Department of Gynecologic Oncology, Hoag Hospital Cancer Center, Newport Beach, CA, USA

Definition

A biopsy is a medical examination entailing the removal of cellular tissue via a needle or surgical resection. In particular, an incisional or core biopsy involves a select sample of tissue, whereas an excisional biopsy necessitates a larger specimen. The biopsy results are typically evaluated microscopically by a pathologist, who determines if a lesion's pathology is benign or malignant. Although histological confirmation of tumor diagnosis can be achieved, a biopsy sampling error can result if the specific tissue section does not contain the most representative cellular features. When the biopsy is abnormal, the cell structure may be unusual and indicative of malignancy. However, further pathological examination is often required to make a definitive diagnosis.

Cross-References

▶ Radiosurgery, Stereotactic Radiosurgery

References and Readings

Yu, X., Liu, Z., Tian, Z., Li, S., Huang, H., Xiu, B., et al. (2006). Stereotactic biopsy for intracranial space-occupying lesions: Clinical analysis of 550 cases. *Stereotactic and Functional Neurosurgery, 75*, 103–108.

Blast Effects

Kayla LaRosa
Educational and Psychological Studies/TBI Model Systems, University of South Florida/J.A. Haley VA, Tampa, FL, USA

Synonyms

Blast injury

Definition

Blast effects are injuries or symptoms resulting from a shock wave or blast caused by high-order or low-order explosives such as dynamite, bombs, or C-4 (CDC 2016). Effects resulting from blasts may vary from auditory problems to brain injury and are classified as primary, secondary, tertiary, or quaternary (CDC 2016). Primary blast effects are unique to high-order explosives and may include injuries such as concussion, eye rupture, or abdominal hemorrhage (CDC 2016). Secondary and tertiary effects may result from bomb fragments, flying debris, or blast wind with any body part being affected. Last, quaternary effects include explosion-related injuries, illness, or disease, such as burns, close or open brain injury, and breathing problems due to toxic fumes, dust, or smoke from a blast.

See Also

▶ Blast Injury
▶ Mild Traumatic Brain Injury
▶ Severe Brain Injury
▶ Traumatic Brain Injury (TBI)

References and Readings

Center for Disease Control Injury Prevention (2016). Explosions and blast injuries: A primer for clinicians. Retrieved from: https://www.cdc.gov/masstrauma/pre paredness/primer.pdf
Lash, M. (2017). Understanding the effects of concussion, blast, and brain injuries: A guide for families, veterans, and caregivers. Brainline Military. Retrieved from: http://www.brainlinemilitary.org/content/2008/11/under standing-effects-concussion-blast-and-brain-injuries-gui de-families-veterans-and-caregi_pageall.html

---

Blast Injury

Bradley J. Hufford
Neuropsychology, Rehabilitation Hospital of Indiana, Indianapolis, IN, USA

Synonyms

This term is highly associated (but technically not synonymous) with mild traumatic brain injury and post-concussive symptoms.

Definition

A trauma sustained as a result of exposure to an explosion or its effects. Technically, blast injury can affect any physical system/function; its neurological effects are highlighted here.

Historical Background

Blast injuries can occur in any setting, civilian or military. However, exposure to the effects of explosive forces is much more associated with military populations and has been since the advent of modern warfare. Awareness of the effect of blast injuries began to emerge in earnest with the phenomenon of "shell shock" during the First World War. That war exposed a staggering number of soldiers to explosive injuries, far more than had previous conflicts. As a result, an ever-increasing number of military personnel presented with vague but incapacitating complaints that prevented them from returning to active (particularly front line) duty. Initially, these symptoms were considered to be secondary to organic central nervous system injury. Over time, however, others favored a more psychological or even intentional (i.e., malingering) explanation, citing the fact that many shell-shocked servicemen did not appear to have been as close to the explosion as would seem necessary to truly be negatively affected. The nature of the shell-shock symptoms was further obscured by the lack of diagnostic methods, absence of a clear definition of the syndrome, and even political factors (e.g., superiors being able to justify returning much-needed soldiers to frontline duty if their complaints reflected psychological or constitutional weaknesses rather than neurological/organic injuries). This debate of "psychological versus neurological" causes has continued throughout subsequent wars and is a particular focus of the recent conflicts in the Middle East, given the high incidence of explosives utilized by terrorists and non-Coalition combatants.

Current Knowledge

With improvements in medical care of trauma and the development of more effective defensive equipment (i.e., body and vehicle armor), a greater number of servicemen and women injured in combat are surviving than ever before: The mortality rate for wounded personnel has declined from approximately 30% during the Second World War to approximately 10% during the recent conflicts in Iraq and Afghanistan. As a result, a greater number of the wounded are surviving with traumatic brain injury than in the past – from under 20% during the Vietnam conflict to perhaps near 50% in the recent conflicts. Overall, it has been estimated that up to 30% of all combat troops in Operations Iraqi Freedom and Enduring Freedom (OIF/OEF) may have incurred an acquired brain injury of some degree. The majority of these combat-related brain injuries are sustained as a result of exposure to an explosion.

Explosions may cause injury through four mechanisms:

1. Primary Blast Injury
   A primary injury is one sustained from exposure to the shock/pressure waves initiated by the explosion. When explosive munitions are detonated, a shock-wave approaching a speed of 8000 m/s is generated. The waves generated from a blast can cause life-threatening injuries when they strike an individual directly or if they reflect off nearby surfaces and then come into contact with the person. The force generated is of such a magnitude that it often results in an instant fatality or in trauma to multiple body systems. Body organs that are relatively solid or fluid-filled tend to sustain a lesser degree of injury than those that are gas-filled or have a gas-liquid interface, such as the tympanic membrane, lung, colon, etc. Although not fully understood, research suggests that the explosion may injure the central nervous system directly, as in a concussion, but may also indirectly affect the brain. The latter case may occur when peripheral somatic areas are impacted by the blast, setting in motion events

that ultimately impact the CNS, such as chemical/metabolic cascades, physical sequelae (i.e., cerebral infarction caused by an air embolism), and/or kinetic events (e.g., transfer of shock/pressure wave energy from the body, up the vasculature into brain tissue). It has been postulated that the severity and number of a person's physical wounds from the primary blasts often overshadow symptoms of traumatic brain injury, delaying diagnosis and treatment for these injuries.

2. Secondary Blast Injury
   Secondary injuries occur when shrapnel, debris, or other objects are caught up by the blast and propelled against/into an individual. Many of these injuries are therefore penetrating in nature.

3. Tertiary Blast Injury
   This type of injury is sustained when the person is caught up and propelled by the blast wind that follows the initial shock wave and is thrown against an object, a structure, the ground, other individuals, etc., often resulting in blunt force wounds.

4. Quaternary Blast Injury
   Quaternary blast injuries arise from the after-effects of an explosion. Examples include being exposed to radiation, fire, chemicals, dust, or toxic substances that were precipitated by the explosive event.

Typically, an individual is exposed to more than one mechanism, making the contributions of one particular mechanism difficult to separate from others.

Approximately 60% of explosion-related injuries in combat lead to an acquired brain injury. As is the case with other etiologies, the majority of brain injuries resulting from explosions are classified as mild in nature. "Mild" traumatic brain injury (mTBI) has not been consistently defined in the literature, which is a substantial limitation in making meaningful comparisons between studies. Despite this, definitions such as that proposed by the American Congress of Rehabilitation Medicine (ACRM) are coming into wider acceptance and have largely been adopted by the military. The ACRM definition of mTBI includes at least one of the following symptoms: less than half an hour of loss of consciousness, less than 24 h of post-traumatic amnesia, any retrograde or anterograde amnesia, mental status changes immediately after injury, and transient/permanent neurological impairments. The literature cautions that a mild TBI from an explosion may not be equivalent to mild TBI from other etiologies (e.g., motor vehicle accidents, sports injuries), as the former may affect the brain more diffusely and tend to involve trauma to other organ systems, thereby complicating the patient's clinical presentation and recovery. However, many studies have indicated that factors such as loss of consciousness, resultant symptom profiles, and recovery courses do not appear to substantially differ between blast victims and those injured by other means, tentatively suggesting that knowledge gleaned from studying these other etiologies has at least some applicability to blast injury survivors.

Cognitive (e.g., memory, attention), somatic (e.g., dizziness, headache, sleep initiation/maintenance difficulties), and emotional (e.g., nervousness, irritability) symptoms are commonly seen initially after blast injuries. In civilian mTBI samples, these symptoms usually resolve quickly, with most individuals showing rapid recovery within the first week. However, over one-third may continue to experience significant post-concussion symptoms, and as many as 15% may continue to experience persistent symptoms after 12 months ("Persistent Post-Concussion Syndrome"). Unfortunately, these persistent symptoms have not been consistently defined, and many point out that the constellation of symptoms present are vague and lack specificity needed to identify them as constituting a true syndrome.

There is debate over whether the more chronic symptom constellation after mild TBI reflects a true neurological condition; this has particular relevance in blast injury, as the brief history of "shell shock" above illustrates. Those favoring a more neurological position cite animal models in which direct and indirect exposure to primary blasts causes structural, chemical, and electrophysiological changes in the brain. Additionally, some studies using functional MRI and diffuse tensor imaging in humans have reported cerebral alterations in some (albeit not all) persons who have sustained blast injuries. Conversely, those weighing psychological factors more heavily in terms of causation point to the mTBI literature that indicates non-neurological factors, such as premorbid psychological coping resources and external stressors, appear to influence the development of concussion symptoms in some individuals. The fact that mTBI symptoms overlap considerably with symptoms seen in disorders such as posttraumatic stress disorder (PTSD) is particularly noteworthy, given the high incidence of PTSD in military personnel who have experienced combat: Gaylord et al. (2008) found that nearly 20% of military persons who incurred blast and burn injuries were appropriate for both mild brain injury and PTSD diagnoses. Hoge et al. (2008) reported that approximately 15% of soldiers surveyed after being returned home might meet criteria for both mTBI and PTSD; these servicemen and women were more likely to have been exposed to a blast injury. In addition, their survey indicated that the presence of affective distress might be the major factor in maintaining chronic health difficulties, including mTBI symptomatology. A compromise position of sorts posits mTBI symptoms are likely neurological in origin but are subsequently maintained by emotional/psychological factors and that the presence of PTSD and similar affective disturbances can complicate healing from and coping with mTBI (and, concomitantly, mTBI symptoms can exacerbate and prolong PTSD symptoms). The fact that PTSD symptoms can arise long after the actual trauma indicates that these emotional disturbances may influence a person at virtually any point in his/her brain injury recovery.

Treatment of blast injuries begins with a thorough diagnostic assessment. The armed services have made significant improvements in their endeavors to standardize comprehensive screening and interviewing methods to identify service personnel who may have experienced an acquired brain injury, beginning on the battlefield and continuing throughout the military's medical system. Efforts have been made to carefully screen every wounded individual for other symptoms (e.g., tinnitus) that place them at higher risk for having sustained a TBI in a blast, to help ensure mTBIs are not underdiagnosed. The assessment process includes a thorough medical evaluation of the patient's current condition and a comprehensive interview that elicits historical information about past psychological treatment/coping, substance use, and combat exposure.

Neuropsychological evaluation is recommended to occur as early as possible to help identify postconcussive symptoms and clarify the diagnostic picture, enabling education and treatment efforts to proceed more quickly. Whereas there are cognitive deficits commonly seen after most mTBIs (e.g., slowed attention and information processing speed, motor slowness, executive dysfunction, and memory difficulties), the profile of cognitive weaknesses can be quite variable, necessitating a broad-based neuropsychological assessment (i.e., a sampling of all major cognitive domains). Additionally, as is the case in sports concussions, the symptom picture for many blast survivors may evolve relatively rapidly, arguing for use of tests that have alternate forms (e.g., California Verbal Learning Test-2nd Edition, Hopkins Verbal Learning Test-Revised). Tracking somatic symptoms (e.g., Neurobehavioral Symptom Inventory, Post-Concussion Scale-Revised) over time may also have utility. Because of the high degree of PTSD and other affective disorders, a thorough psychological evaluation should always be performed (including objective personality measures such as the MMPI-2 or PAI and instruments such as the PTSD Checklist), and observation for these symptoms should be an ongoing effort, not simply one restricted to an initial evaluation. Given the high degree of lowered effort present in civilian mTBI cases, effort testing (e.g., Test of Memory Malingering) is often advocated, with the caveat that poor performance on an effort test should not automatically be interpreted as an indicator of intentional feigning of symptoms, but as a sign that further investigation is warranted as to the cause of the lowered effort.

After a thorough diagnostic assessment has been performed, treatments generally have proceeded along the lines advocated for mild brain injuries attributed to non-blast causes. Specifically, reassurance and education regarding the nature and general recovery of cognitive and other symptoms after mTBI is delivered. Specific treatments need to be tailored to the individual, in recognition that not all mTBIs are expressed identically. For instance, in a cluster analysis performed on 1341 servicemen who had sustained an mTBI in combat over the previous 2 years, Bailie et al. (2016) found four different subtypes: good recovery (low overall cognitive and affective symptoms; 37.8% of the sample), high PTSD but few cognitive symptoms (21.9%), elevated cognitive but few affective symptoms (21.5%), and mixed symptoms (18.6%). These results suggest an array of treatment strategies that is necessary to effectively address appropriate needs. Such treatment strategies would include medication (e.g., analgesics for pain, soporific medication for insomnia, antidepressants for affective symptoms), relaxation strategies for anxiety symptoms, psychotherapy for PTSD symptoms, and evidence-based cognitive rehabilitation.

Future Directions

The research literature in blast injury is still evolving. The following is a partial list of necessary future research efforts: clarifying definitions of mTBI and post-concussive symptom constellations; separation of the effect of different blast mechanisms (e.g., primary, secondary) on the brain; standardization of research methodology with respect to inducing blast injuries in animal subjects; comparison of mTBI symptoms, course, and recovery between blast injury survivors and those who have injuries from other sources; investigation of the effect of multiple blast exposures; and investigation of how PTSD/affective distress differs from and interacts with mTBI. Studies should take into account situational factors such as combat exposure, combat intensity, length and number of deployments, as well as potentially moderating variables on symptom expression and recovery (e.g., substance use, pain intensity, sleep integrity). More prospective research is

clearly needed. Within neuropsychology, development of alternate forms for many tests is encouraged.

See Also

► Concussion
► Mild Traumatic Brain Injury
► Post-concussive Syndrome
► Post-Traumatic Stress Disorder
► Traumatic Brain Injury (TBI)

References and Readings

Bailie, J., Kennedy, J., French, L., Marshall, K., Prokhorenko, O., Asmussen, S., Reid, M., Qashu, F., Brickell, T., & Lange, R. (2016). Profile analysis of the neurobehavioral and psychiatric symptoms following combat-related mild traumatic brain injury: Identification of subtypes. *The Journal of Head Trauma Rehabilitation, 31*(1), 2–12.
Batten, S., Beal, S., Bleiberg, J., et al. (2009). *Defense centers of excellence for psychological health and traumatic brain injury and defense and veterans brain injury center consensus conference on cognitive rehabilitation for mild traumatic brain injury.* Washington, DC.
Bogdanova, Y., & Verfaellie, M. (2012). Cognitive sequelae of blast-induced traumatic brain injury: Recovery and rehabilitation. *Neuropsychological Review, 22,* 4–20.
Cernak, I., Wang, Z., Jiang, J., Bian, X., & Savic, J. (2001). Ultrastructural and functional characteristics of blast injury-induced neurotrauma. *The Journal of Trauma, Injury, Infection, and Critical Care, 50,* 695–706.
Gaylord, K., Cooper, D., Mercade, J., Kennedy, J., Yoder, L., & Holcomb, J. (2008). Incidence of post-traumatic stress disorder and mild traumatic brain injury in burned service members: Preliminary report. *The Journal of Trauma, Injury, Infection, and Critical Care, 64,* S200–S206.
Hoge, C., McGurk, D., Thomas, J., Cox, A., Engel, C., & Castro, C. (2008). Mild traumatic brain injury in U.S. soldiers returning from Iraq. *The New England Journal of Medicine, 358*(5), 453–463.
Jackson, G., Hamilton, N., & Tupler, L. (2008). Detecting traumatic brain injury among veterans of operations enduring and Iraqi Freedom. *North Carolina Medical Journal, 69*(1), 43–47.
Jones, E., Fear, N., & Wessely, S. (2007). Shell shock and mild traumatic brain injury: A historical review. *American Journal of Psychiatry, 164,* 1641–1645.

Blessed Dementia Scale

Avril J. Keller[1], Elisabeth M. S. Sherman[2] and Esther Strauss[3]
[1]Alberta Children's Hospital, University of Calgary, Calgary, AB, Canada
[2]Copeman Healthcare Centre, Calgary, AB, Canada
[3]Department of Psychology, University of Victoria, Victoria, BC, Canada

Synonyms

Blessed dementia rating scale (BDRS); Blessed-Roth DS; Dementia scale (DS); Modified Blessed dementia scale (DS); Newcastle DS; Revised dementia scale (RDS)

Description

The Blessed dementia scale (DS) was developed in 1968 by Blessed and colleagues in an attempt to quantify the "degree of intellectual and personality deterioration" (p. 799) in the elderly.

This rating scale consists of 22 items that reflect (1) changes in performance of everyday activities (8 items; e.g., using money and finding one's way), (2) changes in habits including self-care (3 items; i.e., eating, dressing and continence), and (3) changes in personality, interests, and drives (11 items; e.g., evaluation of rigidity and affect). A close friend or relative is asked to provide these behavior ratings of the examinee over the past 6 months; when unavailable, medical records can be used. The DS is scored on a 0–28-point scale, where higher numbers indicate a larger decrement in functional capacity. On everyday activity items, a score of 1 is given for total inability to perform a task; a score of 0.5 is given for partial, variable, or intermittent inability to perform an activity; and a score of 0 is given if the patient is able to perform the task. The changes

in habits section are scored on a 4-point scale (i.e., 0–3), resulting in a stronger contribution to the total score. Personality changes are scored 1 if present or 0 if absent (Blessed et al. 1968, 1988). A total cutoff score of 4 out of 28 is typically used to differentiate patients with dementia versus those without. Scores of 4–9 indicate mild impairment, whereas scores of 10 or higher suggest moderate to severe impairment (Eastwood et al. 1983). Stern et al. (1987) have suggested 15 as the threshold for moderate impairment.

The original DS also included a second section comprised of a brief battery of simple cognitive tasks, called the information-memory-concentration test (IMCT; Blessed et al. 1968, 1988). Similar to other brief mental status instruments, the IMCT incorporates 12 items of information/orientation, 11 items of long-term memory, a brief test for the 5-min recall of a person's name and address, and 3 sequencing tasks requiring concentration (Blessed et al. 1968, 1988). This sub-component is typically no longer included in the DS.

Historical Background

The original dementia scale (DS) evaluated informant-reported changes in behavior and daily functioning and also included cognitive tasks given to the patient. It was developed by Blessed, Tomlinson, and Roth in 1968 in an attempt to compare the deterioration of intellect and personality with underlying brain neuropathology (Blessed et al. 1968, 1988). The revised dementia scale (RDS) was introduced in 1988 and included only items reflecting informant-rated changes in everyday activities and habits (items 1 through 11; Erkinjuntti et al. 1988). The sensitivity and specificity of the revised scale was higher than that of the original DS, possibly due to lower dementia specificity of the excluded items (i.e., changes in personality, interests, and drive; Lawson et al. 1977). However, the 4-week test-retest reliability for the revised scale was lower ($r = 0.68$) than the original ($r = 0.79$), potentially due to the inclusion of fewer items (Erkinjuntti et al. 1988).

---

†Esther Strauss: deceased.

Items from the DS have been included in the standardized interview with relatives that is part of the Cambridge Mental Disorders of the Elderly Examination (CAMDEX; Roth et al. 1986). Elements of this scale have also been incorporated in the standardized battery of the Consortium to Establish a Registry for Alzheimer's Disease (CERAD; Morris et al. 1988). Additional analysis of the scale has indicated that the items can be subdivided into four groups, each with its own score (cognitive, items 1–7, score range 0–7; personality change, items 12–17, score range 0–6; apathy/withdrawal, 18, 20, and 21, score range 0–3; basic self-care, 9–11, score range 0–3), in order to aid in interpretation (Stern et al. 1990).

Psychometric Data

In community-dwelling individuals, test-retest reliability after 4 weeks was $r = 0.79$; the first 11 items show marginal reliability ($r = 0.68$; Erkinjuntti et al. 1988). Cole (1990) found an interrater reliability of $r = 0.59$ when comparing DS ratings by two independent raters who each interviewed the caretakers of 47 dementia patients.

The initial study employing the DS showed that scores increased as the presence of senile plaques increased ($r = 0.77$; Blessed et al. 1968). Also, the DS showed discriminative validity in identifying senile dementia patients compared with depressed, paraphrenia, delirious, and physically ill patients (Blessed et al. 1968). Others have also noted that the DS is able to discriminate between dementia patients and community residents (Erkinjuntti et al. 1988; Lam et al. 1997). When a cutoff of 4/28 was used, the DS was shown to have a sensitivity of 90% and a specificity of 84% (Erkinjuntti et al. 1988). Moderate to high correlations have been reported with other measures such as the CERAD total score ($r = 0.40$; Chandler et al. 2005), the Mini-Mental State Exam ($r = 0.80$; Hendrie et al. 1988), and the CAMDEX ($r = 0.77$; Hendrie et al. 1988). Additionally, Stern et al. (1987)

reported that disease progression can be monitored using the DS; cognitive deficiencies affecting instrumental activities of daily living (e.g., handling money, remembering short lists) were evident early and worsened throughout the disease course, whereas changes in basic self-care did not occur until 4–5 years into the illness (Stern et al. 1990).

A cutoff of 1.5 on the RDS yields a sensitivity of 93% and a specificity of 97% in discriminating between demented and non-demented subjects, regardless of level of dementia (Erkinjuntti et al. 1988). The RDS is also highly correlated with the Activities of Daily Living Scale, the Instrumental Activities of Daily Living Scale, and the Functional Activities Questionnaire (Juva et al. 1997).

The DS appears minimally affected by demographic factors. Age correlates moderately with DS scores ($r = 0.31$), but when degree of dementia is taken into account, age does not have a significant effect (Erkinjuntti et al. 1988). Education appears unrelated to DS scores (Erkinjuntti et al. 1988). African-American patients score higher on the DS than white patients (Hargrove et al. 1998). The DS has been translated and validated in Chinese, Korean, and Czech (Lam et al. 1997; Lee et al. 1999; Vajdickova et al. 1995).

Clinical Uses

The DS offers a blend of items commonly found on mental status exams, activities of daily living scales, and instrumental activities of daily living scales. It is quick and easy to administer and additionally provides a quantification of the degree of dementia severity. As such, it is ideal for use by general practitioners and specialized medical and mental healthcare professionals to gauge initial status, as well as to track disease progression. The DS may also provide more useful information in a clinical setting than the MMSE and other cognitive assessment scales (Mant et al. 1988) because it measures functional aspects of dementia.

Cross-References

▶ Alzheimer's Disease
▶ Bristol Activities of Daily Living Scale
▶ Clinical Dementia Rating
▶ Dementia
▶ Dementia Rating Scale-2
▶ Lawton-Brody Instrumental Activities of Daily
  Living Scale

References and Readings

Blessed, G., Tomlinson, B. E., & Roth, M. (1968). The association between quantitative measures of dementia and of senile changes in the cerebral gray matter of elderly subjects. *British Journal of Psychiatry, 114*(512), 797–811.

Blessed, G., Tomlinson, B. E., & Roth, M. (1988). Blessed-Roth Dementia Scale (DS). *Psychopharmacology Bulletin, 24*(4), 705–708.

Chandler, M. J., Lacritz, L. H., Hynan, L. S., Barnard, H. D., Allen, G., Deschner, M., et al. (2005). A total score for the CERAD neuropsychological battery. *Neurology, 65*(1), 102–106.

Cole, M. G. (1990). Interrater reliability of the Blessed Dementia Scale. *Canadian Journal of Psychiatry, 35*(4), 328–330.

Eastwood, M. R., Lautenschlaegar, E., & Corbin, S. (1983). A comparison of clinical methods for assessing dementia. *Journal of the American Geriatrics Society, 31*(6), 342–347.

Erkinjuntti, T., Hokkanen, L., Sulkava, R., & Palos, J. (1988). The Blessed Dementia Scale as a screening test for dementia. *International Journal of Geriatric Psychiatry, 3*, 267–273.

Folstein, M. F., Folstein, S. E., & McHugh, P. R. (1975). Mini mental state: A practical method for grading the cognitive state of patients for the clinician. *Journal of Psychiatric Research, 12*(3), 189–198.

Hargrove, R., Stoeklin, M., Haan, M., & Reed, B. (1998). Clinical aspects of Alzheimer's disease in black and white patients. *Journal of the National Medical Association, 90*, 78–84.

Hendrie, H. C., Hall, K. S., Brittain, H. M., Austrom, M. G., Farlow, M., Parker, J., et al. (1988). The CAMDEX: A standardized instrument for the diagnosis of mental disorder in the elderly: A replication with a U.S. sample. *Journal of the American Geriatrics Society, 36*(5), 402–408.

Juva, K., Maela, M., Erkinjuntti, T., Sulkava, R., Yukoski, R., Valvanne, J., et al. (1997). Functional assessment scales in detecting dementia. *Age and Ageing, 26*(5), 393–400.

Lam, L. C. W., Chiu, H. F. K., Li, S. W., Chan, W. F., Chan, C. K. Y., Wong, M., et al. (1997). Screening for dementia: A preliminary study on the validity of the Chinese version of the Blessed-Roth Dementia Scale. *International Psychogeriatrics, 9*(1), 39–46.

Lawson, J. S., Rodenburg, M., & Dykes, J. A. (1977). A dementia rating scale for use with psychogeriatric patients. *Journal of Gerontology, 32*, 153–159.

Lee, D. Y., Yoon, J. C., Lee, K. U., Jhoo, J. H., Kim, K. W., Lee, J. H., et al. (1999). Reliability and validity of the Korean version of Short Blessed Test (SBT-K) as a dementia screening instrument. *Journal of Korean Neuropsychiatric Association, 38*, 1365–1375.

Lezak, M. D., Howieson, D. B., & Loring, D. W. (2004). *Neuropsychological assessment* (4th ed.). New York: Oxford University Press.

Mant, A., Eyland, E. A., Pond, D. C., Saunders, N. A., & Chancellor, A. H. B. (1988). Recognition of dementia in general practice: Comparison of general practitioners' opinion with assessments using the mini-mental state examination and the Blessed Dementia Scale. *Family Practice, 5*(3), 184–188.

Morris, J. C., Mohs, R. C., Rogers, H., Fillenbaum, G., & Heyman, A. (1988). Consortium to establish a registry for Alzheimer's disease (CERAD) clinical and neuropsychological assessment of Alzheimer's disease. *Psychopharmacology Bulletin, 24*(4), 641–651.

Roth, M., Tym, E., Mountjoy, C. Q., Huppert, F. A., Hendrie, H., Verma, S., et al. (1986). CAMDEX: A standardized instrument for the diagnosis of mental disorders in the elderly with special reference to early detection of dementia. *British Journal of Psychiatry, 149*, 698–709.

Stern, Y., Mayeux, R., Sano, M., Hauser, W. A., & Bush, T. (1987). Predictors of disease course in patients with probable Alzheimer's disease. *Neurology, 37*(10), 1649–1653.

Stern, Y., Hesdorffer, D., Sano, M., & Mayeux, R. (1990). Measurement and prediction of functional capacity in Alzheimer's disease. *Neurology, 40*(1), 8–14.

Vajdickova, K., Kolibas, E., Heretik, A., & Kosc, M. (1995). Application of behavioural scale in the diagnosis of dementia of advanced age. *Ceska A Slovenska Psychiatrie, 91*(1), 7–14.

Blindsight

Sophie Lebrecht and Michael J. Tarr
Visual Neuroscience Laboratory, Brown
University, Providence, RI, USA

Short Description or Definition

Blindsight is a neuropsychological disorder that results from damage to the primary visual cortex

(V1). Such localized cortical damage produces localized visual impairment in the patient's visual field contralateral to the site of the damage. Critically, despite the nominal loss of vision, patients with blindsight preserve the ability to detect and discriminate visual stimuli presented in the impaired region of their visual field. Lawrence Weiskrantz's (1986) observation of this ability to "see" stimuli in a "blind" visual field led him to refer to this disorder as "blindsight."

Categorization

There are two types of blindsight, termed Type I and Type II. Patients with Type I blindsight report no conscious awareness of stimuli presented in the damaged region of their visual field, yet preserve the ability to detect stimuli presented there. Patients with Type II blindsight report a faint conscious perception of stimuli in the damaged region of their visual field, yet preserve the ability to detect stimuli with higher precision than their conscious perception.

Epidemiology

Blindsight results from brain damage to the primary visual cortex (V1) located in the posterior region of the occipital cortex, typically caused by a tumor, a hemorrhage, or some sort of brain trauma.

Natural History, Prognostic Factors, and Outcomes

The first cases of blindsight were observed in war veterans with damage to their occipital lobe (Pöppel et al. 1973). These veterans had no conscious perception of stimuli in the damaged portion of their visual field yet were able to track a moving light presented there. The most extensive experimental work in this area was completed with patient DB, who was diagnosed in the 1970s. DB's case is extensively reviewed in the seminal book on blindsight (Weiskrantz 1986).

Neuropsychology and Psychology of. . . (Syndrome/Illness)

The area of impaired vision in the visual field of a blindsight patient is referred to as a scotoma – defined as an island of visual loss surrounded by an area of normal visual acuity (Fig. 1). It is important to note that the visual impairment manifests in the region of the visual field contralateral to the hemisphere where the brain injury has occurred. For example, damage to the left hemisphere of V1 results in impairment to the right visual field. Typically, because early visual brain areas are retinotopically mapped, the extent of the damage to the occipital lobe corresponds to the extent of the impairment in the visual field. For example, if an entire hemisphere's occipital lobe is ablated, then the entire contralateral visual field is damaged – such a condition is termed hemianopia. Likewise, if a quarter of V1 is damaged (i.e., one half of one hemisphere's occipital lobe), a quarter of the contralateral visual field is damaged – such a condition is termed quadranopia. Figure 2 illustrates the pattern of

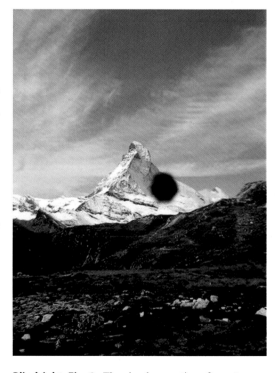

Blindsight, Fig. 1 The visual perception of a scotoma

B

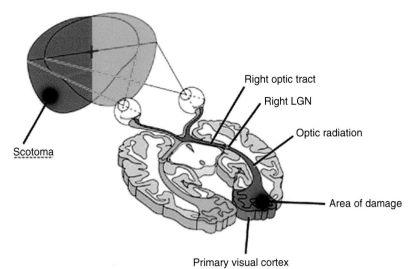

Blindsight, Fig. 2 The relationship between a region of damage in the visual cortex (V1) and the corresponding impairment in the visual field (Adapted from Bear et al. 2006)

Right optic tract

Right LGN

Optic radiation

Scotoma

Area of damage

Primary visual cortex

visual impairment and the corresponding scotoma that arises when only a small region of the occipital lobe is damaged. Although a patient with such a pattern of sparing and loss might experience blindsight in such a restricted scotoma, the most interesting cases of blindsight have been where patients have lost *all* conscious visual experience, that is, there is injury covering early visual brain areas across both hemispheres.

Note that not all patients with scotomas experience blindsight. The functional definition is that despite an absence of conscious perception, patients with blindsight retain the ability to detect and discriminate stimuli presented in their scotoma. For example, patients can localize moving and stationary stimuli using saccades or pointing. They can also discriminate line orientations, detect motion, and recent evidence suggests some patients can even differentiate between different wavelengths of color and form presented simultaneously in their scotoma (Trevethan et al. 2007). Primate studies support the claim that this unconscious perception is not subserved by islands of undamaged tissue. When the striate cortex of primates is cortically ablated, like humans, they have no conscious perception of stimuli presented in their scotoma, but do retain unconscious perception. The strongest neural evidence supporting the existence of blindsight comes from the identification of subcortical connections from the lateral geniculate nucleus

(LGN) directly to the extrastriate cortex. These pathways, unaffected by V1 damage, are potential mediators for the unconscious visual perception observed in blindsight. The identification of this pathway has prompted a fascinating debate regarding the role of V1 in the neural representation of consciousness. Scientists have posited that if there is perception, but not conscious perception, without V1, then V1 must play a critical role as a neural correlate of consciousness; this remains an active area of research (for review see Tong 2003).

Evaluation

Because blindsight patients experience no conscious awareness of stimuli presented in their scotoma, experimenters rely on a two-alternative forced choice (2AFC) procedure to diagnose and evaluate the symptoms of the disorder. The 2AFC procedure, typically used to assess behavioral performance in nonspeaking primates, presents patients with a target stimulus, a probe stimulus (matched to target), and a distractor stimulus (nonmatched to target); the target can be presented either prior to or simultaneously with the paired probe and distractor. The patient must select either the probe or the distractor as matching the target. The patient is not allowed to respond, "I don't know," so in this way the task is a forced-choice. In a variant of this procedure used to assess blindsight, experimenters present an image both to the scotoma and the hemisphere of normal visual acuity then ask subjects to report whether the two stimuli are the same or different (Weiskrantz 1986). Given that chance performance in these procedures is 50%, it is interesting to note that patients estimate their success rate on these tasks to be roughly 50%, but in reality their success rate is closer to 90%, illustrating the disconnect between conscious and unconscious vision in blindsight. Similar results have been observed using a somewhat different procedure designed to measure the unconscious perception of visual motion in blindsight patients: saccades tracking or pointing in which a moving object is presented within the visual field of the scotoma and the patient is asked to track the object with their eyes or with their finger.

Treatment

There is a period of spontaneous recovery for neurovisual lesions, typically up to 3 months post-lesion, but has been reported to extend to up to a year. Following this period, active discrimination of stimuli presented in the scotoma seems to be the best strategy for improvement in humans (Sahraie et al. 2006) and nonhuman primates (Dineen and Keating 1981). As such, blindsight patients that participate as experimental subjects sometimes show large improvements in their visual discrimination abilities. For example, patient DB, the first blindsight patient studied extensively (Weiskrantz 1986), was recently retested, 30 years after his right striate cortex was surgically removed during the treatment of a nonmalignant venous tumor. Patient DB can now discriminate complex circular forms presented in his scotoma, for example, he can discriminate a circle from an oval. Previously the ability to distinguish form was accounted for by DB's ability to distinguish line orientations; however, this explanation cannot account for now-present circular form discrimination (Trevethan et al. 2007). One possibility is that

DB's improvement in form perception is the result of the large number of hours DB spent completing experimental testing.

One point to consider when diagnosing or treating patients with blindsight is that Type I patients have *no* conscious access to the stimuli presented in the scotoma. Consequently, experimenters should be cautious in asking for specific answers when running a 2AFC task in that this task may be distressing to a patient who experiences no conscious visual perception. That is, they may find such a task irrelevant to their personal experience.

Cross-References

▶ Cortical Blindness
▶ Hemianopia
▶ Scotoma
▶ Visual Field Deficit

References and Readings

Bear, M. A., Connors, B. W., & Paradiso, M. A. (2006). *Neuroscience exploring the brain*. Baltimore: Lippincott Williams & Wilkins.

Dineen, J., & Keating, E. G. (1981). The primate visual system after bilateral removal of striate cortex. Survival of complex pattern vision. *Experimental Brain Research. Experimentelle Hirnforschung. Expérimentation Cérébrale, 41*(3–4), 338–345.

Pöppel, E., Held, R., & Frost, D. (1973). Residual visual function after brain wounds involving the central visual pathways in man. *Letters to Nature, 243*, 295–296.

Sahraie, A., Trevethan, C. T., MacLeod, M. J., Murray, A. D., Olson, J. A., & Weiskrantz, L. (2006). Increased sensitivity after repeated stimulation of residual spatial channels in blindsight. *Proceedings of the National Academy of Sciences of the United States of America, 103*(40), 14971–14976.

Tong, F. (2003). Primary visual cortex and visual awareness. *Nature Reviews Neuroscience, 4*(3), 219–229.

Trevethan, C. T., Sahraie, A., & Weiskrantz, L. (2007). Can blindsight be superior to 'sighted-sight'? *Cognition, 103*(3), 491–501.

Weiskrantz, L. (1986). *Blindsight: A case study and its implications*. Net Library, USA: Oxford University Press.

Werner, J. S., & Chalupa, L. M. (2004). *The visual neurosciences*. Cambridge, MA: MIT Press.

Block Design

Brianne Magouirk Bettcher[1,2], David J. Libon[3], Edith Kaplan[4], Rod Swenson[5] and Dana L. Penney[6]
[1]Department of Neurosurgery and Neurology, University of Colorado School of Medicine, Denver, CO, USA
[2]Rocky Mountain Alzheimer's Disease Center, Aurora, CO, USA
[3]Departments of Geriatrics, Gerontology, and Psychology, Rowan University, New Jersey Institute for Successful Aging, School of Osteopathic Medicine, Stratford, NJ, USA
[4]Department of Psychology, Suffolk University, Boston, MA, USA
[5]Department of Psychiatry and Behavioral Science, University of North Dakota School of Medicine, Fargo, ND, USA
[6]Department of Neurology, The Lahey Clinic, Burlington, MA, USA

Synonyms

Kohs blocks

Description

The block design (BD) test is a subtest from the Wechsler corpus of intelligence tests that requires the examinee to use three-dimensional blocks to construct a model from a two-dimensional stimulus card. Blocks consist of sides that are all white, all red, or diagonally half red and white. Performance is timed. Although bonus points are awarded for speed, the score is either all or none, that is, a score is awarded only if the model is correctly produced within the prescribed time limit.

Edith Kaplan: deceased.

Historical Background

Hutt (1925) notes that the first documented use of block construction as a psychological test was by Francis N. Maxfield, working at the University of Pennsylvania Psychology Laboratory and Clinic, who devised a "color cube" test to study "imageability in children." The procedures devised by Maxfield were also used by Clara Town (1921, cited in Hutt 1925). Both of these researchers were interested in studying analytic problem-solving strategies in children. However, it was Samuel Calmin Kohs (1916–1960) who derived the block design (BD) test that was ultimately adapted by David Wechsler. It appears that Maxfield, Town, and Kohs used the same commercially available blocks, that is, all blocks were constructed with four colors – red, white, blue, and yellow. Kohs' procedure differed from Maxfield and Town in that he asked children to use blocks to copy two-dimensional designs printed on stimulus cards rather than from models constructed by the examiner using identical blocks, a method adopted by Wechsler. Kohs (1920), 1923) specifically used block construction as a means to assess intelligence. Consistent with the prevailing views of the day, Kohs viewed intelligence as a unitary or global construct. The Kohs BD test consisted of a series of 17 designs (culled from a corpus of 35 original designs). Kohs (1920), 1923) clearly viewed his test as equal to the existing Binet scales in measuring general intellectual ability. He also viewed the "performance" (Kohs 1920) or nonverbal nature of his test as a means to assess intelligence in children where it was either not possible or problematic to use language or language-related tests. As adopted by Wechsler later, Kohs awarded bonus points for speed. Interestingly, a separate scoring system was also derived to measure "moves" or "each separate and distinct change in the position of the block" (Kohs 1920). All these early researchers readily acknowledged the multidimensional aspect of their block construction procedures and commented on the qualitative features of children's block construction strategies.

Psychometric Data

Successful completion of the BD test requires a host of cognitive abilities (Kramer et al. 1991) including specific analytic and synthetic problem-solving strategies (Schorr et al. 1982). *Analytic strategies* refer to mental segmentation of the stimulus design into individual blocks. After mentally dividing the blocks into segments, blocks are subsequently arranged to match each unit. This strategy might capitalize on the presence of perceptual edge cues and implicit grid information when constructing the design (Kaplan 1988; Kaplan et al. 1991). *Synthetic strategies* emphasize the design as a whole and may not rely on segmentation for test completion. Examinees who utilize this strategy focus primarily on the gestalt or overall form of the design. Specific BD test items tend to "pull" for one strategy versus the other. However, overreliance on either problem-solving approach will ultimately lower an examinee's test score and could be highly suggestive of either focal or lateralized neurological insult.

The BD test is often viewed as a measure of the so-called *constructional apraxia* (Kleist, 1923, cited in Benton and Tranel 1993) and has been naively associated with right parietal brain damage (Kaplan 1988). Clear evidence of the multi-dimensional cognitive skills necessary for optimal performance on the BD test comes from two sources: patients with cerebral disconnection (Geschwind 1979; Kaplan 1988) and patients with focal brain lesions. For example, patients who have undergone a commissurotomy (Geschwind 1979; Kaplan 1988) provided a unique opportunity to study BD problem-solving strategies because these patients serve as their own controls. Since these patients have undergone resection of the corpus callosum and the anterior commissure, sensory information cannot be transferred between the hemispheres. Illustrations provided by Geschwind (1979) and Kaplan (1988) show that when commissurotomized patients use their right hand, that is, when BD constructions are guided by the left hemisphere with no input from the right hemisphere, the inherent 2×2 or 3×3 matrix is violated, and there is a tendency for blocks to pile up on the right side of the design reflecting an inattention of left hemi-space suggestive right hemisphere dysfunction (Kaplan 1988, Figures 1–2). Very different errors occur with commissurotomized patients attempting BD using their left hand, that is, when constructions are guided by the right hemisphere with no input from the left hemisphere. Now, the 2×2 or 3×3 grid matrix is rarely violated. However, blocks tend to be rotated so that the internal details of individual blocks do not match the model. Thus, Geschwind (1979) and Kaplan (1988) show that regardless of which hand is used, commissurotomized patients produce zero point responses, but the underlying brain-behavior relationships responsible for these response strategies are very different. Kaplan et al. (1981) noted that similar behavior occurs in patients with focal right and left hemisphere lesions. Patients with right-sided lesions often break the 2×2 or 3×3 matrix inherent in the stimulus resulting in highly distorted responses, blocks continue to collect on the right side of hemi-space, and constructions are often initiated on the right side with patients working from right to left. Patients with left-sided lesions respect the inherent grid configuration of the BD stimuli. These patients often make single-block, rotational errors or misalign internal details (Kaplan et al. 1991) with responses initiated on the left side of hemi-space.

Clinical Uses

Kaplan and colleagues (Kaplan 1988; Kaplan et al. 1991) have suggested a number of additional testing and scoring procedures to extract detailed information from the BD test performance. These are listed below and are part of the WAIS-R-NI corpus (Kaplan et al. 1991).

1. *Providing Additional Blocks*: Rather than constraining the examinee's performance by providing only four or nine blocks as prescribed by the Wechsler test manual, Kaplan et al. (1991) suggests presenting the patient with nine blocks on all four-block test items and 12 blocks on all nine-block test items. Attempting to construct designs with too few

or too many blocks conveys additional information about possible spatial as well as executive impairment.

2. *Flow Charting*: Documenting the patient's performance with a flow chart is mandatory to the cogent analysis of BD test performance. Examples of the rich data which can be obtained with a flow chart are illustrated by Kaplan et al. (1991, Figure 6). As described above, focal right-hemisphere lesioned patients tend to break the 2 × 2 or 3 × 3 grid configuration of the stimulus matrix and often produce distorted responses. Kaplan et al. (1991) provides examples of BD constructions produced by right-anterior and right-posterior lesioned patients in Figures 6c and 6d, respectively (see p. 90). The 3 × 3 grid configuration is broken by both patients. However, the construction of a patient with a right-posterior lesion is measurably more distorted than the construction produced by a right-anterior lesioned patient suggesting greater perceptual-spatial impairment. Thus, as suggested many years ago by Kohs (1920, 1923), an analysis of BD "moves" provides important information.

3. *Errors Subtypes*: The WAIS-R-NI (Kaplan et al. 1991) suggests a variety of error scores that supplement the traditional total Wechsler scale score. The scoring techniques described below are designed to supplement standardized scoring procedures and help in identifying underlying brain pathology.

   1. **Rotational errors**: Scored when a block's surface coloring is incorrect. This type of internal detail error could be associated with a left hemisphere lesion.
   2. **Broken configuration**: Scored when the 2 × 2 or 3 × 3 grid matrix of the design is violated. As noted above, such errors are often seen in patients with right hemisphere lesions.

While rotational and broken configuration errors often occur in patients with circumscribed stroke, patients with epilepsy (Zip-Williams et al. 2000) or brain injury (Wilde et al. 2000) lateralized to one side of the brain may also make these errors.

1. **Orientation errors**: Scored when a block(s) is incorrectly oriented, that is, when the final product or elements of the final product are shifted or misoriented about 30° in relation to the model. Spatial, perceptual, or executive problems might underlie this difficulty.
2. **Perseverations**: Scored when incorrect block placements persist either within or between successive BD trials. Gross perseverative behavior is often seen in patients with frontal lobe or frontal systems lesions. Less severe perseverative behavior might occur in conjunction with rotational and broken configuration errors and may suggest dysexecutive behavior associated with a specific brain region.
3. **Stimulus bound**: Examples include instances when the examinee is drawn to build their construction either right next to or under the stimulus booklet or even pile blocks on top of the stimulus booklet. Less egregious but no less important stimulus-bound errors occur when patients are aware of but unable to self-correct errors.
4. **Response latency**: Patients with bradyphrenia may ultimately produce a correct construction and might be able to self-correct errors but may complete a correct design only after the time limit as prescribed in the test manual has passed. Such behavior might be associated with subcortical syndromes. However, slow time to completion often occurs in patients with alcohol abuse, brain injury, multiple sclerosis, or epilepsy.
5. **Start position**: Using a flow chart, documenting the start position of the first block also allows for examination of a "preferred" side and can be indicative of lateralized brain dysfunction (Akshoomoff-Haist et al. 1989).

Block Design Use with Additional Populations

Healthy and Pathological Aging

An observed pattern of developmental cognitive change associated with age is the relative stability of verbal abilities coupled with a significant diminution in visuospatial and constructional abilities. Evidence suggests that the BD test differentiates between younger and older adults (Kaufman 1990; Troyer et al. 1994), but the specific cognitive functions that underlie this behavior have been debated. Joy et al. (2001) provided a comprehensive evaluation of the reported age-related decline in BD test performance and offered normative data for the clinical interpretation of BD in healthy older adults. In addition to standard pass-fail scoring, these researchers also utilized proportional scoring methods as well as the supplemental measures detailed in the WAIS-R-NI. Results confirmed a moderate negative correlation between standard BD score and age ($r = 0.455$); however, the use of proportion scores, elimination of time constraints, and termination of time bonuses significantly reduced the documented age differences. These authors interpreted this finding as evidence for less severe age-related impairment in visuospatial and constructional abilities in healthy older adults than traditional scoring techniques suggest. In general, it is important to carefully consider the role of psychomotor slowing and error types when administering the standard block design test to healthy older adults in order to avoid differently penalizing individuals based on age. Older adults diagnosed with a neurodegenerative disorder exhibit different patterns of errors depending upon their neuropsychological profile and diagnosis. Stimulus-bound errors, broken configurations, and psychomotor slowing are all more prevalent in individuals diagnosed with a dementia relative healthy older adult controls.

Cross-References

▶ Constructional Apraxia

References and Readings

Akshoomoff-Haist, N. A., Delis, D. C., & Kiefner, M. G. (1989). Block constructions of chronic alcoholic and unilateral brain-damaged patients: A test of the right hemisphere vulnerability hypothesis of alcoholism. *Archives of Clinical Neuropsychology, 4*, 275–281.

Benton, A., & Tranel, A. (1993). Visuoperceptual, Visuospatial, and Visuoconstructional Disorders. In K. M. Heilman & E. Valenstein (Eds.), *Clinical neuropsychology* (3rd ed.). New York: Oxford University Press.

Caplan, B., & Caffery, D. (1992). Fractionating block design: Development of a test of visuospatial analysis. *Neuropsychology, 6*, 385–394.

Geschwind, N. (1979). Specializations in the human brain. *Scientific American, 241*, 180–199.

Hutt, R. B. W. (1925). Standardization of a color cube test. *The Psychological Clinic, 16*, 77–97.

Joy, S., Fein, D., Kaplan, E., & Freedman, M. (2001). Quantifying qualitative features of block design performance among healthy older adults. *Archives of Clinical Neuropsychology, 16*, 157–170.

Kaplan, E. (1988). A process approach to neuropsychological assessment. In T. Boll & B. R. Bryant (Eds.), *Clinical neuropsychology and brain function: Research. Measurement, and practice: Master lectures.* Washington, DC: The American Psychological Association.

Kaplan, E., Palmer, E. P., Weinstein, C., & Baker, E. (1981). *Block design: A brain-behavior based analysis.* Paper presented at the annual European meeting of the International Neuropsychological Society, Bergen, Norway.

Kaplan, E., Fein, D., Morris, R., & Delis, D. (1991). *The WAIS-R as a neuropsychological instrument.* San Antonio: The Psychological Corporation.

Kaufman, A. S. (1990). *Assessing adolescent and adult intelligence.* Boston: Allyn & Bacon.

Kohs, S. C. (1920). The block design tests. *Journal of Experimental Psychology, 3*, 357–376.

Kohs, S. C. (1923). *Intelligence measurement.* New York: Macmillan.

Kramer, J. H., Kaplan, E., Blusewicz, M. J., & Preston, K. A. (1991). Visual hierarchical analysis of block design configural errors. *Journal of Clinical and Experimental Neuropsychology, 13*, 455–465.

Lezak, M., Howison, D. B., & Loring, D. W. (2004). *Neuropsychological assessment* (4th ed.). New York: Oxford University Press.

Schorr, D., Bower, G. H., & Kiernan, R. (1982). Stimulus variables in the block design task. *Journal of Consulting and Clinical Psychology, 50*, 479–487.

Troyer, A. K., Cullum, C. M., Smernoff, E. N., & Kozora, E. (1994). Age effects on block design: Qualitative performance features and extended-time effects. *Neuropsychology, 8*, 95–99.

Wilde, M. C., Boake, C., & Sherer, M. (2000). Wechsler adult intelligence scale-revised block design broker configuration errors in non-penetrating traumatic brain injury. *Applied Neuropsychology, 7*, 208–214.

Zip-Williams, E. M., Shear, P. K., Strongin, D., et al. (2000). Qualitative block design performance in epilepsy patients. *Archives of Clinical Neuropsychology, 15*, 149–157.

Blood Alcohol Level

Ross Zafonte[1], Brad Kurowski[2] and
Nathan D. Zasler[3]
[1]Department of Physical Medicine and
Rehabilitation, Spaulding Rehabilitation
Hospital, Massachusetts General Hospital,
Brigham and Women's Hospital, Harvard
Medical School, Boston, MA, USA
[2]Department of Physical Medicine and
Rehabilitation, Spaulding Rehabilitation
Hospital, Massachusetts General Hospital,
Brigham and Women's Hospital, Harvard
Medical School, Cincinnati, OH, USA
[3]Concussion Care Centre of Virginia, Ltd.,
Richmond, VA, USA

Synonyms

Blood alcohol concentration; Blood alcohol content

Definition

Measure of alcohol in the blood.

Current Knowledge

Blood alcohol level (BAL) is typically expressed as milligrams or grams of ethanol per deciliter (e.g., 100 mg/dL or 0.10 g/dL). A level of 20–30 mg/dL typically results from the ingestion of one to two drinks. One drink corresponds to 340 mL (12 oz.) of beer, 115 mL (4 oz) of wine, and 43 mL (1.5 oz) of a shot. Blood alcohol levels as low as 20–80 mg/dL can lead to decreased inhibitions and decreased cognitive and motor performance, while levels of 300–400 mg/dL can lead to coma or death. Blood alcohol levels typically correlate inversely with cognitive and motor performance (i.e., as blood alcohol levels increase, cognitive and motor performance decrease). Specifically, increased blood alcohol levels correlate with slower reaction time and inversely correlate with frontal executive

function. The tendency to underestimate one's own blood alcohol level seems to pose an additional risk of impairment and injury risk. Additionally, speed of cognitive performance recovers as alcohol is metabolized and BAL decrease; however, accuracy may continue to remain impaired.

Cross-References

► Coma
► Executive Functioning
► Frontal Lobe

References and Readings

Domingues, S. C., Mendonca, J. B., Laranjeira, R., & Nakamura-Palacios, E. M. (2009). Drinking and driving: A decrease in executive frontal functions in young drivers with high alcohol concentration. *Alcohol, 43*(8), 657–664.

Harrison's Online – *Harrison's principles of internal medicine* (16th edn.). Chapter 372: Alcohol and alcoholism.

Laude, J. R., & Filmore, M. (2016). Drivers who self-estimate lower blood alcohol concentrations are riskier drivers after drinking. *Psychopharmacology (Berl), 233*(8), 1387–1394. https://doi.org/10.1007/s00213-016-4233-x.

Schweizer, T. A., & Vogel-Sprott, M. (2008). Alcohol-impaired speed and accuracy of cognitive functions: A review of acute tolerance and recover of cognitive performance. *Experimental and Clinical Psychopharmacology, 16*(3), 340–350.

Blood Flow Studies

Cindy B. Ivanhoe[1] and Ana Durand Sanchez[2]
[1]Neurorehabilitation Specialists Baylor College of Medicine, The Institute for Rehabilitation and Research, Houston, TX, USA
[2]Physical Medicine and Rehabilitation, Baylor College of Medicine, Houston, TX, USA

Synonyms

Duplex/Doppler ultrasound (US); Vascular ultrasound

Definition

A blood flow study is a noninvasive imaging technique which is used to measure blood flow and pressure through arteries and veins, as well as chambers and valves of the heart. Doppler ultrasound (US) may be used to diagnose vascular conditions such as cerebral vasospasm, cerebral or limb thrombosis, vascular stenosis, valvular heart disease, and peripheral vascular and aneurysmal disease. It may also be used to evaluate the condition of bypass grafts and blood flow to transplanted organs.

Current Knowledge

Blood flow studies are used most often to study blood flow particularly in the legs, neck, and brain. Blood flow studies such as Doppler US uses a transducer that sends high-frequency sound waves which bounce off of solid objects including red blood cells. The sound waves are reflected back to the transducer. Moving objects, such as the red blood cells, cause a change in pitch of the sound waves (also known as the "Doppler effect"). These reflected waves are sent to and processed by a computer which translates the waves into pictures or graphs. The images are representative of the flow of blood through the vessel.

There are different types of Doppler US studies currently being utilized by physicians. Continuous wave Doppler is typically used at the bedside and only produces sound from the transducer which the practitioner uses to listen for blockage or stenosis of the vessel – usually a superficial one. Duplex Doppler produces both a picture of the blood vessel and a graph representing the speed and direction of blood flow (hence the name "duplex"). Color Doppler uses a computer to convert the Doppler sounds into colors and overlay those colors on an image of the blood vessel. Power Doppler is more sensitive than color Doppler in detecting blood flow. It combines the results given by color Doppler with those of duplex Doppler. It is commonly used to evaluate

the flow of blood through vessels within solid organs.

Transcranial Doppler (TCD) is used to measure blood flow through the brain's blood vessels. It is becoming more widely used to evaluate for emboli, stenosis, vasospasm, and the risk of stroke.

Limitations to studies include obesity, cardiac arrhythmias, heart disease, and smoking within an hour of study. Studies are done in the inpatient and outpatient settings monitoring.

Variations in blood flow can affect microvascular and macrovascular beds for a wide range of clinical situations. There are new expanding techniques to study blood flow but ultrasound remains the commonly used techniques in hospital an outpatient clinical settings.

See Also

▶ Cerebral Blood Flow
▶ Doppler Ultrasound
▶ Regional Cerebral Blood Flow
▶ Transcranial Doppler

References and Readings

Blaivas, M. (2007). Ultrasound in the detection of venous thromboembolism. *Critical Care Medicine, 35*(5), S224–S234.

Hamper, U. M., DeJong, M. R., & Scoutt, L. M. (2007). Ultrasound evaluation of the lower extremity veins. *Radiologic Clinics of North America, 45*(3), 525–547.

Roberts, D. R., & Forfia, P. R. (2011). Diagnosis and assessment of pulmonary vasculature disease by doppler echocardiography. *Pulmonary Circulation, 1*(2), 160–181.

Rubens, D. J., Bhatt, S., Nedelka, S., & Cullinan, J. (2006). Doppler artifacts and pitfalls. *Radiologic Clinics of North America, 44*(6), 805–835.

Webb, R. C., Ma, Y., Krishnan, L. Y., Yoon, S., et al. (2015). Epiderman devices for noninvasive, preise, and continuous mapping of macrovascular and microvascular blood flow. *Science Advances, 1*(9), 1–13.

Weber, T. M., Lockhart, M. E., & Robbin, M. L. (2007). Upper extremity venous Doppler ultrasound. *Radiologic Clinics of North America, 45*, 513–524.

Blood Oxygen Level Dependent (BOLD)

Alan Weintraub[1] and John Whyte[2]
[1]Craig Hospital, Rocky Mountain Regional Brain Injury System, Englewood, CO, USA
[2]Moss Rehabilitation Research Institute, Albert Einstein Healthcare Network, Elkins Park, PA, USA

Synonyms

BOLD

Definition

Blood–oxygen-level-dependent (BOLD) imaging is a technique used to generate images in functional MRI (fMRI) studies. The goal of this technique is to discern regional differences in cerebral blood flow in an effort to delineate more specific regional activity. This version of magnetic resonance imaging depends on the different magnetic properties of oxygenated versus deoxygenated hemoglobin and thus, indirectly, on variations in local tissue perfusion. The utility of BOLD imaging for functional magnetic resonance imaging (fMRI) also depends on the physiological phenomenon by which metabolically active cerebral tissue "demands" more perfusion than less-active tissue. Thus, populations of neurons that are particularly active during a cognitive or motor task actually elicit a relative surplus of perfusion, which, in turn, results in an increase in the ratio of oxygenated to deoxygenated hemoglobin, detectable as a change in the BOLD signal.

Historical Background

As early as 1890, Roy and Sherrington noted that regional cerebral blood flow increased in areas of neural activity. This increase in perfusion became detectable in vivo with the advent of positron emission tomography (PET), in which radioactive tracers are injected and their emitted radiation detected. It was not until the discovery of BOLD contrast in 1990 by Ogawa and colleagues at Bell Laboratories that it was possible to measure neuron-mediated changes in blood flow without radiation exposure. While fMRI relies on an evolving understanding of both the physiologic and biophysical origins of BOLD, this technique has become a powerful research modality in mapping brain activation in animals and humans.

Current Knowledge

Because of its dependence on the state of oxygenation of the blood, the BOLD signal is several steps removed from the typical phenomenon of interest: changes in neural activity. All measures of cerebral blood flow are indirect, in the sense that they can be influenced by cardiovascular factors (e.g., changes in cardiac output, vascular resistance) as well as changes in metabolic demand by neuronal and glial tissue. BOLD technique represents the relationship between oxygen delivery and oxygen extraction, rather than oxygen consumption itself – a more direct measure of tissue metabolic activity. The clinician and research scientist should appreciate the delay of several seconds between the changes in neural activity and changes in associated blood flow. Thus, BOLD imaging technique requires mathematical modeling of the "hemodynamic response function" (the increase and subsequent return to baseline of flow associated with a neural event). The derived BOLD signal should correlate to resting neuronal states or in response to specific behavioral and cognitive events that require neural processing. The hemodynamic response function can be modeled in a normative sense (i.e., the shape of the blood flow response in a "typical" organism) or in the individual subject.

Although the BOLD signal is not a direct measure of neuronal activity, its signal detected by fMRI reflects changes in deoxyhemoglobin derived from cerebral mediated changes in blood oxygenation and blood flow. This phenomenon appears to be closely linked to neuronal activity, a process referred to as neurovascular coupling. Research exploring the neurovascular coupling mechanisms and the BOLD signal are opportunities to more completely understand the underlying pathobiological mechanisms underlying brain development, disease states, and aging.

BOLD technique is also an important concept in resting state fMRI studies. These concepts offer a broader understanding of human brain connectivity and especially how it is influenced by a variety of disease states and its inherent underlying pathophysiologic mechanisms. In addition, BOLD imaging techniques and fMRI studies in human neuroscience most often make use of one of the two common experimental designs: blocked or event related (Fig. 1). In the blocked design, the subject is asked to perform a particular cognitive or motor task in blocks that alternate with other blocks of a contrasting task or rest. The BOLD signal is then statistically averaged

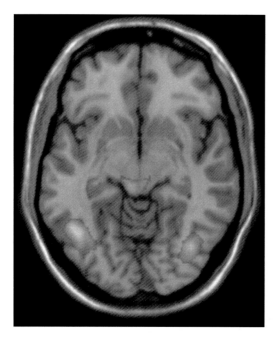

Blood Oxygen Level Dependent (BOLD), Fig. 1 Blood–oxygen-level dependent. This axial slice of the brain shows the areas of most significant BOLD activation across 18 control subjects, obtained while they attended to three randomly moving visual stimuli. Higher visual areas in the occipital cortices (motion areas V5/MT+) and superior colliculi show the greatest activation

across the two types of blocks, and a measure of the difference between them is mapped onto each voxel in the MR image, thus showing those areas of the brain that had the largest change in BOLD signal between the two conditions. A contrasting rest block is typically used when one is interested in the brain areas involved in all aspects of the task, although this method has been criticized because there is no standardization of the subject's mental activity during rest. Alternatively, if one is interested in the brain areas involved with a specific task process, one might alternate the experimental task with a control task that shares most but not all of the features of the experimental task. For example, if a research subject performs alternating blocks of finger tapping in response to a visual signal versus viewing the visual signal without tapping, areas involved in the perception of the visual signal will tend to be canceled out across conditions whereas neural networks specifically involved in the tapping response will be highlighted. In this way, a wide range of cognitive and motor tasks have been studied in normal subjects as a way of localizing the neural networks involved in their performance and in patient subjects, as a way of exploring how that localization may have been altered by pathology or recovery.

In event-related BOLD designs, experimental trials of different types can be delivered in a random sequence and averaged in a time-locked fashion. The timing between trials is sometimes "jittered" (i.e., randomly varied) so that even though the hemodynamic responses from individual trials overlap, their individual effects can be separately modeled (deconvolved), by incorporating the known temporal spacing between them.

More recently, the BOLD signal has been used to understand how activities in different parts of the brain are interrelated. Modern neuroscience posits the presence of distributed neural networks, rather than focal regions, supporting specific cognitive and motor processes. Since considerable distances may separate components of these neural networks, it is of interest to understand how they communicate with each other in the performance of specific cognitive activities. By assessing how strongly changes in the BOLD signal in different regions are correlated over time, one can derive a measure of "functional connectivity," assessed either at rest or during the performance of specific tasks. Measures of functional connectivity do not specify the actual anatomical connections between regions but merely demonstrate the degree to which their activity levels are linked over time.

With any of these experimental designs, the BOLD signal must also be mapped to an anatomical model of the brain. Modeling the signal separately in each voxel of the MRI image and then contrasting the signal in each voxel between the experimental conditions of interest do this. This may require additional manipulations, such as warping each subject's image to a standard template, "smoothing" the signal so that the activity in collections of voxels rather than individual voxels is highlighted, and deriving statistical maps that code the reliability of the change of interest across brain regions and individual subjects. Several forms of computer software are available for processing raw fMRI data into analyzable maps and statistical results.

Conclusions

Although BOLD and other fMRI techniques are extremely powerful research tools, they incorporate a large number of data transformations and assumptions between the raw signal acquisition and interpretations at the level of brain activity and behavior. A crucial perspective in interpreting BOLD and fMRI results must comprehensively consider BOLD's vascular and metabolic underpinnings. This understanding is important to analyze under both resting conditions and in disease states. As noted above, conclusions reached by these techniques can be undermined by alterations in the coupling between neural activity and blood flow, by failure to accurately understand the cognitive and motor processes required by the task and by invalid application of the many analytical and statistical methods that transform the measured BOLD signal into statistical maps of brain activity.

Cross-References

▶ Functional Imaging
▶ Magnetic Resonance Imaging

References and Readings

Barkhof, F., Haller, S., & Rombouts, S. A. (2014). Resting-state functional MR imaging: A new window to the brain. *Radiology, 272*(1), 29–49.

Hillman, E. M. (2014). Coupling mechanism and significance of the BOLD signal: A status report. *Annual Review of Neuroscience, 37*, 161–181.

Kida, I., & Hyder, F. (2006). Physiology of functional magnetic resonance imaging: Energetics and function. *Methods in Molecular Medicine, 124*, 175–195.

Kim, S. G., & Ogawa, S. (2012). Biophysical and physiological origins of blood oxygenation level-dependent fMRI signals. *Journal of Cerebral Blood Flow and Metabolism, 32*(7), 188–1206.

Lee, M. H., Smyser, C. D., & Shimony, J. S. (2013). Resting-state fMRI: A review of methods and clinical applications. *AJNR. American Journal of Neuroradiology, 34*(10), 1866–1872.

Mark, C. I., Mazerolle, E. L., & Chen, J. J. (2015). Metabolic and vascular origins of the BOLD effect: Implications for imaging pathology and resting-state brain function. *Journal of Magnetic Resonance Imaging, 42*(2), 231–246.

Veldsman, M., Cumming, T., & Brodtmann, A. (2015). Beyond BOLD: Optimizing functional imaging in stroke populations. *Human Brain Mapping, 36*(4), 1620–1636.

Yablonskiy, D. A., Sukstanskii, A. L., & He, X. (2013). Blood oxygenation level-dependent (BOLD)-based techniques for the quantification of brain hemodynamic and metabolic properties – Theoretical models and experimental approaches. *NMR in Biomedicine, 26*(8), 963–986.

Blood-Brain Barrier

Nam Tran
Neurosurgery, Virginia Commonwealth University Medical Center, Richmond, VA, USA

Synonyms

Cerebral microvasculature

Definition

The blood-brain barrier (BBB) maintains brain homeostasis by regulating the movement of compounds across the endothelium of cerebral capillaries.

Current Knowledge

BBB serves to maintain brain homeostasis by regulating the influx and efflux of compounds to and from the brain. The presence of a barrier was first documented by Paul Ehrlich in the late nineteenth century. However, it was not until the advent of the electron microscope that the makeup of the BBB was begun to be understood. The brain microvascular endothelium comprises the BBB. In contrast to endothelium from other vascular beds, the morphologic features unique to the brain microvascular endothelium, such as tight junctions, increased electrical resistance, and lack of pinocytic vesicles, provide limited and selective access to this highly specialized organ. Only lipophilic molecules less than 600 Da can passively diffuse through the BBB. This protects the brain from toxins, microorganisms (i.e., bacteria), and peripheral neurotransmitters. This selective barrier can potentially limit the entry of large substances required for normal brain function, including insulin, amino acids, and glucose. In order to circumvent this problem, the BBB has developed highly specialized transport mechanisms on both the luminal and abluminal membrane surfaces, such as Na-K-Cl cotransporter, γ-glutamyl transpeptidase (GGTP), and the GLUT-1 glucose transporter. The protective BBB can be at a disadvantage in that it prevents the entry of pharmacologic agents that are often hydrophilic.

Also unique to the brain microvascular endothelium is their intimate association with astrocytes, forming the glia limitans. Astrocytes are thought to participate in the induction and maintenance of the endothelial BBB phenotype. In vitro studies have shown that astrocytes cocultured with endothelial cells can induce BBB phenotypic features, including tight junctions and increased electrical resistance. Astrocytic membranes and supernatant from astrocytic cultures share similar inductive properties. The mechanisms of this induction and the inductive factor(s) have yet to be fully elucidated.

In addition to its regulatory role, studies of the BBB are beginning to emerge to demonstrate its function in establishing a unique brain milieu. In vitro BBB models have shown decreased tissue plasminogen activator and then anticoagulant protein thrombomodulin expression and increased plasminogen activator inhibitor-1 expression by the brain endothelium compared with the endothelium from the periphery. These findings suggest a procoagulant environment in the brain that may predispose the brain to strokes.

Cross-References

▶ Neuroglia

Body Dysmorphic Disorder

Amma A. Agyemang
Department of Physical Medicine and
Rehabilitation, Virginia Commonwealth
University Medical Center, Richmond, VA, USA

Synonyms

Dysmorphia

Definition

Previously known a dysmorphia, body dysmorphic disorder (BDD) is an obsessive-compulsive disorder (OCD)-related condition characterized by a preoccupation with one or more perceived defects or flaws in one's physical appearance that are not observable or appear slight to others. The disorder is manifested through repetitive behaviors such as excessive grooming, skin picking, or mental acts such as comparing one's appearance to others, in efforts to assuage appearance concerns. Muscle dysmorphia is a subtype of BDD, in which there is a preoccupation with one's body build being too small or insufficiently muscular.

Categorization

The disorder is classified with the obsessive-compulsive and related disorders in the *Diagnostic and Statistical Manual of Mental Disorders* (5th ed.; DSM-5; American Psychiatric Association 2013).

Current Knowledge

Epidemiology
National prevalence rates of BDD range from 1.7% to 2.4%, with higher rates in outpatient (1–8-6.7%) and inpatient (13.1–16%) clinical samples, as well as in patients seeking cosmetic surgery and dermatologic treatments (7.7–24.5%). Risk factors for BDD include childhood neglect and abuse and a family history of OCD. The mean age of onset is 16–17 years and most individuals develop symptoms by age 18. Nevertheless, BDD does occur among the elderly as well, though much less is known about the nature of the disorder in this segment of the population.

Etiology and Clinical Issues
The etiology of BDD is complex, encompassing biological, psychological, and socioenvironmental factors. Biological factors that have been implicated include hyperactivity in the left orbitofrontal cortex and volume abnormalities in the orbitofrontal cortex and anterior cingulate cortex. Additionally, maladaptive beliefs and cognitive biases about physical appearance, reinforced through life experiences, likely play a role. Compared to obsessive-compulsive disorder, BDD tends to be associated with higher suicidal ideation,

greater psychiatric comorbidity, and poorer insight. Associated/comorbid conditions include major depressive disorder, social anxiety disorder, and substance-related disorders.

Assessment and Treatment
With regard to assessment, the primary rule out is eating disorders, however, BDD must also be differentiated from other OCD-related disorders, illness anxiety, depressive and anxiety disorders, and psychotic disorders. It is recommended that patients receiving mental health treatment be screened for BDD, by asking whether individuals are worried or unhappy with their appearance and through use of standardized measures such as the Yale-Brown Obsessive-Compulsive Scale. Effective pharmacologic interventions include serotonin reuptake inhibitors such as escitalopram and fluoxetine. Psychotherapeutic interventions include BDD-specific cognitive-behavioral therapy (CBT). There is emerging evidence for the utility of internet-based CBT.

See Also

▶ Obsessive-Compulsive and Related Disorders

References and Readings

American Psychiatric Association. (2013). *Diagnostic and statistical manual of mental disorders (DSM-5 ®)*. Washington, DC: American Psychiatric Association.

Enander, J., Andersson, E., Mataix-Cols, D., Lichtenstein, L., Alström, K., Andersson, G., ... & Rück, C. (2016). Therapist guided internet based cognitive behavioural therapy for body dysmorphic disorder: Single blind randomised controlled trial. *BMJ, 352*, i241.

Fang, A., Matheny, N. L., & Wilhelm, S. (2014). Body dysmorphic disorder. *Psychiatric Clinics of North America, 37*(3), 287–300.

Harrison, A., de la Cruz, L. F., Enander, J., Radua, J., & Mataix-Cols, D. (2016). Cognitive-behavioral therapy for body dysmorphic disorder: A systematic review and meta-analysis of randomized controlled trials. *Clinical Psychology Review, 48*, 43–51.

Phillips, K. A., & Hollander, E. (2008). Treating body dysmorphic disorder with medication: Evidence, misconceptions, and a suggested approach. *Body Image, 5*(1), 13–27.

Phillips, K. A., Pinto, A., Menard, W., Eisen, J. L., Mancebo, M., & Rasmussen, S. A. (2007). Obsessive–compulsive disorder versus body dysmorphic disorder: A comparison study of two possibly related disorders. *Depression and Anxiety, 24*(6), 399–409.

Phillips, K. A., Keshaviah, A., Dougherty, D. D., Stout, R. L., Menard, W., & Wilhelm, S. (2016). Pharmacotherapy relapse prevention in body dysmorphic disorder: A double-blind, placebo-controlled trial. *American Journal of Psychiatry, 173*(9), 887–895.

Body Schema

John E. Mendoza
Department of Psychiatry and Neuroscience, Tulane Medical School and SE Louisiana Veterans Healthcare System, New Orleans, LA, USA

Synonyms

Somatognosis

Definition

General term for the personal awareness of one's body, including the location and orientation of its various parts and their relative motion in space and time, as well as its functional integrity.

Current Knowledge

Although usually taken for granted, to effectively carry out normal motor activities one needs to appreciate both the static and kinetic state of the body as a whole as well as its individual parts. This information is derived from a number of sensory feedback loops, including signals from receptors in the muscles, tendons, ligaments and the skin (proprioceptive, kinesthetic, and tactile information), the inner ear or vestibular sense (orientation, direction, and speed of movement of the head), and vision. Perhaps as a result of collective experiences with such discrete sensory input, it has been suggested that individuals eventually develop what might be considered a superordinate sense of one's own body, independent of its movement in space or time. This knowledge, at least to some extent, transcends one's own body and allows insights into bodies in general. Because awareness of body schema is such a fundamental operation of the central nervous system, it almost functions at a subliminal level. One is normally only aware of its operation when it becomes dysfunctional.

Disorders of body schema, known as *asomatognosias*, can take on various guises. Although relatively rare, *autotopagnosia* represents what might be considered the quintessential body schema disturbance. This deficit involves difficulties in identifying body parts and/or appreciating their relative relations to one another. Care should be taken to differentiate asomatognosia from unilateral neglect or anomia. In the former, the deficit is restricted to one side of the body; in the latter, difficulties with naming extend beyond just parts of the body. More commonly, autotopagnosia is restricted to difficulty identifying individual fingers, especially the middle three. The deficit is usually bilateral and will frequently involve not only difficulties with regard to the patient's own fingers, but also those of the examiner or pictorial representations of a hand. Deficits are often found whether tested visually or tactually and whether verbal or nonverbal (e.g., matching to a model) responses are required. Unilaterally expressed deficits in finger recognition using only tactile stimulation likely reflect a more basic somatosensory disturbance.

Right-left disorientation, the inability to reliably distinguish the right from the left sides of one's body in the absence of a more generalized aphasic disorder, is another commonly cited example of a disturbance of body schema. As with finger agnosia, difficulties extend beyond the patients themselves to include problems with extrapersonal right-left discriminations. *Anosognosia* and *anosodiaphoria* (a milder form of anosognosia), along with *unilateral neglect* or *hemi-inattention* are sometimes viewed as specialized forms of a body schema disorder. One major difference is that these latter syndromes are generally limited to one side of the body, whereas autotopagnosia, the more restricted finger agnosia, and right-left disorientation affect both sides of the body. The one notable exception to this rule is *Anton's syndrome*, a form of anosognosia in which the patient denies blindness where both right and left visual fields are involved. While there is some potential variability with regard to localizations of lesions, asomatognosia, when bilaterally expressed, is most commonly associated with lesions of the left parietal region, typically involving the inferior parietal lobule. Unilateral neglect or hemiinattention syndromes may occur following anterior or posterior lesions of either hemisphere, although they are most common following right posterior lesions. Anton's syndrome is typically associated with bilateral lesions involving the posterior cerebral arteries.

Cross-References

▶ Allesthesia
▶ Anosodiaphoria
▶ Anosognosia
▶ Autotopagnosia
▶ Cortical Blindness
▶ Finger Agnosia
▶ Hemiinattention
▶ Right Left Disorientation

References and Readings

Adair, J. C., Schwartz, R. L., & Barrett, A. (2003). Anosognosia. In K. M. Heilman & E. Valenstein (Eds.), *Clinical neuropsychology* (4th ed., pp. 185–214). New York: Oxford University Press.

Denburg, N. L., & Tranel, D. (2003). Acalculia and disturbances of body schema. In K. M. Heilman & E. Valenstein (Eds.), *Clinical neuropsychology* (4th ed., pp. 161–184). New York: Oxford University Press.

Goldenberg, G. (2003). Disorders of body perception and representation. In T. E. Feinberg & M. J. Farah (Eds.), *Behavioral neurology and neuropsychology* (2nd ed., pp. 285–294). New York: McGraw-Hill.

Prigatano, G. P., & Schacter, D. L. (Eds.). (1991). *Awareness of deficit after brain injury: Clinical and theoretical issues*. New York: Oxford University Press.

Borderline Personality Disorder

Cynthia Rolston
Department of PM&R, Virginia Commonwealth University-Medical College of Virginia, Richmond, VA, USA

Synonyms

Emotional intensity disorder

Definition

Borderline personality disorder (BPD) is characterized in the *Diagnostic and Statistical Manual of Mental Disorders* (DSM-5; American Psychiatric Association 2013) by pervasive instability in relationships, affect, and self-image, present in adulthood and across contexts. Criteria include frantic avoidance of real or imagined abandonment; impulsivity; self-harm, including self-injury and suicidal behavior; marked emotional reactivity with intense, disproportionate anger; persistent feelings of emptiness; and transient paranoid ideation or dissociation.

Categorization

BPD is classified with the cluster B personality disorders in DSM-5.

Current Knowledge

Prevalence

Rates of BPD are estimated at 1–5.9% in the community, with 75% female. Treatment settings have higher rates: about 6% in primary care, 10% in outpatient mental health clinics, and 20% in inpatient psychiatric programs. Increased risk for BPD is found in first-degree relatives, Native Americans, and Blacks (Tomko et al. 2014).

Diagnostic Considerations

Men with BPD may report greater symptom severity, separation anxiety, and body image concerns in childhood and odd thinking in adolescence (Goodman et al. 2013; Busch et al. 2016). Impulsivity diminishes, but affective reactivity persists with aging (Arens et al. 2013). Symptoms vary across cultures, with self-harm/suicidality more common in developed countries (Jani et al. 2016; Paris and Lis 2013).

Clinical Correlates

BPD has been proposed as a mood disorder, noting similar affective variability, impulsivity, and related limbic dysregulation to bipolar disorder (BD; Sjåstad et al. 2012; Perugi et al. 2013). While comorbidity is high, both BD and BPD exist primarily without the other (Zimmerman and Morgan 2013). Mood disorders, eating disorders, PTSD, ADHD, and other personality diagnoses are frequent comorbid conditions. Premature death, suicide, and significant physical injuries are not uncommon.

Physiology and Neuropsychology

In BPD, the hippocampus, anterior cingulate cortex, dorsolateral prefrontal cortex, and amygdala are implicated (Mak and Lam 2013; O'Neill and Frodl 2012; Ruocco et al. 2016). Prefrontal gray matter deficits may increase with age, while parieto-occipital deficits may be more pronounced in younger individuals (Kimmel et al. 2016). This population may also have atypical sensitivity to stress hormones, dysregulation of the oxytocinergic system, and atypical sleep patterns (Herpertz and Bertsch 2015; Winsper et al. 2016). Neurocognitive findings include increased selective attention to negative stimuli, difficulty with dichotomous thinking, emotional processing, and poor visuospatial working memory (Mak and Lam 2013; Winter et al. 2017; Thomsen et al. 2017).

Treatment

Dialectical behavior therapy (DBT) has been the most frequently studied model of psychotherapy, with mentalization-based therapy (MBT), schema-focused therapy (SFT), and Systems Training for Emotional Predictability and Problem-Solving (STEPPS) also frequently used. No treatment can boast a broad and sound evidence base, and replication studies are desperately needed (Stoffers et al. 2012).

No medication is currently approved for BPD, although common pharmacologic adjunctives may include mood stabilizers, antipsychotics, and antidepressants. When alcohol use disorder co-occurs, anticonvulsants and second-generation antipsychotics may be prescribed. Oxytocin yields some promise, with some studies showing reduced emotional reactivity, while others have found increased interpersonal anxiety and uncooperative behaviors (Amad et al. 2015).

See Also

▶ Personality Disorders

References and Readings

Amad, A., Thomas, P., & Perez-Rodriguez, M. M. (2015). Borderline personality disorder and oxytocin: Review of clinical trials and future directions. *Current Pharmaceutical Design, 21*(23), 3311–3316. doi:CPD-EPUB-68145 [pii].

American Psychiatric Association. (2013). *Diagnostic and statistical manual of mental disorders* (5th ed.). Arlington: American Psychiatric Association Publishing.

Arens, E. A., Stopsack, M., Spitzer, C., Appel, K., Dudeck, M., Volzke, H., ... Barnow, S. (2013). Borderline personality disorder in four different age groups: A cross-sectional study of community residents in Germany. *Journal of Personality Disorders, 27*(2), 196–207. 10.1521/pedi.2013.27.2.196

Busch, A. J., Balsis, S., Morey, L. C., & Oltmanns, T. F. (2016). Gender differences in borderline personality disorder features in an epidemiological sample of adults age 55–64: Self versus informant report. *Journal of Personality Disorders, 30*(3), 419–432. https://doi.org/10.1521/pedi_2015_29_202.

Goodman, M., Patel, U., Oakes, A., Matho, A., & Triebwasser, J. (2013). Developmental trajectories to male borderline personality disorder. *Journal of Personality Disorders, 27*(6), 764–782. https://doi.org/10.1521/pedi_2013_27_111.

Herpertz, S. C., & Bertsch, K. (2015). A new perspective on the pathophysiology of borderline personality disorder: A model of the role of oxytocin. *The American Journal of Psychiatry, 172*(9), 840–851. https://doi.org/10.1176/appi.ajp.2015.15020216.

Jani, S., Johnson, R. S., Banu, S., & Shah, A. (2016). Cross-cultural bias in the diagnosis of borderline personality disorder. *Bulletin of the Menninger Clinic, 80*(2), 146–165. https://doi.org/10.1521/bumc.2016.80.2.146.

Kimmel, C. L., Alhassoon, O. M., Wollman, S. C., Stern, M. J., Perez-Figueroa, A., Hall, M. G., ... Radua, J. (2016). Age-related parieto-occipital and other gray matter changes in borderline personality disorder: A meta-analysis of cortical and subcortical structures. *Psychiatry Research, 251*, 15–25. https://doi.org/10.1016/j.pscychresns.2016.04.005

Mak, A. D., & Lam, L. C. (2013). Neurocognitive profiles of people with borderline personality disorder. *Current Opinion in Psychiatry, 26*(1), 90–96. https://doi.org/10.1097/YCO.0b013e32835b57a9.

O'Neill, A., & Frodl, T. (2012). Brain structure and function in borderline personality disorder. *Brain Structure & Function, 217*(4), 767–782. https://doi.org/10.1007/s00429-012-0379-4.

Paris, J., & Lis, E. (2013). Can sociocultural and historical mechanisms influence the development of borderline personality disorder?. *Transcultural Psychiatry, 50*(1), 140–151.

Perugi, G., Angst, J., Azorin, J. M., Bowden, C., Vieta, E., Young, A. H., & BRIDGE Study Group. (2013). Is comorbid borderline personality disorder in patients with major depressive episode and bipolarity a developmental subtype? Findings from the international BRIDGE study. *Journal of Affective Disorders, 144*(1–2), 72–78. https://doi.org/10.1016/j.jad.2012.06.008.

Ruocco, A. C., Rodrigo, A. H., McMain, S. F., Page-Gould, E., Ayaz, H., & Links, P. S. (2016). Predicting treatment outcomes from prefrontal cortex activation for self-harming patients with borderline personality disorder: A preliminary study. *Frontiers in Human Neuroscience, 10*, 220. https://doi.org/10.3389/fnhum.2016.00220.

Sjåstad, H. N., Grawe, R. W., & Egeland, J. (2012). Affective disorders among patients with borderline personality disorder. *PLoS One, 7*(12), e50930. https://doi.org/10.1371/journal.pone.0050930 [doi].

Stoffers, J. M., Vollm, B. A., Rucker, G., Timmer, A., Huband, N., & Lieb, K. (2012). Psychological therapies for people with borderline personality disorder. *The Cochrane Database of Systematic Reviews, 8*, CD005652. https://doi.org/10.1002/14651858.CD005652.pub2.

Thomsen, M. S., Ruocco, A. C., Uliaszek, A. A., Mathiesen, B. B., & Simonsen, E. (2017). Changes in neurocognitive functioning after 6 months of mentalization-based treatment for borderline personality disorder. *Journal of Personality Disorders, 31*(3), 306–324.

Tomko, R. L., Trull, T. J., Wood, P. K., & Sher, K. J. (2014). Characteristics of borderline personality disorder in a community sample: Comorbidity, treatment utilization, and general functioning. *Journal of Personality Disorders, 28*(5), 734–750. https://doi.org/10.1521/pedi_2012_26_093.

Winsper, C., Tang, N. K., Marwaha, S., Lereya, S. T., Gibbs, M., Thompson, A., & Singh, S. P. (2016). The sleep phenotype of borderline personality disorder: A systematic review and meta-analysis. *Neuroscience and Biobehavioral Reviews, 73*, 48–67.

Winter, D., Niedtfeld, I., Schmitt, R., Bohus, M., Schmahl, C., & Herpertz, S. C. (2017). Neural correlates of distraction in borderline personality disorder before and after dialectical behavior therapy. *European Archives of Psychiatry and Clinical Neuroscience, 267*(1), 51–62. https://doi.org/10.1007/s00406-016-0689-2.

Zimmerman, M., & Morgan, T. A. (2013). The relationship between borderline personality disorder and bipolar disorder. *Dialogues in Clinical Neuroscience, 15*(2), 155–169.

Boston Diagnostic Aphasia Examination

Nancy Helm-Estabrooks
Department of Communication Disorders and Sciences, College of Health and Human Sciences, Western Carolina University, Cullowhee, NC, USA

Synonyms

BDAE

Description

Boston Diagnostic Aphasia Examination (3rd ed.) (BDAE-3) Authors: Harold Goodglass, Edith Kaplan, Barbara Barresi, 2001, Publisher: Pro-Ed, 8700 Shoal Creek Blvd, Austin, TX 78757–6897, http://www.proedinc.com. The complete BDAE-3 test kit includes stimulus cards, test booklets for Standard and Short forms, the 60-item Boston Naming Test with record booklets, a DVD, and a hardbound text that contains the test manual.

The Boston Diagnostic Aphasia Examination-3 (BDAE-3; Goodglass et al. 2001a) is a comprehensive, multiple subtests instrument for investigating a broad range of language impairments that are common consequences of brain damage. It is designed as a comprehensive measure of aphasia. The examination provides materials and procedures to evaluate five language-related sections and an additional section on praxis. The five language domains include conversational and expository speech, auditory comprehension, oral expression, reading, and writing. In addition to individual subtest scores, the test yields three broader measures: the Severity Rating Scale (a rating of the severity of observed language/speech disturbance), the Rating Scale Profile of Speech Characteristics (a rating of observed speech characteristics and of scores in two main language domains), and the Language Competency Index (a composite score of language performance on BDAE-3 subtests). The extended version includes a sixth section, "Praxis," which examines natural and conventional gestures, use of pretend objects, and bucco-facial and respiratory movements. The test manual is part of the text by Goodglass et al. (2001b). It provides suggestions for administering, scoring, and interpreting performance on subtests, as well as directions for plotting and interpreting patient profiles. Percentiles or standard scores can be derived for each subtest.

Administration

The 44-page test booklet provides instructions for test administration. The short form and extended form items are specified in the test booklet and are also presented in different typeface; the short form items are presented in bold typeface, and the extended form items appear in italics. The standard administration includes all of the bold short form items in addition to regular typeface items.

Historical Background

The BDAE is designed to meet three goals: to enable diagnosis of aphasia syndromes, to measure the breadth and severity of aphasic disturbance, and to provide a comprehensive assessment of language to guide therapy. Initially published by Goodglass and Kaplan in 1972, it

was revised in 1983 and again in 2001. Changes from the previous edition include the addition of abbreviated and expanded testing formats, incorporation of the Boston Naming Test, addition of a Language Competence Index, and clarification of scoring procedures and definitions. The revision also was designed to integrate recent advances in neurolinguistics research, including methods to assess narrative and discourse complexity, category-specific dissociations in lexical production/comprehension, syntax comprehension, and analysis of grapheme-phoneme conversion during reading. The ultimate goal for the authors in developing the test was clinical utility.

The BDAE-3 consists of more than 50 subtests that can be administered in three different formats: standard, short, and extended. The standard format most closely resembles earlier versions of the BDAE. The new short form of the test provides a brief assessment. The extended version offers a comprehensive neurolinguistic profile that includes evaluation of spontaneous narrative, processing of word categories, syntax comprehension, and reading/writing. The BDAE-3 allows both a quantitative and a qualitative evaluation of language. The examination is based on an assumption that the nature of the aphasic deficit is determined by (1) organization of language in the brain, (2) the location of the lesion causing the aphasia, and (3) interactions among parts of the language system.

The BDAE has been adapted and translated for use in many languages including Spanish, French, German, Italian, Dutch, Greek, Hindi, Finnish, Mandarin Chinese, Japanese, and Portuguese.

Psychometric Data

Norms

Standardization of the BDAE-3 is based on a population of individuals with aphasia (IwA) who were referred concurrently by field examiners working in inpatient, outpatient, and private practice settings. Means and standard deviations for the BDAE-3 subtests for IwA are provided in the test manual. The number of IwA administered the 50 subtests varies from a maximum of 85 to a low of 31. Means are also provided for 15 non-clinical individuals who, on average, failed less than one item per subtest. Rosselli et al. (1990) and Pineda et al. (2000) provide norms for the Spanish version of the BDAE-2 (Goodglass and Kaplan 1986) that is based on 156 healthy individuals living in Columbia, South America.

Reliability

Kuder-Richardson reliability coefficients for subtests reflect variability, ranging between <0.65 and <0.95 with about two-thirds of the coefficients reported in the manual (Goodglass et al. 2001a), ranging from 0.90 upwards. No stability coefficients for test-retest are provided. The authors state that test-retest reliability is difficult to attain with IwA. The current reliability coefficients demonstrate very good internal consistency in terms of what the items within the subtests are measuring (Goodglass et al. 2001b). For most subtests, correlations are very high between the short and standard forms (>0.90; Goodglass et al. 2001b). No reliability information is provided in the BDAE-3 manual regarding the Severity Rating Scale, Language Competency Index, praxis assessment, or Spatial-Quantitative Battery.

Validity

A correlation matrix was obtained for all the scores in the BDAE-3 battery, and the correlation coefficients 0.60 or greater are displayed in the manual (Goodglass et al. 2001a), with severity partialled out, showing intercorrelations between subtests for the standardization sample. Based on these, "a number of sharply defined clusters" are indicated by the authors (p. 16). Strauss et al. (2006), however, pointed out that the lack of data on the entire correlational matrix makes it "difficult to estimate convergent and discriminant validity within and across BDAE-3 clusters" (p. 896) especially given the fact that the more than 50 subtests were administered to just 31–85 subjects. Based on data for earlier versions of the

BDAE, Goodglass and Kaplan (1972) found a strong general language factor and factors covering spatial-quantitative-somatagnostic, articulation-grammatical fluency, auditory comprehension, and paraphasia domains. Goodglass and Kaplan (1983) described a second factor analysis using a sample of 242 adults with aphasia, concluding that auditory comprehension, repetition-recitation, reading, and writing were factors of equal importance. Similar findings in normal individuals were reported by Pineda et al. (2000) for the BDAE-2 Spanish version.

Correlations between earlier versions of the BDAE and other measures have been described. For example, the BDAE oral apraxia task has been correlated with other articulation tasks (Sussman et al. 1986); correlations for the auditory comprehension measure on the BDAE and the Token Test and with respective measures of the Porch Index of Communicative Ability (PICA) have been reported (Divenyl and Robinson 1989). Brookshire and Nicholas (1984) found the BDAE auditory comprehension subtest did not predict auditory paragraph comprehension of independent standardized material.

Goodglass and Kaplan designed the BDAE to assess various components of language function for the purpose of discriminating among different patterns of CNS lesions indicative of types of aphasia. Studies to date have not determined decision rules for the diagnosis of individual subtypes of aphasia (Crary et al. 1992; Reinvang and Graves 1975).

Ecological validity of the BDAE for predicting progress with aphasia therapy has been described by various authors (e.g., Davidoff and Katz 1985; Marshall and Neuburger 1994).

Clinical Uses

The BDAE is derived from samples of 85 adult individuals with stroke and 15 elderly nonclinical volunteers. Therefore, it is most useful when assessing adult populations with language impairments resulting from strokes, but it may be used effectively with persons who have sustained traumatic brain injury (e.g., Theodoros et al. 2008) and forms of dementia (e.g., Tsantali et al. 2013). The BDAE offers a comprehensive look at language function from a neuropsychological perspective. Complete administration of this battery requires approximately 90 min. The short form requires approximately 40–60 min. The BDAE is one of the most popular batteries for use by speech-language pathologists for evaluation of aphasia and other neurologic language impairments. In addition to its strength as a comprehensive assessment of language, the BDAE provides useful instructions for observing and recording specific types of error responses (e.g., paraphasia) found in individuals with aphasia, reflecting what has been termed the "Boston school" approach to aphasia classification. The detailed examination of conversational and expository speech is an important and unique aspect of the BDAE and is well described in the manual (Goodglass et al. 2001b).

BDAE results can be used to guide aphasia treatment programs (Helm-Estabrooks et al. 2014) and to measure the effects of treatment (Robey 1998).

Cross-References

▶ Anomic Aphasia
▶ Aphasia
▶ Boston Naming Test
▶ Broca's Aphasia
▶ Conduction Aphasia
▶ Praxis
▶ Wernicke's Aphasia

References and Readings

Brookshire, R. H., & Nicholas, L. E. (1984). Comprehension of directly and indirectly stated main ideas and details in discourse by brain-damaged and non-brain-damaged listeners. *Brain and Language, 21,* 21–36.

Crary, M. A., Wertz, R. T., & Deal, J. L. (1992). Classifying aphasias: Cluster analysis of western aphasia battery and Boston diagnostic aphasia examination. *Aphasiology, 6,* 29–36.

Davidoff, M., & Katz, R. (1985). Automated telephone therapy for improving comprehension in aphasic adults. *Cognitive Rehabilitation, 3,* 26–28.

Divenyl, P. L., & Robinson, A. J. (1989). Nonlinguistic auditory capabilities in aphasia. *Brain and Language, 37,* 290–326.

Goodglass, H., & Kaplan, E. (1972). *Boston diagnostic aphasia examination (BDAE).* Philadelphia: Lea & Febiger.

Goodglass, H., & Kaplan, E. (1983). *The assessment of aphasia and related disorders* (2nd ed.). Philadelphia: Lea & Febiger.

Goodglass, H., & Kaplan, E. (1986). *La evaluacion de la afasia y transformos relacionados* (2nd ed.). Madrid: Editorial Medica Panamericana.

Goodglass, H., Kaplan, E., & Barresi, B. (2001a). *Boston diagnostic aphasia examination* (3rd ed.). Austin: Pro-Ed.

Goodglass, H., Kaplan, E., & Barresi, B. (2001b). *The assessment of aphasia and related disorders* (3rd ed.). Austin: Pro-Ed.

Helm-Estabrooks, N., Albert, M. L., & Nicholas, M. (2014). *Manual of aphasia and aphasia therapy* (3rd ed.). Austin: Pro-ED.

Marshall, R. C., & Neuburger, S. I. (1994). Verbal self-correction and improvement in treated aphasia clients. *Aphasiology, 8,* 535–547.

Pineda, D. A., Rosselli, M., Ardila, A., Mejia, S. E., Romero, M. G., & Perez, C. (2000). The Boston diagnostic aphasia examination-Spanish version: The influence of demographic variables. *Journal of the International Neuropsychological Society, 6,* 802–814.

Reinvang, I., & Graves, R. (1975). A basic aphasia examination: Description with discussion of first results. *Scandinavian Journal of Rehabilitation Medicine, 7,* 129–135.

Robey, R. R. (1998). A meta-analysis of clinical outcomes in the treatment to aphasia. *Journal of Speech, Language, and Hearing Research, 41*(1), 172–188.

Rosselli, M., Ardila, A., Florez, A., & Castro, C. (1990). Normative data on the Boston diagnostic aphasia evaluation in a Spanish speaking population. *Journal of Clinical and Experimental Neuropsychology, 12,* 313–322.

Spreen, O., & Risser, A. H. (Eds.). (2003). *Assessment of aphasia.* New York: Oxford University Press.

Strauss, E., Sherman, E. M. S., & Spreen, O. (2006). *A compendium of neuropsychological tests* (3rd ed.). New York: Oxford University Press.

Sussman, H., Marquardt, T., Hutchinson, J., & MacNeilage, P. (1986). Compensatoryarticulation in Broca's aphasia. *Brain and Language, 27,* 56–74.

Theodoros, D., Hill, A., Russell, T., Ward, E., & Wootton, R. (2008). Assessing acquired language disorders in adults via the internet. *Telemedicine Journal and E-Health, 14*(6), 552–559.

Tsantali, E., Economidis, D., & Tsolaki, M. (2013). Could language deficits really differentiate mild cognitive impairment (MCI) from mild Alzheimer's disease? *Archives of Gerontology & Geriatrics, 57*(3), 263–270.

Boston Naming Test

Carole R. Roth[1] and Nancy Helm-Estabrooks[2]
[1]Otolaryngology Clinic, Speech Division,
Naval Medical Center, San Diego,
CA, USA
[2]Department of Communication Disorders and
Sciences, College of Health and Human Sciences,
Western Carolina University, Cullowhee,
NC, USA

Synonyms

BNT

Description

Boston Naming Test (2nd (BNT-2)

   Authors: Kaplan, Edith, Goodglass, Harold, Weintraub, Sandra

   Second edition 2001

   Publisher: Pro-Ed, 8700 Shoal Creek Blvd, Austin, TX 78757–6897

   http://www.proedinc.com

   Also available as part of the revised BDAE-3 (Goodglass et al. 2001) from Pro-Ed.

   The Boston Naming Test (BNT) is a widely used tool for assessing confrontation naming ability. The BNT consists of 60 black and white line drawings of objects that are ordered according to vocabulary word frequency from *bed* to *abacus*. The order of the pictured stimuli takes into account the finding that individuals with dysnomia often have greater difficulties with the naming of low frequency objects. Thus, instead of a simple category of anomia, naming difficulties may be rank ordered along a continuum.. This type of picture-naming vocabulary test is useful in the evaluation of children with learning disabilities and adults with brain injury or dysfunction. When used in conjunction with the Boston Diagnostic Aphasia Examination, inferences can be drawn regarding language facility and possible localization of cerebral damage.

Administration

The Boston Naming Test assesses naming abilities of children, adults with aphasia, and nonclinical adults. The drawings are shown to the examinee one at a time, and the examinee is asked to name each of them. Item familiarity decreases as the test progresses. Following presentation of each picture stimulus, two types of cues may be presented when there is an error response: a "stimulus cue" (descriptive, e.g., "used by a carpenter" for *saw*) and a "phonemic cue" (the beginning sound of the target word, e.g., "s …" for saw) A stimulus cue is presented when the examinee clearly misperceives the picture (e.g., "worm" for *pretzel)* or indicates a lack of recognition of the picture. A phonemic cue is presented after each error response, including following a stimulus cue. The examinee is given up to 20 s to respond following each stimulus presentation and after the cues. All responses are recorded as a "correct response" or as an error with the actual error response written verbatim for later coding by type. Types of cues ("stimulus cue" or "phonemic cue") presented are noted. Response latencies in seconds are also documented. The total correct score is the sum of the accurate spontaneous responses given within 20 s of picture presentation or following a stimulus cue. Correct responses following a phonemic cue are not included in the total correct score.

Historical Background

The test was originally published by Kaplan and colleagues in 1978 as an experimental version with 85 items. It was revised to a 60-item test in 1983. The current version (BNT-2) retains the same 60 items and includes a short 15-item version as well as a multiple-choice version. Short forms of the BNT have been developed to reduce test time. These include Fastenau et al. (1998), Graves et al. (2004), Lansing et al. (1999), Mack et al. (1992), Saxton et al. (2000), Teng et al. (1989), and Williams et al. (1989). The 15-item short-form 4 (Mack SF4) developed by Mack et al. (1992) was adopted by the authors of the

BNT-2 and can be found at the beginning of the stimulus booklet and answer sheet. The Mack et al. 15- item version has been adopted by the Consortium to Establish a Registry for Alzheimer's Disease (CERAD).

In a 2011 study, Hobson, et al. explored whether the 15-item BNT/CERAD version and two 30-item (even and odd) versions could predict scores earned on the 60-item version by participants with and without AD. Estimated 60-item scores created from the shorter versions were then correlated with actual scores. The 60-item scores estimated from the 30-item versions had good predictive value for actual 60-item BNT scores and the 15-item version less so.

The new BNT-2 also includes a multiple-choice version that can be administered following the standard presentation, specifically to further assess the examinee's recognition of the lexicon for items previously missed. The BNT-2 is available separately and as part of the revised BDAE-3. The BNT has been adapted and translated for use in at least a dozen languages including a 30-item adaptation for Spanish-speaking people in the United States.

Psychometric Data

Reliability, Validity, and Norms

Reliability
Internal consistency for the 60-item form has been reported to range between 0.78 and 0.96. Reliability coefficients have been lower for the abbreviated versions; for example, the Mack SF4 version ranges between 0.49 and 0.84. Test-retest reliability is high over short intervals. For longer time intervals, such as 11–12 months, test-retest reliability was marginal to high; for example, in a healthy, elderly Caucasian adult population, test-retest reliability ranged between 0.62 and 0.89 (Mitrushina and Satz 1995); and high retest reliability (0.92) in a normal or neurologically stable adult population (Dikmen et al. 1999). In 2012, Sachs and colleagues published a BNT reliability study of 844 cognitively unimpaired, Caucasian adults who were over age 55. The BNT was

readministered between 9 and 24 months after the baseline exam. During a 9–15-month retest period, a 4-point decline occurred. A 6-point decline occurred during a 16–24-month retest period. The participant's age and family history of dementia further characterized the cutoff values for reliable changes in BNT performance.

Validity
The BNT has been shown to correlate highly with other language-related measures, including the visual naming test of the Multilingual Aphasia Examination (Axelrod et al. 1994; Schefft et al. 2003), as well as with measures of intelligence, including the Verbal Comprehension Factor of the WAIS-R and the Standard Raven Progressive Matrices in children aged 6–12 years (Storms et al. 2004).

Poor performance on the BNT has been described in subjects with neurologic disease, including left-hemisphere and brainstem strokes, anoxia, multiple sclerosis, Parkinson's disease, Alzheimer's disease, and closed head injuries.

Norms
The norms available in the test booklet are limited to small groups of adults ranging in age between 18 and 79 ($N = 178$) and of children ranging in age between 5.0 years and 12.5 years ($N = 356$). Information about geographical region, ethnicity, or time reference for this normative data is not provided.

Data on BNT norms for children is limited. The BNT record form presents norms for ages 5 years and 0 months (5-0) through 12-5, based on small groups in successive 6-month age increments. The data were collected in 1987 and the normative data are believed to be largely from Caucasian boys and girls who were attending public and private schools and living with middle-class families in suburban or urban areas of the northeastern United States.

Martielli and Blackburn (2015) collected normative BNT-2 data for 100 male and 100 female adolescents aged 15–18 years. None of the 200 participants had neurologic, psychiatric, or academic problems. No statistically significant differences in BNT scores based on gender, age, or grade occurred. Martielli and Blackburn provide normative means and standard deviations, collapsed across age and gender.

Cross-sectional studies suggest that age (Heaton et al. 2004; Ivnik et al. 1996; MacKay et al. 2005; Mitrushina et al. 2005) and verbal intelligence affect the BNT scores (Killgore and Adams 1999; Steinberg et al. 2005; Tombaugh and Hubley 1997). Gender has been reported to be unrelated to BNT performance (Henderson et al. 1998; Ivnik et al. 1996; Lucas et al. 2005; Riva et al. 2000). Other studies suggest men outperform women in older samples, possibly because of male-biased items (Randolph et al. 1999). Reading vocabulary is strongly correlated with BNT performance (Graves and Carswell 2003; Senior et al. 2001). Geographic region and ethnicity have been shown to affect performance (Heaton et al. 2004; Lucas et al. 2005). Linguistic background also affects test scores according to Roberts et al. (2002).

It can be found in the literature a number of normative reports for adult English speakers (see pp. 905–907, Strauss et al. 2006). For example, Heaton et al. (2004) reviewed studies over a 25-year period and presented age, gender, and educational norms for two ethnicity groups: Caucasians and African Americans. Mitrushina et al. (2005) compiled data from 14 studies, comprising a total of 1,684 educated participants with above-average intelligence who were administered the 60-item version. Their data was presented in 5-year increments, ranging from ages 25–84 years. The data is considered to be similar to those provided by Kaplan et al. (2001) and may overestimate expected performance for individuals with lower educational and intellectual levels. Ivnik et al. (1996) provided age-corrected norms for 663 primarily Caucasian individuals older than 55 years of age, derived from the Mayo Older Americans Normative Studies (the MOANS projects). Raw scores are converted to age-corrected scaled scores having a mean of ten and a standard deviation (SD) of three (Strauss et al. 2006). Additional studies have expanded the utility of the MOANS project by providing age- and IQ-adjusted percentile equivalents of MOANS age-adjusted BNT scores, for individuals over 55 years (Steinberg et al. 2005), and age- and education-adjusted normative data based on African Americans from the Mayo Older African American Normative studies (MOAANS) project (Lucas et al. 2005; Strauss et al. 2006).

Pedraza and colleagues (2009) used item response theory (IRT) and methods to detect differential item functioning (DIF) of BNT items with 336 Caucasian and 334 African American participants. Twelve items were shown to have DIF between the two groups. Additional analyses showed that six of these items (*dominoes, escalator, muzzle, latch, tripod,* and *palette*) represent the strongest evidence for race-/ethnicity-based DIF. This study demonstrates that psychometric and sociocultural factors can lead to BNT score discrepancies between groups.

Zec and colleagues (2007a) published the results of a BNT study conducted with 1111 "normal elderly" adults aged 50–101 years and 61 younger adults aged 20–49 years. They found both significantly lower scores and increasing variability among increasing age groups and with lower educational levels. In a subsequent study (Zec et al. 2007b), BNT raw scores earned by 1,026 participants ranging in age from 50–95 were converted to scaled scores and percentiles.

Zec and colleagues present these norms and recommend them for use in assessing people with suspected dementia.

Clinical Uses

The BNT, a visual confrontation naming test, is recommended as a supplement to the Boston Diagnostic Aphasia Examination. It can be used to assess naming abilities of children, individuals with aphasia a, and typical adults, although there is limited and poorly described normative data and no test-retest reliability for children.

In their 2013 chapter on using a process approach to aphasia, Helm-Estabrooks and Nicholas describe the clinical and diagnostic utility of response patterns to the BNT. Responses typical of a person with Broca's aphasia and a person with

Wernicke's aphasia are used to illustrate the clinical value of looking beyond BNT scores to analyzing transcribed responses.

Cross-References

▶ Anomia
▶ Boston Diagnostic Aphasia Examination

References and Readings

Axelrod, B. N., Ricker, J. H., & Cherry, S. A. (1994). Concurrent validity of the MAE visual naming test. *Archives of Clinical Neuropsychology, 9*, 317–321.

Dikmen, S. S., Heaton, R. K., Grant, I., & Temkin, N. R. (1999). Test-retest reliability and practice effects of expanded Halstead-Reitan neuropsychological test battery. *Journal of the International Neuropsychological Society, 5*, 346–356.

Fastenau, P. S., Denburg, N. L., & Mauer, B. A. (1998). Parallel short forms for the Boston Naming Test: Psychometric properties and norms for older adults. *Journal of Clinical and Experimental Neuropsychology, 20*, 828–834.

Goodglass, H., Kaplan, E., & Barresi, B. (2001). *Boston diagnostic aphasia examination* (3rd ed.). Austin: Pro-Ed.

Graves, R. E., Bezeau, S. C., Fogarty, J., & Blair, R. (2004). Boston Naming Test Short Forms: A comparison of previous forms with new item response theory based forms. *Journal of Clinical and Experimental Neuropsychology, 26*, 891–902.

Heaton, R. K., Miller, S. W., Taylor, M. J., & Grant, I. (2004). *Revised comprehensive norms for an expanded Halstead Reitan Battery: Demographically adjusted neuropsychological norms for African American and Caucasian adults.* Lutz: PAR.

Helm-Estabrooks, N., & Nicholas, M. (2013). The process approach to aphasia. In L. Ashendorf & D. J. Libon (Eds.), *Neuropsychological assessment using the Boston process approach: A practitioner's guide* (pp. 170–199). New York: Oxford Press.

Hobson, V. L., Hall, J. R., Harvey, M., Munro Cullum, C., Lacritz, L., Massman, P. J., Waring, S. C., & O'Bryant, S. E. (2011). An examination of the Boston Naming Test: Calculation of "estimated" 60-item score from 30- and 15-item scores in a cognitively impaired population. *International Journal of Geriatric Psychiatry, 26*, 351–335.

Ivnik, R. J., Malec, J. F., Smith, G. E., Tangalos, E. G., & Peterson, R. C. (1996). Neuropsychological test norms above age 55: COWAT, BNT, MAE Token, WRAT-R Reading, AMNART, Stroop, TMT, and JLO. *The Clinical Neuropsychologist, 10*, 262–278.

Henderson, L. W., Frank, E. W., Pigatt, T., Abramson, R. K., & Houston, M. (1998). Race, gender and educational level effects on Boston Naming Test scores. *Aphasiology, 12*, 901–911.

Kaplan, E., Goodglass, H., & Weintrab, S. (1978, 1983). *The Boston naming test: Experimental edition (1978).* Boston: Kapan & Goodglass. (2nd ed.) Philadelphia: Lea & Febiger.

Kaplan, E., Goodglass, H., & Weintrab, S. (2001). *The Boston naming test* (2nd ed.). Austin: Pro-Ed.

Killgore, W. D. S., & Adams, R. L. (1999). Prediction of Boston Naming Test performance form vocabulary scores: Preliminary guidelines for interpretation. *Perceptual and Motor Skills, 89*, 327–337.

Lansing, A. E., Ivnik, R. J., Cullum, C. M., & Randolph, C. (1999). An empirically derived short form of the Boston Naming Test. *Archives of Clinical Neuropsychology, 14*, 481–487.

Lucas, J. A., Ivnik, R. J., Smith, G. E., Ferman, T. J., Willis, F. B., Petersen, R. C., & Graff-Radford, N. R. (2005). Mayo's older African Americans normative studies: Norms for Boston Naming Test, controlled oral word association, category fluency, animal naming, Token test, WRAT-3 reading, trail making test, stroop test, and judgment of line orientation. *The Clinical Neuropsychologist, 19*, 243–269.

Mack, W. J., Freed, D. M., Williams, B. W., & Henderson, V. W. (1992). Boston Naming Test: Shortened version for use in Alzheimer's disease. *Journal of Gerontology, 47*, 164–168.

MacKay, A., Connor, L. T., & Henderson, V. W. (2005). Dementia does not explain correlation between age and scores on Boston Naming Test. *Archives of Clinical Neuropsychology, 20*, 129–133.

Martielli, T. M., & Blackburn, L. B. (2015). When a funnel becomes a martini glass: Adolescent performance on the Boston Naming Test. *Child Neuropsychology: A Journal on Normal and Abnormal Development in Childhood and Adolescence, 1–13.*

Mitrushina, M., & Satz, P. (1995). Repeated testing of normal elderly with the Boston Naming Test. *Aging Clinical and Experimental Research, 7*, 123–127.

Mitrushina, M. M., Boone, K. B., Razani, J., & D'Elia, L. F. (2005). *Handbook of normative data for neuropsychological assessment* (2nd ed.). New York: Oxford University Press.

Morris, J. C., Mohs, R. C., Rogers, H., Fillenbaum, G., & Heyman, A. (1988). Consortium to establish a registry for Alzheimer's disease (CERAD) clinical and neuropsychological assessment of Alzheimer's disease. *Psychopharmacology Bulletin, 24*, 641–652.

Neils, J., Baris, J. M., Carter, C., Dell'aira, A. L., Nordloh, S. H., & Weiler, E. (1995). Effects of age, education, and living environment on Boston naming test performance. *Journal of Speech and Hearing Research, 38*, 1143–1149.

Nicholas, L. E., Brookshire, R. H., MacLennan, D. L., Schumacher, J. G., & Porrazzo, S. A. (1988). The Boston naming test: Revised administration and scoring procedures and normative information for non-brain-damaged adults. *Clinical Aphasiology, 18*, 103–115.

Pedraza, O., Graff-Radford, N. R., Smith, G. E., Ivnik, R. J., Willis, F. B., Petersen, R. C., & Lucas, J. A. (2009). Differential item functioning of the Boston Naming Test in cognitively normal African American and Caucasian older adults. *Journal of the International Neuropsychological Society, 15*, 758–768.

Randolph, C., Lansing, A., Ivnick, R. J., Cullum, C. M., & Hermann, B. P. (1999). Determinants of confrontation naming performance. *Archives of Clinical Neuropsycology, 14*, 489–496.

Roberts, P. M., Garcia, L. J., Desrochers, A., & Hernandez, D. (2002). English performance of proficient bilingual adults on the Boston Naming Test. *Aphasiology, 16*, 635–645.

Sachs, B. C., Lucas, J. A., Smith, G. E., Ivnik, R. J., Peterson, R. C., Graff-Radford, N. R., & Pedrazal, O. (2012). Reliable change on the Boston Naming Test. *Journal of International Neuropsychological Society, 18*, 375–378.

Saxton, J., Ratcliff, G., Munro, C. A., Coffery, C. E., Becker, J. E., Fried, L., & Kuller, L. (2000). Normative data on the Boston Naming Test and two equivalent 30-item short-forms. *The Clinical Neuropsychologist, 14*, 526–534.

Schefft, B. K., Testa, S. M., Dualy, M. F., Privitera, M. D., & Yeh, H. S. (2003). Preoperative assessment of confrontation naming ability and intrictal paraphasia production in unilateral temporal lobe epilepsy. *Epilepsy and Behavior, 4*, 161–168.

Steinberg, B. A., Beiliauskas, L. A., Smith, G. E., Langellotti, C., & Ivnik, R. J. (2005). MAYO's older Americans normative studies: Age- and IQ-adjusted norms for the Boston Naming Test, the MAE Token test, and the judgment of line orientation test. *The Clinical Neuropsychologist, 19*, 280–328.

Storms, G., Saerens, J., & De Deyn, P. P. (2004). Normative data for the Boston Naming Test in native Dutch-speaking Belgian children and the relation with intelligence. *Brain and Language, 91*, 274–281.

Strauss, E., Sherman, E. M. S., & Spreen, O. (2006). *A compendium of neuropsychological tests: Administration, norms, and commentary* (3rd ed.pp. 901–915). New York: Oxford University Press.

Teng, E. L., Wimer, C., Roberts, E., Damasio, A. R., Eslinger, P. J., Folstein, M. F., Tune, L. E., Whitehouse, P. J., Bardolph, E. L., Hui, H. C., & Henderson, V. W. (1989). Alzheimer's dementia: Performance on parallel forms of the dementia assessment battery. *Journal of Clinical and Experimental Neuropsychology, 11*, 899–912.

Tombaugh, T. N., & Hubley, A. (1997). The 60-item Boston Naming Test: Norms for cognitively intact adults aged 25 to 88 years. *Journal of Clinical and Experimental Neuropsychology, 19*, 922–932.

Van Gorp, W., Satz, P., Kiersch, M., & Henry, R. (1986). Normative data on the Boston naming test for a group of normal older adults. *Journal of Clinical and Experimental Neuropsychology, 8*, 702–705.

Welch, L. W., Doineau, D., Johnson, S., & King, D. (2002). Educational and gender normative data for the Boston naming test in a group of older adults. *Brain and Language, 53*(2), 260–266.

Williams, B. W., Mack, W., & Henderson, V. W. (1989). Boston naming test in Alzheimer's disease. *Neuropsychologia, 27*, 1073–1079.

Zec, R. F., Burkett, N. R., Markwell, S. J., & Larsen, D. L. (2007a). A Cross-sectional study of the effects of age, education, and gender on the Boston Naming Test. *The Clinical Neuropsychologist, 21*(4), 587–616.

Zec, R. F., Burkett, N. R., Markwell, S. J., & Larsen, D. L. (2007b). Normative data stratified for age, education, and gender on the Boston Naming Test. *The Clinical Neuropsychologist, 21*(4), 617–637.

Boston Process Approach

Shahal Rozenblatt
Advanced Psychological Assessment, P. C., Smithtown, NY, USA

Synonyms

BPA

Definition

Born out of the work of A. R. Luria (e.g., Higher Cortical Function in Man, 1966), the Boston process approach (BPA) to neuropsychological testing is a method of exploring the patient's approach to a task and the process involved in attaining a specific test score (Loring 1999). Its aim is to provide a more accurate characterization of neuropsychological function and dysfunction and the nervous system components involved (Kaplan 1988; Strauss et al. 2006).

Current Knowledge

According to Edith Kaplan (1988, 1990), the "achievement"-oriented approach to assessment, where performance is based on the scores obtained on a particular test, is flawed in that it assumes that the scores obtained are reflective of an underlying unitary mechanism. As an example, two individuals could arrive at a similar score via distinctly different processes that are dependent on distinctly different neural structures and/or pathways. The inherent loss of data that occurs by focusing on composite or total scores resulted in the development of an approach that focused on how a specific result was obtained. This led to the Boston process approach (BPA). In addition to careful observation of the strategies used during the completion of a task, the BPA emphasizes the importance of demographic variables (e.g., age, gender, socioeconomic status, education, and occupational status), medical history, and mental health history, as each of these variables can influence a patient's performance. According to Kaplan (1990), the BPA differs from the fixed and flexible battery approaches to testing in that the final score is deemphasized, that is, whether a response is right or wrong is less important than how it was attained. In addition, the test may be administered differently from the standardized approach, and additional measure may be introduced in order to better understand the component processes that influence or are involved in a particular task. Modified materials may also be used to gain a better understanding of the errors or unusual approaches that were noted on a task (Milberg et al. 1986).

While right or wrong answers are deemphasized in the BPA, Kaplan (1990) felt that it was essential for the qualitative observations to be quantifiable and subjected to statistical analyses. This led to the development of a wide variety of measures including the NEPSY – Second Edition (Korkman et al. 2007) and Delis-Kaplan Executive Function System (Delis et al. 2001). Each of these measures provides a number of standard scores, enabling comparisons with a normative sample. In addition, they provide the clinician with a way of understanding the patient's approach to the task, enabling complex processes to be broken down into simpler components, so that the area(s) of weakness and strength can be more readily identified.

Despite the growing popularity of the BPA, there have been criticisms. As outlined by Strauss et al. (2006), criticisms of the approach include insufficient norms, limited information about reliability and validity, and problems with readministration due to nonstandard initial administration. This can result in practice effects but can also change how the patient approaches the test when it is readministered.

See Also

▶ Fixed Battery
▶ Flexible Battery
▶ Hypothesis Testing Approach to Evaluation

Further Readings

Delis, D. C., Kaplan, E., & Kramer, J. H. (2001). *Delis-Kaplan executive function system*. San Antonio: The Psychological Corporation.

Kaplan, E. (1988). A process approach to neuropsychological assessment. In T. Boll & B. K. Bryant (Eds.), *Clinical neuropsychology and brain function: Research, measurement, and practice*. Washington, DC: American Psychological Association.

Kaplan, E. (1990). The process approach to neuropsychological assessment of psychiatric patients. *Journal of Neuropsychiatry, 2,* 72–87.

Korkman, M., Kirk, U., & Kemp, S. L. (2007). *NEPSY II. Administrative manual*. San Antonio: Psychological Corporation.

Loring, D. W. (1999). *INS dictionary of neuropsychology*. New York: Oxford University Press.

Luria, A. R. (1966). *Higher cortical function in man*. New York: Basic Books.

Milberg, W. P., Hebben, N., & Kaplan, E. (1986). The Boston process approach. In I. Grant & K. M. Adams (Eds.), *Neuropsychological assessment of neuropsychiatric disorders*. New York: Oxford University Press.

Strauss, E., Sherman, E. M. S., & Spreen, O. (2006). *A compendium of neuropsychological tests: Administration, norms, and commentary* (3rd ed.). New York: Oxford University Press.

Brachytherapy

Bram Goldstein
Department of Gynecologic Oncology, Hoag Hospital Cancer Center, Newport Beach, CA, USA

Synonyms

Internal radiation therapy

Definition

Brachytherapy is a form of radiation therapy and often indicated for the treatment of specific, recurrent brain tumors and head or neck cancers. The procedure involves the placement of radioactive (e.g., iridium-192, palladium-103, or iodine-125) seeds inside or adjacent to a targeted lesion. The primary advantage of brachytherapy is that the treatment allows for a higher radioactive dose to be delivered to the tumor bed without damaging the surrounding, healthy brain tissue (Sneed, Prados, Phillips, Weaver, and Wara 1992). In particular, high-dose rate brachytherapy utilizes catheters to mitigate exposure and accelerate the treatment time. Intracavitary brachytherapy is another subtype that involves the use of a balloon catheter which delivers localized radiation therapy to the affected area. Following the completion of radiotherapy, the radiation source and balloon catheter are then removed. Brachytherapy is a safe procedure, although reported side effects include infection, seizures, and headaches.

References and Readings

Sneed, P. K., Gutin, P. H., Prados, M. D., Phillips, T. L., Weaver, K. A., Wara, W. M., et al. (1992). Brachytherapy of brain tumors. *Stereotactic and Functional Neurosurgery, 59*, 157–165.

Bradykinesia

Anna DePold Hohler[1] and Marcus Ponce de Leon[2]
[1]Boston University Medical Center, Boston, MA, USA
[2]Madigan Army Medical Center, Tacoma, WA, USA

Definition

Bradykinesia is a slowness of movement. It is often seen in parkinsonian individuals and is a cardinal feature of Parkinson's disease. It can be seen in movements of small muscles when an individual is asked to rapidly open and close a hand, tap a finger, or move an arm back and forth to grab an object. It can involve any limb in isolation, such as decreased arm swing during gait evaluation or the entire body at once, evident in the abnormal stillness of a patient with Parkinson's disease. It may fluctuate during the day depending on fatigue and medication levels in the case of Parkinson's disease.

Cross-References

► Parkinson's Disease

References and Readings

Fahn, S., & Jankovic, J. (Eds.). (2007). Parkinsonism: Clinical features and diagnosis. In *Movement disorders* (pp. 79–100). Philadelphia: Churchill Livingstone Elsevier.

Brain Abscesses

Michael R. Villanueva and Susan K. Johnson
Department of Psychology, University of North Carolina at Charlotte, Charlotte, NC, USA

Definition

Brain abscesses are an intracranial mass of immune cells, pus (i.e., collection of dead neutrophils), and other materials stemming from a bacterial or fungal infection.

Current Knowledge

Etiology
Brain abscesses may arise by direct infection of organisms, local extension from adjacent focal areas, or distribution by way of the bloodstream. Moreover, they form as an inflammatory response

to bacteria or fungal infections within the brain. This inflammatory response leads to a localization of infected brain cells, immune cells, and microorganisms within an area of the brain (Kumaret al. 2014). This area becomes encapsulated by an abscess wall, which is formed by adjacent cells to prevent further infection of neighboring structures. This results in the formation of an encapsulated, purulent (pus-filled) mass within the brain. While this inflammatory response can serve to protect the brain from further injury, it can also have significant negative consequences. If the abscess ruptures, it can lead to inflammation of the ventricles (i.e., fluid-filled cavities containing cerebral spinal fluid) within the brain in addition to inflammation of the meninges (i.e., membranes that surround the brain and spinal cord). If the brain begins to swell, the mass may raise intracranial pressure and promote progressive herniation within the brain, which can be fatal (Kumar et al. 2014).

Symptoms

Clinically, cerebral abscesses can be devastating and often lead to an increase in intracranial pressure and localized deficits (Kumar et al. 2014). Additionally, symptoms associated with brain abscesses can develop slowly (i.e., within a 2-week period) or suddenly. A nonexhaustive list of symptoms may include the following: headaches, gait disturbances, disequilibrium, changes in mental status, vomiting, and stiffness/aching of the neck, shoulders, or back.

Prognosis

If brain abscesses are left untreated, death is the most likely outcome. On the other hand, treatment can significantly reduce the mortality rate to about 10%. Earlier treatment predicts a better outcome, although long-term neurological deficits may persist despite all intervention approaches (Kumar et al. 2014 and http://www.nlm.nih.gov/medlineplus/ency/article/000783.htm).

Treatment

Brain abscesses are treated as medical emergencies and may require hospitalization. If the infectious agent is bacterial in nature, antibiotics are usually the treatment of choice. However, if the infection is determined to be of fungal origin, then antifungal medications may be prescribed. Surgery is usually indicated if intracranial pressure continues to increase, medications fail to reduce the size of the abscesses, or the abscesses are at risk of rupture (www.nlm.nih.gov/medlineplus/ency/article/000783.htm).

Cross-References

▶ Brain Swelling
▶ Cyst
▶ Inflammation

References and Readings

Kumar, V., Abbas, A., & Fausto, N. (2014). *Robbins and Cotran pathologic basis of disease* (9th ed.). Philadelphia: W.B. Saunders Company.

Brain Death

Tiffany L. Powell
Department of Neurosurgery, Virginia Commonwealth University, Richmond, VA, USA

Synonyms

Death

Definition

Brain death is the irreversible loss of all brain function. Including the lack of capacity for consciousness and respirations (Presidents Commission for the Study of Ethical Problems in Medicine 1981). Brain death is equivalent to traditional circulatory death, which is defined by cessation of tissue perfusion and the absence of pulses. However, with brain death the heart will continue to beat and spinal cord reflexes may persist for a short time (Canadian Neurocritical Care Group 1999).

Current Knowledge

History of the Definition of Brain Death

In 1959, Mollaret and Goulon first introduced the term *coma dépassé* (beyond coma) to describe irreversible brain damage (Mollaret and Goulon 1959). The modern scientific concept of brain death is largely based on this original description of 23 comatose patients who exhibited loss of brainstem reflexes, respirations, and flat electroencephalograms (EEG). Several years later, the Harvard ad hoc committee formalized the definition of brain death using neurological criteria and published their landmark article in *1968*. These publications helped to define current practice guidelines, now widely accepted by clinicians, involved in the diagnosis of brain death.

Criteria for the Diagnosis of Brain Death in Adults

The determination of brain death is largely a clinical diagnosis. Any experienced physician should be able to make the diagnosis; however, in some states, a specialist in the field of neuroscience is required to make the assessment. Certain criteria should be met before a diagnosis of brain death is considered in order to determine the presence of unequivocal neurologic devastation. These include interpreting relevant imaging studies and excluding the presence of conscious altering drugs. (Table 1, Wijdicks 2000).

When the assessment for neurologic devastation is complete, a focused and methodical clinical examination should follow with emphasis on the documentation of coma, absence of brainstem reflexes, and demonstration of apnea following maximal stimulation of respiratory centers (Table 2).

In some instances, the clinical determination of brain death is not possible because of a patients' extreme hemodynamic or respiratory instability. In these cases, certain confirmatory testing can be completed to make the diagnosis.

Brain Death, Table 1 Assessment of neurologic devastation

Clinical or radiographic evidence of catastrophic and irreversible brain injury
Exclusion of drug intoxication, sedatives, or paralytic agents
Correction of severe electrolyte, acid-base, or endocrine disturbances
Core body temperature $> 32\,^{\circ}\mathrm{C}$

Brain Death, Table 2 Clinical criteria for brain death

1. Coma, profound state of unconsciousness
2. Pupils fixed at midposition and dilated
3. Absence of papillary response to light
4. Absence of pupil movement with head manipulation or injection of cold water into the EAC (external auditory canal)
5. Absence of motor response
6. Absence of corneal and gag reflexes
7. Absence of coughing in response to tracheal suctioning
8. Absence of respiratory drive at $Paco_2$ 60 mmHg or 20 mmHg above patients baseline[a]

[a]$Paco_2$ is the partial pressure of arterial carbon dioxide
(Reprinted from Wijdicks (2001) with permission)

These often include cerebral angiography, transcranial doppler, electroencephalography (EEG), or nuclear imaging. These tests are not required for the standard diagnosis of adult brain death.

References and Readings

Ad Hoc Committee of the Harvard Medical School. (1968). A definition of irreversible coma. Report of the Ad Hoc Committee of the Harvard medical school to examine the definition of brain death. *Journal of the American Medical Association, 205*, 337–340.

Canadian Neurocritical Care Group. (1999). Guidelines for the diagnosis of death. *Canadian Journal of Neurological Sciences, 26*, 64–66.

Mollaret, P., & Goulon, M. (1959). Le coma dépassé. *Revue Neurologique, 101*, 3–15.

President's Commission for the Study of Ethical Problems in Medicine. (1981). Guidelines for the determination of death. *Journal of the American Medical Association, 246*, 2184–2186.

Wijdicks, E. F. (2000). *Brain death*. Philadelphia: Lippincott Williams & Wilkins.

Wijdicks, E. F. (2001). The diagnosis of brain death. *New England Journal of Medicine, 344*, 1215–1221.

Brain Injury Association of America

Thomas R. Wodushek and Michael R. Greher
School of Medicine, Department of Neurosurgery,
University of Colorado, Aurora, CO, USA

Synonyms

BIAA

Membership as of 2016

The Brain Injury Association of America (BIAA) consists of more than 27 divisions and state affiliates across the USA, as well as hundreds of local chapters and support groups. A portion of the individuals involved at these various levels subscribe to the national mailing list which includes the names of approximately 25,000 individuals. Approximately two-thirds of the list members are traumatic brain injury (TBI) survivors and their family members, while the remaining represents a wide variety of professional providers and researchers (Ayotte, personal communication, February, 2016).

Major Areas or Mission Statement

"Our mission is to advance brain injury prevention, research, treatment and education and to improve the quality of life for all individuals impacted by brain injury. Through advocacy, we bring help, hope and healing to millions of individuals living with brain injury, their families and the professionals who serve them" (www. biausa.org).

Landmark Contributions

The BIAA, formerly the National Head Injury Foundation, was founded in 1980 by Marilyn and Marty Spivack and other family members of brain injury survivors. Among BIAA's landmark contributions was its success in securing congressional approval of the 1996 Traumatic Brain Injury Act (PL 104–166), later reauthorized as Title XIII of the Children's Health Act of 2000 (PL 106–310), the S. 793 TBI Act of 2008, and most recently the TBI Reauthorization Act of 2014 (S. 2539). The original bill created the federal TBI program to address the struggles of many persons with TBI in gaining access to appropriate community-based care. It is the only federal law that addresses the millions of Americans who suffer permanent disability as a result of traumatic brain injury. The ability to achieve successive appropriation bills has been due in part to the work of the BIAA and others to persuade approximately 100 members of the congress to join the Congressional Brain Injury Task Force. The latest version of the bill provided new emphasis on brain injury management in children by tasking the CDC to study TBI care in children and identify potential opportunities for new research. The BIAA, in cooperation with the Mount Sinai Brain Injury Research Center, published a 2013 position paper on this topic (Gordon et al. 2013).

In 1992, the BIAA was integral in shaping the Defense and Veterans Head Injury Program, later renamed the Defense and Veterans Brain Injury Center (DVBIC). This organization's mission is to serve veterans and active-duty military TBI victims via clinical care, research initiatives, and ongoing education of victims, families, providers, and policy makers. The program has nearly tripled in size from its 6 initial locations in 1992 to 16 that now offer specialized care; it acts as the operational component of the Defense Centers of Excellence for Psychological Health and Traumatic Brain Injury.

In 1996, the BIAA founded the Academy of Certified Brain Injury Specialists (ACBIS) which to date has certified over 6500 members. The mission of ACBIS is to improve the care provided to individuals with brain injury through enhanced education and training of their health-care providers. Training is provided by volunteers and based primarily upon *The Essential Brain Injury Guide*, which is now published in its fifth edition (Academy for the Certification of Brain Injury Specialists 2016). Certification is granted to those with appropriate work experience who have successfully completed the training and written examination.

In 1999, the US Supreme Court decided the case of *L.C. & E.W.* vs. *Olmstead*. The court held that under Title II of the Americans with Disabilities Act "states are required to place persons with mental disabilities in community settings rather than in institutions. . ." when appropriate. The ruling tasked the states to plan reforms in treatment, transportation, housing, education, and social support, in order to integrate brain injury survivors (among others) into the least restrictive setting possible. To aid state agencies working toward compliance, the BIAA partnered with Independent Living Research Utilization to provide regional training workshops regarding the content of the Olmstead decision. Although the BIAA is no longer doing trainings specifically for this purpose, their advocacy and legislative efforts continue to be driven toward increasing access to medical care, including rehabilitation, for all brain injury survivors. In 2006, these efforts included the publication *Cognitive Rehabilitation: The Evidence, Funding, and Case for Advocacy of Brain Injury* (Katz et al. 2006), which included ten recommendations to increase access and delivery of cognitive rehabilitation services across the nation.

In 2000, the BIAA in coordination with the Brain Trauma Foundation, the American Association of Neurological Surgeons, and other professional contributors developed and published *Guidelines for the Management of Severe Brain Injury* (2000). The BIAA was also involved in authoring *Management and Prognosis of Penetrating Brain Injury* (Aarabi et al. 2001). These publications were created to provide up-to-date, evidence-based guidelines and protocols to improve the outcome of TBI patients. The BIAA's newest effort involves partnering with the Icahn School of Medicine at Mount Sinai to provide recommendations for post-acute TBI care; this will be the first guideline focused upon treatment efforts after the inpatient stage. These guidelines should be published by 2017 and will address outpatient rehabilitation efforts as well as chronic disease management for those suffering from moderate to severe TBI.

Major Activities

The BIAA has demonstrated a long-term commitment to shaping public policy and partnering with governmental agencies. It has repeatedly worked to preserve and expand rehabilitation options for persons with brain injury, particularly Medicare and Medicaid beneficiaries. It has worked to secure federal funding for research and public education on brain injury. The BIAA remains active in disability advocacy and has provided consultation and assistance in developing numerous legislative proposals that benefit those who have sustained brain injury. Encouraging private/public partnerships, particularly to facilitate clinical care for military service-related brain injury, has been a crucial area of intervention. Public policy initiatives have also sought to address trauma care, child abuse prevention, transportation safety, brain injury education, and respite care (Ayotte, personal communication, February, 2016).

The BIAA views brain injury prevention and awareness as a primary component of its mission. The association has distributed information kits, produced public service announcements, and provided access to subject matter experts for a number of media outlets. In recent years it has focused on Internet-friendly methods for disseminating information and connecting survivors with educational materials and possible providers. The BIAA also publishes *TBI Challenge!*, a quarterly newsletter with a distribution that includes 25,000 households. It continues to host/cohost educational meetings and conferences and has added both live and recorded webinars to its array of education options. This webinar series, free to survivors, included topics geared toward survivors and caregivers, as well as professional providers and researchers. BIAA continues to maintain a comprehensive website and makes electronically available the National Directory of Brain Injury Rehabilitation Services. On an annual basis, the BIAA responds to over 100,000 requests for assistance through either its national information call center or its website.

See Also

▶ Traumatic Brain Injury (TBI)

References and Readings

Aarabi, B., Alden, T. D., Chestnut, R. M., Downs J. H., Ecklund, J. M., Eisenberg, H. M., ... Walters, B. C. (2001). Management and prognosis of penetrating brain injury – Guidelines. *Journal of Trauma, Injury, Infection and Critical Care, 51*, S1–S86.

Academy of certified brain injury specialists. (2016). *The essential brain injury guide* (5th ed.). McLean: Brain Injury Association of America.

Brain Injury Association of America. (2005). *Academy of certified brain injury specialists (ACBIS)*. Retrieved from http://www.aacbis.net/index.html.

Brain Injury Association of America. (n.d.). *Brain injury association USA home page*. Retrieved from http://www.biausa.org.

Brain Trauma Foundation, American Association of Neurological Surgeons, Joint Section on Neurotrauma and Critical Care. (2000). Guidelines for the management of severe traumatic brain injury. *Journal of Neurotrauma, 17*, 451–627.

Defense and Veterans Brain Injury Center. (n.d.). *Defense and veterans brain injury center: Home of defense and veterans head injury program*. Retrieved from http://www.dvbic.dcoe.mil.

Gordon, W. A., Oswald, J. M., Vaughn, S. L., Connors, S. H., & Brown, M. (2013). *States of the states: Meeting the educational needs of children with traumatic brain injury*. Retrieved from www.biausa.org/biaa-position-papers.htm.

Katz, D. I., Ashley, M. J., O'Shanick, G. J., & Connors, S. H. (2006). *Cognitive rehabilitation: The evidence, funding, and case for advocacy of brain injury*. McLean: Brain Injury Association of America.

Brain Plasticity

Jennifer Sue Kleiner
Department of Psychology, University of Arkansas for Medical Sciences Blandford Physician Center, Little Rock, AR, USA

Definition

Plasticity refers to the brain's ability to change its structure in response to development, the environment, or injury.

Current Knowledge

Brain plasticity, or neuroplasticity, refers to the brain's ability to change in response to development, to the environment (including learning), and in response to injury or aging. While it was once conceptualized that once the brain ceases development, that it would then be resistant to change, or in effect be static. Research over the last several decades has demonstrated that the brain continues to be capable of change, or restructuring, throughout the life span. While much research with respect to brain plasticity focuses on outcomes following injury, brain plasticity also refers to developmental changes that occur in the brain throughout the life span, including synaptic changes that occur in response to the acquisition of new learning and memories. As such, plasticity is seen as an intrinsic property of the central nervous system in that the brain is constantly restructuring and reorganizing in response to new learning. Specifically, studies of learning new behaviors, such as learning Braille, result in the rapid, but transient onset of cortical enlargement that gives way to a more stable but less dramatic cortical enlargement associated with plasticity.

Research has demonstrated that a variety of factors affect plasticity of neural reorganization and proliferation. One such environment includes the richness of the environment in which an organism is grown. Specifically, organisms that grow in a richly stimulating environment in which a variety of experiences are encountered have greater plasticity than individuals who are reared in less-stimulating environments. Empirical experimentation in humans and animals alike have demonstrated that the dendrite length as well as the density of synapses in organisms with enriched motor and sensory environments surpass those raised in less-stimulating environments. However, these differences appear only to exist with early learning environments, as adolescents and adults show no such sensitivity to environmental factors. Both gender and hormone differences also appear to play a role in neural plasticity, with specific respect to cortical areas; for example, while males are more sensitive to experience related to the visual cortex, females are more sensitive to development in the hippocampal area.

However, the concept of brain plasticity may be best understood by examining the processes by which the brain changes in response to injury. Responses to injury may result in the loss of a previously held behavior, release of a previously suppressed behavior, the assumption of a function by a neighboring neuronal network, or the development of new behaviors (which may be adaptive or maladaptive). Physiologically, reorganization can occur by changing the balance between excitatory and inhibitory synaptic and membrane responses as well as by strengthening or weakening synaptic connections. Brain plasticity can also involve the growth of new dendrites and axons to form new synaptic connections. Research suggests that the age of onset of the injury is critical in the development of new connections, as long connections are more difficult to form in the mature brain, whereas the young brain may be more capable of forming long connections due to the existence of excess connectivity. Changes in connectivity can occur through the strengthening or weakening of synaptic density or the rearrangement of synaptic connections. While the concept of neuroplasticity does at times result in recovery of adaptive behavioral changes, plasticity may also lead to unmasking of previous suppressed and maladaptive behaviors as well as the development of dysfunctional behaviors.

Brain plasticity may occur via multiple difference mechanisms. Perhaps the most common, and best understood, mechanism includes the expansion of a specified area of circuitry or the recruitment of either a local or distal area of circuitry. Such reorganization of function is a common post-injury response and occurs shortly following the injury and continues to develop years following the injury as the organism adapts. Remodeling or reorganization occurs both at the cortical and subcortical level, and can occur both within and between functional modalities. For example, much literature exists examining the reorganization of neuronal circuitry in response to blindness. Early onset blindness results in the functional

loss of a large area of the brain. The learning of alternative communication techniques, such as Braille, requires the adaptation of new behavior; research has demonstrated that individuals who have learned Braille have larger sensory maps related to the finger pad used in reading as compared to the contralateral equivalent or as compared to individuals who do not read Braille. Furthermore, not only do blind individuals develop enlarged corresponding sensory maps, it has also been demonstrated that the occipital, or visual, cortex is subsequently recruited for tactile information processing, as well as auditory information processing.

The advancement of technology has furthered our understanding of the existence of, and mechanisms behind, neuroplasticity. The ability to specify and characterize brain function via visualization of glucose and oxygen metabolism has allowed for exploration of mechanisms of plasticity. Processes of functional neuroimaging, including positron emission tomography as well as functional magnetic resonance imaging, allows for indirect visualization of synaptic activity; experimentation involving tasks being performed while the brain is being imaged allows for examination of synaptic changes. Magnetic resonance spectroscopy is thought to be a promising technique that allows for analysis of the connection between neurochemical changes and behaviors. Electroencephalography and magnetoencephalography allows to direct measurement of neuronal activity; however, it lacks structural specificity. Transcranial magnetic stimulation also allows for direct analysis of neural activity by temporarily suppressing brain regions, allowing for direct assessment of brain-behavior relationships in conjunction with functional neuroimaging techniques.

References and Readings

Galaburda, A., & Pascual-Leone, A. (2003). Mechanisms of plasticity and behavior. In T. E. Feinberg & M. J. Farah (Eds.), *Behavioral neurology & neuropsychology* (2nd ed., pp. 57–70). New York: McGraw-Hill.
Kolb, B. (1995). *Brain plasticity and behavior*. Mahwah: Erlbaum.

Kolb, B., Gibb, R., & Robinson, T. E. (2003). Brain plasticity and behavior. *Current Directions in Psychological Science, 12*(1), 1–5.

Kolb, B., & Whishaw, I. Q. (1998). Brain plasticity and behavior. *Annual Review of Psychiatry, 49,* 43–64.

Nelson, C. A., & Luciana, M. (2001). *Handbook of developmental cognitive neuroscience.* Boston: Massachusetts Institute of Technology.

Brain Reserve Capacity

Glen E. Getz
Department of Psychiatry, Allegheny General Hospital, Pittsburgh, PA, USA

Synonyms

Global reserve; Reserve

Definition

Brain reserve capacity is the brain's resilience to pathological damage or changes. The greater the brain reserve capacity, the less likely an individual will demonstrate behavioral disturbance associated with a disease.

Historical Background

Research has attempted to understand the role of various factors involved in cognitive decline. Frequent central nervous system disorders occur in the elderly, which increase the likelihood of cognitive decline. Age, in itself, is a factor known to alter cognitive functioning. Brain reserve capacity is the brain's ability to effectively manage the increasing changes in normal aging and to cope with pathological damage.

Postmortem examination of elderly individuals provides evidence that there is a discrepancy between the clinical manifestation of Alzheimer's disease and the neuropathology of the disorder (Katzman et al. 1988). Specifically, this early study found that a subset of individuals whose brains were found to have a high degree of pathology associated with Alzheimer's disease did demonstrate minimal clinical symptoms associated with the disease. Interestingly, the results from this study suggested that the weight of the brains in this subset of patients was higher. These patients were also found to have more neurons. It was subsequently concluded that perhaps these patients' larger brains and their possession of more neurons were protective against dementia symptoms. While subsequent studies have been inconclusive, many studies have suggested that head circumference, brain volume, intracranial volume, and genetic influences also play an important role in brain reserve capacity (Stern et al. 2006).

Current Knowledge

Research consistently demonstrates that the underlying neuropathology is not consistent with behavioral disturbance caused by dementia. Brain reserve capacity partially explains this phenomenon. Symptomatic behaviors are less likely to be prevalent in individuals with greater brain reserve capacity. Research has consistently found that cognitive reserve capacity, that is, the lifestyle approaches that encourage cognitive activity, plays an important role in functional ability despite neuropathological changes. Brain reserve capacity, such as increased amount of neurons and neuronal connections, is at least in part due to behaviors that encourage cognitive reserve capacity, such as education and occupation. It has also been argued that innate intelligence of life experiences, including educational and professional achievements, may increase cognitive reserve by helping a set of behavioral skills that allow people to manage their behaviors better (Vasile 2013).The interplay among cognitive activity, physical activity, diet, and brain reserve capacity is being carefully studied in an attempt to understand the complex relationship.

Future Directions

Identifying factors that increase the likelihood of brain reserve capacity has the possibility of being an invaluable tool toward improving the quality of elderly people's lives and potentially reducing the risk of developing Alzheimer's disease and other types of dementia. The National Institute of Aging and other federally funded programs have invested millions of dollars to better understand the factors in improving brain reserve capacity. Studies will continue to better understand factors that increase brain cells, synaptic connections, and other neurophysiological markers. The implementation and advancement of technology will assist in providing a clearer understanding of these factors as well.

Cross-References

▶ Alzheimer's Disease
▶ Cognitive Reserve

References

Katzman, R., Terry, R., DeTeresa, R., Brown, T., Davies, P., Fuld, P., et al. (1988). Clinical, pathological and neurochemical changes in dementia: A subgroup with preserved mental status and numerous neocortical plaques. *Annals of Neurology, 23,* 138–144.
Stern, Y. (2006). In L. Bieliauskas (Ed.), *Cognitive reserve, theory and application.* New York: Psychology Press.
Vasile, C. (2013). Cognitive reserve and cortical plasticity. *Procedia – Social and Behavioral Sciences, 78,* 601–604.

Brain Swelling

Beth Rush
Psychiatry and Psychology, Mayo Clinic, Jacksonville, FL, USA

Definition

Expansion of the size of the brain that occurs following head trauma and brain injury.

Current Knowledge

Brain swelling can elevate intracranial pressure immediately following brain injury and can continue hours or days after the onset of brain injury. Once intracranial pressure is elevated, oxygen, glucose, and blood have difficulty reaching all portions of the brain. Blood vessels are no longer efficient in carrying blood, oxygen, and nutrients throughout the brain. As a consequence, increased intracranial pressure complicates the degree of brain injury and also the brain's natural response to trauma.

Brain swelling can occur in 15–20% of severe brain injuries. The exact mechanism that leads to brain swelling is poorly understood, but once trauma is sustained, the brain tissue swells to compress harder and harder against the rigid skull. Brain swelling must be managed emergently following brain injury because patients experiencing brain swelling are at a higher risk of death. The brain may swell to a point in which portions of the brain herniate through openings in the skull. Brain swelling may compress the brainstem, the area of the brain that maintains consciousness, and critical life functions, such as cardiac function and respiration. Mitochondrial function is now thought to be directly related to brain edema. Acute management of brain swelling is important at the gross and molecular level. Methods of managing brain swelling involve administering medications to constrict blood vessels, drilling a burr hole or conducting decompressive craniotomy to relieve pressure, temporarily removing a portion of the skull in a decompressive craniectomy to relieve pressure (and replacing the skull fragment once pressure is normalized), placing an external drain to relieve pressure and excess fluid from the surface of the brain, placing the patient on artificial respirator so that carbon dioxide does not accumulate in the brain, inducing hypothermia, administering medications to reduce potential oxidative stress, and using an electronic intracranial pressure monitor with a valve to adjust pressure over time.

B

Cross-References

▶ Edema
▶ Intracranial Pressure

References and Readings

Marmarou, A. (2007). A review of progress in understanding the pathophysiology and treatment of brain edema. *Neurosurgery Focus, 22,* E1.
Vlodavsky, E., Palzur, E., Shehadeh, M., & Soustiel, J. F. (2015). Post-traumatic cytoxic edema is directly related to mitochondrial function. *Journal of Cerebral Blood Flow and Metabolism, 37* (1):166–177.

Brain Training

John DeLuca
Research Department, Kessler Foundation, West Orange, NJ, USA

Synonyms

Brain games

Brain training is a term used primarily by companies which market cognitive intervention products or by the lay public, rather than clinicians or researchers. The term is somewhat of a misnomer as only a very small fraction of published studies have assessed neural activity directly. Companies use this term to refer to "... practicing core cognitive abilities with the goal of improving performance on other cognitive tasks, including those involved in everyday activities..." (Simons et al. 2016, pp. 105). Support for the term and particularly its effectiveness is highly controversial, and scientific effectiveness should be differentiated from marketing and other claims. Care should be used in that the term brain training is not synonymous with concepts like cognitive training or cognitive rehabilitation.

Cross-References

▶ Cognitive Rehabilitation

References and Readings

Simons, D. J., Boot, W. R., Charness, N., Gathercole, S. E., Chabris, C. F., Kambrick, D. Z., & Stine-Morrow, A. L. (2016). Do "brain-training" programs work? *Psychological Science in the Public Interest, 17*(3), 103–186.

Brain Tumor

Ethan Moitra[1] and Daniel Smith[2]
[1]Department of Psychiatry and Human Behavior, Brown University, Providence, RI, USA
[2]Department of Psychology, Drexel University, Philadelphia, PA, USA

Definition

An abnormal mass of tissue in which some cells (glial or non-glial) grow and multiply uncontrollably. A tumor can be benign or malignant. It is associated with damage or mutation to the TP53 gene on human chromosome 17. P53 regulates the cell cycle and functions in tumor suppression. A tumor can cause damage by increasing pressure in the brain, by shifting the brain or pushing against the skull, and by invading and damaging nerves and healthy brain tissue. Some tumors may be truly indolent in their growth, growing so slowly that they are present for an unknown length of time because symptoms are less gross and disruptive. Those that are actively growing may be more likely to present with the following symptoms, depending on tumor locus: headaches; nausea or vomiting; seizures or convulsions; difficulty in thinking, speaking, or finding words; personality changes; weakness or paralysis in one part or one side of the body; loss of balance; vision changes; confusion and disorientation; and memory loss (Levin et al. 2001; Price et al. 2007).

Cross-References

▶ Astrocytoma
▶ Glioma
▶ Neuroblastoma
▶ Neurocytoma

References and Readings

Levin, V. A., Leibel, S. A., & Gutin, P. H. (2001). Neoplasms of the central nervous system. In V. T. DeVita, S. Hellman, & S. A. Rosenberg (Eds.), *Cancer: Principles and practice of oncology* (pp. 2100–2160). Philadelphia: Lippincott, Williams, & Wilkins.

Price, T. R. P., Goetz, K. L., & Lovell, M. R. (2007). Neuropsychiatric aspects of brain tumors. In S. C. Yudofsky & R. E. Hales (Eds.), *The American Psychiatric Publishing textbook of neuropsychiatry and behavioral neurosciences* (5th ed., pp. 735–764). Washington, DC: American Psychiatric Association.

Brainstem Auditory Evoked Responses

Flora M. Hammond and Sheryl Katta-Charles
Department of Physical Medicine and
Rehabilitation, Indiana University School of
Medicine, Indianapolis, IN, USA

Synonyms

Auditory brainstem responses (ABR); Auditory brainstem response audiometry; Auditory evoked response (AER); BAER; Brainstem auditory evoked potentials (BAEP); Brainstem response (BSR)

Definition

Brainstem auditory evoked responses (BAER) test the function of the auditory nerve and auditory pathways of the brain by measuring the electrophysiologic responses to repeated clicks presented to each ear. The response time of electrical waves generated from different anatomical parts of the brain-ear system are plotted as summarized below (Lew et al. 2007):

Wave I: Cochlear nerve (CN VIII)
Wave II: Cochlear nucleus (CN VIII)
Wave III: Superior olivary complex
Wave IV: Lateral lemniscus
Wave V: Inferior colliculus

Waveform morphology and interwave differences are compared to healthy controls to establish abnormality in function along the auditory pathway. Unilateral delays suggest a lesion to cranial nerve VIII along its pathway or in the brainstem. BAER may be abnormal in acoustic neuroma, demyelinating disease, migraine headaches, multiple sclerosis, brainstem tumor, brainstem stroke, or brain injury of various etiologies. Common uses of BAER include infant hearing screening, acoustic neuroma detection, multiple sclerosis diagnosis, and intraoperative monitoring during cerebellopontine angle tumor resection. Magnetic resonance imaging (MRI) may provide greater anatomic detail and would be preferable for detecting a small lesion. However, BAER may be particularly useful in an individual who cannot undergo MRI.

Current Knowledge

BAER results are generally not affected by the effect of anesthesia and medications or peripheral vestibular pathology. BAER is sometimes used for prognostic purposes after brain injury, but its use is limited for this purpose. Complete absence of responses is considered an ominous sign (Lew et al. 2007), and abnormal BAER may confirm suspicion of brainstem injury, while normal BAER simply indicates preservation of the auditory pathways through the brain. BAER does not reveal information about damage that may have occurred elsewhere in the brain, and thus, normal BAER does not necessarily predict good outcome (Lew et al. 2007; Zafonte et al. 1996).

Cross-References

▶ Evoked Potentials

References and Readings

Huszar, L. (2006). Clinical utility of evoked potentials. *eMedicine*. Retrieved 9 July 2007 from http://www.emedicine.com/neuro/topic69.htm. Accessed 23 Mar 2017.

Lew, H. L., Lee, E. H., Pan, S. S. L., & Chiang, J. Y. P. (2007). Electrophysiologic assessment techniques: Evoked potentials and electroencephalography. In N. D. Zasler, D. I. Katz, & R. D. Zafonte (Eds.), *Brain injury medicine* (p. 158). New York: Demos.

Lew, H. L., Tanaka, C., Hirohata, E., & Goodrich, G. L. (2016). Auditory, vestibular and visual impairments. In D. X. Cifu (Ed.), *Physical medicine and rehabilitation* (pp. 1137–1161). Philadelphia: Elsevier.

Luauté, J., Fischer, C., Adeleine, P., Morlet, D., Tell, L., & Boisson, D. (2005). Late auditory and event-related potentials can be useful to predict good functional outcome after coma. *Archives of Physical Medicine and Rehabilitation, 86,* 917–923.

Luaute, J., Maucort-Boulch, D., Tell, L., Quelard, F., Sarraf, T., Iwaz, J., Boisson, D., & Fischer, C. (2010). Long-term outcomes of chronic minimally conscious and vegetative states. *Neurology, 75,* 246–252.

Vernet, M., Bashir, S., Enam, S. F., Kumru, H., & Pascual-Leone, A. (2012). Electrophysiologic techniques. In N. D. Zasler, D. I. Katz, & R. D. Zafonte (Eds.), *Brain injury medicine* (pp. 236–238). New York: Demos.

Zafonte, R. D., Hammond, F. M., & Peterson, J. (1996). Predicting outcome in the slow to respond traumatically brain-injured patient: Acute and subacute parameters. *NeuroRehabilitation, 6,* 19–32.

Brainstem Glioma

Robert Rider
Department of Psychology, Drexel University, Philadelphia, PA, USA

Synonyms

Midbrain glioma; Pontine glioma

Definition

Brainstem gliomas are highly aggressive tumors of the central nervous system occurring more frequently in children than in adults (Fig. 1). This type of tumors often originates from the left side and typically involves one of three anatomical locations within the brainstem. Pontine brainstem gliomas are associated with the poorest prognosis

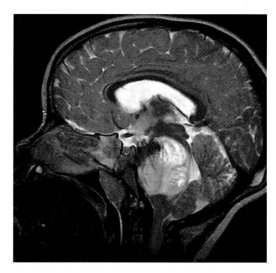

Brainstem Glioma, Fig. 1 (Picture credit: Michael Phillips and Peter C. Fisher)

for survival, while tectal and cervicomedullary gliomas are associated with longer survival. Tectal brainstem gliomas are often associated with hydrocephalus as a result of compression of the fourth ventricle. Typical manifestations of cervicomedullary tumors include dysphagia, unsteadiness, nasal speech, and sensory loss in the face. Pontine brainstem gliomas are associated with cranial nerve or long tract symptoms, including problems with the control of facial muscles, ocular movements, and swallowing. Diffuse brainstem gliomas, once thought to be a single entity, are now thought to comprise a group of tumors with varying courses and outcomes. Brainstem gliomas can also occur in the cervicomedullary junction, pons, midbrain, and tectum; prognosis is worse and very grim for diffuse brainstem gliomas. Diffuse brainstem gliomas do not typically enhance on MRI. They are not responsive to radiotherapy, and treatment is usually limited to chemotherapy.

References and Readings

Albright, L., Pollack, I., Adelson, P., Humphreys, R., George, T., Painter, M., et al. (2007). *Principles and practice of pediatric neurosurgery* (2nd ed.). New York: Thieme.

Donaldson, S., Laningham, F., & Fisher, P. (2006). Advances toward an understanding of brainstem gliomas. *Journal of Clinical Oncology, 24*(8), 1266–1272.

Brainstem Strokes

Elliot J. Roth
Department of Physical Medicine and
Rehabilitation, Northwestern University,
Feinberg School of Medicine, Chicago, IL, USA

Definition

A stroke that is caused by ischemia or hemorrhage in the midbrain, pons, or medulla is called a "brainstem stroke." There are many brainstem stroke clinical syndromes, the presentation of each depending on the specific location in the brain stem that is involved. Most brainstem stroke syndromes result from ischemia due to partial blockage or complete occlusion of arteries in the vertebrobasilar system located at the posterior region of the brain.

Current Knowledge

Localization of the brainstem lesion can usually be made by recognizing the specific pattern of clinical deficits and understanding the anatomical basis for these clinical manifestations. Many of these strokes cause dysfunction of one or more of the many cranial nerves that originate from the brain stem. The specific clinical dysfunction, typically involving head and neck functions, localizes the tissue injury to the side that is ipsilateral to the clinical deficit. Some also involve motor or sensory deficits of the body, which localize the injury to the side that is contralateral to the clinical deficit. When cerebellar signs such as ataxia and discoordination are present in association with other brainstem findings, this localizes the lesion to the ipsilateral side, and usually to the pons. When unilateral facial and contralateral body sensory deficits exist, this also localizes the lesion to the brain stem. Other symptoms, such as vertigo, double vision, nausea, and selected tremors, are also reflective of dysfunction of certain specific brainstem structures. Because the brain stem also contains the life support centers that control respiration, blood pressure, and heart rate, a brainstem stroke has the potential to be fatal.

In its most severe form, an infarction of the ventral pons can interrupt the function of all motor pathways, causing locked-in syndrome, in which the patient can receive and understand sensory stimuli, but has no motor control, resulting in complete total body paralysis and inability to speak, while maintaining awareness and sensation.

MRI scanning usually facilitates the diagnosis of brainstem stroke.

Cross-References

▶ Basilar Artery
▶ Cerebrovascular Disease
▶ Lacunar Infarction
▶ Locked-In Syndrome
▶ Posterior Cerebral Artery
▶ Posterior Communicating Artery
▶ Pure Motor Stroke
▶ Thalamic Hemorrhage
▶ Vertebrobasilar System

References and Readings

Chua, K., & Kong, K. (1996). Functional outcome in brain stem stroke patients after rehabilitation. *Archives of Physical Medicine and Rehabilitation, 77*, 194–197.
Dauby, J.-D. (1996). *The diving bell and the butterfly: A memoir of life in death.* New York: Vintage.
Nelles, G., et al. (1998). Recovery following lateral medullary infarction. *Neurology, 50*, 1418–1422.

Brexipiprazole

Efrain Antonio Gonzalez
College of Psychology, Nova Southeastern
University, Fort Lauderdale, FL, USA
Utah State University, Logan, UT, USA

Generic Name

Brexipiprazole

Brand Name
Rexulti

Class
Atypical Neuroleptic, Serotonin-Dopamine Modulators (SDAM)

Proposed Mechanism(s) of Action

The efficacy of brexpiprazole may be mediated through a combination of partial agonist activity as serotonin 5-HT1A and dopamine D2 receptors, and antagonist activity at serotonin 5-HT2A receptors.

Indication

Schizophrenia, adjunctive treatment of major depressive disorder

Off Label Use

No common offlabel use

Side Effects

Serious
Increased risk of death in elderly people with dementia-related psychosis, CVA among elderly patients, hyperglycemia, low white blood cell count, orthostatic hypotension, seizures.

Common
Headache, weight gain, somnolence, dyspepsia, constipation, fatigue, dizziness, anxiety, restlessness, increased appetite.

References and Readings

Physicians' desk reference (71st ed.) (2017). Montvale: Thomson PDR.

Additional Information
CenterWatch: https://www.centerwatch.com/drug-information/fda-approved-drugs/drug/100084/rexulti-brexpiprazole.
http://www.drugs.com/drug_interactions.html.
Drug Molecule Images: http://www.worldofmolecules.com/drugs/.
Free Drug Online and PDA Software: www.epocrates.com.
Free Drug Online and PDA Software.
Gene-Based Estimate of Drug interactions: http://mhc.daytondcs.com: 8080/cgi bin/ddiD4?ver=4&task=getDrugList.
Medscape Psychiatry.
Pill Identification.: http://www.drugs.com/pill_identification.html.
https://rexulti.com/us/mdd.

Brief Cognitive Rating Scale

Megan Becker and Daniel N. Allen
Department of Psychology, University of Nevada, Las Vegas, NV, USA

Synonyms

BCRS

Description

The Brief Cognitive Rating Scale (BCRS; Reisberg and Ferris 1988) is used to assess functional and cognitive abilities in both normal aging and progressive dementia. The BCRS is part of the Global Deterioration Scale Staging System (GDS; Reisberg et al. 1993) which is composed of three separate rating scales that include the GDS, the Functional Assessment Staging (FAST; Reisberg 1988), and the BCRS. The BCRS is comprised of two parts and provides objective ratings for a number of domains which include cognitive functions, functional abilities, mood, and behavior. Part I includes ratings for concentration, recent memory, remote memory, orientation, and functioning and self-care, while Part II allows for ratings of speech and language abilities, motoric capacities, mood and behavior, praxis ability, calculation ability, and feeding capacity.

Each of the domains is rated on a 1–7-point scale that ranges from normal (rating of 1) to profound impairment (rating of 7). For each domain, a behavioral anchor is provided for each point on the rating scale. The authors provided examples of questions that might be used to elicit information needed to complete the BCRS as well as guidelines for scoring each domain. Ratings are completed based on interviews with the patient and an informant who is knowledgeable regarding the patient's day-to-day activities and functioning. Interviews may be conducted in person or over the telephone. The BCRS has been translated into a number of languages including Chinese, French, Polish, Spanish, and Swedish, among others.

Current Knowledge

From a psychometric standpoint, the BCRS has excellent interrater reliability when completed by trained clinicians and high test-retest reliability (Foster et al. 1988; Reisberg et al. 1989). Validity studies indicate that the BCRS has strong correlations with the GDS, the Mini-Mental State Examination, some neuropsychological measures of memory abilities, and measures of activities of daily living and quality of life. Relationships have also been demonstrated between BCRS scores and neuropathology measured using a variety of techniques (EEG, PET, SPECT, neurological examination). BCRS scores are sensitive to the progression of Alzheimer's disease, with significant declines in scores as the disease progresses (Ihl et al. 1992). The BCRS has been used with elderly persons in India and compared to the Hindi Cognitive Screening Test (HCST) during its development, which correlates with the BCRS total score ($r = -0.87$) and composite axes (Tripathi and Tiwari 2013). Thus, the BCRS is useful in both research and clinical settings where it can provide valuable information regarding progression of cognitive decline, as well as the impact that such decline has on behavior and function.

Cross-References

▶ Alzheimer's Dementia

▶ Alzheimer's Disease
▶ Modified Mini-Mental State Examination
▶ Multi-infarct Dementia

References and Readings

Foster, J. R., Sclan, S., Welkowitz, J., Boksay, I., & Seeland, I. (1988). Psychiatric assessment in medical long-term care facilities: Reliability of commonly used rating scales. *International Journal of Geriatric Psychiatry, 3*, 229–233.
Ihl, R., Frölich, L., Dierks, T., Martin, E., & Maurer, K. (1992). Differential validity of psychometric tests in dementia of the Alzheimer type. *Psychiatry Research, 44*, 93–106.
Reisberg, B. (1988). Functional assessment staging (FAST). *Psychopharmacology Bulletin, 24*, 653–659.
Reisberg, B., & Ferris, S. H. (1988). Brief cognitive rating scale (BCRS). *Psychopharmacology Bulletin, 24*, 629–636.
Reisberg, B., Ferris, S. H., de Leon, M. J., & Crook, T. (1988). Global deterioration scale (GDS). *Psychopharmacology Bulletin, 24*, 661–663.
Reisberg, B., Ferris, S. H., Steinberg, G., Shulman, E., de Leon, M. J., & Sinaiko, E. (1989). Longitudinal study of dementia patients and aged controls. In M. P. Lawton & A. R. Herzog (Eds.), *Special research methods for gerontology* (pp. 195–231). Amityville: Baywood.
Reisberg, B., Sclan, S. G., de Leon, M. J., Kluger, A., Torossian, C., Shulman, E., Steinberg, G., Monteiro, I., McRas, T., Mackell, J., & Ferris, S. H. (2007). The GDS staging system. In A. J. Rush (Ed.), *Handbook of psychiatric measures* (pp. 431–435). Washington, DC: American Psychiatric Publishers.
Tripathi, R. K., & Tiwari, S. C. (2013). Cognitive functioning of community dwelling urban older adults with reference to socio-demographic variables. *Indian Journal of Clinical Psychology, 40*(2), 92–102.

Brief Psychiatric Rating Scale

Edward E. Hunter
Department of Psychiatry and Behavioral Sciences, University of Kansas Medical Center, Kansas City, KS, USA

Synonyms

BPRS

Definition

The Brief Psychiatric Rating Scale (BPRS) (Overall and Gorham 1962, 1988) consists of a series of 18 items assessing the following psychiatric symptoms: somatic concern, anxiety, emotional withdrawal, conceptual disorganization, guilt feelings, tension, mannerisms and posturing, grandiosity, depressive mood, hostility, suspiciousness, hallucinatory behavior, motor retardation, uncooperativeness, unusual thought content, blunted affect, excitement, and disorientation. The instrument takes approximately 5–10 min to rate, following an interview with the patient. The clinician rates each item on a scale ranging from 1 (not present) to 7 (extremely severe). The inventory is geared toward severe psychopathology.

Current Knowledge

The BPRS continues to be a very commonly used instrument. Between 2013 and 2015, there were well over 300 articles cited in MedLine which employed the BPRS in clinical and experimental studies. Expanded versions of the BPRS have been developed. These include behavioral anchors and structured interview questions (Woemer et al. 1988). The BPRS has a well-established history of acceptable psychometric properties. For instance, using a behaviorally anchored 24-item version and no specific interview format or rater training, Lachar et al. (2001) obtained weighted kappa agreement between psychiatrists on the majority of items at above 0.75. Furthermore, scores on the BPRS are highly correlated with those of other similar instrument constructs although, as with all such clinician-rated scales, relationships with external criteria are modest (Mortimer 2007).

In neuropsychological practice, the BPRS can enable the clinician to organize and quantify observations of psychotic symptoms or other seriously disordered behavior, both as part of an evaluation and in tracking to course of the clinical condition over time. It is most commonly used with psychotic disorders such as schizophrenia (e.g., Samara et al. 2015; Dunayevich et al. 2006),

but is appropriate with other psychiatric conditions, including bipolar disorder (Picardi et al. 2008) and major depression (Zanello et al. 2013). It can also be useful with persons having neurological conditions with psychotic or other psychiatric symptoms including Alzheimer's disease, dementia with Lewy bodies, Parkinson's disease (Cummings et al. 2007; Devanand 1998; Tariot et al. 2004), and traumatic brain injury (Diaz et al. 2012).

Versions of the BPRS are widely available and may be found online at http://uwaims.org/files/measures/BPRS.pdf (18-item version) and http://www.public-health.uiowa.edu/icmha/outreach/documents/BPRS_expanded.PDF (24-item expanded version).

See Also

► Affective Disorder
► Alzheimer's Disease
► Anxiety
► Clinical Interview
► Dementia with Lewy Bodies
► Parkinson's Disease
► Psychosis
► Psychotic Disorder
► Structured Clinical Interview for DSM-IV (SCID-I/SCID-II)

References and Readings

Cummings, K. R., Raman, R., & Thai, L. (2007). Quetiapine for agitation or psychosis in patients with dementia and parkinsonism. *Neurology, 68,* 1356–1363.

Devanand, D. P. (1998). A randomized, placebo-controlled dose-comparison of a trial of haloperidol for psychosis and disruptive behaviours in Alzheimer's disease. *American Journal of Psychiatry, 155,* 1512–1520.

Diaz, A. P., Schwarzbold, M. L., Thais, M. E., Hohl, A., Bertotti, M. M., Schmoeller, R., Nunes, J. C., Prediger, R., Linhares, M. N., Guarnieri, R., & Walz, R. (2012). Psychiatric Disorders and Health-Related Quality of Life after Severe Traumatic Brain Injury: A Prospective Study. *Journal of Neurotrauma, 29*(6):1029–1037

Dunayevich, E., Sethuraman, G., Enerson, M., Taylor, C. C., & Lin, D. (2006). Characteristics of two alternative schizophrenia remission definitions: Relationship to clinical and quality of life outcomes. *Schizophrenia Bulletin, 86,* 300–308.

Lachar, D., Bailley, S. E., Rhoades, H. M., Espandas, A., Aponte, M., Cowan, K. A., Gummattira, P., Kopecky, C. R., & Wassef, A. (2001). New subscales for an anchored version of the Brief Psychiatric Rating Scale: Construction, reliability and validity in acute psychiatric admissions. *Psychological Assessment, 13*, 384–395.

Mortimer, A. M. (2007). Symptom rating scales and outcome in schizophrenia. *The British Journal of Psychiatry Supplement, 50*, s7–14.

Overall, J. E., & Gorham, D. R. (1962). The brief psychiatric rating scale. *Psychological Reports, 10*, 790–812.

Overall, J. E., & Gorham, D. R. (1988). The Brief Psychiatric Rating Scale (BPRS): Recent developments in ascertainment and scaling. *Psychopharmacology Bulletin, 24*, 97–99.

Picardi, A., Battisti, F., de Girolamo, G., Morosini, P., Norcio, B., Bracco, R., & Biondi, M. (2008). Symptom structure of acute mania: A factor study of the 24-item Brief Psychiatric Rating Scale in a national sample of patients hospitalized for a manic episode. *Journal of Affective Disorders, 108*, 183–189.

Samara, M. T., Leucht, C., Leeflang, M. M., et al. (2015). Early improvement as a predictor of later response to antipsychotics in schizophrenia: A diagnostic test review. *American Journal of Psychiatry, 172*, 617–629.

Tariot, P. N., Profenno, L. A., & Ismail, M. S. (2004). *Journal of Clinical Psychiatry, 65*(Suppl 11), 11–15.

Woerner, M. G., Mannuzza, S., & Kane, J. M. (1988). Anchoring the BPRS. *Psychopharmacology Bulletin, 24*, 112–117.

Zanello, A., Berthoud, L., Ventura, J., & Merlo, M. C. (2013). The Brief Psychiatric Rating Scale (version 4.0) factorial structure and its sensitivity in the treatment of outpatients with unipolar depression. *Pssychiatry Research, 15*, 626–633.

Brief Symptom Inventory

Joseph F. Rath and Lisa M. Fox
NYU Langone Medical Center, Department of Psychology, Rusk Institute of Rehabilitation Medicine, New York, NY, USA

Synonyms

BSI; BSI-18

Description

The BSI (Derogatis and Melisaratos 1983) is a shortened, 53-item version of the Symptom Checklist-90 (SCL-90; Derogatis et al. 1973) that measures emotional-behavioral functioning in nine dimensions: somatization, obsessive-compulsive, interpersonal sensitivity, depression, anxiety, hostility, phobic anxiety, paranoid ideation, and psychoticism. Four additional items not specific to any one domain load on several different dimensions. In addition, three global indices – Global Severity Index (GSI), Positive Symptom Total (PST), and Positive Symptom Distress Index (PSDI) – provide more general assessment of psychological well-being. The BSI-18 (Derogatis 2000), an 18-item short form of the BSI intended as a screen for psychiatric disorders and psychological distress, consists of three 6-item subscales: somatization, depression, and anxiety. A GSI also can be calculated.

Not intended for use as diagnostic tools, both instruments are designed to identify psychological symptoms in medical populations, psychiatric patients, and community non-patients, with separate norms for males and females. Written at a sixth grade reading level and available in over 24 languages, these self-report measures can be hand- or computer-administered to individuals ages 13 and older (BSI) or 18 and older (BSI-18). Respondents rate the extent to which a specific problem has distressed them in the past 7 days (although evaluations over other time intervals may be specified), using a 5-point scale (0 = *not at all* to 4 = *extremely*). Administration is straightforward, taking 4 (BSI-18) to 8–10 min (BSI) to complete.

Scores are determined by summing values for each symptom dimension and then dividing by number of items endorsed in the respective dimension. A GSI can be calculated for either measure by adding the scores for all subscales, as well as the additional items (in the BSI), and then dividing by number of responses. For the BSI only, the PST is determined by counting the number of items endorsed with a positive (nonzero) response, and the PSDI is derived by dividing the sum of the item values by the PST. Raw scores can be converted to standardized T scores, generating a profile that graphically illustrates a respondent's current psychological symptom presentation. Interpretation of the BSI can be done at three levels: global scores, primary symptom dimensions, and discrete symptoms (Derogatis and Melisaratos 1983). Computer administration, scoring, and interpretation programs are available for both instruments.

Advantages of the BSI and the BSI-18 are that they can be completed quickly and used for repeated assessments. Also, both measures are reported to be sensitive to mild-to-severe psychological distress, making them useful with many populations. Limitations include typical concerns associated with self-report measures, such as possible patient response bias and over- or underreporting, as well as limited utility with some medical populations (e.g., neurologic), given the paucity of acceptable norms and concerns that certain items on the BSI may be closely related to physical and cognitive symptoms (Slaughter et al. 1999).

Historical Background

In response to the need for briefer evaluation tools relevant in a variety of assessment settings, including medical and industrial research studies, the BSI and BSI-18 were derived from the SCL-90, a 90-item checklist that includes the same nine symptom dimensions and three global indices as the BSI. The SCL-90, itself, was developed in 1973 (Derogatis et al. 1973) and was derived from the Hopkins Symptom Checklist (Derogatis et al. 1974). The BSI was published in 1983 (Derogatis and Melisaratos 1983), and the BSI-18 followed in 2000 (Derogatis 2000).

Psychometric Data

The most recent BSI manual (Derogatis 1993) provides normative data from four samples: (1) 1,002 heterogeneous psychiatric outpatients, (2) 914 adult non-patients, (3) 423 psychiatric inpatients, and (4) 2,408 adolescent non-patients. The BSI-18 was normed on two samples: (1) 1,134 community adults and (2) 1,543 adult cancer patients. Additional norms have been developed for such diverse samples as older adults (Hale et al. 1984), college students (Cochran and Hale 1985), individuals

with spinal cord injury (Heinrich et al. 1994), British psychiatric outpatients (Ryan 2007) and community-dwelling adults (Francis et al. 1990), Israeli adolescents (Canetti et al. 1994), and others (see Derogatis 1993). Internal consistency coefficients are strong for both the BSI (0.71–0.83) and BSI-18 (0.74–0.89). Test-retest reliability also is good, ranging from 0.68–0.91 (BSI) to 0.68–0.84 (BSI-18).

BSI and BSI-18 manuals cite a variety of studies supporting validity in a range of settings and populations, including psychoneuroimmunology, psychopathology, pain assessment and management, HIV research, student mental health, and general clinical studies. For example, in symptomatic adults, convergent validity between the BSI and the Minnesota Multiphasic Personality Inventory (MMPI) was shown to be 0.30–0.72 (Derogatis and Melisaratos 1983) for the Wiggins content scales (i.e., 13 scales tapping content areas such as social maladjustment and authority conflict) and Tryon cluster scales (i.e., seven scales assessing conceptual clusters such as social introversion and bodily symptoms). Convergent validity also has been demonstrated between the BSI and several other scales in predicting affective status among chronic pain patients (Kremer et al. 1982). High correlations were also found between the SCL-90 and the BSI (0.92–0.96; Derogatis 1993) and BSI-18 (0.91–0.96; Derogatis 2000). In terms of predictive validity, the BSI has been shown to be a good predictor of psychopathology in several populations, including a community unipolar depression cohort (Amenson and Lewinsohn 1981), drug-using adults (Buckner and Mandell 1990), and the elderly (Hale et al. 1984). Screening studies completed with medical cohorts (e.g., Kuhn et al. 1988) found the BSI to be a strong and reliable predictor of psychological distress, whereas the BSI-18 has been demonstrated to predict levels of distress in cancer patients (e.g., Recklitis et al. 2006).

Some concern has been raised about the factor structure and discriminant validity of the BSI and BSI-18. For example, Boulet and Boss (1991) found that BSI subscales correlated with non-analogous scales on the MMPI, suggesting poor discriminant validity. In terms of factor structure, moderate to high intercorrelations were found among BSI subscales, with one factor explaining over 70% of the variance in a principal components analysis (Boulet and Boss 1991). Several cross-cultural studies of the BSI-18 (e.g., Asner-Self et al. 2006) found only the GSI (versus the three subscales) to be a valid indicator of psychological distress. These researchers suggested that the BSI and BSI-18 assess the degree, but not the exact nature of psychopathology, and therefore GSI scores should be considered the most useful indicator of psychological distress derived from the measures.

Clinical Uses

The BSI and BSI-18 are widely used measures of psychological distress employed with a variety of populations including inpatient and outpatient medical and psychiatric patients, individuals receiving treatment for substance abuse, and college students. Individuals who are of extremely low intelligence, delirious, and psychotic or have motivation to distort their responses are not good candidates for either measure. Given factor structure concerns noted above (e.g., Boulet and Boss 1991), the instruments may be used most appropriately as screening tools to alert clinicians to elevated levels of psychological distress, rather than as diagnostic indicators. According to the BSI manual (Derogatis 1993), the measures are "most useful in clinical and research settings where time is a major limiting variable."

Both measures can be used as onetime assessments or administered repeatedly to evaluate treatment efficacy or trends over time. Both are reported to have been used successfully in primary care settings to assess significant changes in psychological distress and symptoms in patients with medical problems. The measures can be used in nonclinical populations (e.g., to assess caregiver distress) as well.

Both the BSI and BSI-18 may be useful tools for inclusion in neuropsychological assessments, given their brevity and utility for repeated administrations. The BSI-18 was reported to be a valid screening measure for the overall level of psychological distress in both inpatients and outpatients with traumatic brain injury (TBI; Meachen et al. 2008). The Federal Interagency TBI Outcomes Workgroup recommends the BSI-18 as a core common data element for use in TBI research as an indicator of psychological status and response to treatment (Hicks et al. 2013; Wilde et al. 2010). However, the observation that most items in the BSI obsessive-compulsive scale are more reflective of cognitive complaints (e.g., concentration and memory problems) than classic obsessive-compulsive disorder traits (Slaughter et al. 1999) highlights an issue of particular concern to neuropsychologists. Given the overlap between many items and cognitive and physical symptoms, clinicians are urged to interpret elevations cautiously and remain vigilant against misusing scale names for diagnostic purposes. It is crucial not to rely on psychiatric interpretations of elevated scales in neurological patients who have no history of emotional difficulties; instead, BSI and BSI-18 item responses might best be examined individually and used to guide treatment.

Cross-References

► Beck Anxiety Inventory
► Beck Depression Inventory
► Brief Psychiatric Rating Scale
► Center for Epidemiological Studies: Depression
► Geriatric Depression Scale
► Hamilton Depression Rating Scale
► Millon Clinical Multiaxial Inventory
► Minnesota Multiphasic Personality Inventory
► Personality Assessment Inventory
► Self-Report Measures
► Symptom Checklist-90-Revised
► Zung Self-Rating Depression Scale

References and Readings

Amenson, C. S., & Lewinsohn, P. M. (1981). An investigation into the observed sex difference in prevalence of unipolar depression. *Journal of Abnormal Psychology, 90*, 1–13.

Asner-Self, K. K., Schreiber, J., & Marotta, S. A. (2006). A cross-cultural analysis of the Brief Symptom Inventory-18. *Cultural Diversity and Ethnic Minority Psychology, 12*, 367–375.

Boulet, J., & Boss, M. W. (1991). Reliability and validity of the brief symptom inventory. *Psychological Assessment, 3*, 433–437.

Buckner, C. J., & Mandell, W. (1990). Risk factors for depressive symptomatology in a drug-using population. *American Journal of Public Health, 80*, 580–585.

Canetti, L., Shalev, A. Y., & De-Nour, A. K. (1994). Israeli adolescents' norms of the Brief Symptom Inventory (BSI). *Israel Journal of Psychiatry and Related Sciences, 31*, 13–18.

Cochran, C. D., & Hale, W. D. (1985). College student norms on the Brief Symptom Inventory. *Journal of Clinical Psychology, 41*, 777–779.

Derogatis, L. R. (1993). *Brief Symptom Inventory (BSI): Administration, scoring, and procedures manual* (3rd ed.). Minneapolis: National Computer Systems.

Derogatis, L. R. (2000). *Brief Symptom Inventory-18 (BSI-18): Administration, scoring, and procedures manual.* Minneapolis: National Computer Systems.

Derogatis, L. R., & Melisaratos, N. (1983). The Brief Symptom Inventory: An introductory report. *Psychological Medicine, 13*, 595–605.

Derogatis, L. R., Lipman, R. S., & Covi, L. (1973). SCL-90: An outpatient psychiatric rating scale: Preliminary report. *Psychopharmacology Bulletin, 9*, 13–28.

Derogatis, L. R., Lipman, R. S., Rickels, K., Uhlenhuth, E. H., & Covi, L. (1974). The Hopkins Symptom Checklist (HSCL): A self-report inventory. *Behavioral Science, 19*, 1–15.

Francis, V. M., Rajan, P., & Turner, N. (1990). British community norms for the Brief Symptom Inventory. *British Journal of Clinical Psychology, 29*, 115–116.

Hale, W. D., Cochran, C. D., & Hedgepath, B. E. (1984). Norms for the elderly on the Brief Symptom Inventory. *Journal of Clinical and Consulting Psychology, 52*, 321–322.

Heinrich, R. K., Tate, D. G., & Bucklew, S. P. (1994). Brief Symptom Inventory norms for spinal cord injury. *Rehabilitation Psychology, 39*, 49–56.

Hicks, R., Giacino, J., Harrison-Felix, C., Manley, G., Valadka, A., & Wilde, E. A. (2013). Progress in developing common data elements for traumatic brain injury research: Version two–the end of the beginning. *Journal of Neurotrauma, 30*, 1852–1861.

Kremer, E. F., Atkinson, J. H., & Ignelzi, R. J. (1982). Pain measurement: The affective dimensional measure of the McGill pain questionnaire with a cancer pain population. *Pain, 12*, 153–163.

Kuhn, W. F., Bell, R. A., Seligson, D., Laufer, S. T., & Lindner, J. E. (1988). The tip of the iceberg: Psychiatric consultations on an orthopaedic service. *International Journal of Psychiatry in Medicine, 18*, 375–382.

Meachen, S. J., Hanks, R. A., Millis, S. R., & Rapport, L. J. (2008). The reliability and validity of the Brief Symptom Inventory-18 in persons with traumatic brain injury. *Archives of Physical Medicine and Rehabilitation, 89*, 958–965.

Recklitis, C. J., Parsons, S. K., Shih, M., Mertens, A., & Robison, L. L. (2006). Factor structure of the Brief Symptom Inventory-18 in adult survivors of childhood cancer: Results from the childhood cancer survivor study. *Psychological Assessment, 18*, 22–32.

Ryan, C. (2007). British outpatient norms for the Brief Symptom Inventory. *Psychology and Psychotherapy: Theory, Research and Practice, 80*, 183–191.

Slaughter, J., Johnstone, G., Petroski, G., & Flax, J. (1999). The usefulness of the Brief Symptom Inventory in the neuropsychological evaluation of traumatic brain injury. *Brain Injury, 13*, 125–130.

Wilde, E. A., Whiteneck, G. G., Bogner, J., Bushnik, T., Cifu, D. X., Dikmen, S., . . ., & von Steinbuechel, N. (2010). Recommendations for the use of common outcome measures in traumatic brain injury research. *Archives of Physical Medicine and Rehabilitation, 91*, 1650–1660.e1617.

Brief Test of Attention

Molly E. McLaren[1] and Adam J. Woods[2,3,4]
[1]Center for Cognitive Aging and Memory, Department of Clinical and Health Psychology, University of Florida, Gainesville, FL, USA
[2]Department of Clinical and Health Psychology, College of Public Health and Health Professions, University of Florida, Gainesville, FL, USA
[3]Center for Cognitive Aging and Memory, McKnight Brain Institute, University of Florida, Gainesville, FL, USA
[4]Department of Neuroscience, University of Florida, Gainesville, FL, USA

The Brief Test of Attention (BTA) is a test of attention based on Cooley and Morris's conceptualization of attentional processes (Cooley and Morris 1990; Schretlen et al. 1996a). It was developed to be a pure measure auditory divided attention, and as such attempts to eliminate possible confounds of other attentional tasks such as motor and reasoning component (Schretlen et al. 1996a). It has also been suggested the BTA may be a useful embedded measure of cognitive effort (Busse and Whiteside 2012). The BTA has been used to assess attention in a variety of populations including Parkinson's disease, sleep apnea, cancer, and traumatic brain injury (TBI; Aloia et al. 2003; Butler et al. 2008; Rao et al. 2010; Tröster et al. 1997; Wong 1999). Of note, the BTA is not intended to measure normal attention but instead to be a screening tool for attentional deficits (Schretlen 1997; Strauss et al. 2006). Additionally, the BTA does not assess visual attention (Strauss et al. 2006).

The BTA takes approximately 10 min to administer and has two parts (Schretlen 1997; Strauss et al. 2006). In both parts, individuals are asked to listen to a voice on a recording read 10 lists of letters and numbers. The length of each list ranges from 4 to 18 items. In the first part, individuals are asked count how many numbers are read, ignoring the letters in each list. In the second part, individuals count how many letters are read, ignoring the number for each list. The specific numbers and letters do not need to be recalled, just the total amount read per list. One point is given for each correctly counted trial. Possible scores range from 0 to 20 points. Normative data is available for individuals age 6–14 and 17–82 (Strauss et al. 2006). Recently, normative data of the BTA was published for Spanish speaking adults in 11 Latin America countries (Rivera et al. 2015).

The BTA has been shown to correlate most strongly with other known attentional test, and specifically may be more related to more complex attentional tasks (Trails B; digit backwards; Schretlen et al. 1996a). Initial validity and reliability measures for the BTA indicate acceptable internal consistency (coefficeint $\alpha = 0.82$) in adults (Schretlen et al. 1996a). When both clinical and healthy populations were combined internal consistency was high (coefficient $\alpha = 0.91$; Schretlen et al. 1996a). There have been variable results from examination of test-retest reliability for the BTA. In one study of adolescent girls tested 3 months apart, test-retest reliability was low ($r = 0.45$), however it was suggested that limited range may have contributed to this finding (Schretlen 1997). In contrast, an examination of older adults assessed at baseline and 9 months reported adequate test-retest reliability ($r = 0.70$; Schretlen 1997). While practice affects appear to be small or nonexistent, there have been concerns regarding a ceiling effect in the test (Schretlen

1997; Strauss et al. 2006). Age is the largest demographic variable predicting performance on the BTA, with older age associated with poorer performance (Schretlen 1997; Schretlen et al. 1996a; Strauss et al. 2006). Other demographic variables that may contribute to BTA performance include ethnicity, education level, and gender (Schretlen et al. 1996a; Schretlen 1997; Strauss et al. 2006). Demographic variables as a whole account for 17.5% of the variance in scores on the BTA, with age being the largest contributor to variance (Schretlen 1997).

BTA has been shown to be sensitive to individuals with mild head injury (Wong 1999). A report examining the validity of the BTA in Huntington's disease patients found this group performed significantly worse than controls on the BTA. In contrast, a small group on amnestic patients were not found to perform differently from controls on the BTA, suggesting intact memory function may not be needed to successfully complete the BTA (Schretlen et al. 1996b).

Overall, the BTA appears to be a valid and relatively consistent measure of divided auditory attention. More research examining validity and reliability in minority populations is needed, as is further evaluation of test-retest reliability in different populations.

References

Aloia, M. S., Ilniczky, N., Di Dio, P., Perlis, M. L., Greenblatt, D. W., & Giles, D. E. (2003). Neuropsychological changes and treatment compliance in older adults with sleep apnea. *Journal of Psychosomatic Research, 54*(1), 71–76. https://doi.org/10.1016/S0022-3999(02)00548-2.

Busse, M., & Whiteside, D. (2012). Detecting suboptimal cognitive effort: Classification accuracy of the Conner's continuous performance test-II, brief test of attention, and trail making test. *The Clinical Neuropsychologist, 26*(4), 675–687. https://doi.org/10.1080/13854046.2012.679623.

Butler, R. W., Copeland, D. R., Fairclough, D. L., Mulhern, R. K., Katz, E. R., Kazak, A. E., Noll, R. B., Patel, S. K., & Sahler, O. J. Z. (2008). A multicenter, randomized clinical trial of a cognitive remediation program for childhood survivors of a pediatric malignancy. *Journal of Consulting and Clinical Psychology, 76*(3), 367.

Cooley, E. L., & Morris, R. D. (1990). Attention in children: A neuropsychologically based model for assessment.

Developmental Neuropsychology, 6(3), 239–274. https://doi.org/10.1080/87565649009540465.

Rao, V., Bertrand, M., Rosenberg, P., Makley, M., Schretlen, D. J., Brandt, J., & Mielke, M. M. (2010). Predictors of new-onset depression after mild traumatic brain injury. *The Journal of Neuropsychiatry and Clinical Neurosciences, 22*(1), 100–104. https://doi.org/10.1176/appi.neuropsych.22.1.100.

Rivera, D., Perrin, P. B., Aliaga, A., Garza, M. T., Saracho, C. P., Rodriguez, W., Justo-Guillen, E., Aguayo, A., Schebela, S., Gulin, S., Weil, C., Longoni, M., Ocampo-Barba, N., Galarza-del-Angel, J., Rodriguez, D., Esencarro, L., Garcia-Egan, P., Martinez, C., & Arango-Lasprilla, J. C. (2015). Brief test of attention: Normative data for the Latin American Spanish speaking adult population. *Neuropsychological Rehabilitation, 37*, 663–676.

Schretlen, D. (1997). *Brief test of attention professional manual.* Odessa: Psychological Assessment Resources.

Schretlen, D., Bobholz, J. H., & Brandt, J. (1996a). Development and psychometric properties of the brief test of attention. *The Clinical Neuropsychologist, 10*(1), 80–89. https://doi.org/10.1080/13854049608406666.

Schretlen, D., Brandt, J., & Bobholz, J. H. (1996b). Validation of the brief test of attention in patients with Huntington's disease and amnesia. *The Clinical Neuropsychologist, 10*(1), 90–95. https://doi.org/10.1080/13854049608406667.

Strauss, E., Sherman, E. M. S., & Spreen, O. (2006). *A compendium of neuropsychological tests: Administration, norms, and commentary.* New York: Oxford University Press.

Tröster, A. I., Fields, J., Wilkinson, S., Pahwa, R., Miyawaki, E., Lyons, K., & Koller, W. (1997). Unilateral pallidal stimulation for Parkinson's disease: Neurobehavioral functioning before and 3 months after electrode implantation. *Neurology, 49*(4), 1078–1083.

Wong, T. M. (1999). Validity and sensitivity of the brief test of attention with acute brain injury and mild head injury patients. *Archives of Clinical Neuropsychology, 14*(8), 617–818. [Abstract].

Bristol Activities of Daily Living Scale

Jessica Fish
Medical Research Council Cognition and Brain Sciences Unit, Cambridge, UK

Synonyms

Bristol ADL scale (BADLS); Revised Bristol activities of daily living scale (BADLS-R)

Description

The Bristol ADL scale is an informant-rated measure that covers 20 ADLs, both basic and instrumental. Items are rated on a four-point scale (from totally dependent to totally independent, with an additional "not applicable" option).

Historical Background

The BADLS was developed specifically for use in people with dementia, as existing scales were felt to be insensitive to change in this group, having been designed for healthy older adults or people with physical disabilities. Initially, 22 items were included based on the rationale that they appeared in at least two existing ADL measures. Caregivers of people with dementia completed the questionnaire by mail, including feedback on the relevance and importance of the items and response options. Some modifications were made to the scale, with the next version incorporating different response options. Two items on which participants scored at floor and ceiling respectively were removed, leading to the final 20-item version. Bucks and Haworth (2002) stated that the measure is regularly used in 58% of memory clinics in the United Kingdom, but that a revision was needed in order to increase sensitivity to mild cognitive impairment and to reflect changes in understanding of disability (particularly in light of the 2001 WHO framework) since the scale was developed. Bucks and Haworth (2002) also stated that studies evaluating a revised BADLS are underway, but no papers reporting these studies have been published to date (information correct as of 02.06.09).

Psychometric Data

The 22-item preliminary version of the BADLS had good test-retest reliability ($r = 0.95$, for kappa scores; for individual items, see Bucks et al. 1996), and evidence of its validity was found through correlations between the BADLS and MMSE scores ($r = 0.55$) and between BADLS and observed performance ratings ($r = 65$). The

final 20-item version of the BADLS, completed
by 50 caregivers of people with dementia (mixed
diagnoses), found estimates of reliability and
validity consistent with the previous version,
with BADLS-MMSE scores correlating at 0.67.
Principal components analysis identified a four-
factor structure consisting of instrumental ADLs
(seven items explaining 40.3% of variance), self
care (six items explaining 10.3% of variance),
orientation (five items explaining 7.5% of variance), and mobility (two items explaining 7% of
variance). Byrne et al. (2000) found that the
BADLS was a good measure of change in ADL
proficiency over time in people with Alzheimer's
disease (AD) receiving anticholinesterase inhibitors, as judged by its correlations with MMSE and
ADAS-Cog scores and sensitivity of 74% and
specificity of 65% in detecting improvement/sta-
bility versus decline, in comparison with
clinician-rated judgments.

A recent systematic review of 12 instrumental
ADL scales for persons with dementia (Sikkes et al.
2009) concluded that the BADLS was of "moderate
quality," the highest rating awarded in the review,
which was given to only two measures, BADLS and
the Disability Assessment for Dementia.

Clinical Uses

Wicklund et al. (2007) noted that the Bristol ADL
scale is heavily weighted toward basic ADLs
rather than instrumental ADLs, so this should
be borne in mind when considering using
it. Nonetheless, the BADLS has been used as a
primary or secondary outcome measure in a number of clinical trials, including those of pharmaceutical and psychosocial interventions in people
with dementia. Recent examples include open-
label and controlled trials on the safety of aspirin
(AD2000 Collaborative Group 2008) and neuroleptic treatments (Ballard et al. 2008) in people
with AD, a comparison of cholinesterase inhibitor
and glutamate agonist treatment in moderate-
severe AD (Jones et al. 2009), and RCTs of reminiscence therapy (Woods et al. 2009) and interpersonal psychotherapy (Burns et al. 2005) for
people with Alzheimer's disease and other

dementias. Bucks and Haworth (2002) have
noted that completing the questionnaire may be
in itself helpful for caregivers, as it can help them
to understand the effects of dementia in real-life
terms.

Cross-References

▶ Activities of Daily Living Questionnaire
▶ Alzheimer's Disease Cooperative Study ADL Scale
▶ Disability Assessment for Dementia
▶ Lawton-Brody Instrumental Activities of Daily Living Scale

References and Readings

AD2000 Collaborative Group. (2008). Aspirin in Alzheimer's disease (AD2000): A randomised open-label trial. *Lancet Neurology, 7*, 41–49.
Ballard, C., Lana, M. M., Theodoulou, M., Douglas, S., McShane, R., Jacoby, R., et al. (2008). A randomised, blinded, placebo-controlled trial in dementia patients continuing or stopping neuroleptics (the DART-AD trial). *PLoS Medicine, 5*, 587–599.
Bucks, R. S., & Haworth, J. (2002). Bristol activities of daily living scale: A critical evaluation. *Expert Reviews in Neurotherapeutics, 2*, 669–676.
Bucks, R. S., Ashworth, D. L., Wilcock, G. K., & Siegfried, K. (1996). Assessment of activities of daily living: Development of the Bristol activities of daily living scale. *Age and Ageing, 25*, 113–120.
Burns, A., Guthrie, E., Marino-Francis, F., Busby, C., Morris, J., Russell, E., et al. (2005). Brief psychotherapy in Alzheimer's disease. *British Journal of Psychiatry, 187*, 143–147.
Byrne, L. M. T., Wilson, P. M. A., Bucks, R. S., Hughes, A. O., & Wilcock, G. K. (2000). The sensitivity to change over time of the Bristol activities of daily living scale in Alzheimer's disease. *International Journal of Geriatric Psychiatry, 15*, 656–661.
Jones, R., Sheehan, B., Phillips, P., Juszczak, E., Adams, J., Baldwin, A., et al. (2009). DOMINO-AD protocol: Donepezil and memantine in moderate to severe Alzheimer's disease – A multicentre RCT. *Trials, 10*, 57.
Sikkes, S. A. M., de Lange-de Klerk, E. S. M., Pijnenburg, Y. A. L., Scheltens, P., & Uitdehaag, B. M. J. (2009). A systematic review of instrumental activities of daily living scales in dementia: Room for improvement. *Journal of Neurology Neurosurgery and Psychiatry, 80*, 7–12.
Wicklund, A. H., Johnson, N., Rademaker, A., Weitner, B. B., & Weintraub, S. (2007). Profiles of decline in

activities of daily living in non-Alzheimer's dementia. *Alzheimer's Disease and Associated Disorders, 21*, 8–13.

Woods, R. T., Bruce, E., Edwards, R. T., Hounsome, B., Keady, J., Moniz-Cook, E. D., et al. (2009). Reminiscence groups for people with dementia and their family carers: Pragmatic eight-centre randomised trial of joint reminiscence and maintenance versus usual treatment: A protocol. *Trials, 10*, 64.

Broca, Pierre Paul (1824–1880)

Michael J. Larson
Brigham Young University, Provo, UT, USA

Name and Degrees

Pierre Paul Broca received a bachelor's degree of letters (a subject that includes history and literature) in 1840 from his hometown Sainte-Foy-la-Grande College and subsequently received a Bachelor of Science degree in mathematics. He began his study of medicine in 1841 at the age of 17 at the Faculty of Medicine at the University of Paris. He completed his formal medical training there in 1848. Broca was studious and progressed rapidly during his medical studies. He was named *externe* of the Faculty of Medicine hospitals following a competitive application in 1843, *interne* in 1844, and *interne laureate*, with a 1-year extension in 1847. He competed successfully to receive the positions of Anatomy Assistant of the Faculty of Medicine in 1846 and Prosector of Anatomy to the Faculty in 1848. His mentors included such renowned individuals as François Leuret at the Bicêtre, Philippe Ricord at the Hôpital du Midi, Langier at the Hôpital Beaujon, Pierre Nicolas Gerdy at the Faculty of Medicine (Paris), and Philippe-Frédéric Blandin at the Hôtel-Dieu.

Major Appointments

- Following the completion of his medical studies, Broca served as a lecturer at the Faculty of

Medicine in Paris. He lectured on topics in anatomy and surgery until a formal competition for a professorship at the Faculty of Medicine opened in 1853. That year, at the age of 29, Broca successfully competed to achieve the distinction of Professor Agrégé and Chirurgien du Bureau Central (also known as Chirurgien des Hôpitaux or Surgeon of the Hospitals) at the Faculty of Medicine. In 1867, he was selected to chair the *pathologie externe*. Broca received the distinction of a professor of clinical surgery in 1868. That same year, he was elected a member of the Académie de Médicine and resigned his chair of the *pathologie externe* in order to accept the chair of Clinical Surgery. He held this position until his death. During his tenure as the chair of Clinical Surgery, Broca worked in several Parisian hospitals, including the Hôpital St. Antoine, the Pitié, the Hôtel des Cliniques, and the Hôpital Necker.

Major Honors and Awards

- Broca became widely recognized throughout France for his work. In 1865, he was elected president of the Paris Société de Chirurgie. In 1868, he was appointed to the Académie de Médicine and named a member of the French Legion of Honor. He was elected to a permanent seat in the French Senate in 1880, just before his death. Broca also received many posthumous honors, including the eponymous naming of Broca's area, Broca's aphasia, and the diagonal band of Broca.

Landmark Clinical, Scientific, and Professional Contributions

Early Career

- Although Broca is best known for his work on speech and the localization of brain functions, he first established his reputation as a physician and scientist using the microscope to study diseases (Finger 2004). He described in detail the histology of articular cartilage (the type of cartilage that covers the end of bones) and the histology of Rickets and demonstrated that muscular dystrophy is primarily a disease of the muscles. Broca was among the first to use a microscope to show that cancer cells can penetrate the venous and lymphatic systems as they metastasize. In the early 1850s, he performed the first experiment in Europe using hypnotism as surgical anesthesia.

- Broca was a prolific writer. He wrote several medical classics early in his career, including an extensive treatise on brain aneurysms, *Des aneurysms et de leur traitment*, published in 1856 and a memoir on cancer, *Memoir sur l'anatomie pathologique du cancer*, published in 1850.

Speech and Localization of Function

- Broca's most well-known observations were made in 1861 and the several years that followed. During that time, there was considerable fervor regarding the plausibility of cortical localization of functions, as Franz Joseph Gall's early nineteenth-century phrenology had fallen out of favor. Gall, based on his observations of skull shape, placed the ability to speak and recall words in the inferior aspect of the frontal lobes. Jean Baptiste Bouillaud followed Gall's localizationist views and hypothesized that the anterior lobes of the brain contained a center for speech production. Bouillaud even offered a prize to the first individual who reported a case with loss of speech without lesion to the frontal lobes.

- In February 1861 at a meeting of the Société d'Anthropologie de Paris, a heated debate ensued when Pierre Gratiolet, another well-respected scientist of the time, proposed total brain volume as a meaningful correlate of intelligence and indicated that the functions of all parts of the brain were essentially identical. These views were vehemently opposed by Bouillaud and his student and son-in-law Simon Alexandre Ernest Aubertin. Broca was present during these debates as the secretary of the Société d'Anthropologie. As he considered the views presented, Broca eventually sided with Bouillaud and Aubertin and became less

willing to accept the idea that all parts of the cerebral hemispheres function in the same way (Finger 2000).

- On April 12, 1861, a Monsieur Leborgne was admitted to Broca's surgical service at the Bicêtre for cellulitis and gangrene of the right leg. Affected by epilepsy since childhood, Leborgne developed considerable limitations in his ability to speak along with right hemiparesis at age 30. He could comprehend speech and communicate using pantomime, but his speech output was limited to the monosyllabic phrase "tan," which became his nickname.

- Leborgne died due to complications from the cellulitis and gangrene on April 17, 1861. Broca quickly completed an autopsy and presented his preliminary findings at the meeting of the Société d'Anthropologie de Paris the following day. He reported atrophy of both hemispheres of Leborgne's brain, with extensive softening of left-frontal areas originating from the third left-frontal convolution. He further examined Leborgne's brain specimen and presented his in-depth findings at the Société in August 1861. His presentation included a description of Leborgne's epilepsy and physical difficulties, including right-sided paralysis and loss of speech, along with a description of the growth of a lesion from the third left-frontal convolution to other areas of the brain. Over time, the area of the third left-frontal convolution became known as "Broca's area" as a result of this case.

- Later in 1861, Broca's surgical service was referred a Monsieur Lelong who had fractured his left femur after a fall. Lelong was an 84-year-old man who had been admitted to the Bicêtre 8 years previously for "senility." In the spring of 1860, Lelong had suddenly collapsed and fallen unconscious. Upon recovery, he was able to produce only four French words: "*oui*," "*non*," "*toujours*," and "*trios*," though his pantomimes were nearly always correct (Lee 1981). Lelong lived for only 12 days after he was referred to Broca's service. Following Lelong's death, Broca performed an autopsy and found lesions in

B

the second and third frontal convolutions. Presenting the findings from the case of Lelong to the Société d'Anthropologie de Paris in November 1861, Broca indicated that the findings confirmed those from his study of Leborgne and hypothesized Lelong's left-frontal lesion was due to an old hemorrhage that had occurred at the time Lelong lost his speech in 1860 (Lee 1981).

• Broca called the inability to produce language in the context of intact comprehension, as seen in the cases of Leborgne and Lelong, "aphémie" (Armand Trousseau subsequently renamed such disturbances "aphasia" in 1864). Broca published several additional cases of aphémie with lesions to the left hemisphere. For example, in 1863, he published a series of eight cases showing primarily left-frontal lesions with language production deficits. In an 1865 manuscript, Broca firmly asserted that the left hemisphere is the dominant seat for language production.

• Broca's declaration that the left hemisphere is predominantly responsible for language is among the clearest and most dramatic examples of localization of neural functions. Broca continues to receive the primary credit for reporting on the localization of language functions, although there were others who may have preceded him. In 1836, Marc Dax presented a work indicating that disturbances in language production were due to lesions of the left hemisphere. Dax's work remained largely unknown until his son Gustave Dax presented and published his deceased father's work in the years after 1863 (see Buckingham 2006 and Finger 2000).

Surgery

Broca focused heavily on the relation between the skull and the brain. In June 1871, he treated a 38-year-old laborer who was kicked in the left-frontal region of the skull by a horse. There was no fracture; nevertheless, the patient showed difficulties with speech production after approximately 1 month. He eventually lost his full ability to express himself through speech and lapsed into a coma. Broca suspected an abscess in the area of the third frontal convolution and performed a craniotomy at this approximate location based on his hypothesis. He successfully drained the abscess, but the patient slipped back into coma after approximately 11 h and died. Autopsy revealed a left-sided, predominantly frontal, meningoencephalitis (Jay 2002). This surgery based on Broca's findings regarding the localization of speech functions is likely the first practical application of the theory of cortical localization (Finger 2004; Stone 1991).

Anthropology

From approximately 1866 until his death, Broca focused the majority of his efforts on the advancement of anthropology. Indeed, due to his interest in anthropology and the remains of early humans, he did not write any papers at all on speech and the brain after 1877 (Finger 2000). Broca's initial interest in anthropology was piqued after serving on a commission examining excavations in the cemetery of the Celestins in 1847. The discovery of Neanderthal Man in 1856, the publishing of Charles Darwin's controversial ideas in *On the Origin of Species* in 1859, and the subsequent controversy on the origins of man furthered Broca's desire to study anthropology.

Much of Broca's anthropological research focused on the comparative study of skulls and the cranium circumference across ethnic groups. He devised various instruments, standardized techniques, and methods to examine the structure and topography of the brain based on measurements from prehistoric craniums. He invented at least 27 instruments to determine the relation between the brain and skull, including a goniometer (instrument to measure angles), craniograph (instrument used to depict the outline of the skull), and several stereographic instruments (Cowie 2000).

In 1869, Broca published the first description of the Gibraltar skull. Discovered in 1848, the Gibraltar skull was among the earliest skeletal remains identified as belonging to the early species of *Homo sapiens neanderthlensis*. Broca was also fascinated with the topic of neolithic trephination, the process, whereby a hole is scraped or drilled into the skull. His interest in trephination began in 1867 after he examined an Incan skull with cross-hatched cuts. He hypothesized that the operations were performed to treat "internal maladies" in children (Finger 2004) and was among the first to speculate that trephination was a therapeutic practice that was survived postoperatively based on the signs of inflammation at the wound margins (Cowie 2000).

Broca was very active in the study of anthropology during the final years of his life. Indeed, he was known to spend many hours per day in the École d'Anthropologie he founded. During the last two decades of his life, Broca published over 240 papers and monographs on anthropological topics (Schiller 1992), including a five-volume work entitled, *Mémoires d'Anthropologie*, published in 1871.

Short Biography

Pierre Paul Broca was born on June 28, 1824, in Sainte-Foy-la-Grande, a small town near Bordeaux, France. He was raised under the Calvinist Protestant tradition. His maternal grandfather, in addition to serving as mayor of Bordeaux during the French revolution, was a pastor. His mother, Annette Thomas, was the sister of a Protestant minister. His father, Jean Pierre (known as Benjamin) Broca, was a physician who served for several years as a surgeon in the French Army and was present at the Battle of Waterloo (Finger 2000).

Following his undergraduate education, Broca sought to study engineering at the École Polytechnique in Paris (Schiller 1992). The death of his only sibling, a sister named Léontine, in 1840, along with pressure from his parents to remain closer to home and follow his father's career path, led to his decision to change his course of study to medicine in 1841.

Broca showed considerable interest in the scientific societies that prevailed in Paris both during his study of medicine and throughout his career. He joined the Société Anatomique (Anatomical Society) in 1847 and the Société de Chirurgie (Surgical Society) in 1849. He also founded several societies, schools, and laboratories. In 1848, he established a society of free-thinking individuals, many of whom were sympathetic to Charles Darwin's controversial theories. He started the anthropology laboratory at the École des Hautes Études in Paris in 1858, the Société d'Anthropologie de Paris, the first-known anthropological Société in the world, in 1859, the Revue d'Anthropologie in 1872, and the École d'Anthropologie in Paris in 1876. Broca held leadership positions in many of these societies, including secretary of the Société Anatomique, general secretary of the Société d'Anthropologie de Paris, president of the Société de Chirurgie, and director of the École d'Anthropologie.

Broca married Lugol Augustine, the daughter of Dr. Jean Guillaume Auguste Lugol, who propagated the use of iodine in the treatment of disease, on July 6, 1857. The couple had three children, one daughter and two sons. Just as Broca followed in his father's footsteps by becoming a physician, his two sons succeeded him as well-respected medical scientists.

Pierre Paul Broca died on July 9, 1880, in Paris at the age of 56. Autopsy showed that all organs were apparently sound, although some have speculated his cause of death to be heart disease (Finger 2000, 2004). Following his autopsy one of his students remarked, "We shall probably not be far from the truth in attributing the catastrophe to cerebral exhaustion, arising from too protracted a course of severe intellectual exertion" (Memoir of Paul Broca 1881). He was buried at the Montparnasse Cemetery in Paris. In his life, Broca published over 500 books and articles. His influence on ideas regarding cortical localization, speech, and anthropology endures today. Indeed, many scientists would agree that the foundations of modern neuropsychology and cognitive neuroscience were laid by Pierre Paul Broca (Dronkers et al. 2007).

Cross-References

- Aphasia
- Broca's Aphasia
- Localization
- Speech
- Tan
- Wernicke's Aphasia

References and Readings

Broca, P. P. (1850). Memoire sur l'anatomie pathologique du cancer. *Bulletin de la Societe Anatomique de Paris, 25*, 45.

Broca, P. P. (1856). *Traite des anevrismes et leur traitement*. Paris: Labe & Asselin.

Broca, P. P. (1861a). Sur le principe es localisations cerebrales. *Bulletin de la Societe d'Anthropologie, 2*, 190–204.

Broca, P. P. (1861b). Nouvelle observation d'aphemie produite par une lesion de la moitie posterieure de deuxieme et troisieme circonvolution frontales gauches. *Bulletin de la Societe Anatomique, 36*, 398–407.

Broca, P. P. (1863). Localisations des fonctions cerebrales. *Siege de la faculte du language articule. Bulletin de la Societe d'Anthropologie, 4*, 200–208.

Buckingham, H. W. (2006). The Marc Dax (1770–1837)/Paul Broca (1824–1880) controversy over priority in science: Left hemisphere specificity for seat of articulate language and for lesions that cause aphemia. *Clinical Linguistics & Phonetics, 20*, 613–619.

Clower, W. T., & Finger, S. (2001). Discovering trepanation: The contributions of Paul Broca. *Neurosurgery, 49*, 1417–1425.

Cowie, S. E. (2000). A place in history: Paul Broca and cerebral localization. *Journal of Investigative Surgery, 13*, 297–298.

Dronkers, N. F., Plaisant, O., Iba-Zizen, M. T., & Cabanis, E. A. (2007). Paul Broca's historic cases: High resolution MR imaging of the brains of Leborgne and Lelong. *Brain, 130*, 1432–1441.

Finger, S. (1994). *Origins of neuroscience*. New York City: Oxford University Press.

Finger, S. (2000). *Minds behind the brain*. New York City: Oxford University Press.

Finger, S. (2004). Paul Broca (1824–1880). *Journal of Neurology, 251*, 769–770.

Greenblatt, S. H. (1970). Hughlings Jackson's first encounter with the work of Paul Broca: The physiological and philosophical background. *Bulletin of the History of Medicine, 44*, 555–570.

Grodzinsky, Y., & Amunts, K. (2006). *Broca's region*. New York City: Oxford University Press.

Hothersall, D. (2004). *History of psychology* (4th ed.). New York City: McGraw-Hill.

Jay, V. (2002). Pierre Paul Broca. *Archives of Pathology and Laboratory Medicine, 126*, 250–251.

Lee, D. A. (1981). Paul Broca and the history of aphasia: Roland P. Mackay award essay, 1980. *Neurology, 31*, 600–602.

Memoir of Paul Broca. (1881). *The Journal of the Anthropological Institute of Great Britain and Ireland, 10*, 242–261.

Schiller, F. (1983). Paul Broca and the history of aphasia. *Neurology, 33*, 667.

Schiller, F. (1992). *Paul Broca: Founder of French anthropology, explorer of the brain*. New York: Oxford University Press.

Schreider, E. (1966). Brain weight correlations calculated from original results of Paul Broca. *American Journal of Physical Anthropology, 25*, 153–158.

Stone, J. L. (1991). Paul Broca and the first craniotomy based on cerebral localization. *Journal of Neurosurgery, 75*, 154–159.

Broca's Aphasia

Lyn S. Turkstra
School of Rehabilitation Science, McMaster University, Hamilton, ON, Canada

Synonyms

Anterior aphasia; Expressive aphasia; Motor aphasia

Short Description or Definition

It is a type of aphasia that is characterized by speech that is effortful, sparse, and halting, and impaired repetition, with relatively intact language comprehension. The spoken output of individuals with Broca's aphasia often is described as telegraphic, as it contains primarily content words and lacks functors, bound morphemes, and other grammatical elements. Paraphasic errors are also present. Reading and writing performance generally mirrors that of auditory comprehension and oral expression. Some individuals with Broca's aphasia have agrammatism, a lack of grammatical structure in their extemporaneous or repeated output that is often associated with impaired comprehension of grammatical structures. Personality and intelligence are typically intact, and, in general, nonlinguistic cognitive functions are relatively preserved, but this is difficult to test the given role of language in cognitive functions.

Categorization

Broca's aphasia is a type of aphasia that is characterized by speech that is effortful, sparse, and halting, with impaired repetition and relatively intact language comprehension.

Natural History, Prognostic Factors, and Outcomes

The prognosis for recovery of functional communication in individuals with Broca's aphasia depends on the underlying cause of the aphasia as well as factors such as the size of the lesion and the patient's age, premorbid language skills, and comorbid health conditions. Individuals who initially present with Broca's aphasia often evolve to a clinical profile of anomic aphasia, with relatively good auditory and reading comprehension, and deficits primarily in word-finding and the comprehension and production of complex syntax.

Neuropsychology and Psychology of Broca's Aphasia

Broca's aphasia has been traditionally associated with lesions to Brodmann's areas 44 and 45 in the frontal lobe of the dominant (typically left) hemisphere. Autopsy data and neuroimaging studies, however, have shown both the absence of Broca's aphasia in individuals with lesions in this region and also the reverse (Yang et al. 2008). The debate about localization of Broca's aphasia is part of a larger theoretical discussion of the modularity of language and other cognitive functions, in which localizationist views are contrasted with processing accounts (e.g., that Broca's aphasia results

from slow lexical activation) (Patil et al. 2016). For the treatment implications of this debate, see discussion in Basso and Marangolo (2000).

Depression is a common psychological consequence of aphasia and is significantly more common after anterior left-hemisphere lesions (including those associated with nonfluent aphasia) than lesions in other areas (Carson et al. 2000). The most commonly used tools for evaluation of depression rely heavily on language processes and thus have limited utility for individuals with aphasia (Turner-Stokes and Hassan 2002). Scales designed to limit verbal demands, such as the Cornell Depression Scale (Alexopoulos et al. 1988), have been used in studies of aphasia but have not been validated for this population (Townend et al. 2007). A systematic review of measures of depression in aphasia (Townend et al. 2007) indicated that adaptation of existing scales and use of other informants were common approaches to the diagnosis of depression in individuals with aphasia and recommended collaboration between mental health and language experts in the diagnostic process.

Evaluation

Aphasia is typically evaluated using a combination of standardized language tests and careful observation of extemporaneous communication. Assessment of cognitive functions such as attention, memory, and executive functions is challenging in this group, given both the verbal demands inherent in the structure of most neuropsychological tests and the complex interplay of language and other cognitive functions. Cognitive tests considered to have relatively low language demands (e.g., the Cognitive Linguistic Quick Test, Helm-Estabrooks 2001; or Raven's Standard Progressive Matrices, Raven 1938, included in the Western Aphasia Battery) are sometimes used to test cognitive abilities other than language, with the caveat that language impairments are likely to influence performance on these tests as well (Beeson et al. 1993).

The specific tests and measures used depend on the goals of the assessment (e.g., diagnosis

B

vs. prediction of functional performance vs. treatment planning), the time postonset (e.g., comprehensive test batteries are not appropriate in the context of acute stroke), and the patient's clinical presentation. As lesions typically associated with Broca's aphasia affect motor structures in the frontal lobe, many patients with Broca's aphasia also have apraxia of speech and hemiplegia or hemiparesis, which poses a particular challenge in assessment of language and other cognitive functions.

Treatment

There is a wide variety of validated treatment techniques for nonfluent aphasia, particularly for Broca's aphasia. These range from traditional stimulation-type therapies, which have been the staple of aphasia therapy since the Second World War, to current treatments such as conversational script training (Manheim et al. 2009), constraint-induced aphasia therapy (Cherney et al. 2008), training of communication partners (Kagan et al. 2001), and direct training of underlying grammatical structures (Thompson and Shapiro 2005). Most of the treatment literature has focused on individuals with vascular disorders, primarily stroke. For these patients, speech-language therapy interventions have been found to be effective in improving both impairments and functional communication ability even several years after the stroke.

Cross-References

▶ Aphasia
▶ Nonfluent Aphasia
▶ Paraphasia
▶ Speech-Language Therapy

References and Readings

Academic of Neurologic Coaammunication Disorders and Sciences. *Evidence-based practice guidelines* (*association*). www.ancds.org. Retrieved 1 Oct 2008.

Alexopoulos, G. S., Abrams, R. C., Young, R. C., & Shamoian, C. A. (1988). Cornell scale for depression in dementia. *Biological Psychiatry, 23*(3), 271–284.

Basso, A., & Marangolo, P. (2000). Cognitive neuropsychological rehabilitation: The emperor's new clothes? Special issue: Cognitive neuropsychology and language rehabilitation. *Neuropsychological Rehabilitation, 10*(3), 219–229.

Beeson, P. B., Bayles, K. A., Rubens, A. B., & Kaszniak, A. W. (1993). Memory impairment and executive control in individuals with stroke-induced Aphasia. *Brain and Language, 45*, 253–275.

Carson, A. J., MacHale, S., Allen, K., Lawrie, S. M., Dennis, M., House, A., et al. (2000). Depression after stroke and lesion location: A systematic review. *Lancet, 356*(9224), 122–126.

Cherney, L. R., Patterson, J. P., Raymer, A., Frymark, T., & Schooling, T. (2008). Evidence-based systematic review: Effects of intensity of treatment and constraint-induced language therapy for individuals with stroke-induced Aphasia. *Journal of Speech, Language, and Hearing Research, 51*(5), 1282–1299.

Goodglass, H. (1993). *Understanding aphasia*. San Diego: Academic.

Helm-Estabrooks, N. (2001). *Cognitive linguistic quick test* (1st ed.). San Antonio: Psychological Corporation.

Kagan, A., Black, S., Duchan, J., Mackie, N., & Square, P. (2001). Training volunteers as conversation partners using "supported conversation for adults with Aphasia" (SCA): A controlled trial. *Journal of Speech, Language, and Hearing Research, 44*, 624–638.

Manheim, L. M., Halper, A. S., & Cherney, L. (2009). Patient-reported changes in communication after computer-based script training for aphasia. *Archives of Physical Medicine and Rehabilitation, 90*(4), 623–627.

Patil, U., Hanne, S., Burchert, F., De Bleser, R., & Vasishth, S. (2016). A computational evaluation of sentence processing deficits in aphasia. *Cognitive Science, 40*(1), 5–50.

Raven, J. C. (1938). *Progressive matrices: A perceptual test of intelligence*. London: H.K. Lewis.

Thompson, C. K., & Shapiro, L. P. (2005). Treating agrammatic aphasia within a linguistic framework: Treatment of underlying forms. *Aphasiology, 19*(10/11), 1021–1036.

Townend, E., Brady, M., & McLaughlan, K. (2007). A systematic evaluation of the adaptation of depression diagnostic methods for stroke survivors who have aphasia. *Stroke, 38*(11), 3076–3083.

Turner-Stokes, L., & Hassan, N. (2002). Depression after stroke: A review of the evidence base to inform the development of an integrated care pathway. Part 1: Diagnosis, frequency and impact. *Clinical Rehabilitation, 16*(3), 231–247.

Yang, Z. H., Zhao, X. Q., Wang, C. X., Chen, H. Y., & Zhang, Y. M. (2008). Neuroanatomic correlation of the post-stroke aphasias studied with imaging. *Neurological Research, 30*(4), 356–360.

Brodmann's Areas of the Cortex

Kimberle M. Jacobs
Department of Anatomy and Neurobiology,
Virginia Commonwealth University, Richmond,
VA, USA

Definition

Brodmann's areas of the cortex refer to 52 regions of the cerebral cortex that were identified in 1909 by German Neurologist, Korbinian Brodmann, based on cytoarchitectonic (cell size, spacing or packing density, and lamination) differences. Brodmann's areas are typically shown on a map of the brain surface, but each region is continued through the depth of cerebral cortex. These regions were originally identified based on Nissl-stained sections of human brain; however, Brodmann believed that they applied to all mammals.

Current Knowledge

In some cases, the boundary identified by Brodmann is also a functional boundary. For instance, primary visual cortex is contained in Brodmann's area 17. Brodmann's area 18 is considered to be higher-order visual cortex. Somatosensory functions are associated with Brodmann's areas 3, 1, and 2, with part of area 3 being recognized as primary somatosensory cortex. Brodmann's areas 41 and 42 are associated with audition (hearing). Primary motor cortex (the output for motor commands) is associated with Brodmann's area 4, while premotor cortex (where the decision to move likely arises) is found in Brodmann's area 6.

A different interpretation of cytoarchitechtonic regions (107 areas) was published by Constantin von Economo and Georg N. Koskinas in 1925.

Cross-References

▶ Auditory Cortex
▶ Cerebral Cortex
▶ Neocortex
▶ Somatosensory Cortex
▶ Visual Cortex

References and Readings

Brodmann, K. (2005). *Brodmann's: Localisation in the cerebral cortex* (trans: Carey L. J.). Berlin: Springer.
Falk, D., & Gibson, K. R. (Eds.). (2008). *Evolutionary anatomy of the primate cerebral cortex.* Cambridge: Cambridge University Press.

Bromocriptine

David J. Libon
Departments of Geriatrics, Gerontology, and
Psychology, Rowan University, New Jersey
Institute for Successful Aging, School of
Osteopathic Medicine, Stratford, NJ, USA

Definition

Bromocriptine is one of the groups of medicines classified as ergot alkaloids. Bromocriptine acts to block the release of prolactin which is produced by the pituitary gland. Bromocriptine is used to treat a variety of medical conditions including problems with menstruation, infertility, Parkinson's disease, neuroleptic malignant syndrome, and pituitary adenomas. When used in conjunction with diet, bromocriptine can also be used to treat type 2 diabetes.

References and Readings

Ropper, A. H., & Samuels, M. A. (2009). *Adams and victor principles of neurology* (9th ed.). New York: McGraw Hill.

Brown-Séquard Syndrome

John E. Mendoza
Department of Psychiatry and Neuroscience,
Tulane Medical School and SE Louisiana
Veterans Healthcare System, New Orleans,
LA, USA

Synonyms

Hemisection of spinal cord

Definition

Brown-Séquard syndrome is a neurological condition in which, as a result of a lesion affecting one half of the spinal cord, there is paralysis and loss of proprioception, vibration, and fine tactile discrimination on one side of the body and loss of pain and temperature on the other.

Current Knowledge

To fully appreciate this syndrome, it is helpful to understand some basic anatomy of the spinal cord. Recall that the *lateral corticospinal* tract, which carries voluntary motor impulses originating in the cortex, descends in the lateral portion of the cord after having crossed the midline (decussated) in the medulla. On the sensory side, fibers that mediate position sense (*proprioception*), fine tactual discrimination (*stereognosis*), and vibration enter the cord through the dorsal nerve roots and, without synapsing, travel up the same side of the cord from which they enter (via the posterior columns or *lemniscal system*) until they synapse in the medulla. By contrast, those dorsal root (sensory) fibers that carry information regarding pain and temperature synapse in the dorsal horn of the cord on the same side in which they entered. From there, their second-order neurons cross the midline of the cord in the ventral while commissure and then ascend contralaterally as the ventral and lateral spinothalamic tracts (*anterolateral system*).

Thus, a lesion that transects one-half of the spinal cord will cause motor symptoms on the same side of the body as a result of severing the lateral corticospinal tract on that side. This will result in residual upper motor neuron type deficits below the level of the lesion (e.g., spastic paralysis, hyperreflexia, clonus, loss of superficial reflexes, and a positive Babinski). As the lesion also affects the ventral horns, lower motor neuron signs (flaccid paralysis, severe atrophy, hyporeflexia, and fasciculations) are potentially discernable at the level of the lesion. Because the posterior columns are affected, the individual will also demonstrate a loss of proprioception, fine tactual discrimination, and vibratory sense below the level of the lesion on that same side. Finally, as a result of a disruption of the ascending spinothalamic tracts, there will be a loss of pain and temperature. However, because these latter tracts represent sensory information that has crossed over from the opposite side of the cord, the loss of pain and temperature will be contralateral to the lesion (and one of the sides opposite to the motor and posterior column symptoms). Because the fibers carrying signals for pain and temperature ascend and descend a couple of spinal segments before decussating, the level of loss of pain and temperature will be slightly below that of proprioception and stereognosis.

A Brown-Séquard syndrome usually results from a penetrating injury as might be found in a knife or bullet wound. Because such wounds lack anatomical precision, exactly one half of the cord is rarely severed, but the term is applied if the clinical picture generally matches that which was described above.

Cross-References

▶ Anterolateral System
▶ Posterior Columns

Brunel Balance Assessment

Tamara Bushnik
Inter-Hospital Research and Knowledge
Translation, Rusk Rehabilitation, New York,
NY, USA

Synonyms

BBA

Definition

The Brunel Balance Assessment (BBA) clinical assessment tool is designed as an outcome measure to assess balance before and after stroke physiotherapy interventions. It consists of 12 items that progress from easy to difficult in a hierarchical manner to form an ordinal scale. The easiest item is "static sitting balance with upper limb support"; a mid-range item is "dynamic standing balance"; the hardest item is "advanced change of the base of support." Each item is assessed by evaluating performance on a specific task with task-specific criteria for succeeding; for example, dynamic standing balance is assessed by evaluating the distance that the individual can reach beyond arm's length. Success at this task is set at a minimum reach of 7 cm. Each item is scored using a pass/fail criteria based upon task-specific performance or time standards. The BBA items are arranged into three subscales which can be used individually: sitting, standing, and stepping balance.

Current Knowledge

Homogeneity of the scale: All items have item-total correlations of more than 0.20. Cronbach's alpha, a measure of internal consistency, was 0.93 (Tyson and DeSouza 2004). Therefore, the scale was deemed homogeneous and internally consistent.

Reliability: Test-retest reliability was assessed using observations on consecutive days, while inter-rater reliability was assessed using two independent raters. There was 100% agreement for both forms of reliability (Tyson and DeSouza 2004).

Validity: Criterion validity was assessed by comparison with the sitting section of the Motor Assessment Scale (sitting balance), the Berg Balance Test (standing balance), and the Rivermead Mobility Index (stepping balance/functional mobility). The correlation coefficients were 0.83 (Motor Assessment Scale), 0.97 (Berg Balance Test), and 0.95 (Rivermead Mobility Index). Predictive validity was assessed by comparing BBA scores during in-hospital admission within 2–4 weeks after stroke to scores on the Barthel Index and Rivermead Mobility Index at 3 months poststroke in 102 individuals (Tyson et al. 2007). Individuals who had limited sitting balance during hospitalization showed little recovery of functional mobility independence. Individuals who were able to walk (with or without assistive equipment) during hospitalization were mostly independent at 3 months poststroke in transfers, walking, and stairs. For those individuals with limited standing balance during hospitalization, the majority regained the ability to walk, conduct transfers, and navigate stairs, although more of these individuals required assistance.

Minimal Clinically Important Difference (MCID): Due to the hierarchical nature of the scale, the MCID is considered to be a change of one level.

Cross-References

► Barthel Index
► Berg Balance Scale
► Motor Assessment Scale
► Rivermead Mobility Index

References and Readings

Tyson, S. F., & Connell, L. A. (2009). How to measure balance in clinical practice. A systematic review of the psychometrics and clinical utility of measures of balance activity for neurological conditions. *Clinical Rehabilitation, 23*, 824–840.

Tyson, S. F., & DeSouza, L. H. (2004). Development of the Brunel Balance Assessment: A new measure of balance disability post stroke. *Clinical Rehabilitation, 18*, 801–810.

Tyson, S. F., Hanley, M., Chillala, J., Selley, A. B., & Tallis, R. C. (2007). The relationship between balance, disability, and recovery after stroke: Predictive validity of the Brunel Balance Assessment. *Neurorehabilitation and Neural Repair, 21*, 341–346.

Bulimia Nervosa

Kristin M. Graham
Department of Physical Medicine and Rehabilitation, Virginia Commonwealth University, Richmond, VA, USA

Synonyms

Bulimia

Definition

Bulimia nervosa is defined in the *Diagnostic and Statistical Manual of Mental Disorders* (5th ed.; *DSM-5*; American Psychiatric Association 2013) as a feeding and eating disorder characterized by episodes of binge eating that occur during a discrete period of time and are accompanied by a sense of lack of control. Behaviors to expel food eaten (e.g., self-induced vomiting, laxatives) and/or restrictive caloric intake behaviors typically follow binge eating episodes. Additionally, individuals engage in inappropriate behaviors to prevent weight gain, and self-evaluation is disproportionately influenced by body shape and weight. Individuals typically experience fear of gaining weight and a desire to lose weight, as is common in anorexia nervosa.

Categorization

The disorder is classified with the Feeding and Eating Disorders in DSM-5.

Current Knowledge

Development and Course

The development of bulimia nervosa is common during adolescence and young adulthood and is often associated with stressful life events or the occurrence of binge eating behavior during or following a period of dieting. The disorder is 10 times more common in females than males, with a prevalence of approximately 1–3% (APA 2013). Risk of suicidal ideation or behaviors is greater in individuals with this disorder.

Associated Features and Current Research

Individuals with bulimia nervosa are typically within the normal weight to overweight range (body mass index ≥18.5 and <30). The disorder can produce a number of medical problems, including amenorrhea, electrolyte imbalance, and gastrointestinal dysfunction, and there is a significant risk of mortality. A wide range of functional limitations, such as social disturbances, are associated with bulimia nervosa. Additionally, studies have identified neuropsychological impairments in the areas of attention and executive functioning that are associated with bulimia nervosa (Lauer 2002). Common comorbid conditions include mood disorders, anxiety disorders, substance abuse, and personality disorders (most commonly borderline personality disorder).

Assessment and Treatment

Diagnosis typically involves psychiatric assessment, physical examination, and laboratory testing for associated medical conditions. Course of treatment is also impacted by the information gathered in the diagnostic phase, as well as factors such as interpersonal history and functioning, medical and psychiatric comorbidity, and previous treatment attempts. Treatment often combines pharmacological (e.g., antidepressants) and psychological interventions. Cognitive behavioral therapy has emerged as the superior treatment approach (McGilley and Pryor 1998). Differential diagnoses include anorexia nervosa, binge eating disorder, major depression, and borderline personality disorder.

See Also

▶ Anorexia Nervosa
▶ Binge-Eating Disorder
▶ Body Dysmorphic Disorder
▶ Feeding and Eating Disorders
▶ Rumination Disorder

References and Readings

American Psychiatric Association. (2013). *Diagnostic and statistical manual of mental disorders (DSM-5®)*. Washington, DC: American Psychiatric Association.

Jenkins, P. E., Luck, A., Cardy, J., & Staniford, J. (2016). How useful is the DSM-5 severity indicator in bulimia nervosa? A clinical study including a measure of impairment. *Psychiatry Research, 246*, 366–369.

Lauer, C. J. (2002). Neuropsychological findings in eating disorders. In *Biological psychiatry* (pp. 1167–1172). New York: Wiley.

McGilley, B. M., & Pryor, T. L. (1998). Assessment and treatment of bulimia nervosa. *American Family Physician, 57*(11), 2743–2750.

Wonderlich, S. A., Peterson, C. B., Crosby, R. D., Smith, T. L., Klein, M. H., Mitchell, J. E., & Crow, S. J. (2014). A randomized controlled comparison of integrative cognitive-affective therapy (ICAT) and enhanced cognitive-behavioral therapy (CBT-E) for bulimia nervosa. *Psychological Medicine, 44*(03), 543–553.

Bupropion

Cristy Akins[1] and Efrain Antonio Gonzalez[2,3]
[1]Mercy Family Center, Metarie, LA, USA
[2]College of Psychology, Nova Southeastern University, Fort Lauderdale, FL, USA
[3]Utah State University, Logan, UT, USA

Generic Name

Bupropion, Bupropion hydrobromide

Brand Name

Wellbutrin, Wellbutrin SR, Wellbutrin XL, Zyban, Aplenzin, Buproban, Budeprion SR, and Forfivo XL

Class

Antidepressants, smoking cessation aids, and dopamine reuptake inhibitors

Proposed Mechanism(s) of Action

Increases norepinephrine/noradrenaline and dopamine, blocks norepinephrine reuptake pump, may increase dopamine neurotransmission in the frontal cortex, and blocks dopamine reuptake pump.

Indication

Major depressive disorder, seasonal affective disorder, and smoking cessation.

Off-Label Use

Bipolar disorder, ADHD, and neuropathic pain.

Side Effects

Serious
Seizures, hypomania, induction of mania, and activation of suicidal ideation (controversial).

Common

Dry mouth, constipation, nausea, weight loss, insomnia, dizziness, headache, agitation, tremor, abdominal pain, tinnitus, tremor, palpitation, anorexia, urinary frequency, and sweating.

References and Readings

Physicians' Desk Reference (71st ed.). (2017). Montvale: Thomson PDR.

Stahl, S. M. (2007). *Essential psychopharmacology: The prescriber's guide* (2nd ed.). New York: Cambridge University Press.

Additional Information

Centerwatch: https://www.centerwatch.com/drug-information/fda-approved-drugs/drug/986/aplenzin-bupropion-hydrobromide.
Drug Interaction Effects: http://www.drugs.com/drug_interactions.html.
Drug Molecule Images: http://www.worldofmolecules.com/drugs/.
Free Drug Online and PDA Software: www.epocrates.com.
Free Drug Online and PDA Software: www.medscape.com.
Gene-Based Estimate of Drug interactions: http://mhc.daytondcs.com:8080/cgibin/ddiD4?ver=4&task=getDrugList.
Pill Identification: http://www.drugs.com/pill_identification.html.

Burden of Proof

Moira C. Dux
US Department of Veteran Affairs, Baltimore, MD, USA

Synonyms

Standards of proof

Definition

This refers to the duty to provide evidence for allegations raised in the context of legal action. The standard of proof is the degree of proof needed in a legal action to persuade the court (e.g., judge or jury) that a given allegation is indeed founded or true. There are three main types of standards of proof: beyond a reasonable doubt, clear and convincing evidence, and a preponderance of the evidence. Artificial percentages have been associated with each of these standards of proof with beyond reasonable doubt coinciding with 90–95% certainty, clear and convincing evidence of 75%, and a preponderance of the evidence associated with just over 50%. Each of these standards is used during different inquiries in criminal procedure (e.g., insanity defense, competency to stand trial, and competency to be executed), and there are other standards used by appellate courts when reviewing trial court records. Under the current *Mental Penal Code* standard for insanity, "The defendant has the burden of providing the defense of insanity by clear and convincing evidence."

Cross-References

▶ Beyond a Reasonable Doubt
▶ Clear and Convincing Evidence
▶ Preponderance of the Evidence

References and Readings

Denney, R. L. (2005). Criminal forensic neuropsychology and assessment of competency. In G. Larrabee (Ed.), *Forensic neuropsychology: A scientific approach*. New York: Oxford University Press.
Melton, G. B., Petrila, J., Poythress, N. G., & Slobogin, C. (2007). *Psychological evaluations for the courts: A handbook for mental health professionals and lawyers* (3rd ed.). New York: Guilford Press.

Buspirone

Efrain Antonio Gonzalez
College of Psychology, Nova Southeastern University, Fort Lauderdale, FL, USA
Utah State University, Logan, UT, USA

Generic Name

Buspirone

Brand Name

BuSpar, Buspirex, Bustab, and Linbuspirone

Class

Antianxiety agents, anxiolytics, and nonbenzodiazepines

Proposed Mechanism(s) of Action

Serotonin 1A partial agonist, thus diminishing the overall serotonergic activity at those receptor sites.

Indication

Anxiety disorders.

Off-Label Use

Mixed anxiety and depression, treatment-resistant depression, and smoking cessation.

Side Effects

Serious
Very rare cardiac symptoms.

Common
Dizziness, sedation, nervousness, and nausea.

References and Readings

Physicians' Desk Reference (71st ed.). (2017). Montvale: Thomson PDR.

Stahl, S. M. (2007). *Essential psychopharmacology: The prescriber's guide* (2nd ed.). New York: Cambridge University Press.

Additional Information
Drug Interaction Effects: http://www.drugs.com/drug_interactions.html.

Drug Molecule Images: http://www.worldofmolecules.com/drugs/.

Free Drug Online and PDA Software: www.epocrates.com.

Free Drug Online and PDA Software: www.medscape.com.

Gene-Based Estimate of Drug interactions: http://mhc.daytondcs.com:8080/cgibin/ddiD4?ver=4&task=getDrugList.

Pill Identification: http://www.drugs.com/pill_identification.html.

Butters, Nelson (1937–1995)

Meryl A. Butters and James T. Becker
Department of Psychiatry, University of Pittsburgh School of Medicine, WPIC, Pittsburgh, PA, USA

Major Appointments

- NIMH Postdoctoral Research Fellow at the Neuropsychology Section of NIMH, Bethesda, MD (1964–1966)
- Instructor, College of General Studies, George Washington University (1965–1966)
- Assistant Professor, Ohio State University (1966–1967)
- Lecturer in Psychology, Antioch College (1966–1967)
- Lecturer in Psychology, Wellesley College (1967–1968)
- Lecturer in Psychology, University of Massachusetts (Boston) (1967–1983)
- Research Career Scientist, Boston Veterans Administration Medical Center (1967–1983)
- Professor of Neurology (Neuropsychology), Boston University School of Medicine (1967–1983)
- Senior Lecturer, Northeastern University, University College (1967–1983)
- Affiliate Professor of Psychology, Clark University (1973–1983)
- Chief, Psychology Service, San Diego Department of Veteran Affairs Medical Center (1983–1995)
- Professor of Psychiatry, University of California School of Medicine (San Diego) (1983–1995)

Major Honors and Awards

- Phi Beta Kappa, Summa Cum Laude, A.B.. with Honors
- NIH Predoctoral Research Fellowship (1961–1964)
- NIMH Postdoctoral Research Fellowship (1964–1966)

- Member of the Collegium of the Distinguished Alumni of the College of Liberal Arts of Boston University (elected 1974)
- Fellow, American Association for the Advancement of Science
- American Psychological Association (Fellow Divisions 3, 6, 40; President of Division 40 1982–1983; Representative to APA Council 1990–1992)
- International Neuropsychological Society (Secretary-Treasurer 1974–1977; Board of Governors 1978–1981; Treasurer 1980–1983; President, 1984–1985)
- National Academy of Neuropsychology (Fellow; President 1992–1993)
- American Psychological Society (Fellow, 1988)
- American Board of Clinical Neuropsychology (Founding Fellow, Vice-President 1991–1993)
- Distinguished Clinical Neuropsychologist Award from the National Academy of Neuropsychology (1991)
- Meritorious Service Award from the Department of Veteran Affairs (1993)
- Distinguished Service Award from the American Board of Professional Psychology (1993)

Landmark Clinical, Scientific, and Professional Contributions

- Nelson Butters authored or coauthored over 200 peer-reviewed scientific articles, 60 invited monographs and book chapters, and reams of abstracts. He coedited or coauthored six books and delivered a multitude of invited lectures and presentations. Butters expended much professional energy demonstrating the existence of distinct dissociations among cognitive functions, especially memory, within and between patients with various forms of cerebral dysfunction. He was unusually successful (perhaps uniquely so) at integrating neuroanatomy and cognitive theory with applied neuropsychology. As a result, one of the most distinguishing features of his career was that his work was very highly regarded by cognitive and clinical researchers as well as practicing clinicians. He was especially proud of this "cross-professional" appeal.
- Butters' earliest work was conducted in primates. Two tests in particular could reveal memory loss in monkeys – the delayed response (DR) and delayed alternation (DA) tasks. For both DR and DA, the animals had to hold information in memory for a short time before making a response to obtain a reward. Lesions in the prefrontal cortex, in particular along the sulcus principalis, severely disrupted the monkeys' ability to either perform or learn the tasks. In 1969, Butters, in collaboration with Deepak Pandya, demonstrated that the middle third of the sulcus principalis was the critical region associated with impairments of DR and DA. In 1971, they described functional differentiation along the axis of the sulcus principalis; the middle third differed from the anterior and posterior portions with regard to their efferent (outgoing) projections of the prefrontal cortex. In 1972, with their student Gary Van Hoesen, they reported on the afferent (incoming) projections to the entorhinal cortex around the hippocampus – another brain region critical for memory functions.
- At the same time, Butters was working closely with Donald Stein and Jeffrey Rosen on recovery of function following frontal lobe lesions in nonhuman primates. They showed that if one removed sections of the frontal lobes in monkeys in serial fashion, that is, over a series of operations, the resulting deficit was less than that exhibited by monkeys who experienced the same lesion, in one step. They concluded that these results demonstrated at least partial recovery of function. This finding in adult monkeys was important because, at the time, it was believed that if a brain lesion occurred after 12 months of age (in the monkey), recovery was not possible. Patricia Goldman was showing that infant macaques with brain lesions could fully recover some functions, but not others – the data from the Rosen, Stein, and Butters series shed light on the question of whether, and by how much, older animals (and by extension,

humans) could recover function after a brain lesion.

- One of his earliest human studies (published with Melvin Barton in 1970) on the role of the frontal and parietal lobes in concrete operations shaped much of Butters' philosophy of neuropsychology and laid the groundwork for his career examining the brain structures that mediate abnormal cognition. They took concepts and methods that were popular in human cognition at that time and used them to examine the role of various brain structures in these cognitive processes. For example, humans with damage to the parietal lobes have difficulty reversing – or changing – their behavior. That is, once taught a rule, they have difficulty deviating from that rule. What was unclear at the time was whether this deficit was a fundamental deficit in reversal or a consequence of a deficit in retention – the ability to remember the old rule or learn the new one. The results of these experiments not only informed investigators on the nature of the behavioral and cognitive changes that follow focal brain damage but lent insight into the cognitive processes themselves.

- Butters made exemplary use of what Hans-Lukas Teuber referred to as the "natural fracture lines of behavior." That is, when a patient suffers a brain injury, behavior and cognition fail neither completely nor in a random manner. Rather, the breakdown occurs at points where different cognitive processes intersect. By comparing and contrasting the nature and extent of changes in cognition across patients with different forms of brain damage, we advance our understanding of the neuroanatomical basis of the cognitive process in question, the organization of the process itself, and how these affect the individual patient. This concept became a theme – sometimes explicit and sometimes implicit – that was woven into the fabric of Butters' research career.

- An early series of studies in the 1970s with Ina Samuels exemplified this approach. Together they systematically examined visual and auditory short-term memory in individuals with a variety of lesions. In the early 1970s, cognitive

psychologists were debating the relative merits of serial versus parallel processing in normal human memory. Butters' work with Laird Cermak on patients with amnesic disorders was among the first to examine this and other central topics of cognitive psychological research. The Butters and Cermak collaboration was particularly fruitful because it directly influenced the development of models of normal human memory – particularly the notion that memory is neither a serial nor parallel process but rather that the *type* or *intensity* of the processing was what was critical (i.e., "levels of processing" argument espoused by Fergus Craik).

- While in Boston, Butters and his colleagues made great strides in elucidating the neuropsychological effects of alcoholism. The papers that emanated from studies of chronic, non-amnestic alcoholics (in collaboration with Christopher Ryan, James Becker, Kathleen Montgomery, and Barbara Jones) had a lasting influence on the way that the neuropsychology of alcoholism was viewed and studied. Butters' work also focused on the amnesic syndrome associated with chronic, severe alcoholism. With Laird Cermak, his systematic series of studies focused on the role of interference and encoding in the short-term memory defects of patients with alcoholic Korsakoff's syndrome. It is noteworthy that Butters developed personal relationships with many of these patients, venturing out to their homes (sometimes state hospitals or nursing homes) and repeatedly reevaluating them for different projects. This work was important not only because of what it revealed about both normal and pathological memory but also because it clearly demonstrated that a long-term consequence of alcoholism can be an amnestic disorder (a matter that was hotly debated at the time). Perhaps the most enduring legacy of Butters and Cermak's work from this period was the 1980 publication of *Alcoholic Korsakoff's Syndrome: An Information Processing Approach to Amnesia*. The title was not an accident – they wanted to emphasize the role of neuropsychology in analyzing information processing and how this research informed our models of normal memory and memory systems. The publication of this text marked the beginning of the modern era of "cognitive neuroscience."

- Another trend in Butters' research during the middle to late 1970s was prompted by his desire to better understand retrograde amnesia, which had not yet been studied in any systematic way, due, in part, to the lack of suitable test instruments. He collaborated with Marilyn Albert, who took on the task of developing the Boston Retrograde Amnesia Battery, which became the first carefully validated and well-normed retrograde memory battery applicable to individuals of various ages. This productive collaboration, which later included Jason Brandt and Donald Stuss, firmly established that the retrograde memory impairment exhibited by Korsakoff's patients had a clear temporal gradient, suggesting that the neural substrates of memory change with the passage of time. That is, over time, episodic memories mediated by the hippocampal circuitry are actively recalled, thereby losing their spatial and temporal markers, becoming part of semantic memory, stored elsewhere (likely the temporal-parietal association cortices).

- During his last years in Boston, Butters devoted considerable time to studying the cognitive effects of Huntington's disease (HD), demonstrating a functional dissociation between the locus of the lesions in HD (the basal ganglia) and those found in Korsakoff's syndrome (the limbic system). This research predated the identification of the HD gene and development of a test to determine whether the offspring of HD patients were destined to develop the disease. As part of the "Center Without Walls," Butters worked with people "at risk" for HD (i.e., who had a parent with the disease) to determine whether measures of cognition administered earlier in life could predict those who would ultimately develop the disease.

- In 1983 Butters accepted an offer to join the Department of Psychiatry at the University of California-San Diego (UCSD), where he relished the opportunity to develop a clinical service with neuropsychologists who conducted research as well as provided clinical care. In addition to developing a first-rate psychology service, Butters maintained his prolific research publication rate. Soon after arriving in San Diego, UCSD was designated an Alzheimer's Disease Research Center, which provided Butters with the opportunity to expand his research on memory. His studies now included Alzheimer's disease, which he considered the prototypical "cortical" dementia. In San Diego his work with David Salmon, William Heindel, William Beatty, Munro Cullum, Eric Granholm, Alexander Troster, Agnes Chan, Andreas Monsch, and a host of other students and colleagues focused on three main areas, yielding a significant scientific contribution in each.

- Butters' work with David Salmon and their colleagues demonstrated that the memory disorders of cortical and subcortical dementias are dissociable, with Alzheimer's disease characterized by poor consolidation and rapid forgetting due to limbic damage and Huntington's disease by poor retrieval associated with fronto-striatal dysfunction. Butters' work with trainee Mark Bondi and others in his research group was among the first to show that the neuropsychological characteristics of very early Alzheimer's disease differed from the benign cognitive changes of normal aging and could therefore be used for the early and even preclinical detection of the disease, presaging similar findings in HD. Finally, researchers were beginning to investigate the phenomenon of implicit memory, and Butters' work with William Heindel, David Salmon, Jane Paulsen, and others showed that various forms of implicit memory could be dissociated in Alzheimer's disease, Huntington's disease, and Parkinson's disease. These studies were the first to dissociate priming and procedural learning in the brain, showing that procedural learning deficits were associated with basal ganglia dysfunction while priming deficits were linked with neocortical damage that occurs in Alzheimer's disease. Any one of these contributions would have been impressive; together they represent a truly remarkable accomplishment.

- In 1986 the American Psychological Association (APA) acquired the journal *Neuropsychology*, and Butters was appointed editor. APA tradition allows new editors to choose the colors of the journal's binding – and Butters chose a white background with (Boston) Celtic green for the text (he was a lifelong fan of his hometown basketball team). Butters' goal for the journal was that it should become one of the journals of record for basic, applied, *and* clinical research in neuropsychology. This will be another of his lasting legacies.

- Most important to Butters were his students – his academic children (and in some cases grandchildren) were almost as important to him as his biological children, Meryl, Paul, and Lisa. His attraction was international (e.g., John Hodges, Narinder Kapur, Matti Laine), and his mentees continue to lead the field (e.g., Kathie Welsh-Bohmer, Terry Jernigan).

- A narrative of Butters' contributions to neuropsychology would be woefully incomplete without a personal description. He possessed tremendous internal drive and held both his students and colleagues to the high standards he applied to himself. Every Butters' student carries distinct memories of the red ink and blunt reviews accompanying their manuscript drafts. His academic rigor notwithstanding, Butters was universally known as an involved, supportive mentor and colleague. His role extended to that of job broker, and he devoted an inordinate amount of time and energy to assisting and advising a vast array of students and colleagues about both professional and personal matters. He was described as being biologically incapable of tolerating an unhappy "student" (a term that he applied quite broadly); he had to help make things right (even if the student did not immediately appreciate his wisdom). In his later years, he took tremendous pleasure in referring to himself as the "Godfather of Neuropsychology."

- Butters was blunt, brash, and famously irreverent. While his lifestyle was decidedly mainstream, he reveled in characterizing himself as something of a rebel. He was unendingly curious about those who walked to the beat of a different drummer. His personal role models included Marlon Brando, Lenny Bruce, and Woody Allen. He had a keen sense for and appreciation of the absurd and ironic and found humor in the darker side of life, though he never took himself too seriously. On more than one occasion, he was heard saying: "If I hadn't become a neuropsychologist, I would've been a comedian." At every APA and INS meeting social hour, Butters could be found, beer in hand, listening to and recounting hilarious stories about friends, colleagues, and family. Most of the time, he played a leading role in these comedic tales. In sum, Butters' rare combination of intellectual creativity, drive, irreverence, and appreciation of satire allowed him to make his mark both in the field of neuropsychology and in the hearts of his contemporaries.

Short Biography

Nelson Butters was born on May 7, 1937, in Boston, MA. He initially attended public school in Brookline, MA, and then Worcester Academy, a private boarding school, graduating first in his class. He was an accomplished athlete and scholar. A concussion sustained playing football left him with lifelong anosmia, an irony not lost on him when he later published articles on the importance of assessing olfaction in brain-damaged patients. In addition to his obvious academic talent, he took great pride in his carefully crafted image as a motor scooter-riding "bad boy," emulating James Dean and Marlon Brando. Later in life, he took great pleasure in recounting tales of his friendship with his classmate, the late social and political activist Abbie Hoffman. Butters particularly enjoyed retelling stories of "drag racing" against Hoffman from Worcester to Boston, MA, and attending wild parties at Hoffman's home. Somehow surviving high school, he went on to attend the University of Chicago and Boston University.

Butters was at first unsure of his professional goals. His parents had pushed for him to become a physician or lawyer, but neither profession held much appeal. Public speaking came rather easily to him, and he was excited by the idea of being a positive influence in the lives of college students. Therefore, during the second or third year of college, he decided to become a psychology teacher.

Butters entered the doctoral program in psychology at Clark University in the fall of 1960. At the time Clark had one of the leading psychology programs in the world. He was awarded a Woodrow Wilson Fellowship for his first year of graduate school because of his commitment to college teaching. During his second or third year in graduate school, he ran across a research article by Mortimer Mishkin and H. Enger Rosvold about delayed alternation, reversal learning, and the frontal lobes in monkeys. Butters became fascinated with the concept that one could examine the neurological structures that underlie cognitive and psychological processes. At the time he was particularly interested in what went on in the brain and what brain structures played a part in the development of concrete or formal operations in the thinking processes of children.

At the end of his third year of graduate school, Butters wrote to Hal Rosvold, a researcher at the National Institutes of Health (NIH), asking whether he would consider taking him as a postdoctoral fellow. A visit to Rosvold's lab led to a postdoctoral fellowship with Rosvold and Mishkin from 1964 to 1966. His work at the NIH focused on the roles of the septal nuclei, basal forebrain, and caudate nucleus in reversal learning and delayed alternation performance. Butters was fulfilling his plan to spend "a couple of years" studying physiological psychology and perhaps do "a few studies" on the neurological bases of cognition before resuming the path toward his teaching career.

Butters resumed his teaching path in 1966 by taking teaching positions at Wright State University and Antioch College in Ohio. However, the "few studies" he had conducted while at NIH caught the attention of Harold Goodglass and Norman Geschwind of the Boston Veterans Administration Hospital and Department of Neurology of the Boston University School of Medicine. Moreover, Butters and Goodglass had become acquainted during the former's years at Clark. The personal relationship, combined with Butters' cutting-edge animal work, led to an invitation from Geschwind and Goodglass to join their burgeoning Aphasia Research Center. Butters eagerly accepted the opportunity to join this exciting group and to return home to Boston. While he initially studied nonhuman primates, he took the opportunity to learn about human neuropsychology from the early pioneers, many of whom resided in Boston. In addition to Geschwind and Goodglass, he reveled in learning from and exchanging ideas with the likes of Edith Kaplan, Marlene Oscar Berman, Howard Gardner, Edgar Zurif, and many others. The unparalleled atmosphere at the Boston VA Hospital led to Butters' first studies in human neuropsychology. During 1967–1970 he conducted both animal and human research, and after 1970 his work focused exclusively on human cognition.

In 1983 Butters moved to San Diego, CA, to join the Department of Psychiatry at UCSD, where he continued to flourish. Continuing his research program, Butters also built a psychology service with a particular emphasis on training. He surrounded himself with superb colleagues including, among others, Robert Heaton and Dean Delis.

In early 1993 Butters developed oral motor weakness, and by March 1993 it was clear that he had amyotrophic lateral sclerosis. He was 55 years old and at the height of his career. He handled his nearly 3-year battle with ALS in typical Butters fashion, continuing to work and socialize until the week before his death. He took the opportunity to tell his students, colleagues, and family how grateful he was to have had them in his life. When he lost the ability to speak, he used adaptive computer equipment to communicate. The week before he died, he was still telling off-color and self-deprecating jokes by laboriously typing with his big toe, irreverent and irrepressible until the end.

Cross-References

References and Readings

Albert, M. S., Butters, N., & Brandt, J. (1981). Patterns of remote memory in amnesic and demented patients. *Archives of Neurology, 38*(8), 495–500. PMID: 6454407.

Brandt, J., Butters, N., Ryan, C., & Bayog, R. (1983). Cognitive loss and recovery in long-term alcohol abusers. *Archives of General Psychiatry, 40*(4), 435–442.

Butters, N. (1966). The effect of LSD-25 on spatial and stimulus perseverative tendencies in rats. *Psychopharmacologia, 8*(6), 454–460.

Butters, N. (1984). The clinical aspects of memory disorders: Contributions from experimental studies of amnesia and dementia. *Journal of Clinical Neuropsychology, 6*(1), 17–36. PMID: 6230375.

Butters, N. (1992). Memory remembered: 1970–1991. *Archives of Clinical Neuropsychology, 7*(4), 285–295. PMID:14591284.

Butters, N. (1996). Memoirs, in Nelson Butters remembered. *APA Division 40 Newsletter, 14*(3), 1, 3–7.

Butters, M. A., & Butters, N. M. (2002). Nelson M. Butters: One step ahead. In A. Y. Stringer, E. L. Cooley, & A. L. Christensen (Eds.), *Pathways to prominence: Reflections of 20th century neuropsychologists*. New York: Psychology Press.

Butters, N., & Cermak, L. S. (1974). The role of cognitive factors in the memory disorders of alcoholic patients with the Korsakoff syndrome. *Annals of the New York Academy of Sciences, 233*, 61–75. PMID: 4523804.

Butters, N., & Pandya, D. (1969). Retention of delayed-alternation: Effect of selective lesions of sulcus principalis. *Science, 165*(3899), 1271–1273. PMID: 4979528.

Butters, N., & Rosvold, H. E. (1968). Effect of caudate and septal nuclei lesions on resistance to extinction and delayed-alternation. *Journal of Comparative and Physiological Psychology, 65*(3), 397–403. PMID: 4970002.

Butters, N., Lewis, R., Cermak, L. S., & Goodglass, H. (1973). Material-specific memory deficits in alcoholic Korsakoff patients. *Neuropsychologia, 11*(3), 291–299. PMID: 4792180.

Butters, N., Tarlow, S., Cermak, L. S., & Sax, D. (1976). A comparison of the information processing deficits of patients with Huntington's chorea and Korsakoff's syndrome. *Cortex, 12*(2), 134–144. PMID: 133786.

Butters, N., Wolfe, J., Martone, M., Granholm, E., & Cermak, L. S. (1985). Memory disorders associated with Huntington's disease: Verbal recall, verbal recognition and procedural memory. *Neuropsychologia, 23*(6), 729–743. PMID: 2934642.

Butters, N., Granholm, E., Salmon, D. P., Grant, I., & Wolfe, J. (1987). Episodic and semantic memory: A comparison of amnesic and demented patients. *Journal of Clinical and Experimental Neuropsychology, 9*(5), 479–497. PMID: 2959682.

Butters, M., Becker, J. T., & Brandt, J. (1996). A legend in his own time: tribute to Nelson Butters, in Nelson Butters remembered. *APA Division 40 Newsletter, 14*(3), 2, 7–8.

Cermak, L. S. (Ed.). (1994). *Neuropsychological explorations of memory and cognition: Essays in honor of Nelson Butters*. New York: Plenum.

Chan, A. S., Butters, N., Paulsen, J. S., Salmon, D. P., Swenson, M. R., & Maloney, L. T. (1993). An assessment of the semantic network in patients with Alzheimer's disease. *Journal of Cognitive Neuroscience, 5*(2), 254–261. https://doi.org/10.1162/jocn.1993.5.2.254. PMID: 23972157.

Granholm, E., & Butters, N. (1988). Associative encoding and retrieval in Alzheimer's and Huntington's disease. *Brain and Cognition, 7*(3), 335–347. PMID: 2969744.

Heindel, W. C., Salmon, D. P., Shults, C. W., Walicke, P. A., & Butters, N. (1989). Neuropsychological evidence for multiple implicit memory systems: A comparison of Alzheimer's, Huntington's, and Parkinson's disease patients. *The Journal of Neuroscience, 9*(2), 582–587. PMID: 2521896.

Hodges, J. R., Salmon, D. P., & Butters, N. (1990). Differential impairment of semantic and episodic memory in Alzheimer's and Huntington's diseases: A controlled prospective study. *Journal of Neurology, Neurosurgery, and Psychiatry, 53*(12), 1089–1095. PMID: 2149861.

Jernigan, T., & Butters, N. (1989). Neuropsychological and neuroradiological distinctions between Alzheimer's and diseases. *Neuropsychology, 3*, 283–290.

Moss, M. B., Albert, M. S., Butters, N., & Payne, M. (1986). Differential patterns of memory loss among patients with Alzheimer's disease, Huntington's disease, and alcoholic Korsakoff's syndrome. *Archives of Neurology, 43*(3), 239–246. PMID: 2936323.

Rosen, J., Stein, D., & Butters, N. (1971). Recovery of function after serial ablation of prefrontal cortex in the rhesus monkey. *Science, 173*(3994), 353–356. PMID: 4997798.

Shimamura, A. P., Salmon, D. P., Squire, L. R., & Butters, N. (1987). Memory dysfunction and word priming in dementia and amnesia. *Behavioral Neuroscience, 101*(3), 347–351. PMID: 2955793.

Tröster, A. I., Butters, N., Salmon, D. P., Cullum, C. M., Jacobs, D., Brandt, J., & White, R. F. (1993). The diagnostic utility of savings scores: Differentiating Alzheimer's and Huntington's diseases with the logical memory and visual reproduction tests. *Journal of Clinical and Experimental Neuropsychology, 15*(5), 773–788. PMID: 8276935.